Deer's Treatment of Pain

Timothy R. Deer • Jason E. Pope
Tim J. Lamer • David Provenzano
Editors

Deer's Treatment of Pain

An Illustrated Guide for Practitioners

Springer

Editors
Timothy R. Deer
The Spine and Nerve Center of the Virginias
Charleston, WV
USA

Jason E. Pope
Evolve Restorative Center
Santa Rosa, CA
USA

Tim J. Lamer
Department of Anesthesiology
and Perioperative Medicine
Mayo Clinic
Rochester, MN
USA

David Provenzano
Pain Diagnostics and Interventional Care
Sewickley, PA
USA

ISBN 978-3-030-12280-5 ISBN 978-3-030-12281-2 (eBook)
https://doi.org/10.1007/978-3-030-12281-2

This Springer imprint is published by the registered company Springer Nature Switzerland AG
The registered company address is: Gewerbestrasse 11, 6330 Cham, Switzerland

This book is possible due to the support and love of my wife Missy, who has been by my side for many wonderful years. I also dedicate this book to God, who has blessed me through grace well beyond my greatest expectations. I also thank my children, Morgan, Taylor, Reed, and Bailie, for inspiring me in so many ways. Lastly, to our patients, I am eternally grateful for your trust and am hopeful that my work will impact your life in a way that is meaningful.

Timothy R. Deer, MD, DABPM, FIPP

To Emily, my wife, CHRO, and partner. Thank you for your unwavering support, grace, and the selflessness through the many years we have spent together. I love you more than words can express and humbled by your hard work you put in every day for our family and our practice. We are together in all adventures.

To my daughter Vivienne. Thank you for your kindness. You are growing up into a kind and talented girl and I enjoy all we do together.

To my twins Liam and Olivia. Thank you for your love and adventurous, brave outlook. It reminds me anything is possible.

To my father and mother. Thank you for your unyielding love and advice as I navigate the balance of father, son, husband, and work.

To my twin brother, who always humbled me with his intellect and perspective and leading by example.

To Eric Bruntlett, Steven Falowski, and Michael Fishman, for their friendship, candor, advice, and guidance.

To my entire Evolve Restorative Center family. Thank you for your willingness to help patients and going the extra mile to make sure our patients are cared for and supported. We are building something great.

To Timothy Deer, my brother, thank you for your friendship, support, advice, and partnership. We will continue to work towards globalization of pain care to improve safety and outcomes. We are not victims of circumstance.

To Springer, for their continued work in making this text edition a reality.

Finally, thank you to God, for making all things possible.

Jason E. Pope, MD, DABPM, FIPP

To my wife Halena, my best friend, advisor, and counselor. Your love, support, and companionship are so cherished and appreciated by me. And to our amazing children, Olivia, Tyler, Elizabeth, and Allison. We are so grateful for your love and watching you grow into the wonderful and exceptional young adults that you have all become is the most important and inspirational part of our lives.

To my patients, whom I have had the honor and pleasure of caring for over the past 30 plus years. I have learned more from you than all of my 30 plus years of training and education.

To my Mayo Clinic colleagues. It is an honor to work with such a dedicated and talented group of people in an amazing medical facility.

To all of the students, residents, and fellows that I have been honored to help teach and mentor. Watching your evolution into successful physicians and individuals is both gratifying and inspirational.

Tim J. Lamer, MD

To Dana, Nora, and Marco. Thank you for all your support and understanding (Another project that kept me in the study!).

To all my previous educators. Without your guidance and instruction, I would have never acquired the knowledge required to pursue this project.

Finally, to our patients. It is an honor to help you deal with the challenges of pain. I continue to learn from these experiences daily.

David Provenzano, MD

Foreword

I am honored to write this foreword for *Deer's Treatment of Pain: An Illustrated Guide for Practitioners.* As an interventional pain management specialist, I have devoted my career to the treatment of patients with pain and share Tim Deer's passion for patient care, clinical research, and education of the next generation of pain physicians. I have known Dr. Deer for two decades as a friend and colleague and have watched with admiration and respect as he has become among the most highly regarded figures in the field. His leadership in interventional pain is internationally recognized, and he is directly responsible for much of the sentinel work in many areas of pain therapy, particularly neuromodulation and intrathecal drug delivery.

Dr. Deer is an accomplished triathlete. His charitable work with the Ironman Foundation exemplifies the generosity and integrity he brings to all that he does, including the publication of this important textbook, which establishes a new standard reference for our field. This comprehensive resource includes over 100 chapters written by today's thought leaders in every area of pain treatment. It provides the reader with the basic science, anatomy, physiology, and practical treatment considerations necessary to successfully navigate the ever-increasing complexity of interventional pain management.

A recent study by the National Institutes of Health's National Center for Complementary and Integrative Health indicates that nearly 50 million American adults experience significant chronic pain or severe pain [1]. Because pain is one of the most common reasons patients seek help from healthcare providers, it is critical that physicians are well versed in its diagnosis and management. I commend Timothy R. Deer and his colleagues, Jason E. Pope, Tim J. Lamer, and David Provenzano, for assembling this comprehensive volume which details the current understanding of both pain and its treatment. Sections address both pharmacologic and interventional approaches to pain control, as well as neuromodulation, intrathecal drug delivery systems, regenerative therapies, and minimally invasive structural surgeries. Well-placed illustrations and other graphics serve to enhance the text, further increasing the book's value. In summary, the expertise presented in *Deer's Treatment of Pain* provides us with an authoritative reference work that belongs on the desk of every student, clinician, and scientist involved in the study and treatment of pain.

Aaron Calodney, MD, FIPP, ABIPP, DABPM
Director, Clinical Research, Precision Spine Care
Clinical Associate Professor of Anesthesiology
Louisiana State University Medical School, Shreveport
Shreveport, LA
USA

Reference

1. Nahin RL. Estimates of pain prevalence and severity in adults: United States, 2012. J Pain. 2015;16(8):769–80.

Preface

Chronic pain is an international issue that impacts the well-being of all nations for numerous reasons. In the past decade, we have come to the realization that the opioid epidemic is a tremendous challenge and has taken a huge toll on society. In that same complex setting, we also have the challenge of an aging population, traumatic injuries, disease progression, and sports-related ailments all of which cause chronic pain syndromes that require solutions. It is in this complicated time that we feel new guidance is needed for the physician or healthcare provider who is attempting to do an optimal job in treating this patient population. This is the environment that created the need for *Deer's Treatment of Pain*.

This textbook has been created with a number of committed physicians who are striving to improve therapeutic efficacy, patient safety, and ethical medical treatment. This is intended to merge a comprehensive text with an atlas feeling where you can visually learn best treatment options for your patient. The physician who embraces these options of an algorithmic treatment approach based on best evidence, expert opinion, and clinical experience will enhance their ability to provide optimal care to those who suffer and seek a remedy.

In developing this educational material, I had the honor of working with Tim Lamer, MD; David Provenzano, MD; and Jason E. Pope, MD. This team of dedicated physicians has created a group who shaped the contents, edited the materials, suggested additions, and used the highest standards to make a commitment to creating an optimal learning experience for the reader.

I wish each of you the best of success as you raise the standard of care in your community by continuing to strive to learn new options and methods. It is my belief that by working together, we can truly offer solutions that will better the human experience.

Charleston, WV, USA — Timothy R. Deer

Contents

Contributors

Rishi Raj Agarwal, MD Department of Anesthesiology, Northwestern University, Feinberg School of Medicine, Chicago, IL, USA

Anuj Aggarwal, MD Department of Anesthesiology, Perioperative and Pain Medicine, Stanford University, Redwood City, CA, USA

Yamah Amiri, MBBS Pain Management, Ochsner Health System, New Orleans, LA, USA

Hamed Asadi, PhD, FRANZCR, CCINR, EBIR Interventional Neuroradiology Service, Department of Radiology, Austin Hospital, Melbourne, Australia

School of Medicine, Faculty of Health, Deakin University, Waurn Ponds, Australia

Interventional Neuroradiology Unit, Monash Imaging, Monash Health, Melbourne, Australia

Javid Baksh, DO, MD Premier Pain Solutions, Asheville, NC, USA

G. Baranidharan, FRCA, FFPMRCA Leeds Pain and Neuromodulation Centre, Leeds, UK

Markus A. Bendel, MD Mayo Clinic, Rochester, MN, USA

Nicholas J. Bremer, MD, D.ABA Center for Pain Relief, Spine and Nerve Centers of the Virginias, Charleston, WV, USA

Randall P. Brewer, MD Department of Anesthesiology, Duke University School of Medicine, Durham, NC, USA

Departments of Neurology and Anesthesiology, Louisiana State University School of Medicine, Shreveport, LA, USA

River Cities Interventional Pain Specialists, Shreveport, LA, USA

Taylor Brittan, BS Neurosurgery Department, Ochsner Health System, New Orleans, LA, USA

Abram H. Burgher The Pain Center of Arizona, Peoria, AZ, USA

Lucas W. Campos, MD, PhD Interventional Pain Physicians, Chico, CA, USA

Alexios G. Carayannopoulos Department of Physical Medicine and Rehabilitation, Rhode Island Hospital, Providence, RI, USA

Comprehensive Spine Center: Rhode Island Hospital, Providence, RI, USA

Newport Hospital, Newport, RI, USA

Warren Alpert Medical School, Brown University, Providence, RI, USA

American Society of Interventional Pain Physicians, Rhode Island Chapter, Paducah, KY, USA

Jonathan D. Carlson, MD Hawaii Pain & Spine, Kailua, HI, USA

Midwestern Medical School, Glendale, AZ, USA

Hawaii Pain & Spine, Arizona Pain, Kailua, HI, USA

Nicole S. Carter Faculty of Medicine, Nursing and Health Sciences, Monash University, Melbourne, Australia

Ronil V. Chandra Faculty of Medicine, Nursing and Health Sciences, Monash University, Melbourne, Australia

Interventional Neuroradiology Unit, Monash Imaging, Monash Health, Melbourne, Australia

Shamard Charles, MD Harvard T.H. Chan School of Public Health, NBC News Group, New York, NY, USA

Tony Y. Chon, MD Division of General Internal Medicine, Mayo Clinic, Rochester, MN, USA

Seth Christian, MD, MBA Paradigm Orthopedics and Sports Medicine, Slidell, LA, USA

Steven P. Cohen, MD Department of Anesthesiology and Critical Care Medicine, Johns Hopkins School of Medicine, Baltimore, MD, USA

Department of Physical Medicine and Rehabilitation, Johns Hopkins School of Medicine, Baltimore, MD, USA

Department of Anesthesiology, Uniformed Services University of the Health Sciences, Bethesda, MD, USA

Department of Physical Medicine and Rehabilitation, Uniformed Services University of the Health Sciences, Bethesda, MD, USA

Stephen D. Coleman, MD Anesthesia, Perioperative and Pain Medicine, Stanford University, Stanford, CA, USA

David Copenhaver, MD, MPH UC Davis Cancer Pain Management and Supportive Care, University of California, Davis Division of Pain Medicine, Davis, CA, USA

Alan Gonzalez Cota, MD, FIPP A.I.M. Interventional Spine Division, Rockville, MD, USA

Legacy Pain Management Rehabilitation, Bethesda, MD, USA

KureSmart Pain Management, Annapolis, MD, USA

Timothy R. Deer, MD, DABPM, FIPP The Spine and Nerve Center of the Virginias, Charleston, WV, USA

Didier Demesmin, MD University Pain Medicine Center, Somerset, NJ, USA

Rutgers Robert Wood Johnson Medical School, Piscataway, NJ, USA

JFK Johnson Rehabilitation Institute, Edison, NJ, USA

Pain Medicine Department, Saint Peter's University Hospital, New Brunswick, NJ, USA

University Clinical Research Center, Somerset, NJ, USA

Daniel R. Denis, MD, FRCS(C) Ochsner Health System, Kenner, LA, USA

Mehul J. Desai, MD, MPH International Spine, Pain & Performance Center, Washington, DC, USA

George Washington University, School of Medicine, Washington, DC, USA

James Dierkes, MD Department of Anesthesiology, Duke University Medical Center, Durham, NC, USA

Dan DuBose, MD

Sam Eldabe, MBChB, FRCA, FFPMRCA Department of Pain and Anaesthesia, James Cook University Hospital, Middlesbrough, UK

Jennifer L. Erian, MD Expert Pain P.A., Department of Anesthesiology, McGovern Medical School, The University of Texas Health Science Center at Houston, Houston, TX, USA

Steven Falowski, MD Functional Neurosurgery, Neurosurgical Associates of Lancaster, Lancaster, PA, USA

Kris Ferguson, MD Aspirus Hospital, Wausau, WI, USA

Christina E. Fitch, DO, MPH University of Massachusetts Medical School- Baystate Campus, Springfield, MA, USA

Alexander Fontenot, MD Anesthesiology Department, Ochsner Health system, New Orleans, LA, USA

Rishi Gaiha, MD Department of Anesthesiology, Northwestern University, Feinberg School of Medicine, Chicago, IL, USA

Christopher Gates Velentium LLC, Katy, TX, USA

Halena M. Gazelka, MD Division of Pain Medicine, Department of Anesthesiology and Perioperative Medicine, Mayo Clinic College of Medicine and Science, Rochester, MN, USA

Tony George, DO University Pain Medicine Center, Somerset, NJ, USA

Christopher Gilligan, MD, MBA Brigham and Women's Hospital, Boston, MA, USA

Vitaly Gordin, MD Department of Anesthesiology and Perioperative Medicine, Pennsylvania State University, Hershey, PA, USA

Yuri Gordin, MD Department of Physical Medicine and Rehabilitation, Pennsylvania State University, Hershey, PA, USA

Edna Gouveia, MD Neurosurgery Department, Ochsner Health System, New Orleans, LA, USA

Patrick D. Grace, MD Department of Anesthesiology and Pain Medicine, The University of Kansas Health System, Kansas City, KS, USA

Karina Gritsenko, MD Albert Einstein College of Medicine/Montefiore Medical Center, Montefiore Multidisciplinary Pain Program, The Bronx, NY, USA

Alba Guevara, MD Department of Anesthesiology and Perioperative Medicine, Pennsylvania State University, Hershey, PA, USA

Maged Guirguis, MD Pain Management, Ochsner Health System, New Orleans, LA, USA

Interventional Pain Management, Department of Anesthesiology & Critical Care Medicine, Ochsner Health System, New Orleans, LA, USA

University of Queensland Ochsner Medical School, Brisbane, QLD, Australia

Louisiana State University School of Medicine, New Orleans, LA, USA

Ochsner Medical Center, Jefferson, LA, USA

Ashish Gulve, FFPMCAI, FCARCSI, MD Department of Pain Management, The James Cook University Hospital, Middlesbrough, UK

Osama Hafez, MD Department of Anesthesiology, Moffitt Cancer Center, University of South Florida, Tampa, FL, USA

Jonathan Hagedorn, MD Department of Pain Medicine, Mayo Clinic, Rochester, MN, USA

Nameer Haider, MD, FAAPMR-AQPM, DABPM Spinal & Skeletal Pain Medicine, Utica, NY, USA

Ian Hakkinen, MBBS Pain Management, Ochsner Health System, New Orleans, LA, USA

Joshua Hanna, MD Neurosurgery Department, Ochsner Health System, New Orleans, LA, USA

Joshua A. Hirsch, MD Neuroendovascular Program, Massachusetts General Hospital, Boston, MA, USA

Harvard Medical School, Boston, MA, USA

Yasmine Hoydonckx, MD, FIPP Department of Anesthesia, Toronto Western Hospital, Toronto, ON, Canada

Christy Hunt, DO, MS Department of Physical Medicine and Rehabilitation, Mayo Clinic, Rochester, MN, USA

Corey W. Hunter, MD Department of Rehabilitation Medicine, Icahn School of Medicine at Mount Sinai, New York, NY, USA

Ainsworth Institute of Pain Management, New York, NY, USA

Kenneth Ike, MD Department of Anesthesia, Pain Management Clinic, Grady Hospital, Atlanta, GA, USA

Marilyn S. Jacobs, PhD, ABPP Department of Psychiatry and Biobehavioral Sciences, David Geffen School of Medicine at UCLA, Los Angeles, CA, USA

Sameer Jain, MD Department of Pain Medicine, Pain Treatment Centers of America, Little Rock, AR, USA

Piotr K. Janicki, MD, PhD Department of Anesthesiology and Perioperative Medicine, Penn State College of Medicine, MS Hershey Medical Center, Hershey, PA, USA

Gabriel P. Jasper Jasper Spine Institute, Brick, NJ, USA

Jasper Spine Learning Institution, Jersey Shore University, Neptune, NJ, USA

Navdeep Jassal, MD Department of Neurology, University of South Florida, Tampa, FL, USA

Mihir M. Kamdar, MD MGH Divisions of Palliative Care and Anesthesia Pain Medicine, Massachusetts General Hospital, Boston, MA, USA

Dost Khan, MD Department of Anesthesiology, Northwestern University Feinberg School of Medicine, Chicago, IL, USA

Chong H. Kim, MD MetroHealth/Case Western Reserve University, Department of PM&R, Cleveland, OH, USA

Chase A. Kissling, MD Walter Reed National Military Medical Center, Bethesda, MD, USA

Narayan R. Kissoon, MD Division of Headache, Department of Neurology, Mayo Clinic, Rochester, MN, USA

Division of Pain, Department of Anesthesiology, Mayo Clinic, Rochester, MN, USA

Kiran K. Koneti, FRCA, EDRA Department of Anaesthetics, Sunderland Royal Hospitals, Sunderland, UK

Brian Harris Kopell, MD Center for Neuromodulation, Department of Neurosurgery, Mount Sinai Health System, New York, NY, USA

Bryan K. Lai, MD Expert Pain P.A., Department of Anesthesiology, McGovern Medical School, The University of Texas Health Science Center at Houston, Houston, TX, USA

Tim J. Lamer, MD Division of Pain Medicine, Department of Anesthesiology and Perioperative Medicine, Mayo Clinic, Rochester, MN, USA

Luke A. Law, MD Department of Anesthesiology, Mayo Clinic, Rochester, MN, USA

Eric T. Lee, MD, MA Musculoskeletal Care and Regenerative Medicine, St Charles Spine Institute, Thousand Oaks, CA, USA

Michael S. Leong, MD Stanford Pain Management Center, Redwood City, CA, USA

Thabele Leslie-Mazwi, MD Neuroendovascular Program, Massachusetts General Hospital, Boston, MA, USA

Harvard Medical School, Boston, MA, USA

Clarence T. Li, MD Departments of Neurology, Mayo Clinic, Rochester, MN, USA

Sean Li, MD Premier Pain Centers, An Affiliate of National Spine and Pain Centers, Shrewsbury, NJ, USA

Susan Lim, MD Brigham and Women's Hospital, Boston, MA, USA

Tiffany Lin, MD Department of Anesthesiology and Critical Care, The University of Chicago, Chicago, IL, USA

Paul J. Lynch, MD, DABA Arizona Pain Specialists, Scottsdale, AZ, USA

Ankit Maheshwari, MD Case Western Reserve University, Cleveland, OH, USA

University Hospitals of Cleveland, Cleveland, OH, USA

Julian Maingard, MBBS, BMedSci Interventional Neuroradiology Service, Department of Radiology, Austin Hospital, Melbourne, Australia

School of Medicine – Faculty of Health, Deakin University, Waurn Ponds, Australia

Samia Malik, MD Department of Neurology, University of South Florida, Tampa, FL, USA

Mark N. Malinowski, DO, DABA Adena Spine Center, Chillicothe, OH, USA

Amanda Markow New York Presbyterian Brooklyn Methodist Hospital, New York, NY, USA

Tory L. McJunkin, MD, DABA Arizona Pain Specialists, Scottsdale, AZ, USA

W. Porter McRoberts, MD FAAPMR ABPMR ABA/Pain, University of Miami School of Medicine, Miami, FL, USA

Pankaj Mehta, MD, DABA, DABPM Pain Specialists of Austin, Killeen, TX, USA

Daniel Morgan, PhD Department of Anesthesiology and Perioperative Medicine, Pennsylvania State University, Hershey, PA, USA

Michael Mueller, MD, MPH Department of Anesthesiology and Perioperative Medicine, Pennsylvania State University, Hershey, PA, USA

Geeta Nagpal, MD Department of Anesthesiology, Northwestern University, Feinberg School of Medicine, Chicago, IL, USA

Andrew Ng Department of Anesthesiology, Jefferson Pain Center, Thomas Jefferson University Hospital, Philadelphia, PA, USA

Lynn K. Ngai, MD Stanford University, Stanford, CA, USA

Eric V. Ngo, MD Expert Pain P.A., Department of Anesthesiology, McGovern Medical School, The University of Texas Health Science Center at Houston, Houston, TX, USA

Tyler Nix, MD, MPH Anesthesiology Department, Ochsner Health System, New Orleans, LA, USA

Devang Padalia, MD Interventional Pain Department, Moffitt Cancer Center, University of South Florida, Tampa, FL, USA

Dipan Patel, MD, DABA Garden State Pain Control Center, Clifton, NJ, USA

Residents & Fellows Society, North American Neuromodulation Society (NANS), Jersey City, NJ, USA

Vikram B. Patel, MD Phoenix Interventional Center for Advanced Learning, Algonquin, IL, USA

Sanket Pathak, MD Department of Anesthesiology, Thomas Jefferson University Hospital, Philadelphia, PA, USA

Denis G. Patterson, MD Nevada Advanced Pain Specialists, Reno, NV, USA

Christian Peccora, MD Texas Pain Consultant Associates, Houston, TX, USA

Philip Peng, MBBS, FRCPC Department of Anesthesia, Toronto Western Hospital, Toronto, ON, Canada

Jeffrey Peterson, BA COO, Center for Pain Relief, Inc. & The Spine and Nerve Centers of the Virginias, Charleston, WV, USA

Julie G. Pilitsis, MD, PhD Department of Neuroscience and Experimental Therapeutics, Neurosurgery, Albany Medical College, Albany, NY, USA

Thomas P. Pittelkow, DO, MPH Division of Pain Medicine, Department of Anesthesiology and Perioperative Medicine, Mayo Clinic College of Medicine and Science, Rochester, MN, USA

Jason E. Pope, MD, DABPM, FIPP Evolve Restorative Center, Santa Rosa, CA, USA

Lawrence R. Poree, MD, MPH, PhD Department of Anesthesia and Perioperative Care, University of California at San Francisco, San Francisco, CA, USA

Jose Posas III Pain Management, Ochsner Health System, New Orleans, LA, USA

Chane Price, MD Interventional Pain Physician, University of Miami, Coral Gables, FL, USA

David Provenzano, MD Pain Diagnostics and Interventional Care, Sewickley, PA, USA

Sascha Qian, MD Spinal & Skeletal Pain Medicine, Utica, NY, USA

Xiang Qian, MD, PhD Department of Anesthesiology, Perioperative and Pain Medicine, Stanford University, Stanford University Pain Management Center, Redwood City, CA, USA

Wenchun Qu, MD, PhD Department of Physical Medicine and Rehabilitation, Division of Pain Medicine, Spine Center, Mayo Clinic, Rochester, MN, USA

Maunak V. Rana, MD Department of Anesthesiology and Critical Care, The University of Chicago, Chicago, IL, USA

Corey Reeves, MD Department of Physical Medicine and Rehabilitation, University of South Florida, Tampa, FL, USA

Dustin Reynolds, MD Expert Pain P.A., Department of Anesthesiology, McGovern Medical School, The University of Texas Health Science Center at Houston, Houston, TX, USA

Tina Rivenbark, MHA, CMPE Advanced Practice Solutions, Wilmington, NC, USA

Mathew Roberts, MS Medical University of South Carolina, Charleston, SC, USA

Daniel Rothstein, MD University Pain Medicine Center, Somerset, NJ, USA

Rutgers Robert Wood Johnson University Hospital, New Brunswick, NJ, USA

Pain Medicine Department, Saint Peter's University Hospital, New Brunswick, NJ, USA

Jeffery Rowe, MD Main Line Spine & Main Line Spine Surgery Center, King of Prussia, PA, USA

Vafi Salmasi, MD Department of Anesthesiology, Perioperative and Pain Medicine, Systems Neuroscience and Pain Laboratory, Stanford University School of Medicine, Redwood City, CA, USA

Rebecca A. Sanders, MD Department of Pain Management, Kansas Spine and Specialty Hospital, Wichita, KS, USA

Puneet Sayal, MD International Spine, Pain & Performance Center, Washington, DC, USA

Dawood Sayed, MD The University of Kansas Health System, Kansas City, KS, USA

Vikram Sengupta, MD Spinal & Skeletal Pain Medicine, Utica, NY, USA

Anish Sethi, DO Chronic Pain Medicine, Department of Anesthesiology, Thomas Jefferson University Hospital, Philadelphia, PA, USA

Ann Cai Shah, MD Department of Anesthesia and Perioperative Care, Anesthesia and Pain Medicine, University of California at San Francisco, San Francisco, CA, USA

Bunty J. Shah, MD Penn State Milton S. Hershey Medical Center, Hershey, PA, USA

Jay M. Shah, MD Department of Pain Medicine, Weill-Cornell Tri-Institutional Pain Program, New York, NY, USA

Neal Shah, MD Interventional Pain Department, Moffitt Cancer Center, University of South Florida, Tampa, FL, USA

Aanchal Sharma, MD Expert Pain P.A., Department of Anesthesiology, McGovern Medical School, The University of Texas Health Science Center at Houston, Houston, TX, USA

Jaspreet Singh, MD Department of Neurology, University of South Florida, Tampa, FL, USA

Elena E. Skaribas Southern Methodist University, Dallas, TX, USA

Ioannis M. Skaribas, MD, DABA Expert Pain P.A., Department of Anesthesiology, McGovern Medical School, The University of Texas Health Science Center at Houston, Houston, TX, USA

Lee-Anne Slater, FRANZCR, CCINR Faculty of Medicine, Nursing and Health Sciences, Monash University, Melbourne, Australia

Interventional Neuroradiology Unit, Monash Imaging, Monash Health, Melbourne, Australia

Kevin Smith, PhD Kevin G. Smith, Ph.D. and Associates, P.C., Houston, TX, USA

Sadie E. Smith, MD Department of Anesthesiology and Perioperative Medicine, Penn State Health/Penn State College of Medicine, Hershey, PA, USA

Andrew So, MD Albert Einstein College of Medicine/Montefiore Medical Center, New York City, NY, USA

Lisa Stearns, MD Center for Pain and Supportive Care, Phoenix, AZ, USA

Roger Strachan, MD, FRCSE, FRCS(SN) Department of Neurosurgery, James Cook University Hospital, Middlesbrough, UK

Geoffrey Stricsek, MD Neurological Surgery, Thomas Jefferson University, Philadelphia, PA, USA

William A. Stuart, RPh Hartley Medical Center Pharmacy, Inc., Long Beach, CA, USA

Edward L. Swing, PhD Arizona Pain Specialists, Scottsdale, AZ, USA

Reda Tolba, MD Wake Forest Baptist Medical Center, Winston Salem, NC, USA

Hiep Tran, MD Department of Anesthesiology, Baylor Scott and White Health, Temple, TX, USA

Texas A&M University College of Medicine, Killeen, TX, USA

Katherine D. Travnicek, MD Pain Institute of Nevada, Las Vegas, NV, USA

Ned Urbiztondo, MD Spinal & Skeletal Pain Medicine, Utica, NY, USA

Elias Veizi, MD, PhD Case Western Reserve University, Cleveland, OH, USA

Louis Stokes VA Medical Center, Cleveland, OH, USA

Amy Wachholtz, PhD Department of Psychology, University of Colorado-Denver, Denver, CO, USA

Atul A. Walia, DO Integris Pain Management, University of Oklahoma Health Sciences Center, Oklahoma City, OK, USA

Torin Walters, MD Department of Diagnostic Radiology, Joan C. Edwards School of Medicine, Marshall University, Senior Partner Radiology Inc, Huntington, WV, USA

Dajie Wang, MD Chronic Pain Medicine, Department of Anesthesiology, Thomas Jefferson University Hospital, Philadelphia, PA, USA

James C. Watson, MD Departments of Neurology, Mayo Clinic, Rochester, MN, USA

Departments of Anesthesiology, Pain Medicine, Mayo Clinic, Rochester, MN, USA

Brian H. Wetherington, MD Department of Anesthesiology and Pain Medicine, The University of Kansas Health System, Kansas City, KS, USA

Simon Willis, MD Department of Anesthesiology, University of Virginia School of Medicine, Charlottesville, VA, USA

Nicole Wolfgram, RN, FNP-BC Aspirus Hospital, Wausau, WI, USA

Kurt A. Yaeger, MD Department of Neurosurgery, Icahn School of Medicine, Mount Sinai Hospital, New York, NY, USA

Ajax Yang, MD Department of Rehabilitation Medicine, Icahn School of Medicine at Mount Sinai, New York, NY, USA

Part I

Introduction

The Disease-Based Treatment of Pain

1

Andrew So and Karina Gritsenko

Introduction

The concept of pain has been an implicit variable in the equation of human life for many centuries. As one of the oldest universal phenomena, pain and its effects have asserted varying degrees of influence on religion, philosophy, and politics over time. Most notably, however, the phenomenon of pain has challenged physicians in their treatment planning and methodology; despite its ubiquitous existence, pain has never been universally understood due to its differing definitions across societies, beliefs, and contexts. Subsequently, medical professionals have been continuously tasked with redefining the phenomenon of pain.

Today, pain is one of the leading motivations for patients to seek physician treatment, as it is a component of many disease states; some would even argue that pain has evolved into a disease state in and of itself. This designation is the product of centuries of research that have resulted in various theories attempting to define pain as a complex biological process integrating the roles of anatomy, function, and external experience. With each new theory, the scope of pain's definition has expanded, and physicians have created new approaches to treatment.

As medical professionals' definition and understanding of the pain phenomenon has changed over time, treatment methods have evolved into multimodal approaches designed to attack the various components of this complex disease pathway. To better understand today's pain management techniques, it is important to familiarize oneself with the historical theories of pain, the current pain model, and the available treatments that have crafted the current approach.

A. So (✉)
Albert Einstein College of Medicine/Montefiore Medical Center, New York City, NY, USA

K. Gritsenko
Albert Einstein College of Medicine/Montefiore Medical Center, Montefiore Multidisciplinary Pain Program, The Bronx, NY, USA

Background and Historical Perspective

As it is regarded today, pain has not always been considered a biological phenomenon. In the prehistoric times, pain was thought to be a means of punishment that arose from an external experience of the spiritual world. In Ancient Chinese philosophy, pain was believed to be an imbalance between the vital forces of yin and yang, the complementary/opposing forces of life.

Early Greek philosophers also had their own postulations on the sensation of pain, as evident in the text of the *Iliad* by Homer (eight century to mid-fourth century BC), who used terms such as *penthos* and *algos* to describe different forms of physical and moral pain. The philosopher Aristotle designated the heart as the center of pain and sensation and believed that pain stemmed from the sensitivity of human organs.

Religion has also been used to explain the concept of pain, particularly in the Middle Ages. With the spread of Christianity, there seemed to be a preoccupation on the crucifixion of Christ and therefore a greater emphasis on bodily suffering. From this preoccupation emerged the idea that pain was a form of divine retribution, as demonstrated with martyred saints and the concept of purgatory.

The Shift to the Anatomical Basis of Pain

Over the centuries, the concept of pain slowly registered a paradigm shift from a philosophical and theological ideology to a more anatomical explanation. The works of Herophilus and Galen contributed to this pivotal shift. Herophilus studied the anatomy of the brain in the third century and laid early foundations in the understanding of the human nervous system and its anatomy. Approximately 1500 years later, the works of the physician Claudius Galen (130–201 AD) would suggest the existence of two sets of nerves with different roles: motor and sensation. Galen also demonstrated that the complete transection of the spinal cord caused sensory and

T. R. Deer et al. (eds.), *Deer's Treatment of Pain*, https://doi.org/10.1007/978-3-030-12281-2_1

motor deficits and theorized that the spinal column was the connection between the brain and other organs. Galen's work demonstrated one of the earliest pathways that suggest pain required an organ to receive information from the outside world, a connecting passageway, and an organizing center to transform outside sensory information to perception.

During the Renaissance, philosopher Rene Descartes would describe a detailed somatosensory pathway. In his 1662 manuscript, *Treatise of Man*, Descartes builds on Galen's theories, describing the existence of nerves in the human body that convey both sensory and motor information. Descartes proposed the existence of gates between the brain and nerves, from which arouse the idea of mechanism; this theory compares the human body to a machine and describes pain as a consequence of damage to said hypothetical machine. Descartes' work showed that pain was an internal process organized by the human brain, rather than an external presence that entered the body, as was historically believed. In many ways, Descartes initiated the proposition of a human physiological process of pain.

In the years that followed these early anatomical studies, several important theories, which will be discussed in the next section of this chapter, would expand on these anatomical findings and be pivotal in constructing our modern-day knowledge of the pain pathway.

The Early Pain Theories

The current working definition of pain, as defined by the International Association for the Study of Pain, is "an unpleasant sensory and emotional experience associated with actual or potential tissue damage." The IASP's definition further describes pain as an integrative experience with both biological and psychosocial components. While there have been numerous theories proposed to explain pain, this chapter will focus on the most prevalent and influential theories of the past.

The Specificity Theory (1811)

The specificity theory was one of the first modern pain theories to suggest a separate anatomical neural pathway for pain perception. Maximilian von Frey postulated that the human body had five sensations (touch, heat, cold, pleasure, and pain), each with their own dedicated receptors and pathways to the brain. He theorized that noxious stimuli activated their own specialized receptors and were relayed by individualized pain fibers. Adding to the specificity theory, Charles Bell later suggested the idea of specialized spinal nerve roots with different functions. He hypothesized that the ventral nerve roots were responsible for motor and sensory activity in the dorsal nerve roots.

From the specificity theory stems some of our modern ideas of the pain pathway – the ideas of specialized pain nociceptors, specialized nerves that carry varying pain signals (i.e., alpha-delta and C-nociceptive fibers), and a specialized spinothalamic tract in the spinal cord dedicated to nociception.

Pattern Theory (1894)

The Pattern theory, proposed by Alfred Goldscheider in 1894, suggests that the perception of pain is not the product of just one stimulation site transmitting to the brain, as proposed by the specificity theory, but rather an aggregate of multiple stimulation sites. It also postulates that the frequency of stimulation is responsible for variance in the intensity of pain. Goldscheider theorized that if a pain stimuli was applied repeatedly in higher frequency (temporal summation), it would appear more intense to the individual. Similarly, he suggested that pain could be spread over a large area and that such stimuli applied to a greater body area would convey a more intense pain (spatial summation).

Gate Control Theory of Pain (1965)

In 1965, Ronald Melzack and Charles Patrick would propose the gate control theory, which answered some of the limitations of its predecessor theories and ultimately revolutionized the field of pain medicine. The research behind the gate control theory of pain is rooted in the notion that pain signals are transmitted from the peripheral nervous system via small afferent pain fibers (alpha-delta and c fibers) to the dorsal horn of the spinal cord, which eventually leads to the brain. Along this pathway lie hypothetical "gates" that can be closed by varying mechanisms in order to inhibit the propagation of pain signals.

The gate control theory outlines two inhibitory pathways. First, it describes the ability of large nerve fibers (alpha-beta fibers), which carry non-noxious information and are located in the substantia gelatinosa of the spinal cord, to inhibit smaller afferent nerve fibers carrying nociceptive information. This proposed mechanism explains the theory behind the practice of rubbing or caressing a painful area of the body in order to alleviate pain. This idea is also the fundamental foundation behind the concepts of neuromodulation and transcutaneous electrical nerve stimulation (TENS).

The second inhibitory pathway is a descending inhibitory mechanism from the brain centered in the reticular formation. The theory states that heightened activity of this descending efferent pathway from the reticular system leads to an increased likelihood of gate closure and the subsequent inhibition of pain. This explains the theory behind hypnosis and why patients many times ignore the presence of painful stimuli while hypnotized.

Summarized, the overall perception of pain was said to be a balance between the two inhibitory mechanisms and the activity of the small noxious fibers. The gate control theory was important in showing the role of both the central and peripheral nervous systems in the perception of pain and was the first to explain the ability for non-noxious stimuli to modulate and change one's pain perception. As stated, it would also serve as the foundation of neuromodulation, a technique commonly used today for pain management.

Sensitization Models

Although the previous models laid the foundation for the neural pathway of pain, they failed to explain why pain could persist after the removal of the original stimuli, as demonstrated in chronic pain syndromes. The idea of sensitization (which includes both peripheral and central sensitization) would provide an answer to this phenomenon.

The term peripheral sensitization refers to the situation in which a nerve has increased excitability and therefore increased signal transmission. Peripheral sensitization can be applied to the pain pathway as commonly demonstrated following tissue injury, when inflammatory messengers including prostaglandins, cytokines, leukotrienes, and bradykinin are released. These inflammatory messengers cause changes in the voltage-gated sodium channels of neurons, which produce reduced activation potential and increased excitability. Subsequently, peripheral pain receptors are "sensitized" to have a lower threshold for firing, which results in increased response to noxious stimuli and can even result in a response to non-noxious stimuli.

Central sensitization is the idea that persistent pain transmission over time from the peripheral nervous system can cause the pain pathways in the spinal cord and brain to make new, stronger synapses (known as use-dependent plasticity). These new synapses cause a modulated pain transmission containing prolonged responses, or windup. Furthermore, the central sensitization model theorizes that increased activity from brain areas implicated in pain have the ability to modulate pain perception. Central sensitization can be used to explain hyperalgesia, allodynia, and spontaneous pain. There have been more detailed models proposed to explain its mechanism; the details behind these, however, are not the focus of this chapter.

Biopsychosocial Model

Although these historical theories appropriately suggested a biomedical mechanism to pain, the biopsychosocial model, which was proposed in 1977 by Engel, was the first to suggest that psychosocial factors can affect pain perception and maintenance of pain. This refuted the then-traditional view that pain was merely a sensation. Similarly, the Institute of Medicine in 2011 stated its belief that "pain arises in the nervous system, but represents a complex and evolving interplay of biological, behavioral, environmental, and social factors...."

There is not one singularly accepted scientific explanation behind psychology's role in the pain pathway, but many theories rest on the foundation that psychological factors may sensitize both peripheral and central nerve pathways, causing a heightened sensitivity to pain which ultimately affects the cognitive processing of the pain stimulus in the brain. The biopsychosocial model illustrates that pain is the product of a biomedical pathway (activation and transmission of noxious stimuli) and an integration of psychosocial influences, such as beliefs, cognition, mental state, and society.

This model can be used to explain why chronic pain patients often develop negative coping mechanisms (e.g., catastrophizing perceived helplessness and low self-efficacy), which ultimately influence pain severity and prolong a patient's symptoms. Similarly, depression has been found to be highly associated with chronic pain, with a prevalence rate between 30 and 54% and often serving as a prognostic indicator for greater disability. The biopsychosocial model draws further support from evidence that patients with chronic pain often benefit from cognitive- and behavioral-based interventions. Ultimately, the biopsychosocial model helped to evolve pain treatment approaches to more holistic ones, encompassing treatments for both the body and the mind.

Overview of the Current Pain Pathway

When considered in aggregate, these early pain theories provide substantial evidence in illustrating pain as a biological process with a dedicated pathway in the nervous system. This section will bring together these theories to outline the current scientific thinking of nociception and its mechanism, which is an important consideration in understanding the various treatment modalities of today. Future chapters will also provide more detailed information on the various components of the pain pathway.

The pain pathway starts with dedicated receptors and nociceptors, which respond to local tissue damage including mechanical (pressure and pinch), heat, and chemical. If an original stimulus exceeds the activation threshold, nociceptors convert the original stimulus into an electrical signal that is transmitted to the central nervous system for processing. When activated, these nociceptors produce a cascade of inflammatory mediators, which only further activate and sensitize them (a process known as peripheral sensitization).

Examples of these mediators include prostaglandins, bradykinin, and histamine.

From here, the transduced electrical signal is carried via A-delta (Aδ) and C fibers, which serve as the primary afferent nerve fibers in the pain pathway. Thinly myelinated Aδ fibers are responsible for sharp and stinging pain sensations, whereas C fibers typically convey duller pain. These fibers carry signal to the spinal cord where they eventually terminate in the dorsal horn and synapse with second-order neurons. The signal then travels up to the brain along the spinothalamic and spinoreticular tracts, which are located in the anterolateral white matter of the spinal cord. Once in the brain, the signal is processed by the thalamus and projected to the somatosensory cortices, insula, anterior cingulate cortex, and prefrontal cortex, all of which are important for pain perception. The lateral system is thought to be responsible for analyzing pain location, duration, intensity, and quality, whereas the medial system is thought to be responsible for perception.

Throughout the pathway lie mechanisms that can inhibit the propagation of pain signal. Information about non-noxious stimuli are carried by alpha-beta fibers and travel adjacent to the alpha-delta and C fibers; as postulated by the gate control theory, these non-noxious fibers may inhibit the fibers of nociception if activated simultaneously. Furthermore, the signal can be modulated by a variety of spinal mechanisms, which include endogenous opioids and cannabinoid systems, as well as inhibitory aminos such as GABA and nitric oxide. Lastly, the signal can be inhibited by descending pathways from the brain. These descending pathways are mediated by noradrenaline and serotonin; the two parts of the brain most important in the descending inhibition pathway are the periaqueductal gray and the nuclei raphe magnus.

Permanent lesions or persistent damage to different parts of the pain pathway can lead to central and peripheral sensitization. The modulation of the pathway via sensitization can also lead to many different types of pain, including chronic pain states and hyperalgesia.

Types of Pain

To better understand the treatment of pain as a disease state, one should first understand the various types of pain we know to exist today. With continued and increasingly advanced research within the field of pain medicine, physicians have developed more standardized methods in classifying the many different types of pain; one way to identify pain type is to analyze its characteristics of duration, anatomic source, and etiology. In 2002, the SCI Pain Task Force of the International Association of the Study of Pain developed a taxonomy to subdivide the various pain states, which is now one of the most common methods used to classify pain. This classification system uses a physiological/etiological approach, stratifying pains by the physiological mechanism behind each type based on etiology. In this method of pain classification, three types of pain can be identified. The first two types, known as nociceptive and neuropathic, carry distinguishing characteristics, while the third type (mixed) combines characteristics of both nociceptive and neuropathic pain.

Nociceptive Pain

Nociceptive pain describes pain that typically arises from the injury of somatic structures such as the skin, muscles, tendons, ligaments, bones, and joints. Nociceptive pain is the consequence of the transduction of noxious stimuli by A-delta and C fibers, as previously described in this chapter. Nociceptive pain can be further subdivided into somatic pain and visceral pain.

A. Somatic pain is pain associated with peripheral tissue damage sensed by cutaneous nociceptors. Specialized nociceptors sense somatic pain in response to various harmful stimuli, most notably thermal (hot vs. cold), chemical (such as those produced by cuts and the inflammatory mediators produced by damaged tissues), and mechanical (e.g., stretching and pinching). Somatic pain can be thought of as a protective mechanism; it allows the body to localize tissue damage and withdraw itself from the source.

B. While somatic pain is typically associated with external stimuli, visceral pain draws on information from internal organs (more specifically and most typically, the mucosal lining of hollow organs). In further contrast, somatic pain withdraws the body from potential harm, where visceral pain is the inner organs' defense mechanism to signal danger given their inability to elicit motor activity and move away from the pain signal. For example, the mucosal lining of the GI tract contains receptors with the ability to detect harmful changes such as dangerously high/low pH levels or the overstretching of the organ, which in turn produce symptoms of nausea and bowel distention and lead to defecation, vomiting, etc. Simplistically, visceral pain can be viewed as an attempt to maintain an internal homeostasis of the body.
Visceral pain is the product of vagal and spinal visceral afferent neurons. In contrast to somatic pain, there are no dedicated centers in the central nervous system specifically concerned with the transmission of visceral pain signals. This broadly explains why patients with visceral pain often have difficulty localizing the exact location of their pain. Furthermore, visceral pain can be felt in loca-

tions distant from the source of the stimulation, which is termed referred pain. The exact mechanism of referred pain is not known. One hypothesis suggests that sensory afferents supply multiple locations and that the stimulation of one location activates its other branches which in turn obscures the exact localization of the original stimulus.

Neuropathic Pain

Neuropathic pain is pain caused by damage of either the peripheral or central nervous system. The International Association of the Study of Pain formally defines neuropathic pain as "pain caused by a lesion or disease of the somatosensory nervous system." Central neuropathic pain is sourced from lesions within the spinal cord or brain. Some common disease states implicated in central neuropathic pain include spinal cord lesions, multiple sclerosis, transverse myelitis, and syringomyelia. In contrast, peripheral neuropathic pain is caused by lesions within the small unmyelinated C fibers and the myelinated A fibers. The peripheral neuropathies can be further subdivided based on distribution. Most peripheral neuropathies generally fall within two categories: peripheral focal/multifocal lesions and peripheral generalized lesions. Some examples of focal and multifocal lesions include entrapment syndromes, post-traumatic neuralgia, postherpetic neuralgia, and diabetic mononeuropathy; generalized lesions include polyneuropathies associated with diabetes mellitus, alcoholism, and HIV.

Research reveals a complex pathophysiology behind the etiology of neuropathic pain. In general, however, it can be stated that the peripheral nervous system responds to the presence of noxious stimuli when, in the absence of such stimuli, it would otherwise remain dormant. With lesion/damage/chronic disease, these nerves are sensitized (as detailed previously) and develop pathological baseline activity that causes neuropathic pain, even in the absence of noxious stimuli.

Acute Versus Chronic Pain

Pain can also be categorized by duration; these designations include acute and chronic pain. Acute pain is normally described as pain that extends for less than 3 days. It is the consequence of a specific disease or injury and is normally self-limited. For example, patients often experience a degree of pain in the days immediately following surgery, but this pain tends to subside thereafter with the passage of a moderate amount of time. Conversely, chronic pain is pain that persists beyond the expected healing period for a specific injury or disease; typically pain greater than 3 months is defined as chronic pain. Chronic pain is hypothesized to be the result of permanent changes within the nervous system (central and peripheral sensitization, as discussed previously), and the associated syndromes of chronic pain are typically the focus of pain management and treatment. Some examples include chronic lower back pain, headache, myofascial pain, and fibromyalgia. These chronic pain syndromes comprise components of both neuropathic and nociceptive pain and are marked by distinguishing biological etiologies.

Treatment: A Multimodal Approach

Today's approach to pain treatment is the result of many decades of research into the effectiveness and efficiencies of treatment methods and reflects the depth of the patient pool currently seeking treatment. It has been estimated that roughly 100 million adults suffer from chronic pain and that chronic pain is responsible for 90 million physician visits, 14% of all prescriptions, and 50 million lost workdays annually. The total healthcare cost associated with pain treatment in the United States is estimated to be $650 billion dollars per year. With such a prevalent burden on both society and medicine, the American Board for Hospital Accreditation has adopted pain as the "fifth vital sign." Similarly, Canada added pain assessment and management to its Achieving Improved Measurement Standards in 2005. Continued increases in the number of patients seeking treatment for pain have led to the formal protocolization of pain assessment and treatment in the inpatient setting.

The task of developing efficacious and cost-effective treatment methods has challenged physicians and scientists for decades. A well-received and widely utilized solution was developed by anesthesiologist John J. Bonica, who pioneered the multidisciplinary approach to pain treatment. As a physician who treated chronic pain in soldiers after World War II, Bonica was one of the first physicians to consult experts from different disciplines (neurology, psychiatry, surgery) in an attempt to find more effective and all-encompassing treatments for his patients. Utilizing this multidisciplinary approach, Dr. Bonica witnessed vast improvements in his patients' pain ratings and led him to open the first multidisciplinary pain clinic in 1950. This multidisciplinary approach to treatment produced greater patient satisfaction and decreased healthcare costs.

Since the landmark events of Dr. Bonica's multidisciplinary approach to treatment, physicians have accepted the multifaceted mechanism involved in the generation, adaptation, and chronicity of pain, as illustrated throughout this chapter. With this acceptance, pain management has evolved into a multimodal approach, and pain treatment now often encompasses a combination of pharmaceutical, surgical, behavioral, and alternative treatments. Utilizing a multidisciplinary approach, the goal of pain management today is not only to reduce a patient's pain symptoms but to improve the individual's overall physical function, better manage chronic diseases, and improve psychological well-being in relation to a patient's pain in the hopes of creating an improved overall general state.

This section of the chapter serves as an introduction to the current modalities of pain treatment and the diseases they treat. Pain treatment can be simplified into two broad categories: pharmacological and nonpharmacological strategies. Future chapters will be dedicated to more detailed descriptions and analyses of each of the modalities.

Pharmacological Treatments

Pharmacological treatment is one of the oldest methods of pain treatment that is still widely used today. Specific pharmacological algorithms, which will be discussed in a future chapter, have been proposed to aid practitioners in treating pain. When implementing pharmacological strategies, it is important to consider the type of pain that is being treated, whether it be nociceptive, neuropathic, or mixed; specific classes of medication treat different types of pain with varying efficacies. Furthermore, a multimodal approach to pharmacological treatment is considered most beneficial for patients. The aim of a multimodal approach is to use medications that act on different receptors and/or parts of the pain pathway to create synergistic effects and consequently stronger pain relief. Some of the most commonly utilized pharmacological treatments include nonsteroidal anti-inflammatory drugs (NSAIDS), antidepressants, anticonvulsant medications, and opioids.

Nonsteroidal Anti-inflammatory Drugs (NSAIDS)

Nonsteroidal anti-inflammatory drugs (NSAIDS) are one of the most popular agents in the treatment of multiple pain states, most notably inflammatory pain. NSAIDS provide pain relief via anti-inflammatory mechanisms by inhibiting prostaglandins-producing enzymes, which are present in both the central and peripheral parts of the pain pathway. Prostaglandins are produced by the COX class of enzymes, with COX-1 and COX-2 being the most pertinent isoforms to the pain pathway [62]. Although NSAIDS inhibit both COX-1 and Cox-2, it has been suggested that most of its analgesic properties arise from its COX-2 inhibition. Nonselective COX agents inhibit both COX-1 and Cox-2 isoforms; some examples of nonselective inhibitors include aspirin, paracetamol, ibuprofen, and naproxen. Selective COX inhibitors, or those that only inhibit COX-2, were later designed to prevent the common side effects associated with nonselective agents (most notably GI intolerance and renal injury). Examples of selective COX inhibitors include celecoxib, meloxicam, and rofecoxib. It is important to note that NSAIDS, although frequently used in the treatment of neuropathic pain, have been shown to have little utility in the treatment of nociceptive pain. NSAIDS have been found most effective in treating diseases with an inflammatory mechanism such as osteoarthritis and rheumatoid arthritis.

Antidepressants

Antidepressants, although originally intended for the treatment of psychiatric illnesses, have also been found effective in pain treatment. Antidepressant medications work by inhibiting the reuptake of certain neurotransmitters, most notably serotonin and norepinephrine, causing a buildup that potentiates inhibitory pain pathways in the spinal cord.

The three classes of antidepressants most commonly utilized in pain management are tricyclic antidepressants (TCAs), selective serotonin reuptake inhibitors (SSRIs), and serotonin-norepinephrine reuptake inhibitors (SNRIs). Tricyclic antidepressants were the first class to be used in pain medicine and work by blocking the reuptake of serotonin and noradrenaline. TCAs have been found beneficial in the treatment of neuropathic pain, fibromyalgia, and headaches. However, notable side effects of TCAs include cardiac arrhythmia and hypertension.

Selective serotonin reuptake inhibitors, unlike tricyclic antidepressants, only inhibit the reuptake of serotonin and were developed in an attempt to avoid the side effects of TCAs. There has also been increased research on newer SNRI drugs, which inhibit the reuptake of serotonin and noradrenaline, showing their helpfulness in treatment of neuropathic pain and fibromyalgia.

Anticonvulsant Medications

Anticonvulsant medications have been effective in the field of chronic pain management since their inception in the 1960s due to their neuromodulating properties. Anticonvulsants assert their activity by enhancing the inhibitory pathway of the gamma-aminobutyric acid (GABA) pathway; gabapentin and pregabalin are the most researched and most commonly utilized anticonvulsants in the field of pain management. These drugs have become clinically favored as adjunct agents in the treatment of chronic neuropathic pain, particularly in postherpetic neuralgia and diabetic neuropathy. Carbamazepine, also in this class of drugs, is considered a mainstay in the treatment of chronic neuropathic pain associated with trigeminal neuralgia. The popularity of anticonvulsants has risen over time because of their wide safety margin. The most common side effect of anticonvulsants is dose-dependent sedation.

Opioids

Opioids are one of the oldest, most potent, and most popular drug classes used in pain management and treatment. Opiates is the term used to encompass naturally occurring derivatives of opium such as morphine and codeine; opioids is a broader term used to describe any drug that produces morphine-like actions, whether they be naturally occurring (opiates) or artificially synthesized (as with fentanyl, heroin, and methadone). The effectiveness of these drugs in treating pain, particularly acute pain within the first 6 weeks of an acute pain trigger, is undisputed, but there is currently no proven data to show efficacy beyond the acute pain period. In addition, adverse effects have been a significant source of scrutiny in the medical field; due to the current rise in opioid misuse, addiction, and overprescribing, there has been a sway in the pendulum of pain treatment to minimize the use of opioids at this time.

Opioids exert their desired effects via G-coupled protein receptors, which are subclassified as mu, kappa, and delta receptors. Simplistically, opioid receptors inhibit adenylyl cyclase, which subsequently inhibit cyclic AMP (cAMP) and the release of certain neurotransmitters implicit in pain production and perception. Opioids for chronic pain treatment are usually prepared in either oral or transdermal forms.

Although many would accept their role in the management of acute pain, opioids have been highly scrutinized in the context of chronic pain management, predominantly due to their adverse side effects and potentially abusive qualities. The primary side effects of opioids are reported to be constipation, nausea, and sedation. More serious side effects, such as hypogonadism, amenorrhea in women, and impairment in neuropsychological function, have also been associated with chronic opioid use. Furthermore, opioids have been shown to have addictive properties, and the concepts of drug addiction, tolerance, and dependence must be addressed with patients when administered for prolonged use in the treatment of chronic pain.

Interventional Techniques

Although pharmacological and noninvasive techniques are typically the first and primary line of defense in the treatment of chronic pain, it has been estimated that approximately 10% of patients cannot be adequately treated with these methods. In these select patients, the role of interventional techniques has been explored to find potential solutions in the treatment and management of their pain. Interventional techniques are usually utilized when a patient's pain arises from a spinal etiology, such as discogenic or sacroiliac joint pain. Interventional techniques have been used to both help alleviate pain, as well as to locate and diagnose the source of a patient's pain. Common interventional techniques include injection therapy, intrathecal drug delivery, and discography.

Injection Therapy

Injection therapy encompasses a wide array of injection types used in the treatment of chronic pain and were first reported to be utilized in 1901. With the development of modern techniques, injection therapy has become an accepted tool in treating pain patients.

Peripheral injection therapies include trigger point and intra-articular joint injections. Trigger point injections involve dry needling into tender muscle points, which attempts to elicit a twitch in the targeted muscle and subsequently alleviate any painful preexisting muscle contractures. The dry needling can also be supplemented with concomitant injections of local anesthetics, though this has not been scientifically proven effective. Anecdotally, physicians have witnessed the benefits of trigger point injections in the treatment of myofascial pain, while intra-articular joint injections have been utilized in the treatment of chronic joint pain. These injections are performed with corticosteroids, which are aimed at reducing inflammation in the joint.

Central injection therapies include intrathecal therapy, epidural injections, and radiofrequency ablation. In the United States, epidural steroid injections are the most common intervention form of this type utilized in pain treatment. Epidural steroid injections achieve their pain-alleviating properties by reducing inflammation of nerve roots and their surrounding environment and have been shown to be useful in the treatment of radiculopathies caused by disc pathology such as disc herniation. Traditionally, epidural steroid injections had been administered via the interlaminar approach, where the injection is placed in the space between two laminae. Other approaches, such as caudal and transforaminal, have also become more common with the advancement of technique and the advent of fluoroscopic-guided practices.

Radiofrequency ablation (RFA) is the process by which a generated radio frequency wave is injected via an insulated needle to produce heat energy from the induction of ion oscillation. The heat energy produced subsequently causes the thermal ablation of the surrounding environment. In relation to pain treatment, RFA has been targeted at dorsal root ganglions and nerve plexus in various diseases in an attempt to cause nerve denervation and block pain signal propagation. RFA has been shown helpful in the treatment of trigeminal neuralgia (gasserian ganglion), cluster headaches (sphenopalatine ganglion), and postherpetic neuralgia (percutaneous dorsal root ganglions). The most common use of radiofrequency ablation has been witnessed in the treatment of facet-mediated back pain, given RFAs particular effectiveness in its ability to denervate medial branch nerves.

Neuromodulation

Neuromodulation is one of the newest emerging treatment concepts in the field of pain management. Although largely still considered an evolving treatment, the foundation of neuromodulation originated in the mid-1960s with Melzack and Wall's gate control theory of pain, which states that the transmission of pain depends upon the opening and closing of a "gate" by large and small fibers. Neuromodulation functions under the assumption that it may be possible to alter the activation of these large and small fibers in different parts of the pain pathway, resulting in the inhibition pain. The alteration of these fibers can be achieved via two forms: electrical and chemical neuromodulation.

Electrical neuromodulation is accomplished by placing implantable electrodes, attached to a generator, in the peripheral and central nervous system to generate a pulse onto the targeted nerves. Different types of electrical neuromodulation include spinal cord stimulation (SCS), peripheral nerve stimulation (PNS), occipital nerve field stimulation (ONFS), deep brain stimulation (DBS), and motor cortex stimulation (MCS).

Spinal cord stimulation has been most frequently implemented in the treatment of persistent back pain following failed back surgery. Spinal cord stimulation has also been used in the treatment of ischemic leg pain from peripheral vascular disease, unstable angina, and complex regional syndrome. Deep brain stimulation, similar to spinal cord stimulation, asserts its pain-alleviating effects through the electrical stimulation of subcortical structures. Although not completely understood, the stimulation of the periaqueductal and periventricular gray matter of the thalamus may cause the release of endogenous opiates that provide pain relief. Motor cortex stimulation has been indicated in the treatment of central post-stroke pain.

Neuromodulation can also be accomplished through chemical means by delivering drugs directly into the central nervous system. Chemical neuromodulation is most commonly accomplished via intrathecal drug delivery systems.

Psychological Treatment of Pain

As defined by the biopsychosocial model, pain is not solely a biological mechanism but can also be influenced by an individual's environment and mental well-being. Pain can often produce anxiety in patients and has been shown to ultimately worsen the overall perception of pain. Thus, it is not surprising that today's treatment protocols often include components aimed at assessing and treating the psychological impacts of pain.

The most common technique used to treat the psychological effects of pain is cognitive behavioral therapy (CBT). Cognitive behavioral therapy identifies the negative perceptions, emotions, and beliefs an individual associates with his or her physical pain, which often cause increased stress and anxiety. Furthermore, CBT seeks to identify any negative coping mechanisms individuals have learned or developed to cope with pain. Once identified, CBT attempts to equip patients with new techniques and positive tools to cope, adapt, and manage their pain independently, counteracting the previously held negative beliefs and ineffective coping mechanisms. Cognitive behavioral therapy has been shown effective in improving patients' moods, quality of life, and treatment satisfaction.

Conclusion: Putting It All Together

The concept of pain remains a medical phenomenon. Today's definition of pain is complex and continues to evolve with new scientific discoveries and the overall advancement of medicine. Given the dynamic nature of pain, its definition is likely to continue to change over time; it remains well established, however, that pain is an integrative process comprising an interplay between the human anatomy/physiology, psychological factors, and external environment. Under the current definition, it is also widely accepted that many types of pain and a multitude of pain states exist. With such diversity among the mechanics and types of pain, the field of pain management has evolved to encompass multimodal and multidisciplinary approaches to treatment. As physicians continue to seek a full understanding of pain in an effort to better serve patients, it is expected that treatments will continue to evolve and new modalities will be pioneered. Nevertheless, the historical context provided in this chapter serves as the foundation of today's treatment methods and provides a strong base for future developments in the field of pain management.

Recommended Reading

1. Anwar K. Pathophysiology of pain. Dis Mon. 2016;16(9):324–9.
2. Ashburn M, Staats P. Management of chronic pain. Lancet. 1999;353(9167):1865–9.
3. Baron R. Mechanisms of disease: neuropathic pain—a clinical perspective. Nat Clin Pract Neurol. 2006;2(2):95–106.
4. Bashir U, Colvin LA. The place of pharmacological treatment in chronic pain. Anaesth Intensive Care Med. 2013;14(12):528–32.
5. Beissner F, Brandau A, Henke C, et al. Quick discrimination of A delta and C fiber mediated pain based on three verbal descriptors. Ikeda K, ed. PLoS One. 2010;5(9):e12944.
6. Binshtok AM. Mechanisms of nociceptive transduction and transmission: a machinery for pain sensation and tools for selective analgesia. Int Rev Neurobiol. 2011;97:143–77.
7. Bittar RG, Teddy PJ. Peripheral neuromodulation for pain. J Clin Neurosci. 2009;16(10):1259–61.
8. Braz J, Solorzano C, Wang X, Basbaum AI. Transmitting pain and itch messages: a contemporary view of the spinal cord circuits that generate gate control. Neuron. 2014;82(3):522–36.
9. Buyten JP. Radiofrequency or neuromodulation treatment of chronic pain, when is it useful? Eur J Pain Suppl. 2008;2(S1):57–66.
10. Campbell LC, Clauw DJ, Keefe FJ. Persistent pain and depression: a biopsychosocial perspective. Biol Psychiatry. 2003;54(3):399–409.
11. Chapman CR. New directions in the understanding and management of pain. Soc Sci Med. 1984;19(12):1261–77.
12. Cheatle MD. Biopsychosocial approach to assessing and managing patients with chronic pain. Med Clin N Am. 2016;100(1):43–53.
13. Chen J. History of pain theories. Neurosci Bull. 2011;27:343.

14. Chen M, Hoshino H, Saito S, Yang Y, Obata H. Spinal dopaminergic involvement in the antihyperalgesic effect of antidepressants in a rat model of neuropathic pain. Neurosci Lett. 2017;649:116–23.
15. Cohen S, Raja S. Goldman's Cecil medicine. 24th ed. Philadelphia: Elsevier; 2012 . Chapter 29, Pain. p. 133–40.
16. Colloca L, Ludman T, Bouhassira D, Baron R, Dickenson A, et al. Neuropathic pain. Nat Rev Dis Primers. 2017;3:17002.
17. Craig AD. Pain mechanisms: labeled lines versus convergence in central processing. Annu Rev Neurosci. 2003;26(1):1–30.
18. Dale R, Stacey B. Multimodal treatment of chronic pain. Med Clin N Am. 2016;100(1):55–64.
19. Dedeli O, Kaptan G. Spirituality and religion in pain and pain management. Health Psychol Res. 2013;1(3):e29.
20. Deer TR. An overview of interventional spinal techniques. Semin Pain Med. 2004;2(3):154–66.
21. Dietrich J. Psychology and chronic pain. Anaesth Intensive Care Med. 2011 Feb;12(2):42–3.
22. D'Mello R, Dickenson AH. Spinal cord mechanisms of pain. Br J Anaesth. 2008;101(1):8–16.
23. Doleys DM. Chronic pain as a hypothetical construct: a practical and philosophical consideration. Front Psychol. 2017;8:664.
24. Dowell D, Haegerich TM, Chou R. CDC guideline for prescribing opioids for chronic pain – United States, 2016. MMWR Recomm Rep. 2016;65(RR-1):1–49.
25. Duan B, Cheng L, Ma Q. Spinal circuits transmitting mechanical pain and itch. Neurosci Bull. 2018;34(1):186–93.
26. Dubin AE, Patapoutian A. Nociceptors: the sensors of the pain pathway. J Clin Invest. 2010;120(11):3760–72.
27. Dworkin RH, O'Connor AB, Audette J, et al. Recommendations for the pharmacological management of neuropathic pain: an overview and literature update. Mayo Clin Proc. 2010;85(3 Suppl):S3–S14.
28. Finnerup NB, Haroutounian S, Kamerman P, Baron R, Bennett DL, Bouhassira D, et al. Neuropathic pain. Pain. 2016;157(8):1599–606.
29. Grichnik KP, Ferrante FM. The difference between acute and chronic pain. Mt Sinai J Med. 1991;58(3):217–20.
30. Hadidi S, Baranidharan G. Implantable technology for pain management. Anaesth Intensive Care Med. 2016;17(11):536–42.
31. Hamann MCJ, Tsai EC, Tator CH, Shoichet MS. Novel intrathecal delivery system for treatment of spinal cord injury. Exp Neurol. 2003;182(2):300–9.
32. Handwerker H. Itch hypotheses. Itch Front Neurosci. 2014:1–8.
33. High KNW. Pain pathways: peripheral, spinal, ascending, and descending pathways. In: Rajs practical management of pain. Elsevier Inc. 2008. p. 119–34. https://doi.org/10.1016/B978-0-323-04184-3.X5001-8.
34. Hillinger MG, Wolever RQ, Mckernan LC, Elam R. Integrative medicine for the treatment of persistent pain. Prim Care. 2017;44(2):247–64.
35. Hoffert M. The gate control theory re-revisited. J Pain Symptom Manag. 1986;1(1):39–41.
36. Honey CM, Tronnier VM, Honey CR. Deep brain stimulation versus motor cortex stimulation for neuropathic pain: a minireview of the literature and proposal for future research. Comput Struct Biotechnol J. 2016;14:234–7.
37. Kansal A. Visceral pain. Anaesth Intensive Care Med. 2016;17(11):543–7.
38. Keele KD. Anatomies of pain. Oxford: Pl. XIII. Blackwell Scientific Publications; 1957.
39. Kremer MCA, Salvat E, Muller A, Yalcin I, Barrot M. Antidepressants and gabapentinoids in neuropathic pain: mechanistic insights. Neuroscience. 2016;338:183–206.
40. Kroenke K, Krebs EE, Bair MJ. Pharmacotherapy of chronic pain: a synthesis of recommendations from systematic reviews. Gen Hosp Psychiatry. 2009;31(3):206–19.
41. Lima D. Endogenous pain modulatory system in the light of the gate control theory. Pain Forum. 1996;5(1):31–9.
42. Lynch ME, Watson CPN. The pharmacotherapy of chronic pain: a review. Pain Res Manag. 2006;11(1):11–38.
43. Maixner W, Fillingim RB, Williams DA, Smith SB, Slade GD. Overlapping chronic pain conditions: implications for diagnosis and classification. J Pain. 2016;17(9):T93–107.
44. Manworren RC. Multimodal pain management and the future of a personalized medicine approach to pain. AORN J. 2015;101(3):307–18.
45. Marchand S. The phenomenon of pain. Seattle: IASP Press; 2012.
46. Mcdonald J, Lambert DG. Opioid mechanisms and opioid drugs. Anaesth Intensive Care Med. 2016;17(9):464–8.
47. Melzack R. From the gate to the neuromatrix. Pain. 1999;82:S121–6.
48. Melzack R, Wall PD. Pain mechanisms: a new theory. Pain Forum. 1996;5(1):3–11.
49. Mendell LM. Constructing and deconstructing the gate theory of pain. Pain. 2014;155(2):210–6.
50. Mendis V, Mottaleb R, Fung M. Radiofrequency techniques in pain management. Anaesth Intensive Care Med. 2016;17(11):564–7.
51. Moayedi M, Davis KD. Theories of pain: from specificity to gate control. J Neurophysiol. 2012;109(1):5–12.
52. Nasmerow L, Kutner E, Wakefiled E, Rzepski B, Sahl R. Pain amplification syndrome: a biopsychosocial approach. Semin Pediatr Neurol. 2016;23(3):224–30.
53. Nijs J, Wilgen CPV, Oosterwijck JV, Ittersum MV, Meeus M. How to explain central sensitization to patients with 'unexplained' chronic musculoskeletal pain: practice guidelines. Man Ther. 2011;16(5):413–8.
54. Ochs S-A. History of nerve functions: from animal spirits to molecular mechanisms. Cambridge: Cambridge University Press; 2004.
55. Ossipov MH, Dussor GO, Porreca F. Central modulation of pain. J Clin Invest. 2010;120(11):3779–87.
56. Pearce JMS. Von Frey's pain spots. J Neurol Neurosurg Psychiatry. 2006;77(12):1317.
57. Penney JN. The biopsychosocial model of pain and contemporary osteopathic practice. Int J Osteopathic Med. 2010;13(2):42–7.
58. Pergolizzi J, Ahlbeck K, Aldington D, Alon E, Coluzzi F, Dahan A, et al. The development of chronic pain: physiological CHANGE necessitates a multidisciplinary approach to treatment. Curr Med Res Opin. 2013;29(9):1127–35.
59. Perl ER. Pain mechanisms: a commentary on concepts and issues. Prog Neurobiol. 2011;94(1):20–38.
60. Pleuvry B. Non-opioid analgesics. Anaesth Intensive Care Med. 2005;6(1):25–9.
61. Rey R. The history of pain. Cambridge, MA: Harvard Univ. Press; 1998.
62. Roe M, Sehgal A. Pharmacology in the management of chronic pain. Anaesth Intensive Care Med. 2016;17(11):548–51.
63. Sanchis MN, Lluch E, Nijs J, Struyf F, Kangasperko M. The role of central sensitization in shoulder pain: a systematic literature review. Semin Arthritis Rheum. 2015;44(6):710–6.
64. Serpell MG, Makin A, Harvey A. Acute pain physiology and pharmacological targets: the present and future. Acute Pain. 1998;1(3):31–47.
65. Seth B, Gray LD. Genesis of chronic pain. Anaesth Intensive Care Med. 2016;17(9):431–5.
66. Sousa MVPD, Ferraresi C, Magalhães ACD, Yoshimura EM, Hamblin MR. Building, testing and validating a set of home-made von Frey filaments: a precise, accurate and cost effective alternative for nociception assessment. J Neurosci Methods. 2014;232:1–5.
67. Stanos S, Tyburski M, Harden NR. Braddom's physical medicine and rehabilitation. 5th ed. Philadelphia: Elsevier; 2015. Chapter 37, Chronic Pain. p. 809–17.
68. Steeds C. The anatomy and physiology of pain. Surgery – Oxford International Edition. 2009;27(12):507–11.
69. Stein C. Opioids, sensory systems and chronic pain. Eur J Pharmacol. 2013;716(1–3):179–87.

70. Tashani O, Johnson M. Transcutaneous Electrical Nerve Stimulation (TENS) a possible aid for pain relief in developing countries? Libyan J Med. 2009;4(2):62–5.
71. Taylor LEV, Stotts NA, Humphreys J, Treadwell MJ, Miaskowski C. A biopsychosocial-spiritual model of chronic pain in adults with sickle cell disease. Pain Manag Nurs. 2013;14(4):287–301.
72. Tompkins DA, Hobelmann JG, Compton P. Providing chronic pain management in the "Fifth Vital Sign" Era: historical and treatment perspectives on a modern-day medical dilemma. Drug Alcohol Depend. 2017;173:S11–21.
73. Turk DC, Wilson HD, Cahana A. Treatment of chronic non-cancer pain. Lancet. 2011;377(9784):2226–35.
74. Wolff BB. Gate control theory and the brain. Pain Forum. 1996;5(2):147–9.
75. Woolf CJ. Central sensitization: implications for the diagnosis and treatment of pain. Pain. 2011;152(3 Suppl):S2–15.
76. Wrigley P, Siddall P. Wall & Melzack's textbook of pain. 6th ed. Philadelphia: Elsevier/Saunders; c2013. Chapter 68, Pain following Spinal Cord Injury. p. 978–89.

Algorithms of Pain Treatment

2

Andrew So and Karina Gritsenko

Introduction

Chronic pain is one of the most common symptoms for which patients seek medical attention. It is estimated that up to 11.2% of adults in the United States suffer from chronic pain [1] and that patients in the United States alone spend between $560 billion and $635 billion on chronic pain treatment annually [2]. Chronic pain also remains widely prevalent due to its ubiquitous nature; it is associated with a plethora of conditions, such as cancer, lower back pain, and neuropathic pain conditions [3].

At present, there is not one universally accepted formula to treat chronic pain, and many times treatment is based on anecdotal outcomes and non-evidence-based personal experiences [4]. Dr. John Bonica, who was a trained anesthesiologist during World War II, was one of the first physicians to formalize the treatment of chronic pain, leading to the eventual transformation of chronic pain into its own subspecialty. Dr. Bonica was also one of the first physicians to treat pain in a multidisciplinary way in an attempt to formalize a more effective approach to pain treatment [5]. Since then, numerous societies have been established that are dedicated to the fields of pain treatment and management.

Even with the advent of a multidisciplinary approach by Dr. Bonica, it remains impossible to create a single set of criteria to treat the wide array of pain states and disease mechanisms. Various tools and guidelines have been set forward to aid physicians in their treatment approaches and to streamline a more protocolized approach to the treatment of pain. As such, pain physicians should understand the current approach to treating chronic pain patients and the tools that are available to aid in this journey.

To provide a better understanding of the common algorithms used in chronic pain treatment, this chapter will discuss the importance of the initial patient evaluation in the treatment process and highlight several effective tools physicians can implement. It will also highlight the currently accepted treatment guidelines for some pain states most commonly encountered by physicians.

Assessment Algorithm

Although treatment algorithms typically vary depending upon the type of pain being treated (cancer, neuropathic, lower back pain, etc.), a macro-level analysis of pain algorithms reveals strong underlying points of commonality, including the importance of the initial evaluation of a chronic pain patient. Therefore, we begin our analysis of pain algorithms by exploring the initial process of patient assessment and its role in framing overall treatment plans.

A comprehensive initial assessment provides vital information on an individual's pain and aids in treatment decision-making that will provide the best suited outcome for individual patients [6]. In formulating their Pain Taxonomy framework, the American Pain Society defines the importance of a reliable and valid pain assessment in the treatment of chronic pain patients; this initial assessment functions as a vital tool in helping determine the severity of pain, surveying the course of the pain, and establishing the pathophysiology of the pain. With this information, physicians are equipped with a better understanding of the patient and thus are more ably prepared to craft effective treatment plans [7]. There is a myriad of literature focused in detail on the specific domains that should be investigated in the initial pain assessment, but given the purpose and scope of this chapter, this section will focus on the most highlighted domains. Each of these domains is discussed in brief below.

A. So (✉)
Albert Einstein College of Medicine/Montefiore Medical Center, New York City, NY, USA

K. Gritsenko
Albert Einstein College of Medicine/Montefiore Medical Center, Montefiore Multidisciplinary Pain Program, The Bronx, NY, USA

T. R. Deer et al. (eds.), *Deer's Treatment of Pain*, https://doi.org/10.1007/978-3-030-12281-2_2

History

Nearly all pain treatment algorithms emphasize the importance of an initial history review. Gathering and understanding a detailed, holistic background on a patient and his/her medical history often supply practitioners with significant information that eventually aids in treatment planning. The result of this initial interview can guide a practitioner in making medical diagnoses, determining a need for further workup, and/or assessing potential treatment options [6].

In their most recently published Practice Guidelines for Chronic Pain Management, the American Society of Anesthesiologists (ASA) recommends that the initial evaluation of a chronic pain patient includes a detailed medical history with specific focus on the chronology of the pain. Attention should be paid to obtaining details such as the intensity, quality, location, duration, and distribution of a patient's reported pain. In addition to symptom history, social history (with a focus on abuse), surgical history, and family history should also be investigated and recorded. Furthermore, the ASA recommends a review of previous diagnostic tests, medication lists (both past and present), and any other previously implemented treatments to investigate their historical effectiveness [8].

Physical Exam

A thorough physical exam is also a fundamental component of the initial evaluation. The aim of the physical exam is to elicit information to help make a proper diagnosis and may also help eliminate underlying and treatable pathology [9]. In general, a physical exam should follow that of a normal generalized comprehensive human systems exam. Particular attention should be given to the system under which the initial chief complaint falls. Furthermore, special attention should be paid to the musculoskeletal and neuromuscular system, as the majority of chronic pain falls under this system [10]. Eliciting symptoms, such as focal weaknesses, site tenderness, and neurological deficits may help providers make accurate diagnosis.

Pain Intensity: Pain Intensity Rating Scales

As covered, one purpose of the initial interview is to determine the intensity of a patient's pain, which some argue to be the most important dimension investigated in the initial pain assessment [11]. With an understanding of pain intensity, clinicians are better prepared to gauge the severity of a patient's pain and its realistic impact/burden on the patient's functional capacity. Furthermore, clinicians can make more informed treatment decisions based on a patient's pain intensity and, even more importantly, assess the efficacy of a treatment by evaluating positive/neutral/negative changes in reported intensity [12].

An objective and accurate system of measuring pain intensity remains difficult to define, predominantly due to the multitude of factors that can influence a patient's perception of pain, from pathophysiological to psychosocial aspects [13]. Given its subjective nature and with only a limited amount of time for clinicians to ascertain a patient's pain intensity, the role of pain measurement scales has proven to be essential. The verbal rating scale (VRS), the visual analog scale (VAS), and the numerical rating scale (NRS) are among the most commonly used pain measurement scales in clinical practice. While all of these scales have proven to be helpful, distinct advantages and disadvantages can be identified for each [14].

The verbal rating scale has been implemented in practice since the 1940s and consists of a list of qualitative descriptors used to define various levels of pain intensity. An example of a verbal rating scale would be no pain, mild pain, moderate pain, and severe pain. Each adjective is also assigned a numeric value in an ascending order of pain intensities; in the previous example, no pain = 0, mild pain = 1, and so forth [15]. Patients are asked to select the term from the rating scale which best correlates to their perceived pain intensity, and the numeric value associated with that adjective is then assigned. A major advantage of the verbal rating scale is its relative simplicity and easy implementation [13]. Some criticize the verbal rating scale since patients may have to be familiar with the terms to properly use it.

The visual analog scale is a linear model anchored at one end by the non-existence of pain symptoms and opposed at the other by the worst imaginable pain. A numerical value is also plotted on the line to coincide with the various pain intensity descriptors, with 0 equating to no pain and 10 with the worst imaginable pain [16]. Patients are asked to mark where on the line their pain intensity lies. The biggest advantage of the VAS noted is its high degree of "sensitivity" when compared to the other scale rating systems [17]. However, the VAS has been characterized as more complex and may be difficult to implement for patients with cognitive impairments.

The numeric rating scale consists of a numerical scale, usually 0 to 10 (0 = no pain and 10 = most severe pain ever). Patients are instructed to pick a number that best reflects their pain intensity. The numeric rating scale has been seen to be easier to use than the visual analog scale [7].

Pain Quality: The McGill Pain Questionnaire

Along with the varying pain intensities discussed previously, pain can also be characterized by its perceived qualities. Even though two varying pain symptoms may be ranked as having the same intensity (e.g., 9/10), individuals may characterize the pain differently with descriptors such as shooting, sharp, dull, etc. Therefore, it is important physicians gather information on the sensory and effective quality of a patient's pain perception [7].

The McGill Pain Questionnaire is one of the most widely utilized tools to help provide a qualitative measure of clinical pain [18]. Having been developed by Melzack and Torgerson based on the gate control theory of pain, the McGill Pain Questionnaire was first published in 1975 [19] and consists of descriptors grouped into three main dimensions: sensory, affective, and evaluative [20]. The sensory component aims to reveal information regarding pain location, intensity, and quality, while the affective component examines any fear and/or anxiety that may be associated with an individual's pain. Lastly, the evaluative component attempts to analyze the overall subjective pain experience of a patient [18].

The McGill Pain Questionnaire can be administered in two different forms. The first, and longer, form contains 78 descriptors, while the second is a more abbreviated version with only 15 descriptors. Patients are presented with sets of grouped descriptors from each domain and asked to select the descriptors which most accurately describe their pain [18].

In its original summation, Melzack theorized that the total number of words chosen or the pattern of words chosen by an individual could help physicians decipher between different pain conditions; he believed each pain condition would possess a unique pattern, similar to a pain fingerprint [21]. Since its creation, the McGill Pain Questionnaire has been shown to possess strong reliability and validity in helping clinicians differentiate various pain conditions, determine pain pathophysiology, and even monitor treatment responses [18, 21].

Psychological Considerations

As the biopsychosocial model explains, pain cannot be characterized as a mere physiological experience; rather, pain is an integrative process influenced by both the body and the mind. As such, the initial evaluation of a pain patient should also include a psychological assessment. Chronic psychological states, such as depression and emotional distress, have been proven to significantly affect patients' perception of pain. It has been estimated that about 50% of people with chronic pain also suffer from depression [22]. Common symptoms of depression and emotional distress include unwanted stress, fatigue, and lowered activity states [1], all of which can heighten the perception of pain severity. Furthermore, studies have shown that depression and anxiety often contribute to lowered pain thresholds.

In response, pain physicians have implemented various scales used to assess the presence and degree of depression in patients into initial pain evaluations, such as the Beck Depression Inventory and the Center for Epidemiological Study for Depression Scale [23, 24] during the initial screening process, certain yellow flags, such as symptoms of depression, patient beliefs of pain as harmful, and a history of passive/uninterested involvement in treatment have been predictors for increased probability of long-term patient disability.

The World Health Organization Analgesic Ladder for Cancer Pain

Dr. John Bonica, one of the founders of and innovators in the multidisciplinary pain medicine field, reported that up to 70% of cancer patients cite pain as the most severe disease-associated symptom. With up to three million patients per year being treated for cancer pain worldwide [25], it is not surprising that the optimization of cancer pain treatment has been placed at the forefront of pain management algorithms.

In 1986, the World Health Organization (WHO) published a document entitled "Cancer Pain," which proposed a stepwise management tool for the treatment of chronic cancer pain [26]. This proposed protocol later became popularly known as the World Health Organization analgesic ladder and has become proliferative in cancer patient care and one of the most used treatment guides in the field of pain management. The protocol has been translated into 22 different languages around the world.

At the ladder's time of conception, a negative stigma surrounded the prescription of opioids. Both medical practitioners and the government alike feared that such prescriptions could ultimately result in higher rates drug addiction, abuse, and tolerance; in extreme scenarios, epidemic levels were feared. However, many patients continued to suffer from poorly treated cancer pain. Therefore, the WHO's analgesic ladder was an attempt to formally remove the negative stigma surrounding opioid prescriptions by providing practitioners a tool, which created a protocol with an accepted stepwise opioid prescription algorithm [26, 27].

The analgesic ladder was constructed on expert opinion, rather than quantitative data, and sought to integrate inexpensive medications in order to make its implementation more feasible and applicable worldwide [28]. The ladder utilizes four different drug classes: non-opioids, weak opioids, strong opioids, and adjuvants. In simplicity, the ladder functions under the foundation that a patient should be prescribed these medications in a sequential manner, with non-opioids utilized first. Over time, and as a patient's pain intensity increases, he/she is incrementally progressed to the next and more aggressive medication, with strong opioids being the end of the spectrum and used with only the most severe pain. The ladder also accepted the risk of addiction, instead prioritizing a patient's comfort during the final stages of life [29].

The three steps, which were obtained from the WHO initial article, will be summarized below [30].

Step 1: For mild pain, physicians should start with a non-opioid with/without adjuvant:

Non-opioid analgesics:

Aceteminiphen
ASA
NSAIDS

(adjuvants: anxiolytics, antidepresants, hypotics, anticonvulsants, sodium channel blockers, cannabinoids, steroids)

If pain persists or intensifies, escalate to Step 2.

Step 2: Add a weak opioid to a non-opioid with/without adjuvant.

Weak opioid:

Codeine
Tramadol
Buprenorphine
Oxycodone
+non-opioid and adjuvant

If pain continues to persist or intensify, escalate to Step 3.

Step 3: Switch to a strong opioid with a non-opioid with/without adjuvant.

Strong opioid:

Morphine
Fentanyl
Methadone
Hydromorphone [30]

The WHO also provides many recommendations for implementing the analgesic ladder. It recommends that oral administration should be preferred over all other routes of administration. Furthermore, it states that analgesic medication should be given at regular intervals. Lastly, analgesic medication and dosing should be based on a patient's subjective rating of his/her pain intensity [30].

Criticisms

At its initial implementation, the ladder was widely deemed a success, and it was estimated that it achieved satisfactory pain relief in up to 90% of patients with cancer pain [31]. Despite its success in a high percentage of patients, many providers remain critical of its effectiveness and implementation. A common criticism of the ladder is that it was not formulated on concrete data but rather expert opinion. Many also believe there remains a lack of strong evidence to support the efficacy of the ladder [26], while still others criticize the validity of Step 2 in the ladder; meta-analysis comparing the use of non-opioids to non-opioids in conjunction with a weak opioid has shown no statistical difference in treating moderate pain [32]. Additional, some believe that the ladder fails to highlight the importance of non-pharmacological and interventional therapies, suggesting the addition of a fourth step to encompass these therapies [31].

Some critics believe the ladder is in part responsible for ushering in the current opioid epidemic. Given its perceived success in terminally ill patients, the ladder legitimized the once stigmatized use of opioids in chronic non-cancer pain. Its effects were notable in the United States, which saw a fourfold increase in opioid prescriptions between the years of 1999 and 2010 [29].

Opioid Epidemic

Although the WHO ladder was intended for use in cancer pain patients, the use of opioids for the treatment of non-cancer pain became highly prevalent. Influenced by James Campbell's concept as pain as the fifth vital sign, the 1990s saw a large push to evaluate and treat pain more effectively [33]. The Department of Veterans Affairs further provoked this movement by emphasizing the importance of pain evaluation and treatment as a standard of care [34], while the Joint Commission on Accreditation of Healthcare Organizations also stressed the importance of chronic pain treatment when they began to assess pain management as a requirement for accreditation [35].

With this newly emphatic focus on pain treatment, pharmaceutical companies pushed the marketing of opioids as a safe interventional tool in the treatment of chronic pain. With both the increased marketing of opioids in the treatment of chronic non-cancer pain and the increased emphasis on pressure to effectively treat pain patients, prescription opioid use boomed [36]; between 1999 and 2000, the use of opioids quadrupled [37]. Opioid use became so prevalent that the Centers for Disease Control and Prevention reported that by 2006, more unintentional overdoses were caused by prescription opioids than by heroin and cocaine combined [38]. Slowly the pain community has seen the harms of over-prescriptions of opioids, and practice has slowly swung away from opioids to alternative interventions [39, 40].

Opioid Guidelines

Much debate surrounds the appropriate use of opioids in chronic pain management. Regardless of the reason behind their use, many societies have issued safety guidelines and measurements in an effort to streamline and create a more safe use of prescription opioids. The American Society of Interventional Pain Physicians outlines basic principles for prescribing opioids in its guide entitled, "Opioids in the Management of Chronic Non-Cancer Pain." The guide emphasizes the importance of a comprehensive medical evaluation and interval patient assessments to ascertain the efficacy of opioid therapy and to monitor for abusive behaviors. Furthermore, they focus on the importance of patient adherence to controlled substance agreements set for by his/her provider [41]. In 2016, the Centers for Disease Control and Prevention published guidelines regarding the prescription of opioids for chronic pain. These recommendations were aimed at primary care clinicians (family physicians and internists) to provide recommendations for the prescribing of opioid pain medication for patients 18 and older in primary care settings, as this population represents a large majority of opioid prescribing. Recommendations focus on the use of opioids in treating chronic pain, pain that is defined as lasting greater than 3 months or past the time of normal tissue healing, excluding active cancer treatment, palliative care, and end-of-life care. This is an important document as it has received national support through the CDC [42]. There have been multiple societies including the American Society of Interventional Pain Physicians (ASIPP), APS (American Pain Society), and the American Society of Regional Anesthesia and Pain Medicine (ASRA) that have shown support for a more conservative approach to opioid prescribing as we are in the midst of an opioid epidemic and evidence to support long-term opioid therapy is limited.

Furthermore, it has been suggested that the DIRE score may provide a useful rating scale in determining the appropriateness of opioid use in particular patients. The DIRE score assigns numerical values for Diagnosis (how advanced the patient's condition is), Intractability (how many treatments have been tried), Risks (evaluates a patient's ability to abuse medications such as mental health history, reliability, and current social support), and Efficacy (how well opioids provide pain relief and improvement in patient function). The scores for each subsection are then summed, and the score is used to predict the appropriateness of opioid use for that individual [43].

Treatment Algorithms and Guidelines

Armed with a better understanding of the common tools used in patient evaluation and treatment, we will now mention a focus on some of the most few commonly encountered pain syndromes and diseases in the field of pain management. This section will serve as an introduction to treatment guidelines by highlighting key factors of each pain state; please refer to the perspective guidelines for more information.

Lower Back Pain

Lower back pain is one of the most common reasons patients seek medical attention. It is estimated that most primary care physicians see at least one patient with chronic lower back pain per week. Furthermore, the economic burden of lower back pain in the United States is estimated at between 12.2 and 90.6 billion dollars [44]. Due to its widespread occurrence and high economic burden, providers across many different specialties have been tasked with finding effective treatment options for patients. At this time, there is not one accepted treatment algorithm for chronic lower back pain, despite efforts by various societies and task forces to develop a protocol for treatment strategies.

The American Academy of Family Physicians (AAFP) published "Chronic Lower Back Pain: Evaluation and Management," which discusses a possible approach to treating a patient with chronic lower back pain. In its recommendations, the AAFP stresses the importance of the initial evaluation of patients presenting with lower back pain. In short, the AAFP recommends that physicians conduct an initial evaluation (with thorough medical history) and physical in an attempt to categorize patients' pain into one of the following: (1) nonspecific low back pain, (2) back pain associated with radiculopathy or spinal stenosis, (3) back pain referred from a non-spinal source, or (4) back pain associated with another specific spinal cause. Furthermore, the AAFP recommends that imaging not be included in the initial workup, unless there is a suspicion for infection, fracture, or cauda equina syndrome or unless required before invasive interventions [45].

The AAFP also concentrates on the pharmacological and non-pharmacological management of chronic lower back pain. The AAFP recommends that treatment begin with the use of nonsteroidal anti-inflammatory drugs (NSAIDS) and acetaminophen. If acetaminophen and/or NSAIDS fail, adjuvant medications, such as tramadol and opioids, should be utilized. The AAFP also discusses non-pharmacological options such as acupuncture, exercise therapy, and behavior therapy and how each modality may play a role in providing pain relief [45].

Lastly, the AAFP provides a potential algorithm when treating patients with chronic lower back pain (please review the complete AAFP review guidelines for a more detailed explanation). In summarizing their approach, the AAFP delineates three scenarios where further workup beyond the initial evaluation should be pursued. These are covered below with the corresponding intervention suggested:

1. Red flags for cauda equina syndrome: immediate workup and/or emergency department referral
2. Fracture suspected: plain-film radiography
3. Progressive neurological symptoms: magnetic resonance imaging

If none of these scenarios are suspected, the AAFP recommends a trial of conservative care, which includes multimodal treatment, utilizing the medications discussed above;

weight loss, exercise, and the use of cognitive behavioral therapy are also suggested solutions. If all previous treatment attempts fail, the AAFP recommends a surgical evaluation as the last step in their approach [46].

In February 2017, the American College of Physicians published its own evidence-based clinical practice guidelines for noninvasive treatments of acute, subacute, and chronic lower back pain. The American College of Physicians based their guidelines on a systematic review of randomized, controlled trials and a review of previously published guidelines. Similarly to the AAFP, the American College of Physicians suggests a conservative initial approach to treatment, such as acupuncture, massages, and spinal manipulation. If non-pharmacological measures fail, the use of NSAIDS and muscle relaxants as the first line of pharmacological treatment is also recommended. The use of opioids is the final method of treatment if all other previous stated modalities fail, though the guidelines stress the importance of weighing the risks and benefits for each individual patient [47].

The American College of Physicians and the American Pain Society published a joint clinical practice guideline on the treatment of low back pain. The guidelines include stepwise algorithm, which contains similar recommendations to those previously covered. The first step in the algorithm emphasizes the importance of conservative management; patients encouraged to stay physically active. Pharmacological treatments should include acetaminophen, muscle relaxants, tricyclic antidepressants, and gabapentin. Non-pharmacological interventions should also be considered and include physical therapy, acupuncture, massage, and behavior therapy. The second step of the algorithm focuses on a reassessment of the patient 4 to 6 weeks after the initial consultation. If the pain is controlled on original therapy, the patient should continue with current treatment plan. If the pain is not controlled, and radiculopathy and/or spinal stenosis is suspected, then one should consider ordering a magnetic resonance imaging. If significant nerve root impingement is present, one should consider pain physician referral, surgical evaluation, and/or other invasive treatments [48].

Neuropathic Pain

Though no one set algorithm exists for the treatment of neuropathic pain, most of the review articles do agree that pharmacological treatment should be the mainstay for treatment of patients with neuropathic pain.

Robert Dworkin and colleagues conducted a systematic literature review and published their own guidelines on the pharmacological management of neuropathic pain, which was later endorsed by the American Pain Society (APS). In its review, Dworkin recommends that the first step in treating neuropathic patients, as emphasized in previous sections of this chapter, should include a thorough patient evaluation, where a diagnosis of neuropathic pain must be established. Next, they recommend that initial therapy be initiated with first-line agents, which include secondary amine tricyclic antidepressants, selective serotonin and norepinephrine reuptake inhibitors, and calcium channel ligands (gabapentin and/or pregabalin). The use of topical lidocaine for patients with peripheral neuropathic pain is also recommended, as adjuvants to the previously stated pharmacological treatments.

If the patient experiences only partial pain relief, then a second first-line agent should be added to the regimen. If different combinations of first-line agents fail, second-line drugs, such as opioids and tramadol, should be considered and/or referral to pain management [49].

Fibromyalgia

Fibromyalgia is a chronic condition that affects mainly females. Although its pathogenesis is not completely understood, it is classically described as generalized pain with multiple, distinct tender points all over the body and associated with changes in neurotransmitters such as serotonin, substance p, growth hormone, and cortisol leading to central sensitization [50, 51]. Common associated symptoms include fatigue, sleep problems, and psychological disorders. It has been estimated that fibromyalgia affects between 0.2 and 6.6% of women in the United States [52].

The common treatment methods for fibromyalgia include both pharmacologic and non-pharmacologic interventions. Multiple guidelines have been published to aid physicians in treatment decision-making. The three most commonly cited guidelines were those published by the European League Against Rheumatism (EULAR), the Association of the Scientific Medical Societies in Germany (AWMF), and the Canadian Fibromyalgia Guideline Committee [53].

The EULAR 2016 guidelines, which involved participation by 12 European countries, conducted a systematic review with a primary goal of treating the pain associated with fibromyalgia. Exercise therapy is given the highest degree of recommendation as the initial treatment for fibromyalgia. Furthermore, the guidelines emphasize the importance of patient education during initial treatment planning. If these measures fail, pharmacological treatment should be added. Some of the pharmacological treatments, with varying strength recommendations, include amitriptyline, anticonvulsants, muscle relaxants, nonsteroidal anti-inflammatory agents, and serotonin reuptake inhibitors [54].

The Association of the Scientific Medical Societies in Germany also developed guidelines for the treatment of fibromyalgia through a systematic literature review. In its guidelines, the importance of patient education is highlighted, as well as the importance of developing treatment goals in tandem with the patient and appropriately managing expectations. Similar to the EULAR guidelines, it favors the use of physical activity treatment as the initial treatment option [55]. Similarly, the Canadian Fibromyalgia Guideline Committee produced guidelines that also emphasize the importance of physical activity in treatment, giving it the highest level of recommendation. It does state the role of pharmacological interventions that can be utilized but cites evidence that these produce only moderate pain relief [56].

Conclusion: Putting It All Together

Though pain remains one of the most common symptoms for which individuals seek medical attention, there is not one established method to treatment. Over time, physicians have sought answers on how best to treat pain, attempting to establish a streamlined, methodical treatment approach. However, it would be impossible to create one set algorithm to treatment given the many different types of pain and multitude of pain states that exist. Nevertheless, various guidelines, such as the WHO analgesic ladder, have been created to aid clinicians in their quest for optimal pain treatment. While it is important that clinicians understand existing algorithms, it is equally critical that physicians remain open-minded in their treatment approaches. Pain treatment approaches remain fluid in nature, and it is likely that the algorithms to pain treatment will continue to change over time as clinicians discover new, more effective treatment technologies and techniques.

References

1. Nahin RL. Estimates of pain prevalence and severity in adults. United States, 2012. J Pain. 2015;16(8):769–80.
2. Livshits G, Malkin I, Freidin MB, Xia Y, Gao F, Wang J, et al. Genome-wide methylation analysis of a large population sample shows neurological pathways involvement in chronic widespread musculoskeletal pain. PAIN. 2017;158(6):1053–62.
3. Gereau RWIV, Sluka KA, Maixner W, Savage SR, Price TJ, Murinson BB, et al. A pain research agenda for the 21st Century. J Pain. 2014;15(12):1203–14.
4. Varrassi G, Müller-Schwefe G, Pergolizzi J, Orónska A, Morlion B, Mavrocordatos P, et al. Pharmacological treatment of chronic pain – the need for CHANGE. Curr Med Res Opin. 2010;26(5):1231–45.
5. Seymour J, Clark D, Winslow M. Pain and palliative care: the emergence of new specialties. J Pain Symptom Manage. 2005;29(1):2–13.
6. Dansie EJ, Turk DC, et al. Assessment of patients with chronic pain. Br J Anaesth. 2013;111(1):19–25.
7. Fillingim RB, Loeser JD, Baron R, Edwards RR. Assessment of chronic pain: domains, methods, and Mechanisms. J Pain. 2016;17(9 Suppl):T10–20.
8. Practice Guidelines for Chronic Pain Management An Updated Report by the American Society of Anesthesiologists Task Force on Chronic Pain Management and the American Society of Regional Anesthesia and Pain Medicine. Anesthesiology. 2010;112(4):810–33.
9. Searle RD, Bennett MI. Pain assessment. Anaesth Intensive Care Med. 9(1):13–5.
10. Herr KA, Garand L. Assessment and measurement of pain in older adults. Clin Geriatr Med. 2001;17(3):457–78, vi.
11. Green L, McGhie J. Assessment of acute and chronic pain. Anaesth Intensive Care Med. 2001;12(1):9–11.
12. Chien C-W, Bagraith KS, Khan A, Deen M, Strong J. Comparative responsiveness of verbal and numerical rating scales to measure pain intensity in patients with chronic pain. J Pain. 14(12):1653–62.
13. Frampton CL, Hughes-Webb P. The measurement of pain. Clin Oncol. 2011;23(6):381–6.
14. Ferreira-Valente MA, Pais-Ribeiro JL, Jensen MP. Validity of four pain intensity rating scales. PAIN. 2011;152(10):2399–404.
15. Jensen MP, Karoly P, Braver S. The measurement of clinical pain intensity: a comparison of six methods. Pain. 1986;27(1):117–26.
16. Scott J, Huskisson EC. Graphic representation of pain. Pain. 1976;2(2):175–84.
17. Carlsson AM. Assessment of chronic pain. I. Aspects of the reliability and validity of the visual analogue scale. Pain. 1983;16(1):87–101.
18. Melzack R. The McGill Pain Questionnaire: Major properties and scoring methods. PAIN. 1975;1(3):277–99.
19. Ngamkham S, Vincent C, Finnegan L, Holden JE, Wang ZJ, Wilkie DJ. The McGill pain questionnaire as a multidimensional measure in people with cancer: an integrative review. Pain Manag Nurs. 2012;13(1):27–51.
20. Dworkin RH, Turk DC, Trudeau JJ, Benson C, Biondi DM, Katz NP, et al. Validation of the Short-Form McGill Pain Questionnaire-2 (SF-MPQ-2) in acute low back pain. J Pain. 2015;16(4):357–66.
21. Dudgeon BJ, Ehde DM, Cardenas DD, Engel JM, Hoffman AJ, Jensen MP. Describing pain with physical disability: narrative interviews and the McGill Pain Questionnaire. Arch Phys Med Rehabil. 2005;86(1):109–15.
22. Romano JM, Turner JA. Chronic pain and depression: does the evidence support a relationship? PAIN. 1985;23(3):315.
23. Turk DC, Okifuji A. Assessment of patients' reporting of pain: an integrated perspective. Lancet. 1999;353(9166):1784–8.
24. Beck AT, Ward CH, Mendelson MM, Mock JJ, Erbaugh JJ. An inventory for measuring depression. Arch Gen Psychiatry. 1961;4(6):561–71.
25. Ventafridda V, Tamburini M, Caraceni A, De Conno F, Naldi F. A validation study of the WHO method for cancer pain relief. Cancer. 1987;59(4):850–6.
26. Reid C, Davies A. The World Health Organization three-step analgesic ladder comes of age. Palliat Med. 2004;18(3):175–6.
27. Ahmedzai SH. Window of opportunity for pain control in the terminally ill. Lancet. 2001;357(9265):1304–5.
28. Vargas-Schaffer G. Is the WHO analgesic ladder still valid? Twenty-four years of experience. Willowdale: College of Family Physicians of Canada; 2010. p. 514–7, e202 p.
29. Ballantyne JC, Kalso E, Stannard C. WHO analgesic ladder: a good concept gone astray. BMJ. 2016;352:i20.
30. World Health Organization. Cancer pain relif and palliative care. Geneva: WHO; 1990.
31. Mercadante S, Fulfaro F. World Health Organization guidelines for cancer pain: a reappraisal. Ann Oncol. 2005;16(suppl_4):iv132–iv5.
32. Twycross R, Lickiss N. Pain control and the world health organization analgesic ladder. JAMA. 1996;275(11):835.
33. Gallagher EJ, Esses D, Lee C, Lahn M, Bijur PE. Randomized clinical trial of morphine in acute abdominal pain. Ann Emerg Med. 2006;48(2):150–60, e1–4.
34. Alam A, Juurlink DN. The prescription opioid epidemic: an overview for anesthesiologists. Can J Anaesth. 2016;63(1):61–8.

35. Harden RN. Chronic pain and opiates: a call for moderation. Arch Phys Med Rehabil. 2008;89(3 Suppl 1):S72–6.
36. Wilkerson RG, Kim HK, Windsor TA, Mareiniss DP. The opioid epidemic in the United States. Emerg Med Clin North Am. 2016;34(2):e1–e23.
37. Manchikanti L, Helm S 2nd, Fellows B, Janata JW, Pampati V, Grider JS, et al. Opioid epidemic in the United States. Pain Physician. 2012;15(3 Suppl):Es9–38.
38. Vital signs: overdoses of prescription opioid pain relievers-United States, 1999–2008. MMWR Morb Mortal Wkly Rep. 2011;60(43):1487–92.
39. Knight KR, Kushel M, Chang JS, Zamora K, Ceasar R, Hurstak E, et al. Opioid pharmacovigilance: a clinical-social history of the changes in opioid prescribing for patients with co-occurring chronic non-cancer pain and substance use. Soc Sci Med. 2017;186:87–95.
40. Kennedy-Hendricks A, Busch SH, McGinty EE, Bachhuber MA, Niederdeppe J, Gollust SE, et al. Primary care physicians' perspectives on the prescription opioid epidemic. Drug Alcohol Depend. 2016;165:61–70.
41. Trescot AM, Helm S, Hansen H, Benyamin R, Glaser SE, Adlaka R, et al. Opioids in the management of chronic non-cancer pain: an update of American Society of the Interventional Pain Physicians' (ASIPP) guidelines. Pain Physician. 2008;11(SPEC. ISS. 2):S5–S62.
42. Dowell D, Haegerich TM, Chou R. CDC guideline for prescribing opiods for chronic pain United States, 2016. MMWR Recomm Rep. 2016;65(1):1–49.
43. Jamison RN, Serraillier J, Michna E. Assessment and treatment of abuse risk in opioid prescribing for chronic pain. Pain Res Treat. 2011;2011:941808.
44. Haldeman S, Dagenais S. A supermarket approach to the evidence-informed management of chronic low back pain. Spine J. 2008;8(1):1–7.
45. Last AR, Hulbert K. Chronic low back pain: evaluation and management. Am Fam Physician. 2009;79:1067–74.
46. Herndon CM, Zoberi KS, Gardner BJ. Common questions about chronic low back pain. Am Fam Physician. 2015;91(10):708–14.
47. Qaseem A, Wilt TJ, McLean RM, Forciea M, for the Clinical Guidelines Committee of the American College of P. Noninvasive treatments for acute, subacute, and chronic low back pain: a clinical practice guideline from the american college of physicians. Ann Intern Med 2017;166(7):514–530.
48. Chou R, Qaseem A, Snow V, et al. Diagnosis and treatment of low back pain: a joint clinical practice guideline from the american college of physicians and the american pain society. Ann Intern Med. 2007;147(7):478–91.
49. Dworkin RH, O'Connor AB, Audette J, Baron R, Gourlay GK, Haanpää ML, et al. Recommendations for the pharmacological management of neuropathic pain: an overview and literature update. Mayo Clin Proc. 2010;85(3 Suppl):S3–S14.
50. Padin Galea JM, Fernandez-Acenero MJ, de la Fuente JLM. Characteristics of patients with fibromyalgia. Foot (Edinburgh, Scotland). 2017;32:27–9.
51. Jahan F, Nanji K, Qidwai W, Qasim R. Fibromyalgia syndrome: an overview of pathophysiology, diagnosis and management. Oman Med J. 2012;27(3):192–5.
52. Marques AP, Santo AS, Berssaneti AA, Matsutani LA, Yuan SL. Prevalence of fibromyalgia: literature review update. Rev Bras Reumatol Engl Ed. 2017;57(4):356–63.
53. Ablin J, Fitzcharles M-A, Buskila D, Shir Y, Sommer C, Häuser W. Treatment of fibromyalgia syndrome: recommendations of recent evidence-based interdisciplinary guidelines with special emphasis on complementary and alternative therapies. Evid Based Complement Alternat Med. 2013;2013:485272.
54. Macfarlane GJ, Kronisch C, Dean LE, Atzeni F, Häuser W, Fluß E, et al. EULAR revised recommendations for the management of fibromyalgia. Ann Rheum Dis. 2017;76(2):318–28.
55. Häuser W, Arnold B, Eich W, Felde E, Flügge C, Henningsen P, et al. Management of fibromyalgia syndrome – an interdisciplinary evidence-based guideline. GMS Ger Med Sci. 2008;6:Doc14.
56. Fitzcharles M-A, Ste-Marie PA, Goldenberg DL, Pereira JX, Abbey S, Choinière M, et al. 2012 Canadian Guidelines for the diagnosis and management of fibromyalgia syndrome: executive summary. Pain Res Manag. 2013;18(3):119–26.

3 The Opioid Epidemic and the Need for a Pain Strategy

Tory L. McJunkin, Paul J. Lynch, and Edward L. Swing

Introduction

Opioids are one of the most commonly used treatments for chronic pain in the USA, with over 250 million prescriptions written each year. Approximately 38 percent of the US population receives an opioid prescription in a given year. Opioids are generally regarded as effective and appropriate for acute pain as well as cancer pain, but considerable controversy exists about the appropriateness of long-term opioid use for chronic noncancer pain. In addition to concerns about the efficacy of long-term opioid therapy, there is concern about the potential for patients to abuse opioids, with harmful or even fatal consequences. An estimated 64,000 Americans died of drug overdose in 2016, with opioids causing the vast majority of these deaths. Opioids are now responsible for more deaths than traffic accidents. Though many of these deaths are the result of illicit opioids (e.g., heroin, non-pharmaceutical fentanyl), opioid prescribers still bear a special responsibility as many opioid abusers became addicted to prescription opioids before turning to illicit opioids due to the cost or difficulty of obtaining prescription opioids. Opioids remain a useful therapy for some chronic pain patients, but there is a clear need for a strategy for delivering opioid therapies.

When opioids are used for treating chronic noncancer pain, it should be as part of a comprehensive pain management approach including conservative care (rest, icing), physical treatments (chiropractic care, physical therapy), non-opioid medications (NSAIDs, membrane stabilizers, muscle relaxants), psychological treatments (cognitive therapy, biofeedback), interventional treatments (nerve blocks, epidural steroid injections, nerve radiofrequency ablations), regenerative treatments (platelet rich plasma and stem cell injections), and implanted device therapies (spinal cord stimulators). Most or all of these therapies are lower risk than opioids. A comprehensive approach has the potential to provide greater pain relief in conjunction with opioids as well as reduce patient risk by lowering opioid doses or discontinuing opioids altogether. Additionally, an effective and responsible approach to prescribing opioids should include safety practices such as dosage limits, repeated urine drug testing, and the use of state prescription drug monitoring programs. Such practices help identify possible opioid abuse, allowing providers to discontinue opioid therapy for patients who are unable to safely use these drugs. These patients may continue to receive other pain treatments, including nonnarcotic medications, injection treatments, and implanted device therapies.

Background and Historical Perspective

The first evidence for the cultivation of poppies and the isolation of opium from them is found among the Sumerians (in modern day Iraq) dating back to the third millennium BCE. The Sumerian word for poppies means "plant of joy." Initial uses of opium included religious rituals, medicinal purposes, and recreational use. The use of opium is described by Greek writers (e.g., Theophrastus) by 300 BCE. Ancient physicians used opium treatments such as spongia somnifera (sponges soaked in opium used to relieve pain during surgery), though some were wary of these treatments because the potency and absorption rate could not be controlled, making them dangerous. By the eight or ninth century CE, Arab traders had brought opium to India and China and to various parts of Europe between the tenth and thirteenth century CE.

Morphine, the active ingredient in opium, was first isolated and named by Sertürner in 1806, with codeine following a few years later. The invention of the hypodermic syringe in the 1850s enabled morphine to be used in minor surgical procedures as well as for chronic and postoperative pain. When heroin was developed in 1898, it was felt that, as

T. L. McJunkin · P. J. Lynch · E. L. Swing (✉)
Arizona Pain Specialists, Scottsdale, AZ, USA
e-mail: DrMcJunkin@PainDoctor.com; DrLynch@PainDoctor.com; TedS@PainDoctor.com

T. R. Deer et al. (eds.), *Deer's Treatment of Pain*, https://doi.org/10.1007/978-3-030-12281-2_3

a more potent drug than morphine, doses could be better controlled, therefore making it less addicting. This claim has been repeated for other opioids developed since, though in each case it remains unsupported by the available evidence. Various synthetic and semisynthetic opioids (synthetic drugs affecting the same receptors as natural opiates) were developed during the twentieth century, including oxymorphone (1914), oxycodone (1916), hydrocodone (1920), hydromorphone (1922), methadone (1946), fentanyl (1959), and buprenorphine (1969).

Prior to the 1990s, the use of opioids in the USA was largely limited to acute pain (e.g., from trauma or surgery) and cancer pain. During the 1990s, many physicians were taught that chronic noncancer pain was undertreated and that opioids were a safe and appropriate therapy for treating such pain. Between 1990 and 2000, the rate of opioid prescriptions rose from 8 percent of physician visits to 16 percent. Prescription opioid use in the USA has continued to grow since 2000, from an equivalent morphine dose of 46,946 kg to 148,316 kg in 2014. Prescription opioids appear to have peaked in the USA in 2012 at 165,525 kg, declining somewhat since. Opioid-related deaths, on the other hand, have continued to rise, from about 3 per 100,000 in 2000 to 9 per 100,000 in 2014.

This increase includes two separate trends – (1) an increase in deaths caused by prescription opioids (e.g., morphine, oxycodone, and methadone) and (2) an increase in deaths linked to illicit opioids (e.g., heroin and fentanyl). Deaths from prescription opioids have been relatively steady since 2012, whereas deaths from illicit opioids (fentanyl in particular) have risen dramatically over that time period. In many cases, states that have implemented policies to restrict prescription opioid abuse have seen increases in illicit opioid use as some opioid users switch from prescription to illicit opioid use. The shift of some individuals from prescription opioids to illicit opioids represents a challenge for reducing opioid deaths. Nevertheless, efforts among US physicians to implement policies and systems that can limit the harmful consequences of opioids remain important as medical prescriptions remain a major factor in the development of opioid addiction.

Uses and Indications

Studies have found that approximately 18% of patients receiving opioids demonstrate aberrant medication taking behavior. This includes testing negative for prescribed opioids, testing positive for non-prescribed opioids or other prescription drugs, and testing positive for illicit drugs. One study found that, among those taking opioids non-medically, approximately 71% received them from a friend or family member (with 79% of those friends/family members having received the opioids from a doctor's prescription). Given this significant risk of diversion and abuse, when opioids are used for chronic, noncancer pain, a number of practices should be taken to reduce these risks.

The US Centers for Disease Control and Prevention (CDC) issued guidelines for primary care physicians initiating opioid therapy for chronic noncancer pain, including:

- Setting realistic goals for opioid therapy
- First trying non-opioid therapies
- Discussing the risks and benefits of opioids with the patient
- Evaluating the risk of harm or misuse
- Starting with a low dose of a short-acting opioid

Additionally, the CDC recommends that patients receiving ongoing opioid therapy continue to be evaluated for risk of harm or misuse with:

- Urine drug testing (both to confirm the presence of prescribed medications and the absence of any non-prescribed or illicit drugs)
- Checking the state prescription drug monitoring program for opioid prescriptions from other sources
- Offering naloxone, an opioid antagonist that can be used to reverse an opioid overdose, to patients taking moderate doses (≥50 MME)
- Avoiding doses of greater than or equal to 90 MME

Evidence for Efficacy

The clinical evidence offers support for the short-term use of opioids as an effective treatment for chronic pain. A meta-analysis found that the short-term use of opioids relieved an average of 28% of pain, compared with 7% for placebo. Patient and physician expectations for the outcome of opioid therapy should be tempered by this finding. Thus, patients experiencing partial pain relief (e.g., 30%) from opioids should generally not have the dosage increased. Higher doses increase the risk of death: patients taking more than 100 milligram morphine equivalent (MME) have approximately nine times the risk of a fatal overdose compared with patients taking less than 100 MME. Further, higher opioid doses may increase the risk of opioid-induced hyperalgesia, a condition in which opioids actually sensitize the patient to pain, leading to greater pain associated with the underlying condition.

The evidence for the efficacy of long-term opioid therapy is much more limited. The vast majority of randomized, blinded trials of opioids lasted less than 16 weeks. A few studies have examined longer time periods (e.g., 6–18 months). These studies found that patients receiving long-term opioid therapy experienced an average of 63% less pain. This finding is qualified by the fact that these studies tend to experience very high dropout rates (between 52% and 88%) due to a combination of reasons, such as adverse events or insufficient pain relief. These findings are thus more difficult to interpret. It appears that at least some patients continue to get pain relief from long-term opioid therapy. However, given the substantial risks associated with opioid use, they should be utilized as part of a comprehensive pain management approach including appropriate restrictions (e.g., a dosage limit) and precautions (e.g., urine drug testing).

Pearls and Pitfalls

- High doses of opioids are associated with higher risk of overdose or death.
- Set an upper limit for highest level of opioids to be prescribed for chronic noncancer pain.
- Concurrent use of benzodiazepines, barbiturates, psychiatric medications, or other sedating medications significantly increases the risk associated with opioids
- One must risk stratify patients (e.g., low, moderate, or high) currently on opioids and test for use, misuse, and abuse.
- Patients and physicians must have realistic expectations for efficacy (30–40% reduction in pain) when using opioids chronically.
- Opioids should be thought of as a "high-risk" therapeutic option, and other more conservative approaches should be maximized or exhausted before chronic use.
- Observe and follow state and national guidelines and recommendations.

Recommended Reading

1. Bloodworth D. Issues in opioid management. Am J Phys Med Rehabil. 2005;84(3 Suppl):S42–55.
2. Brownstein MJ. A brief history of opiates, opioid peptides, and opioid receptors. Proc Natl Acad Sci U S A. 1993;90:5391–3.
3. Centers for Disease Control and Prevention. Checklist for prescribing opioids for chronic pain. Accessed 11/21/2017 from https://www.cdc.gov/drugoverdose/pdf/pdo_checklist-a.pdf.
4. Manchikanti L, Kaye AM, Knezevic NN, et al. Responsible, safe, and effective prescription of opioids for chronic non-cancer pain: American Society of Interventional Pain Physicians (ASIPP) guidelines. Pain Physician. 2017;20:S3–S92.
5. Noble M, Tregear SJ, Treadwell JR, Schoelles K. Long-term opioid therapy for chronic noncancer pain: a systematic review and meta-analysis of efficacy and safety. J Pain Symptom Manag. 2008;35(2):214–28.
6. Paulozzi LJ, Jones CM, Mack KA, Rudd RA. Vital signs: overdoses of prescription opioid pain relievers—United States, 1999–2008. CDC Morb Mortal Wkly Rep. 2011;60(43):1487–92.
7. Sehgal N, Manchikanti L, Smith HS. Prescription opioid abuse in chronic pain: a review of opioid abuse predictors and strategies to curb opioid abuse. Pain Physician. 2012;15(3S):ES67–92.

Part II

Anatomy and Physiology of Pain

4 Nerve Function and Neurons

Tony George and Didier Demesmin

Introduction

Nerves are a basic unit of life with channels, pumps, and receptors imbedded in their membrane and neurotransmitters packaged in vesicles near nerve terminals for the passages of ions to help us perceive and respond to stimuli. Nerves and their supportive glia help regulate and maintain homeostasis inside and outside the cell membrane. Nerves individually have a preset defined functional role; however, when viewed collectively they process complex sensory and motor information. Nerves can be grouped by their methods of transmission, morphology of nerve fibers, tissue they innervate, rate of electrical discharge, and order of neurons. They can be classified as motor, sensory, or mixed nerves or can be classified by its direction of transmission as in an ascending, descending, or facilitating interneuron. They are described as somatic or autonomic based on the tissue they innervate and can be described by their appearance such as myelinating or un-myelinating and unipolar or bipolar. Nerves have unique adaptive properties and are able to modify their roles and responses to changing external stimuli. A nerve can be a uniquely designated nerve for a special function or could be grouped in fascicular bunches with other nerves to execute a collective function.

T. George (✉)
University Pain Medicine Center, Somerset, NJ, USA

D. Demesmin
University Pain Medicine Center, Somerset, NJ, USA

Rutgers Robert Wood Johnson Medical School, Piscataway, NJ, USA

JFK Johnson Rehabilitation Institute, Edison, NJ, USA

Pain Medicine Department, Saint Peter's University Hospital, New Brunswick, NJ, USA

University Clinical Research Center, Somerset, NJ, USA
e-mail: DDemesmin@longcall.com

Basic Function

Nerves are in a constant state to maintain equilibrium within the cell by removing ions and passively permitting ions entry into the cell. The nerve is selective in allowing ions to diffuse through its membrane. It permits the larger potassium ion to pass through the membrane while limiting the smaller sodium ion entry. The nerve membrane has active transmembrane pumps which pump three sodium ions out for every two potassium ions into the cell. Once net equilibrium is attained, there is no movement of ions across the cell and is in a polarized state. In its polarized state, it has a net negative potential, also known as a resting potential. The nerves resting potential is at −70 mV. The matrix inside and outside the cell called the intracellular and extracellular matrix are charged and have the ability to conduct. External stimuli either innocuous or nociceptive disrupt this equilibrium and cause this matrix to conduct. A nerve can be stimulated but may not necessarily depolarize. In order to depolarize a minimum electric stimulus called a threshold potential is required. An action potential occurs once a threshold potential has been reached which triggers a cascade of further depolarization by opening more sodium channels through a positive feedback mechanism. An action potential is an all or none response where the nerve is completely depolarized. This depolarization activity continues until the sodium channels become inactivated and cannot transmit anymore sodium ions. This period of inactivation is called the refractory period where no depolarization can occur for a defined period of time until it has reset itself. Repeat stimuli during this refractory period do not trigger any new action potential.

Morphology (Fig. 4.1)

Nerves, during fetal development, originate from the ectoderm, the outer layer of the three embryonic germ layers. Nerves have dendrites, soma, axons, synaptic terminals, and myelin which form its basic structure. Chemical, thermal,

T. R. Deer et al. (eds.), *Deer's Treatment of Pain*, https://doi.org/10.1007/978-3-030-12281-2_4

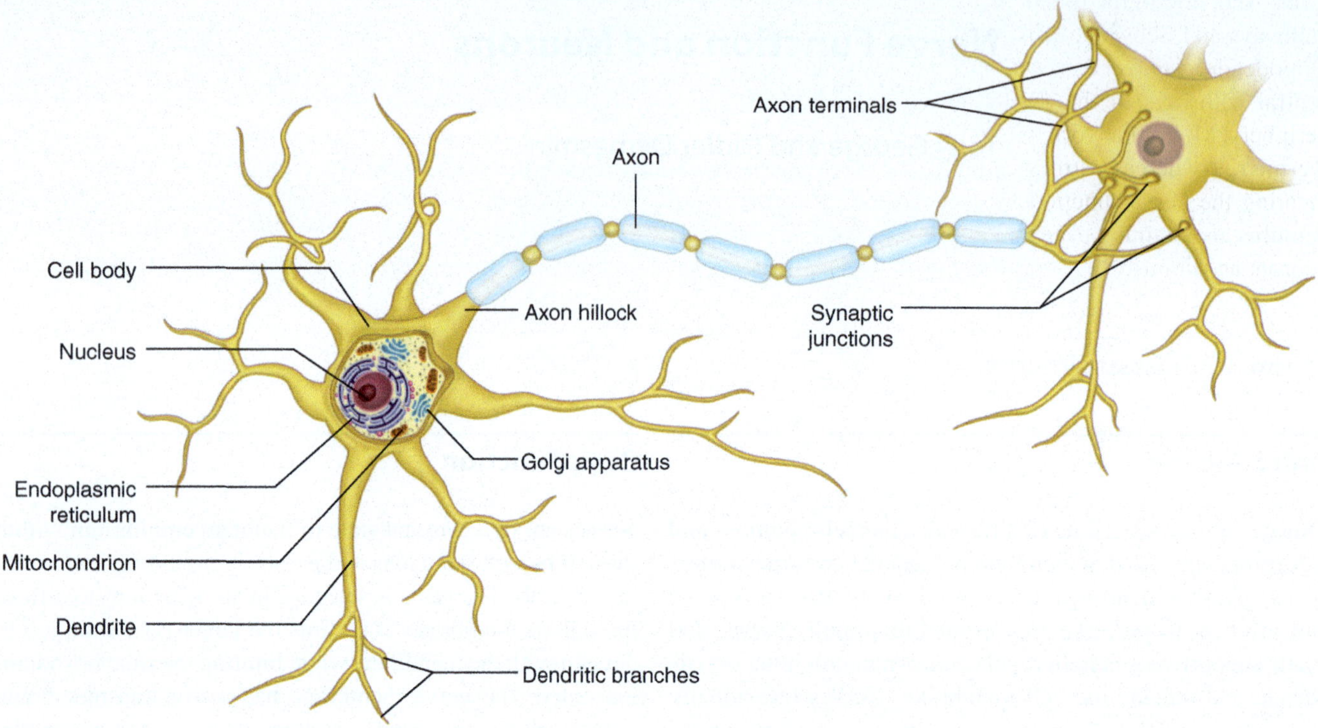

Fig. 4.1 Nerve basic morphology

pain, or pressure stimuli are picked up by receptors on dendritic processes and converted to miniature electric signals. These miniature electric signals from different dendrites travel through the dendritic spines toward the soma where they converge, and their signals are summated. If the summated electric signals are sufficient for threshold stimulus, an action potential is triggered at the axon hillock. This action potential now travels through the myelinated axons through saltatory conduction and finally reach the presynaptic terminals where the potential is converted back to chemical responses through neurotransmitter release. Neurotransmitters packaged in vesicles in the presynaptic membrane transfer this signal to the next cell which continues to propagate the signal received by the preceding nerve.

Some sensory and motor nerves have insulated concentric sheaths covering their surface called myelin. These are provided by Schwann cells in the peripheral neural networks and oligodendrocytes in the central neural networks. Schwann cells typically envelop an individual nerve axon, whereas oligodendrocytes have the ability to envelope multiple neurons simultaneously. Myelination of a nerve allows for faster conduction of a peripheral stimulus. Electric currents jump between fixed points in between myelinated segments called nodes where there are higher concentrations of depolarizing sodium channels. This is called saltatory conduction where myelinated nerves do not require current to travel through the length of the nerve. As a result they are able to conduct faster with faster conduction velocities through the neuron.

Orientation

Nerves can be grouped on their structural appearances such as the orientation of the axon and dendrites with respect to the cell body and can be classified as unipolar, bipolar, and multipolar cells. A unipolar neuron has a unidirectional axon ending with branching dendrites. A unique variant of the unipolar neuron is the pseudounipolar neuron which has two short branches, one serving as the axon and the other as dendritic endings. A bipolar neuron has bidirectional axons with branching dendrites. The majority of the neurons however are multipolar, and these neurons have one axon with several branching dendrites. A Purkinje cell found in the cerebellum is an extreme variant of multipolar cells with large networks of branching dendrites allowing it to receive and integrate complex information.

Support Structures

The nerves are aided by supporting glial cells which assist in carrying out its function and help with neuromodulation processes. Glial cells are made up of astrocytes, oligodendrocytes, and microglia found in the spinal and supraspinal pathways and Schwann cells found in peripheral pathways. Oligodendrocytes serve as the myelinating counterpart in the central pathways to the Schwann cell and its role in the periphery. Microglia work to remove debris and dead cells in the matrix, whereas astrocytes play an import role in augmenting the nerve function by regulating its response to a stimulus, maintaining the extracellular matrix adjacent to the neuron, and contribute to forming the blood-brain barrier.

Connective Tissue Relation

Nerves travel in units and rarely in isolation. During their course they are protected by layers of connective tissue which act as diffusion barriers and provide tensile strength. The endoneurium envelops each unmyelinated or myelinated axon. The perineurium envelops bundles of nerves wrapped in endoneurium, and finally the epineurium envelops fascicles of perineurium. These connective tissues give integrity to the nerve by preventing it from loosely flailing through its intended pathway and by providing significant tensile strength where it is able to withstand significant stretch and multangular forces and act as a diffusion barrier preventing crossover discharges of the nerve. These nerve bundles are intertwined with vascular endothelium creating a blood-nerve barrier.

Sensory and Motor Nerves

Sensory Nerves

The three sensory nerve types include the A-delta, A-beta, and C fibers. Of the three the A-beta nerve has the largest diameter, is the fastest conducting, and has the most myelinated fibers. Second in magnitude, speed, and myelination is the A-delta fiber, and lastly the smallest, slowest, and devoid of myelin is the C fiber. The A-delta and C nerves are implicated in pain processing and modulation, whereas the A-beta nerves process light touch, pressure of varying intensity, and cutaneous hair movement. At the periphery hair follicles, skin follicles and joint receptor provide the respective stimuli for the A-beta nerves. The A-delta and C fibers have transducing channels which are receptive to ranges of temperature from cold, warm, and hot and are able to recognize changes in acidity. They have receptors that are able to sense local tissue injury and its sequelae including inflammation and extracellular changes. Their velocities range from 2 m/s for the C fibers to 5–20 m/s for the A-delta fibers. A-beta the fastest among the three sensory fibers have velocities ranging from 25 to 70 m/s but do not transmit pain. Their transmission velocities create unique pain perceptions patterns where the slower C fiber pain is perceived as a slow and burning pain, whereas the faster A-delta fiber pain is perceived as a sharp, stabbing, electric, and tingling pain. A peripheral tissue injury, for example, is immediately perceived through the sensory myelinated A-delta fiber as a sharp or electric sensation. Several second later this injury is perceived by the individual as a burning sensation through the sensory slow-conducting signals provided by the unmyelinated C fibers. The ratio of C fibers outnumber A-delta fibers by more than 2:1 in the periphery.

Motor Nerves

The three motor nerve types include A-alpha, A-beta, and A-gamma motor neurons. Motor neurons are relatively larger and faster than sensory neurons. In comparison to sensory nerves, the velocities of A-alpha fibers are 50–120 m/s and A-gamma fibers are 10–50 m/s. A-beta fibers have dual sensory and motor function and have velocities ranging from 25 to 70 m/s. The A-alpha fibers are important in the muscle stretch reflex. They have peripheral nerve endings originating from muscle spindles. Their cell bodies are located in the anterior horn cell. They terminate to attach to structures on the muscles such as intrafusal and extrafusal fibers through the neuromuscular junction. The alpha motor neuron attaches to extrafusal fibers on the skeletal muscle. The gamma motor neuron attaches to the intrafusal fibers on the muscle spindle and the beta neurons attach to both extrafusal and intrafusal fibers.

A motor nerve action potential triggers a sequence of neurotransmitter-induced chemical changes which take place at the neuromuscular junction, the meeting point of motor nerves and muscle fibers. The terminal end of the axon merges with a muscle fiber at the neuromuscular junction to transmit electrical impulses. During a depolarization potential, there is an influx of calcium through voltage-gated channels which stimulate acetylcholine-containing vesicles. At the presynaptic membrane or the terminal end of the motor nerve, round vesicles filled with acetylcholine fuse with the presynaptic membrane and release acetylcholine into the synaptic cleft. These in turn bind to receptors on the postsynaptic membrane of the muscle fiber to open ion channels. This triggers an end plate potential through the muscle fiber causing the actin and myosin filaments of the muscles to move.

Motor units are a defined number of muscle fibers innervated by a single alpha motor neuron. A neuron can innervate a few fibers such as 10 muscle fibers or a multitude of fibers such as over a 1000. Innervation ratio is the ratio of muscle units to a single nerve. Fine motor control fibers have lower innervation ratios, whereas gross motor control fibers have larger innervation ratios. For example, extraocular eye movement has smaller motor units than hamstring muscles which have much larger motor units innervated by a nerve. Nerves can have a highly specific defined function requiring pairing with a selective few muscle fibers or gross function attaching to several hundreds of muscle fibers.

Nerve Signal Processing (Fig. 4.2)

Nerve function is communicating information from the primary peripheral site to a central command center and being able to respond to the stimuli appropriately. Raw information is processed along the pathway and modulated so the higher centers have accurate information and are able to respond appropriately. For example, an isolated pin prick is processed differently than a chronic 4-month-old nerve tissue injury after foot surgery even though peripherally both may appear as noxious stimuli. Sensory information from the primary site to the brain is first transduced, then transmitted, next modulated, and finally perceived as an innocuous non-nociceptive or nociceptive stimulus with or without an emotional component to each individual.

Transduction is the process of converting an external energy into electric activity through action potentials in a nerve. External stimuli through mechanical, chemical, heat, or cold stimulus are picked up by receptors on the surface of primary afferent neurons. The next step, transmission, involves transferring the electric signal from its source in the periphery through the ascending pathways in the spinal cord, brainstem, and brain, then processing a response to the stimulus in these higher centers, and transmitting that response through the descending pathway to the terminal nerves to perform a motor or sympathetic function. Modulation an adaptable ability of nerves to modify a stimulus by amplifying or diminishing a signal influences the response to a stimulus as it transmits through the signal pathway loop. Modulation is influenced at the dorsal root ganglion, supraspinal pathways, and even in the periphery. The ability of nerves to modulate a response is being tapped to modify painful states through spinal cord stimulation of the dorsal columns and dorsal root ganglion. Finally, perception of this signal involves both a sensory and emotional component as both the somatosensory regions of the brain and limbic regions are involved in processing sensory signals. The limbic emotional influence and modulation of nerve signals primarily influence the variability of perception of each type of stimulus among individuals. The subjective sensation of this stimulus is what we call pain. The various descriptions of painful stimuli such as hyperalgesia, allodynia, hyperesthesia, hypoesthesia, and dysesthesia all describe various perceptions of these painful states.

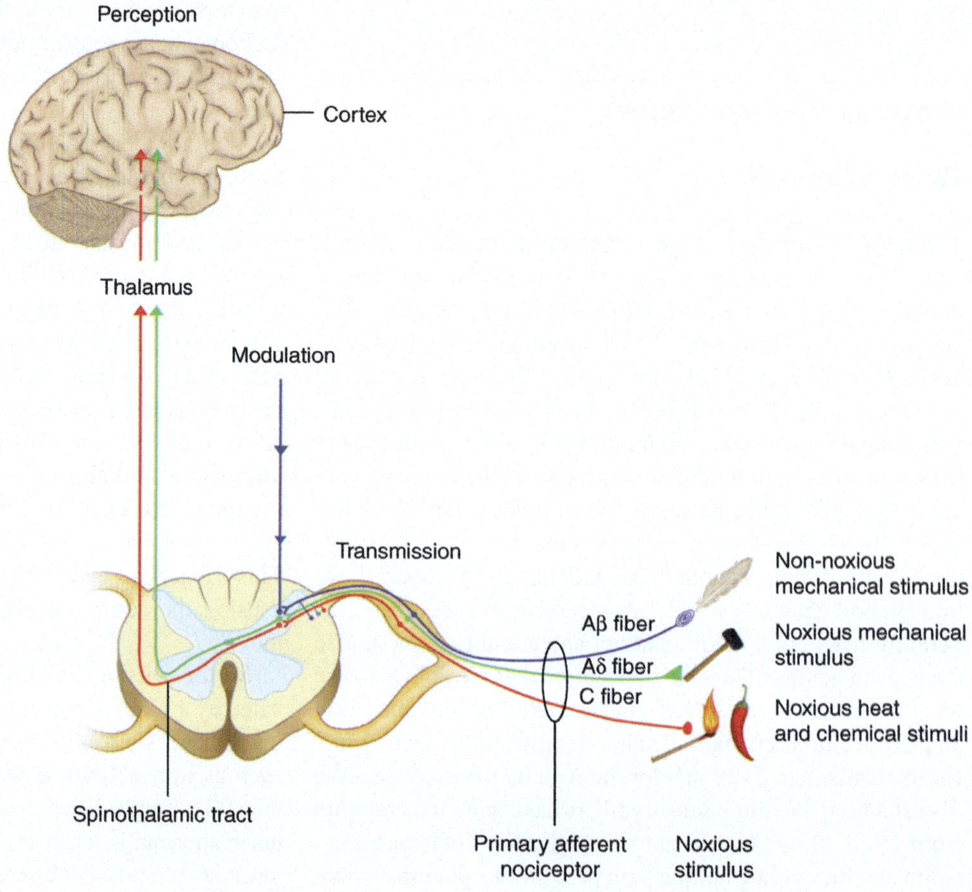

Fig. 4.2 Nerve signal processing

Neurotransmitters

At the cellular level, nerves attempt to maintain homeostasis within the cell. Nerve endings are equipped with channels, pumps, and receptors which selectively allow the passage of charged and uncharged particles and permit the stimulation of nerve endings. Nerve endings have different densities of receptor proteins and channels based on the type of nerve and location. A somatic afferent nerve ending, for example, may have a larger concentration of mechanoreceptors on the skin surface in comparison to a visceral afferent on the liver. Even among pain processing A-delta and C fibers, there are different densities and types of receptors expressed on their surfaces. Nerves have to self-regulate their activities in order to maintain voltage homeostasis. The proteins making up the channels and pumps are created centrally in the body of the nerve cell and transported peripherally through axon transport system. Due to the lack of protein creating molecules including ribosomes in the periphery, most protein creation occurs around the nucleus of the cell body itself.

The role of neurotransmitters, signaling molecules, and receptors are paramount in coordination of stimulus response and modulation of nerve signaling (Fig. 4.3). Molecules such as lipids, peptides, and nerve growth factors play a pivotal role in initiating and mediating nerve response. Two groups of neurotransmitters emerge the small-molecule, rapidly acting neurotransmitters and the large-molecule, slower-acting neurotransmitters. The former include the amino acids such as glutamate, the amines such as norepinephrine, acetylcholine, and nitric oxide, and the latter include the neuropeptides and growth factors. The rapidly acting small-molecule neurotransmitters trigger immediate responses from initiation of sensory stimuli to execution of motor response, whereas the slower-acting large-molecule neuropeptides influence long-term changes in the cell receptor distribution, potentiation of stimulus, and strengthening of synaptic connections. Among

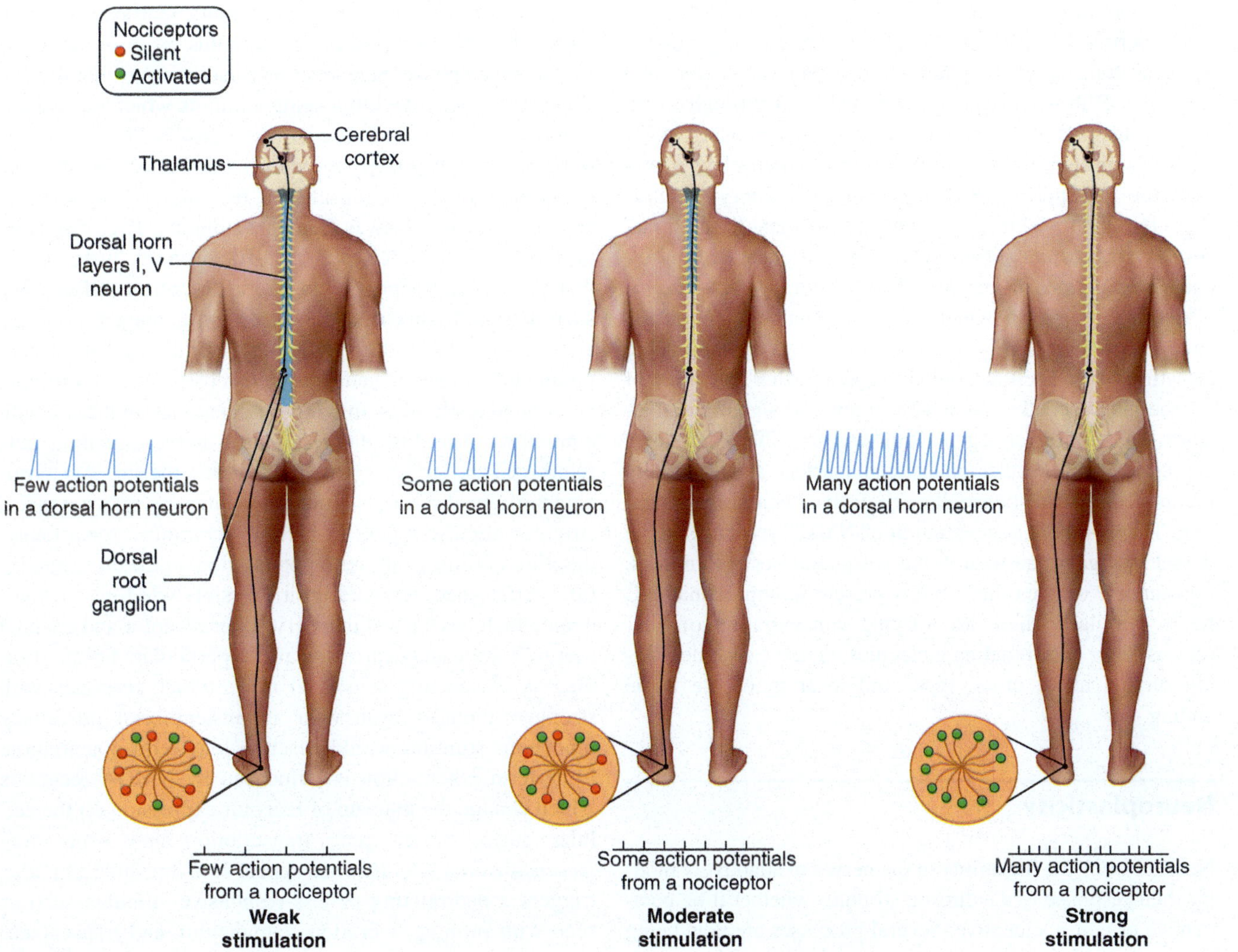

Fig. 4.3 Stimulus response

these small-molecule neurotransmitters, glutamate and nitric oxide work as excitatory neurotransmitters, while GABA, glycine, dopamine, and serotonin work as inhibitory neurotransmitters. Norepinephrine works as predominantly excitatory but also has inhibitory roles. Large-molecule neuropeptide neurotransmitters mediate long-term changes in neurons to facilitate or inhibit stimuli. Neuropeptide has a greater role on the long-term effects of nerve function and plays an important role in neuromodulation.

A neurogenic stimulus is evoked when allogenic signaling molecules are released into the extracellular fluid after a tissue injury. Damaged tissues and cells in the vicinity of injury such as mast cells and basophils release molecules including bradykinin, serotonin, histamine, and substance P which activate peripheral somatic or visceral nociceptors. Tissue injury triggers inflammatory mediators around the injury site where a cascade of activation involving bradykinin, prostaglandin, serotonin, and nerve growth factor create a zone of inflammation initiating transduction through peripheral nociceptors. Substance P and calcitonin gene-related peptide trigger vasodilation and plasma extravasation in the periphery. Transmission of this stimulus is mediated by neurotransmitters calcitonin gene-related peptide and substance P in the peripheral terminals and through excitatory glutamate and aspartate in central terminals. GABA works as an inhibitory neurotransmitter which plays a pivotal role in suppressing or permitting excitatory stimulus flows through its inhibitory activity on neurons. At the spinal cord level, norepinephrine, serotonin, and encephalin influence modulation of peripheral and supraspinal systems. NMDA receptor is known to influence spinal modulation and have a particular role in activating neuropeptides and nerve growth factors. Their activation triggers further activation of intracellular second messenger systems and signaling molecules and ultimately gene transcription. This modifies expression of molecules on the nerve surface and ultimately modulates nerve response through delayed central sensitization. There is more concentration of NMDA receptors in the dorsal root ganglion than in the peripheral nerve terminals. Substance P on the other hand is present in unmyelinated C fibers. Similarly there are varying concentration of neurotransmitter and signaling molecules on nerve cells depending on the nerve order, type, and location of the nerve ending.

Neuroplasticity

Neuroplasticity is the ability of the nerves to adaptively modify their response to a recurring stimulus whether it be nociceptive or non-nociceptive. Several processes are now being understood about the dynamic nature of neurons. By the end of the nineteenth century, the understood theory stated neurons were hard-wired structures without adaptive properties. Landmark opposing theories such as the gate control theory by Melzak and Wall helped change this perception and understand the neuroplasticity of nerves and their ability to adapt and modify a stimulus.

Sensitization

Nerve cells are dynamic in their ability to respond to stimuli. On creation, sensory nerves have an innate preset threshold of response to a stimulus and can be grouped as high-threshold and low-threshold fibers. However their thresholds can adapt to the nature of stimulus by responding sooner and often or conversely delayed and sparingly. For example, low-threshold C fibers are typically fatigue and respond less with stimulus, whereas high-threshold C fibers lower their threshold by responding earlier and with more intensity. The former is a desensitization process, whereas the latter is a sensitization process.

Sensitization is the process of attuning neurons to respond more accurately to a perceived stimulus by reinforcing the signal and response. Sensitization can occur peripherally and centrally. A negative influencing stimulus which has caused or has the potential to cause harm is translated by the neuron to respond appropriately to address the damaging influence of the stimulus by feedback and feedforward mechanisms and direct the tissue away from that stimulus. They discharge impulses often, intensely, and furthermore there is an increase in the receptive field size of the sensitized neurons such that the tissues near the vicinity of damaged tissue are also sensitized. Wind-up phenomenon and long-term potentiation are immediate and delayed mechanisms of sensitizing neurons to a stimulus. In wind-up phenomenon theory, with continuing stimulus, the responding nerve signaling gets reinforced and stronger and subsides after the signal is terminated. A repeat stimulus of the same intensity may not give a stronger impulse unless as before it continues for a longer duration of time. Long-term potentiation on the other hand is time-established, temporarily irreversible wind-up phenomenon which has ensued in a nerve after receptor and channel reorganization and expression after a particular chronic stimulus. A chronically sensitized nerve which responds with stronger impulses even with a transient brief previously innocuous stimulus would describe long-term potentiation. Long-term potentiation is influenced by NMDA receptors which change the makeup of receptor expression on the cellular surface after gene transcription and expression. Desensitization occurs when repeat low-threshold stimulus triggers a neutralizing or less responsive stimulus such as seen with rubbing, vibration acupuncture, and transcutaneous electric nerve stimulation and is the underlying principle by which spinal cord stimulation devices operate.

Sensitization causes a nerve to respond earlier and intensely. Nerves located at or around tissue injury are sensitized to tactile and thermal stimuli where previous innocuous stimuli are now perceived as nociceptive and a zone of primary hyperalgesia is created. After a bruise or a paper cut, light touch of the injured tissue could be perceived as painful. The area surrounding the primary zone is called zone of secondary hyperalgesia. This is a sensitized area which extends beyond the primary zone and is mediated by low-threshold tactile afferent nerves. Unlike the primary zone, these nerves are not influenced by thermal stimuli. This response could be mediated by the ordering of wide-dynamic range and nociceptive sensing neurons into laminae in the spinal cord which may play a role in sensitizing these afferent neurons to stimuli in the periphery.

Peripheral sensitization can occur if there is an increased pool of algesic substances near nerve endings in the peripheral surface, an increase in sensitization of peripheral nociceptors created by tissue injury and inflammation, or an increase in segmental reflexes provoked by peripheral tissue injury. The dorsal root ganglion, an essential contributor in peripheral sensitization, is a complex relay center between the central pathways originating from the spinal cord and peripheral pathways. It is part of the peripheral circuitry having complex synaptic associations where stimuli from the periphery converge providing a positive or negative summative effect.

Central sensitization occurs in the central pathways of the brain and spinal cord where complex processing occurs. A multitude of changes take place intrinsically within a neuron at the spinal level to modulate their function to future stimuli. A sustained nociceptive response peripherally increases the radius of the receptive field size in the spinal pathway such that a nociceptive signal can be picked up earlier by the spinal neuron. Next, the threshold for stimulation is lowered. Innocuous stimuli which were previously disregarded by nociceptive neurons are now activated by them. Furthermore the spinal neuron duration of activation are longer, and their magnitude of response is larger. The enhanced responsiveness of a peripheral nerve to noxious stimuli can have a profound influence such that it affects the adjacent non-nociceptive neurons in the spinal cord to respond as well. Strong sustained peripheral nerve stimulation affects the nociceptive responsive nerves and exerts a response from the preganglionic nerve in the spinal cord. These preganglionic nerves convey the stimulus to postganglionic nerves which stimulate afferent nociceptors in the periphery and reinforce the loop of enhanced pain perception. Postganglionic nerves could also influence afferent nociceptors further from the site of tissue injury as seen in visceral-mediated pain. The premise of referred pain works through the same principle reversely where visceral pain reaches postganglionic neurons which can stimulate a response on afferent neurons in the periphery. Modulation can be assisted through the responses of adjacent neurons as well. Delayed central sensitization, previously discussed as long-term potentiation, also occurs through intracellular changes at the level of gene transcription which occurs in the nucleus of cell bodies in the dorsal root ganglion. These changes are not immediately apparent but play a pivotal role in influencing effects of chronic pain perception. Sensory nerves from the periphery and preganglionic nerves or extensor motor neurons sometimes have common meeting points where they converge and influence eccentric responses such as seen in the case of referred pain and with the stretch reflex, a mechanism referred to as convergence.

Nerve Organization in the Spinal Cord

Nerves travel in fascicles inside the perineurium and epineurium. Each individual nerve picks up a stimulus in the periphery and ascends through their pathway to become organized within fascicles as first-order neurons which terminate in the spinal cord. Here the second-order neurons get organized into different layers as they pass through higher processing centers. In the spinal cord, neurons are organized into different laminae or tracts. These are graded from I to X. The C fibers terminate in I and II, and the A-delta fibers terminate in III, IV, and V. The thickly myelinated A-beta fibers terminate in III to V. The alpha motor neuron of the descending tract terminates in IX, whereas the interneurons terminate in VII and VIII.

This grouping of neurons into distinct layers creates two distinct neuron bundles classified as wide-dynamic range (WDR) neurons and nociceptive-specific (NS) neurons. Wide-dynamic range neurons are located from laminae III to V where they are activated by both nociceptive and non-nociceptive stimuli. These three laminae have varying concentration of A-beta, A-delta, and C fibers. Nociceptive sensitive neurons are located in laminae I–II which are activated exclusively by noxious stimuli and have A-delta and C fiber neurons. The WDR neurons create a distinct histogram of activation distinct from NS range neuron activation. Their nonselective activation of innocuous and non-innocuous stimulus has been utilized to guide spinal cord stimulator devices to selectively stimulate the WDR neurons and overpower the nociceptive response from the NS range fibers.

Neuromodulation and gate control theory have its premise that nerve responses can be altered by external stimulus through excitatory and inhibitory effects of nerves. Larger dense fibers like the A-beta fibers are inhibitory, whereas smaller fibers like the A-delta and C fibers are excitatory. An excitatory nociceptive response from tissue injury or inflammation can be suppressed or overpowered by a stronger inhibitory response from the larger fibers through their stimulation of mechanoreceptors in the periphery. The gate serves as the hypothetical checkpoint selectively allowing inhibitory responses to go through the gate whereas preventing excitatory responses from going through. This landmark study was published by Melzack and Wall in 1965 and is the foundational principle for neuromodulation through an external TENS devices and internal spinal cord stimulator devices.

Other Modulation Mechanisms

Silent nociception is the concept of recruiting nerves on standby, trained for a role but dormant until the need arises. This akin to reserve forces in the army which are trained for a purpose but do not respond until their services are required. These nerves begin to respond after a certain threshold of mechanical or thermal stimuli where more nerve recruitment is required. They stay dormant but connected to the second-order neurons where a primary first-order neuron is recruited to correspond with the second-order neuron. If the primary first-order neuron is damaged or destroyed, the dormant neuron takes over its function.

Collateral sprouting can occur at nerve terminals centrally in the spinal cord level and also occur at nerve terminals in the neuromuscular junction. It is a way for establishing or enhancing connections caused by severed nerves or weak connections. For example, A-beta fibers establish connections with A-delta and C fibers to enhance their responsiveness after a nerve injury. Similarly at neuromuscular junctions, denervated muscles are reinnervated by collateral sprouting of healthy adjacent motor units which try to reestablish muscle activity in denervated motor units. The new connections established are weaker than and not as uniform as the former connections established before the injury; however its work to reestablish its former connection speaks of the innate ability of nerves to adapt to changing circumstances.

Interneurons also play a critical role in mediating quick responses required in spinal reflexes and in modulating nerve responses to sustained input. Interneurons are located in central processing centers of the brain and spinal cord and play a pivotal role in neuromodulation through the effects of glutamate and GABA receptors. A-alpha nerves the fastest of the sensory nerves which originate in muscle spindle help avert noxious stimuli by triggering a quick motor reflex response through the facilitating interneuron in the spinal cord. In a knee jerk reflex, for example, sensory stimuli reach the interneurons where excitatory glutamate receptors activate the quadriceps motor neuron to contract, whereas inhibitory GABA receptors inhibit the antagonist hamstring muscle and cause it to relax creating the knee jerk response. Similarly the interneuron plays a role in modulating nociceptive stimulus by reducing the inhibitory role of GABA and contributing to central sensitization or conversely increasing the inhibitory role of GABA and contributing to desensitization of stimulus.

Summary

Nerves serve as messengers of communication. They are dynamic structures which can adapt to accommodate varying external stimuli. Their summative efforts help us sense, perceive, and respond to stimuli. Sometimes injury unravels this network and creates disarray and malfunctioning signaling pathways. The nerves attempt to restore homeostasis through modulation of stimulus and modifying perception to respond appropriately. However, when it is unable to restore itself to synchrony, painful states develop and require treatment to restore to its native state.

Recommended Reading

1. Arle JE, et al. Essential neuromodulation. London: Elsevier; 2011.
2. Cousins MJ, et al. Neural blockade in clinical anesthesia and pain medicine. Philadelphia: Wolters Kluwer; 2008.
3. Honorio B, et al. Essentials of pain medicine. 3rd ed. Philadelphia: Elsevier; 2011.
4. Hall JE. Guyton and hall textbook of medical physiology. 13th ed. Philadelphia: Elsevier; 2016.
5. McMahon SB, et al. Wall & Melzack's textbook of pain. 6th ed. Philadelphia: Elsevier; 2013.
6. Preston DC. Electromyography and neuromuscular disorders. 2nd ed. Philadelphia: Elsevier; 2005.
7. Raj PP. Pain medicine a comprehensive review. St. Louis: Mosby; 1996.
8. Winn HR. Youmans and Winn neurological surgery. Philadelphia: Elsevier; 2017.

Peripheral Nerve Anatomy

5

Daniel Rothstein and Didier Demesmin

Spinal Nerves

Arising from the spinal cord at each vertebral level are the dorsal and ventral roots. The dorsal root contains afferent sensory fibers. The ventral root contains both efferent motor fibers and autonomic fibers. The dorsal and ventral roots unite to form a spinal nerve. Therefore, spinal nerves are mixed nerves, carrying both sensory and motor innervation. There are 31 pairs of spinal nerves: 8 cervical (C1–C8), 12 thoracic (T1–T12), 5 lumbar (L1–L5), 5 sacral (S1–S5), and 1 coccygeal.

Spinal nerves exit the vertebral column via the intervertebral foramina. The first cervical nerve exits the spinal column between the occipital bone and the C1 vertebral body (atlas). The second cervical nerve exits between the C1 vertebral body and C2 vertebral body (axis), at the C1/C2 foramen. The eighth and final cervical nerve leaves at the C7/T1 foramen because there are seven cervical vertebral bodies. The first thoracic nerve exits at the T1/T2 foramen and so on down the spinal canal.

The spinal nerve divides into ventral (anterior) and dorsal (posterior) rami. The ventral rami supply the anterior and lateral regions of the trunk and limbs. The dorsal rami supply facet joints of the vertebral column, muscles of the back, and overlying integument. The ventral rami of spinal nerves go on to form distinct plexi of nerves. The ventral rami of C1 to C5 form the cervical plexus, ventral rami of C5 to C8 and T1 form the brachial plexus, and the ventral rami of L1-S4 form the lumbosacral plexus. Note that the thoracic spinal nerves give rise to intercostal nerves, rather than forming a plexus.

Cervical Plexus

The cervical plexus (Fig. 5.1) is situated in the neck and innervates structures in the head, neck, and shoulders. As noted above, the cervical plexus is formed from the ventral rami of the spinal nerves C1 to C5. The plexus then divides into superficial cutaneous, deep muscular, and communicating branches.

The superficial cutaneous branches give rise to the ascending lesser occipital nerve, greater auricular nerve, and transverse cervical nerve, as well as the descending supraclavicular nerve. The lesser occipital nerve originates from the ventral ramus of C2 (and sometimes C3) and supplies the skin of the posterolateral neck and upper portion of the external ear. The greater auricular nerve originates from C2 and C3 and supplies the skin of the rest of the external ear as well as the skin in the region of the mastoid, parotid gland, and angle of mandible. The transverse cervical nerve arises from C2 and C3 and supplies the skin on the anterolateral neck and underside of the chin. The supraclavicular nerve originates from C3 and C4 and descends under the platysma muscle and deep cervical fascia. It supplies the skin of the upper and posterior shoulder, anterior chest, and lower aspect of the anterolateral neck.

The deep muscular and communicating branches provide primarily motor innervation and can be categorized into lateral and medial branches. The lateral muscular branches supply the sternocleidomastoid (C2, C3, C4), trapezius (C2, C3), levator scapulae (C3, C4), and scalene muscles (C3, C4). The lateral branches also communicate with the spinal

D. Rothstein (✉)
University Pain Medicine Center, Somerset, NJ, USA

Rutgers Robert Wood Johnson University Hospital, New Brunswick, NJ, USA

Pain Medicine Department, Saint Peter's University Hospital, New Brunswick, NJ, USA

D. Demesmin
University Pain Medicine Center, Somerset, NJ, USA

Rutgers Robert Wood Johnson Medical School, Piscataway, NJ, USA

JFK Johnson Rehabilitation Institute, Edison, NJ, USA

Pain Medicine Department, Saint Peter's University Hospital, New Brunswick, NJ, USA

University Clinical Research Center, Somerset, NJ, USA
e-mail: ddemesmin@longcall.com

T. R. Deer et al. (eds.), *Deer's Treatment of Pain*, https://doi.org/10.1007/978-3-030-12281-2_5

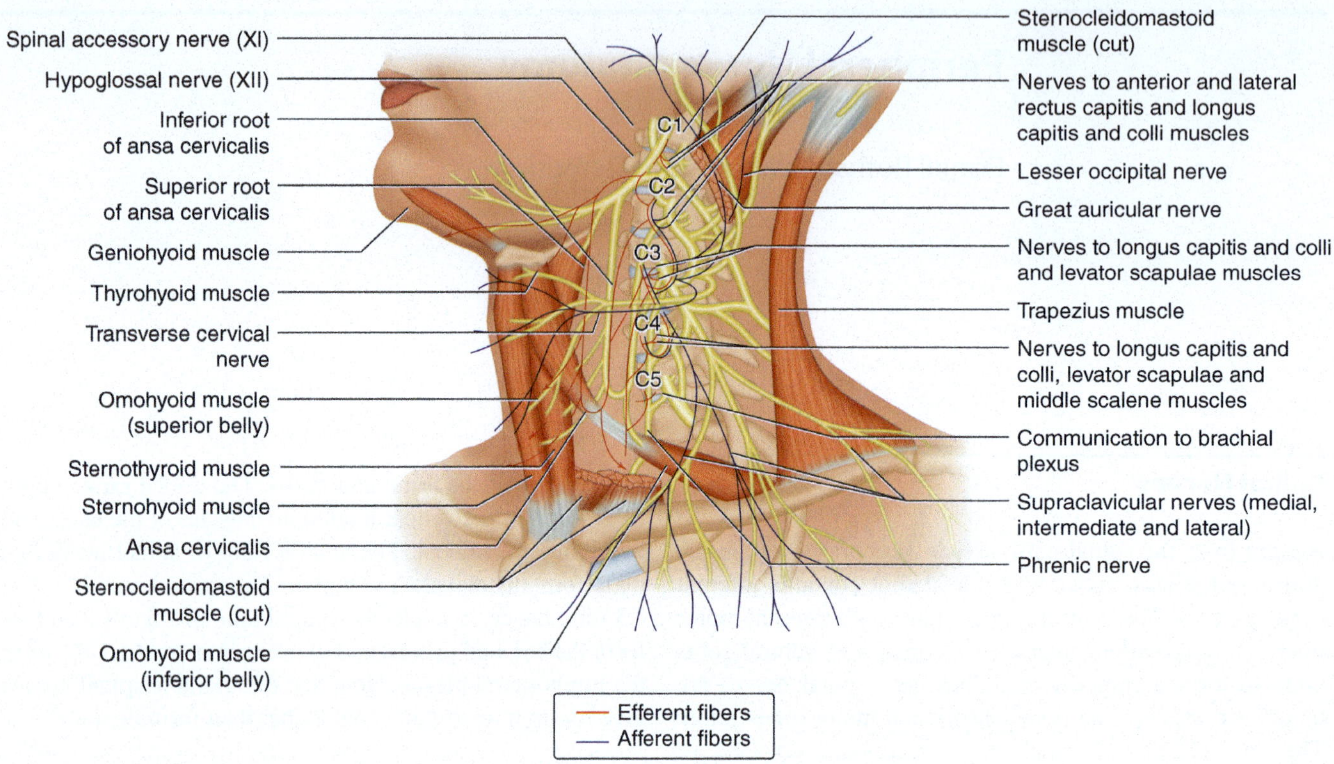

Fig. 5.1 Cervical plexus

accessory nerve (C2, C3, C4). The medial muscular branches innervate the omohyoid, sternohyoid, and sternothyroid muscles via the ansa cervicalis (C1, C2, C3), the prevertebral muscles of the neck, and the diaphragm via the phrenic nerve (C3, C4, C5). The phrenic nerve supplies both motor and sensory innervation to the diaphragm. Medial branches also communicate with the hypoglossal nerve, vagus nerve, and sympathetic nerves.

Brachial Plexus

The brachial plexus (Fig. 5.2) originates in the neck, extends into the axilla, and proceeds into the arm, supplying cutaneous and muscular innervation to the entire upper extremity and pectoral region. The brachial plexus arises from the ventral rami of C5–C8 and T1. The upper roots (C5–C7) generally supply lateral structures in the upper extremity, and the lower roots (C8, T1) usually supply medial structures. All five roots contribute in supplying posterior structures.

After emerging from the intervertebral foramina, these five nerve roots (C5–C8 and T1) course between the anterior and middle scalene muscles, enter the base of the neck, and converge to form three trunks. C5 and C6 join to form the upper trunk; C7 forms the middle trunk; and C8 and T1 join to form the lower trunk. The trunks are named according to their anatomic position. The trunks course laterally through the posterior triangle of the neck and give rise to three anterior and three posterior divisions. The divisions exit the posterior triangle and enter the axilla to form three cords. The anterior divisions of the upper and middle trunk unite to form the lateral cord; the anterior division of the lower trunk forms the medial cord; and all three posterior divisions combine to form the posterior cord. Branches from the anterior divisions typically innervate flexors muscles, while branches from posterior divisions typically innervate extensor muscles.

The cords derive their name based on their position relative to the axillary artery. The three cords then give rise to five terminal branch peripheral nerves. The ulnar nerve arises from the medial cord. The median nerve arises from both the medial and lateral cords. The musculocutaneous nerve arises from the lateral cord. The radial and axillary nerves arise from the posterior cord.

The terminal branch peripheral nerves provide motor and sensory innervation to the upper extremity. The musculocutaneous nerve (C5, C6, C7) innervates the brachialis, biceps brachii, and coracobrachialis muscles. It supplies sensation to the lateral half of the anterior forearm via the lateral cutaneous branch of the forearm. The axillary nerve (C5, C6) provides motor fibers to the teres minor and deltoid muscles and sensation to the inferior deltoid region. The median nerve (C6–T1) is responsible for motor function of most of the forearm flexors muscles, the thenar muscles, and the lat-

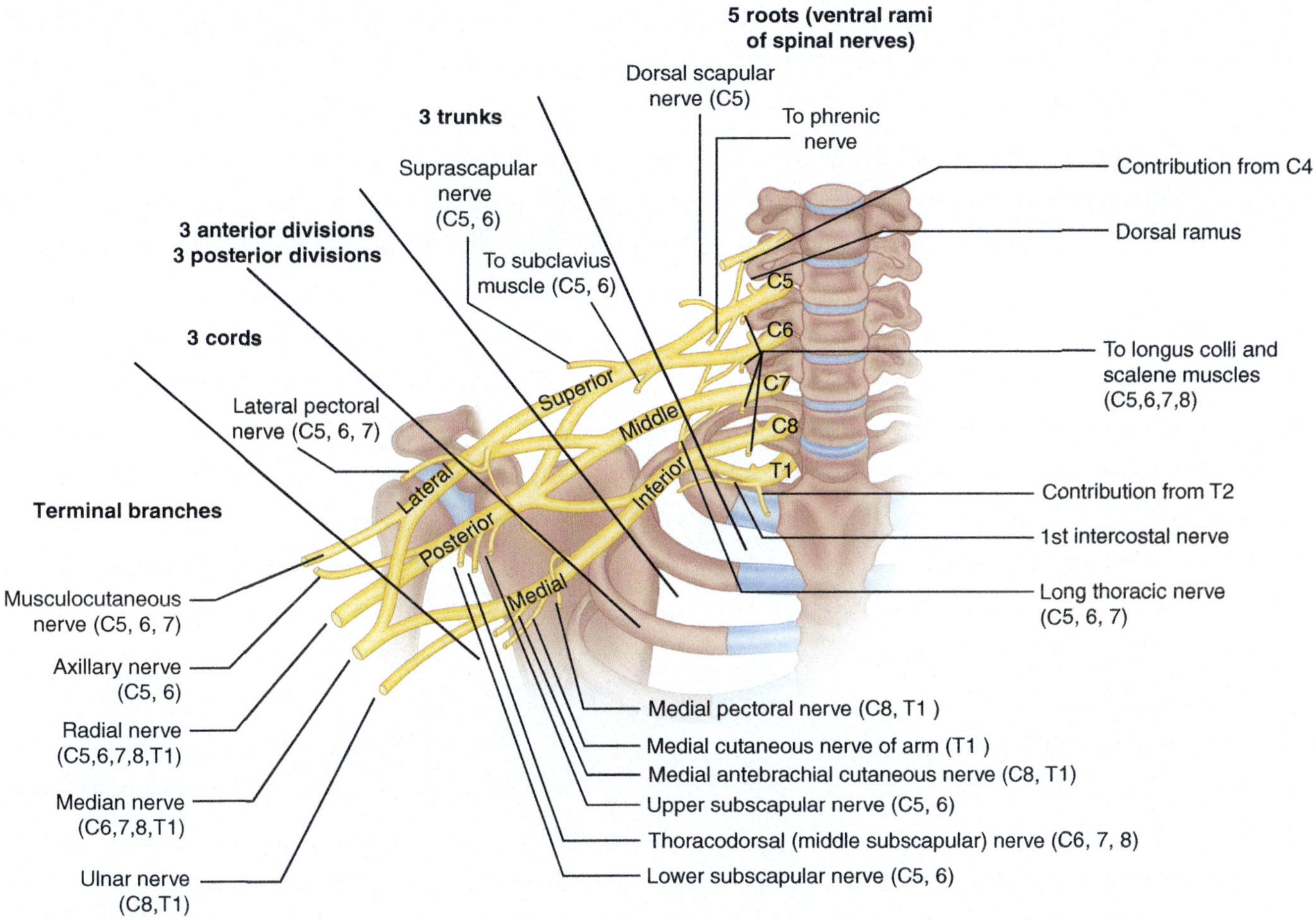

Fig. 5.2 Brachial plexus

eral two lumbricals. It provides sensory innervation to the lateral aspect of the palm via the palmer cutaneous branch and the anterior aspect of the lateral three and a half fingers via the digital cutaneous branch. The radial nerve (C5–T1) supplies the triceps and the extensor muscles in the posterior forearm and provides sensation to the posterior arm, forearm, and posterolateral hand. Finally, the ulnar nerve (C8, T1) provides motor innervation to the flexor carpi ulnaris and medial aspect of the flexor digitorum profundus and the hand muscles aside from the thenar and lateral two lumbrical muscles. The ulnar nerve supplies the skin of the 5th and medial 4th fingers and the associated palmar aspect of the hand.

In addition, numerus preterminal nerves branch off at various points along the brachial plexus. The dorsal scapular nerve and long thoracic nerve branch off at the root level. The dorsal scapular nerve (C5) innervates the rhomboid major and minor muscles, while the long thoracic nerve (C5, C6, C7) descends below the axilla to innervate the serratus anterior muscle. The nerve to subclavius muscle (C5, C6) is derived from the upper trunk, as is the suprascapular nerve (C5, C6), which supplies the supraspinatus and infraspinatus muscles of the rotator cuff. At the cord level, the lateral pectoral nerve (C5, C6, C7) and the medial pectoral nerve (C8, T1) are derived from the lateral cord and medial cord, respectively. Although the lateral pectoral nerve primarily innervates the pectoralis major muscle and the medial pectoral nerve primarily innervates the pectoralis minor muscle, commonly these two nerves combine as a single unit and distribute fibers to both muscles. The medial brachial cutaneous nerve (C8, T1) comes off the medial cord and supplies sensation to the inferior medial aspect of the arm. The medial antebrachial cutaneous nerve (C8, T1) also arises from the medial cord and supplies the skin of the lower portion of the anterior arm as well as medial forearm.

Lumbar Plexus

The lumbar plexus (Fig. 5.3) provides motor and sensory innervation to the abdominal wall, pelvis, and anterior and medial aspects of the lower extremity. There

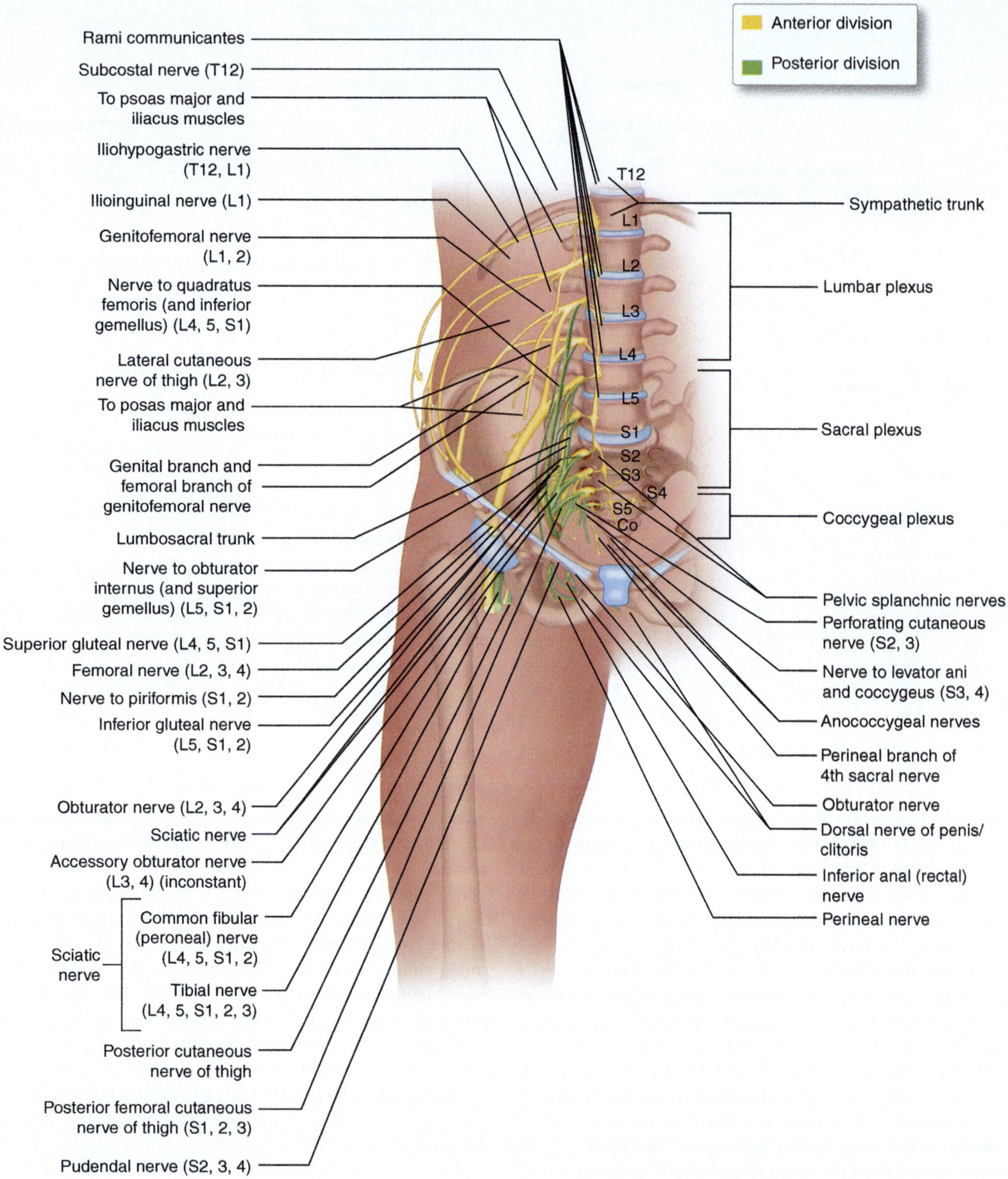

Fig. 5.3 Lumbosacral plexus

are five lumbar nerve roots on each side of the spinal column, each exiting via its respective intervertebral foramen. L1 exits between the first and second lumbar vertebrae (L1/L2 foramen), and L5 exits between the fifth lumbar vertebrae and the first sacral vertebrae (L5/S1 foramen).

After exiting the intervertebral foramina, the lumbar nerves separate into dorsal and ventral rami. The dorsal rami run posteriorly between the transverse processes and divide into medial and lateral branches. The medial branches run medially, innervating the facet joints and multifidus muscles. The lateral branches run laterally, supplying the erector spinae and intertransverse muscles and providing sensation to the skin of the gluteal region.

The ventral rami run anteriorly along the sides of the vertebral bodies, communicate with the lumbar sympathetic trunk via rami communicantes, and innervate the psoas and quadratus lumborum muscles. The ventral rami of the upper four lumbar roots form the lumbar plexus. The fourth and fifth ventral rami form the lumbosacral trunk. The ventral rami of the fifth lumbar and first four sacral roots, with a branch from the fourth lumbar root, contribute to the formation of the sacral plexus.

As noted above, the lumbar plexus is formed by the ventral rami of L1, L2, L3, and L4, with varying contribution from the ventral ramus of T12. It is located anterior to the lumbar transverse processes, within the psoas major muscle. Although there is some variability among individuals in the arrangement of the lumbar plexus, terminal branch nerves arise from one or more spinal nerve roots.

The iliohypogastric nerve (T12, L1) runs from the posterior boarder of the psoas muscle, across the quadratus lumborum to the iliac crest. It innervates the muscles of the posterior abdominal wall: internal oblique and transversus abdominis. It also provides sensation to the skin of the upper lateral gluteal region.

The ilioinguinal nerve (L1) follows a similar path to the iliohypogastric nerve, also innervating the internal oblique and transversus abdominis muscles. It then courses through the superficial inguinal ring and distributes to the skin of the anteromedial thigh, the scrotum in males, and labia majora and mons pubis in females.

The genitofemoral nerve (L1, L2) emerges from the substance of the psoas muscle and descends along its medial boarder, dividing into the genital and femoral branches. The genital branch passes through the internal inguinal ring and, in males, accompanies the spermatic cord to the scrotum, innervating the cremaster muscle. In females, the genital branch accompanies the round ligament but does not innervate any specific muscles. The femoral branch descends along the external iliac artery, courses under the inguinal ligament, and enters the sheath of the femoral vessels situating lateral to the femoral artery. It supplies the skin of the superior half of the anterior thigh.

The lateral femoral cutaneous nerve (L2, L3) is a purely sensory nerve. It courses from the lateral boarder of the psoas muscle, across the iliacus muscle to the anterior superior iliac spine. It then passes under the inguinal ligament and supplies cutaneous innervation of the anterior and lateral thigh down to the level of the knee.

The obturator nerve (L2, L3, L4) emerges from the medial boarder of the psoas muscle, descends posterior to the common iliac arteries, and passes along the lateral wall of the pelvis to the obturator foramen. At the obturator foramen, it gives off an articular branch to the hip joint. It then enters the thigh via the obturator canal and divides into an anterior and posterior branch. The anterior branch innervates the adductor longus, adductor brevis, gracilis, and, occasionally, the pectineus muscles. It then pierces the fascia lata and is distributed to the skin of the middle part of the medial thigh. The posterior branch supplies the adductor externus and adductor magnus muscles and sends an articular branch to the knee joint.

The femoral nerve (L2, L3, L4) emerges from the inferior lateral boarder of the psoas muscle and passes beneath the inguinal ligament into the thigh. It descends through the femoral triangle lateral to the femoral artery and lies beneath the fascia iliaca, where it supplies articular branches to the hip and knee joints. The femoral nerve supplies muscular branches to the anterior thigh, innervating the hip flexors (pectineus, iliacus, and sartorius) and knee extensors (quadriceps: rectus femoris, vastus lateralis, and vastus intermedius). The femoral nerve provides sensation to the lower extremity via anterior cutaneous branches proximally and the saphenous nerve distally. The anterior cutaneous branches come off in the femoral triangle and innervate the integument of the anteromedial thigh. The saphenous nerve is the largest cutaneous branch of the femoral nerve. It descends along the femoral artery through the adductor canal, down the medial thigh and leg, supplying the skin of the medial leg, ankle, and foot.

Sacral Plexus

The sacral plexus (Fig. 5.3) provides motor and sensory innervation to the pelvis and lower limb. There are five sacral nerves on each side of the sacral canal, with the four upper nerves each exiting via their respective sacral foramina and the fifth sacral nerve exiting between the sacrum and coccyx. As in the rest of the spine, each sacral nerve divides into dorsal and ventral rami. The dorsal rami of S1, S2, and S3 divide into medial and lateral branches. The medial branches innervate the multifidus muscle and the lateral branches, along with contributions from L4 and L5, supply the posterior sacral ligament, sacroiliac joint, and skin over the posterior gluteal region. The dorsal rami of S4 and S5 do not divide into medial and lateral branches and join the coccygeal nerve to innervate the skin over the coccyx.

The ventral rami of the sacral nerves emerge from the anterior sacral foramina and communicate with the sacral sympathetic ganglia. The ventral rami of S1–S4, with contributions from L4 and L5 (lumbosacral trunk), go on to form the sacral plexus. The sacral plexus is located anterior to the piriformis muscle on the posterior pelvic wall. The lumbosacral trunk, S1, S2, and part of S3 then combine to form the upper (larger) cord, while the remainder of S3 and part of S4 form the lower (smaller) cord. From the cords, five major terminal nerves arise: superior gluteal, inferior gluteal, sciatic, posterior femoral cutaneous, and pudendal.

The superior gluteal nerve (L4, L5, S1) arises from the pelvis through the greater sciatic foramen at the superior aspect of the piriformis muscle, together with the superior gluteal artery and vein. It supplies the gluteus minimus and gluteus medius muscles and the tensor fascia lata. The inferior gluteal nerve (L5, S1, S2) also arises from the pelvis through the greater sciatic foramen but at the inferior aspect of the piriformis muscle. It innervates the gluteus maximus muscle.

The sciatic nerve (L4–S3) is the largest peripheral nerve in the body measuring up to 2 cm in width. It supplies sensation to most of the leg and foot and motor function to all the muscles of the posterior thigh and the entire leg and foot. The sciatic nerve exits the pelvis via the greater sciatic foramen inferior to the piriformis muscle and descends along the posterior thigh. It sends branches to the hamstring muscles (semimembranosus, semitendinosus, and biceps femoris) and hamstring portion of the adductor magnus. At the top of popliteal fossa or above (varies among individuals), the sciatic nerve bifurcates into the tibial and common fibular nerves.

The tibial nerve descends down the leg posterior to the tibia. It innervates all the calf muscles, gastrocnemius, soleus, and plantaris, in the superficial compartment and popliteus, flexor hallucis longus, flexor digitorum longus, and tibialis posterior in the deep compartment. The tibial nerve continues to descend down the ankle, winding posterior and inferior to the medial malleolus and distributing sensation to the plantar foot. At the popliteal fossa, branches of the tibial and common fibular nerve combine to form the sural nerve, supplying sensation to the posterolateral leg and foot.

After bifurcating from the sciatic nerve, the common fibular nerve runs lateral and inferior along the inner boarder of the biceps femoris muscle, winds around the neck of the fibula, and enters the lateral compartment of the leg where it divides into the deep fibular and superficial fibular nerves. The deep fibular nerve supplies muscles of the anterior compartment of the leg (tibialis anterior, extensor digitorum longus, and extensor hallucis longus) as well as the intrinsic muscles of the foot. The superficial fibular nerve supplies the muscles of the lateral compartment of the leg (fibularis longus and brevis). The deep fibular nerve provides sensation to the web space between the first and second toes, whereas the superficial fibular nerve innervates the rest of the dorsum of the foot and anterolateral leg.

The posterior femoral cutaneous nerve (S1, S2, S3) exits through the greater sciatic foramen inferior to the piriformis muscle. It runs posterior to the gluteus maximus muscle passing down the back of the thigh and supplying cutaneous innervation to the posterior thigh and leg as well as the perineum. As with the lateral femoral cutaneous nerve, the posterior femoral cutaneous nerve has no motor innervation.

The pudendal nerve (S2, S3, S4) also exits the pelvis via the greater sciatic foramen inferior to the piriformis; however, it then reenters the pelvis through the lesser sciatic foramen. It courses anteriorly and superiorly along the ischiorectal fossa, gives off the inferior anal nerve, and bifurcates into the perineal nerve and the dorsal nerve of the penis or clitoris. As such, the pudendal nerve provides cutaneous innervation to the penis and the clitoris and much of the perineum. Muscular branches are sent to muscles of the perineum, levator ani, external urethral sphincter, and external anal sphincter.

Autonomic Nervous System

The autonomic nervous system (ANS) controls involuntary actions and maintains homeostasis throughout the body by regulating multiple organ systems including respiratory, cardiovascular, digestive, urinary, and reproductive. Visceral sensory (afferent) fibers send input to the ANS, while visceral motor (efferent) fibers innervate exocrine glands, cardiac muscle, and smooth muscle. The autonomic nervous system is composed of the sympathetic and parasympathetic nervous systems (Fig. 5.4), each with differing and often opposite functions. The sympathetic nervous system generally produces a catabolic effect, whereas the parasympathetic nervous system generally produces an anabolic effect.

Sympathetic preganglionic cell bodies are located in the intermediolateral column of the spinal cord from the first thoracic segment until the second lumbar segment (T1–L2). These neurons then exit the spinal canal as myelinated fibers together with the ventral roots, branch off from the spinal nerves, and travel to the paravertebral ganglia, also known as the sympathetic trunk, located on the anterolateral aspect of the vertebral body. Paired ganglia extend the length of the spinal column with 3 cervical, 12 thoracic, 4 lumbar, and 4 or 5 sacral ganglia. Preganglionic neurons can synapse at, above, or below the corresponding paravertebral ganglia. Postganglionic neurons track from the paravertebral ganglia to their target organs.

Some sympathetic preganglionic fibers pass through the paravertebral ganglia without synapsing, instead continuing as splanchnic nerves. These nerves synapse in preverterbral ganglia located anterior to the vertebral body. The preverte-

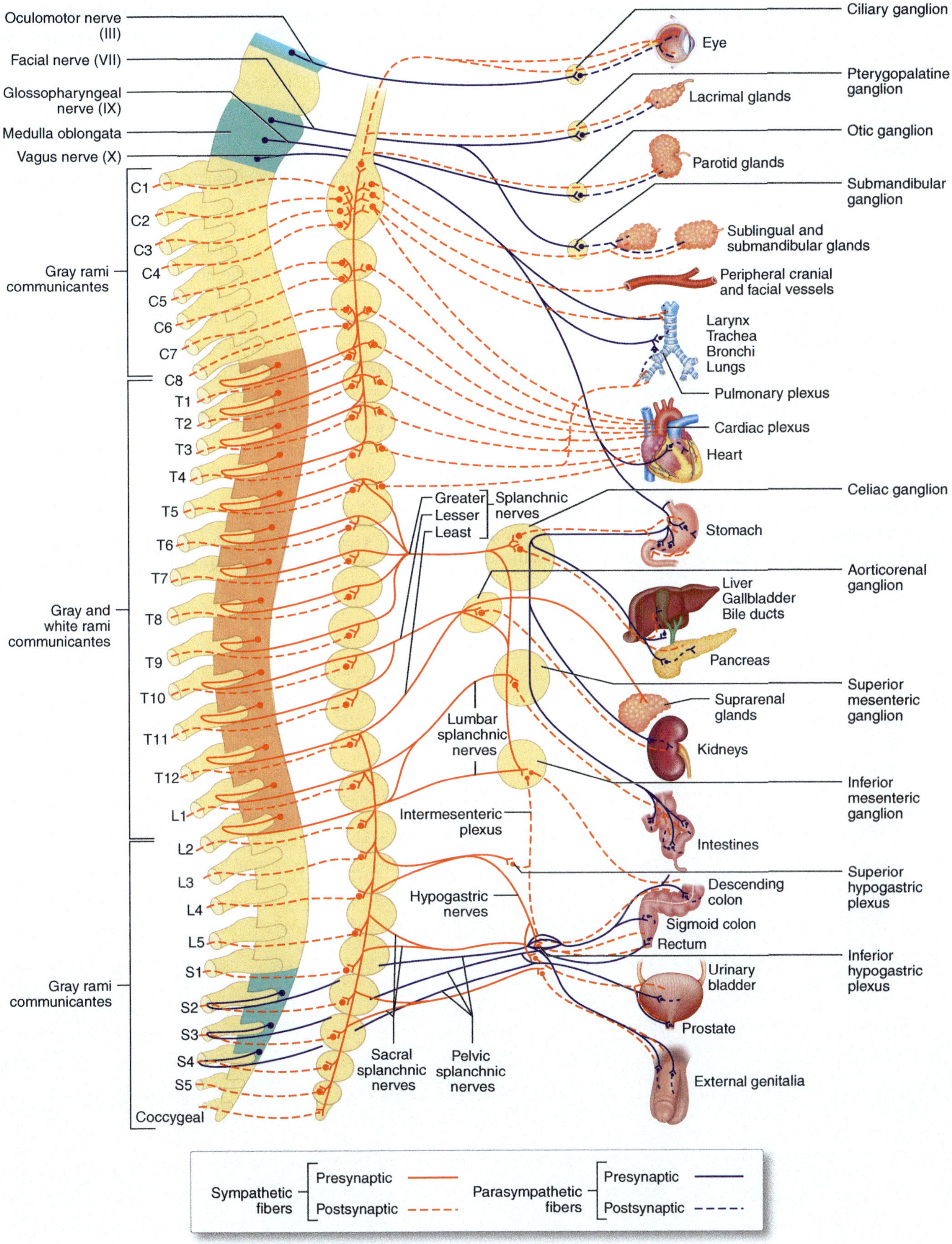

Fig. 5.4 Autonomic nervous system

bral ganglia are located in clusters around major arteries in the abdomen and pelvis and are named according to these arteries (e.g., celiac plexus). Postganglionic fibers originating in prevertebral ganglia course to their target organs. Characteristically in the sympathetic nervous system, the preganglionic fibers are short, and the postganglionic fibers are long.

Parasympathetic preganglionic fibers originate in the nuclei of the brain stem as well as the second through fourth sacral levels (S2–S4) of the spinal cord. These neurons extend to synapse at parasympathetic ganglia located close to the target organs. Postganglionic neurons then synapse on the target organs. Therefore, in the parasympathetic nervous system, the preganglionic fibers are long, and the postganglionic fibers are short.

Parasympathetic innervation to the head is mediated through cranial nerves III (oculomotor), VII (facial), and IX (glossopharyngeal). The oculomotor nerve carries preganglionic parasympathetic fibers to the ciliary ganglion where they synapse with postganglionic fibers to innervate pupillary constrictor muscles. The facial nerve carries parasympathetic fibers via the pterygopalatine ganglion and submandibular ganglion to control salivary, tear, and nasal glands. The glossopharyngeal nerve carries parasympathetic fibers via the otic ganglion that control salivation. Cranial nerve X (vagus) conveys parasympathetic innervation for thoracic and most abdominal organs. The vagus nerve sends preganglionic fibers to multiple plexi including cardiac, esophageal, and pulmonary. Postsynaptic fibers innervate the liver, pancreas, kidneys, ureter, stomach, intestines, and part of the colon.

Parasympathetic outflow from the spinal cord occurs only at the sacral level. Preganglionic fibers from sacral segments S2, S3, and S4 form pelvic splanchnic nerves that track to the inferior hypogastric plexus. Postsynaptic nerves go on to innervate the remainder of the colon, rectum, bladder, and reproductive organs.

Recommended Reading

1. Agur A, Dalley A. Grant's atlas of anatomy. 14th ed. Philadelphia: Wolters Kluwer; 2017.
2. Gray H. Gray's anatomy: the Unabridged Running Press Edition of the American Classic. Philadelphia: Running Press; 1974. p. 762–810.
3. Netter F. Atlas of human anatomy. 6th ed. Philadelphia: Saunders; 2014.
4. Stranding S. Gray's anatomy: the anatomical basis of clinical practice. 41th ed. Europe and United States: Elsevier; 2015. p. 762–75.

Spinal Cord Anatomy

6

Alan Gonzalez Cota

Introduction

The spinal cord, located inside the vertebral canal, transmits nerve impulses to 31 pairs of spinal nerves, allowing communication between the brain and peripheral nerves. Of clinical relevance, this transmission is achieved through two basic functions: afferent signals, in which sensations that arise from the nervous tissue of the trunk, neck, and forelimbs are transmitted to the brain, and efferent signals, in which the brain transmits signals to the trunk, neck, and limbs to effector organs, stimulating them to perform certain actions. The functions of the spinal cord also include control of immediate and vegetative movements, such as the reflex act, the central nervous system, and the sympathetic and parasympathetic systems.

External Anatomy

The spinal cord is one of most extensive networks of nervous tissue in the human body. The axons of these neurons can reach up to one meter in length. With a weight of approximately 30 grams, in its complete development, the spinal cord reaches an average length of 44 cm inside the spinal canal (from the foramen magnum to the first or second lumbar vertebra). In the newborn, the marrow can reach to L3, and embryonic tissue is found to the base of the coccyx.

Morphologically, the spinal cord is cylindrical in the upper cervical and lumbar segments and ovoid, with a transverse diameter greater than the anteroposterior diameter, in the lower cervical and thoracic segments. The spinal cord is also asymmetric in almost 80% of humans; of those, the right side is larger in 75%. This asymmetry is due to the fact that more fibers from the descending corticospinal tracts cross (decussate) from left to right.

A. Gonzalez Cota (✉)
A.I.M. Interventional Spine Division, Rockville, MD, USA

Legacy Pain Management Rehabilitation, Bethesda, MD, USA

KureSmart Pain Management, Annapolis, MD, USA

The spinal cord has two surfaces and two borders: an anterior surface, two lateral borders, and a posterior surface (Fig. 6.1). The anterior aspect of the midline of the spinal cord represents the anterior middle groove and is laterally bordered by the anterior collateral grooves. These collateral grooves are the origins of the motor or efferent nerve roots of the spinal nerves and also separate them from the lateral borders. The posterior surface presents a mid-posterior sulcus that extends through a partition all the way into to the central gray matter (discussed later) and is limited to the sides by the posterior collateral sulci corresponding to the origins of the sensory or afferent nerve roots of the spinal nerves. Between them there is a paramedian groove that superficially divides the marrow into two parts that correspond to the fasciculus gracilis (or tract of Goll) and fasciculus cuneatus (or tract of Burdach). Of importance for neuromodulation, these two tracts occupy the posterior white column of the cord, the tract of Goll being medial to the tract of Burdach. They carry sensations of conscious proprioception, light touch, and vibration. Nerve fibers from the coccygeal, sacral, lumbar, and lower thoracic segments ascend in the tract of Goll, while the nerve fibers from the upper thoracic and cervical segments run in the tract of Burdach. This pathway carrying conscious proprioceptive and stereognosis is termed the dor-

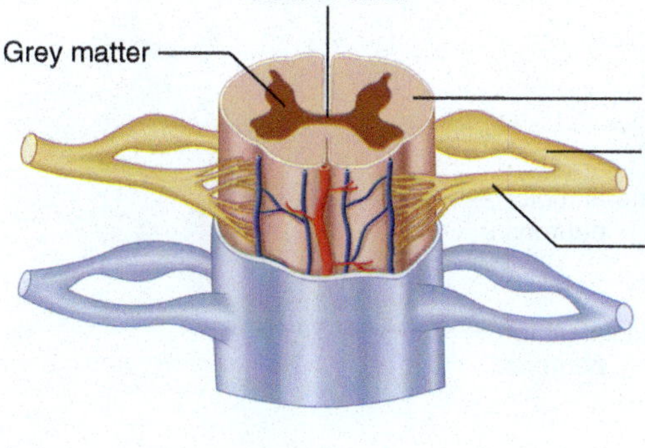

Fig. 6.1 Spinal cord cross-sectional anatomy

T. R. Deer et al. (eds.), *Deer's Treatment of Pain*, https://doi.org/10.1007/978-3-030-12281-2_6

sal column and connects to the thalamus and cerebral sensory cortex via the medial lemniscus pathway.

The spinal cord has two higher caliber segments or enlargements, one cervical and one lumbosacral. The cervical enlargement extends from the C4 to T1 and is due to the entry of nerve roots into the spinal cord that transmit nerve signals to and from the upper limbs. The lumbar enlargement extends from T11 to L1 and is due to the entry of nerve roots into the spinal cord that transmit nerve signals to and from the lower limbs and pelvis. The lower portion of the cord tapers and ends with a cone-shaped tip known as the conus medullaris. Inferiorly it is continuous with the terminal filum that extends to the bottom of the dural sac at the level of the second sacral vertebra, which is connected to the coccygeal filament and inserts into the coccyx.

Longitudinally, the spinal cord is divided into 31 segments, one for each pair of spinal nerves – 8 cervical, 12 thoracic, 5 lumbar, 5 sacral, and, more rarely, 1 coccygeal. Each segment has two pairs of symmetrically located roots, dorsal and ventral.

Three meningeal membranes wrap concentrically with the spinal cord: the pia mater, the arachnoid, and the dura mater. The pia mater inserts into the multiple grooves of the spinal cord and directly protects the spinal cord. Between the pia mater and the arachnoid is a space filled with cerebrospinal fluid, the subarachnoid space. Outside this space is the arachnoid, the most dense and distinguishable of the meningeal membranes. The arachnoid is a thin, transparent, lax network; it does not insert into the grooves of the spinal cord. In some sections of the spinal cord, it is difficult to differentiate the pia mater from the arachnoid, hence the term pia-arachnoid. The dura mater is the strong fibrous outermost meningeal layer. Between the arachnoid and the dura is a virtual space called the subdural space.

The spinal cord is attached to the medulla oblongata in its most cranial segment. It is stabilized in the center by conjunctive extensions that adhere to the dura mater and by connective tissue found between the nerve rootlets to the pia mater, the denticulate ligaments. Caudally, it is stabilized by an extension of the dura that surrounds the filum terminale, attaching to the base of the coccyx. The clinically relevant vascular supply is discussed at the end of this chapter.

Internal Anatomy

In a cross section of the spinal cord, the center contains the gray matter, which has a butterfly shape, with white matter in the periphery – the reverse of the brain configuration.

Gray Matter

The relatively thin posterior extensions that almost reach the posterior sulcus are the posterior horns; the anterior horns are the more rounded extensions (Fig. 6.2). The three-dimensional arrangement of the ventral and dorsal horns forms true columns that run through the spinal cord to form the gray anterior and posterior columns. The dorsal

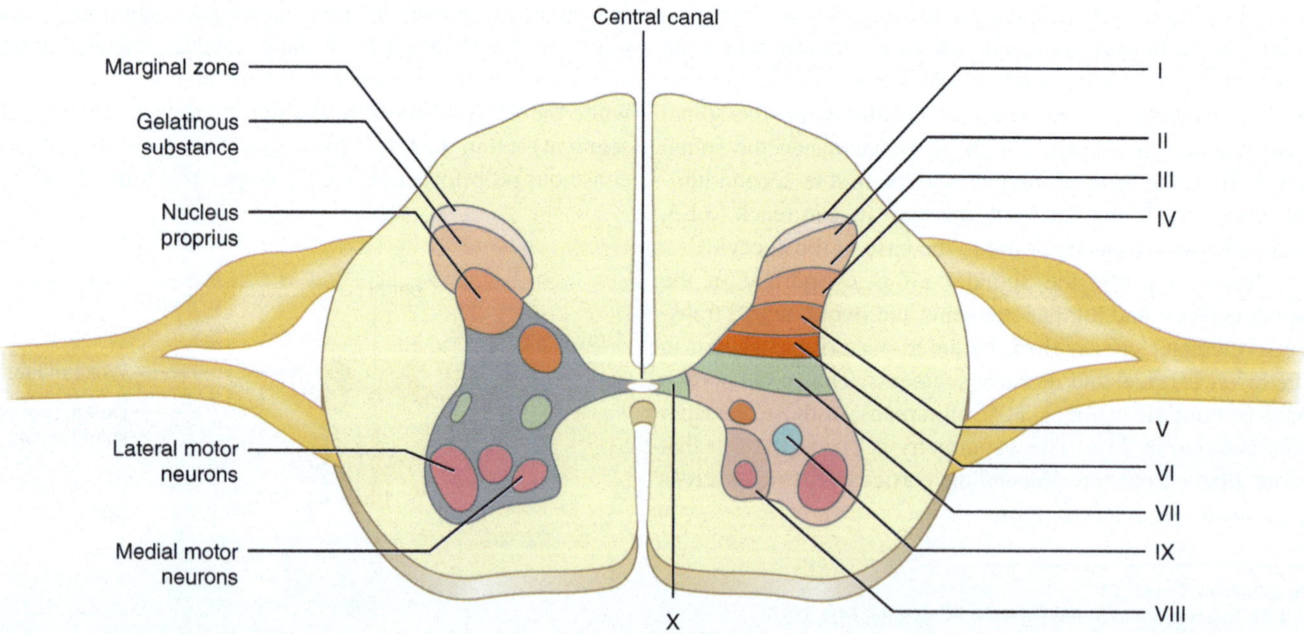

Fig. 6.2 Spinal cord gray matter cross-sectional view

horns, functionally somatosensitive, are formed by sensory neurons that receive impulses from the dorsal roots. The ventral horns, functionally somatomotor, are comprised of motor neurons whose axons leave the spinal cord via the ventral roots. In the upper thoracic and lumbar segments, there is a small lateral horn that emerges from the junction of the ventral horn with the dorsal horn that contains sympathetic visceral neurons. In the lateral part of the base of the dorsal horn of the upper cervical segments, it is difficult to distinguish the boundary between the gray matter and the white matter because nerve cells and fibers are mixed – this is the reticular formation that travels cephalad in the brain stem.

The gray matter is composed mainly of neuronal bodies and immunomodulatory cells (neuroglia). The two ventral and dorsal horns are connected by the gray commissure. This gray commissure is divided into posterior and anterior segments by a small central hole called the ependymal conduit or canalis centralis, a vestige of the primitive neural tube. At the thoracic and lumbar levels are also lateral horns in the form of wedges, corresponding to neurons that form the autonomous sympathetic or thoracolumbar system (intermediolateral nucleus). The consistency is fairly uniform, although the substance surrounding the ependymal duct is more transparent and soft, so it has been given the name of substantia gelatinosa. The spinal cord gray matter can be further divided into:

- *Dorsal horn*: The posterior horn receives axons from the dorsal ganglia through the homonymous roots and contains sensory beams. It comprises the nucleus of Clarke's column, where fibers transmit unconscious deep sensitivity; the gelatinous substance of Rolando, where synapses are made of fibers that transmit pain and temperature; and the nucleus proprius, where the first synapse of the spinothalamic tract occurs.
- *Intermediate-lateral horn*: Only found in the upper thoracic and lumbar segments (L1, L2, and sometimes L3) of the spinal cord. Contains sympathetic preganglionic neurons.
- *Ventral horn*: The anterior horn, composed of axons of motor neurons. It comprises the anterolateral system (the limbs) and the antero-internal nucleus destined for the dorsal muscles of the trunk and the neck.
- *Intermediate zone*: Contains a large number of interneurons.

White Matter (Fig. 6.3)

The white matter of the spinal cord is composed of a large number of nerve fibers, neuroglia, and blood vessels. In a cross-section, its arrangement around the gray matter is observed. The white color is due to the presence of myelin

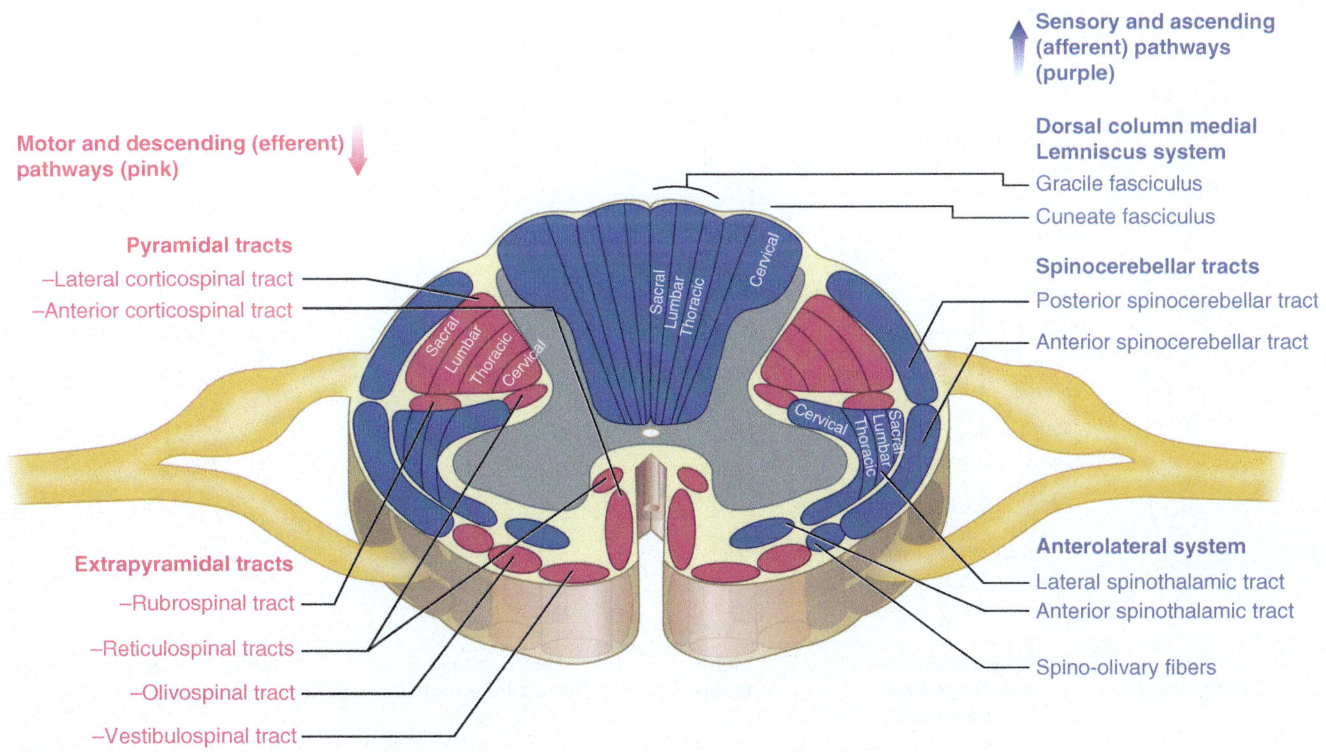

Fig. 6.3 Spinal cord white matter cross-sectional view

fibers that run longitudinally. The nerve fibers of the white matter bind the medullary segments together, and the spinal cord with the brain.

- *The dorsal column system* (*posterior spinal cord*) contains ascending sensory pathways (whose neuronal bodies are in the dorsal root ganglia) that participate in two modes of proprioception – kinesthesia (pressure and vibration) and epicritic touch (differentiation of two points and recognition of forms). It consists of two fascicles (both in pairs): the gracile fascicle of Goll (medial – carries information from the lower body) and the cuneate fascicle of Burdach (lateral – carries information from the upper body). It has small motor fibers which are in charge of reflex arcs: between the two fascicles of Goll is the septomarginal fascicle (oval bundle) and between the Goll and the Burdach, the semilunar fascicle.
- *The lateral spinal cord* contains ascending and descending pathways. The ascending fibers relay stimuli of pain, temperature, and gross touch (protopathic) and are comprised of the spinocerebellar, spinothalamic, spinoreticular, and spinotectal fascicles. In contrast, the descending fibers are motor and control voluntary movements. They are comprised of the corticospinal, rubrospinal, and reticulospinal fascicles.
- *The anterior cord* contains ascending and descending pathways. The ascending pathway has three tracts, and each relays different information: the spinotectal is responsible for reflex movements of eyes and head when visual information arrives, the spino-olivary sends light touch information to the cerebellum, and the ventral spinothalamic relays sensation of deep touch and pressure. The descending pathways (motor) are responsible for movement control and are comprised of the medial reticulospinal, vestibulospinal, and anterior corticospinal tracts.

The Sites of Crossing Over

In addition to knowledge of the location of the white matter of different tracts, it is vital for the clinician to know the sites of contralateral crossing over. There are three major sensory systems within the spinal cord: pain-temperature, proprioception-vibration (stereognosis), and light touch (Fig. 6.4). The tract for pain-temperature enters the spinal cord, crosses over within 1–2 segments, ascends to the thalamus in the other side, and then moves to the brain cortex. Injury to the spinothalamic tract will result in loss of pain-temperature sensation in the contralateral side, below the level of the injury.

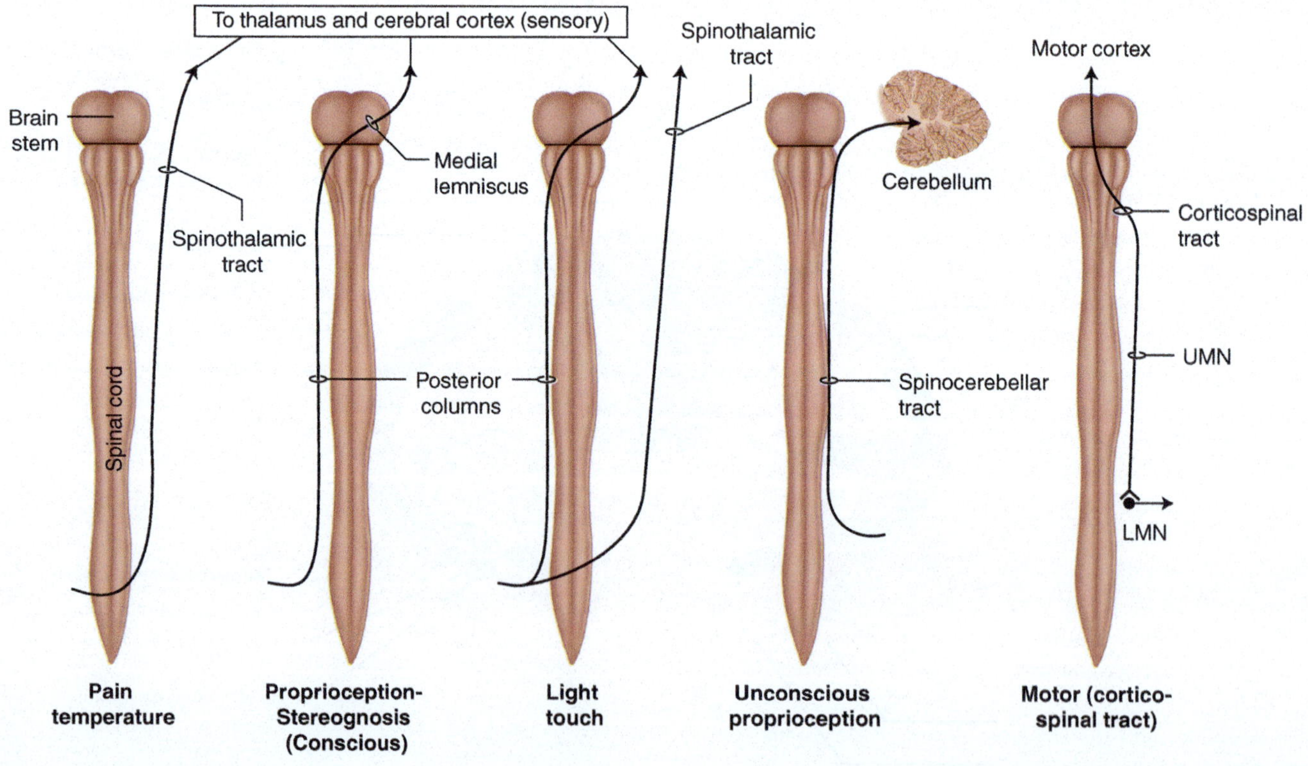

Fig. 6.4 Schematic of the spinal cord ascending and descending pathways

The tract for conscious proprioception (dorsal columns) initially remains in the same side of the spinal cord, crossing over at the junction between the spinal cord and the brain stem. A lesion of the dorsal columns results in loss of proprioception-vibration of the ipsilateral side, below the level of injury.

The two tracts described above carry the information for light touch. The tract for light touch remains partially uncrossed until it reaches the brain stem (dorsal columns) and partially crosses at lower levels (spinothalamic tract). This is the reason why light touch is preserved in unilateral spinal cord injury.

All sensory pathways eventually cross over and terminate in the thalamus. From there, they project into the sensory cortex of the brain. Injury to the thalamus or sensory cortex may result in loss of all sensations in the contralateral side of the body. There is also an unconscious proprioception tract, the spinocerebellar pathway, which reaches the ipsilateral side of the cerebellum only (not up to the thalamus and sensory cortex), thus never crossing. The motor pathway (corticospinal tract, descending) extends from the brain cortex through the brain stem, crossing over at this level (medial lemniscus).

Blood Supply of the Spinal Cord

There are three main arterial systems: a single anterior spinal artery, two posterior spinal arteries, and multiple segmental (or radicular) arteries (Fig. 6.5).

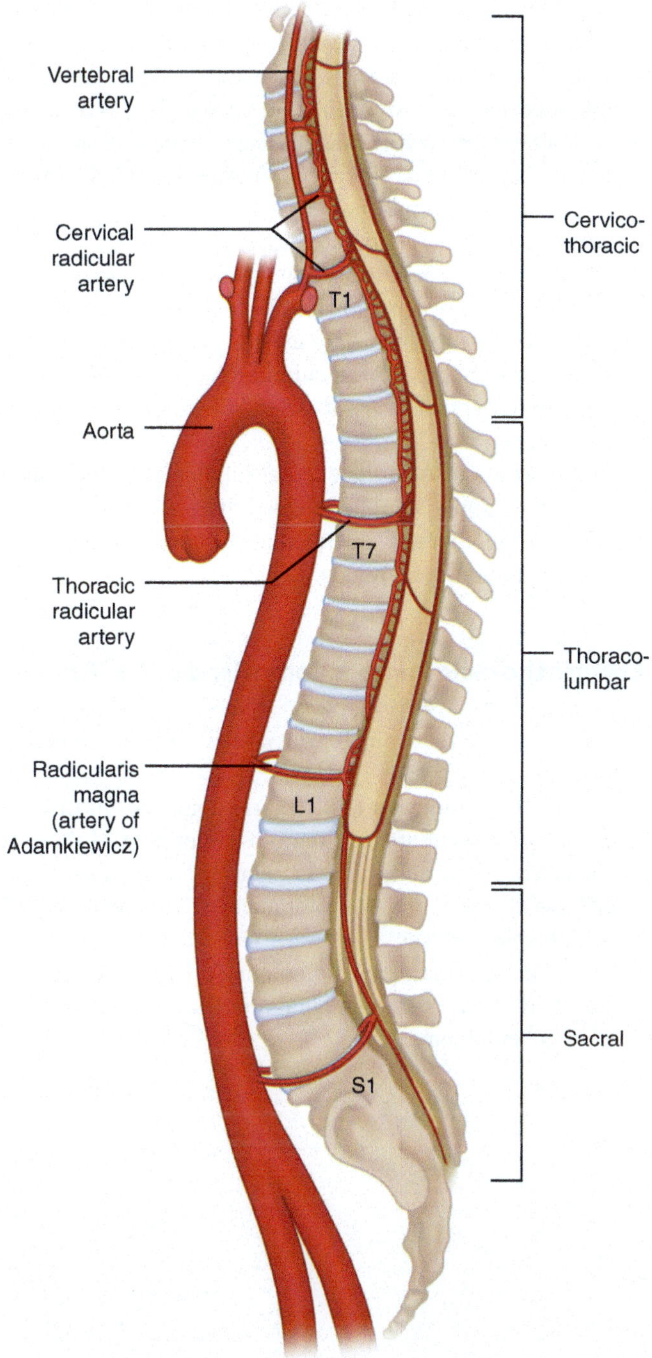

Fig. 6.5 Spinal cord relevant vascular anatomy for the spine interventionist

- *The anterior spinal artery* originates from branches of the two vertebral arteries, receives blood from the anterior segmental medullary arteries (including the radicular artery magna or artery of Adamkiewicz), and runs along the anterior aspect of the spinal cord. It does not have any major branches. This vessel is located in the pia mater along the anterior medial fissure; it irrigates that membrane, as well as the substance of the spinal cord, and has branches in its inferior portion that are distributed toward the cauda equina. It descends in front of the spinal cord and anastomoses with a series of small branches that enter the vertebral canal through the intervertebral foramina. These branches are derived from the vertebral artery, the ascending cervical artery (a branch of the lower thyroid artery in the neck), the intercostal arteries in the thorax, the lumbar artery, the iliolumbar artery, and the lateral sacral arteries in the abdomen and pelvis. Compromise of the anterior spinal artery leads to a syndrome of bilateral involvement of the corticospinal tract, producing motor deficits, and bilateral involvement of the spinothalamic tract, producing sensory deficits in the form of loss of sensitivity to pain and temperature. Cauda equina syndrome (loss of lower limb function; loss of smooth muscle tone of the bowel or bladder) can also occur as a result of a compromised anterior spinal artery.
- *The posterior spinal arteries* originate from the vertebral arteries at the brain stem level and often from the posterior

inferior cerebellar arteries. They then descend via the mid-posterior sulcus, located in front of the nerve roots. Along this path they anastomose with a series of radicular (segmental) branches, which enter the vertebral canal through the inter-vertebral foramina, forming a plexus. The posterior spinal arteries continue as two main trunks descending to the lower part of the spinal cord, toward the cauda equina. Near its origin, each posterior spinal artery emits an ascending branch, terminating ipsilaterally near the fourth ventricle. Branches of the posterior spinal arteries form anastomoses around the dorsal roots of the spinal nerves and travel to the contralateral side (by means of very tortuous transverse branches).

- *The radicular arteries* only exist at certain levels of the spinal cord. Six to ten radicular arteries anastomose with the anterior spinal artery at different levels (see below).

To better understand the clinical implications, the spinal cord blood supply can be divided into three functional regions: cervicothoracic, intermediate or upper thoracic, and the thoracolumbosacral region:

Cervicothoracic Region: Comprised of C1–T2

- C1–C4: anterior spinal artery, few or no radicular arteries
- C5–T2: large radicular (2–4) arteries, branches of the vertebral or cervical arteries; the most important of these is the artery of the cervical enlargement that enters the spinal canal along the neuroforamen of the seventh and eighth spinal nerves.
- In addition, multiple radiculomedullary arteries are attached to the posterior spinal arteries, especially in the cervical enlargement.

Intermediate or Thoracic Region

- T3–T8 are poorly vascularized by radicular arteries than branch from the intercostal arteries. It receives a single radicular artery that enters the spinal canal along the path of the T7, T8, or T9 neuroforamina.

Thoracolumbosacral Region

- T8 – cauda equina: a rich blood supply from the radicular branches from the intercostals and lumbar arteries. The Adamkiewicz artery (or lumbar enlargement artery) plays an important role in thoracolumbosacral blood supply. It enters the spinal canal predominately on the left side and at the T9, T10, T11, T12, L1, or L2. In addition to the aforementioned arteries, there are multiple posterior radicular arteries that partially supply the dorsal columns, anterior and posterior roots, and meninges.

Recommended Reading

1. Mendoza JE, Foundas AL. The spinal cord and descending tracts. In: Mendoza JE, Foundas AL, editors. Clinical neuroanatomy. A neurobehavioral approach. New York, NY: Springer-Verlag; 2008. p. 1–22.
2. Noback CH, Strominger NL, Demarest RJ, Rugiero DA. Motoneurons and motor pathways. In: Noback CH, Strominger NL, Demarest RJ, Rugiero DA, editors. The human nervous system: structure and function. Totowa, NJ: Humana Press; 2005. p. 193–206.
3. Noback CH, Strominger NL, Demarest RJ, Rugiero DA. The spinal cord. In: Noback CH, Strominger NL, Demarest RJ, Rugiero DA, editors. The human nervous system: structure and function. Totowa, NJ: Humana Press; 2005. p. 129–140.

Anatomy of the Brain and Brain Stem

7

Mark N. Malinowski

Introduction

The brain is also referred to as the encephalon. Globally, the brain is composed on the cerebrum (forebrain, FB), the cerebellum, and the brain stem (BS) in a rostral to caudal organization, respectively. The central nervous system (CNS) as a whole consists of the brain and spinal cord (SC). Commonly, the mistake is made to refer to the cerebrum as the brain independently of the brain stem, but they are not considered mutually exclusive in general anatomical terms.

Brain Stem and Ascending Input

The brain stem is composed on the mesencephalon or midbrain (MB), the pons, and the medulla oblongata (MO) and arises from the most cephalad portion of the cervical SC. There are three longitudinal layers of the brain stem and from dorsal to ventral include the tectum, the tegmentum, and the basis. However, the tectum is predominantly associated with the midbrain, whereas the pons and medulla are known to consist of the pontine and medullary tegmenta and pontine and medullary bases. The dorsal aspect of the pons, dorsal to the pontine tegmentum, is the floor of the fourth ventricle. Dorsal to the brain stem is the cerebellum, and this structure is attached to the BS by two peduncles each containing a superior, middle, and inferior component. Dorsal to the midbrain is two pairs of colliculi (superior and inferior) known as the quadrigeminal plate.

The BS is the main conduit for ascending and descending pathways from the SC. The brain stem is also a source of ascending and descending pathways as well as the location of many nuclei, or collections of cell bodies of neurons of the CNS.

M. N. Malinowski (✉)
Adena Spine Center, Chillicothe, OH, USA

The MO is known to have rostral and caudal components, and this is determined by the location or absence of the fourth ventricle, respectively. Paramount to the somatosensory system is the dorsal column pathway (DCP) providing information of two-point discrimination, fine touch, and proprioception. Ascending fibers of DCP from the gracile and cuneate tracts terminate on the gracile and cuneate nuclei (dorsal column nuclei), respectively, in the lower MO. These second-order target cells then project contralaterally, forming the internal arcuate tract (lemniscal decussation), of which then creates the medial lemniscus that projects to the thalamus (Fig. 7.1). The MO is also known to contain ascending information from the ventrolateral (spinothalamic) tract and spinoreticular tract known for transmission of sharp pain, hard touch, and temperature from the skin. These remain ipsilateral having already decussated at the level of the dorsal horn.

The MO also contains second-order neurons associated with the spinocerebellar tract. Input from mechanoreceptors is relayed to the nucleus dorsalis (lumbar/sacral) and accessory cuneate nucleus (upper extremities) from the dorsal spinocerebellar tract that ascends to the cerebellum through the inferior cerebellar peduncle. The ventral spinocerebellar tract is composed of second-order neurons that arise from the Rexed laminae in the lumbosacral regions and enter the cerebellum through the superior peduncle.

The MO also contains fibers associated with descending pathways. The corticospinal pathway (CSP) consists of neurons from the motor cortex crosses at the junction of the medulla and the cervical cord. This area is known as the pyramidal tract within the MO. Other descending tracts within the MO include the descending tract of cranial nerve (CN) V that relay pain, temperature, and touch from the trigeminal distribution in the face to the pars caudalis or spinal nucleus of CN V in the inferior portion of the medulla. In the dorsal aspect of the rostral component of the MO near the ventral aspect of the fourth ventricle lays the medial longitudinal fasciculus (MLF). This area is known to mediate signals associated with head motion and gaze. This area is

T. R. Deer et al. (eds.), *Deer's Treatment of Pain*, https://doi.org/10.1007/978-3-030-12281-2_7

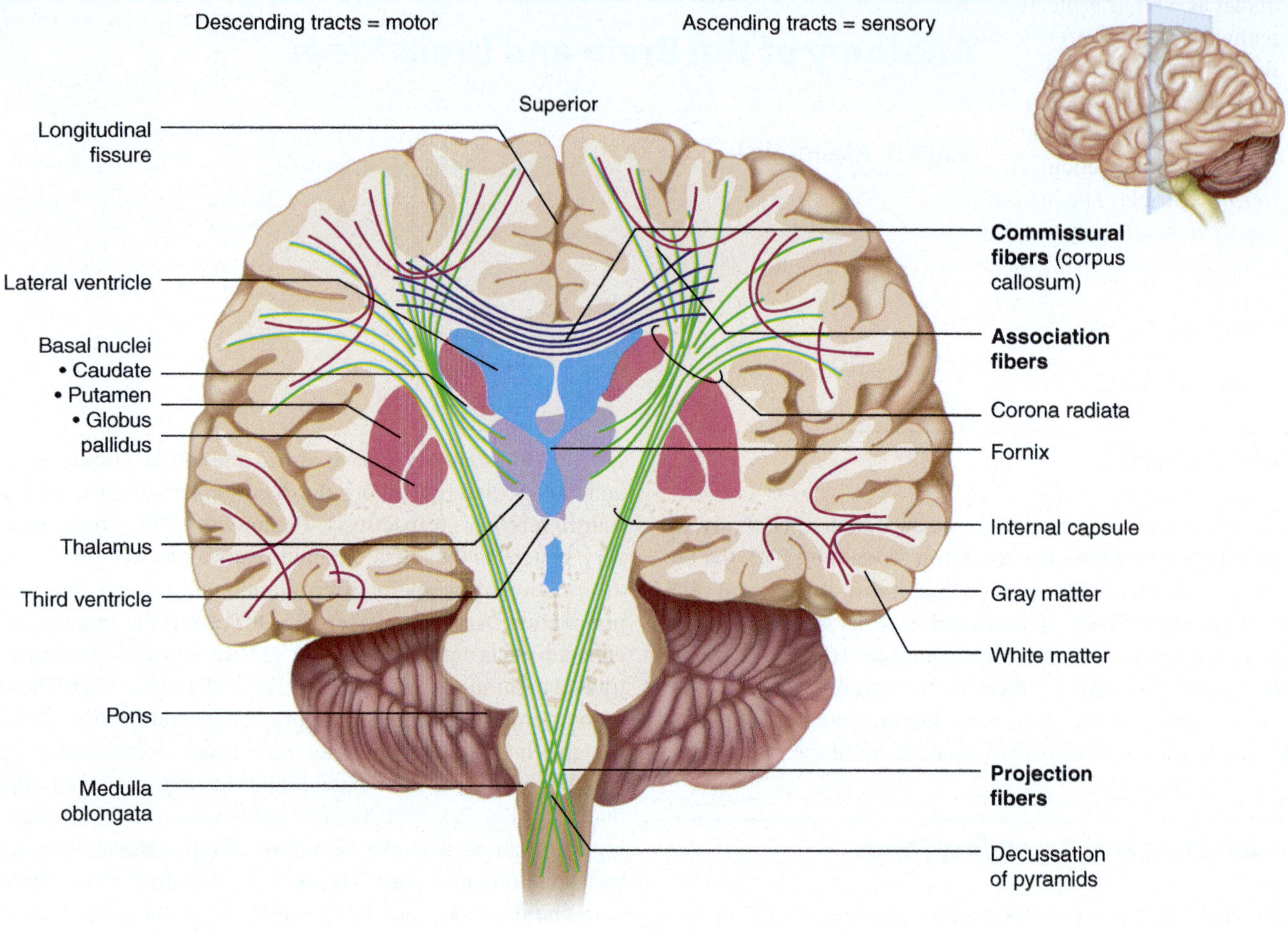

Fig. 7.1 Lemniscal decussation. Ascending fibers decussate at the level of the medulla and project via the internal capsule to the contralateral cortex

associated with the vestibular nuclei of the pons as well as fibers from nuclei associated with eye movement (the abducens, trochlear, and oculomotor centers). Similarly, neck movement due to visual cues emanates from the superior colliculus (in the MB) through the MO by way of the tectospinal tract to the cervical cord and below. In close approximation to the MLF as well as the fourth ventricle are the solitary nucleus (SN) and tract (ST) and the hypoglossal nucleus (CN XII, tongue movement). The nucleus of CN XII sends fibers anteriorly to exit as the hypoglossal nerve. The SN is an important structure in nociception as it receives information from CNs VII, IX, and X that synapse on the ST. In addition to taste (rostral SN), this tract is important in relaying information associated with visceral sensation. Also contained in the MO is the dorsal motor nucleus of CN X. This sends parasympathetic control to the heart, lungs, and abdomen through CNs IX and X. Nearby is the superior salivatory nucleus that provides parasympathetic tone to the submandibular glands, lacrimal glands, and pterygopalatine ganglia. Other nuclei of the MO are the vestibular and cochlear nuclei. The vestibular nuclei (superior, inferior, medial, and lateral) are near the fourth ventricle, while the cochlear nuclei are present laterally near the inferior cerebellar peduncle, and these are associated with balance and hearing, respectively. The inferior cerebellar peduncle is mostly closely associated with the MO.

The pons is rostral to the MO in the brain stem and, as previously mentioned above, contains base and tegmentum components. The pons is also ventral to the cerebellum, and it is most closely associated with the middle cerebellar peduncle. The base of the pons (BP) is known to house the continuity of the corticospinal tracts, but these begin to scatter and move laterally in order to form more cohesive and independent tracts in the MB. Similarly, the BP is also known to house the raphe nuclei, an area most importantly associated with the serotonergic pain pathways that send fibers to the cortex, basal ganglia, and thalamus, among others. The tegmentum of the pons (PT) contains several cranial nerve-associated nuclei as well as projections from ascending and descending pathways. In the inferior-most portion of the PT, the nuclei for CN VI (abducens) and CN VII (facial) are present. The projection fibers from the CN VII nucleus are known to loop medially around the nucleus of CN VI. In close association are the pontine reticular formation and, more dorsally, the fourth ventricle. The medial lemniscus appears still medially, but as it ascends it gradually moves laterally. In addition, other structures such as the superior olivary nucleus that is associated with the auditory pathway are present and communicate with CN VIII.

The more superior portion of the PT harbors the central trigeminal nuclei (CN V). The trigeminal nerves project information associated with fine touch, pain, and temperature as well as proprioceptive information. The three branches of the trigeminal nerve (V1, V2, V3) project to the trigeminal ganglia whereby sensory information is relayed to one of the three structures based on type of stimulus (Fig. 7.2). The main sensory nucleus of V receives information on fine touch. Fibers from this nucleus decussate and project to the contralateral thalamus. Pain and temperature are sent to the descending spinal tract of V. Projection fibers from the descending tract project to the medulla (pars caudalis) or to the pars interpolaris or pars oralis. Proprioceptive information is relayed to the mesecephalic tract and nucleus within the MB. The masticatory nucleus medial to the main nucleus provides input to the muscle of mastication and tensor tympani. Therefore, the muscles of the face are controlled by CN VII except most of the muscle of mastication by way of CN V3.

The MB is the structure just rostral to the pons and also ventral to the cerebellum. Therefore, the MB is most closely associated with the superior cerebellar peduncle. The basis of the MB contains large bundles (crus cerebri) that house the corticospinal (CSP), corticobulbar (CBP), and corticopontine (CPP) pathways. The CSP and CBP are tracts that originate from the sensorimotor cortex (SMC) with some contribution from other areas of the cortex. The CBP pathway

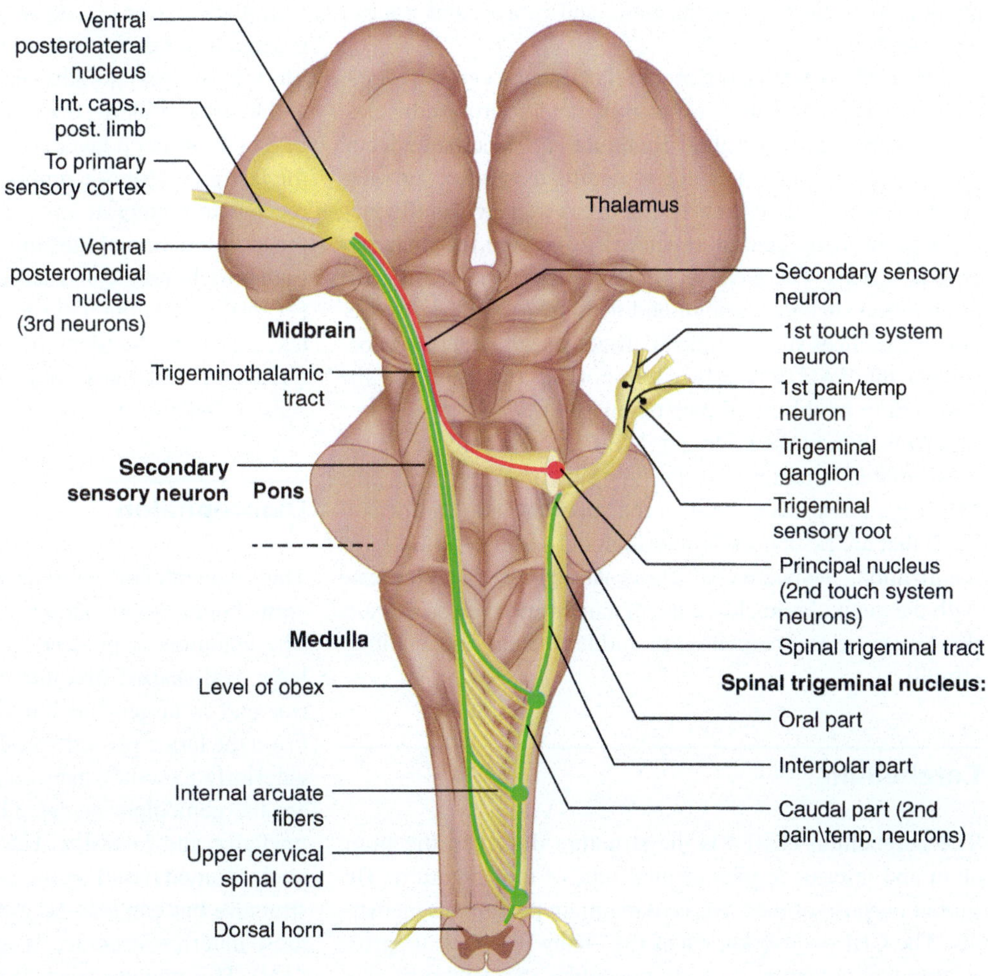

Fig. 7.2 The trigeminal pathway. Ipsilateral first-order fibers synapse at the corresponding trigeminal nucleus. Second-order neurons decussate and project to the contralateral VPM thalamic nucleus

arises from the area of the SMC associated with the face and descends to the crus cerebri to somatic and brachial efferent nuclei (i.e., to control muscles of the face and tongue). The oculomotor nuclei (CN III) fibers are also located near the cerebral peduncles and exit from the basis. The CSP pathway continues to the pyramids of the MO and descends to the corticospinal tract within the spinal cord. Finally, the basis of the MB also contains the substantia nigra, an area that receives input from the cortex and striatum and has an important role in the control of movement. Disease of this area is the basis for Parkinson's disease.

The tegmentum of the MB (TMB) is the area dorsal to the basis. The TMB is a conduit for many of the aforementioned ascending and descending pathways. The TMB also contains the red nucleus, the trochlear nucleus (CN IV), the oculomotor nucleus (CN III), and the Edinger-Westphal nucleus. While the nuclei of CN III and CN IV are involved with somatic motor control of the eye, the Edinger-Westphal nucleus mediates the parasympathetic reflex associated with pupillary constriction due to light stimulus. The red nucleus is associated with motor coordination as input from the cerebellum is triaged to the thalamus and rubrospinal tract of the spinal cord.

The TMB also is also closely related to the cerebral aqueduct, the conduit between the third and fourth ventricles. Circumscribing the cerebral aqueduct is the periaqueductal gray matter (PAG). The locus coeruleus nuclei are also nearby, and these noradrenergic neurons exert wide influence throughout many central structures to include the thalamus among others. The PAG is an important structure for the modulation of pain through endogenous as well as exogenous substances such as opiates. Together with the locus coeruleus, the PAG is likely an important structure for the descending inhibition of pain pathways.

The tectum of the midbrain (MBT) is considered to be the most dorsal structure of the longitudinal layers of the MB. This is known to contain the superior and inferior colliculi that are associated with visual and auditory stimuli and localization, respectively. These structures communicate with the genicular nuclei of the thalamus and created circuits that integrate the responses to sudden visual and auditory stimuli.

Cerebellum

The cerebellum (CBL) is the structure dorsal to the brain stem and inferior to the occipital lobe of the cerebrum. The global purpose of the CBL is to maintain postural homeostasis. The CBL is also known as the "baby brain" as its gross anatomical construct strongly resembles the cerebrum. The CBL has two lobes separated by the vermis. The lobes have a cortical layer and the cerebellar white matter. The CBL is connected to the brain stem through three tracts on each side, the superior, medial, and inferior peduncle. The inferior peduncle mainly consists of ascending input from the spinal cord and inferior aspect of the brain stem. The middle peduncle receives input from the pontine nuclei and the cerebrum. While the superior peduncle receives some input from the spinocerebellar tract, it mainly contains output fibers targeting the thalamus, rubrospinal tract, and other parts of the spinal cord.

The CBL cortex has three layers, the molecular, Purkinje, and granular layer. Within the granule layer are the granule cells, and these cells project to the Purkinje layer and run parallel to these cells and provide excitatory input. The Purkinje cells innerve the cells of the cerebellar deep layers. In the molecular layer exist the basket cells, the Golgi cells, and the stellate cells. The basket and stellate cells provide inhibition to the Purkinje cells, while the Golgi cells inhibit the granule cells. Basket, stellate, and Golgi cells all receive excitatory input from granule cells that have branched to become parallel cells in the molecular layer of the cortex. Afferent input to the CBL arises from either climbing fibers from the inferior olivary nucleus or from mossy fibers from the spinal cord or pontine nuclei. Similarly, there is strong serotonergic and noradrenergic input from the raphe nucleus and locus coeruleus, respectively.

The CBL deep layer consists of four pairs of deep nuclei, the fastigial, globose, emboliform, and dentate. These nuclei receive and integrate input from multiple sources to include the aforementioned Purkinje cells, spinal cord pathways, and both noradrenergic and serotonergic cells. These nuclei project to the rubrothalamic tracts and contralateral motor cortex. Similarly, the deep nuclei also project to the vestibular nuclei, the reticular formation, and the spinal cord to provide sense of balance homeostasis.

Diencephalon

The diencephalon consists of the thalamus, hypothalamus, epithalamus, subthalamus, and geniculate bodies (Fig. 7.3). The thalamus is present in each half of the brain and is a large oval-shaped structure that is not symmetric. The posterior end is larger and bulbous and known as the pulvinar. From the larger posterior end, the thalamus tapers as it moves anteriorly to somewhat of a point. Posteriorly and inferiorly are the geniculate nuclei (GN) that sit in a satellite fashion medially and laterally. The thalamus is a large cluster of nuclei named based on the corresponding position within the structure but can also be grouped based upon function. The most anterior structure is aptly named the anterior nuclei (AN). This nucleus spans both the dorsal and ventral aspects of the thalamus. However, the thalamus is then further divided into dorsal and ventral groups until the pulvinar.

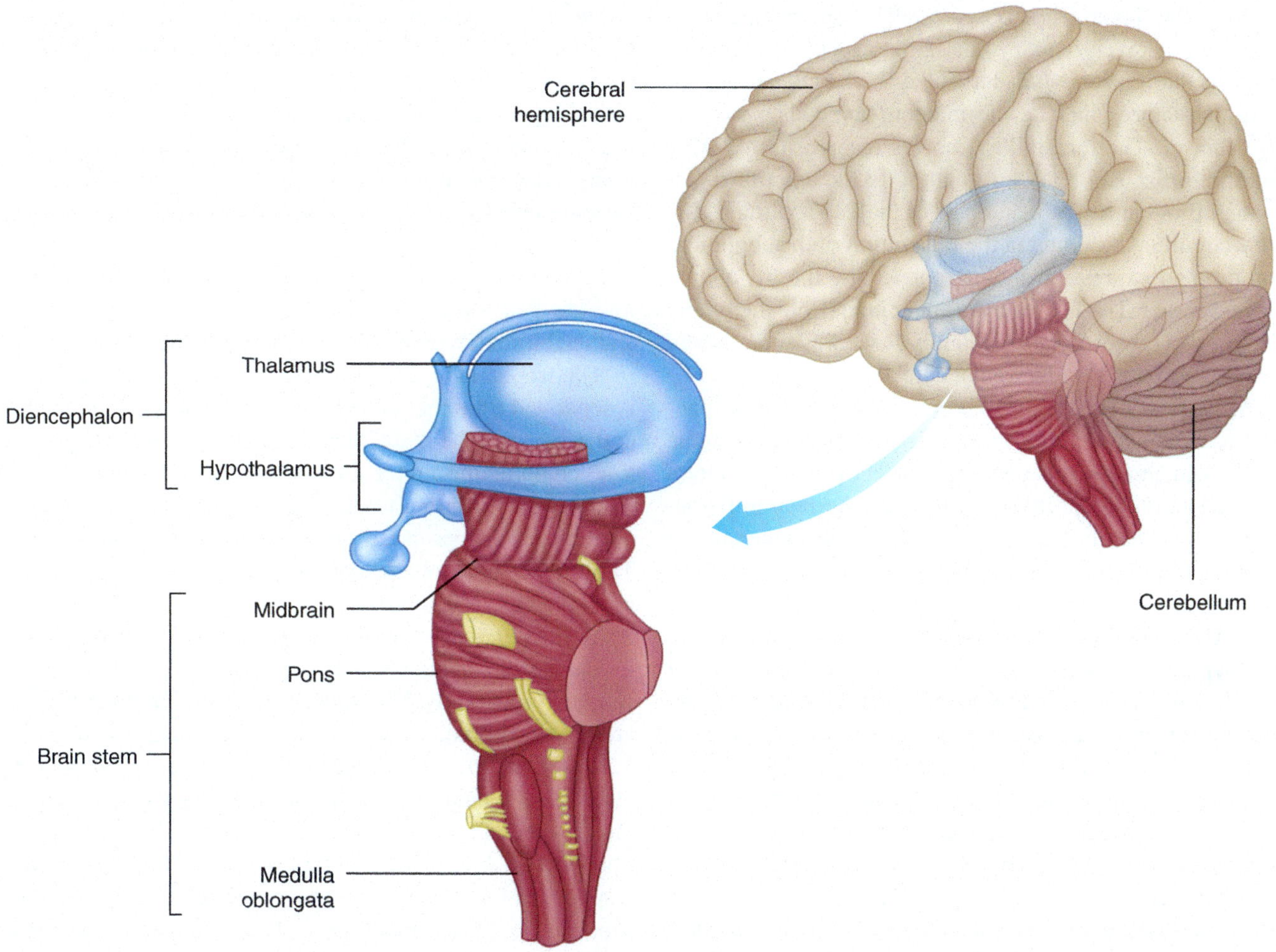

Fig. 7.3 Anatomy of the diencephalon. The diencephalon consists of the thalamus, hypothalamus, epithalamus, subthalamus, and geniculate bodies

Ventrally, there exists the ventral anterior nucleus (VAN), the ventrolateral nucleus (VLN), and the ventral posterior nucleus (VPN). The VPN can further be divided into the ventral intermediate (VIN), the ventroposteriomedial nucleus (VPMN), and ventroposteriolateral nucleus (VPLN). Medial to the VPN exists the arcuate nucleus. Dorsally, there are two nuclei, specifically the lateral dorsal nucleus (LDN) and the medial nucleus (that also ranges dorsal to ventral). The posterior aspect of the lateral dorsal nucleus is the lateral posterior nucleus (LPN). The median nuclei (MN) are midline and associated with the third ventricle and interthalamic adhesion. The medial nuclei (MLN) are medial to the internal medullary lamina. Posteriorly, the pulvinar nucleus (PN) is positioned and spans the dorsal to ventral dimension of the thalamus with the exception of the lateral and medical geniculate nuclei (LGN, MGL) present on its lateral and medial undersurface, respectively. Groups of medial and lateral nuclei are separated by an internal lamina providing obvious demarcation, whereby the internal medullary lamina bifurcates anteriorly into the external medullary lamina.

The thalamus can be divided into five functional subtypes – sensory, motor, limbic, multimodal, and intralaminar groups. The intralaminar nuclei include the intralaminar and reticular nuclei and are not well understood. The multimodal nuclei include the PN, LDN, and LPN and have significant communication with the parietal lobe of the cerebrum whereby sensory and sensory association areas exist. The functional sensory nuclei are best known as the VPL and VPM nuclei as well as the GNs. These are critical target sites for the ascending sensory pathways from the head and body as well as taste and hearing. Functional sensory nuclei are relay point to the primary sensory cortex for ascending pain signals to be further discriminated. The limbic nuclei are the AN and dorsal MLN. These receive input from the olfactory cortex and amygdala. This connection suggests its function in the affective responses to sensation with integration of the prefrontal cortex and hypothalamus.

The hypothalamus (HT) is positioned anterior and inferiorly from the thalamus. It is composed of several nuclei to include the paraventricular, supraoptic, and preoptic nuclei as well as the ventromedial, dorsomedial, and arcuate nuclei. Nearby structures include the mammillary bodies and the optic chiasm. The mammillary bodies receive strong input from the fornix and relay information to the anterior thalamus and provide a significant part of the Papez circuit. The Papez circuit is important in the integration of the cognition, emotion, and expression by interconnecting the hypothalamus and cortex. The HT receives major input from the limbic system, the cortex, and the thalamus as well as somatic and visceral afferents from the spinal cord.

The purpose of the HT is to promote autoregulatory functions such as eating, temperature, water balance, circadian rhythm, and emotional expression. The HT provides efferent communication to the thalamus through the mammillothalamic tract (as part of Papez circuit) and to the tegmentum of the brain stem via the mammillotegmental tract. A significant amount of emission from the HT affects the pituitary gland. The adenohypophysis (anterior pituitary, AP) and the neurohypophysis (posterior pituitary, PP) receive hormones and direct axonal input, respectively. The AP receives input from the HT through hormonal secretion to the blood in the portal hypophyseal system. These are releasing or inhibitory hormones. In contrast, the PP receives direct fibers from the supraoptic and paraventricular neurons (magnocellular neurons) that in turn release oxytocin and vasopressin into the general circulation.

The subthalamus is inferior to the thalamus and borders the tegmentum of the MB. The subthalamic nuclei are an elongated structure that approximates the substantia nigra and the internal capsule. The subthalamus receives input from the basal ganglia, specifically from the globus pallidus, and reciprocates. The start of the efferent pathway from the striatum (caudate and putamen) begins with this interconnection. The basal ganglia are a major component for the control of movement.

The epithalamus is composed of the pineal gland, habenular trigones, and the habenular commissure that joins them. The habenular trigones flank the third ventricle and contain the habenular nuclei. The pineal gland lays interposed between the superior colliculi. The global function of these structures is not well understood.

Cerebrum

The cerebrum (telencephalon) is composed of two cerebral hemispheres, each of which contains six lobes (frontal, parietal, occipital, temporal, insular, and limbic) and is separated by a deep median longitudinal cerebral fissure. Underlying the cortex is the cerebral white matter and the gray matter structures known as the basal ganglia. The cerebrum is composed of convolutions (gyri) separated by depressions called sulci or fissures depending on depth. The lateral cerebral fissure divides the temporal lobe from the frontal and parietal lobes. The circular sulcus divides the insular cortex from surrounding structures. The central sulcus separates the frontal lobe anteriorly from the parietal lobe posteriorly. The parieto-occipital fissure traverses the medial surface of the posterior hemisphere and separates the parietal lobe from the occipital lobe. The corpus callosum is the large, white commissure that runs longitudinally along the cerebral fissure and enables intercommunication between the hemispheres.

The frontal lobe (FL) is anterior to the central sulcus and is separated from the posterior parietal lobe (PL) and the lateral temporal lobe at the lateral cerebral fissure. The frontal lobe contains the motor cortex but also is responsible for judgment, motivation/initiative, reasoning and creativity, and inhibition of inappropriate behavior (prefrontal cortex, PFC). The PFC is in close association with the limbic system and the thalamus. Together with the association cortex, the PFC turns thought process into motivation and coordinated action.

The FL is composed of the superior, middle, and inferior frontal gyri laterally. The inferior gyrus is composed of three areas, the orbital, triangular, and the opercular portions. Medially, the PL is composed of the cingulate gyrus and the paracentral lobule. The FL houses the primary motor cortex most commonly known as Area 4 of Brodmann's classification system. Area 4 is located in the precentral gyrus and is responsible for voluntary muscle movement and largely contributes the corticospinal tract. The homunculus has been widely used to demonstrate the distribution of motor control in the body based on location along Area 4 (Fig. 7.4). In addition, Area 44 and 45 are very important in the control of speech. Known as Broca's area, disease of this area may lead to Broca's aphasia whereby the patient is unable to vocalize in spite of knowing what to say.

The parietal lobe (PL) is located between the lateral cerebral fissures laterally and is posterior to the central sulcus but anterior to the parieto-occipital sulcus. Several gyri are found within the PL to include the postcentral, supramarginal, angular, cingulate, and precuneus gyri. The PL is predominantly somatosensory located in Areas 3, 1, and 2 of the lobe. The predominant input to this sensory cortex is the thalamus, specifically the VPM and VPL areas. Classically, the sensory cortex is often represented by the homunculus (Fig. 7.4). Medially and deep within the lobe, the sensory cortex represents the foot. Moving more superficial and from medial to lateral, the cortex represents the proximal extremities to the hand and then the face, lips, and tongue until the lateral sulcus delineates the lateral most border of the cortex.

Posterior to the parieto-occipital cortex lays the occipital lobe. This lobe is composed of two general areas, the primary visual cortex (Area 17) and the visual association

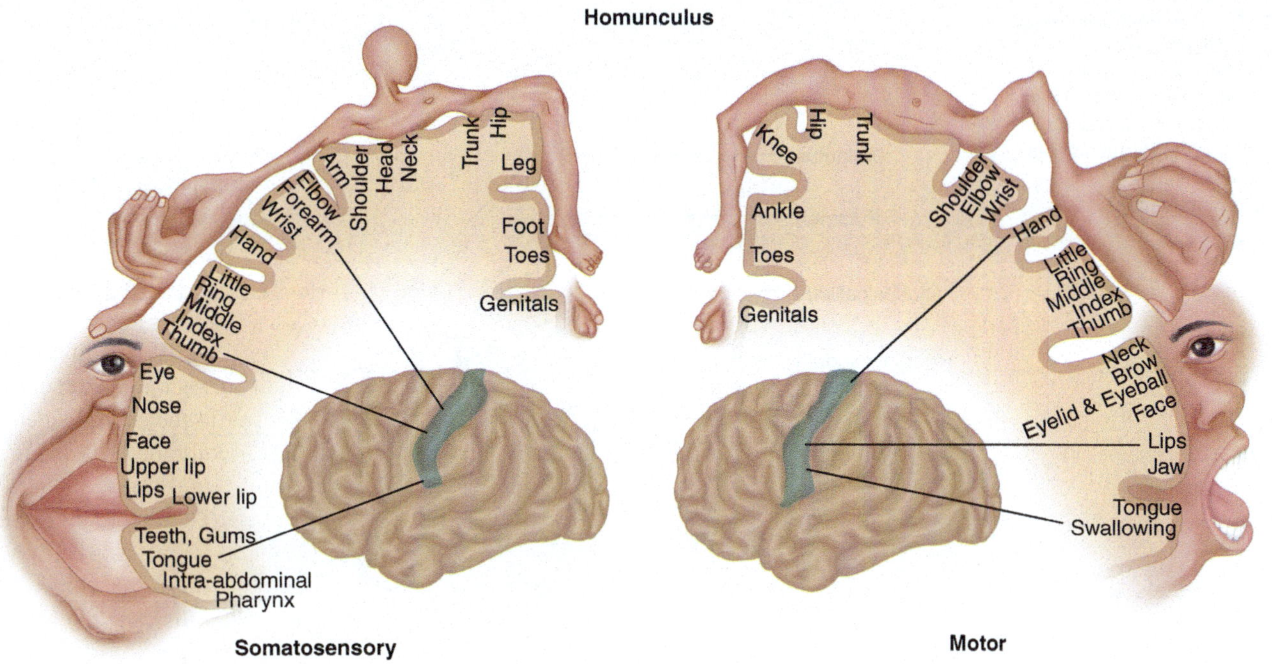

Fig. 7.4 The homunculus. Relative sensory and motor representations within the cortex

cortex (Area 18 and 19). The calcarine fissure lies underneath the lobe and divides it into the cuneus and lingual gyrus. Visual stimulus is relayed to Area 17 where the upper retina is represented by the upper visual cortex. Areas 18 and 19 are associated with the visual association areas and are responsible for visual details such as shape or color.

The temporal lobe (TL) is located on the lateral aspect of each cerebral hemisphere below the level of the lateral cerebral fissure. The lateral temporal lobe has three major areas and is composed of superior, middle, and inferior gyri. Other gyri of note are the transverse temporal, fusiform, and parahippocampal gyrus. Lastly, the uncus is the large, curved structure at the most anterior and medial aspect of the lobe. The TL contains the primary and associative auditory cortex, Areas 41 and 41, respectively. Nearby is the planum temporale that is involved with language and music. Area 22, anterior to the associative auditory cortex in the superior gyrus, is Wernicke's area. This is responsible for language comprehension. The limbic system is the cortical areas that make up the cingulate, parahippocampal, and subcallosal gyri and the hippocampal formation. This area is associated with some of the most primitive functions such as the fight or flight mechanism as well as aggression, feeding behaviors, and sexual behaviors. More detail on this area will be discussed below.

Within the cerebrum are several association areas. Each sensory system consists of a primary and secondary, modality-specific association areas. These multimodal association areas receive input from a variety of areas in the cortex to encode for the attributes of a stimulus. For instance, association areas can take the sound of a sizzling hamburger and associate the visualization of a hamburger, its taste, and the feeling of holding it.

Movement and the Basal Ganglia

The control of movement is a complex integration of several structures of the CNS and begins in the motor component of the sensorimotor cortex near the central sulcus. The primary and premotor cortices (areas 4 and 6) both provide the majority of the input, but the primary sensory cortex from the parietal lobe also provides strong input (areas 3, 1, 2). Additionally, Betz cells of layer V in area 4 contribute to the descending tracts. The additional components of the motor system include the various tracts (corticobulbar, corticospinal, corticopontine, rubrospinal, reticulospinal and vestibulospinal, and tectospinal), the cerebellum, and the basal ganglia (Fig. 7.5).

The corticospinal tract arises primarily from the precentral motor cortices and descends through the posterior aspect of the internal capsule and into the medullary pyramid. Most of these upper motor neuron descending fibers enter the pyramid and then decussate to the contralateral side where they continue toward their lower motor neuron targets in the spinal cord via the lateral corticospinal tract. The corticobulbar tract descends from the sensorimotor cortex that is responsible for the face and targets brachial and efferent nuclei of the brain stem.

The extrapyramidal system (EPS) is composed of several structures important for essential motor controls. The basal ganglia (BG) are areas of gray matter in the deeper layers of

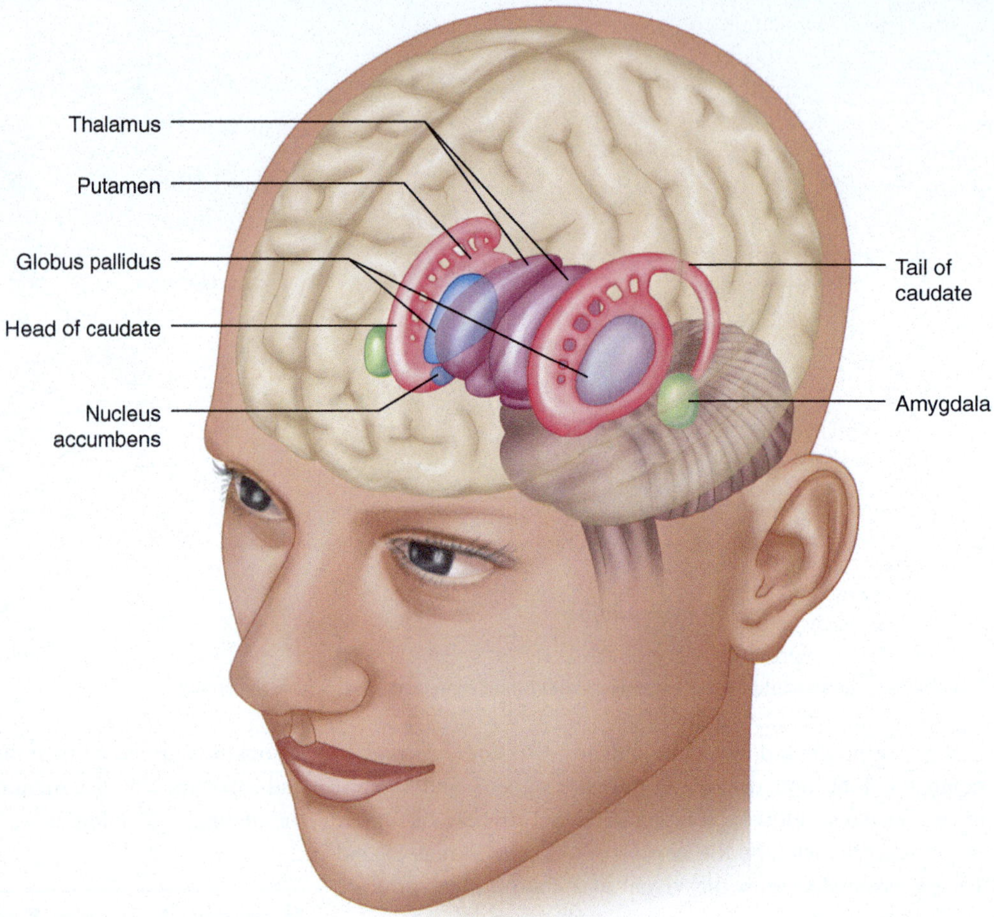

Fig. 7.5 The basal ganglia. The basal ganglion is composed of the caudate nucleus, putamen, and globus pallidus. The basal ganglion receives a significant amount of input from the sensorimotor cortex

the cerebral hemispheres. The BG is composed of the caudate nucleus, the putamen, and the globus pallidus (collectively, "corpus striatum"). The lenticular nuclei are the putamen and globus pallidus in reference to their lens-like shape. The internal capsule is the area of the brain that separates the lenticular nuclei from the caudate and thalamus. It contains an anterior and posterior component or limb. The anterior limb is contains tracts between the thalamus and the cortex. The posterior limb contains the corticospinal and corticobulbar tracts as well as the ascending and descending pathways with the most posterior as containing third-order sensory neurons from the thalamus to the sensory cortex.

The caudate and putamen are the primary input structures of the basal ganglia. These areas receive a significant amount of excitatory input from the sensorimotor cortex through the corticostriate projections. Other structures send input to these structures to include some structures of the limbic system as well as the substantia nigra (SN). Inhibitory input is sent to the inner globus pallidus, which then sends inhibitory signals to the thalamus (ventral nuclei), the substantia nigra (striatonigral pathway), and the cerebellum. The substantia nigra sends input back to the striatum where they both modulate movement using both excitatory and inhibitory synapses on dopamine cells. Disease of the substantia nigra is a major etiology of Parkinson's disease. The SN and the globus pallidus send inhibitory input to the ventral thalamus and to the sensorimotor cortex as well as to the limbic system. Some input from the striatum to the substantia nigra is relayed past the BG to modulate head and eye movements.

The subthalamus is also a target of the globus pallidus in a feedback loop. The cortex sends information to the globus that in turn is relayed to the subthalamic nuclei and back again. The subthalamus together with the red nucleus, cerebellum, and motor cortex acts as a convergent center that relays information to the spinal cord to modulate musculoskeletal muscle tone.

The overarching theme is that the BG provides complex feedback loops that affect motor control. Damage to negative feedback loops within the basal ganglia can lead to disease states that are characterized by repetitive, uncontrolled movements. These diseases include tremors and hemiballismus.

Subcortical pathways are important for movement that results from unconscious control. The muscles of the limbs and trunk are under the control of the reticulospinal, vestibulospinal, and tectospinal tracts. As previously mentioned, the rubrospinal tract arises from the red nucleus and provides tone to skeletal muscles. Sensorimotor information that is from the cortex is relayed to the reticular formation (reticular activating system) and emits information through the reticulospinal tract. The reticular formation is responsible for the state of arousal and consciousness in a nonspecific, generalized fashion. In addition to ascending projections from the brain stem to the cortex, the reticular formation sends descending signals via this tract to modulate spinal reflex activity, sensory input, and autonomic activity.

Input from the cerebellum and vestibular nerve synapses on the vestibular nucleus in the floor of the fourth ventricle. Information is relayed to the vestibulospinal tract from this nucleus to the spinal cord to modulate reflex loops associated with alpha and gamma motor neurons. Influence of these reflex loops allows for the maintenance of upright posture and opposition to gravity.

The tectospinal tract emanates from the superior colliculus. This tract descends within the MO and anterior spinal cord to affect control of reflexes of the upper trunk, neck, and eyes in response to visual stimuli.

Limbic System

The limbic system is one of the most fundamental aspects of the central nervous system. The limbic system is responsible for basic survival mechanisms of life as well as the expression of emotion. Functions of the limbic system include visceral output like sexual drive, rage, fear, aggression, eating behavior, and control of visceral emotional responses (e.g., piloerection, pupillary changes, etc.). The limbic system is composed of the limbic lobe, the amygdala, and the hippocampal formation. The limbic lobe exists superficial to the corpus callosum. The limbic lobe is composed of the parahippocampal, cingulate, and subcallosal gyri. The hippocampal formation (HF) is a group of structures closely associated with the thalamic region. This formation is composed of the hippocampus, the dentate gyrus, the supracallosal gyrus, the fornix, and the septal area (Fig. 7.6).

The olfactory system is very closely related to the limbic system and provides a significant amount of input. Receptors in the mucous membranes transmit signals to the olfactory bulb by way of the olfactory nerves. The olfactory bulb neurons project posteriorly by way of the medial and lateral olfactory striae. The lateral striae project to the olfactory area of the cortex that is composed of the amygdala, pyriform, and entorhinal cortices. The pyriform cortex projects to the frontal lobe where sensory discrimination occurs. The medial striae project to the limbic lobe, specifically subcallosal gyrus. Some projections reach the anterior olfactory nucleus that reciprocates input back to the olfactory bulb and is associated with smell sensation. Others project to the anterior perforated substance and extend the optic tract and mediate a reflex mechanism of the sense of smell and the eyes.

The HF is located deep within the parahippocampal gyrus. As described above, the HF is composed of five structures. The dentate gyrus is located on the upper portion of the parahippocampal gyrus. This area is a major receiving area of the HF from many other cortices by way of the entorhinal

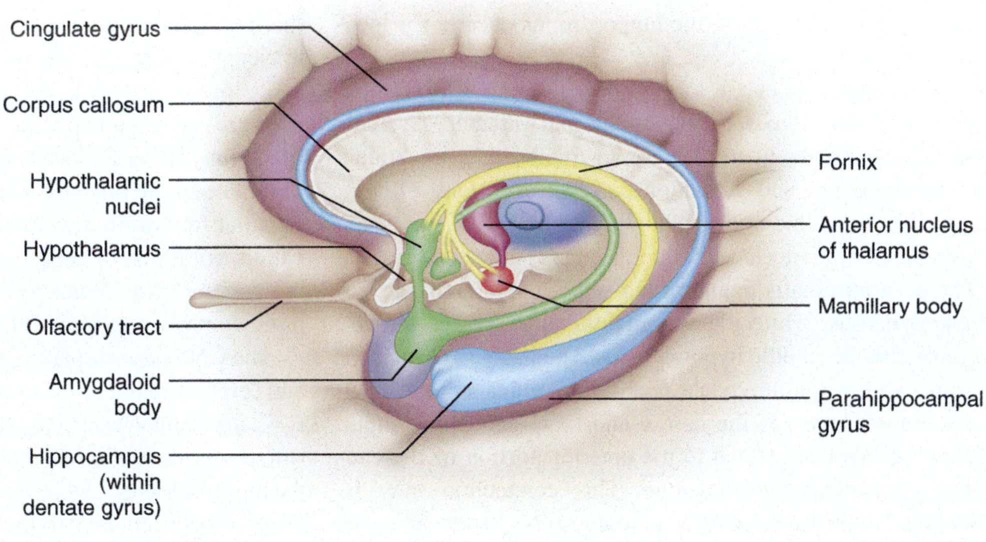

Fig. 7.6 The hippocampal formation (HF) is a group of structures closely associated with the thalamic region. This formation is composed of the hippocampus, the dentate gyrus, the supracallosal gyrus, the fornix, and the septal area

cortex, a component of the olfactory system. The dentate gyrus is known to undergo neurogenesis beyond youth. The hippocampus is a curved structure that lays beneath the floor of the fourth ventricle and is covered by the parahippocampal gyrus. It is known to have three sections, CA1, CA2, and CA3. Axons from the perforant and alvear pathways emanate from the entorhinal cortex to reach the dentate gyrus and hippocampus. Mossy fiber cells of the dentate gyrus project to cells within CA3 where some cells project posteriorly, while others project to CA1.

The hippocampus continues posteriorly to become the fornix. The fornix is the major efferent tract from the hippocampus. It extends to the thalamic region as well as the septum. The fornix begins as the alveus, forms the fimbria of the fornix, and loops around the thalamus to form the crus of the fornix. The crus is connected on each side by the hippocampal commissure. Efferent fibers within the fornix target the mammillary bodies, the septal area, or the anterior thalamus. The Papez circuit is formed by input that begins in the parahippocampal gyrus and projects through the hippocampus and fornix to the anterior thalamus by way of the mammillothalamic tract. The anterior thalamus projects to the cingulate gyrus and back to the parahippocampal gyrus. This forms a feedback loop that is extremely important for the cognition and the experience and expression of emotion. Other cortical areas project to the Papez circuit to include the supracallosal and subcallosal gyri, aptly named due to their close proximity to the corpus callosum.

The hippocampus is widely known to be responsible for learning and memory. Damage to this structure is known to cause anterograde amnesia. Together with the thalamus and temporal lobes, among other structures, the hippocampus allows for the conversion of information from short-term to long-term memory. Furthermore, the hippocampus is known to contain cells that provide memory for spatial arrangement and navigation. Similarly, specialized cells from the entorhinal cortex that project to the hippocampus encode for location information.

The septal nuclei are located near the anterior commissure, and other areas of the limbic and olfactory systems heavily innervate them. The septal nuclei are the brain's pleasure center, and activation can lead to strong efferent stimulation of the diencephalon and MB. Similarly, the amygdala is connected to, among others, the septal nuclei. The stria terminalis connects the septal nuclei and anterior hypothalamus, while the amygdalofugal pathways directly connect to the middle hypothalamus. The basolateral nuclear group within the amygdala receives significant input from association areas of the cortex and reciprocates the input. They are also connected to the anterior portion of the caudate, putamen, and thalamus. This connection may be involved with associating a stimulus type to the affective response. The corticomedial nuclear group receives strong input from the olfactory system and relays responses to the diencephalon and brain stem. The amygdala may be responsible for control of, among others, sexual behavior and oral intake.

The autonomic nervous system (ANS) is composed of the sympathetic and parasympathetic nerve system. The ANS is completely under unconscious control implicating the reason for its name. Full review of the ANS is beyond the scope of this chapter, but some important points should be made. The sympathetic nervous system (SNS) arises from the thoracic and lumbar (when present) areas of the spinal cord as projections from cells that contain cell bodies within the intermediolateral cell columns. It also includes the adrenal medulla. The parasympathetic nervous system (PNS) is composed of cells that arise from cranial and sacral regions of the nervous system. The cranial fibers specifically arise from the brain stem at the Edinger-Westphal nucleus, the medial aspect of the oculomotor nucleus, and the superior and inferior salivatory nuclei. The sacral fibers emanate from the S2, S3, and S4 levels and synapse on target cells in the viscera plexus of Meissner and plexus of Auerbach. In the head, there are four ganglia that contain fibers of the SNS, PNS, and somatic fibers emanating from the trigeminal nerve. These are the ciliary, pterygopalatine, otic, and submaxillary ganglia of which only the PNS synapses on the cells of the ganglion.

Visceral pain signals ascend through either the SNS or PNS and are dependent on the organ. The vagus nerve carries pain impulses from the esophagus, larynx, and trachea, while the SNS carries pain afferents from the organs of the chest cavity and abdomen, specifically the heart, upper digestive system, kidneys, bladder, and gall bladder. Pelvic pain is generally associated with sacral fibers of S2, S3, and S4. This includes the rectum, prostate, urethra, cervix, and vagina. It should be noted that the bladder is dually innervated by both the SNS (upper) and PNS (lower). Similarly, the lung pleura receive dual innervation from somatic fibers (parietal pleura) and SNS fibers (visceral pleura). Non-nociceptive input to the brain stem occurs from the vagus and glossopharyngeal nerves, relaying information such a pressure or chemospecific input to modulate autonomic functions. These fibers are found in the tractus proprius and terminate in the nucleus tractus solitarius. Together with the reticular formation, involuntary reflex arcs exist such as salivation, vomiting, or gagging. The pons also contains input to the pneumotaxic center to control respiration, and the midbrain controls pupillary reflex.

The CNS has extensive systems whereby the flow of blood and cerebral spinal fluid is managed. Deep to the cerebrum are two large lateral ventricles (LVs). The LVs contain the anterior, posterior, and inferior horns. These LVs are connected to the third ventricle (TV) by interventricular foramen of Monroe. Wedged between the two thalamic regions, the TV is in very close proximity to the optic recess and hypothalamus.

The cerebral aqueduct connects the TV to the fourth ventricle (FV). The FV extends between the pons and medulla and dorsally at the cerebellum. CSF from the cerebellum communicates with the FV laterally (foramen of Luschka) and medially (foramen of Magendie). The choroid plexus is found throughout the LV, TV, and FV as specialized extensions of the pia mater. The pia mater is one of three coverings of the CNS and is most adhered to the brain. The arachnoid mater forms the next most superficial layer and creates a fluid-filled space above the pia mater to allow free flow of CSF. The dura mater is the most superficial covering and envelops the brain and spinal cord, the deeper meninges, and vascular supply. The dura mater lays just deep to the skull, and it also creates various septa that provide natural separations of the cerebrum and cerebellum. These layers are important in creating the blood-brain and blood-CSF barriers.

The vascular supply to the brain is extensive. Arterial supply to the brain and brain stem arises from two sources, the internal carotid arteries (ICAs) and the vertebral arteries (VAs). The ICAs arise from the common carotid arteries, and the VAs extend from the subclavian arteries. The circle of Willis (CoW) is a misshaped halo of arteries that are created by the ICAs and VAs whereby the ICAs communicate anteriorly (anterior communicating artery [ACA]) and the VAs posteriorly through the posterior cerebral artery (PA) and associated posterior communicating arteries (PCA). After entering the cranial vault, the ICA forms the carotid siphon and then provides supply to the ophthalmic artery and anterior choroidal artery. The ACA connects both ICAs and thus both hemispheres. The VAs enter the skull base and converge to become the basilar artery (BA). The BA diverges to become two posterior cerebral arteries. Along the way, the BA provides tributaries in pairs to provide blood supply to the cerebellum, the thalamus, and the brain stem.

Venous drainage from the CNS is less complex. Superior cerebral veins drain to the superior sagittal sinus, while inferior cerebral veins drain to the middle cerebral vein or transverse sinus. Drainage from deeper structures ultimately drains to the great cerebral vein or inferior sagittal sinus that become confluent at the straight sinus. The straight sinus joins the superior sagittal sinus at the confluence of sinuses posteriorly, which then form the transverse sinuses that drain to the internal jugular vein.

The neuroanatomic components of the brain are complex. Both higher processes and more primitive functions require a significant amount of integration. The pain matrix involves many critical areas of the brain and brain stem (Fig. 7.7). Pain processing and the human response are a fundamental example of the interrelationship between cognitive-affective processes, survival mechanisms, and learning and memory.

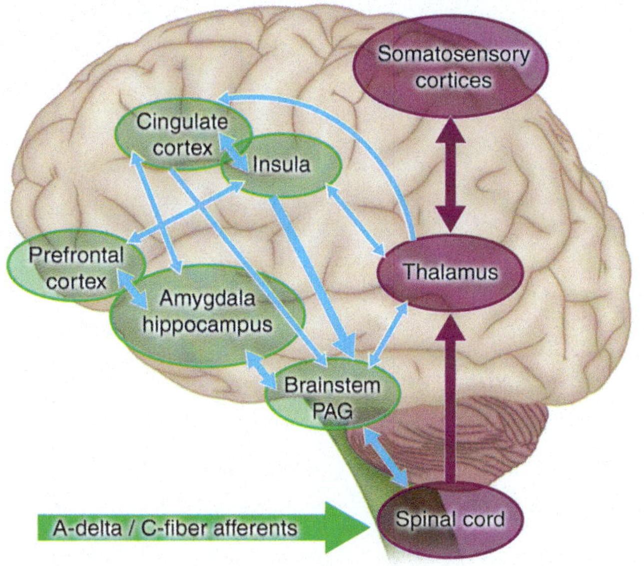

Fig. 7.7 The pain matrix involves many critical areas of the brain and brain stem

Key Points

1. Ascending nociceptive pathways arrive and the sensorimotor cortex through two routes, the pyramidal system and the ventrolateral pathways.
2. The thalamus is a key moderator to the pain response and serves to coordinate many other areas of the brain.
3. The cognitive-affective aspect of the pain experience not only includes the sensory cortex, but also the limbic system. The limbic system is the area responsible for the human behavior toward, and memory of, the experience of painful stimuli.
4. The sensorimotor cortex is somatotopically organized, and some crossover in function exists.
5. Feedback loops exist, and the basal ganglia coordinate the functional response to noxious stimuli.

Recommended Reading

1. Felton D, O'Banion M, Maida M. Netter's atlas of neuroscience. 3rd ed. Philadelphia: Elsevier; 2016. p. 51–460.
2. Haines D. Neuroanatomy in clinical context: an atlas of structures, sections, systems and syndromes. 9th ed. Philadelphia: Lippincott Williams and Wilkins; 2015. p. 189–288.
3. Kandel E, Schwartz J, Jessell J, Siegelbaum S, Hudspeth A. Principles of neural science. 5th ed. New York: The McGraw-Hill Companies; 2013. p. 337–932.
4. Waxman S. Clinical neuroanatomy. 28th ed. New York: The McGraw-Hill Companies; 2017. p. 77–256.

Mediators of Pain and Pain Processing

8

Mark N. Malinowski

Background and Historical Perspective

The mechanisms of pain processing are well researched, but significant anatomic and neurobiological unknowns still exist. The perception of pain by the human body involves complicated interconnections between several different areas of the spinal cord, brainstem, and brain. There are well-defined pathways that assimilate and disseminate noxious input, while other more elusive pathways exist that integrate the body's response to tissue damage and determination of the longevity of the pain experience.

Primary Processing of Pain

Ascending Pain Pathways

Nociception, or the perception of pain, occurs through sensory input from the vast neuronal network known as the somatosensory nervous system (SSNS). The SSNS is not just responsible for nociception as it also senses pressure, light touch, tactile discrimination (e.g., course or smooth), vibration, and body position. The SSNS also codes for graphesthesia, stereognosis, and two-point discrimination. The anatomy of the SSNS is often discussed in terms of first-, second-, and third-order neurons that are responsible for the reception of, integration of, and the coordinated response to the painful stimulus, respectively.

First-order neurons are peripheral pseudo-unipolar neurons that detect pain through specialized nociceptors. A nociceptor is a receptor on a free nerve ending associated with the peripheral branch of the first-order neuron. Pseudo-unipolar neurons have cell bodies in the dorsal root ganglion (DRG) and have only one axon that bifurcates into a peripheral branch that ends in a sensory receptor and a central branch that leaves the DRG and communicates with the spinal cord. The DRG is a structure that is formed by a large cluster of peripheral neuron cell bodies and other cells and neuromatrix (see Fig. 8.1). The DRG is located just distal to the spinal nerve and rootlets and is located just outside of the neuroforamen in most levels.

M. N. Malinowski (✉)
Adena Spine Center, Chillicothe, OH, USA

Receptor Activation

Reception of the nociceptive stimulus involves transduction of the stimulus in the periphery from the initial form of noxious stimulus to a neuronal signal that is transmitted rostrally. This is accomplished through a variety of receptors in the ending of first-order neuron. Membrane proteins such as the transient receptor potential (TRP) family of ion channels are a well-characterized group of specialized nociceptors (Fig. 8.2). TRP receptors respond to noxious, chemical or thermal stimuli, or to changes in pH. The TRP-1 receptor is one that has been identified to be sensitive to capsaicin, to thermal changes as well as pH changes associated with tissue damage. TRP-2 is activated by extreme temperature elevations, and TRP-8 is known to respond to cold stimuli. Other ion channel receptors include SCN9A, a receptor classified as tetrodotoxin-resistant Na2+ channels. Genetic deletion of this receptor is found in those patients who are completely unable to sense pain. Some receptors are known to have purinergic ionotropic binding sites (e.g., adenosine/ATP) that are coupled to Mas-related receptor family that sensitize receptors after tissue damage.

First-Order Neurons

Nociceptive first-order neurons (FONs) (aka peripheral nociceptive afferents, PNA) can be divided into two classes: A-delta ("fast") and C fibers ("slow"). "Fast" pain and "slow" pain is often temporally referred to as the "first wave" and "second wave" of a painful event, respectively. For example, a hammer to thumb event may initially be conveyed as a sharp signal (first wave), but delayed sensations (second wave) may be perceived as a throbbing sensation. A-delta type I neurons respond to fast pain that is well defined and

T. R. Deer et al. (eds.), *Deer's Treatment of Pain*, https://doi.org/10.1007/978-3-030-12281-2_8

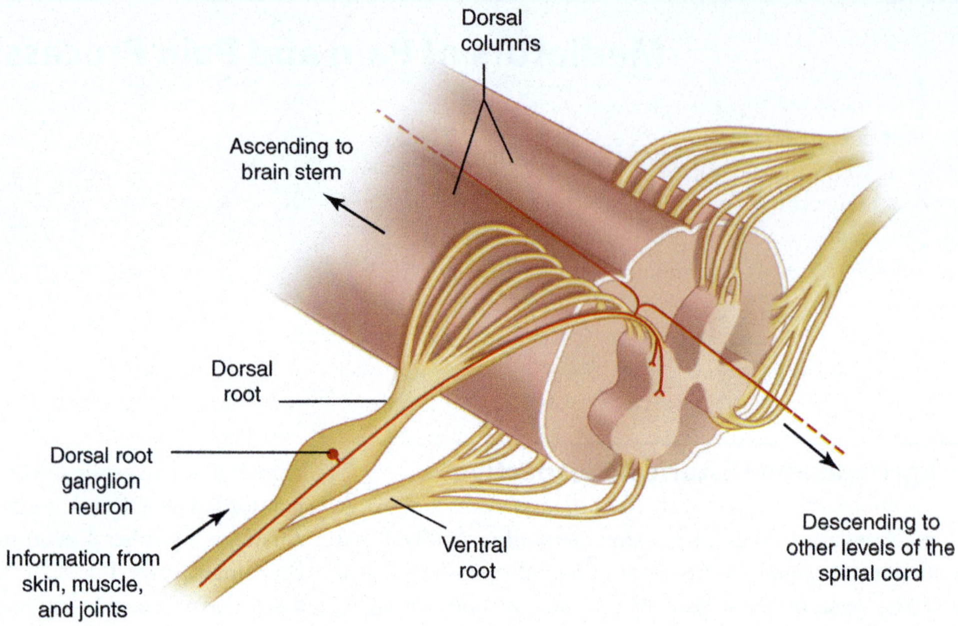

Fig. 8.1 The dorsal root ganglion. The dorsal root ganglion is the collection is unipolar neuron cell bodies. The dorsal root ganglion is responsible for the synthesis of the neuromatrix and associated species responsible for proper function of the neuron

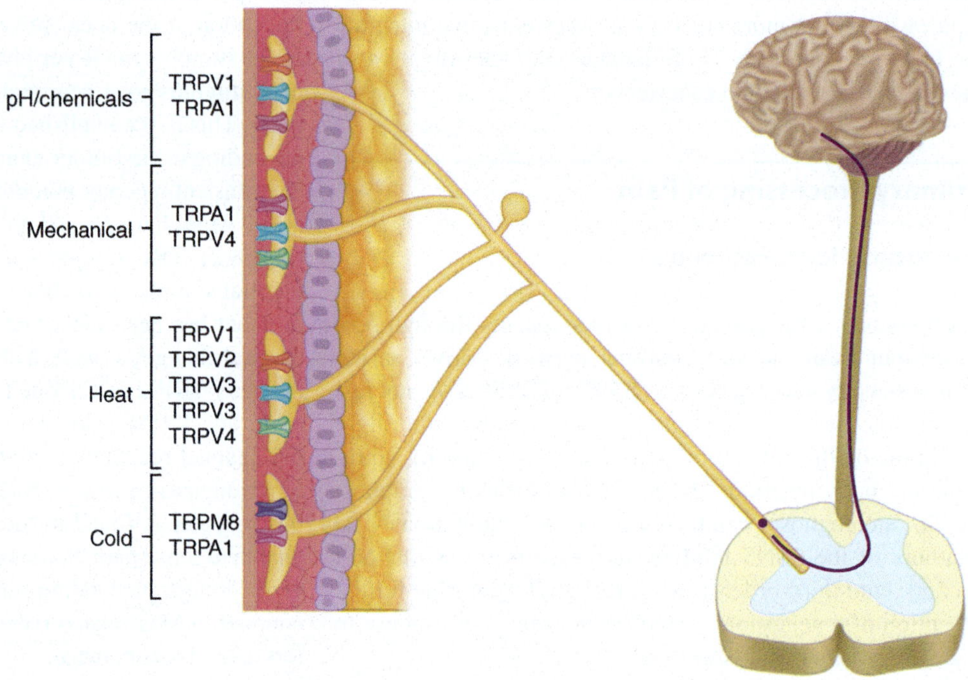

Fig. 8.2 Peripheral nociceptors of the TRPA and TRPV families. There are multiple receptor subtypes associated with one type of stimulus, and signal transduction is relayed to an action potential in the unipolar neuron to the dorsal horn

localized. A-delta-1 neurons are responsive to heat after prolonged or repetitive exposure, but they are initially poor responders to temperature. Initial response to heat is received by type 2 A-delta neurons.

On the contrary, C fibers are neurons that transmit "slow pain" that is not well localized usually as a result of tissue injury. Slow pain can be characterized as a diffuse burning or throbbing sensation. C fibers are responsive to chemical, thermal, and mechanical stimuli although they can have subspecialized roles by containing more than one receptor type. High-threshold receptor C fibers respond to noxious thermal and/or mechanical stimuli (e.g., "polymodal"). Visceral and deeper somatic FONs are exceptional as they can be associated with autonomic activation and associated negative effects.

A-beta fibers are a third type of FON that merits special mention. Under normal conditions they are responsible for mechanical sensation that is not painful. However, A-beta fibers may be responsible for mechanical allodynia under pathological conditions associated with injury.

Upon activation, FONs transmit the signal to the gray matter of the spinal cord. The area of the spinal cord segment is known as the dorsal horn (DH), whereas the corresponding locations ventrally are referred to the ventral horn (VH). FONs associated with touch, vibration, or limb position synapse in the dorsal columns (DCs) of the spinal cord at specific areas. The gracilis funiculus is the area of the DC that received sensory input from the mid thoracic and caudal body regions, whereas the cuneate funiculus is the target input from the mid thoracic and cephalad structures. These FONs branch into the DH as they unilaterally ascend for the purpose of reflex pain feedback mechanisms.

The rexed lamina (RL) are anatomical layers within the gray matter of the spinal cord, and each layer appears to contain a variety of target cells. Similarly, it is important to understand that each lamina is not exclusive to one cell type as intercommunication between layers occurs. Generally, lamina I receives input from predominantly A-delta and some C fibers in response to noxious stimuli, with some of these specializing in intense temperature (C fiber derived) or both noxious and non-noxious mechanical stimuli. Lamina II (substantia gelatinosa) receives mainly C-fiber input with some A-delta fibers, and it contains a mix of inhibitory and excitatory interneurons mediating both painful and non-painful inputs. Lamina II also receives input from A-beta fibers. Lamina III and IV generally do not mediate painful stimulus input but instead receive a significant amount of input from A-beta FONs, although some A-delta fibers are also present. A-beta fiber input with some A-delta and C fibers synapse in Lamina V. Laminae VII and VIII are not well defined. These likely receive innocuous input. Lamina VII appears unique in that it received input from stimulation from either body side and could be associated with bilateral painful conditions. Lamina X receives input from C fibers, A-delta fibers, and unmyelinated visceral FONs. Laminae II, III, and IV are the only layers that contain non-nociceptive inputs. FONs target either silent neurons that behave in a binary capacity (either on or off) or wide-dynamic range (WDR) neurons that demonstrate a broad capability. WDR neurons respond in a graded response rather than a binary response as above. WDR neurons provide FON stimulation the ability to elicit a divergent response but also receive multiple inputs from a heterogeneous source of both noxious and innocuous FONs, but some also contain wide-dynamic range (WDR) interneurons (lamina IV) or both WDR neurons and nociceptive-specific neurons (lamina II). WDR neurons are predominantly found in laminae IV, V, and VI (see below).

Nociceptive FONs release a wide variety of neurotransmitters (NTs) onto targets in the DH. There are several NTs to include glutamate, substance P, calcitonin gene-related peptide (CGRP), adenosine triphosphate (ATP), nitric oxide (NO), and prostaglandins among others. In terms of classification, PNAs are sometimes viewed in terms of the NT they release. However, PNAs may release one or more than one NT, and the relative quantities may vary based on tissue type, characteristics of initial stimulus (i.e., brief vs. prolonged), or the presence of a pathological condition. Lastly, PNAs may also be grouped into subsets based on their sensitivities to known toxins (i.e., capsaicin).

The response within the spinal cord to PNA activation and transmission is dependent not only on the characteristics of stimulus or type of NT but also on the second messenger systems involved. Second messenger systems are known to be G-protein-mediated intracellular responses that lead to a wide variety of outcomes within the target cell. Second messenger systems may be G-protein-specific stimulatory or inhibitory, leading to activation or inhibition of the intracellular second messenger or an associated ion channel. Similarly, receptors may be associated with a variety of tissue-specific second messenger systems. For example, peptidergic C fibers release the excitatory amino acid glutamine as well as other NTs such as tachykinins, substance P (SP), neurokinin A, and CGRP. Neurokinin A and SP may both activate neurokinin receptors and are associated with the second messenger system phospholipase C (PLC). In contrast, CGRP is associated with the second messenger adenylyl cyclase (AC). Glutamate and EAA aspartate activate glutamate receptors that demonstrate a broad post-activation capability (metabotropic glutamate receptors vs. ion channel receptors AMPA and NMDA). These glutamate receptors of the NMDA subclass are found in abundance in the DH. In addition to glutamate, these receptors require glycine to activate the receptor. This receptor is an ion channel for calcium (Ca2+) permeability of the membrane. Similarly, AMPA glutamate receptors predominantly exist on nociceptive neurons through the spinal cord, and they determine the permeability of Ca2+ at their targets. Generally these receptors have less affinity to glutamate, are kinetically quicker, and transmit sodium ion (Na2+) rather than Ca2+ through their channels. Alternatively, metabotropic glutamate receptors have a number of receptor subtypes and are present throughout SSNS pathways. At the dorsal horn, receptor subtypes mGLU1 and mGLU5 predominate in the transmission of nociceptive input through second messenger systems such as PLC and AC. Others subtypes may act on gene transcription or modify K+ channels.

The PNA-DH synapse is known to demonstrate synaptic plasticity. Synaptic plasticity is known as the ability for neurons to demonstrate autoregulation at the synaptic junction. Synaptic plasticity can occur presynaptically or postsynaptically. Presynaptic modulation can result in the facilitation or inhibition of neurotransmitter release from the axon terminal. For example, presynaptic NMDA receptors at junctions that release EAAs and SP may demonstrate further presynaptic release of these NTs. In contrast, some presynaptic mGLU receptor subtypes are thought to suppress their own release through inhibitory second messenger systems. Similarly, both postsynaptic and presynaptic facilitation may occur. For example, in some cells SP not only activates NK-type receptors postsynaptically but also may facilitate its own release through presynaptic mechanisms. Ultimately, the effects of different NTs upon target cells depend on the NT, the type of PNA and support cells (glia, interneurons), the wide variety of receptor types as associated local target cells, and associated second messenger systems involved. However, synaptic transmission within the spinal cord is further complicated by the presence of a vast array of target cells to include interneurons and projection neurons.

Second-Order Neurons

Dorsal horn neurons receiving input from PNAs may fall into three broad classifications: silent neurons, wide-dynamic range (WDR) neurons, and non-nociceptive neurons. These neurons communicate within each segment, among segments, or at supraspinal levels. Projection neurons (PN) are DH neurons that communicate with supraspinal targets and are found predominantly in lamina I, V, and VI. Interneurons (IN) communicate locally and are responsible for local modulation and integration of signals from PNAs. These INs are generous in lamina II, and they may be excitatory or inhibitory, but some IN function in both capacities.

Excitatory interneurons (EIN) in lamina II may indirectly facilitate transmission of PNAs through activation of PN in lamina I when targeted by PNAs. Similarly, EINs targeted by PNAs can also facilitate transmission of PNAs by reflexively stimulating the terminals of PNAs in a feedback loop fashion. EINs from lamina II may influence PNs from deeper lamina V through dendrites from these layers that reach to lamina II. In particular, A-beta fibers project to lamina V as do some C fibers. EIN may play a role of intercommunication between these fibers in some disease states that require A-beta and C fiber facilitation. EAAs involved may include SP, glutamate, and vasoactive intestinal peptide (VIP).

Inhibitory interneurons (IIN) act to suppress the activity of their target cells. These antinociceptive INNs utilize a wide variety of neurotransmitters (NT) that have receptors coupled to ion channels to hyperpolarize a target cell or work by G-protein-coupled second messenger systems in a cascade-like fashion to induce suppression. These receptors (with corresponding neurotransmitters) include predominantly muscarinic cholinergic (acetylcholine), opioidergic (endogenous opiate peptides, enkephalins, dynorphin), and GABAergic (gamma-aminobutyric acid [GABA]). The IIN cohabitate with antinociceptive NTs (e.g., substance P) or pro-nociceptive (e.g., nitrous oxide). This cohabitation of NTs complicates any suggestion that INs are mutually exclusive to one role or another. Lastly, IINs act presynaptically on target PNA or postsynaptically on target PN. In addition, PNA cells also directly target IINs that reciprocate stimulation in an antinociceptive feedback loop.

Other support cells exist in and around the dorsal horn and throughout the CNS. Glial cells and immunocompetent microglia secrete local chemical mediators and play an important role in the modulation of pain signals in the presence of central or peripheral tissue damage.

Glial cells are known to be support cells for local homeostasis within the central nervous system (CNS). Not only do they possess channels for Ca2+, the cell membrane hosts a variety of receptors to NTs that are involved in the transmission of pain. Glial cells receive synaptic transmission (glutamate) promoting the release of chemical mediators (NO, prostaglandins [PGs], adenosine triphosphate [ATP], cytokines) that facilitate nociception in the presence of central or peripheral inflammation. Cytokines appear to have dual roles, however. In some cases (IL-6) cytokines may induce or facilitate allodynia and hyperalgesia, while other cytokines (IL-1beta) may promote inhibition of nociceptive signals in the dorsal horn or inhibit long-term potentiation in central sensitization.

Projection neurons (PN), as opposed to interneurons, by definition leave their segment of origin. These sensory pathways may be organized into monosynaptic pathways (MSP) and polysynaptic pathways (PSP). The former group is composed of PN that synapse directly onto specific central targets. Known MSP include the spinothalamic tract (STT), spinomesencephalic tract (SMT) (spinoparabrachial tract [SPT]), spinohypothalamic tract (SHT), and the spinoreticular tract (SRT). Polysynaptic pathways include the spinocervical pathway (SCP), the postsynaptic dorsal column pathway (PDCP), and second-order neurons that arise from connections in higher centers such as the lateral cervical nuclei (SCP) and the cuneate and gracile nuclei (PDCP) in the medulla. These pathways are predominantly non-nociceptive with some exception.

The main purpose of ascending pathways is to transmit nociceptive information to higher centers in the brain from the skin, musculoskeletal system, and the viscera. A wide range of pathways and NTs exist to accomplish this. It is somewhat helpful to understand ascending pathways by discussing them in the context of regions of the spinal cord rather than as independent pathways. The prevailing concept to understand the organization and function of afferent nociceptive transmission is that it is dynamic and multimodal and is determined by the physiological or pathological circumstances present (Fig. 8.3).

The PSDCP is located in the dorsal midline of the spinal cord. These dorsal columns (dorsal funiculi) predominantly contain fibers that are non-nociceptive (position, vibratory). However, PSDCP may receive input from other known pain

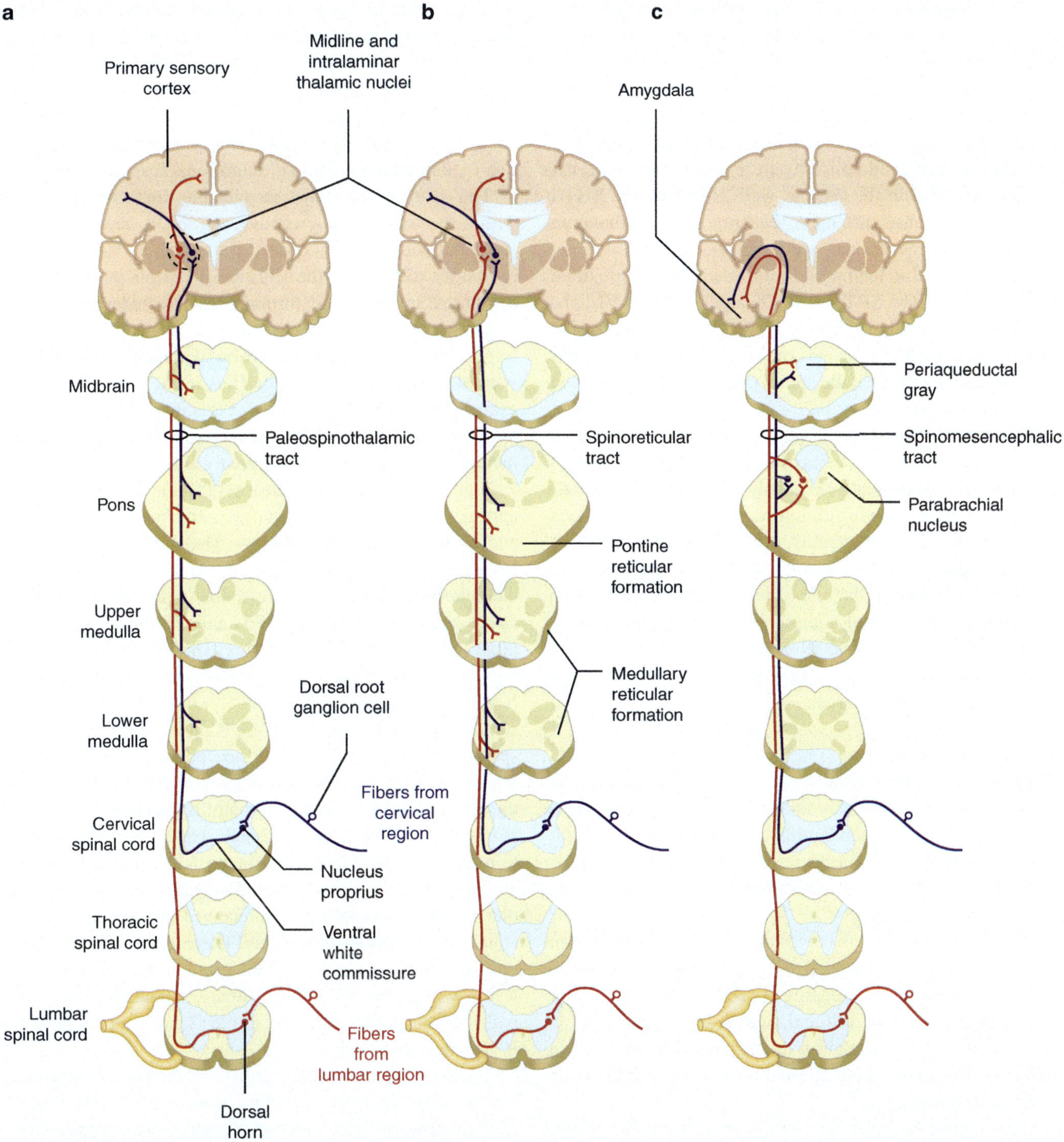

Fig. 8.3 Ascending pathways. While most non-nociceptive information is relayed through the dorsal horns, nociceptive stimuli are relayed to the ventrolateral horn associated with some ascending tracts. Unipolar neurons transmitting nociceptive information synapse with secondary neurons that decussate to the ventrolateral columns. Ascending tracts are polysynaptic. Branches to structures within the brainstem en route to the primary somatosensory cortex provide integration of the response to nociceptive stimuli

pathways such as the spinothalamic, spinomesencephalic/spinoparabrachial, and spinocervical pathways found in the dorsolateral funiculus (DLF). In particular, neurons from lamina I associated with the STT connect to a dorsal spinothalamic tract in addition to its known tract in the ventrolateral funiculus. Therefore, due to the polysynaptic nature of the PSDCP, it may be strongly involved in the pathological state of mechanical allodynia.

The monosynaptic pathways project contralaterally whereby PNAs synapse on PNs that either decussate immediately or at direct adjacent levels to the ventrolateral funiculus. The ventrolateral funiculus (VLF) is organized such that fibers emanating most cephalad are medial whereas fibers originating in the caudal regions are more medial. The STT and SHT ascend predominantly in the VLF, but some PNs are also included in the DLF as well. However, the SHT is unique in the sense that upon reaching the hypothalamus, PNs ascend and decussate once again to contralateral targets in the diencephalon lending it to impose transmission at targets bilaterally. The SRT and SMT largely use the VLF, but the SRT also contributes PNs to the DLF that remain ipsilaterally, while the SMT ascends on the contralateral side. The SPT appears to traverse the spinal cord dorsally in the contralateral DLF as well.

The overall experience of pain is determined by the interaction between the two categories of ascending pathways. The sensory-discriminative pathways are responsible for the identification of a painful stimulus and encoding of the location, intensity, duration, quality, duration, etc. The affective-cognitive pathways are responsible for the psychological aspect of the pain and the role of mood, memory, toleration, and coping with painful stimuli. No single pathway likely predominates, and the overall experience of pain is dependent on the character of signal input to, and integration within, the supraspinal targets.

Third-Order Neurons

The concept of a single pathway for the transmission of pain stimuli to the brain is likely an oversimplification given the known complexity of the lamina and corresponding ipsilateral and contralateral trajectories of their PNs. However, the interrelationship of these tracts appears to begin within the nuclei of the thalamus.

The thalamus serves to communicate to the limbic system and integrates the emotional experience of pain with the sensory-discriminative component. The thalamus is a bilateral structure with the left and right sides appearing to be mirror images. The thalamus is an organized cluster of nuclei that serve to receive, integrate, and relay noxious input to the cortex and limbic system.

The ventroposterolateral (VPL), ventroposterior medial (VPM), and ventroposterior inferior (VPI) nuclei are key nuclei in the receipt and processing of noxious stimuli. The ventral STT preferentially innervates the VPL and VPM nuclei, while the dorsal STT appears to preferentially innervate the VPI nucleus. The VPL and VPM neurons appear to have small receptor field and therefore appear to be predominantly involved in the sensory-discriminative aspect of pain. The posterior thalamus to include the posterior division of the ventromedial nucleus (VMpo), the pulvinar and posterior nucleus also receives input from the dorsal STT, and it is involved with the integration of nociceptive and thermal stimuli. Lastly, the ventral caudal position of the medial thalamus receives dorsal STT input and communicates to the striatum among others and may be involved in the escape mechanism from painful stimuli. The VPI, VMpo, and the ventral caudal medial thalamus may also integrate the attention to, and understanding of, emotional response to pain.

The neurotransmitters responsible for communication within the thalamic nociceptive and WDR neurons are not clear, but some trends conserved the lamina. EAAs play an excitatory role within the VPL and VPM nuclei where their responses are mediated through NMDA and metabotropic glutamate receptors, and their cortical projections appear to be similar. A significant proportion of the thalamus also consists of GABAergic IINs. The IINs in the thalamus subdue excitatory output. Dysfunction of this inhibitory mechanism may lead to unopposed pro-nociception. This may be a core mechanism in chronic pathological pain.

Thalamic projection neurons (TPNs) to higher centers appear to be arranged into sensory-discriminative pathways and affective-cognitive pathways. The somatosensory cortex I/II, inferior and anterior parietal cortex, the insular cortex, the anterior cingulate, and prefrontal cortex all appear to be target sites for TPNs. The VPL and VPM provide a large input to the somatosensory cortex. The VPI provides a large input to the secondary somatosensory cortex. While TPNs from the VPL and VML widely innervate the primary somatosensory cortex, local WDR and central nociceptive-specific neurons within this cortex possess small contralateral receptive fields. Small fields provide the ability to narrow the location and intensity of painful input, and repetitive stimulation of WDR neurons may lead to central sensitization. While some TPNs from the posterior thalamic nucleus also project to the primary somatosensory cortex, the secondary somatosensory cortex received input predominantly from VPI and posterior nucleus. There are studies that show that experience pain is present even in the presence of a lesion within the STT-VPL-primary somatosensory cortex pathway; the acceptance of a single ascending pain pathway is no longer reasonable.

There are other cortical regions involved in the interpretation of pain. While the primary cortex receives very specific encoding information, other areas such as the secondary cortex, inferior parietal cortex, or anterior cingulate gyrus are more specific to the emotional component of the pain. Input to these areas and the associated response are dependent on the thalamic nuclei from which they receive input.

The limbic system is composed of the limbic lobe (the annular area of the cortex), the amygdala, and the hippocampal formation. The limbic system is responsible for primal functions of the brain to include, but limited to, activation of "fight or flight" responses and emotional states. Since the limbic system is composed of several CNS structures, their interrelationship and activation patterns through WDR and nociceptive neuron input determine the complicated emotional/behavioral response to painful stimuli.

The limbic system receives input both directly and indirectly. Indirectly, areas of the cortex that are part of ascending tracts also relay information back to the thalamus and to the limbic system in a reciprocal manner to affect cognition and mood. Direct input to the limbic system occurs both from the PBN and the periaqueductal gray (PAG) as it is relayed via the SMT. The cingulate gyrus of the limbic lobe and the insular cortex receive significant nociceptive input, whereas insula receives input directly from the VPM nucleus and is associated with the autonomic component of pain.

The ascending integration of pain processing consists of several pathways that cannot be considered mutually exclusive. The ventral lateral fasciculus and ventral STT relay information to the VPL area of the thalamus and are integral in the interpretive precision of the painful stimulus (location, intensity, etc.). The emotional experience of the painful stimulus appears to be mediated through the dorsal STT and the PSDCP as ascending nociception reaches the VPI and VMpo and relayed to the cortex and limbic system. Similarly, the PAG, amygdala, and PBN among other areas receive direct input from areas other than the ventral STT and influence or be influenced by the emotional component of pain as seen in clinical scenarios where pain leads to depression or anxiety, and the presence of these mood states worsens clinical symptoms of pain.

Descending Pathways

Descending modulation of nociception is thought to occur in the dorsal horn rexed laminae. Descending influence can lead to facilitation or inhibition of ascending pain pathways. Descending fibers arise from many sites in the supraspinal compartment and project fibers to the dorsal horn. Similarly, both DI and DF fibers may have common sites of origin. As with ascending pathways, DI and DF exert their influence and are dependent not only on the type of neurotransmitter but also milieu of receptor phenotypes and postsynaptic target cell types.

The connectivity of descending pathways is very complex. In general, some pathways may originate from one supraspinal source but traverse different areas of the spinal cord as they descend and may have entirely divergent functions (e.g., DI and DF). Neurons may descend within the spinal cord through the dorsolateral or ventrolateral funiculi. Whether inhibition or facilitation of a pain signal occurs may depend on whether the neuron directly synapses on the terminal of the PNA or mediates its effects through IINs. For example, DI pathways may act directly onto the PNA to release inhibitory NTs onto the terminal itself thereby decreasing synaptic transmission by the PNA onto the PN. Similarly, the DI pathways may release excitatory NTs directly onto an IIN whereby activation of this IIN leads to synaptic depression at the PNA-PN synapse either pre- or postsynaptically. Furthermore, DF may occur in similar mechanisms by either facilitating PNA synaptic transmission by direct presynaptic potentiation or by activation of EINs. During baseline function of the body, the counterbalance between DI and DF prevents the exaggeration of signals received from the periphery. However, under pathological conditions, this balance may be disrupted.

Several supraspinal regions participate in the descending modulation of nociception. These include the hypothalamus, parabrachial nucleus (PBN), nucleus tractus solitarius (NTS), rostroventromedial medulla (RVM), nucleus raphe magnus (NRM), dorsal reticular nucleus of the medulla (DRN), periaqueductal gray (PAG), and the cerebral cortex.

The hypothalamus holds a significant role in the autonomic response to and cognition of pain. Afferent pathways heavily target the hypothalamus. However, it exerts descending indirectly through intermediaries and not directly onto the dorsal horn. These structures include the NTS, PAG, RVM, and the limbic system, and they are integrated with the hypothalamus to coordinate both affective and cognitive aspects to painful stimuli. Similarly, the amalgamation nuclei and "centers" that compose this structure differentiate themselves through distinct targets and NT pathways. For instance, the medial preoptic nucleus of the hypothalamus is closely connected to the PAG and may suppress nociception through autonomic activation, while other parts of the hypothalamus (e.g., lateral hypothalamus) may activate descending noradrenergic pathways affecting the DH cells.

As described above, the PBN is known to play a role of pain cognition and emotion as well, and it functions similar to the hypothalamus in response to predominantly visceral nociceptive input. The PBN is known to mediate its effects by projecting to structures similar to the hypothalamus, and activation of the PBN may lead to suppression of nociception in the superficial layers of the DH.

The PBN shares similarity with the NTS in the mediation of visceral pain. The NTS is responsive to visceral afferents largely through input from the vagus nerve but also via DH fibers. The PBN and NTS are both heavily interlinked with limbic structures, the hypothalamus, and the cortex. The NTS ultimately projects not only to the PAG but also mediates nociception directly in the DH or through other adrenergic and serotonergic nuclei-associated projections in the modulation of nociception.

The RVM houses several nuclei associated with descending modulation of nociception and provides a signal conduit for input from other supraspinal areas. The heterogeneity of this structure lends itself to roles of both DF and DI, and this dual ability is underscored by the diverse structures that provide input to the RVM (e.g., PBN, NTS). The RVM nuclei are a major contributory center to the mediation of pain associated with tissue and nerve injury.

The DRN of the medulla receives both somatic and visceral input. The DRN appears to be involved in the mediation of pain through descending pathways that terminate in the DH. Similarly, the DRN itself is targeted by DH afferents. Communication between targets in the SC and the DRN appears to mediate hyperalgesia, and in response to tissue damage, the DRN is activated to provide a response that leads to antinociceptive analgesia.

The PAG is also strongly associated with the limbic system, hypothalamus, NTS, and PBN in the mediation of pain and emotion (Fig. 8.4). In addition to supraspinal structures, the PAG also receives direct input from the periphery via PNs. The PAG houses receptors for a variety of neurotransmitters, to include opioid agonists and cannabinoids among a variety of others. The PAG appears to be under tonic inhibition from IINs, and resolution of tonic inhibition by, for example, mu-opioid agonists may lead to the facilitation of descending inhibition through at least in part the descending noradrenergic system. Therefore, the PAG serves as what appears to be a central clearinghouse for the integration of multiple signals to include influence by structures that may or may not provide descending input (i.e., amygdala) (See Fig. 8.5).

Lastly, descending modulation of nociception appears to be mediated not just through subcortical structures (i.e., PAG) but also through a lesser-known pathway involving the dorsal column nucleus. Descending pathways exit from the cortex to the dorsal column nucleus and may play a significant role in the facilitation of neuropathic and visceral pain. Similarly, some cortical areas appear to project to the RVM to include the NRM as well as to the PAG, thereby promoting influence on the DH. Thus, cortical areas appear to provide both direct and indirect influence on nociception through either monosynaptic or polysynaptic means.

As previously alluded, there are multiple descending pathways and their associated neurotransmitters. Norepinephrine (NE, aka *noradrenaline (NA), noradrenergic*) and serotonin (5-HT, *serotonergic*) are well researched, but other pathways exist to include dopamine (DA), acetylcholine (ACh, *cholinergic*), endorphins, adenosine, and glutamate, to name a few. However, the target receptors and

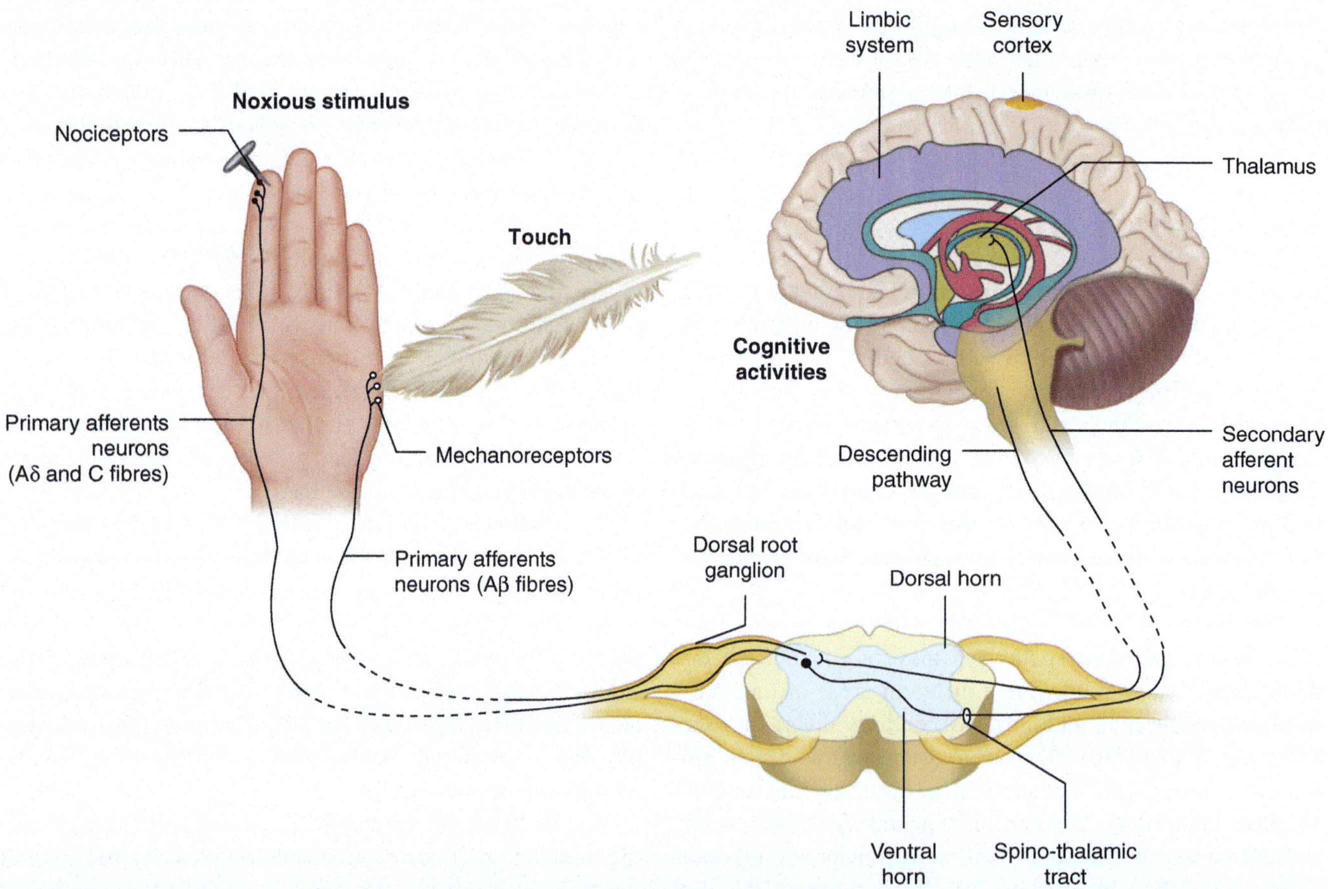

Fig. 8.4 Cognitive-affective pathways. Complicated integration of ascending pathways with the thalamus and limbic system is an important determinant of the outward display of pain. The cognitive-affective dimension of pain may further determine the plasticity of the pain response

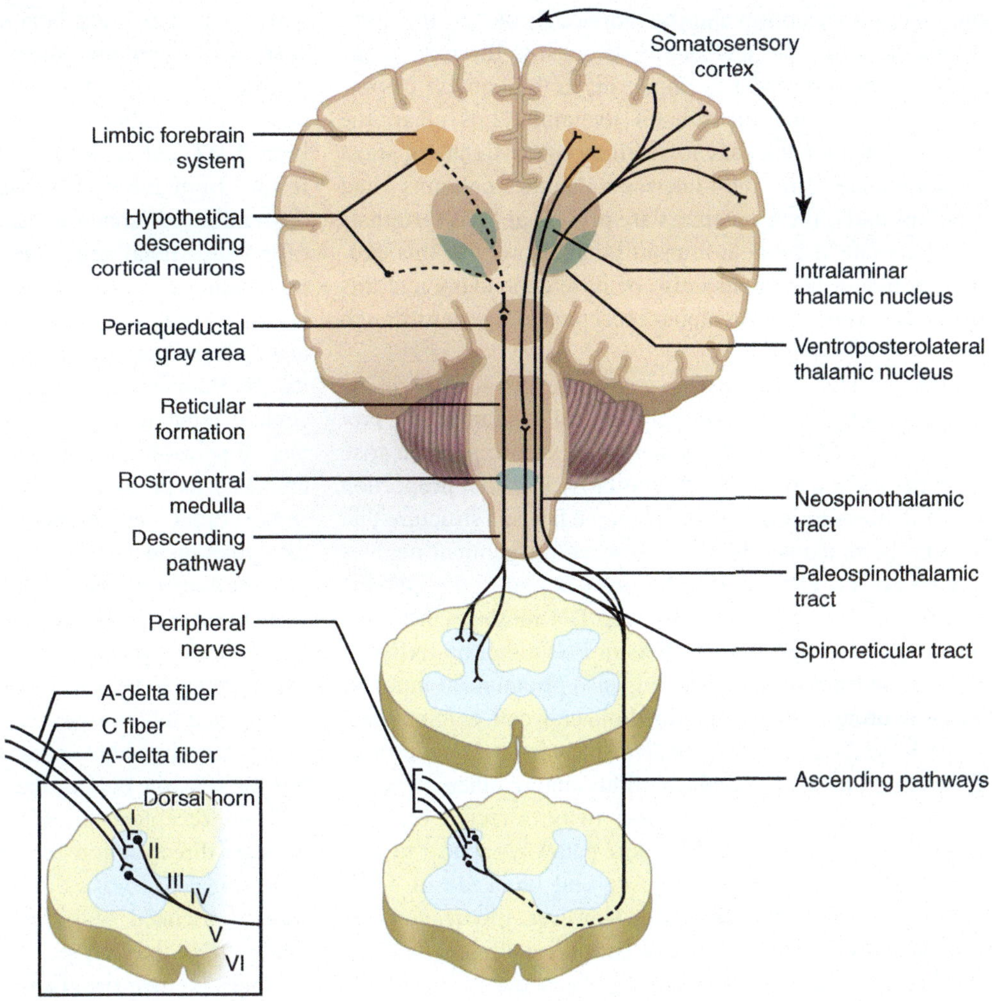

Fig. 8.5 Ascending pathways and descending pathways. Both ascending nociception and non-nociceptive input are relayed centrally through the medulla to the thalamus, limbic system, and the sensory cortex. Descending controls exert their influence through potential facilitation or inhibition through common structure such as the periaqueductal gray area and the thalamus. Cortical descending control mechanisms also may exist

associated second messenger systems provide NTs with diverse and often divergent responses under normal or pathological conditions.

The descending noradrenergic pathway is a well-studied pathway, and it is well known to modulate nociception under normal conditions as well as stress-induced and pathological states. Centers in the medulla and pons may provide descending input through the intermediolateral columns and ventral horn. Medullary nuclei and areas of the locus coeruleus are known sources of these descending NA pathways. These structures are under tonic inhibition from gamma-aminobutyric acid (GABA)-related pathways, a site of possible antinociception for cannabinoids and opioids. Opioid activation in the PAG may also lead to the increased activity of NA by release of inhibitory influence.

The NA descending pathway role is likely determined by circumstances associated with stimulus input. The influence of the NA descending pathway is subtle under normal conditions. However, with increasing stimulus intensity, the role of this pathway changes at least in the acute phase of nociception. Further painful stimulus involving injury or inflammation may lead to recruitment of more neurons of the NA pathway and segue to bridge nociception and the cardiovascular system response to pain. The NA pathway is also known to exhibit influence on the RVM, the heterogeneity of which may influence both DI and DF.

The DI effect of NA is mediated likely through the role of the alpha-adrenoceptor. This receptor is present in significant quantities in the DH as well as in sufficient amounts in the dorsal root ganglion (DRG). NA provides significant suppression of nociception through presynaptic inhibition of PNA NT release in the DH although the extent varies upon location in the CNS. The alpha-2 receptor targets in the rexed laminae lead to target cell inhibition through G-protein mediation target cell hyperpolarization (increased K+ influx) and inhibition of AC. Under certain conditions, volume transmission, or bulk flow of large quantities of NA, can also play a role in mass receptor activation. Furthermore, NA is co-localized with other NTs such as ACh, GABA, adenosine, and others. Although NA promotes DI by the specific activation of alpha-2 adrenoreceptors, there is a preponderance of evidence to suggest that NA more broadly modulates nociception and the individual roles of the other transmitters directly and indirectly. Lastly, the role of the alpha-1 adrenoreceptor is important in the context of pro-nociception. While the role of the alpha-2 is clear, the alpha-1 receptor appears to facilitate pain signaling most predominantly in the intermediolateral columns and VH. Similarly, these receptors are present at PNA terminals and facilitate their neurotransmission. However, this pro-nociceptive influence may also be dose dependent, and this may pose a quandary for alpha-2 receptor analgesics through crossover binding.

The serotonergic pathways within the spinal cord appear to entirely originate from the supraspinal structures. The preponderance of 5-HT in the dorsal spinal cord appears to arise from the RVM and the NRM. Similarly, a smaller proportion of 5-HT fibers may also come from the DRN, a structure that affects the thalamus, hippocampus, and trigeminal nucleus among others. These 5-HT neurons descend to the DH and synapse in the superficial and deep DH in abundance, and they may affect their target PNAs or PNs either by ININs or by volume transmission. There is also pronounced input by 5-HT neurons into the intermediolateral cell columns and ventral horn. These areas receive input from 5-HT projections from the nucleus raphe pallidus among others.

Serotonergic pathways appear to be affected by both acute and chronic pain. In fact these pathways appear to play a role in stress-induced analgesia, and blockade of 5-HT pathways reduces this response. However, this response is also decreased in the presence of peripheral afferent damage. Furthermore, some studies suggest that there is a dual role whereby the serotonergic pathways are involved in both DI and DF, as receptor-specific responses and receptor location are the determinants of this response. This duality appears to depend at least in part on stimulus parameters, with high-frequency and low-frequency stimulation of the RVM leading to DI and DF, respectively. These cells within the RVM are not associated with supraspinal morphine-mediated descending pathways of DF "ON" cells (stimulated by pain, inhibited by opioids) or DI "OFF" cells (stimulated by opioids, deactivated by pain) through central or systemic administration of morphine. However, kappa-opioid receptors are known to mediate the serotonergic response to nociception in the RVM. Kappa receptors are known to directly inhibit primary serotonergic cells, and these cells are also indirectly inhibited by activation of secondary GABAergic cells. Mu- and delta-opioid receptor activation disinhibits these secondary cells, and kappa receptors on these secondary cells lead to disinhibition of GABAergic inhibition (e.g., facilitation) leading to serotonergic DI. Thus, central opioidergic pathways may indirectly mediate descending serotonergic pathways in the DH through a diversity of opioid receptor subtypes. Similarly, there is a variety of other pathways that, as to be discussed later, lead to modulation of the 5-HT pathways. These include beta-endorphins, prostaglandins, and acetylcholine among others.

The dual role of the serotonin pathway in the mediation of pain can be attributed not only to the variety of receptors that bind 5-HT but also to the second messenger system that results from receptor activation. Modalities of control by descending serotonergic pathways include action on neurons of the superficial and deep layers of the DH and associated transmitter release, on the target cell resting state or activation by PNA input, and on the influence of pro-nociceptive NTs and influence upon wide-dynamic range neurons or individual PNAs or interneurons. The temporal pattern of the nociceptive input may also determine the role of 5-HT in the overall perception or prolonged perception of pain with some evidence to point to its poor role in antinociception in the spinal cord in the presence of prolonged neuropathic pain and the depletion of 5-HT in the spinal cord leading to attenuation of pain transmission. Nonetheless, receptor subtype appears to dictate the overall role of 5-HT in nociception. The receptor 5-HT1A is present in significant concentration in the DH and suppresses neuronal firing through the facilitation of K+ current and inhibition of Ca2+ currents. The 5-HT1A receptor appears to mediate hyperalgesia likely through the activation of IINs on PNs in the DH not on PNA terminals. The 5-HTA1 receptor may also play a role in antinociception through direct action on some PNA terminals or through supraspinal pathways emanating from the opioidergic pathways associated with the PAG. Similarly, 5-HT1A may inhibit IINs that suppress NA transmission or presynaptic feedback on their own facilitation of IINs' action on descending NA pathways from the NRM and others. The 5-HT1B receptor is also known to facilitate K+ currents and is found throughout the DH. The 5-HT1B promotes antinociception by negative feedback loop autoreceptors as serotonergic on serotonergic terminals. Similarly, 5-HT1B receptors also appear to medicate antinociception through reduction in the release of CGRP and SP, with 5-HT1D predominant in the cerebral blood vessels. Receptors 5-HT1B, 5-HT1D, and 5-HT1F appear to mediate antinociception in the presence of migraine headache. The 5-HT2 receptor class contains three subtypes with evidence demonstrating that at least 5-HT2A and 5-HT2C are pro-nociceptive in the DH. The receptor 5-HT2A appears to be associated with facilitation of central sensitization at PNA terminals but may also have a role in antinociception through IIN pathways. The 5-HT3 receptor is also an ion channel. It is found in abundance in the superficial laminae. This receptor is known to play an excitatory role in the facilitation of inflammatory pain transmission through modulation of central terminals on PNAs. However, 5-HT3 may also be antinociceptive as well similar to 5-HT2A through an IIN process, but this may include co-localization with other central NT-mediated processes. 5-HT3 receptor may also mediate pain from visceral origin through local mechanisms mediated through vagal afferents. Other serotonergic receptor classes include 5-HT4, 5-HT5, 5-HT6, and 5-HT7. 5-HT4 receptors appear to be related to pro-nociception as mediated through C fiber PNAs. The 5-HT5A receptor appears to mirror the role of 5-HT1A with a heavy correlation with cerebral structures associated with descending NA pathways. The role of the remaining subclasses of 5-HT receptors although present in the DH (5-HT5, 5-HT6, and 5-HT7) is not well defined.

The dopaminergic pathway appears to play a role in the descending modulation of nociception, but it is much less researched. Origins of DA in the nervous system predominantly include the substantia nigra, the paraventricular nucleus of the hypothalamus, and the A11 region of the hypothalamus. DA receptors are organized into the D1 and D2 receptor families with D1 receptors representing the abundance in the spinal cord. Agonist studies appear to represent that D2 receptors mediate antinociception while D1 receptors are the antithesis. No clear mechanism is known to regulate the descending influence of DA in the CNS, but some studies suggest the roles of the PAG. The A11 regions of the hypothalamus appear to reduce the behavioral response to pain, while D2 receptors on target PNAs or PNs in various rexed laminae reduce their excitatory output.

Other Mediators of Pain Processing: Histamine, Endogenous Opioid Peptides, Nitric Oxide, Cannabinoids, and Other Neuropeptides

Several other transmitters exist in the mediation and transmission of pain processing. These transmitters play an important role not only at the level of the DH but also throughout known pathways involved in DI and DF. As with many species involved in neurotransmission, the mechanisms may be facilitatory or inhibitory, and this is dependent on the receptor subtype and the corresponding second messenger system in place. Furthermore, nociception under normal states and pathological conditions play an important role.

Histamine and its associated receptors are known to be present in the CNS whereby histamine is synthesized by cells in the hypothalamus. These cells project to other areas of the brain and brainstem whereby they exert their effects in a receptor-dependent manner. The histamine receptors are known as H1, H2, H3, and H4 whereby H1 and H2 are known to be excitatory and H3 mediates an inhibitory pathways. In the DH PNA terminals, histamine appears to lead to a pro-nociceptive response with peripheral nerve injury leading to expression of histamine receptors. Histamine appears to exhibit differentiating effects on the serotonergic and noradrenergic pathways in the CNS with the response once again dependent on receptor subtype and location. H2 receptors on the average appear to facilitate DI (possibly in association with opioidergic mechanisms of the PAG) whereby H1 receptors appear to promote nociception. In the DH, H3 receptors at least in part appear to mediate pro-nociception through inhibition of presynaptic NT release in a negative feedback manner. Centrally, activation of H3 autoreceptors reduces overall histamine load and promotion of nociception.

Endogenous opioid peptides (EOPs) are a family of peptide with several known receptors in the CNS. These receptors include mu-, delta-, and kappa-opioid receptors. These peptides are cleaved from parent molecules into biologically active substances and byproducts of yet to be determined significance.

Enkephalins (ENK) are a family of peptides to include met- and leu-enkephalin, and these are cleaved from the parent pre-pro-enkephalin. Globally, these substances are known to promote DI either through direct receptor activation or potentiation of other descending pathways that mediate DI. As with the other EOPs, activation of encephalin receptors leads to antinociception through the promotion of K+ currents and the suppression of C2+ currents through negative G-protein mediation of adenylyl cyclase. Cells containing enkephalins are found in significant quantities of the PAG, and there are significant populations of ENK receptors associated with IINs of the DH.

Dynorphins (DYN) are another group of EOPs, and they are formed from the cleavage of pre-pro-dynorphin. DYN is unique to the class of EOPs in that it may play both pro- and antinociceptive roles. Kappa-opioid receptors are known to mediate the antinociceptive mechanisms of DYN both centrally and in the DH through IINs. However, in the DH, DYN can promote nociception through non-Kappa-mediated mechanisms (i.e., NMDA receptors) or interfere with the actions of DI pathways. Centrally, DYN mediates DI through both kappa receptor-mediated pathways in the PAG and amygdala, but in other supraspinal structures, DYN may potentiate DF or interfere with DI pathways. The antinociceptive role of DYN has to be postulated to, at least, in part, be responsible for hyperalgesia and tolerance associated with clinical opioid therapy.

Endorphins are found in several areas of the brain important in descending modulation to include several aforementioned structures such as the medullary nuclei, PAG, and amygdala. Similarly, endomorphin-2 is found in significant quantities in the DH among particular local networks. Mu receptors are known to mediate their intense analgesic effect.

Pro-opiomelanocortin (POMC) is a large protein that is precursor to beta-endorphin and a group of other products collectively referred to as melanocortins. Beta-endorphin is found in cell bodies of some hypothalamic cells, NTS, and within the DH DRG. Within the hypothalamus, these neurons project to the PAG to provide significant input and lead to mu-opioid receptor-mediated DI as well as in part DI mediated through descending noradrenergic pathways. The role for descending NTS tracts as well as local beta-endorphin-containing cells in the DH and receptors in the DRG is not clear although the role may be inferred as antinociceptive.

Melanocortins are the second known group of products of POMC cleavage, and they include various subtypes of melanocyte-stimulating hormone and adrenocorticotrophin-releasing hormone. Although several receptors have been identified, there is relatively little known of their bioactivity sans the MC4 receptor. The mechanism of melanocortins as mediated through the MC4 receptor appears to be AC-mediated facilitation and pro-nociception. This receptor is produced by cells that do not produce POMC and coexists in the proximity of POMC-mediated antinociceptive receptors. MC4-containing cells are found throughout the PAG, medullary nuclei and NTS, locus coeruleus, and the DH. Activation of the MC4 receptor is thought to attenuate endogenous analgesic mechanisms and promote allodynia.

Nociceptin (aka orphaninFQ) and nociceptin originate from the same precursor polypeptide. OrphaninFQ is an endogenous opioid formed from a pre-pro-peptide that works through its receptor ORL1 that is widely found throughout the CNS. The receptor is homologous to known other EOP receptors, but receptor binding to orphaninFQ results in the mediation of nociception antithesis to known opioidergic mechanisms in spite of documented homologous neurochemistry. OrphaninFQ is found in the PAG and RVM as well as sites in the DH laminae. In the DH, orphaninFQ may act in a pro-nociceptive or antinociceptive dose-dependent manner either by direct action at the PNA terminal or through an intermediary mechanism (i.e., IINs). However, orphaninFQ modulates a diffuse inhibitory effect on DI mechanisms with possible influence on both opioidergic and non-opioidergic pathways. Nocistatin is a peptide product of the parent protein that gives rise to the orphaninFQ molecule. Nocistatin appears to work through different receptors, and its action spinally and in higher centers antagonizes those of orphaninFQ by unknown mechanisms of action.

Galanin (GAL) is a neuropeptide known to exert its influence through three known receptors aptly named GAL-1, GAL-2, and GAL-3. The neuropeptide GAL is known to exhibit a duality of mechanisms remaining in common theme to other species discussed, and this duality is determined by receptor subtype. GAL is found both in the supraspinal and spinal compartments, and it plays a role in both resting and pathological states. In the brain, GAL is found in neurons in the PAG, PBN, NTS, and locus coeruleus, and it is known to be present in the noradrenergic and histaminergic tracts. In the DH, GAL is found in intrinsic DH neurons. A consensus appears to exist that GAL is antinociceptive whereby it facilitates the DI of the NA and 5-HT pathways, but its role is dependent on the site of stimulus and presence of GAL receptor subtype as well as location of action (PNA, PNs, etc.). GAL is also thought to be released from NA cells themselves whereby it may be involved in negative feedback of NA neurons through autoreceptors on terminals from cells of the locus coeruleus.

Pools of nitric oxide (NO) are found throughout the CNS and are significantly involved in nociception at a variety of sites. Whether NO arises from descending sources or from local neurons in the DH, it appears to be a mediator of DF in the presence of inflammation or tissue injury. The action of NO may be through the facilitation of glutamate or through attenuation of DI systems at the DH. Similarly, NO may influence nociception through influence of NMDA pro-nociception or interruption of central DI mechanisms.

Lastly, cannabinoids are species of significant interest both scientifically as well as politically. Endogenous ligands to cannabinoid receptors CB-1 and CB-2 arise from membrane phospholipids. CB-1 is predominantly found in the CNS while CB-2 within the immune system. In fact, receptors for cannabinoids are found at nearly every level of the pain pathway. There is substantial support for the strong mechanism of antinociception not only supraspinally but also segmentally and peripherally in the presence of peripheral inflammation and neuropathic pain. Agonist studies demonstrate that peripheral sensitization is reduced with local administration in the hind paw rodent model, and antagonists block this response. Spinal mechanisms are mediated by CB receptors synthesized in the DRG and distributed to both axon terminals and dendrites. Activation of CB receptors may suppress local pro-nociceptive NTs in the DH or interfere with nociceptive transmission in PNs. Similarly, cannabinoids are thought to reduce the receptor fields of WDR neurons in the presence of persistent input. Supraspinal CB receptors are found in the PAG although these receptors are in anatomically different areas than the corresponding opioids, and this underscores their pathways as independent of the opioid-mediated pathways. Other sites of action involve the RVM whereby CB receptor-mediated activation of DI may occur. The influence of DI by cannabinoids appears to be particular to the NA pathway and less associated by mechanisms involving 5-HT receptors.

Key Points

1. Peripheral nociceptive afferent neurons target cells within the spinal cord that can lead to a significantly broad response in the central nervous system, and this is dependent on the tissue type, neurotransmitters, receptors, and second messenger systems involved.
2. The organization and function of afferent nociceptive transmission is dynamic and multimodal and is determined by the physiological or pathological circumstances present.

3. Independent nociceptive ascending tracts are an oversimplification, and the intercommunication between various ascending tracts is an important part of understanding the processing of pathological pain states.
4. The overall experience of pain is determined by the interaction between the two categories of ascending pathways, the sensory-discriminative and affective-cognitive.
5. The thalamus contains several nuclei that receive peripheral nociception and disperse it to a variety of higher centers involved in both the cognitive and subconscious response to pain. Dysfunction of innate inhibitory mechanisms within these higher centers may lead to pathological, unopposed pro-nociception.
6. Determinants of descending inhibition or descending facilitation are influenced by neurotransmitter concentrations and receptor subtype activation.
7. Descending modulation of nociception is complex and is dependent on a variety of mediators, some of which yet to be understood. Known mechanisms such as the noradrenergic and serotonergic pathways may have dual functions and are dependent on normal physiologic or pathological conditions in the periphery as well as supraspinal influences. Stimulus parameters and emotional-cognitive states strongly influence outcomes.

Recommended Reading

1. Gebhart G. Descending modulation of pain. Neurosci Biobehav Rev. 2004;27:729–37.
2. Heinricher M, Tavares I, Leith J, Lumb B. Descending control of nociception: specificity, recruitment and plasticity. Brain Res Rev. 2009;60:214–25.
3. Kandel E, Schwartz J, Jessell J, Siegelbaum S, Hudspeth A. Principles of neural science. 5th ed. New York: The McGraw-Hill Companies; 2013. p. 449–555.
4. Lau B, Vaughan C. Descending modulation of pain: the GABA disinhibition hypothesis of analgesia. Curr Opin Neurobiol. 2014;29:159–64.
5. Llorca-Torralba M, Borges G, Neto F, Mico J, Berrocoso E. Noradrenergic locus coeruleus pathways in pain modulation. Neuroscience. 2016;338:93–113.
6. Martins I, Tavares I. Reticular formation and pain: the past and future. Front Neuroanat. 2017;11(51):1–14.
7. Millan M. The induction of pain: an integrative review. Prog Neurobiol. 1999;57:1–164.
8. Millan M. Descending control of pain. Prog Neurobiol. 2002;66:355–474.
9. Pertovaara A. Noradrenergic pain modulation. Prog Neurobiol. 2006;80:53–83.
10. Pertovaara A. The noradrenergic pain regulation system: a potential target for pain therapy. Eur J Pharm. 2013;716:2–7.
11. Rainville P. Brain mechanisms of pain affect and pain modulation. Curr Opp Neurobiol. 2002;12:195–204.
12. Steeds C. The anatomy and physiology of pain. Surgery. 2013;31(2):49–53.
13. Taylor B, Westlund K. The noradrenergic locus coeruleus as a chronic pain generator. J Neurosci Res. 2017;95:1336–46.
14. Vanegas H, Schaible H. Descending control of persistent pain: inhibitory or facilitatory? Brain Res Rev. 2004;46:295–309.
15. Viguier F, Michot B, Hamon M, Bourgoin S. Multiple roles of serotonin in pain control mechanisms – implications of the 5-HT7 and other 5-HT receptor subtypes. Eur J Pharm. 2013;716:8–16.

Taxonomy of Pain

9

Nicholas J. Bremer

Terminology

Pain is a type of sensation defined by the World Health Organization as an unpleasant sensory and emotional experience associated with actual or potential tissue damage or described in terms of such damage. A key feature in this consensus definition is that pain can exist notwithstanding the absence of an obvious proximal cause. That is, while a noxious stimulus is usually associated with pain, a stimulus need not be present at all for existence of pain. Another key feature of this definition is that no actual physical change need be apparent for the term pain to be applied.

There is no objective test for the existence or degree of pain other than the patient's report; likewise, for that matter, neither is there any test for what qualifies as noxious stimulus in the first instance. Indeed, pain may be the singular entity in the whole of medical practice wherein both the subjective and objective are one in the same. Pain is necessarily, however, an unpleasant emotional and psychological state. The treatment of pain, as a result, has moved to more objective measures and scales of functionality, a related concept, to monitor objective improvement in pain.

Sensation, more generally, can be a described generally as either epicritic or protopathic. Epicritic sensibility is concerned with fine discrimination of touch and temperature and is transmitted by large, myelinated, fast-conduction A Delta (δ) fibers for sharp, well-localized sensation. Epicritic pain can occur in response to thermal and mechanical stimuli. Protopathic sensibility is concerned with pain and temperature and is transmitted by small, unmyelinated, slow-conduction C fibers for dull, achy, poorly localized sensation. Protopathic pain is more common than epicritic pain, and protopathic pain is more responsive to opioid therapy. Protopathic pain results from noxious stimuli, meaning stimuli causing actual or potentially causing tissue damage.

If pain is resultant from activation of nociceptive affect fibers from actual tissue damage, such as C fibers in protopathic sensibility, then it is described as nociceptive pain. On the other hand, if no tissue damage is ongoing and pain is resultant from either a central or peripheral nervous system lesion or dysfunctional state, then it is described as neuropathic pain.

Understanding of descriptive terminology is useful to accurately describe painful symptoms—the very symptoms that themselves may be ambiguous. Proper use of these terms is also essential for diagnosis and clear communication among colleagues. When describing sensation, paresthesia refers simply to an abnormal sensation, whether evoked or spontaneous, such as the tingling associated with a traditional, tonic spinal cord stimulator trial. An unpleasant abnormal sensation, either evoked or spontaneous—that is, an unpleasant paresthesia—is referred to as a dysesthesia, such as the radicular pain associated with a lumbar disc herniation causing radiculitis.

Hypoesthesia (or hypesthesia) refers to diminished pain in response to a normally painful stimulus, such as with the microvascular disease commonly associated with diabetic neuropathy, causing increasing diminished pain response. Anesthesia refers to lack of all sensation altogether in a particular area, such as after a peripheral nerve block performed by a regional anesthesiologist prior to surgery.

Hyperesthesia, on the other hand, refers to increased pain in response to a normally painful stimulus, such as the increased response to a normally mildly painful stimulus in a patient with a specific peripheral neuropathy. Allodynia refers to pain due to a stimulus that does not normally provoke pain, such as the pain associated with lightly touching an affected limb of a patient suffering from complex regional pain syndrome.

The term hyperpathia describes a syndrome and may incorporate one or several terms listed above. This syndrome is characterized by an abnormally painful reaction to a stimulus,

N. J. Bremer (✉)
Center for Pain Relief, Spine and Nerve Centers of the Virginias, Charleston, WV, USA
e-mail: Nicholas.Bremer@CenterforPainRelief.com

T. R. Deer et al. (eds.), *Deer's Treatment of Pain*, https://doi.org/10.1007/978-3-030-12281-2_9

Table 9.1 Stimulus-dependent taxonomy of pain terms related to threshold and response

Term	Threshold	Response
Allodynia	Decreased	Increased
Hyperesthesia	Increased	Increased
Hyperpathia	Variable	Increased
Hypoesthesia	Decreased	Decreased
Analgesia	Decreased	Decreased

especially a repetitive stimulus, as well as an increased in threshold. It may occur in the setting of allodynia, hyperesthesia, hyperalgesia, dysesthesia, or a combination thereof. In addition, faulty identification and localization of the stimulus, delay, radiating sensation, and aftersensation may be present, and the pain is often explosive in character. Table 9.1 summarizes the stimulus-dependent terms with respect to the minimum intensity of a stimulus that is perceived as painful or pain threshold.

Acute and Chronic Pain

The temporal relationship to the stimulus, if any, and the onset and duration of pain are helpful in diagnosis and treatment. In contradistinction to the superordinate category of pain in general, definitions of what constitutes acute or chronic pain are less well defined. Acute pain is pain resulting from nociceptor activation resulting from tissue damage, which typically resolves once healed. Acute pain is universally agreed to serve an adaptive purpose, the warning of injury, for example. Chronic pain is pain that outlasts any acute pain, often with more severe symptoms than the original insult and tissue damage would portend. While the duration of pain is inherent in what might constitute chronic pain, the exact duration for the diagnosis thereof is unsettled, with authors generally supposing anywhere from 3 to 6 months. Chronic pain, in contrast to acute pain, has no obvious biological value or adaptive purpose and, for these reasons, may well be considered a maladaptive entity.

Chronic pain is often associated with sensitization. Sensitization is the increased responsiveness of nociceptive neurons to normal input, or recruitment of a response to normally subthreshold inputs, or both. When occurring in the periphery, there is increased responsiveness and reduced threshold of nociceptive neurons to the stimulation of their receptive fields; in the central nervous system, there is increased responsiveness of nociceptive neurons to their normal or subthreshold afferent input. The mechanisms by which these phenomena occur are complex and discussed in detail elsewhere, but the result is that, in both cases, the pain threshold, or the minimum intensity of a stimulus that is perceived as painful, is reduced.

Pain Syndromes

Neuropathy is a disturbance of function or pathological change in a nerve: in one nerve, mononeuropathy; in several nerves, mononeuropathy multiplex; if diffuse and bilateral, polyneuropathy. Neuralgia refers to pain originating from a nerve, while neuritis is the special case of the inflammatory process affecting nerves, which is commonly manifest by pain.

Radicular pain is pain arising from activation of nociceptive afferent fibers in spinal nerves or roots, which is usually lancinating and travels along dermatomes. Radiculitis is a state of inflammation of those spinal nerves or roots, which is thought to be the major contributor to radicular pain. Radiculopathy is the state of affairs wherein an objective neurologic deficit in motor or sensory function is found on examination or diagnostic tests such as electromyogram in the distribution of a specific spinal nerve or its roots.

Complex regional pain syndrome (CRPS) is a syndrome with four categories of signs and four categories of symptoms, with diagnostic criteria published by the International Association for the Study of Pain (IASP) as a result of a 2003 consensus meeting in Budapest. These Budapest Criteria for CRPS come in a more stringent research flavor, favoring specificity (requiring four symptom categories and two sign categories), as well as a less stringent clinical flavor, favoring sensitivity (requiring three symptom categories and two sign categories). CRPS I, formally known as reflex sympathetic dystrophy (RSD), is a syndrome that develops after an initiating noxious event. CRPS II, formally known as causalgia, is a syndrome that develops after a nerve injury. Clinically, both are typically treated with the same.

Anesthesia dolorosa is pain that occurs in a region without sensation (anesthesia). The treatment of trigeminal neuralgia with microvascular decompression or radiofrequency therapy can result anesthesia dolorosa. This is a dreaded complication in the treatment of facial pain.

Referred pain is pain perceived in one area of the body but actually originating in another. Phantom pain is a type of neuropathic pain occuring in the distribution of a missing limb or deafferentiated body part. While phantom pain is a true neuropathic pain entity, other forms of postamputation pain often confound proper diagnosis and treatment. For example, residual limb pain, a type of nociceptive pain, can present in a similar fashion to phantom limb pain and have neuropathic elements. Residual limb pain can be secondary to ill-fitting prosthesis, neuromas, inflammation, infection, or other problems, making identification of the particular underlying issue at hand of paramount importance. Therefore, a careful history is essential in these cases to ensure a proper diagnosis and treatment plan whenever phantom pain is suspected.

Central pain is regional pain caused by a central nerve system primary lesion or dysfunction, usually associated with abnormal temperature sensation. Deafferentation pain refers to pain due to loss of input into the central nervous system, such as lesions to or injury of peripheral nerves. Somatic pain is carried along sensory fibers and is usually discrete and intense. Visceral pain is carried along sympathetic fibers and is diffuse and poorly localized.

Pain physicians who prescribe opioid therapy to patients will need to be aware of certain aspects of addictionology and even legal terminology. Tolerance refers to the need for increasing dosages to obtain the same effect. Dependence refers to the need to keep taking a substance to avoid a withdrawal syndrome. Abuse refers to taking illicit drugs or legally prescribed medications in a manner not prescribed. Diversion is both a medical and legal concept, involving the transfer of any legally prescribed controlled substance from the individual for whom it was prescribed to another person for any illicit use. Addiction is a primary condition manifesting as uncontrollable cravings, inability to control drug use, compulsive drug use, and use despite doing harm to oneself or others. Opioid-induced hyperalgesia is a syndrome characterized by increasing dosages of opioids causing higher levels of pain, which can be difficult to tell apart from tolerance or inadequate control of pain.

Pain Psychopathology

Chronic pain seems to be comorbid with high rates of depression and anxiety, as well as having other negative consequences, such psychological distress, financial burden, occupational distress, and social isolation. Historically, as Katz noted, pain without an apparent anatomical or neurophysiological origin was labelled as psychopathological. The diagnostic criteria for pain disorder in the Diagnostic and Statistical Manual for Mental Disorders IV Text Revision (DSM-IV-TR) have been eliminated. Instead, in the DSM-V a broader category of diagnostic criteria is included called somatic symptom and related disorders. Internationally, the somatoform disorder criteria described in the DSM-IV-TR along with the World Health Organization International Classification of Diseases 10th Revision (ICD-10) is used, but in practice many chronic pain patients would fit into either iteration. The pain psychologist can be an integral part of interdisciplinary patient care.

Disability

Disability is a term referring to the loss of ability to perform a specific task in the usual or standard manner. The term also carries specific legal implications and alternate or more specific definitions, which vary by agency.

Main Points

1. A challenging aspect of pain medicine is that, by definition, the objective physician evaluation is solely based on subjective patient report.
2. Proper use of nomenclature makes for effective diagnosis and treatment of patients, as well as effective communications among colleagues.
3. Definitions of what constitute acute and chronic pain are not unanimous.
4. The descriptive terminology used in pain is attempt to make ambiguous presentations clearer.
5. Inflammation of nerves typically results in pain, while nerve injury can result in sensory or motor dysfunction and objective findings.
6. CRPS is a diagnosis based on a set of specific criteria based on consensus opinion and may occur with or without a specific nerve injury.
7. Tolerance, opioid-induced hyperalgesia, and inadequate treatment of pain are difficult to distinguish clinically but need to be considered in the differential diagnosis.
8. Physicians prescribing opioid therapy ought to be aware of terminology in addictionology as well as the legal realm.
9. Many pain patients may meet criteria for psychological pain states, and the pain psychologist is an important member of the interdisciplinary care team.
10. Disability status is determined by formal processes that vary by agency.

Recommended Reading

1. American Psychiatric Association. Diagnostic and statistical manual of mental disorders. 5th ed. Arlington: American Psychiatric Publishing; 2013.
2. Benzon H, Raja S, Fishman S, et al. Essentials of pain medicine. 3rd ed. Philadelphia: Elsevier Saunders; 2011.
3. Benzon H, Rathmall J, Wu C, et al. Practical management of pain. 5th ed. Philadelphia: Elsevier; 2014.
4. Demyttenaere K, Bruffaerts R, Lee S, et al. Mental disorders among persons with chronic back or neck pain: results from the World Mental Health Surveys. Pain. 2007;129(3):332–42.
5. Katz J, Rosenbloom B, Fashler S. Chronic pain, psychopathology, and DSM-5 somatic symptoms disorder. Can J Psychiatr. 2015;60(4):160–7.
6. Merskey H, Bogduk N. International association for the study of pain classification of pain. 2nd ed. Seattle: IASP Press; 1994. (online section update 2012).
7. Von Korff M, Crane P, Lane M, et al. Chronic spinal pain and physical-mental comorbidity in the United States: results from the National Comorbidity Survey Replication. Pain. 2005;113(3):331–9.

Pain-Relieving Mechanisms in Neuromodulation

10

Vikram Sengupta, Sascha Qian, Ned Urbiztondo, and Nameer Haider

Introduction

Since its inception more than 50 years ago, the forms and applications of modern neuromodulation have undergone tremendous expansion. The International Neuromodulation Society defines neuromodulation as "the alteration of nerve activity through targeted delivery of a stimulus, such as electrical stimulation or chemical agents, to specific neurological sites in the body," most commonly to reduce pain or improve neurologic function. All forms of neuromodulation are reversible. Neurostimulation is the most common form of neuromodulation technology used today, and it refers to the use of electrical or electromagnetic stimuli upon target tissues to elicit a therapeutic response. Although the focus of this chapter will be on neurostimulation, other non-electrical therapies, such as intrathecal drug delivery systems, may fall into the category of neuromodulation.

On August 10, 2017, the CDC recommended that the opioid epidemic should be declared a national emergency. In light of these circumstances, neuromodulation, which is relatively safe, effective, and validated in the treatment of chronic neuropathic pain, is emerging as an important alternative to opioid therapy. Conversely, chronic high-dose opioid therapy is not validated, is often ineffective, and carries a substantial risk of dependence, abuse, addiction, and other morbidity and mortality. High-dose medication is also theorized to induce opioid-induced hyperalgesia, and these drugs may therefore increase the perception of pain.

In this chapter, we will introduce the broad and ever-expanding panoply of neuromodulation and its applications, describing what is known of the mechanisms of action through which it works. Although similar electrical stimuli may often be delivered, the prevailing mechanism of action will vary based on the pathophysiology of the underlying painful disease state being treated. Although clinical evidence will be provided, more exhaustive summaries of the clinical data will be reserved for later chapters in Part VI, each of which is dedicated to the clinical aspects of a particular form of neuromodulation.

V. Sengupta · S. Qian (✉) · N. Urbiztondo · N. Haider
Spinal & Skeletal Pain Medicine, Utica, NY, USA
e-mail: vsengupta@thrivewellinfusion.com; drhaider@killpain.com

Background and Historical Perspective

The earliest documented use of electrical current for the treatment of pain was around 63 AD, when the Mesopotamian physician, Scribonius Largus, discovered that shocks delivered by the electrical torpedo fish could relieve bodily aches and pains. In the eleventh century, the Islamic philosopher Avicenna used cranial shocks delivered by the electric catfish to treat epilepsy. In the 1600s, the natural philosopher, William Gilbert, reported using the magnetic lodestone to treat headaches and psychiatric illness.

In 1745, Ewald Georg von Kleist and Pieter van Musschenbroek independently invented the world's first capacitor, known as the Leyden jar. Subsequently in 1747, Jean Jallabert used electrical stimulation to increase blood flow, and to provoke muscle contraction and growth, thereby restoring function to the paralyzed limb of a locksmith. Also in the mid-eighteenth century, Benjamin Franklin used his electrostatic generator to treat paralysis and various painful conditions. Some of his treatments achieved transient improvement. However, his use of high voltages caused burns and nerve injuries, leading him to abandon the practice.

The true inception of modern neurostimulation can be traced to three major developments in the mid-twentieth century: (1) the advent and success of the implantable cardiac pacemaker in the late 1950s; (2) the 1965 publication of Melzack and Wall's seminal article, *Pain Mechanisms: A New Theory*, in which they first proposed the gate control theory of pain, postulating that activation of large-diameter sensory nerve fibers could block transmission of pain signals conveyed by small diameter fibers; and (3) the first clinical application of gate control theory by the neurosurgeon

T. R. Deer et al. (eds.), *Deer's Treatment of Pain*, https://doi.org/10.1007/978-3-030-12281-2_10

Norman Shealy in 1967, when he implanted the first spinal cord stimulator (SCS) to successfully treat chronic neuropathic pain.

In 1958, Medtronic released the first implantable pacemaker, followed in 1958 with the first battery-operated wearable pacemaker. The revenue from these early successes was then used to subsidize research and development that repurposed pacemaker technology to meet the growing demand for devices specialized for neural applications. Indeed, the first spinal cord stimulator was a Medtronic cardiac pacemaker with leads modified for intrathecal placement.

In the decades that followed, neuromodulation blossomed into one of the most fascinating and dynamic fields of medicine, with new improvements and applications emerging every year. Monopolar platinum leads have evolved into multi-contact titanium leads. Paddle leads have been developed for insertion by surgical laminotomy. Internal pulse generator (IPG) batteries are smaller and longer-lived. Rechargeable versions are now available. Every year, programs multiply, while the list of validated and experimental applications expands.

The Gate Control Theory of Pain

In 1965, Melzack and Wall first articulated the gate control theory of pain modulation in their seminal article *Pain Mechanisms: A New Theory*, published in the journal *Science*. They hypothesized that stimulation of large myelinated Aβ sensory fibers carrying touch and vibratory information to the dorsal horn could block the transmission of nociceptive stimuli conveyed by small unmyelinated C fibers and thinly myelinated Aδ fibers, thereby closing a conceptual gate to painful afferent stimuli located in the spinal cord. Their model originated from several observations on the sensory neural circuitry located in a crescent-shaped zone capping the dorsal horn known as the substantia gelatinosa (SG).

Pseudounipolar neurons of the dorsal root ganglion (DRG) conveyed painful stimuli along Aδ and C fibers from the periphery into the SG where they formed (1) excitatory synapses with secondary sensory neurons of the spinothalamic tract known as tract cells (TCs) and (2) inhibitory synapses with SG interneurons (INs) that in turn formed inhibitory synapses with TCs. These fibers therefore promoted transmission of painful signals via TCs by way of (1) direct excitation and (2) disinhibition.

Meanwhile, Aβ fibers carrying non-nociceptive signals bound for the dorsal columns (DC) were also observed to send collateral projections into the SG where they formed excitatory synapses with TCs and INs, both of them excitatory. It had been empirically demonstrated that early direct excitation of TCs at the Aβ-TC synapse was quickly overdriven by TC inhibition caused by excitatory signaling at the Aβ-IN synapse. Hence, the net effect of Aβ signaling in the dorsal horn was to block nociceptive transmission to secondary sensory neurons (TCs) of the spinothalamic tract through a mechanism of interneuron (IN)-mediated inhibition, thereby "closing the gate."

On the basis of these observations, Melzack and Wall speculated that by administering exogenous electrical stimulation to Aβ fibers, the spinothalamic gate could be closed as therapy for neuropathic pain. Figure 10.1 depicts a schematic of the gate control circuit similar to the one presented in the original article by Melzack and Wall.

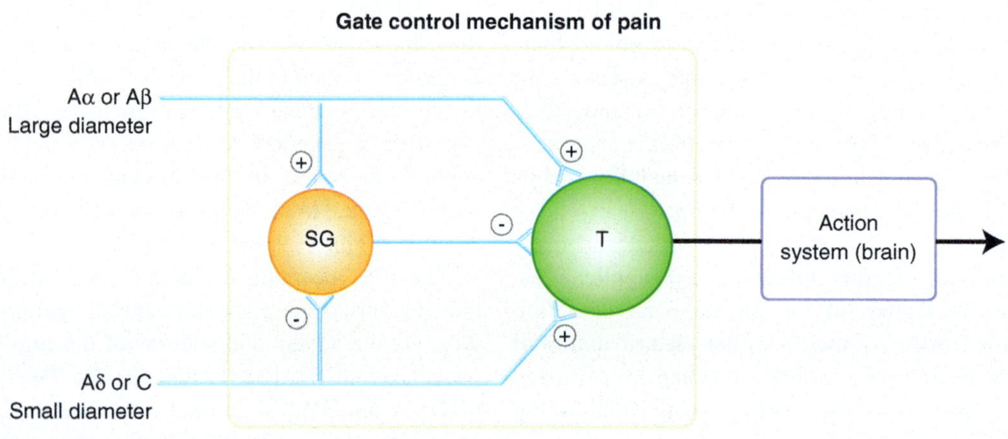

Fig. 10.1 Gate control schematic depicting large-diameter mechanoreceptive Aα and Aβ fibers and small-diameter Aδ and C fibers carrying pain and temperature signals, all entering the dorsal horn from the periphery in parallel, each synapsing on inhibitory interneurons of the substantia gelatinosa (SG) and secondary sensory spinothalamic neuron known as the tract cells (TCs) to form the gate circuitry. The net effect of input from the large fiber afferents is tract cell inhibition, which closes the gate to painful signals. The net effect of the small fiber afferents is TC excitation, which opens the gate to painful signals bound for the brain

Central Neuromodulation and Mechanisms of Action

Deep Brain Stimulation (DBS)

Deep brain stimulation (DBS) is a form of neuromodulation in which current is delivered through electrodes stereotactically implanted into the parenchyma of subcortical brain structures. DBS was first introduced by Benabid et al. when in 1985 they successfully treated symptoms of Parkinson's disease (PD) by combining thalamotomy with neurostimulation of the bilateral ventral intermediate (VIM) thalamic nuclei. In addition to PD, DBS has subsequently been used to control symptoms of dystonia, epilepsy, depression, obsessive-compulsive disorder (OCD), and cluster headaches.

Although the exact mechanism of action remains elusive, DBS is thought to act via three mechanisms: (1) by inhibition, (2) by depolarization blockade, and (3) by adjustment of neural activity. In the first model, neurostimulation depolarizes axons in the target brain structure, thereby causing the release of inhibitory neurotransmitters. In the second model, neurostimulation depresses activity in the target tissue by hyperpolarizing neurons and therefore the electrical threshold needed to produce an action potential. Finally, DBS may induce a more regular and consistent firing in target tissue where electrical activity has become disordered by disease.

DBS has been used to effectively treat a wide swath of neuropsychiatric diseases with varying and often unknown cellular pathophysiology. For each clinical entity, a constellation of functionally linked neuroanatomic loci has been identified. Many single structures, however, have been shown to play crucial roles in multiple diseases. Although there is not yet FDA approval for the treatment of pain, research in DBS has shown it to be effective in the treatment of several types of centrally mediated pain syndromes. For example, the hypothalamus was a promising target for treatment of cluster headaches. Indeed, vigorous hypothalamic activation is known to occur during cluster headache, short lasting unilateral neuralgiform headache with conjunctival injection and tearing, hemicrania continua, and paroxysmal hemicranias. Although all of these entities have been treated successfully with DBS, the hypothalamus has been largely abandoned as a target due to the high rate of morbidity associated with hypothalamic lead deployment.

Motor Cortex Stimulation (MCS)

Electrical stimulation of the cerebral motor cortex via overlying electrodes is known as motor cortex stimulation (MCS). MCS has been used in the treatment of burning central pain by removing the contralateral postcentral gyrus and the ipsilateral precentral gyrus when the pain returned, leading to the conclusion that both gyri were involved in mediating the pain. Although the exact mechanism of action is unclear, MCS is known to inhibit pain signal transmission in patients with central neuropathic pain. Positron-emission tomography (PET) scans using radiolabeled glucose as an index of cerebral blood flow have implicated the ventral, lateral, and medial thalamus as key structures. Other locations that experience increased blood flow under MCS are the anterior cingulate, the orbitofrontal cortices, the anterior insula, and the upper brainstem. It has therefore been hypothesized that MCS diminishes the perception of pain both by modulating the affective-emotional component of chronic pain and by activating descending inhibition of pain impulses through the brainstem.

Transcranial Magnetic Stimulation

Transcranial magnetic stimulation (TMS) is the use of the electromagnetic field generated by an electrical current to generate an electrical current in the target area of the brain by the physical process of electromagnetic induction. A coil placed over the scalp induces an electrical field, which can then be manipulated either to excite or inhibit the target tissue. Theoretical mechanisms of action for TMS on chronic pain include modulation of descending inhibition circuits in addition to effects on limbic circuitry. One significant limitation for TMS is the transient duration of analgesia; it is currently unclear whether TMS results in any permanent neuroplastic changes in pain processing.

Spinal Cord Stimulation (SCS)

Overview

Spinal cord stimulation is neurostimulation via electrodes placed into the epidural space, either percutaneously or by surgical laminotomy, and positioned to overlie the dorsal columns of the spinal cord. SCS is FDA approved for use in chronic intractable pain of the trunk and/or limbs, post-laminectomy syndrome, complex regional pain syndrome I and II (CRPS), chronic radiculopathy, painful neuropathies, chronic refractory angina, and peripheral ischemic limb pain, but it has been used to successfully treat many other pain entities. A more comprehensive list of the indications can be found in Table 10.1. SCS is thought to act via three broad classes of mechanisms, (1) neurophysiological, (2) neurochemical, and (3) vascular.

Neurophysiologic mechanisms are generally attributed to inhibitory control at the level of the dorsal horn and to supraspinal brainstem or thalamocortical mechanisms. Neurochemical mechanisms are thought to restore the

Table 10.1 Uses and indications for neurostimulation

Modality	Common indications	Other indications
Deep brain stimulation (DBS)	Parkinson's disease *Δ Essential tremor *Δ Obsessive-compulsive disorder *Δ Dystonia *Δ	Epilepsy Δ Depression Headaches Addiction disorder Severe obesity
Vagal nerve stimulation (VNS)	Drug-refractory epilepsy * Unipolar and bipolar depression * Cluster headache *	Migraine Δ Hemicrania continua Δ Medication-overuse headache Δ
Spinal cord stimulation (SCS)	Chronic intractable pain of the trunk and/or limbs, including post-laminectomy syndrome * Complex regional pain syndrome I and II * Chronic radicular pain * Painful neuropathies Refractory angina Δ Peripheral ischemic limb pain, refractory or not amenable to surgical bypass Δ	Intercostal neuralgia Spinal cord injury Arachnoiditis Central pain Nerve root avulsion Postherpetic neuralgia Phantom limb pain Abdominal pain Pelvic pain
Dorsal root ganglion (DRG) stimulation	Lower extremity pain secondary to complex regional pain syndrome I and II *Δ Chronic radicular pain	Perineal pain Phantom limb pain Chronic postsurgical knee pain Chronic visceral pain Upper limb neuropathic pain Painful diabetic neuropathy
Peripheral nerve stimulation (PNS)	Chronic pain of peripheral nerve etiology *Δ, including occipital neuralgia	Craniofacial pain Cluster headache Postherpetic neuralgia
Peripheral nerve field stimulation (PNFS)		Axial back pain Abdominal pain Pelvic pain Atypical facial pain

Single asterisk denotes current US Food and Drug Administration (FDA)-approved indications
Single triangle denotes an indication which has received Conformité Européenne (CE) mark

balance of inhibitory and excitatory neurotransmitters both at the segmental level as in the case of gamma-aminobutyric acid (GABA) and glutamate and via descending inhibitory pathways that release serotonin, substance P, and norepinephrine into the dorsal horn. Finally, vascular mechanisms are most pertinent in vascular diseases such as peripheral arterial disease and chronic refractory angina where SCS is thought to relieve pain by restoring the supply of oxygen through vasodilation and by reducing sympathetic tone.

Neurophysiologic Mechanisms of SCS

Stimulation of large myelinated primary sensory neurons in the dorsal cord provokes action potentials that originate at a node of Ranvier and propagate bidirectionally away from the stimulus. Antidromic impulses travel in the opposite direction of natural physiologic impulses. Orthodromic impulses travel in the same direction as natural physiologic impulses. In the case of SCS, orthodromic impulses are those that travel in a rostral direction toward supraspinal structures where Aβ fibers from the dorsal column synapse in the cuneate and gracile nuclei of the medulla, with subsequent impulses traveling to the thalamus and periaqueductal gray (PAG) (Figs. 10.2 and 10.3).

In the case of SCS, antidromic impulses travel in a caudad direction, back into the dorsal horn where they act in a spinal segmental manner by activating inhibitory neurons which then block transmission of nociceptive signals from C and Aδ fibers to secondary neurons known as tract cells. This spinal segmental mechanism is thought to be the primary mechanism by which classical SCS causes relief of neuropathic pain.

Orthodromic impulses are responsible for modulating supraspinal neurophysiologic mechanisms responsible for SCS-mediated pain control. These impulses are also responsible for the paresthesia experienced by patients undergoing SCS.

It is important to note that the paresthesias in and of themselves are not likely causing pain relief. In light of recent computational models conceptualizing the thalamus as a parallel processor for ascending sensory signals, one might speculate that the paresthesia generated in classic SCS causes a profusion of neutral sensory signals that "drown out" the perception of painful stimuli through lateral inhibition and direct signal competition in the thalamus. This, however, is unlikely because classic tonic stimulation typically produces mostly subthreshold presynaptic potentials in the thalamus,

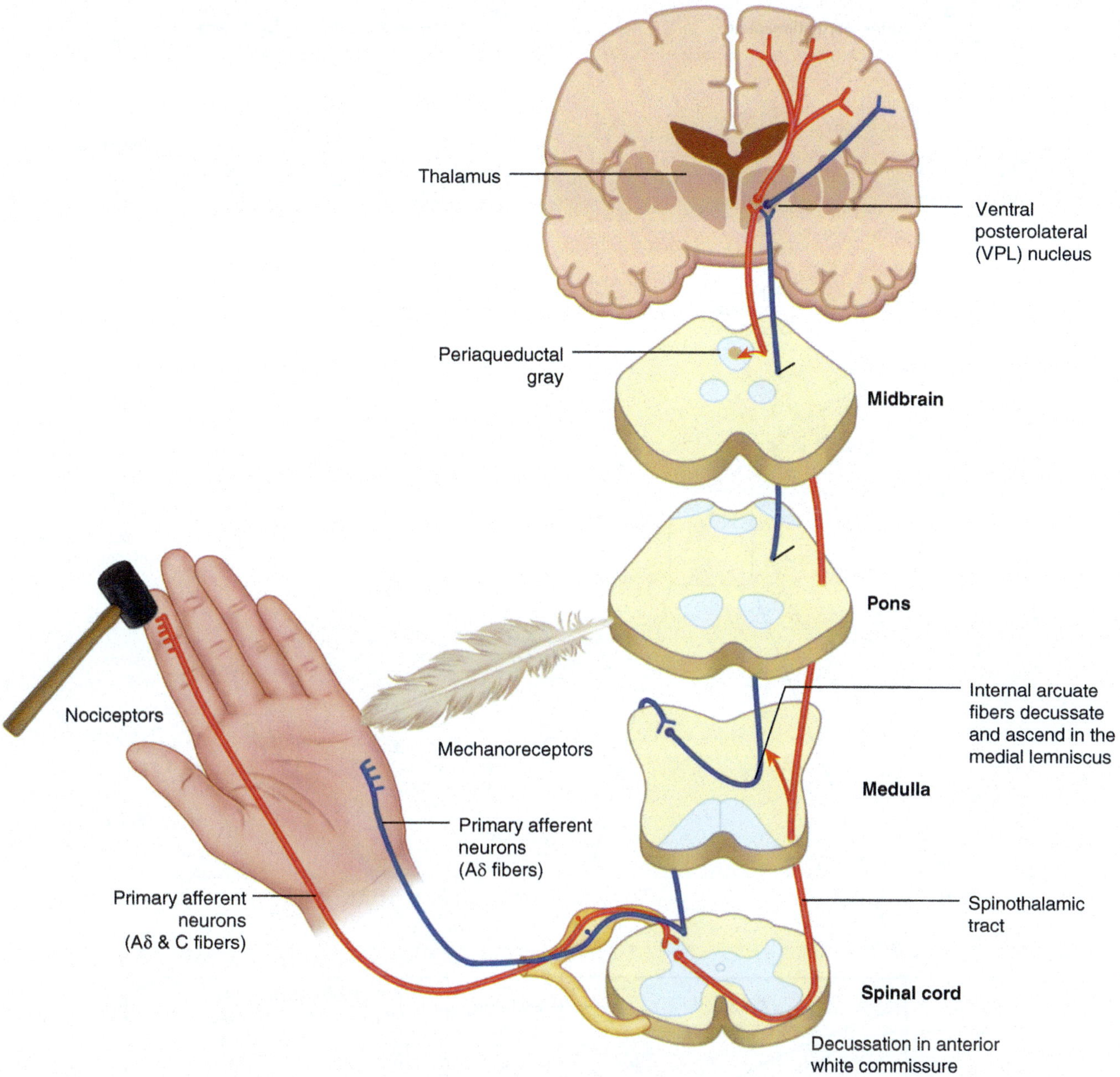

Fig. 10.2 Ascending sensory pathways: the dorsal column and spinothalamic tract. *Dorsal column (blue)*: the axons of pseudounipolar neurons of the DRG carrying fine touch, vibration, pressure, and proprioception along from the periphery along Aα and Aβ fibers enter the white matter tracts of the ipsilateral dorsal column and travel to the medulla where they synapse on second-order neurons in the gracile and cuneate nuclei. These secondary neurons then decussate as internal arcuate fibers to form the medial lemniscus and travel through the pons and form synapses with third-order sensory neurons in the thalamus. Axons coming from the body synapse in the ventral posterolateral nucleus and those from the head synapse in the ventral posteromedial nucleus. Axons of thalamic third-order neurons then travel to the primary somatosensory cortex. *Spinothalamic tract (red)*: the axons of pseudounipolar sensory neurons of the dorsal root ganglion carrying pain and temperature stimuli along Aδ and C fibers project into the dorsal horn and typically rise one to two spinal segments via Lissauer's tract where they synapse on secondary neurons known as tract cells in the substantia gelatinosa or the nucleus proprius. These tract cells give off axons which decussate via the anterior white commissure and then travel to the anterolateral quadrant of the spinal cord where fibers carrying pain and temperature enter the lateral spinothalamic tract and fibers carrying crude touch and firm pressure enter the anterior spinothalamic tract. These axons then travel up the spinal cord, through the rostral ventromedial medulla, and into the thalamus where they synapse with third-order neurons in several thalamic nuclei, including the medial dorsal, ventral posterior lateral, and ventral posterior medial nuclei. These signals are then conveyed to the cingulate cortex, the primary somatosensory cortex, and the insular cortex, respectively. These thalamocortical projections are functionally divided into two subsystems known as the direct system, for the conscious appreciation of pain, and the indirect system, which is responsible unconscious processing of pain. The indirect system is divided into spino-reticulo-thalamo-cortical circuits responsible for arousal and the spino-mesencephalic-limbic circuits responsible for the affective impact of pain

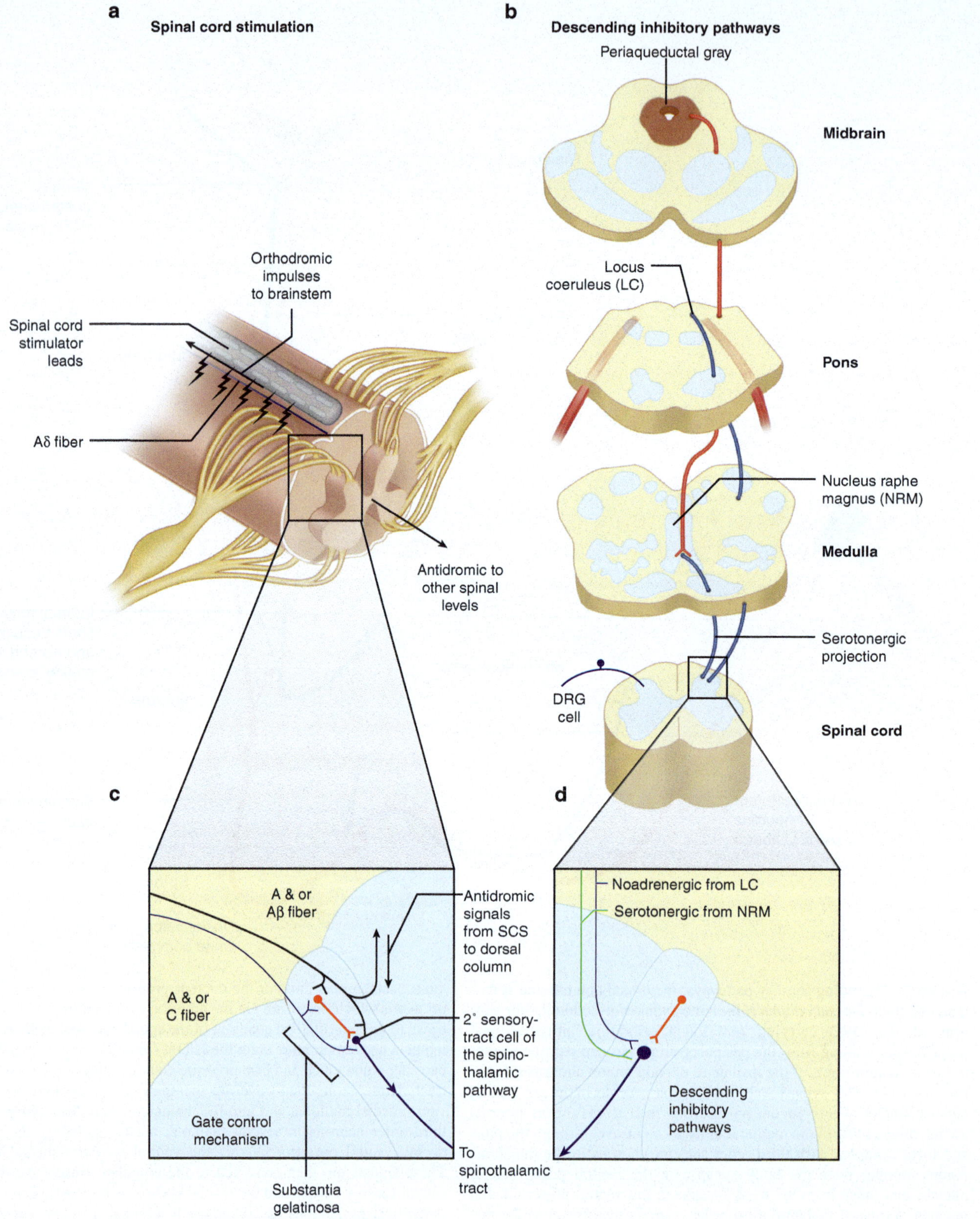

Fig. 10.3 (**a**) Spinal cord section with SCS leads overlying the dorsal columns triggering an ascending orthodromic impulse bound for the medulla and a descending antidromic impulse descending along the same Aβ fiber and into the dorsal horn, thereby closing the gate. (**b**) Gate control neurocircuitry in situ. (**c**) Descending supraspinal inhibitory pathways originating in the periaqueductal gray (PAG) and the medulla where noradrenergic and serotonergic neurons of the locus ceruleus (LC) and the nucleus raphe magnus (NRM) are located, respectively. Through caudad projections that descend along the dorsal columns and terminate in the dorsal horn, these nuclei exert supraspinal neurochemical pain control by secreting inhibitory substance P, norepinephrine, and serotonin into the SG, thereby stabilizing the gate. (**d**) Inhibitory fibers synapsing on a tract cell in the dorsal horn

suggesting that the need for overlap is more of an incidental phenomenon which at most can serve as a perceptual marker that the antidromic signals closing the gate in the dorsal horn have been correctly mapped to the affected dermatomal distribution. Indeed, in order to close the gate on a particular distribution of aberrant nociceptive C and Aδ fibers, Aβ fibers that directly form circuits with those neurons in the dorsal horn and therefore originate in the same dermatome must be stimulated.

However, there are supraspinal mechanisms through which classical SCS is thought to achieve pain relief. One experimental study performed by El-Khoury achieved pain relief by stimulation of sites rostral to various spinal cord lesions, thereby preventing the contribution of an antidromic process to analgesia. This finding implicates higher-order pain relief caused by modulation of sensory-discriminatory elements of pain at the level of the brainstem and also modulation of affective-emotional elements of pain at the level of thalamocortical circuits.

Ultimately, the experimental and clinical data suggest that classical SCS relieves neuropathic pain predominantly through modulation of gating mechanisms at the spinal segmental level. Indeed, one experimental pain model found that DC SCS at the level where an injured sciatic nerve entered the spinal cord was more effective than more rostral stimulation. This notion has been empirically supported through the mapping of the most effective sites for electrode placement.

Neurophysiologic Mechanisms of SCS: Subthreshold Versus Suprathreshold Stimulation

In the context of this topic, any neurostimulation delivered at amplitude that fails to create paresthesia is considered to be *subthreshold*. Likewise, any electrical stimulus with an amplitude sufficient to generate paresthesia is considered to be *suprathreshold*.

Subthreshold SCS at high frequency (10 kHz) has been shown to reduce the excitability of lamina I pain projection neurons when compared to sham in an in vivo model, but its exact mode of action remains unclear. Although this form of SCS has performed well in several large prospective clinical trials, as of the writing of this chapter, the PROCO trial has just released data suggesting there is no clinical benefit conferred by high-frequency stimulation.

In addition to the mechanisms described above, suprathreshold SCS may also work through orthodromic signals that activate frank motor activity in peripheral motor nerves in patients with low-thoracic SCS systems. Efferent motor traffic has been observed even with low-intensity stimulation and is thought to be mediated by monosynaptic facilitation of spinal motor reflexes strong enough to generate orthodromic action potentials.

Neurophysiologic Mechanisms of SCS: Tonic Versus Burst Stimulation Patterns

Classical SCS utilizes tonic stimulation with single pulses in sequence, each with the same pulse width, pulse rate, and amplitude. However, single action potentials do not typically trigger enough central neurons to cause modulation at the level of the thalamus. Indeed, these central neurons must integrate the input from multiple presynaptic neurons in a process known as spatial summation in order to reach threshold. In this context, *threshold* is defined as the membrane voltage required to elicit an action potential. Hence, tonic pulse stimulation is most likely filtered out at the level of the thalamus as noise, only rising to thalamocortical circuits as isolated somatosensory signals. Therefore, classical SCS most likely exerts its main effects by affecting gating in the dorsal horn.

In contrast, it has been observed that through a process known as temporal summation or facilitation, short clusters of action potentials known as "bursts" can lead to the stacking of intracellular calcium concentration in a single presynaptic bouton causing sufficient neurotransmitter release to monosynaptically trigger a postsynaptic central neuron, thereby leading to meaningful signaling either through long-term potentiation (LTP) or long-term depression (LTD). One large prospective, RCT known as the SUNBURST trial found that burst stimulation as described by DeRidder is generally more effective than tonic stimulation and is associated with higher patient satisfaction. Burst stimulation received FDA approval in October 2016. Although its long-term efficacy has yet to be established, burst stimulation is a promising form of SCS which may lead to a new generation of paresthesia-free spinal cord stimulators acting both through pre-existing mechanisms and by a novel supraspinal mechanism, possibly at the level of the thalamus.

Neurochemical Mechanisms of SCS

In addition to the neurocircuitry-mediated gating mechanism described above, antidromic and orthodromic impulses from SCS also relieve neuropathic pain by spinal segmental and supraspinal mechanisms by restoring the balance of inhibitory and excitatory molecules in the neurochemical milieu of the dorsal horn to stabilize the gate via suppression of hyperexcitable nociceptive neurons.

At a spinal segmental level, antidromic impulses propagating along Aβ fibers enter the dorsal horn provoking release of inhibitory GABA, and reducing the release of glutamate, thereby restoring a neurochemical balance that more effectively suppresses the hyperexcitability of wide dynamic range (WDR) neurons that is thought to contribute substantially to central sensitization. These findings have been corroborated by a number of biochemical and anatomical studies of the dorsal horn.

SCS impulses propagated orthodromically along rostral dorsal column projections activate descending supraspinal inhibitory pathways originating in the periaqueductal gray (PAG) and medulla where aminergic neurons of the locus ceruleus (LC) and the nucleus raphe magnus (NRM). Through caudad projections that descend along the dorsal columns and terminate in the dorsal horn, these nuclei exert supraspinal neurochemical pain control by secreting inhibitory norepinephrine, serotonin, and substance P into the SG, thereby further stabilizing the gate.

Vascular Mechanisms of SCS

In the case of vascular diseases such as chronic refractory angina and peripheral artery disease, SCS acts by peripheral vasodilation and downregulation of efferent sympathetic activity. SCS has been shown to increase blood flow in dermatomes corresponding to the spinal segmental level of stimulation. This observation by Cook et al. was subsequently applied in the treatment of peripheral vascular disease and chronic refractory angina. Furthermore, Linderoth and Meyerson found that these effects were mediated both by antidromic activation of small-diameter fibers and by inhibition of sympathetic outflow. Later studies revealed that low-intensity SCS triggers antidromic action potentials along Aβ fibers which, acting indirectly through interneurons, trigger antidromic action potentials in unmyelinated afferent fibers that then migrate to the periphery where they cause the release of a powerful vasodilator known as calcitonin gene-related protein (CGRP) at peripheral nerve terminals. CGRP then activates endothelial nitric oxide synthesis and release, resulting in vascular smooth muscle relaxation and an increase in blood flow to the affected limb.

In the treatment of angina pectoris, SCS reduces anginal pain by redistributing coronary blood flow and by decreasing myocyte oxygen demand. Clinically, this is observed as an increase in the time to angina during exercise, an increased resistance to critical ischemia, and an anti-arrhythmic effect achieved through modulation of cardiac neurons. Notably, SCS does not mask the perception of true myocardial infarction. SCS has been shown to reduce cardiac nociceptive pain transmission, stabilize the cardiac conduction system, reduce infarct size through coronary flow redistribution, and reduce sympathetic outflow. In addition to reduced infarct size, the beneficial effect of SCS manifests as a reduced magnitude of ST segment changes during active ischemia and fewer atrial arrhythmias.

Higher-Order Supraspinal Mechanisms: The Pain Matrix

In addition to the brainstem and subcortical structures discussed above, SCS is thought to interact with and modulate a broader constellation of higher-order structures implicated in the modulation of pain. This group of functionally related, reciprocally interacting brain structures is known as the "pain matrix." The pain matrix consists of the anterior cingulate cortex (ACC), posterior cingulate cortex (PCC), prefrontal cortex (PFC), parietal somatosensory cortex, insula, thalamus, hypothalamus, amygdala, hippocampus, and periaqueductal gray (PAG). It is involved both in modulating the sensory-discriminatory element of pain at the level of the brainstem and in modulating the affective-emotional elements of pain at cortical and subcortical levels.

SCS has been shown to influence the activity of neurons in many of these structures, including the thalamus and somatosensory cortices. One PET study of nine patients with chronic neuropathic lower extremity pain revealed increases in cerebral blood flow to the contralateral thalamus, bilateral parietal association cortices, the anterior cingulate gyrus, and the prefrontal cortex, all components of the pain matrix. In the thalamus and parietal association cortices, SCS is thought to affect pain threshold. In the ACC and prefrontal areas, it may regulate the affective-emotional aspects of pain.

Another study used fMRI to examine the cortical and subcortical effects of SCS on ten patients with chronic pain, concluding that SCS reduces the affective component of pain by reducing the connectivity between somatosensory and limbic structures of the pain matrix, thereby disconnecting the purely sensory signals from structures known to attach affective-emotional salience to the pain.

SCS for Chronic Visceral Abdominal Pain

Chronic visceral abdominal pain evolves by similar mechanisms to those involved in peripheral sensitization in which tonic nociceptive stimulation leads to enlargement of receptive fields, increased recruitment of peripheral fibers, increase in the number of suprathreshold responses to sensory inputs, and spontaneous activation of neurons that are typically silent in response to nociceptive stimuli. The dorsal column has also been shown to transmit some visceral nociceptive afferents and can also amplify visceral pain.

Overall, the mechanism by which SCS achieves visceral abdominal pain relief is quite similar to that in somatic pain control. One unique mechanism, however, is that SCS suppresses the visceromotor response caused by colonic distention, thereby reducing the discomfort caused by gastrointestinal hypermotility and dysmotility. Both thoracic and lumbar lead placement in rat models have been shown to ablate the visceromotor response.

Clinically, SCS has been used to successfully treat mesenteric ischemic pain, esophageal dysmotility, gastroparesis, IBS, chronic pancreatitis, familial Mediterranean fever, posttraumatic splenectomy, generalized chronic abdominal pain, and chronic pelvic pain. However, there is a paucity of prospective, randomized controlled trial data to support widespread use at this time.

Mechanisms of SCS Non-responsiveness

Non-responsiveness to SCS in neuropathic pain is poorly understood. In the setting of CRPS, it occurs in roughly 1/3 of patients and has been reliably connected to the severity of allodynia. It is thought that severe allodynia arises from extreme depletion of the inhibitory neurotransmitter GABA in the dorsal horn. This has been demonstrated in a rat model where experimental depletion of inhibitory neurotransmitters caused severe allodynia that could not be alleviated by SCS. In another experimental study, the intrathecal delivery of the GABA-B agonist baclofen was shown to convert SCS non-responders into SCS responders.

The timing of SCS placement also appears to play a crucial role in its chances of success. Indeed, it has been clinically observed that SCS is most effective when started 7 months to 1 year after the onset of neuropathic pain. Central sensitization appears to play a role in the evolution of SCS non-responsiveness, as it is likely a progressive process mediated in part by the depletion of neurotransmitters essential to SCS responsiveness. One study found that SCS works in part by reversing GABA depletion and glutamate excess known to occur during early central sensitization. Another found that GABA supplementation soon after central cord injury could reverse hyperalgesia but could not do so later in the process. This model of central sensitization as a progressive disease process is borne out in the natural history of neuropathic pain syndromes. For example, after a period of rapid progression lasting around 1 year, the symptoms of CRPS I typically stabilize, thereafter progressing quite slowly or not at all.

The level of mechanical allodynia is a clinical predictor of SCS non-responsiveness. This observation may be related to the fact that mechanical allodynia is conveyed not by C or Aδ fibers, but by large myelinated Aβ fibers, only a small fraction of which are activated by SCS.

Finally, SCS failure may be attributable to suboptimal physical and technical factors, including but not limited to the inaccurate placement of electrodes and excessive thickness of the highly conductive intervening dorsal CSF layer, which can cause dorsal root fiber activation through lateral dispersion of the SCS current. The target site for stimulation depends on the neuroanatomy. Caudally, the dorsal column afferents are located at the surface of the cord, but more rostrally, they course ventrally, which typically makes caudal sites more sensible locations for electrode placement.

Dorsal Root Ganglion (DRG) Stimulation

With dorsal root ganglion (DRG) stimulation, pain control is achieved by placing an electrode, typically by an anterograde percutaneous approach, into the lateral recess of the neural foramen directly over the dorsal root ganglion. These leads are slim and flexible, allowing their placement without compression of the DRG itself.

Neuroanatomically, there are a number of factors that make the DRG an apt target for the neuromodulation of pain. First, it is a site where the bulk of ascending pain inputs, most of them bound for the spinothalamic tract, as well as neutral mechanoreceptive stimuli bound for the dorsal column, converge before somatotopically diverging to ventral and dorsal zones of the spinal cord. Its superficial dorsal location along a relatively thin overlying layer of dura mater and CSF and low surrounding tissue impedances render the DRG more susceptible to stimulation with lower energy levels that average around 15% of the power output required for dorsal column stimulation. The convergence of all sensory pathways at this point allows the stimulation of spinothalamic fibers that are typically inaccessible because they travel in close proximity to the descending motor neurons of the corticospinal tract. Targeting a single nerve root permits greater anatomic specificity for pain control, allowing the stimulator to focus on a foot or toe rather than an entire limb. Finally, paresthesia fields in DRG tend not to vary with position, a benefit that occurs because the lead is deployed into a bony vertebral foramen that is oriented at a 90-degree angle to the spinal cord.

DRG stimulation is thought to actively reduce the net nociceptive activity to the spinal cord by restoring the neural filtration function served by the normal DRG. Notably, this mechanism is distinct from the gate control mechanism by which activation of large-diameter sensory fibers blocks transmission of pain signals in small-diameter fibers at the level of the dorsal horn. Indeed, DRG stimulation appears to normalize peripheral input before it arrives at the gate.

DRG stimulation has demonstrated 1-year efficacy in the treatment of a number of clinical entities, including radicular pain, failed back surgery syndrome, complex regional pain syndrome of the lower extremities, and chronic postsurgical pain. The targeted nature of DRG stimulation allows the treatment of pain in subdermatomal distributions with precisely sculpted paresthesia fields. Examples include the treatment of foot and post-herniorrhaphy groin pain. Other case reports have described DRG stimulation as therapy for low back pain, postherpetic neuralgia, phantom limb pain, visceral pain, somatic body wall pain, upper extremity pain, complex regional pain syndrome of the knee, and postsurgical knee pain.

Peripheral Neuromodulation and Its Mechanisms of Action

Peripheral neuromodulation is possibly the most diverse and rapidly expanding area of neuromodulation. It is comprised of a variety of techniques including peripheral nerve stimulation, peripheral nerve field stimulation, transcutaneous electrical nerve stimulation, and functional electrical stimulation. Since the first percutaneous stimulator was used for chronic headaches in 1999, peripheral neuromodulation has been used to treat an ever-expanding variety of nerves and nerve plexuses to treat neuropathic, visceral, cardiac, abdominal, low back, and facial pain.

Peripheral Nerve Stimulation (PNS)

Peripheral nerve stimulation is a neuromodulation technique in which electrodes are placed percutaneously directly along the course of peripheral nerves and electrical current is applied to alleviate chronic pain. The prevailing hypothesis for the mechanism of pain-relieving action by PNS is via dorsal horn gate closure provoked by orthodromic action potentials that travel along Aβ fibers, entering the dorsal horn from the periphery. Just as with central neuromodulation, however, the mechanism likely varies based on the clinical entity being treated and its unique underlying physiology. PNS may also cause analgesia by neurochemical mechanisms by influencing the local concentration of neurotransmitters, neuromodulators, and inflammatory molecules that mediate the pain response. Animal studies have revealed that repeated stimulation of peripheral nerves results in decreased C-fiber response to pain at the level of the spinal cord.

At low-frequency stimulation, PNS is believed both to modulate downstream nociceptors and to promote favorable central pain processing upstream. Low-frequency stimulation of Aδ fibers in a rat model caused long-term depression of monosynaptic and polysynaptic excitatory postsynaptic potentials in the substantia gelatinosa. In a cat model, stimulation of the posterior tibial and sciatic nerves resulted in decreased C-fiber response to pain at the level of the spinal cord, thereby implicating a spinal pathway. At ultrahigh stimulation frequencies, PNS is thought to cause direct blockade of the peripheral nerve.

A promising development in the field of PNS has been the discovery that, unlike SCS, it may have antinociceptive properties extending beyond ischemic pain. Ellrich and Lamp used laser infrared stimuli to activate Aδ and C fibers in the superficial radial nerves of human subjects. Laser stimulation provoked painful prickling sensations, and associated cortical evoked potentials were observed. However, when peripheral stimulation was applied, the same painful stimulus provoked a diminished perception of pain and was associated with reduced evoked potentials and latencies.

Headache: Occipital Nerve Stimulation for Occipital Neuralgia, Chronic Migraine, and Cluster Headache

The mechanism of action of ONS in occipital neuralgia and chronic migraine relies on the anatomic convergence of trigeminal, dural, and cervical afferents in the brainstem. Experimentally, it has been shown that activation of afferents from the caudal trigeminal nucleus at the level of C2 can induce pain in the trigeminal and cervical distributions. Therefore, electrical stimulation of the occipital nerves, which is superficial and easily accessed branch of C2, can be used to modulate pain in those distributions. A PET study of eight patients with chronic migraines treated with ONS demonstrated changes in regional blood flow to the dorsal rostral pons, the anterior cingulate cortex, and the cuneus, all structures involved in central pain processing. The clinical efficacy of ONS has been evaluated by three large controlled studies, the ONSTIM and PRISM trials, and another randomized study with mixed results.

Sphenopalatine Ganglion (SPG) Stimulation for Cluster Headaches

Another target of interest for PNS in the treatment of refractory cluster headaches is the sphenopalatine ganglion (SPG), which lies in the pterygopalatine fossa providing postganglionic innervation and sensation to the facial, meningeal, and cerebral blood vessels. Local ischemia caused by vasospasm of these vessels is thought to underlie the pain caused by cluster headaches. Furthermore, cluster headaches have been successfully treated by SPG blockade and radioablation, and animal models have shown that SPG stimulation can increase regional blood flow, thereby reversing vasospastic ischemia.

Trigeminal, Facial, and Mandibular Nerve Stimulation for Facial Pain

PNS has been used to treat facial pain in a variety of conditions and involves stimulation of the peripheral nerves that provide sensory innervation to the painful area. Electrodes have also been placed in the V1, V2, and V3 trigeminal distributions to achieve pain relief in trigeminal neuralgia. Direct stimulation of the trigeminal ganglion has also been performed for trigeminal neuralgia, poststroke pain, peripheral nerve injury, and postherpetic neuralgia.

One case series studied PNS for poststroke facial pain and postherpetic neuralgia with five of seven in the poststroke group experiencing relief and none of those in the postherpetic neuralgia group experiencing pain relief.

Single Nerve and Nerve Plexus Pain

Through the use of motor stimulation, ultrasound, and anatomical landmarks, percutaneous electrodes can now safely be placed along any number of painful peripheral nerves or nerve plexuses. The first reports included supraorbital implantation, but an expanding variety of single peripheral nerves have now been reported including median, ulnar, sciatic, genitofemoral, and ilioinguinal.

Peripheral Nerve Field Stimulation (PNFS)

Many patients have neuropathic pain occurring in non-dermatomal distributions, instead of occurring in areas that either span multiple dermatomes or where the receptive fields of several peripheral nerves overlap. In such cases, SCS and PNS can fail to capture the irregular pain patterns, while PNFS can at times provide relief. PNFS does not target a specific nerve or sensory distribution. Instead, the lead is positioned within the tissue in order to stimulate the network of cutaneous afferents that delineate an area of pain. PNFS is thought to cause analgesia either by orthodromic Aβ-mediated gating mechanisms in the dorsal horn or by provoking the release of endorphins. By placing the electrode at the epicenter of pain, relief can often be provided to an entire painful area.

Transcutaneous Electrical Nerve Stimulation (TENS)

TENS is a form of neuromodulation in which electrical stimulation is delivered by adhesive leads placed on the skin over painful areas. More recently, TENS has emerged as a moderately effective treatment for pain. TENS is thought to act via local, spinal, and supraspinal pathways. Low-frequency TENS (<10 Hz) appears to promote signaling via u-opioid, GABA, serotonin, M1, and M3 receptors. The evolution of tolerance to TENS suggests the involvement of descending inhibitory pathways as well.

Functional Electrical Stimulation (FES)

Functional electrical stimulation (FES) is the transcutaneous application of controlled electrical stimulation to generate contractions and functional movement in paralyzed muscles, thereby facilitating and improving the mobility of limbs, and other body functions lost due to injury, including respiratory, sexual, bladder, and bowel function. This is an emerging technology recently improved with brain-computer interfacing that is thought to reduce pain and improve function by work by restoring the activity of deconditioned and unused muscles.

Vagal Nerve Stimulation (VNS)

Vagal nerve stimulation (VNS) is electrical stimulation of the left vagal nerve. VNS has a well-established role in the treatment of epilepsy, but a possible application in the treatment of pain has emerged more recently. Its mechanism of action is unknown, but is thought to be related to synchronization and desynchronization of vagal sensory afferents with cerebral activity.

Medial Branch of the Dorsal Rami of Spinal Nerves

The medial branches of the dorsal rami of spinal nerves provide sensation to the facet joints and motor innervation of the multifidi, small deep spinal muscles known to play a role in local segmental spinal stability and proprioception. Ultrasound and EMG studies have shown that multifidi atrophy and fail to fire appropriately after back injuries. These changes are thought to cause instability that renders subjects more susceptible to repeated back injuries and chronic pain. A new device is being developed to electrically stimulate these muscles with the hope of treating axial back pain by restoring dynamic spinal stability.

Key Points

- The use of electrical stimulation to treat pain is a century-old practice.
- To understand the mechanisms of neuromodulation, it is crucial to first understand the neurophysiological, neurochemical, and vascular processes and the neuroanatomy pertinent to the transmission of pain, both in disease and in health.
- Spinal cord stimulation and other forms of neuromodulation work through multiple mechanisms which can be categorized by type of process (neurophysiological, neurochemical, and vascular) and also by anatomy (local, spinal segmental, and supraspinal).
- The prevailing mechanism of action leading to neurostimulation-mediated pain relief often varies based on the pathophysiology of the underlying painful disease state.
- Gate control theory postulates that activation of large-diameter sensory fibers could block the transmission of pain signals conveyed by small-diameter fibers and is the target of action for multiple forms of central and peripheral neurostimulation.
- There is a preponderance of data to support the efficacy of neurostimulation and to corroborate its underlying mechanisms of action, but much investigation still needs to be done. The most well-validated form of neuromodulation is spinal cord stimulation.
- Neurostimulation is likely to continue to expand in importance over the coming years.

Recommended Reading

1. Ashkan K, Rogers P, Bergman H, Ughratdar I. Insights into the mechanisms of deep brain stimulation. Nat Rev Neurol. 2017;13:548.
2. Chang Chien GC, Mekhail N. Alternate intraspinal targets for spinal cord stimulation: a systematic review. Neuromodulation. 2017;20:629–41.
3. Gildenberg PL. History of pain management. In: A history of neurosurgery. Park Ridge: American Association of Neurological Surgeons; 1997. p. 439–64.
4. Goroszeniuk T, Pang D. Peripheral neuromodulation: a review. Curr Pain Headache Rep. 2014;18(5):412.
5. Imran TF, Malapero R, Qavi AH, Hasan Z, de la Torre B, Patel YR, Yong RJ, Djousse L, Gaziano JM, Gerhard-Herman MD. Efficacy of spinal cord stimulation as an adjunct therapy for chronic refractory angina pectoris. Int J Cardiol. 2017;227:535–42.
6. Lee S, Abd-Elsayed A. Some Non-FDA approved uses for neuromodulation: a review of the evidence. Pain Pract. 2016;16(7):935–47.
7. Liem L. Stimulation of the dorsal root ganglion. In: Stimulation of the peripheral nervous system, vol. 29. Basel: Karger Publishers; 2016. p. 213–24.
8. Melzack R, Wall PD. Pain mechanisms: a new theory. Surv Anesthesiol. 1967;11(2):89–90.
9. Shamji MF, De Vos C, Sharan A. The advancing role of neuromodulation for the management of chronic treatment-refractory pain. Neurosurgery. 2017;80(3S):S108–13.
10. Shealy CN, Mortimer JT, Resnick JB. Electrical inhibition of pain by stimulation of the dorsal columns: preliminary clinical reports. Anesth Analg. 1967;46(4):489–91.
11. Vallejo R, Bradley K, Kapural L. Spinal cord stimulation in chronic pain: mode of action. Spine. 2017;42:S53–60.

Part III

Psychology of Pain

The Normal Response to Pain

11

Randall P. Brewer

Introduction

Under normal physiological, and psychological, conditions, the presence of pain is concurrent with significant physical injury or the presence of physical conditions which will become injurious if an appropriate defensive action or a *normal response to pain* does not occur. According to the International Association for the Study of Pain, pain is "an unpleasant sensory and emotional experience associated with actual or potential tissue damage, or described in terms of such damage," so the appropriate response to pain would necessarily include (1) optimal utilization of the sensory experience to identify and distinguish potential versus presence of tissue damage, (2) while engaging physiological, psychological, and sociological resources to reduce unpleasantness, and (3) the development and implementation of an action plan that both ensures the recovery from the injury and prevents the development of subsequent harm.

The biological role of pain during a threat to the integrity of an individual's existence can be summarized by the three P's: (1) protect, (2) preserve, and (3) prevent. *Protection* is made possible via the acute stress response of "fight or flight," while the ensuing normal pain response allows for *preservation* (restoration of the individual and function of injured tissue) and the *prevention* of future injury (or threat) manifested in future behaviors resulting from learned adaptions. Thus, the normal response to pain is to provide optimum conditions for an individual to restore physical, physiological, and psychological homeostasis. Following a brief period of stress associated with pain, without serious tissue damage, the normal response to pain is the efficient restoration of homeostasis and the complete elimination of both the sensory and emotional experience of pain. Following periods of more significant tissue injury, where there is a need for resources to mount a sustained recovery, the normal experience of pain is shaped by a myriad array of physical, psychological, and sociological factors which, under normal circumstances, allows the individual the most optimal opportunity for the return to pre-injury function without ongoing physiological stress, including the experience of pain. The process of regular physiologic maintenance during conditions of chronic biological stress has been termed allostasis. In many respects, the condition of chronic pain is the process of nervous system allostatic regulation of the very important protective function of pain.

Background and Historical Perspective

The historical study of the response to pain followed centuries of biological inquiry into the more objective realms of human disease, with pain considered an inseparable entity from underlying causative disease states. Not until 1911 was the cerebral cortex believed to play a major role in pain perception in both the continued presence of pain responsiveness following traumatic brain injury 5 and during early epilepsy surgery 9. Head and Holmes also put forth the idea that the thalamus was responsible for pain "perception" and the role of the cerebral cortex was that of pain discrimination and modulation. Dejerine and Roussy offered the contrasting opinion that pain "perception" was mediated by the cerebral cortex. Melzack and Casey, in 1965, further refined that the nature of the brain's response to pain by acknowledging both sensory/discriminative and emotional/affective components of the pain experience and the brain's response to pain involved the simultaneous activation of multiple brain regions which determined the individual's experience of pain. Wall and Melzack further postulated the spinal modulatory response to pain with their famous theory of the "Gate Control Theory of Pain"

R. P. Brewer (✉)
Department of Anesthesiology, Duke University School of Medicine, Durham, NC, USA

Departments of Neurology and Anesthesiology, Louisiana State University School of Medicine, Shreveport, LA, USA

River Cities Interventional Pain Specialists, Shreveport, LA, USA
e-mail: brewer.randall@duke.edu

T. R. Deer et al. (eds.), *Deer's Treatment of Pain*, https://doi.org/10.1007/978-3-030-12281-2_11

that later became substantiated as a major founding principle in the understanding and treatment of pain through the natural adaptive phenomenon of pain modulation.

A discussion of the history of the physiological response to pain directs learners to the discovery of the autonomic nervous system, much attributed to Galen, and the neurohormonal response to stress which was championed by Hans Selye. While the psychological components of the human pain experience continue to undergo vast research and refinement of traditional assumptions, the contributions of pioneers such as Dennis Turk continue to represent the fundamental pillars upon which stands our growing understanding of the normal, or more appropriately "typical," response to persistent pain.

Normal Nociception and Its Physiological Response

In clinical practice, an understanding of the individual's "normal response" to pain must be approached not only by a thorough understanding of the pathological process(es) threatening or generating "tissue damage" but also through the individual's unique physical, psychological, and sociological factors which, in large part, govern the allostatic process of recovery and re-injury prevention.

The Peripheral Response to Pain

The response of the peripheral nervous system to pain involves the activation of peripheral nociceptors by painful stimuli. The type of nociceptor activation depends upon the degree of stimulation and the ensuing nature of the pain-eliciting condition. For mechanical pain, high-threshold mechanoreceptors become activated with sufficient mechanical or physical injury or stress to mechanically sensitive tissues, such as the muscle, connective tissue, and bone. In the normal state, the mechanical pain thresholds vary according to tissue type, for example, the mechanical thresholds for nociception lower substantially on sensitive tissues, such as the cornea, and tympanic membrane compared to thresholds in body regions where discriminative sensation is important for normal function, such as the hands and feet. In the presence of chemical mediators of pain, substances released in response to tissue injury (prostaglandins, bradykinin, adenosine triphosphate, protons, epinephrine, histamine, serotonin, nerve growth factor), the thresholds for nociceptor activation, become lowered in the area of injury and inflammation. The duration and spread of nociception from an initial injury depend upon many factors, such as the presence of secondary injury, and host factors such as immune status and hereditary factors. In normal conditions of tissue injury, the phenomenon of peripheral sensitization occurs which lowers the threshold for the subsequent experience of pain in the region of injury. This process of primary and secondary hyperalgesia, mediated by changes in peripheral nociceptor sensitivity with the additional recruitment of spinal pain facilitating pathways, allows the individual the best opportunity for rapid recognition of tissue threat or injury and allows the central nervous system to take immediate action to mitigate harm and promote recovery.

Transduction, Transmission, and Modulation

The normal response to pain transduction is the transmission of pain via the peripheral and central nervous system for "pain processing." Normally, pain processing entails the rapid localization of the pain stimulus and a simultaneous, accompanying behavioral or "motor" response (such as the spinal pain withdrawal reflex) offering the greatest opportunity for the organism to take action to avoid (further) injury and promote recovery. Following transmission into the dorsal horn of the spinal cord, the normal response occurs at the level of both ascending and descending neural responses aimed to both facilitate and modulate an ongoing pain stimulus. Transmission of pain signals occurs primarily via small myelinated and unmyelinated peripheral sensory axons into the dorsal horn of the spinal cord where a complex process of *pain projection* determines the relative weight of peripheral information transmitted via dorsal column pathways, such as the spinothalamic tract, into the pain processing regions of the brainstem and cerebrum for further refinement and processing. This process of information transmission is subject to *modulation* of the information which includes both the enhancement of the strength of the pain information (facilitation or enhancement) and suppression of the peripheral information (suppression or inhibition).

The Response of the Brain to Pain The normal response to acute pain stimuli, in humans, has been documented in numerous studies utilizing functional brain imaging techniques, such as functional magnetic resonance imaging, electroencephalographic dipole analysis, positron emission tomography, and single-photon emission computed tomography. From these studies, an extensive cortical-subcortical network of pain perception and processing has emerged that includes sensory, limbic, associative, and motor areas of the cerebral hemispheres. Activated regions include the insular cortex, somatosensory cortex, prefrontal cortex, anterior cingulate cortex (ACC), thalamus, and cerebellum. From spinal cord projections into the brainstem and thalamic nuclei, numerous cortical regions receive both direct and indirect nociceptive input. The primary somatosensory cortex receives input from the somatosensory (ventral posterior) thalamus, conveying the discriminative aspects of nociception, such as spatial, temporal, and intensity aspects of pain. Medial thalamic nuclei, as well as other ventral and interlaminar thalamic nuclei, project nociceptive input into the anterior cingulate cortex, a cortical region believed to be important in attention and the emotional/affective experience. The posterior cingulate cortex, receiving direct nociceptive input, projects to the motor cortex and supplemental motor area, providing immediate, direct circuitry for the initiation of behavioral motor responses to painful stimuli. The dorsolateral prefrontal cortex also receives significant nociceptive input from the medial thalamus.

Activated by stress (internal or external), the limbic and paralimbic regions of the paleocortex are believed to play a role in the motivational and affective components of pain. Neurologists have observed individuals with lesions of the somatosensory cortex display pain "unpleasantness" without the accompanying ability to localize or qualify the pain experience. Studies of the anterior cingulate cortex also support a prominent role for this cortical region in "aversive learning" through its role in attention and affective assignment to pain stimuli. Patients without functional interhemispheric connections between the cingulate cortices, such as with agenesis of the corpus callosum, and patients post-cingulotomy display reduced "unpleasantness" associated pain behaviors and attention to pain with retention of discriminative information such as pain location, intensity, and quality.

The insula has been demonstrated to be involved in memory, motor integration, and emotional responses to pain. The posterior insular cortex receives dense nociceptive afferents from spinothalamic input, and the anterior insula is believed to have a role in the subjective (and affective) experience of pain intensity. Stimulation of and lesions involving the posterior insular cortex has been reported to be associated with very specific, localized pain responses. The insular cortex also plays a role in the autonomic response to pain invoking a "homeostatic behavioral drive." Thus the insular cortex functions in the important role of integrating the emotional, behavioral, and autonomic responses to pain with pain intensity and localization. The areas of the insula activated during a pain stimulus can be divided between those areas encoding localization and those encoding magnitude or intensity.

The prefrontal cortex, receiving input from the anterior cingulate, orbitofrontal cortex, and amygdala, is believed to modulate the cognitive response to pain upon the consequences of pain or "suffering" and modulates descending inhibitory input. Reciprocal spinal connections with multiple subcortical structures are important in nociceptive transmission and modulation that include bidirectional spinal cord communication with the cerebellum, caudate nucleus, putamen, nucleus accumbens, parabrachial nucleus, periaqueductal gray (PAG) matter, and amygdala.

Despite the phenomena of "convergence" in pain transmission into the nervous system through consistent pathways from a variety of stimuli, humans are able to distinguish a wide diversity of pain subtypes and assign meaning while integrating pain intensity, quality, and location. This phenomenon occurs despite the activation of similar brain regions from varying types of pain stimuli, such as pressure, cold, heat, visceral, and cutaneous nociception. Temporal assessment of pain occurs primarily at the level of the secondary somatosensory cortex and adjacent insula.

The concept of pain facilitation relates to the facilitation of the initial pain response for further evaluation for a successful action plan to enhance survival and recovery. The initial transmission of "first pain" correlates to activation of the primary somatosensory cortex, whereas "second pain" correlates more closely with activation of the anterior cingulate, with both pain phenomena leading to activation of S2. First pain identifies the presence and location of pain; second pain prepares an individual for action to eliminate the threat of further harm, by activating attention and behavioral responses to limit injury and optimize recovery. With ongoing stimulation, the perception of pain intensity and unpleasantness increases with time. In experimental models, initial activation of the ACC and amygdala occurs during the prediction of a painful stimulus and is followed by activity in the thalamus, basal ganglia, prefrontal cortex (PFC), insula, and supplementary motor area and later activation of association cortex-ventral prefrontal cortex, inferior parietal cortex, and magnitude-coding region of the insula. The initial activation of the amygdala with input pertaining to pain intensity from other regions triggers the subsequent activation, and modulates extent, of the hypothalamic stress response system of autonomic activation. Table 11.1 summarizes the central connectivity of the brain's "pain matrix" governing the pain experience.

Pain Modulation Modulation is a normal response to pain. In situations of life-threatening stress with ongoing, concurrent autonomic activation, such as during combat or extreme physical activity, it has been well established that significant tissue damage may coexist with minimal or no associated perception of "pain." It is the modification of the various factors giving a pain stimulus context that determines the subsequent behavioral context of pain. Cognitive, affective/behavioral context, and memory (past experience of pain) functions are integrated which enable the prioritization of nociceptive stimulation. The presence of both pain facilitation and pain inhibitory influences allows for the affective/behavior and cognitive/evaluative responses to pain to best match the external circumstances such that avoidance of further harm via escape (inhibition) may be weighed against the need to rest and attend to the injury (facilitation) for necessary care or mitigation of secondary harm, i.e., protection, preservation, and prevention.

Table 11.1 The major brain structures, connectivity, and functional roles in pain processing

Cortical regions	Cortical/subcortical inputs	Projections	Role in pain afferent processing	Role in pain behavior
Primary somatosensory	Spinothalamic Thalamocortical (ventral posterior)	Parietal cortex, secondary somatosensory cortex	Sensory-discriminative	Localization, intensity, quality, temporal assignment
Secondary somatosensory cortex	Spinothalamic Thalamocortical (ventral posterior)	Primary somatosensory cortex, posterior cingulate cortex, insula	Sensory-discriminative	Primary receiving area for nociceptive information
Anterior cingulate	Medial and ventral thalamocortical, insula, posterior cingulate cortex, prefrontal cortex	Posterior cingulate cortex, prefrontal cortex, amygdala	Affective-motivational	Unpleasantness Attention
Insular cortex	Spinothalamic Thalamocortical, secondary somatosensory	Amygdala, anterior cingulate	Sensory integration, memory, behavioral	Pain localization, pain intensity/magnitude, autonomic and behavioral responses
Prefrontal cortex	Amygdala, anterior cingulate, orbitofrontal cortex	Anterior cingulate, basal ganglia	Somatic pain perception, cognitive response, emotional modulation	Modulates pain perception, reduces pain "suffering"
Posterior cingulate	Spinothalamic Thalamocortical	Orbitofrontal cortex, insula, anterior cingulate	Spinothalamic input into motor area	Control of motor responses, emotional evaluation, memory processing
Orbitofrontal cortex	Medial thalamus, nucleus accumbens, midbrain nuclei	Amygdala, limbic, sensory, and motor cortex	Processed sensory input	Affective facilitation of pain perception, reward behavior
Amygdala	Parabrachial nucleus, anterior cingulate cortex, insula	Prefrontal cortex, orbitofrontal cortex	Pain affect	Pain behavior
Superior parietal cortex	Sensory cortex, thalamus	Motor association cortex	Attentional modulation	Pain behavior

Modulation of pain occurs initially in the dorsal horn of the spinal cord via intrinsic "gate" mechanisms, as well as descending inhibition from brainstem nuclei, such as the PAG and rostroventral medulla (RVM). Cortical mechanisms contribute to pain modulation via direct influence brainstem modulation and within cortical interconnections. Descending modulation via the release of endogenous opioids through activation of the PAG and RVM occurs via ACC input into the PFC (directly to the PAG) and via the insula through connections to the amygdala.

Psychologically, modulatory states allow for either increased to attention to the painful stimulus or distraction away from the stimulus, depending upon the external circumstances and the need for either direction of attention and behavior toward escape (low attention with aversive behavior) or recovery (high attention state with protective or "guarding" behavior).

The affective, or emotional state, of the individual can influence the initial experience of pain. Experimental pain stimulation of individuals with simultaneous negative emotional state induction results in a disproportionate increase in pain unpleasantness as compared to intensity and discriminative ratings. Functional brain imaging suggests the emotional modulation of the unpleasantness of the pain experience is related primarily to the activation of prefrontal cortex-ACC-PAG circuitry and "attentional" modulation of pain is related to superior parietal cortex activation. Attention (insular cortex and superior, posterior parietal activity) to a painful stimulus preferentially modulates pain intensity via activity in the anterior insular cortex with simultaneous evaluation of pain intensity. The affective state during the pain stimulus is modulated by activity in the PFC and ACC with pain unpleasantness measures correlating with negative affective states.

Functional imaging studies have confirmed that central modulatory circuitry can be activated independently of peripheral input. For example, pain expectation can recreate the brain imaging signature of experimental pain (activation of PAG, PFC, and ventral striatum). Anticipation of pain relief (the placebo response) is associated with a similar pattern of activation that is associated with opioid-induced pain modulation (ACC-PFC-PAG-RVM), and the placebo/opioid pattern of activation is reversed or inhibited by naloxone.

During the acute phase of an injury, the presence of the initial stress response (and environmental context) determines whether the individual is required to attend to the environment (*distraction* away from the painful stimulus) or direct attention toward the injury (directing attention away from the environment and toward the injury). Experimental pain studies have demonstrated that attention to a painful stimulus increases pain intensity and distraction reduces it with descending pathways modulating attention-induced nociceptive facilitation. Likewise, human imaging studies have demonstrated activation of modulatory pathways (ACC and PAG) during distraction-mediated nociceptive suppression.

As noted in clinical experience, the process of modulation following an acute injury is extremely efficient with the acute experience of pain waning over a predictable course, according to the site and extent of tissue injury despite active inflammation and healing such that any occurrence of secondary issue, such as a postoperative infection, allows for the identification of further threats.

The phenomenon of pain *expectation* plays a prominent role in the experience of pain. Anticipation and pain perceptive clues increase pain intensity, imaging reveals activation of the rostral AC and IC, and experimental models suggest central activation of descending pathways in dorsal horn can facilitate or possibly originate a painful experience.

The Role of Key Brainstem Nuclei and Neurotransmitters in the Modulation of Pain

In addition to the processes outlined above, key brainstem nuclei and their neurotransmitter systems play a key central modulatory (bidirectional) role in the dynamic balance between pain facilitation and pain inhibition occurring between peripheral input and the cerebral cortex. The brainstem periaqueductal gray (PAG) matter is a major component of the pain modulatory system that includes its connections with the rostroventral medulla (RVM). Stimulation of the PAG has been consistently demonstrated to produce analgesia in humans an animal models without affecting other nervous system functions, affecting both nocifensive and affective behavior in response to a noxious stimulus. Both endogenous and exogenous opioids play a role in the PAG-RVM pain modulation system. The PAG-RVM system works bidirectionally to both facilitate and inhibit nociceptive signaling from the spinal cord. The RVM primarily serves as a relay of descending inhibitory signals from the amygdala and hypothalamus. The major role of the amygdala, as a primary output of limbic forebrain activity, in response to pain is via the PAG-RVM system. The PAG-RVM also receives sensory input via spinomesencephalic and spinoreticular pathways (including lamina I nociceptive input), projections from the hypothalamus (hypothalamic output can produce facilitation or inhibition of pain), brainstem adrenergic nuclei, and pontomedullary reticular formation nuclei. The major descending projection from the PAG is the RVM where the descending modulation of pain is dependent upon the functional integrity of the PAG-RVM pathways. Rostrally, the PAG projects to the medial thalamus and OFC to complete the bidirectional loop.

Key Brainstem Neurotransmitters and Neuropeptides in Descending Pain Modulation

Therapeutic targets for analgesia commonly include the modulation of the major neurotransmitters and neuropeptides that are key components of endogenous pain modulation. An understanding of the sites and modulatory influences of endogenous neuropeptides such as endogenous opioids, cholecystokinin, and neurotensin, as well as neurotransmitters acting at key modulatory relay nuclei, allows for the development of treatment strategies which may promote modulatory synergy via pharmacological and non-pharmacological methods of pain therapy.

RVM descending output, primarily to the dorsal horn laminae I, II, and V, contains the inhibitory neurotransmitter gamma-aminobutyric acid (GABA), neuropeptides, and serotonin and has both inhibitory and excitatory effects (effected by distinct neuronal groups) on nociceptive transmission in the dorsal horn through synapses upon primary afferents, projection neurons, and interneurons. In the acute pain state, depending upon the severity of the initial stress and autonomic response (where pain suppression is accompanied by the fight or flight response), pain facilitation generally precedes inhibition, simultaneous activation of rostral pathways direct attention, secondary behavioral and physiological responses ascending through RVM outputs to the hypothalamus/preoptic area and amygdala. RVM rostral input includes major input from the PAG (serotonin, endogenous opioids such as enkephalin, glutamate, neurotensin, and substance P) and other brainstem nuclei and reciprocal inputs from the amygdala, hypothalamus/preoptic area, and limbic, infralimbic, and prelimbic cortical areas (ventral and medial prefrontal cortex).

During the process of descending pain inhibitory modulation, the analgesic role of the PAG-RVM system is dependent upon physiologically intact endogenous opioid receptor interactions, with all classes of opioid receptors present in these brainstem nuclei. Experimental data supporting major endogenous opioid influence in brainstem descending modulatory control includes studies demonstrating that the opioid antagonist naloxone reverses stimulation-induced analgesia in PAG-RVM as well as worsens postoperative pain even in the absence of exogenous opioids. The administration of naloxone in the amygdala-PAG-RVM pathway reverses systemic opioid analgesia.

Finally, the PAG-RVM system mediates the analgesic state induced by the psychological phenomenon of conditioned fear which has been demonstrated to be associated with endogenous opioid receptor activation. Studies also suggest a major function of the PAG-RVM system is to implement behavioral decisions about whether to respond to a noxious stimulus. The major reward center associated with central dopamine release in response to various "reward" stimuli, the nucleus accumbens (NAc), connects cortical and subcortical centers associated with motivational processing and ensuing behavior. NAc has bidirectional connections with the multiple pain-related processing centers in the brainstem including dopamine-producing cells in the ventral tegmental area (VTA), reticular formation, hypothalamic nuclei, amygdala, prefrontal cortex, and basal ganglia, and NAc activation is associated with the suppression of nocifensive behavior, mediated by central endogenous opioid release. NAc cell activation has been demonstrated during both internally and externally based reward states and is believed to be a critical subcortical region mediating the sensation of "pleasure" associated with conventional stimuli such as exercise, food, music, and illicit substances, including opioids. An emerging role of dopamine in endogenous modulation has been suggested with experimental models demonstrating the attenuation nocifensive pain behavior with excessive dopamine and hyperalgesia with dopamine deficiency, suggesting a component of the normal response to pain is the modulation of release of dopamine in the striatum (nucleus accumbens, caudate, and putamen). Further, the concept of a "reward deficit" indicating hypoactivity in the VTA-Nac circuitry and its connections may underlie conditions associated with the centralization of pain and the presence of persistent diffuse pain or "chronic widespread pain." The relative activity in these pathways likely contributes to the individual response to new experiences of pain and the ability to engage in the normal process of pain modulation that facilitates successful recovery.

Cannabinoid receptors (CB1) are present in PAG, and cannabinoid-induced nociception is dependent upon CB1 actions in the amygdala-PAG-RVM system. Nicotinic acetylcholine receptors are present in RVM and likely mediate analgesic effects of serotonergic neurons. Neurotensin and CCK are said to "co-distribute" with opioid pain-modulating networks throughout the brainstem. CCK is pronociceptive and anti-opioid at multiple levels in the nervous system. Endogenous CCK limits the analgesic actions of opioids via actions on the CCK2 receptor, as demonstrated in PAG and RVM research. CCK antagonism enhances morphine and placebo analgesia in humans. CCK activates pain-facilitating neurons in RVM at high doses and blocks opioid activation of pain-inhibiting neurons at lower concentrations. Of clinical importance, CCK may play a role in the interaction of anxiety and pain, as CCK is elevated in states of high anxiety. Neurotensin has a biphasic relationship in pain modulation systems with low concentrations inducing pain facilitation and higher concentrations inducing analgesia due to differential actions on the receptors NTR1 (pain facilitation) and NTR2 (pain inhibition) in the RVM pain. Substance P and neurokinin I receptors both promote pain transmission in the RVM (following inflammation) and have a role in analgesia, as NKI receptor density increased with experimental models of inflammation.

Serotonin is present in a significant proportion of RVM neurons (20% of RVM neurons contain serotonin receptors) and plays a prominent role in analgesia. The administration of serotonin inhibits nociceptive transmission in dorsal horn, and serotonin is required for opioid-mediated analgesia in brainstem descending modulatory pathways. Serotonin receptors include both inhibitory and facilitating effects, with 5-HT1 and 5-HT2 likely directly inhibitory and 5-HT3 facilitating action mediated via GABA-ergic inhibitory interneurons in the dorsal horn.

Norepinephrine (NE) is also believed to play a significant role in the pain modulation system; however, the precise role is unknown. NE cell groups are located in the lateral pontine tegmentum, including the locus coeruleus, with descending inhibitory projections into the spinal dorsal horn. Clinically, alpha-2 agonists are analgesic at the spinal level, and there is evidence of bidirectional modulation, with alpha-1 adrenoreceptor activation demonstrating pain facilitation in experimental models. Following nerve injury, descending NE inhibitory systems possibly aid to prevent hyperalgesia. It is likely that supraspinal and spinal NE modulatory systems are capable of independent activation depending upon the pathological state of the injury.

Under some conditions, such as following chronic nerve injury or inflammation, the PAG-RVM system may evoke descending pain inhibition through activation of NE pathways through connections to NE cell groups (RVM reciprocally) as RVM stimulation evokes NE spinal release via descending NE pathways.

Other mediators of pain in disease include glutamate through the N-methyl-D-aspartate (NMDA) receptor and brain-derived neurotrophic factor (BDNF). Glial cell interactions have also shown to be important considerations in chronic pain, with observed evidence of glial activation and cell loss in PAG-RVM in inflammatory and neuropathic experimental pain states.

The "Normal" Response to Chronic Pain

The development of chronic pain is the subject of immense research and interest. For example, the RVM response to a prolonged pain stimulus, even without tissue damage, is a shift from inhibition of ascending pain signals to the facilitation of nociception. This transition from pain inhibition to pain facilitation denotes a shift of attention that has evolved to enhance the likelihood of recovery, from a state of heightened generalized attention and action with focused distraction to a state of focused attention with generalized inaction (rest) in situations requiring the needed time and resources for recovery.

A number of physiologic, pathologic, psychologic, and genetic factors likely interact in a given individual to determine whether, and to what extent, chronic pain develops following an injury. Even in the absence of trauma or injury, multiple individual factors contribute to the likelihood or "risk" of chronic pain development. Factors such as age, gender, and genetic predisposition are inherent conditions which play a role in the likelihood of chronic pain development, while other factors, such as psychological development and pain experiences, psychiatric disorders, psychosocial support, and, in some individuals, nociceptive input sufficient to result in alterations in cerebral pain processing, are seemingly modifiable factors that continue to be the subjects of intense clinical and basic research.

Developmentally, clinical observations suggest that the developing nervous system is quite resistant to the development of chronic pain. For example, chronic pain following neonatal trauma or neurodevelopmental anomalies is much less common compared to a similar degree of nervous system injury in an adult. With further neurological development and maturity, the likelihood of the potential for chronic pain following injury, surgery, or as the result of chronic illness increases linearly with age. In chronic pain states, alterations occur in peripheral, spinal, and supraspinal pain modulatory systems. Additionally, or in some individuals, exclusively, structural (potentially reversible) brain changes occur in the cerebral cortex with chronic pain such that the contribution of peripheral nociceptive input or "threat of tissue damage" has largely abated. Brain imaging studies in chronic pain, in contrast to the acute state, S1 and S2, are less consistently activated, and reduced thalamic activity is noted, indicating less sensory discrimination. Increased activation of the PFC and amygdala is associated with sustained pain and likely relates to activation of both pain-enhancing and pain-inhibiting states. In both chronic and acute pain states, amygdala activation is associated with arousal, pain amplification, and downstream pain facilitation. Experimental models of acute nociception in patients with chronic pain conditions have also demonstrated amplification of the acute pain responses observed in normal individuals, indicating a potential for a state of "heightened awareness" for acute nociceptive input among patients with chronic pain (Table 11.2).

The somatosensory cortex functionally reorganizes after nerve injury, and reorganization may result in increased neuropathic central pain, and brain reorganization can be influenced by successful treatment. For example, the receptive fields of de-afferentiated somatosensory neurons reversibly increased after phantom limb in proportion to the intensity of pain. With chronic pain, gray matter reductions have been noted in the pain processing system, including the ACC, IC, thalamus, frontal cortex, and hippocampus, and decreased gray matter correlates with pain. Cortical gray matter levels return to baseline levels following pain resolution suggesting an active process of synaptic connectivity related to clinical symptoms. In some chronic pain conditions such as chronic widespread pain and fibromyalgia, N-acetyl-aspartate (NAA) and hippocampal volumes decreased creating a potential loss of descending modulation with the pain condition inducing reduced brain connectivity, enhancing nociception. White matter abnormalities have also been described in chronic pain states, with less specificity to cause or effect.

Neurochemically, in studies of functional brain imaging, glutamine reductions are associated with clinical improvement in FM. Demonstrations of reversibly decreased opioid receptor density (opioid binding capacity) and dopamine release in chronic pain states further suggest underfunctioning of the "maintenance" pain suppression systems plays a significant role in the perpetuation of chronic pain.

In summary, during normal conditions, the response to a noxious stimulus undergoes multiple levels of modulatory refinement in the central nervous system such that an individual's response can be matched with immediate and successive ongoing needs for the individual's protection and recovery, if necessary. The process of modulation occurs through multiple parallel and overlapping neural networks which receive rich input from both higher centers regarding the present and past state of the need to respond to the present stress and from peripheral inputs that determine the appropriate levels of behavioral responses, which are contextually manifested by both affective processes such as fear, anxiety, and anger, as well as the cognitive processes of attention, distraction (or counterirritation), expectation, goal setting, learning, and memory. The clinically observed phenomena of both pain suppression and facilitation in both states of disease progression and recovery reflect this vast neural network.

The Systemic Response to Stress: The Sympathoadrenal and Hypothalamic-Pituitary Axis Stress Response Systems Endocrine, autonomic, and immune responses. Vagal afferents and small-diameter sensory axons induce sickness behavior via transmission to the central nervous system. Inflammatory and neuropathic pain results from interactions between the immune and peripheral nervous systems. CNS circuits modulate the immune and inflammatory responses via the sympathetic and adrenal systems of stress response. Sympathetically maintained pain is the result of coupling of sensory and sympathetic systems. Chronic, long-term changes in neuroendocrine function affect nociceptive threshold and hyperalgesia. The immune system and the nervous system are under constant surveillance for threats to ever-changing and potential harms in the environment. Mechanisms of protection undergo regular adaptations to manage threats with responses required whether very rapidly or over extended period of time.

Table 11.2 Conditions altering the response to acute pain conditions

Static conditions	Conditions/examples	Effect on pain response
Age		Altered pain responses in the elderly, developmental pain resistance
Gender	Females	Increase pain sensitivity, increased prevalence of certain pain conditions
Hereditary/genetic factors	Migraine, lower back pain, fibromyalgia	Polygenetic, epigenetic effects on the pain response
Chronic pain and other chronic symptom disorders	Fibromyalgia, lower back pain, migraine, irritable bowel syndrome, temporomandibular joint syndrome, chronic fatigue syndrome	Increased pain sensitivity, disordered affective processing, disordered evaluative processing, pain coping impairment
Neurological disorders		
Peripheral disorders of sensation	Diabetic neuropathy, hereditary sensory neuropathies	Reduced sensation with risk for increased tissue damage +/− concomitant neuropathic pain
Central disorders of sensation	Poststroke, demyelinating disorders, spinal cord injury	Reduced sensation with risk for increased tissue damage +/− concomitant neuropathic pain
Neurocognitive disorders	Dementia, cognitive dysfunction	Altered pain processing (affective, learning, coping)
Psychological disorders		
Affective disorders	Anxiety, panic disorder, bipolar disorder	Heightened pain sensitivity, disordered affective processing
Cognitive/learning disorders	Obsessive compulsive disorder, attention deficit disorder	Disordered affective and/or evaluative processing
Psychotic disorders	Schizophrenia, bipolar disorder	Disordered affective and/or evaluative processing
Addiction and substance disorders	Opioid addiction, substance use disorder, alcoholism	Opioid hyperalgesia, disordered affective and evaluative processing
Personality disorders	Borderline personality disorder, histrionic personality disorder	Altered pain affective perception, altered behavioral responses to pain
Chronic medical illnesses "Allostatic" load	Diabetes, chronic inflammatory illnesses, obesity, smoking	Altered peripheral and central pain resolution/ recovery

Bidirectional Communication Between Brain and Body

The hypothalamus receives constant input regarding homeostasis, such as body temperature, electrolyte status, extracellular fluid osmolality, and blood glucose concentration. Nociceptive afferents, the largest group of afferent neurons, send continuous information, via unmyelinated and small-diameter myelinated axons to the brainstem and hypothalamus as part of normal regulatory input. Afferent signals to the brain also include hormonal status, such as glucocorticoids, cholecystokinin, and sex hormones. Inflammatory cytokines, interleukins, and tumor necrosis factor stimulate neuroendocrine centers in the brain (hypothalamus and brainstem) as well as nociceptive afferents. Gastrointestinal afferent information also includes status of acid, immunoreactive substances such as endotoxin with vagal afferent stimulation triggering illness response. Efferent systems include sympathetic, parasympathetic, HPA, and sympathoadrenal systems. Homeostasis is the maintenance of physiological parameters of electrolytes, temperature, blood pressure, blood glucose, respiration, and oxygenation, the process of maintaining functional stability. Allostasis is the process of adaptation to internal or external environmental stress (exercise, hunger, temperature, physical threat), with physiological changes that occur rapidly, with rapid adjustments according to the needs of the organism. Allostatic processes chronically activated results in stress to nervous system and other tissues. "Allostatic load" may play a role in development of hypertension, diabetes, obesity, atherosclerosis, and hyperlipidemia.

This endogenous hormonal and neural control network is represented in close connection to the brainstem centers for pain modulation (analgesia, hyperalgesia) and serves to link these control systems, metabolic regulation, thermoregulation, sexual function, and defensive behavior. The role of cytokines (immunomodulatory, pro-inflammatory, and regulatory) in the peripheral and central nervous system is to signal pathological tissue stress (versus hormones which are homeostatic), and cytokines are rapidly released from Schwann cells, endothelial cells, leukocytes and macrophages to transiently facilitate pain (hyperalgesia) as determined by tissue damage (release of intracellular contents) and the intensity of nociceptor stimulation. Sickness behavior (experimentally induced by endotoxin intraperitoneal injection and linked to cytokine release) induces fatigue, lethargy, hypersomnolence, anorexia, fever, dysgeusia, decreased socialization, mood depression, cognitive dysfunction, pain, and hyperalgesia. Neurally, products of tissue injury and inflammation interleukins (IL1, IL6) tumor necrosis factor (TNF alpha) and lipopolysaccharide from bacteria (LPS) activate peripheral ganglia in viscera innervated by vagal afferents that synapse in brainstem (nucleus tractus solitarius) with descending pain facilitation and activation of illness responses. Sickness behavior may also be activated via activation of hypothalamus (HT) and limbic system through central processes, giving the potential for the elucidation of a psychological pathway to chronic illness behavior. Afferent vagal impulses and cytokines (which reach the brain via brainstem and hypothalamic transport systems across the blood brain barrier) activate central cytokine networks via glial cells prostaglandin E2 (PG E2) and adenosine triphosphate (ATP) which activate central networks promoting illness behavior. Peripheral release of inflammatory mediators such as TNF alpha induces interleukin and subsequent PG production from cyclooxygenase-2 (CoX-2) activation, which sensitizes nociceptors. Interleukin production also interacts with sympathetic terminals that release NE sensitizing peripheral nociceptors. Circulating glucocorticoids naturally inhibit interleukin-mediated activation of peripheral nociceptors.

Sympathetic modulation of the nervous system occurs via sympathetic efferent activation of the immune system (lymph nodes, spleen, thymus) as well as vasomotor and secretomotor function. The normal physiological response of the sympathetic nervous system to trauma is critical to peripheral sensitization by inflammation-induced release of bradykinin (via PG E2) and nerve growth factor (NGF), and adrenal release of NE sensitizes peripheral nociceptors. The sensitivity of nociceptors (cutaneous) is modulated by adrenaline from the adrenal medulla (which is inhibited by vagal activation). Vagotomy leads to the enhancement of nociception in experimental models. Thus, nociception and pain are under inhibitory control from the visceral domain, maintained by tonic inhibition from vagal afferent input. Vagotomy results in disinhibition of adrenal medulla activation leading to elevated plasma adrenaline. Vagal afferents that modulate sympathoadrenal activity are intestinal afferents (not gastrohepatosplenic – in which vagal activity is pronociceptive). Released adrenaline likely causes nociceptive sensitization via interactions with immune cells to induce release of PGE2.

Illness Behavior: The Appropriate Facilitation of Pain Through Systemic Stress Responses

As indicated above, the slow bidirectional brain-immune communication during illness is coupled with the fast defense and threat/survival system to ensure escape and recovery. The fast response system includes autonomic, HPA, and SA systems. The constant regulation of pain is important in both fast defense and slow recovery phases. The defense system is organized by the HT-mesencephalic system (PAG/RVM) that promotes analgesia, energy availability, and substrate (SA system mobilizes glucose) and HPA activation. In concert with pain facilitation, the fast defense response is associated with activation of CNS centers associated with hypervigilance, attention, and wakefulness. During slow recovery, healing needs to happen that is associated with more pain and hyperalgesia keeping the organism restful. Slow recovery system is modulated by the immune system via afferent vagal/brainstem and CNS (circumventricular) centers. Cytokine activation of nociceptors during inflammation, partly sympathetically mediated, and slow changes in nociceptor sensitivity (or recovery) are linked to sympathoadrenal modulation. The forebrain access to defense systems is able to enhance or initiate fast defense and likely able to initiate slow recovery processes characterized by chronic illness behavior.

In the subacute period following injury or during ongoing physiologic stress due to illness, the normal response for the individual to optimize chances for recovery and functional restoration is manifested in the constellation of phenomena and behaviors considered "illness behavior" or the "sickness response." An understanding of the normal function of this physiological recovery process allows providers to evaluate the behaviors in the context of the pathological burden in various clinical contexts. Unlike many of the features of the pain evaluation (discriminative and affective components), the sickness response includes a constellation of both objective and subjective findings that accompany the hyperalgesic state. The sickness response to injury or infection constitutes of central nervous system response to circulating mediators of infection, inflammation, and physiologic stress, such as endotoxin, leukotrienes, interleukins, and other cytokines. Present to a variable extent, depending upon the level of physiological stress are symptoms of spontaneous pain, allodynia, hyperalgesia, kinesophobia, and malaise. Objectively, individuals display fever (or disordered thermoregulation), fatigue, hypomobility, hypersomnia, mild to moderate cognitive slowing (or encephalopathy in certain situations), and a variable affective component (primarily depression, irritability).

Physiologically, the sickness state is the direct result of HPA activation with elevations of serum cortisol with resulting immunologic and metabolic responses aimed to conserve energy, promote recovery, and prevent re-injury or disallow behaviors which may thwart recovery. In this context, the phenomena of hyperalgesia and fear avoidance behavior are aligned with the long-term existential benefit of the individual. However, in clinical situations characterized by excessive subjective displays of illness behavior and hyperalgesia without accompanying objective signs of physiological stress, providers are faced with reorienting the traditional model of disease-based treatment to that of cognitive, behavioral, and symptomatic management.

Alteration of the Response to Pain in the Developing Brain and the Elderly and the Result of Genetic Influences and Gender Considerations in the Normal Response to Pain

The process of brain maturation includes the early and prominent presence of sufficient peripheral nociception and central nocifensive, behavioral responses, and the requirement for significant external support, i.e., "nurturing" for pain modulation. Despite limited discrimination, the developing brain displays marked resistance to the development of chronic pain, particularly associated with congenital defects (neurological and musculoskeletal) and early childhood trauma compared to their adult counterparts such as phantom limb pain, complex regional pain syndrome, and brachial plexopathy.

Although the likelihood of pain, especially chronic pain, increases with age, research regarding the normal response to pain, in terms of experimental modeling, in the elderly has demonstrated mixed results. Older persons have a high incidence of pain (40%) yet have lower rates of seeking care and lower rates of receiving adequate treatment. Although some data suggests pain "tolerance" is elevated in the elderly, the studies are inconsistent. The result of aging of the peripheral nervous system results in an age-related decrease in mechanosensitive afferents combined with increases in mechanoinsensitive nociceptive afferents. These age-related changes, likely the result of neurotrophic decline, may underpin "idiopathic" peripheral small fiber-related neuropathic pain often observed in the elderly. Psychologically, research has more consistently demonstrated the likelihood of increased rates of depression associated with pain in the elderly, in terms of both reactional depression associated with a chronic pain condition and the "somatization" of affective disorders responding to antidepressant therapy. Pain thresholds and tolerance to pain vary depending upon the type of experimental pain studied. Decreased nociceptors as well as decreased pain modulation and delayed recovery following injury or surgery may lead to increased vulnerability to chronic pain.

Pain as a manifestation of depression in the elderly has been well-documented, and an assessment of depression is part of the standard "pain generator" evaluation in the elderly. Older people have less catastrophizing, and pain avoidance than younger patients, and more likely to use passive coping strategies. The assessment of pain in the elderly must take into account status of physical disabilities as well as the pertinent cognitive and emotional impairments. Clinical research has also demonstrated that older patients with dementia are at even higher risk of undertreatment of pain as a result of multiple factors, including altered autonomic responses, ineffective communication regarding pain, pain behaviors misinterpreted as symptoms of dementia, and the misconception that it is acceptable to undertreat pain in the presence of impaired cognition and memory. When the effective communication of pain is impaired in the elderly, or other special populations, assessments require continual behavioral observations to gauge the effects of treatments for both cognitive-behavioral dysfunction and pain-related behaviors.

Research regarding the genetic influences in pain perception has produced a number of promising avenues of further inquiry and potential therapeutic development pertaining to multiple facets of the response to pain and therapeutic responses to pain treatments. Clinical experience has demonstrated that there is significant individual variability in the sensitivity to pain, the propensity to develop chronic pain, and responses to treatment. Clinical research involving simultaneous brain imaging with experimental pain conditions has indicated that the individual differences in pain largely reflect variations in pain perception. Epidemiological studies have indicated that following injury, the development of chronic pain is quite uncommon for most conditions. Thus, the interplay of genetics, epigenetics, and the environment (type/mechanism of injury with pre-existing established or "primed" central nervous system pathways) determines the individual variability observed in the response to injury or disease and development of chronic pain. Pharmacogenetic studies have elucidated some explanations for the observations that individuals vary with regard to their response to many types of analgesics, including opioids and nonsteroidal anti-inflammatory drugs. Twin studies in pain epidemiology have assisted in the assessment of pain conditions that develop more gradually with little environmental or physical precipitating factors, such as migraine, irritable bowel syndrome, fibromyalgia, chronic tension headache, and somatoform pain disorders. In other disorders, pain studies in twins have found it difficult to distinguish pain perception from the occurrence of a painful condition, as the objectivity of measuring pain relative to the severity of a given condition is quite limited with current technology. As most pain disorders are influenced by multiple environmental factors (culture, lifestyle, stress, trauma), the identification of complex multiple genetic polymorphisms requires very large sample sizes (many thousands of patients) to detect any contributions of heredity in a given disorder. Finally, there is sufficient data to suggest that measures of heredity (of 50% or more concordance) occur in the conditions of back pain, migraine, dysmenorrhea, and irritable bowel syndrome.

Experimental and clinical/epidemiological data have shown gender differences in both the perception of pain and prevalence of chronic pain conditions. Clinical and epidemiological studies indicate women experience a higher frequency of pain-related diagnoses. Then prevalence of headache, widespread pain, temporomandibular joint pain, abdominal pain, and lower back pain is higher in women. The prevalence differences with gender diminish in older age, suggesting a role for hormonal influences in the observed conditions. Experimental studies reveal that, in most, but not all, studies, women report lower thresholds for experimental pain conditions. Women also report higher levels of pain intensity, more frequent episodes of pain, longer durations of pain per episode, and an elevated incidence of more widespread pain. It is estimated that the gender-related phenomena of reporting higher levels of pain and higher likelihood to seek pain treatment may represent some elements of cultural differences related to gender roles and perceived expectations between genders. Gender cultural norms facilitate more pain expression in women, with generally broader social and peer support. Human experimental studies have also demonstrated that gender roles also play a role in pain sensitivity, with masculinity in both males and females associated with reduced pain sensitivity relative to feminine traits. Psychological distress associated with pain is also higher in women compared to men, who report higher levels of catastrophizing. Concomitant conditions associated with heightened pain intensity that have a higher female prevalence, such as anxiety and pain disorder, may also result in some of the disparity in the burden of pain affecting women.

The physiologic basis for reduced pain thresholds and higher incidence of chronic pain in women may be related to differences in gonadal hormones between men and women. Pronociceptive effects of estrogen have been found in animal models, and testosterone has been shown to have antinociceptive properties. With female gonadal hormones, the effects may be due to decreased pain inhibitory processes during periods of estrogen withdrawal. Estrogen also appears to have stimulating effects on both primary pain afferents and dorsal horn pain projection neurons. Opioid-binding studies suggest men have greater activation of the endogenous opioid system during pain conditions, while women may have more baseline activation of endogenous opioid activation with the possibility of less "recruitment" of endogenous opioid inhibition during nociception. Estradiol levels may play a role in endogenous opioid activation in women. Finally, local synthesis of estradiol from testosterone in the central nervous system occurs rapidly and may play a role in rapid pain modulation, particularly facilitation, in women.

The Psychological Response to Pain As indicated above, the processing of nociception by the brain allows for rapid bodily protection as a result of endogenous stress response systems and immediate pain modulation. Psychologically, the complex, mutually interactive, cognitive, and emotional brain networks act initially to maximally engage the individual's support system and subsequently support the individual's successful recovery and future. From birth, the established, innate response to pain automatically displays the "emotional" component conveying to the environment the "unpleasantness" of the stimulus with activation of a community support system alerting to the existence of a potential survival threat. This verbal and behavioral response creates alarm conditions sufficient to mobilize resources for maximal rescue and or protection. (Imagine the response of an infant crying in a theater at the same decibel level as the production.) Over the course of time, and under normal and nurturing conditions, individuals learn the appropriate conditions to sound the alarm to activate the support system through "pain behavior" and the required stimuli to evoke the system by an individual increases over the course of intellectual development such that "pain behavior" is relatively concordant to the potential threat or underlying tissue damage sufficient to activate the system. Thus, under "normal" conditions, the psychological recovery process is overwhelmingly successful; however, it has been demonstrated that high levels of psychological distress, depression, anxiety, and adverse life events are important in the onset of many regional and widespread pain disorders that are characterized by the persistent petition for a community support response. Following an acute injury, at a time when the perception of pain is appropriate, the perception of unpleasantness associated with pain occurs at the subconscious level, and automatic behavior, which becomes learned over time with multiple episodes of nociception during development, is driven to reduce the unpleasant experience of pain while simultaneously learning the cause of nature of the pain as the brain codifies the memory to future occurrences of unpleasantness.

The pain experience is quite diverse among individuals, and the number of potential pain experiences is quite diverse. Pain prediction leads to motivational states, and motivational learning is used to drive decision-making regarding adaptive behaviors when pain is experienced on a frequent basis. In the persistent pain state, behaviors can follow traditional principles of "conditioning" where motivation and reward systems, as opposed to potential or actual tissue damage, determine an individual's response to the pain experience. Further, expectations and beliefs regarding pain directly affect perception and intensity such that an individual's life experience, cognitive status, and underlying state of well-being can determine the extent to which the normal adaptive (associated with recovery and learning) pain response occurs or results in maladaptive behavior.

Psychologically, the perception of intensity is considered an accurate reflection of the nature of pain on a physical/physiological level, whereas the perception of unpleasantness represents the motivational significance of the pain to the individual according to their affective/emotional and cognitive status relative to the pain experience.

The Role of Learning and the Normal Response to Pain During physical and psychological development, reinforcement learning is a very important component of development pertaining to an individual's cognitive and affective ability to overcome and adapt to painful physiologically stressful conditions. Reinforcement learning entails an individual to assign predictive values to pain stimuli based upon prior experience, learning, cognition, and stratify expectations based upon previous experiences. The expectation of complete pain relief, following a course of recovery that is proportional to tissue damage, is consistent with the normal developmental experience and developmentally persists during episodes of intermittent periods of physical pain throughout normal development. Experimental pain research has demonstrated that relief (of experimental pain unassociated with significant systemic stress) has significant rewarding properties, particularly when there is an expectation of ongoing pain (aversiveness), and an individual's expectation of relief has high motivational value based upon these reinforcement models of learning. As such, the expectation of "pain relief" following some period of recovery should be considered the psychologically developmental "normal state," as is the expectation for a motivational "reward" for behaviors that promote recovery and relief. In the normal course of psychological development, the motivational basis for pain relief is the removal of the aversive stimulus and adaptive physical and psychological recovery, rather than other external "rewards" such as passive medical, psychological, or social interventions that may produce reward-reinforcement patterns with concomitant changes on the individual's behavior and motivational perspective. The longer and more severe the aversive state, the more reward or pleasantness is associated with the relief state, information which provides a psychological basis for the persistence of "reward" seeking observed with some individuals with persistent pain. In this context the "reward" sought may consist of medical or pharmacological interventions or simply cognitive resolution for the persistence of the aversive state. Under certain development circumstances, pain is interpreted as punishment, and relief becomes associated with an accentuated "reward" state resulting in more complex behaviors associated with persistent pain.

The phenomenon of instrumental learning is also relevant to the normal psychological response to pain. In the acute state, pain behaviors are relatively simple: aversive, avoidance, escape, defensive, and associated with environmental manipulation to reduce harm. With chronic pain or recurrent episodic pain, more complex systems of behavior are required according to outcomes which may vary with time and motivation, with the need to regularly adjust behaviors to achieve desired outcome (instrumental learning). Goal-directed behavior additionally involves value systems such that pain tolerance may vary according to the relative value of the goal. For example, individuals may be willing to "endure" pain, to various degrees, for the prospect of a desired outcome, such as a return to pre-injury levels of function or to participate in desired recreation or social settings. Additionally, research has indicated that most individuals prefer to "get pain out of the way" or experience pain in a more predictable, controlled fashion as opposed to enduring the affective distress of the potential for the noxious stimulus to be unpredictable in terms of timing, intensity, and duration.

In summary, the normal, adaptive response to pain is a dynamic state of affective and cognitive surveillance that pain results from a set of learned behaviors according to an individual's history of experiences of pain and codification of those individual experiences into a set of beliefs and behaviors centered around the expectations, goals, and concepts of the individual's future. In the adapted state of persistent pain, the ability for the individual to "reassign" the experience from "unpleasant" to another value, such as "tolerable," depends upon multiple psychological systems as well as cultural factors that include innate, learned or habitual, as well as goal-oriented motivational systems.

The Role of Cognition and the Normal Response to Pain Cognitive factors include beliefs about pain, self-efficacy, catastrophizing, coping, attention, and memory. Cognitive processes or "thoughts" about pain influence affective states or "mood," and mood influences thoughts. Behavior is determined by the individuals innate or conditioned response system and their interaction with their environment. Individuals are able to learn to adapt to emotional, cognitive, and behavioral manifestations of pain and can be successfully involved in reversing maladaptive thoughts, feelings, and behaviors, such as the development of negative expectations of their abilities to perform prior levels of function. Negative beliefs reinforce negative feelings that promote enhanced perception of pain. Patients can also become demoralized and believe they have no control over their pain. Another important element of the pain experience is the perception reached by an individual regarding the cause of their pain. Individuals who attribute their pain to a "terrible" or rapidly advancing disease rate higher levels of pain and disability and may consume more resources for "relief" (an innate expectation). Individuals with pre-existing or evolving cognitive states of helplessness and catastrophizing thoughts report higher pain and more utilization of resources. Conversely, individuals with adaptive coping thoughts report less pain and disability. Individuals with adaptive coping understand that pain increases attention/arousal that facilitates higher pain perception and learn to understand that their memory for painful events can increase pain intensity and memory strength, especially with strong affective/emotional content, and may predict future pain intensity of subsequent episodes. Individuals considered to have "adaptive coping" skills are able to alter the physiological (including arousal and affective) responses to memories associated with the pain experience and adjust expectations for outcomes according to objective input rather than moment-to-moment changes which may occur in pain intensity and affective state.

Implicit memory may also play a role in pain facilitation and chronic pain development via somatosensory cortical reorganization and may enhance pain experiences without conscious acknowledgment. Behaviorally, individuals who are able to decrease arousal levels develop habituation or desensitization of pain. Individual's beliefs regarding the meaning of their pain also have direct influences on mood (affecting muscle tension, arousal, and neurochemical/neurohormonal effects). Maladaptive fear avoidance may result from beliefs that the unpleasantness of the pain will reoccur or persist. Beliefs that the persistence or recurrence of the pain is due to worsening of their condition can result in a further cycle of catastrophizing and reinforcement of maladaptive pain behaviors. Adopting beliefs that disability is a normal consequence for their pain, even in the absence of objective disease measures, individuals become ingrained in their beliefs regarding disability that can be reinforced by their environment – family, community, and providers.

It is essential for individuals with chronic pain, especially due to chronic conditions that are not rapidly progressive, to adopt adaptive beliefs to reduce impairment, disability, and suffering (persistent affective distress/unpleasantness) despite the occurrence of pain. The adaptive process includes the restoration of "self-efficacy." Self-efficacy judgments include past performance, performance of others with similar status, verbal influence by others, and self-perception of physical ability. Improving self-efficacy beliefs may activate endogenous opioid system and improve physiological variables. It has been observed that variables of adaptive coping (and lowering of catastrophizing) significantly influence outcomes in both acute and chronic conditions associated with significant pain.

Referred to previously, catastrophizing is a cognitive error that elevates a pain experience beyond reasonable expected outcomes (beliefs that pain will not improve, cannot live with the pain, pain will never end) and negatively influences outcomes. Reduced catastrophizing reduces pain perception and improves pain tolerance and disability. Coping pertains to the self-regulation of pain; overt such as rest, medication, and relaxation; and covert such as distraction, problem-solving, information seeking, and self-assurance. Passive coping, relying upon others and restricting activity, is associated with higher levels of pain, depression, and disability. Coping strategies are often highly individualized and are significantly related to goals. Attention is affected by pain and can lead to hypervigilance to other body sensations with further development of other somatic symptoms, such as the diagnoses of multiple conditions within a single individual that are related to activation of the arousal/affective/attention system, such as fibromyalgia, irritable bowel syndrome, migraine, and temporomandibular joint syndrome.

The Role of Personality and the Normal Response to Pain The cognitive and affective responses to pain are due, in part, to individual traits or "personality" that are more likely than not to be static over time and form a significant component of the psychological framework of an individual's pain experience. Not to go unaccounted for, in terms of estimating the burden of illness related to persistent pain, the various forms of "personality disorders" have frequent representation in the chronic pain population with estimates of over 50% of patients with chronic persistent pain affected by a diagnosable personality disorder, such as borderline personality disorder and histrionic personality disorder. Further, the "pain-prone personality" is characterized by denial of emotional, interpersonal problems, inactivity, depressed mood, guilt, inability to deal with anger and hostility, insomnia, craving for affection and dependency, lack of initiative, and individuals commonly present with a family history of alcoholism, depression, and chronic pain. Many patients with persistent pain report or display the inability to express anger and control intense emotions, while reporting persistently elevated levels of pain. Conversely, chronic pain states may represent the inhibition of affective expression, potentially as a response to persistent pain or a combination of personality traits and the individuals resulting pain experience following injury or illness. Personality characteristics associated with individuals who develop chronic pain also include personal histories of seeking novelty, harm avoidance, behavioral reinforcement, and psychological affirmation/rewards. Finally, it is very important for providers to understand that the majority of the psychological processes occurring in the chronic pain patient are operant, classic conditioning (implicit, non-declarative learning) as opposed to malingering or intentional manipulation of. Pain is a multidimensional experience (physiological, psychological, affective, cognitive, behavioral, and social) with consideration of all facets required for accurate assessment and treatment assignments for optimal outcomes. Providers must understand that individuals inherently predict events based upon past experiences, and behaviors which are either adaptive or maladaptive can be reinforced (learned by individual with pain) by providers, family, and community.

The Role of Acquired Conditions and the Normal Response to Pain The normal response to pain is also subject to the influence of other chronic conditions and psychological states that may affect baseline pain sensitivity and physiological stress responses and influence outcomes. Logically, the normal response to pain is governed by an intact nervous system for the sensation and processing of pain information. Thus, conditions associated with significant impairment to the sensory nervous system, in particular, will alter the experience of pain. As a result, failure of the normal adaptive processes may ensure, resulting in more serious outcomes associated with the condition. The classic example is the Charcot joint associated with severe sensory loss or the loss of an extremity due to severe diabetic neuropathy. Psychologically, individuals with chronic pain, especially multifocal or widespread chronic pain, may manifest altered recovery patterns following illness or injury as a result of "baseline" alterations or "centralization" of the pain processing system. Other psychological factors include the affective disorders such as depression, anxiety, bipolar disorder, and panic disorder as well as past physical and sexual abuse, which may increase the likelihood of the development of chronic pain following injury or illness due to persistent abnormal affective processing of sensory information. Other psychological disorders such as post-traumatic stress disorder, attention deficit disorder, and obsessive-compulsive disorder have a high prevalence in the chronic pain population suggesting altered pain processing leading to the reduce adaptive recovery mechanisms. Addiction and substance use disorders, such as alcoholism and opioid use disorder, have increased rates of chronic pain related to both common conditions such as lower back pain as well as conditions related to the behaviors associated with the disorders, such as infections, trauma, and chronic medical illnesses. Concurrent opioid treatment of chronic pain or opioid use disorder has the potential to alter pain responses due to baseline alterations in opioid receptor sensitivity and hyperalgesic states observed in some individuals undergoing opioid therapy. Chronic pain disorders are increased in psychotic disorders, such as paranoid schizophrenia, with observations of both heightened pain sensitivity, disordered pain coping, and maladaptive learning patterns that are associated with persistent pain and resource utilization. Social factors play a role in the necessary elements of recovery and their influence on the development of chronic illnesses in general. In particular, some pain conditions such as fibromyalgia and chronic widespread pain are significantly more prevalent in regions of lower education, economic deprivation, and unemployment.

The Role of Culture and Social Factors in the Normal Response to Pain

The process of recovery following an injury or illness is strongly influenced by the ability of the individual to mount an adaptive response to the stress associated with the injury and also by the ability of the individual's cultural and social framework to support the individual's recovery. Cross-cultural studies have indicated a prominent role in the culture of an individual in the experience of pain, in terms of cognitive, affective, and social responses. In general, social and cultural support is more consistent with higher burdens of perceived injury or threat to life. With persistent pain, the type of injury or illness, and presence or lack thereof of perceived disability, determines many of the cross-cultural differences observed in the cultures studied. For example, lower back pain, a condition that consumes a significant amount of healthcare resources in many Western cultures, is not considered a condition requiring a medical assessment in some Eastern cultures. Care models that take into consideration the individuals underlying cultural pain beliefs result in improved communication, treatment compliance, and acceptance of outcomes.

The presence of seeking treatment as well as the presence of pain behaviors in the course of private, public, and clinical encounters is strongly influenced by cultural and social factors related to the acceptance of pain as a legitimate medical condition, the acceptance of emotional expression, and the relative value of displays of pain suppression. Abundant research has demonstrated marked improvements in outcomes, including reductions in reported measures of pain, with perceived adequate cultural and social (caregiver and provider) support.

Similar cultural factors influence the responsiveness of providers and others (such as friends, family, and other non-professional caregivers) to an individual's experience of pain. Ethnic factors, such as the perceived burden of illness in minorities, may also influence the responsiveness of a social and medical system to pain. For example, in one research sample, despite higher levels of recorded back pain disability among minority (black) patients compared to majority (white) patients, the minority patients were considered less likely to have significant pathology compared to white patients and were less likely to receive the same level of care, even after controlling for levels of socioeconomic status. These data regarding the role of social, ethnic, and cultural influences that influence the recovery of individuals with pain suggest that health professionals, family members, and the community at large stand to benefit from taking into consideration individuals', providers', and societal beliefs and behaviors in account when evaluating optimal strategies promoting functional recovery and reduced suffering from conditions associated with the complex experience of pain.

Recommended Reading

1. Apkarian AV, Bushnell MC, Schweinhardt P. Representation of pain in the brain. In: Wall and Melzack's textbook of pain. 6th ed. Philadelphia: Elsevier; 2013. p. 111–28.
2. Baliki MN, Petre B, Torbey S, et al. Corticostriatal functional connectivity predicts transition to chronic back pain. Nat Neurosci. 2012;15:1117–9.

3. Basbaum AI, Fields HL. Endogenous pain control systems: brainstem spinal pathways and endorphin circuitry. Annu Rev Neurosci. 1984;7:309–38.
4. Becerra L, Breiter HC, Wise R, et al. Reward circuitry activation by noxious thermal stimuli. Neuron. 2001;32:927–46.
5. Head H, Holmes G. Sensory disturbances from cerebral lesions. Brain. 1911;34(2-3):102–254.
6. Heinricher MM, Fields HL. Central nervous system mechanisms of pain modulation. In: Wall and Melzack's textbook of pain. 6th ed. Philadelphia: Elsevier; 2013. p. 129–12.
7. Patel S, Peacock S. Cultural influences on pain. Rev Pain. 2008;1(2):6–9.
8. Pavlin DJ, Sullivan MJ, Freund PR, Roesen K. Catastrophizing: a risk factor for postsurgical pain. Clin J Pain. 2005;21:83–90.
9. Penfield W, Boldrey E. Somatic motor and sensory representations in the cerebral cortex of man as studied by electrical stimulation. Brain. 1937;60:389–443.
10. Price D. Psychological and neural mechanisms of the affective dimension of pain. Science. 2000;288(5472):1769–72.
11. Seminowicz DA, Wideman TH, Naso L, et al. Effective treatment of chronic low back pain in humans reverses abnormal brain anatomy and function. J Neurosci. 2011;31:7540–50.
12. Wager TD, Atlas LY, Lindquist MA, et al. An fMRI-based neurologic signature of physical pain. N Engl J Med. 2013;368:1388–97.

12 Pain and Suffering

Marilyn S. Jacobs

Introduction

The experience of any type of pain is intrinsically linked to the experience of suffering. Pain can be physical, mental, or social – and these elements usually coincide, no matter the cause. While pain and suffering are distinct phenomena, often, one is prioritized over another or interchanged as being the same. The perception of pain follows bodily intrusion with individual interpretive meanings based upon personal history and emotional and cognitive responses. And, that physical pain causes suffering.

Once a syndrome of pain is established, central sensitization causes interference in normal consciousness which can be accentuated by requisite medical treatments (i.e., side effects from pharmacotherapy), social stress (economic hardship), and unexpected consequences (loss of identity and relationships). Although the development of pain evolves from a myriad of physical etiologies, it frequently is an intrusion such as due to an accident (motor vehicle, industrial), a disease state (disk herniation, diabetes mellitus, cancer), or an ongoing negative social situation (psychological trauma, social dislocation, conditions of wartime, all forms of abuse) which further accentuates the experience.

Pain medicine science and practice has, in the past decades, revolutionized patient care. Advances in pharmacotherapy regimens, surgical techniques, neuromodulation interventions, and multidisciplinary approaches have provided many options for hopeful outcomes. Yet, suffering persists, and its understanding is uneven.

Suffering is a complex experience of fear, distress, uncertainty, and the expectation of loss. Suffering is complex, highly individualized to the person and their history. It denotes the expectation of damage or destruction to identity, social role, value, and future.

M. S. Jacobs (✉)
Department of Psychiatry and Biobehavioral Sciences, David Geffen School of Medicine at UCLA, Los Angeles, CA, USA

The culture of most contemporary healthcare systems is structured according to the emphasis upon basic science, evidence-based treatments, accepted guidelines, the use of technology, and subspecialty collaborations. Also, economic stability has become foundational for medical practice. While humanistic means and the striving for patient-centered care are known approaches, these are often neglected due to these demands of clinical practice. It is increasingly apparent, however, that an understanding of the unique nature of the suffering of each patient with a pain disorder is essential.

Background and Historical Perspective

The subjects of pain and suffering have been a concern of healers and thinkers since the dawn of civilization. Philosophers, religious scholars, psychologists, physicians, and scientists have all considered the experience, the mechanisms, the treatments, and the outcomes. There has been an eternal search for remedies (herbs, opium, and bloodletting) and practices (mesmerism, prayer) to alleviate pain and suffering.

From the viewpoint of philosophy, religion, psychology, and psychoanalysis, suffering is inherent in human life from birth to death. Complete freedom from pain and suffering is unrealistic given the vicissitudes of human existence. There is a long tradition of the acceptance of suffering and reflection of its meaning in the humanities and the social sciences.

The *Book of Job*, in the Judaic and Christian bibles, and the tracts of other religions are examples of religious texts on pain and suffering. In these works, the story of Job and the justice of God in allowing for human suffering are seen as a transitory experience which leads to spiritual enlightenment. C.S. Lewis stated that pain brings the attention of humankind to the meaning of God. Job's suffering and its resolution has similarities to contemporary notions of acceptance, resilience, and prevailing in adversity to both religious and secular ways of being.

T. R. Deer et al. (eds.), *Deer's Treatment of Pain*, https://doi.org/10.1007/978-3-030-12281-2_12

The discovery of anesthesia in the mid-nineteenth century was a medical breakthrough. Controversy emerged. At the onset, its use was questioned due to medical, religious, and ethical concerns. The ethics of anesthesia - i.e., putting a person to sleep while their body was operated upon was questioned. It was questioned as to whether it was useful to interfere with the sensation of pain. These doubts were short-lived. Thus, there may be repercussions to scientific advances for pain and due to the way in which they influence the understanding of the nature of things.

The elaboration of the concept of pain as being tied to perception and not only sensation revolutionized pain medicine. Knowledge in this area accelerated during the twentieth century. Beecher's observations during World War II on Anzio Beach about the meaning of pain led to Melzack and Wall's modeling of the gate control and the neuromatrix theory leading to the multidisciplinary pain medicine practice. These developments have influenced the way in which pain is understood and treated.

From the perspective of historians, pain is a marker in the life of an individual which is one of the many situations which creates subjective reality. It is a phenomenon of being over time. Pain begins as private and is transformed to the social as the individual's experience is met with the categorization. This poses a paradox. Scarry noted that pain is outside of language, personal, and often impossible to communicate. The historian Bourke regards pain as an event made public by the use of language.

All humans will have pain, and all will suffer. It is the relief of pain and suffering more than the cure or removal which is thus the concern of rational thought. It can be said that the attainment of a mature level of consciousness is accompanied by the understanding that these types of limitations, disappointments, and the brevity of all lived moments are to be expected. Yet, the rapidity and availability of technological advances in postmodern life has influenced how these realities are difficult to accept in a culture framed by expectations of immediacy.

A challenge to the notion of pain and suffering being intrinsic to human existence occurs when these occur due to natural disasters, abuse, assault, torture, or political violence. When a pain disorder ensues from such external causes, it may create an existential crisis for many which can shatter beliefs and the just-world hypothesis. Adjustment to these events requires time.

Clinical Implications

Consideration of suffering is essential in the clinical practice of pain medicine. This adage has become a legal and ethical requirement of clinical practice. While technology has advanced, human experience remains the same. The approach of pain management implies that most pain disorders can be ameliorated not cured. There will be residual suffering from the best practices of pain care.

Patients with pain will likely have a pain onset tied to psychological trauma. These beginnings will contain memory traces of hurt and/or harm tied to the physical complaints of tissue damage. Iatrogenic consequences can also be influential.

Pain medicine practitioners are also confronted with challenges due to the population shift to a higher prevalence of chronic illness – a result of more effective treatments for acute conditions. There are now a growing number of patients with chronic conditions for which management is unpredictable, complications common, and suffering persistent. Pain practitioners are now required to become practitioner-healers, supporting their patients overcome the suffering inherent in chronic pain to build new personal meaning, invest in alternative identities, and become empowered toward self-efficacy.

The obstacles of assuming this role for practitioners are significant. To become personally closer to suffering and loss creates countertransference reactions in the provider of care. One can reflect that the suffering that is observed in a person who is the patient could also afflict the person who is providing the care. Physicians and others in medical settings are desensitized from years of seeing traumatic and tragic outcomes. There can be a culture of denial and resistance to sharing bad experiences.

Suffering can be reduced in pain patients if the threats to existence are lessened. Fulfilling involvement with relationships, purpose, and satisfaction in everyday reduces suffering. While suffering cannot always be completely resolved, patients with pain can learn to accept and coexist with it. Patterson's shifting perspectives model of chronic illness suggests that there is no correct way for a patient to view their illness and that acceptance may not be best.

Medical practitioners have an essential role in helping their patients clarify their perspectives about their suffering and providing support and encouragement for behavioral and social changes.

Learning how to talk to patients about suffering is essential. Patients welcome the opportunity to share their stories with medical providers. This interchange opens up the patient's awareness of their psychological world and leads to understand what has happened and what it means. It is existentially necessary to move past a bad experience that the opportunity for emotional disclosure be created. Goleman's concept of emotional intelligence is applicable here. The goal for caregivers would be to be able to identify their own and their patients emotions and use this information to communicate an appreciation of the situation. This type of interaction might enhance the therapeutic interaction and lead to less medical complications and patient/doctor conflicts and lessen burnout of providers of care.

Time constraints and caseload pressures clearly can impede the ability of the pain provider to engage in extended inquiry into the experiences of their patients. It is important to realize that not all patients will need to go deeply into sharing their story. Many patients will have already developed resilience and toleration of suffering and will have a tradition of healing within cultural or religious structures and family relationships.

An integrated approach invites collaboration with other disciplines. Given the time limits of clinical pain medicine practice, referral to mental health practitioners serves as an extension of the healing that physicians and others in the clinic can provide. Although multidisciplinary care is the standard, resources and availability are often limited. Psychotherapy (cognitive behavioral, acceptance commitment, dialectical behavioral, psychodynamic, family, and group) can enlarge the capacity of patients to cope with and understand pain and suffering. Psychopharmacological management can alleviate the concomitant psychological symptoms (anxiety, traumatic stress, depression, addiction) which pain and suffering can cause. Behavioral therapies (hypnosis, meditation, neurofeedback, therapeutic yoga, and relaxation training) are extremely helpful modalities for teaching pain patients self-regulation. Community support groups (12-step, pain coping skills) and family therapy when indicated are also valuable.

In regions where there is a paucity of trained professionals, mid-level practitioners may have the time to undergo training in counseling skills. As well, pastoral counseling is often available as is telehealth for psychological treatments. Patients may also resist a referral to a mental health professional as they may interpret this step as a communication that their pain and suffering are exaggerated or not believed. Emphasis upon the idea of coping skills, the stress of pain, and suffering and emotional disclosure is helpful in the conversation.

Evidence for Efficacy

While its research into pain treatments is straightforward, there are methodological issues in the research of suffering. Pain treatments have a scientific and objectivist basis making them available to clinical trials of efficacy; suffering is difficult to operationalize. The best approach for the study of suffering is qualitative not quantitative. Suffering is an experience for which language falls short. Research into suffering may neglect personal meaning for each sufferer.

The tradition of narrative medicine is a qualitative approach to understand suffering. Suffering is understood by immersion in the patient's story. The skills needed by providers of pain medicine are to be able to identify, accept, interpret, and use the stories which reflect the suffering of their patients. Medical care is enhanced by narrative competence by its practitioners.

Suffering research has found that people who are suffering desire to speak about it – not speaking about suffering increases the experience. The question of whether patients are harmed by being asked to speak about their suffering is answered by the finding that to speak of suffering serves to relieve it. More studies with this approach are needed.

Another relevant area of research has been that of post-traumatic growth, which refers to the development of a higher level of functioning after the experience of adversity. Research has supported this concept as a real possibility for people who have endured difficult life circumstances. Although there has been criticism of post-traumatic growth as lacking in strong evidence, it prevails as a useful paradigm – especially in the context of the burgeoning population of patients with chronic illness. There are specific issues related to posttraumatic growth as this idea applies to physical illness. The reappraisal of life and priorities and the idea that trauma provides opportunities for self-development and reevaluation all are aspects that are specific to the need for survival after illness-related trauma.

Main Points

1. Pain and suffering are both aspects of pain medicine practice and which coincide and require different approaches by providers of pain care.
2. Suffering involves damage to the identity of the person with pain and is highly personal and existential.
3. Pain is an event in a person's life which can be approached by nonmedical means.
4. The care of patients with pain is enhanced by attention paid to the patient's story of illness and its experiential implications and by helping with healing of these consequences.
5. Mental health professionals are essential in the care of pain and suffering when medical treatments are not sufficient but may not be able to alleviate all pain and suffering.
6. Shifting perspectives of health and illness suggest that acceptance is not enough and that a here and now approach to experience is beneficial and may improve coping with the adversity of pain and suffering.

Recommended Reading

1. Arman M, Rehnsfeldt A. How can we research human suffering? Scand J Caring Sci. 2006;20(3):239–40.
2. Bourke J. The story of pain: from prayer to painkillers. London, UK: Oxford University Press; 2013.

3. Cassell EJ. The nature of suffering and the goals of medicine. 2nd ed. New York: Oxford University Press; 2004.
4. Egnew TR. Suffering, meaning and healing: challenges of contemporary medicine. Ann Fam Med. 2009;7(2):170–5.
5. Hefferon K, Grealy M, Mutrie N. Post-traumatic growth and life threatening physical illness: a systematic review of the qualitative literature. Br J Health Psychol. 2009;14(2):343–78.
6. Patterson BL. The shifting perspectives model of chronic illness. J Nurs Scholarsh. 2001;33(1):21–6.
7. Schleifer R. Pain and suffering. New York: Routledge/Taylor & Francis; 2014.
8. Wortham SM. Modern thought in pain: philosophy, politics, psychoanalysis. Edinburgh, UK: Edinburgh University Press; 2015.

Social Impact of Pain Response

13

Alan Gonzalez Cota

Introduction

Despite the consensus of the international medical community that treatment of chronic pain is a human right, approximately 75% of the world's population suffering from chronic moderate-to-severe pain has no access to pain relief treatment.

There is a high prevalence of pain disorders in developed countries, with chronic pain affecting 19–25% of these populations. Half of these receive insufficient treatment, and a third receive no treatment at all, with attendant socioeconomic impacts and labor repercussions. According to the most recent National Health Survey, about 25.3 million of US adults (11%) had pain every day for the previous 120 days. Nearly 40 million adults (17%) had severe pain. The annual monetary cost of chronic pain in the USA pertaining to health resource consumption, disability, and loss of productivity has been estimated at $635 billion.

Analysis of the Pain Question

According to the biopsychosocial model, pain can be described as the interaction between biological factors (genes, physiology, age, sex), psychological factors (cognition, mood, conduct), and social factors (work situation, culture, income, family). From the perspective of the pain practitioner, the most salient of these factors – and the most important to recognize – are the basic concepts: how to approach evaluation of pain, the social impacts of chronic pain, (including impacts on the patient's quality of life), undertreatment of pain (including resulting medicolegal implications of prescription medications), and prevention of pain.

A. Gonzalez Cota (✉)
A.I.M. Interventional Spine Division, Rockville, MD, USA

Legacy Pain Management Rehabilitation, Bethesda, MD, USA

KureSmart Pain Management, Annapolis, MD, USA

Evaluation of Chronic Pain

One of the most important and debated aspects in medicine today in the approach to evaluation of pain is the categorization of pain as a pathologic entity in and of itself. Historically, pain has been viewed by the medical community as an underlying symptom of disease and classified as "chronic" when its duration persists past the expected time of healing from the disease or acute injury. However, clinicians are increasingly voicing the opinion that "chronic pain should be recognized as a disease in its own right…and not only a symptom, and treated with the same priority as an underlying disease".

Supporters for defining pain as disease argue that severe chronic pain is a disabling condition that is associated with increased risk of mortality, independent of sociodemographics and its classification as a disease would allow clinicians to better recognize and address pain in their patients and prescribe more appropriate treatment. But how to arrive at grouping various disparate conditions under the umbrella of a disease entity, chronic pain, is a confounding problem and has been a major hindrance to this effort. A disease is generally characterized by an impairment of normal function, and as having specific symptoms and a distinct etiopathogenesis. Chronic pain is often only recognized by clinicians when patients present with symptoms characterized primarily by pain.

Because of the myriad of complex factors involved in pain, appropriate assessment of pain begins with the initial patient presentation. Acute pain can usually be adequately assessed and treated during the physical exam, but assessment of persistent pain is more time-consuming and may require a more thorough evaluation and follow-up visits. When pain becomes chronic and intractable, referral to a pain specialist may be needed for more comprehensive evaluation and treatment. In addition, some physicians believe that a psychosocial or psychiatric evaluation should also be included in any pain assessment, particularly in the management of chronic pain.

T. R. Deer et al. (eds.), *Deer's Treatment of Pain*, https://doi.org/10.1007/978-3-030-12281-2_13

Current approaches to evaluation of pain include use of tools that attempt to objectivize the patient's perception of pain. The most commonly employed of these instruments include quantitative visual and verbal scales, multidimensional surveys (McGill Melzack, Brief Pain Inventory), and general questionnaires on the impact of pain on quality of life (SF-36 Short Form Survey). The World Health Organization recommends the use of these instruments and stratifying patients into three groups for appropriate pharmacotherapy.

Multiple epidemiological studies have been conducted in various countries across the globe to evaluate the prevalence of pain and satisfaction with current therapies. One large population study, the Pain In Europe study (PIE), used in-depth interviews of 46,394 qualified participants to assess chronic pain in 16 countries across Europe and Israel. Chronic pain was defined by an intensity ≥5 out of 10 on the Numeric Rating Scale (NRS), lasting more than 6 months duration. Results showed an overall prevalence of moderate-to-severe chronic pain of 19% of adult Europeans. Sixty-six percent of total subjects studied had moderate pain (NRS = 5–7) and 34% had severe pain (NRS = 8–10), with an average chronicity of 7 years. The most common medical specialty handling pain by number of visits was primary care (70%) and orthopedics (27%); pain specialists constituted less than 2%. One third of respondents suffering from chronic pain reported receiving no treatment at all, giving reasons ranging from the ability to self-manage pain, reluctance to take pain medication or to simply being resigned to living with chronic pain.

Socioeconomic Impacts of Chronic Pain

The socioeconomic impacts of chronic pain can be evaluated by analysis of direct costs, indirect costs, and intangible costs. Direct costs are those that pertain to healthcare utilization; indirect costs involve disability and loss of work days; and intangible costs pertain to the impacts on the patient's quality of life and costs to caregivers.

Internationally, the cost of chronic pain is 2.2% of the Gross Domestic Product (GDP) in industrialized countries. The most recent reported annual cost of chronic pain in the USA is as high as $635 billion – more than the combined yearly costs for cancer, heart disease, and diabetes.

Indirect costs are defined by the macroeconomic impact of loss of productivity in the workforce. In the USA, an estimated one out of five workers experience difficulties performing job tasks due to chronic pain. In addition, loss of workers due to pain disability or reduced work hours represents a larger economic loss than direct costs. The best estimate of chronic pain direct costs (healthcare utilization) is $368 million US dollars, and the indirect cost related to worker compensation and disability is $4600 million US dollars (93% of total cost).

Intangible costs need to be accounted for as well, such as decreased quality of life, caregiver economical loss, and costs of treating comorbidities associated with chronic pain.

Undertreatment of Pain

The social impacts of undertreatment of pain by clinicians and other healthcare professionals are a topic that is receiving increasing focus in the medical community. Undertreatment is defined as inappropriate or inadequate management of a patient's pain, which occurs for various reasons – clinician knowledge deficits and inadequate pain assessment are the most frequent professional barriers to adequate pain management. Other factors include the fact that pain itself is still frequently viewed as a subjective assessment, and the etiologies of many manifestations of pain are often not fully understood, so pain does not fit the expert knowledge model of disease, as discussed previously. There are numerous etiological pathophysiological events leading to the development of pain; as a result, there are no diagnostic criteria for pain that would fulfill current definitions in evidence-based medicine.

In addition, clinicians should be aware of the legal implications of undertreatment of pain. Inadequate pain management resulting from deviation from accepted medical practice standards can be viewed by the legal system as medical negligence and can result in medical malpractice lawsuits. More clearly defined pain management practices and policy guidelines are now in place to address this issue and will continue to be refined with time as new legal issues arise.

Concern over opioid addiction and adverse effects, coupled with fear of disciplinary action, may cause a clinician to undertreat a patient for whom relief from pain is dependent on them. Although there are many approaches and interventions available in the pain management toolbox, in terms of pharmacologic therapy, the World Health Organization guidelines recommend use of an analgesic ladder, starting with non-opioids (antidepressants, anticonvulsants, bisphosphonates, and corticosteroids, as appropriate) up to opioids as the last option. Treatment can be adjusted using the 4As (analgesia, adverse effects, activities of daily living, and aberrant drug taking) of pain treatment outcomes at each healthcare visit.

Prevention of Chronic Pain

Prevention of both the incidence and prevalence of chronic pain is possible through early identification of risk factors, such as spinal or nervous system surgery, trauma, and comorbidities associated with pain. This would allow for early intervention before pain becomes a chronic condition.

In the USA, the Association of American Medical Colleges (2014) estimate of active pain medicine and pain management specialists is approximately 3500–4000. Even if the majority of chronic pain patients had the financial means and geographical access to these specialists, this number is seriously inadequate to serve the vast numbers of chronic pain sufferers in this population. Further continuing education of primary care and ED physicians in addressing pain assessment and management is needed to help rectify this deficit. Medical schools should also place more time and resources into this increasingly critical issue.

Summary

The social impacts of pain are far-reaching and encompass many aspects of human life in the USA and across the globe. The IOM Report calls for a "cultural transformation" toward more coordinated action in the treatment of pain, stating that "pain patients have long been viewed with skepticism and suspicion, rather than understanding, presenting a barrier to care." According to the National Institutes of Health (NIH), pain is cited as the most common reason Americans access the healthcare system. It is a leading cause of disability and the most common cause of long-term disability, and a major contributor to healthcare costs in the US Pain can be a chronic disease, a barrier to cancer treatment, and can result in comorbidities that also require treatment, such as depression. For these and other reasons discussed in this chapter, the social impacts of pain should be viewed as an increasingly important focus in the overall approach and treatment of pain.

Recommended Reading

1. Breivik H, Collett B, Ventafridda V, Cohen R, Gallacher D. Survey of chronic pain in Europe: prevalence, impact on daily life, and treatment. Eur J Pain. 2006;10:287–333.
2. Gaskin DJ, Richard P. The economic costs of pain in the United States. In: Institute of Medicine (US) Committee on Advancing Pain Research, Care, and Education. Relieving pain in America: a Blueprint for transforming prevention, care, education, and research. Washington, DC: National Academies Press (US); 2011. Appendix C. Available from: https://www.ncbi.nlm.nih.gov/books/NBK92521/.
3. International Association for the Study of Pain. Annual Report. Declaration that access to pain management is a fundamental human right. 2010. https://www.iasp-pain.org/files/Content/ContentFolders/AboutIASP/IASPAnnualReport_2010.pdf.
4. Lohman D, Schleifer R, Amon JJ. Access to pain treatment as a human right. BMC Med. 2010;8:8.
5. McDonnell WM. Special Report: Inadequate pain management: a growing liability risk. 2007 May. Available from: https://www.ahcmedia.com/articles/103364-special-report-inadequate-pain-management-a-growing-liability-risk.
6. NIH factsheets: pain management. NIH Research Portfolio Online Reporting Tools (RePORT). 2013. Available from: https://report.nih.gov/nihfactsheets/ViewFactSheet.aspx?csid=57.
7. Paice JA, Von Roenn JH. Under- or overtreatment of pain in the patient with cancer: how to achieve proper balance. J Clin Oncol. 2014;32:1721–6.
8. Passik SD, Weinreb HJ. Managing chronic nonmalignant pain: overcoming obstacles to the use of opioids. Adv Ther. 2000;17:70–83.
9. Raffaeli W, Arnaudo E. Pain as a disease: an overview. J Pain Res. 2017;10:2003–8.
10. Rosenberg M. Undertreated pain epidemic: multi-modality approach to pain management. J Manag Care Med. 2012;15(1). Available from: http://jmcmpub.org/pdf/15-1/?pdf_page=30.
11. Scoping document for WHO Guidelines for the pharmacological treatment of persisting pain in adults with medical illnesses. 2012. GRC-08-04-0052A. Available from: http://www.who.int/medicines/areas/quality_safety/Scoping_WHO_GLs_PersistPainAdults_webversion.pdf?ua=1.
12. Torrance N, Elliott AM, Lee AJ, Smith BH. Severe chronic pain is associated with increased 10 years mortality. A cohort record linkage study. Eur J Pain. 2010;14:380–6.
13. UN News Centre Report. Over 5 billion people worldwide lacking access to essential medicines, says UN report. 2015 Mar. Available from: http://www.un.org/apps/news/story.asp?NewsID=50230#.WbgiWekg8eE.
14. Zelaya CE, Dahlhamer JM, Lucas JW. QuickStats: age-adjusted percentage of adults aged ≥18 years who were never in pain, in pain some days, or in pain most days or every day in the past 6 months, by employment status — National Health Interview Survey, United States, 2016. MMWR Morb Mortal Wkly Rep. 2017;66:796.

Role of Religion and Spirituality in the Patient Pain Experience

14

Amy Wachholtz and Christina E. Fitch

Introduction

In the United States, as we grapple with the "opioid epidemic" and state-led marijuana legislation, there is increased interest in understanding the experience of pain in greater depth in order to find more effective ways to treat it. Likewise, the biomedical traditional approach to pain management shows improvements in less than half of patients treated. Since 22% of Americans experience moderate to severe pain at least twice a week, medical providers should be seeking auxiliary interventions for the control of pain. Spirituality, as most are aware, is not equivalent to religion. There are multiple different definitions in the research literature, so for the purposes of this chapter, *spirituality* refers to a person's beliefs and practices related to feelings of connectedness and meaning making, whereas *religion* refers to the community-level beliefs and practices. As most research integrates these two definitions, the term R/S is generally used to refer to integrated beliefs and practices in the area of religion, spirituality, and health.

Numerous research studies show chronic pain sufferers in general seek coping mechanisms through R/S beliefs and practices. Strong spiritual well-being is linked with a better ability to cope with pain. Therefore, in the interest of supporting the patient's experience so that they can reduce their pain levels and function at their highest level, it behooves us as providers to assess spiritual and psychological distress. Likewise, this suggests that incorporating spiritual providers into the integrated pain care team would be helpful to support patients in developing strategies to make meaning and connection in their lives.

A. Wachholtz (✉)
Department of Psychology, University of Colorado-Denver, Denver, CO, USA
e-mail: Amy.Wachholtz@UCDenver.edu

C. E. Fitch
University of Massachusetts Medical School- Baystate Campus, Springfield, MA, USA
e-mail: Christina.Fitch@BaystateHealth.org

Background/Historical Perspective

R/S and Health

R/S can have a powerful impact on health in general, both positive and negative. Regular religious attendance (2 × per month or more), even after controlling for multiple possible confounders, was found to have as powerful a positive effect as smoking has a negative effect on health. Additionally, regular religious attendance is correlated with a 7 year longer life span for Caucasians, and 12 years for African-Americans. Alternatively, long-term spiritual struggles can significantly increase morbidity and mortality rates.

While immediately following the terrorist attacks on September 11, 2001, in the United States there was a significant increase in attendance at religious services for approximately 2 years, there since has been a steady decline in regular religious attendance at religious services. Despite this change in practice, a belief in a higher power or some form of spirituality remains high with only 3.1% of Americans identifying themselves as atheistic. During recent years, even while attendance at formal religious services was dropping, individuals increased their use of prayer to address health concerns. This relationship held true even after controlling for socioeconomic status, health status, age, and health insurance status.

R/S and Pain

Among individuals with chronic pain, 61% of patients report regularly using prayer to cope with pain. Prayer is one of the most commonly used religious or spiritual coping strategies when a patient is struggling with chronic pain. When asked how their chronic pain condition affected their religious or spiritual beliefs, 40% of pain patients reported becoming more religious after the onset of their painful condition, while 4% reported becoming less religious or spiritual.

This active use of prayer among religious or spiritual individuals is important, as research has found that the protective

T. R. Deer et al. (eds.), *Deer's Treatment of Pain*, https://doi.org/10.1007/978-3-030-12281-2_14

effects of R/S on health stem more from health-based behaviors rather than only self-identified R/S status. Thus, it is more important to identify how people engage with their R/S beliefs rather than simply how they identify themselves as religious/not religious or spiritual/not spiritual.

R/S strategies are not the common initial response to pain. Instead, acute pain usually elicits a generally self-directed approach. For example, a patient with acute pain will seek out acetaminophen from the medicine cabinet in response to a tension headache. However, R/S practices do become the primary form of coping in response to chronic pain, to poorly controlled, intermittent pain, and when other coping strategies fail. However, it should be noted that for most chronic pain patients, there is a synchronicity to their use of coping mechanisms in that they will often use R/S coping strategies and secular coping strategies simultaneously.

Religious Coping Strategies

Extensive studies have identified four distinct R/S coping strategies related to health, each with unique outcomes on health and pain. Early research studies were limited in their assessment of R/S and assume a simple unidimensional approach to R/S in relation to health (i.e., generally R/S = good or R/S = bad). Additionally, there was a misassumption that R/S coping is equivalent to a passive coping strategy, rather than an active method of addressing pain. Later research has clarified that there is a great deal more complexity to patients' use of R/S coping strategies in relation to health and that R/S coping is indeed an active coping strategy for patients with chronic pain.

There are four types of R/S coping strategies in relation to health.

- The first, *Deferential*, describes the approach where the patient gives all control of a problem over to their higher power. The patient takes little responsibility for his/her own health situation. An example of this form of coping strategy would be a patient saying, "It doesn't matter if I do my home PT exercises or not, if my pain is meant to go away, God will take it away in time." Individuals using this type of strategy generally have lower pain-related self-efficacy and poorer pain outcomes. The exception to this is when the patient actually has very little control over their situation, such as in hospice care. In those types of situations, it appears that reducing futile attempts at controlling health and pain outcomes by engaging in *Deferential* coping styles may conserve energy, reduce pain, and improve quality of life.
- The second type of R/S coping is the *Collaborative* approach. In this paradigm, a patient uses an active joint problem-solving perspective with their higher power to address their pain issue. In this approach, an individual might say, "My higher power will support me and help get me through this, but I have to do my part too." Individuals using this form of coping often have the best pain outcomes, because they actively engage with health professionals and adhere to treatment protocols as part of their responsibility to their higher power. They also feel that they have additional existential support for their efforts.
- The third type of R/S coping is the *Independent* approach. In this scenario, an individual does not engage or rely on a higher power because their belief system does not include a deity. There is no negative emotion associated with this belief, they simply have an atheistic approach to life. An example statement of someone with this viewpoint might be, "I will do it myself because I find the strength within me. I don't believe in God." Individuals using this form of coping generally have positive health outcomes if they adhere to treatment protocols and engage with their health professionals.
- The fourth and final type of R/S coping is the *Abandoned/Punished* approach. In this paradigm, individuals feel that they have been abandoned in their time of need or that their chronic pain is a punishment from their higher power due to a transgression. Their higher power does not provide existential support for these individuals, and there are often a number of powerfully negative emotions related to their relationship with their higher power, such as anger, guilt, and shame. An example statement of someone with the Abandoned/Punished approach might be, "I cheated on my wife so God is punishing me with my chronic pain." This type of R/S coping should be a significant red flag for any medical provider because individuals with this type of coping will generally have far worse functional outcomes, request more pain medications, have higher utilization of medical services, and not use self-directed pain management strategies.

Outside of a formal assessment of these four strategies among their patients, a provider can assess for warning signs that a patient may be engaging in more negative forms of R/S coping techniques in order to refer to a mental health clinician who is familiar in working with R/S struggles (see Table 14.1). While positive R/S is used more frequently than negative R/S among people who have R/S coping strategies, when negative approaches are used, they have a powerful negative impact on mental and physical health outcomes. Individuals who have a personal R/S faith background have better outcomes when using positive R/S coping strategies than individuals who adopt these strategies as a "tool" or "last ditch effort" to control their pain. However, when patients with current faith or practices are encouraged to use positive R/S strategies in response to their chronic pain, there are significant positive mental and physical health outcomes.

Mechanisms of Effects of R/S Coping on Pain

There are a number of psychophysiological mechanisms related to the observed outcome of R/S beliefs on pain (See Fig. 14.1). The hypothalamic-pituitary-adrenal (HPA) axis is stimulated by any physical or emotional distress. The end product of the HPA system is cortisol. Chronic pain affects cortisol levels in that they are high in early chronic pain but lower over years because the axis becomes suppressed. Over time, chronic pain becomes central in nature; the brain's neuroplasticity changes the experience of pain. This process is mediated partially by IL-6, a connection between the nervous and immune systems. The diagram above illustrates the links between spirituality, emotional processing, physiological changes, and the experience of pain.

Pain self-efficacy is an important component of understanding a patient's pain experience as it refers to an individual person's ability to cope and function with their chronic pain. When someone has a strong sense of spiritual distress, pain self-efficacy decreases. Personal resilience and one's confidence in the ability to do enjoyable activities despite pain is fundamental to pain self-efficacy. There may be a positive feedback loop in that those who have confidence that they can do their activities despite pain then receive the benefit of those activities, which in turn give purpose and meaning to their life.

Table 14.1 Empirically validated positive and negative forms of religious/spiritual coping

Positive forms	Negative forms
Seek spiritual connection	Interpersonal religious discontent
Meditation	Punishing God reappraisal
Seek spiritual support	Demonic influence
Religious assistance to forgive others	Spiritual discontent
Asking forgiveness	Reappraisal of God's power
Benevolent religious reappraisal	
Religion as distraction	
Collaborative problem-solving with God	

Since spirituality is a construct of one's connectedness within the universe and the meaning that comes of that connectedness, it is helpful to consider what is occurring when this process is disrupted and the effect it may have on the patient's mood and pain experience. Patients do not become depressed from their pain alone. Through a series of longitudinal and cohort studies, Dezutter and Wachholtz have identified that it is those patients who have moderate to severe pain plus low levels of meaning making who actually develop major depression, which then further impedes actively coping with pain. When chronic pain patients experience a high level of meaning making, they show fewer depressive symptoms and greater life satisfaction regardless of the actual level of their pain. Therefore, it is important to screen for mood and anxiety disorders as well as spiritual coping and style of meaning making.

In clinical practice with chronic pain patients, mental health screening tools that include neurovegetative symptoms in their assessments (e.g., alterations in sleeping, eating, and energy) should be used cautiously. Patients with chronic pain may endorse the neurovegetative symptoms of depression or anxiety (e.g. sleep disruptions, low energy, weight gain), which are caused by the pain itself or iatrogenically due to the medications used to treat the

Fig. 14.1 Pathways to altered pain experience

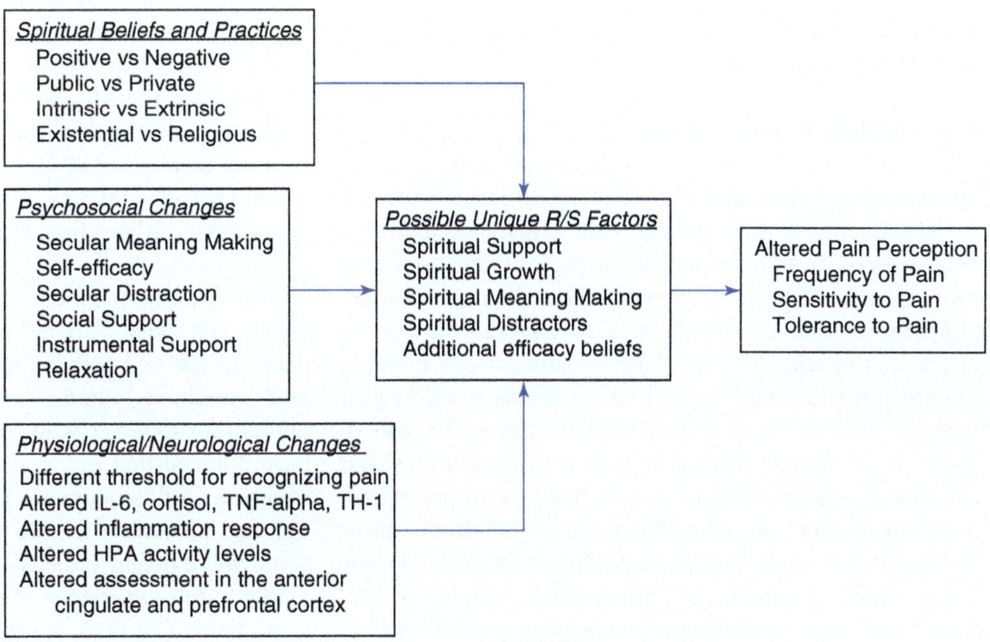

pain. This may artificially elevate depression or anxiety scores on assessments that do not account for the effects of a chronic pain comorbidity. Therefore, using screening tools that focus on emotional and cognitive symptoms of mental health disorders (e.g., Hospital Anxiety and Depression Scale by Zung) is critical when working with chronic pain.

The intent of this data is not to imply that medical caregivers should help patients to find religion in their lives or that those who have regular religious practices or communities will always do better clinically. The notable finding is that those who have a central system of meaning in their lives, despite higher levels of chronic pain, did not have a drop in their life satisfaction. Since the search for and presence of meaning for chronic pain patients seem to be stable over time, it has been postulated that this element may be an inner resource linked to personality and previous life experience that can be utilized for maintenance of well-being and adaptation; in other words, this is a factor of personal resilience that is stable. One could also hypothesize that those who have a personal sense of meaning in their lives deal better with chronic pain because they do not perceive this condition as destabilizing.

The use of opioid analgesia has been shown to dysregulate neural connections so that, via the dopamine system, there forms a desensitivity to rewarding life experiences. In this way, a chronic pain patient using opioids may have a biologically blunted sense of meaning. In a vicious cycle, those who escalate their use of opioids in an effort to treat their "total pain," that is, bio/psycho/social/spiritual/existential pain, may create psychological numbing which does not allow them to work through their existential distress in an effort to make meaning.

Uses and Indications

Importance of Assessment

Spirituality has been shown to be a crucial factor in mood, anxiety, quality of life, and the pain experience among a wide variety of medical patients who experience chronic pain. Spiritual distress was a greater contributor to satisfaction with life than a patient's physical disability in a group of patients in rehabilitation. Among patients with multiple sclerosis, spiritual well-being does not appear to affect pain intensity but does improve pain tolerance, as well as mood, and pain-coping self-efficacy. In a study of those with sickle cell disease, church attendance was linked with lower pain scores even after controlling for health status. Both cancer and spinal cord injury have a serious impact on spiritual well-being, which in turn can affect pain-related quality of life. Spinal cord injury is associated with a lower level of spiritual well-being compared to those without such an injury; in fact, spinal injury caused greater spiritual distress than a diagnosis of cancer. As in other populations, there was found a significant difference in pain intensity in someone with higher spiritual well-being compared to those with lower spiritual well-being – that is, there was on average lower pain in those with greater spiritual well-being. Similarly, if someone has a higher sense of spiritual well-being, that person is less likely to be depressed and more likely to be satisfied with life.

Spirituality in the context of pain management can be important for the clinician to factor in when it affects the way the patient views the provider. Though many spiritual people with a sense of a creator God believe that the Divine is the ultimate healer, there is a corresponding belief that God can use healthcare providers as instruments of healing and grace. It is sometimes challenging for medical providers to assess concretely for spiritual meaning making in the context of pain. However, in the sections below, it will be outlined about how it can be done succinctly, with empirical backing, and without attempting to engage a patient beyond a clinician's scope of practice.

Putting Research into Practice

Case 1: RJ is a 37-year-old man with history of spinal cord injury from an MVA 20 years ago. His brother was driving RJ and two other friends home from a high school soccer game when they were hit by a driver running a red light. One of the friends died, one did not have lasting injuries, and RJ's brother has been wheelchair-bound since the accident but has married. RJ himself has had a spinal cord injury that has made him a quadriplegic.

- What meaning does RJ make of this life event? RJ and his family are Mormons, and they believe that RJ and his brother were spared for a spiritual reason.
- How does this change in his function affect his sense of personhood? That is, is there existential distress? RJ feels loved and valued by his church family despite his disability. He is able to have some level of independence with a motorized wheelchair. He is able to speak and express his emotions.

What has his experience been with chronic pain? Though most quadriplegic patients experience numbness rather than pain, RJ has had pain in his low back for the past 3 years that sometimes becomes severe. He recognizes that this is unusual for someone with quadriplegia, and some caregivers have doubted that this is physiologic but perhaps more an experience of "total pain." This mismatch between expectation and his reality has led to intermittent bouts of depression, where he has socially isolated himself. The pain flares feed into this experience of psychologic suffering in that he is not able to sit in his mechanical wheelchair when he is in pain, so he loses considerable function and ability to connect with others. But his spiritual community and his personal practice of prayer give RJ the hope that he will get through his pain flare.

Assessment Tools

Clinicians report barriers to assessing spirituality in their patients; the most prevalent concern being time constraints. Lack of experience in making the assessment, feeling that such an assessment is not the clinician's responsibility, and concern regarding crossing boundaries where trust will be breached between the provider and patient are additional reasons that prevent spiritual assessments from being regularly conducted. This reticence to inquire about spirituality is interesting considering the evidence discussed above that patients feel it is an important part of their personhood but also because, like the general US population, physicians overall have active spirituality. Approximately 80% of family physicians identify themselves as very or somewhat strong in their beliefs and extremely close to God.

The intent of a spiritual assessment is five-fold:

1. Support patients with empathy and nonjudgmental listening.
2. Document spiritual preferences for the patient's care going forward.
3. Identify potential barriers to well-being in terms of negative spiritual coping so that proper referrals can be made.
4. Ensure the honoring of the patient's faith traditions in the treatment plan.
5. Foster overall wellness by encouraging a patient to access the resources of their community and faith tradition.

There are several commonly used assessment tools in the clinical setting for spiritual assessment. We will discuss the three most prevalent qualitative tools briefly below: "HOPE Questions for Spiritual Assessment," "The FICA Spiritual History Tool," and "OASIS inquiry."

Table 14.2 HOPE questions for spiritual assessment

H: sources of hope	Where do you gain your strength? What are your sources of comfort and peace?
O: organized religion	Are you part of a religious or spiritual community? How does it help you?
P: personal spirituality and practices	Do you have personal spiritual beliefs? What aspects of your spirituality do you find helpful?
E: effects on medical care and end-of-life issues	Is your ability to practice spiritually impaired by your illness? How can I help you access the resources that normally help you? Are there specific practices or restrictions I should know about in that they effect the provision of your medical care?

HOPE

The HOPE screen is an acronym to guide a brief spiritual interview (see Table 14.2). Though the questions are vague, the language is favored by some clinicians in that it does not assume a religious belief system but allows for recording of what a patient finds most important and helpful spiritually.

HOPE Example for a Formal Spiritual Assessment in a Medical Interview

Using the previous case of our 37-year-old patient with spinal cord injury, the HOPE screen might look like this:

- H = RJ finds hope in the belief that his pain will end in this world and that he will not experience suffering in the next life.
- O = His organized religion is the Mormon church, namely, his local ward. He is visited often by Brothers from his ward and prayed over by them as well as his family members.
- P = He prays daily and goes to church and men's Bible study on Sundays. When he is in particularly bad pain, he cries out to God trusting that his suffering will be heard.
- E = RJ feels that his life is a gift from God and he was spared death to bring God's word to others. So, he values his life as it is despite his disability because he is able to witness to his faith. Therefore, he wants life-prolonging treatment including life support.

FICA

The FICA screen is similar to the HOPE survey in that it is also an acronym that gives some framework to spiritual history taking (see Table 14.3).

OASIS

Finally, the Oncologist Assisted Spiritual Intervention Study (OASIS) Patient-Centered Spirituality Inquiry is the only validated screen in both patients and clinicians. The OASIS spiritual assessment is a semi-structured 5–7-minute conversation between physician and patient to understand spiritual concerns as they relate to coping with cancer. Both the interviewers and interviewees found this tool to be helpful and comfortable and allow for timely assessment

Table 14.3 FICA spiritual assessment tool

F	Faith and belief	Do you have spiritual beliefs that help in coping with stress or illness? What gives your life meaning?
I	Importance	Is this belief important to you? Does it influence how you think about health and illness or make decisions for yourself?
C	Community	Do you belong to a spiritual community or would like support in seeking?
A	Address in care	What action or changes do you want? Would it be helpful to see a spiritual counselor?

Table 14.4 OASIS interview

I. Introduce issue in neutral inquiring manner	*When dealing with a serious illness, many people draw on religious or spiritual beliefs to help cope. It would be helpful to me to know how you feel about this.*
II. Inquire further, adjusting inquiry to patient's initial response	(a) **Positive-active faith response**: *What have you found most helpful about your beliefs since your illness?* (b) **Neutral-receptive response**: *How might you draw on your faith or spiritual beliefs to help you?* (c) **Spiritually distressed response** (e.g., anger or guilt): *Many people feel that way . . . what might help you come to terms with this?* (d) **Defensive/rejecting response**: *It sounds like you're uncomfortable I brought this up. What I'm really interested in is how you are coping . . . can you tell me about that?*
III. Continue to explore further as indicated	*I see. Can you tell me more (about . . .)?*
IV. Inquire about ways of finding meaning & peace	*Is there some way in which you are able to find a sense of meaning or peace in the midst of this?*
V. Inquire about resources	*Whom do you have to talk to about this/ these concerns?*
VI. Offer assistance as appropriate and available	*We can arrange for you to talk to someone . . .; there's a support group.*
VII. Bring inquiry to a close	*I appreciate you discussing these issues with me. May I ask about it again?*

(see Table 14.4). This is the only validated assessment tool in that quality of life, spiritual well-being, depression, communication, and acceptability ratings were studied for both the patient and clinician. The OASIS Spiritual Inquiry overall improved the perception of quality care as well as positively impacted the well-being of the patient.

Evidence for Efficacy

In the past 20 years, a number of high-quality spiritually integrated interventions have targeted pain management. Consistently, the outcomes show that for individuals who are interested in accessing spiritual resources to cope with their pain, spiritually integrated interventions can have powerfully positive effects on pain management. The greatest improvements appear to be in the area of pain tolerance rather than pain sensitivity. In other words, it is not about the level of pain a patient is experiencing; it is what that patient can do despite the level of pain and how much medication is required to make them feel they can continue their activities of daily living.

Bormann has completed a series of studies examining the potential role of spiritually based mantram (meaningful word or phrase) repetition among veterans. In a large, multi-site study, she examined how 273 veterans responded to this spiritually based intervention. After 20 minutes a day of focused repetition on the spiritual mantram they chose, after the 8-week study, participants from all sites had multiple positive benefits, including a significant decrease in pain and somatization of emotional experiences.

After following HIV+ patients for 4 years, research found that positive spiritual coping is inversely related to viral load and positively associated with CD4+ counts among individuals with HIV. Individuals using negative spiritual coping were 4 times more likely to have a detectible viral load and CD4 count declined 2.25 times faster compared to those using positive spiritual coping. Lower viral load and higher CD4 counts protect from painful HIV/AIDS opportunistic infections.

This effect has also been found cross-culturally. In Japan, a study taught spirituality based mindfulness therapy to patients and asked them to practice independently every day for 2 weeks. The intervention decreased pain, depression, and anxiety among advanced cancer patients. In a study of Iranian women with breast cancer, a 6-week spiritual therapy intervention had positive effects on pain, spiritual well-being, and quality of life.

Carson and colleagues used the method of Loving-Kindness meditation, a Buddhist spiritual practice. This meditation technique was taught to meditation-naïve participants with low back pain. Carson found that not only were there long-term changes in pre-post assessment of low back pain compared to the usual care group, there was also a short-term pattern that Loving-Kindness practice on any given day resulted in lower pain and anger ratings the following day.

Wachholtz and Pargament completed a series of studies examining spiritual versus non-spiritual forms of meditation and the effect on acute and chronic pain sensitivity and tolerance. In 2005, they compared acute pain response using a cold pressor task [a form of noxious stimuli] among healthy meditation-naive individuals who had been randomly assigned to practice a spiritual meditation, secular meditation, or progressive muscle relaxation for 2 weeks. After 20 minutes/day for 2 weeks of practicing their assigned task, individuals in the spiritual meditation group showed significantly greater pain tolerance than those in the other two groups. In 2008, the same researchers randomly assigned meditation-naïve, frequent migraineurs to one of four meditation tasks: spiritual, secular positive self-statements, secular external neutral-positive statements, and progressive muscle relaxation. Participants practiced 20 minutes/day for 4 weeks. After 4 weeks, participants in the spiritual group had fewer migraine headaches, less severe migraine headaches, greater pain tolerance to acute pain, and less negative affect compared to the other three groups. In 2016, Wachholtz, Malone, and Pargament published a study with frequent migraineurs and found that after 4 weeks of meditation practice, those in the spiritual meditation group used less migraine analgesic or abortive medication than the other groups, even after controlling for migraine frequency and severity.

Wiech and colleagues used fMRI to study the key areas in the brain for modulating pain intensity with 12 Catholics and 12 nonreligious, non-spiritual subjects. They were shown pictures of two women in a similar pose: (1) the Virgin Mary and (2) an unknown woman painted in a similar genre to the Virgin Mary picture. While shown the pictures, they received repetitive mild-moderate electrical shocks. Prior to seeing the pictures, both groups were equally sensitive to the pain. After viewing the pictures, the religious group reported less pain while looking at the picture of the Virgin Mary, whereas the nonreligious group reported the same amount of pain. The fMRI findings found that the right ventrolateral prefrontal cortex (rVLPFC) cluster in the brain was uniquely activated in the religious sample when looking at the Virgin Mary picture. Post-scan self-reports indicated that the Catholic sample used a strategy known as self-focused reappraisal that allowed them to subconsciously downregulate the perceived intensity of the pain when presented with a religious image.

Conclusions

In the care of patients who suffer from chronic pain, spiritual assessment and attention is important to rendering the best care possible. Optimal spiritual support aims to improve feelings of self-efficacy, connectedness, purpose, and personal meaning even in the midst of personal suffering. Studies of small groups of specific populations of people who suffer with chronic pain have contributed to our understanding of spiritual care and pain management. There is certainly sufficient data to spur further research to understand more completely the physiologic effects and neurologic changes of spiritual beliefs and practices on those experiencing pain.

Pearls and Pitfalls

- Spirituality can have a powerful effect on pain, either positive or negative.
- Assessing spiritual health is an important component in a health assessment and subsequent treatment plan.
- It is important to asses for *type* of spiritual coping strategy, not just “yes/no” questions on spiritual beliefs and practices.
- Do not attempt spiritual counseling if you are not adequately trained to do so, but collaborate with professional licensed mental health resources or health-specific chaplains in your local area. Note that most clergy receive minimal training in mental health counseling and no training on health conditions, so strongly encourage referrals to licensed mental health professionals who have training in religious and spiritual forms of psychotherapy or chaplains with training in health chaplaincy.

Recommended Reading

1. Abraido-Lanza AF, Vasquez E, Echeverria SE. En las manos de Dios [in God’s Hands]: religious and other forms of coping among Latinos with arthritis. J Consult Clin Psychol. 2004;72:91–102.
2. Anandarajah G, Hight E. Spirituality and medical practice: using the HOPE questions as a practical tool for spiritual assessment. Am Fam Physician. 2001;63:87.
3. Dezutter J, Wachholtz A, Corveleyn J. Prayer and pain: the mediating role of positive re-appraisal. J Behav Med. 2012;34:542–9.
4. Johnson KS, Elbert-Avila KI, Tulsky JA. The influence of spiritual beliefs and practices on the treatment preferences of African Americans: a review of the literature. J Am Geriatr Soc. 2005;53:711–9.
5. Koenig H, King DE, Carson VB. Handbook of religion and health. 2nd ed. London: Oxford University Press; 2012.
6. Kremer H, Ironson G, Kaplan L, Stuetzele R, Baker N, Fletcher MA. Spiritual coping predicts CD4-cell preservation and undetectable viral load over four years. AIDS Care. 2015;27:71–9.
7. Kristeller JL, Rhodes M, Crope LD. Oncologist assisted spiritual intervention study (OASIS): patient acceptability and initial evidence of effects. Int J Psychiatry Med. 2005;35:329–47.
8. Pargament KI, Koenig HG, Perez L. The many methods of religious coping: development and initial validation of RCOPE. J Clin Psychol. 2000;564:519–43.
9. Pargament KI, Koenig HG, Tarakeshwar N, Hahn J. Religious struggle as a predictor of mortality among medically ill elderly patients. Arch Intern Med. 2001;161:1881–5.
10. Phillips RE, Pargament KI, Lynn Q, Crossley C. Self-directing religious coping: a deistic God, abandoning God, or no God at all? J Sci Study Relig. 2004;43:409–18.
11. Puchalski C. Spiritual assessment in clinical practice. Psychiatric Ann. 2006;36:150–5.
12. Strawbridge WJ, Cohen RD, Shema SJ, Kaplan GA. Frequent attendance at religious services and mortality: a 28 year followup. Am J Public Health. 1997;87:957–61.
13. Wachholtz A, Makowski S. Pain vs. suffering at the end of life. In: Moore RJ, editor. Handbook of pain and palliative care: biobehavioral approaches for the life course. New York: Springer; 2012.
14. Wachholtz AB, Pargament KI. Migraines and meditation: does spirituality matter? J Behav Med. 2008;31:355–61.
15. Wachholtz A, Malone C, Pargament K. Effect of different meditation types on migraine headache medicine use. Behav Med. 2015;43:1–8.
16. Wiech K, Farias M, Kahane G, Shackel N, Tiede W, Tracey I. An fMRI study measuring analgesia enhanced by religion as a belief system. Pain. 2008;139:467–76.

Anxiety and Depression in Patients with Chronic Pain

15

Shamard Charles, Alexios G. Carayannopoulos, and Sanket Pathak

Introduction

Chronic pain management is one of the biggest challenges in healthcare, and its relationship with anxiety and depression is still being explored. This chapter will provide a summary of the intricate relationship between pain, anxiety, and depression, the biological and pathophysiologic interplay between the three, its clinical manifestation, and the most effective treatment options, with an emphasis on the use of nonpharmacological interventions in the treatment of the pain-anxiety-depression continuum.

Background and Historical Perspective

The frequent accompaniment of anxiety and depression with pain and vice versa has long been documented. However, there is considerable controversy, however, regarding the extent to which the three are associated and the genesis or causal nature of each on the other. At one end of the range of beliefs, chronic pain in the absence of organic pathology is a depressive spectrum disorder. At the other end, depression is thought to occur in a relatively small subset of chronic pain patients. Furthermore, some believe that anxiety is a by-product of the two. To further complicate the matter, people who suffer from depression tend to experience anxiety and more severe and longer-lasting pain in comparison to those without depression. So it is reasonable to ask, what is the overlap, if any, between depression and anxiety and pain particularly in the setting of chronic pain syndromes such as fibromyalgia, arthritis, irritable bowel syndrome, low back pain, neuropathic pain, and headache?

The relationship between chronic pain-anxiety-depression is of both practical and theoretical importance. Pain is a controversial syndrome, and its etiology and treatment are a matter of dispute. Anxiety, depression, and pain commonly occur together, and all three can be detrimental to one's personal health and psychosocial well-being. Chronic pain syndromes are notoriously refractory to traditional medical treatments and result in tremendous personal and societal cost. Chronic pain patients frequently display pain behaviors and functional limitations that far exceed "normal" limits. For this reason, chronic pain is a major risk factor for depression and anxiety. Conversely, depression may be a predictor of poor response to treatment for chronic pain. In fact, numerous studies show that patients with pain are at increased risk of a lifetime history of depression, as compared to the normal population. Further, the risk of depression increases when the pain is diffuse, as indicated by the total number of painful sites. This undoubtedly affects quality of life; therefore, an emphasis should be placed on decreasing pain for both amelioration of symptoms and for lessening risk of depression. Increased knowledge about the role of depression in the etiology and maintenance of chronic pain prob-

S. Charles (✉)
Harvard T.H. Chan School of Public Health, NBC News Group, New York, NY, USA

A. G. Carayannopoulos
Department of Physical Medicine and Rehabilitation, Rhode Island Hospital, Providence, RI, USA

Comprehensive Spine Center: Rhode Island Hospital, Providence, RI, USA

Newport Hospital, Newport, RI, USA

Warren Alpert Medical School, Brown University, Providence, RI, USA

American Society of Interventional Pain Physicians, Rhode Island Chapter, Paducah, KY, USA
e-mail: acarayannopoulos@lifespan.org

S. Pathak
Department of Anesthesiology, Thomas Jefferson University Hospital, Philadelphia, PA, USA
e-mail: Sanket.pathak@jefferson.edu

T. R. Deer et al. (eds.), *Deer's Treatment of Pain*, https://doi.org/10.1007/978-3-030-12281-2_15

lems could potentially lead to improved assessment and treatment methods for chronic pain syndromes.

Uses and Indications

Depression and anxiety are extremely common in patients who suffer from chronic pain; therefore, a detailed psychiatric examination is necessary to assess the severity of the underlying depression and to determine the appropriate treatment. According to the World Health Organization (WHO) study, approximately one-fifth of all primary care patients suffer from persistent debilitating pain; they are also four times more likely to have comorbid anxiety or depression than pain-free primary care patients. It has been suggested that serotonin and norepinephrine, neurotransmitters that are located in both the main metabolic pathways involved in both pain transmission and depression, play a significant role in the development and treatment of both conditions. Furthermore, a number of psychotropic agents such as selective serotonin reuptake inhibitors (SSRIs), noradrenergic and specific serotonin receptor antagonist (NaSSa), and serotonin-norepinephrine reuptake inhibitors (SNRIs) have been actively studied and trialed for the treatment of pain disorders or painful somatic symptoms regardless of patients' diagnosis. This has led to the concept of "double-duty" medications, which includes psychiatric medications such as antidepressants and mood stabilizers that are also effective pain relievers. These medications can treat the underlying depression while also alleviating the underlying pain complaint. Because depression and anxiety are frequently found in patients suffering from chronic pain and vice versa, both the pain and underlying psychiatric condition must be addressed to maximize the treatment's success. One cannot be effectively addressed without also looking at the other.

Cognitive behavioral therapy (CBT), hypnosis, and exercise have all been shown to be helpful in anxiety and depression but can also be utilized in patients who suffer from pain. Aggressively addressing the anxiety or depression along with the pain is necessary for recovery to occur. If treatment in one or both lags, a vicious cycle can ensue, whereby pain may exacerbate the underlying anxiety or depression and anxiety or depression may worsen the pain complaints.

Proper diagnosis is essential to treatment. While obvious this cannot be understated. Further, due to the multifactorial nature of pain and depression syndromes, the accompaniment of anxiety, and new discoveries that further elucidate the biological and psychosocial mechanisms involved in both, treatment can be challenging. In most cases it is necessary to use multiple non-pharmacological modalities such as CBT, hypnosis, and exercise alongside pharmacological agents to successfully treat both problems.

Cognitive Behavioral Therapy The symptoms associated with chronic pain and anxiety and depression are demoralizing. Cognitive behavioral therapy (CBT) is a short-term, goal-oriented psychotherapy treatment that takes a hands-on approach to problem-solving. Its goal is to change the way a person feels by encouraging them to reevaluate their patterns of thinking or behavior. CBT is used to help treat a wide range of issues in a person's life, from depression and anxiety to chronic pain and relationship problems. CBT changes one's attitude and behavior by targeting the thoughts, images, beliefs, and attitudes associated with a problem and using focused evaluation and assessment to dissect and to understand how these processes relate to the way a person behaves (Fig. 15.1). CBT is an established treatment for anxiety and depression and is also the best studied psychotherapy for treating pain. Therapists use CBT to help patients learn coping skills so that they can manage, rather than be victimized by, their pain.

It is widely known that depression and anxiety can be effectively treated with selective serotonin reuptake inhibitor medications (SSRI), such as fluoxetine, or with specific forms of psychotherapy, such as cognitive-behavioral therapy (CBT). Anticonvulsants can also be used to stabilize mood as these medications ameliorate nerve hypersensitivity, which is sometimes involved in chronic pain. Monotherapy, which involves that is a single course of any of these treatments, however, leaves between one-third and one-half of the patients insufficiently improved and still depressed (Fig. 15.2). As previously discussed earlier, anxiety-depression and pain are intimately linked, and thus ineffective therapy to treat one likely contributes to ineffective treatment of the other. To increase effectiveness, medication and CBT have been combined (COMB).

In a 2012 systematic review of comparative efficacy of treatments and controls for depression conducted by Arif Khan et al. and published in PLOS, the combination of psychotherapy and antidepressants for depression was found to provide a slight advantage versus antidepressant or psychotherapy monotherapy. This suggests that type of treatment offered is less important than getting depressed patients involved in an active therapeutic program.

Hypnosis Hypnosis uses progressive relaxation techniques through suggestions of calming imagery and sensations, focused attention, and heightened susceptibility to suggestion (Hoi Ning Ngai '00). Patients are able to concentrate on improving their symptoms which often range from chronic pain to anxiety and depression. Many studies have concluded

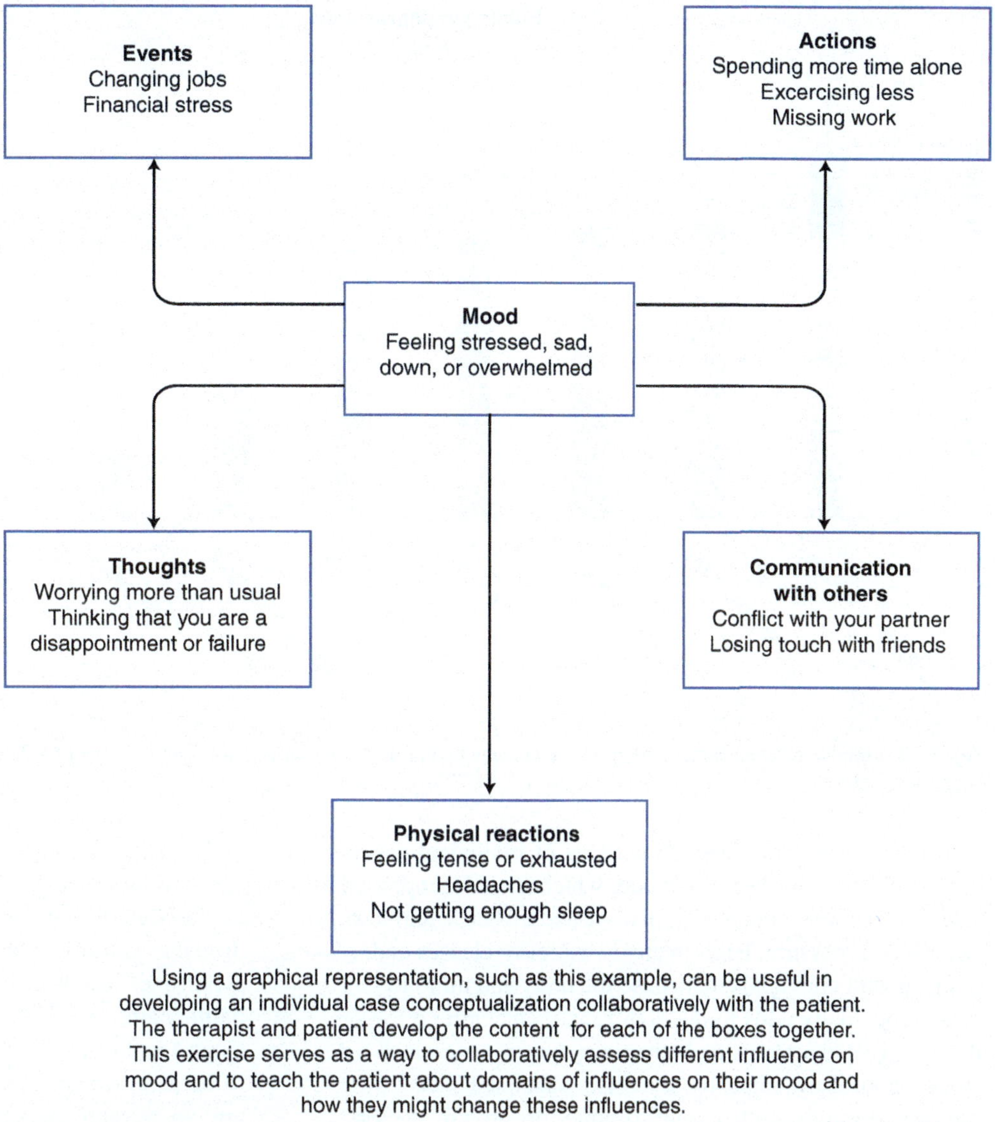

Fig. 15.1 Collaborative case conceptualization worksheet

that hypnosis is a viable intervention in the treatment of chronic pain and depression. In the most comprehensive meta-analysis of measuring outcomes of hypnotic approaches to chronic pain management, hypnosis was deemed to be a "highly promising" although "undeveloped" intervention [2]. Findings from controlled trials indicate that hypnosis is effective for reducing chronic pain intensity on average but that there is also substantial individual variation in outcome. Furthermore, few of any side negative side effects are reported. In fact, "most patients report positive side effects, such as an improved sense of well-being, a greater sense of control, improved sleep, and increased satisfaction with life, independent of whether they report reductions in pain [2]."

Anesthesia may be required for chronic pain syndromes that require surgical intervention. For those with severe anxiety or allergies to the chemical anesthetic, hypnotic analgesia has been used as an effective alternative for sedation and has illustrated short-term pain relief in those who suffer from chronic pain. More importantly, the use of hypnotic analgesia has provided a great deal of pain relief without the use of drugs or other chemicals, while also allowing the patient to be an active participate in their healing process.

Exercise While the evidence behind exercise and pain reduction is not fully elucidated, there's an abundance of research that regular exercise can be as effective at treating depression as medication. Exercise boosts serotonin and endorphins just like antidepressants. This helps to improve mood and to alleviate anxiety. More importantly, a small change in lifestyle can result in major benefits, as maximal results can be felt with 30 to 60 minutes of moderate intensity aerobic activity.

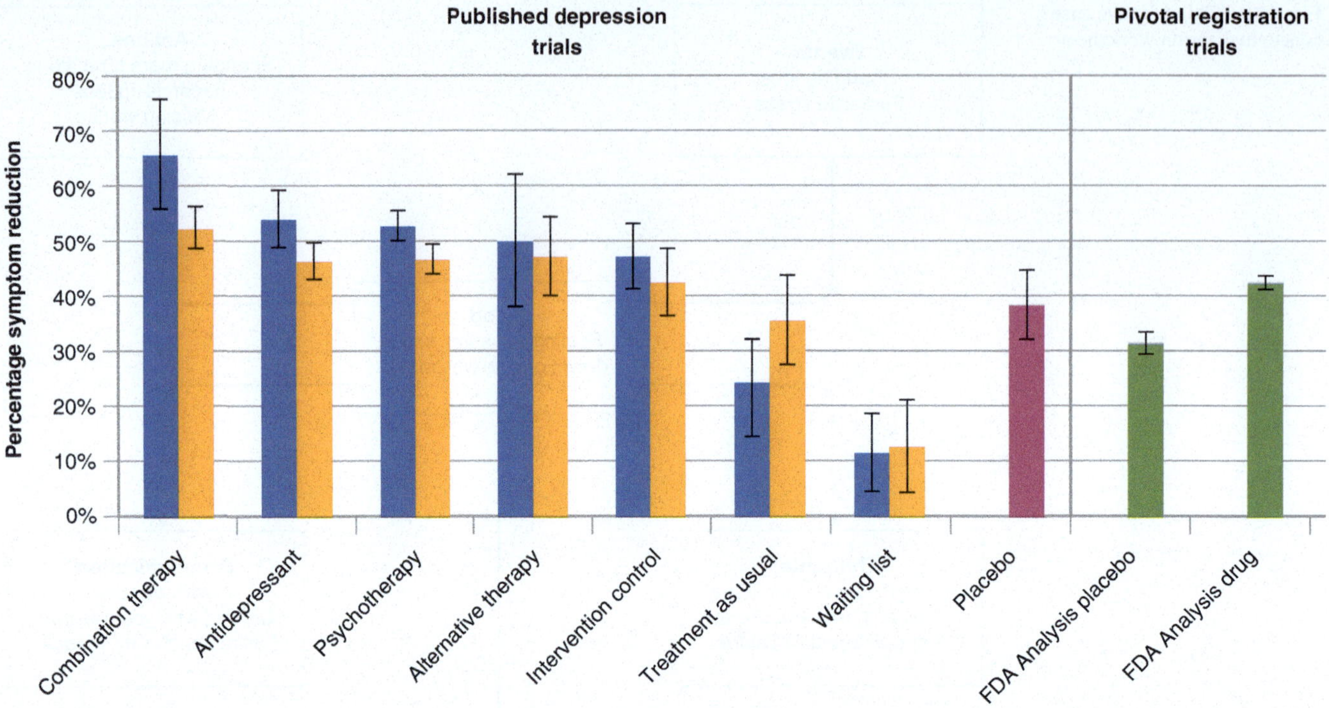

Fig. 15.2 Graphical representation of mean percentage symptom reduction per different treatment modality from FDA unblinded and blinded depression trials

Routine exercising leads to a series of biological events that result in many health benefits which include improved sleep, protection against heart disease and diabetes, and lowering blood pressure. High-intensity exercise releases endorphins, potent chemicals that cause the body and mind to feel good. This likely adds to the high runners feel after a jog or the low-trained athletes feel when they haven't exercised for some time. Low-intensity exercise sustained over time releases proteins called neurotrophic or growth factors, which cause nerve cells to grow and to make new connections. This improvement in brain function makes one feel better and likely contributes to the rewiring of our perception, thoughts, and beliefs about pain.

According to a new study published in a 2014 issue of Medicine & Science in Sports & Exercise, researchers at the University of New South Wales and Neuroscience Research Australia found that regular exercise may alter how a person experiences pain. The more routine exercise is, the new findings suggest, the greater our tolerance for discomfort.

Main Points

- Optimization of chronic pain management is an evolving and sometimes elusive practice and remains one of the most challenging and costly aspects of healthcare.
- The overlap of anxiety, depression, and pain is particularly evident in the following chronic pain syndromes: arthritis, fibromyalgia, irritable bowel syndrome, low back pain, headaches, and neuropathic pain.
- Cognitive behavioral monotherapy has been shown to be as efficacious as pharmacological monotherapy in several studies, but combination therapy remains the most efficacious and thus should be utilized as standard of care.
- Hypnosis has slowly become accepted in traditional medicine as an alternative treatment for anxiety, depression, and chronic pain. Studies have demonstrated a reduction in short-term pain and central nervous system activity during hypnotic procedures that offer promise and preliminary information concerning possible physiological mechanisms of hypnotic analgesia and increased clinical application.
- Exercise is often used as an adjunct therapy for pain relief, but more research needs to be done to elucidate its role in anxiety and depression management.

Recommended Reading

1. Flynn HA, Warren R. Using CBT effectively for treating depression and anxiety. Curr Psychiatry. 2014;13(6):45–53.
2. Jensen MP, Patterson DR. Hypnotic approaches for chronic pain management. Am Psychol. 2014;69(2):167–77.
3. Jones MD, Booth J, Taylor JL, Barry BK. Aerobic training increases pain tolerance in healthy individuals. Med Sci Sports Exerc. 2014;46(8):1640–7.
4. Khan A, Faucett J, Lichtenberg P, Kirsch I, Brown WA. A systematic review of comparative efficacy of treatments and controls for depression. PLoS One. 2012;7(7):e41778.
5. Lépine JP, Briley M. The epidemiology of pain in depression. Hum Psychopharmacol. 2004;19(Suppl 1):S3–7. https://doi.org/10.1002/hup.618.
6. McCaffery M, Pasero C. Pain: clinical manual. 2nd ed. Oulu, Finland: Mosby; 1997. ISBN-13: 978-0815156093.
7. Morris DB. The culture of pain. Berkeley, CA: University of California Press; 1991. ISBN 0520082761.
8. Papolos D, Papolos J. Overcoming depression: the definitive resource for patients and families who live with depression and manic-depression. New York: Harper Perennial; 1997. ISBN-13: 978-0060157562.
9. Sansone RA, Sansone LA. Pain, pain, go away: antidepressants and pain management. Psychiatry (Edgmont). 2008;5:16–9.
10. Wheeler EG, Doce-Lombard J. Living creatively with chronic illness: developing skills for transcending the loss, pain and frustration. Tucson, Arizona: Pathfinder Publishing; 1989. ISBN 0934793174.

16 Psychological Treatments to Improve Outcomes

Marilyn S. Jacobs

Introduction

Psychological evaluation and interventions are an essential aspect of the treatment of pain. The view that the pain experience is perceptual in nature and that emotional and cognitive factors influence the registration of tissue damage by the central nervous system is an established paradigm. Research has confirmed that the extent of tissue damage does not always correlate with the subjective experience of pain. Psychological distress and disorders can establish pain and be caused by pain. Given that chronic pain cannot always be cured and that management of the burden of illness is the most likely direction, the psychological, social, and existential issues which complicate this malady are crucial aspects of care.

Patients with chronic pain can develop the full range of psychiatric diagnoses. Common problems such as depression, anxiety spectrum disorders, cognitive impairment, and addiction are compounded by immersion in the sick role, pain behaviors, loss of identity, and disrupted self-esteem. Other consequences to persistent pain include disorders of homeostasis (sleep, appetite, and sexual functioning), delusional and psychotic disorders, and personality disintegration.

Social morbidity is common when pain is chronic. Economic disruption (loss of ability to maintain employment, depletion of financial resources due to inadequate third-party coverage, and lessened lifestyle), relationship rupture (loss of social network, marital and family discord, loss of role within the family and community), and the inability to function normally in society thus becoming reliant upon social welfare are all too frequent occurrences.

An understanding of the scope of potential problems, interventions, and outcomes in the population of chronic pain patients will enhance patient care and satisfaction and is thus important for comprehensive pain medicine care.

M. S. Jacobs (✉)
Department of Psychiatry and Biobehavioral Sciences, David Geffen School of Medicine at UCLA, Los Angeles, CA, USA

Background and Historical Perspective

For centuries, pain was seen as a sensation due to the impact of a noxious stimulus. Observers and investigators attributed the psychological consequences to moral, personality, or situational causation. The extent to which disruptions in the nervous system caused suffering was mechanistic and line labeled.

It is an underappreciated fact of history that Sigmund Freud discovered psychoanalysis while treating patients with "lesionless pain" – a concern of nineteenth century physicians. Hodgkiss has elaborated how Freud's early works (*Interpretation of Dreams, Project for a Scientific Psychology and Studies in Hysteria*) reflected his realization that somatic pain was not caused by psychological factors but influenced by these elements. Thus, the evolution of psychotherapeutic practices in the twentieth century of all types can be traced to the investigations of pain patients who presented with inexplicable physical complaints that were understood to have psychic components.

At the University of Rochester, Engel and Romano developed the biopsychosocial approach in understanding health, illness, and the provision of medical care. This model was a paradigm shift for clinical practice and was conceived in opposition to the biomedicine of the time. It holds that a biological derangement does not always translate into a disease state, that psychological elements influence illness, that the doctor-patient relationship is very powerful in medical outcomes, and that the meaning of an illness as having a physical cause does not satisfy all patients. This analysis is relevant to the wide range of pain disorders, and furthermore, these factors tend to interact dynamically, changing over time. Recent findings from basic science research and cognitive neuroscience illuminate how psychosocial factors can have more influence than tissue damage in certain patients. The biopsychosocial model has been criticized as being overly reductionist. As well, emerging areas of inquiry have widened the number of variables in health and illness. These include population genetics, social epidemiology, develop-

T. R. Deer et al. (eds.), *Deer's Treatment of Pain*, https://doi.org/10.1007/978-3-030-12281-2_16

mental biology, environmental forces, technology, and the economics of healthcare systems. Complexity theory has been suggested as a more appropriate paradigm; we cannot know all of the inputs on a biological system; thus control is limited.

William Livingston's text *Pain and Suffering* concluded that pain was more than stimulus intensity, i.e., a given patient's sensory input can be influenced by emotional factors from higher brain centers the sum of which is pain perception. His ideas undoubtedly influenced later theories of pain. It became apparent that to understand a patient with pain, one needed to understand the psychology and social circumstances of the patient.

The investigation of biopsychosocial factors is varied and complex. The *Diagnostic Criteria for Psychosomatic Research (DCPR)* is a listing of psychosocial factors which predict outcomes in clinical medicine and are useful in thinking about pain-related variables. These factors are health anxiety, disease phobia, thanatophobia (fear of impending death), illness denial, functional somatic symptoms secondary to a psychiatric disorder, persistent somatization, conversion symptoms, anniversary reaction, type A behavior, irritable mood, demoralization, and alexithymia. Specific to pain management, *Block's Pre-surgical Psychological Screening (PPS) Algorithm* identifies pain sensitivity, depression, anger, anxiety, low self-esteem, excessive guardedness, and catastrophic thinking as risk factors for patient's undergoing invasive pain therapies. Both of these examples illuminate the range of phenomena which may influence pain perception.

Clinical Implications

There is a significant occurrence of psychiatric disorders in patients with chronic pain. Depression is the most common problem followed by anxiety. Knaster found that among 100 patients with chronic pain, 59% had a lifetime incidence of depression, and 39% had a lifetime incidence of anxiety. Comorbid depression and anxiety over the patient's lifetime was 28%. An extensive literature which includes examinations of nationally representative samples confirms these findings. Among the anxiety disorders, post-traumatic stress and related phenomena commonly co-occurs with chronic pain, likely owing to the stress of chronic illness and the traumatic nature of many pain etiologies as well as a history of abuse.

There is a distinction between the onset of a psychiatric disorder such as depression or anxiety in the context of a diagnosable pain disorder (i.e., post-laminectomy syndrome, complex regional pain syndrome) and that of psychological symptoms which occur with medically unexplained symptoms or a somatization disorder. Each psychiatric classification system has used different nosology; hence, these phenomena may be known as psychosomatic, somatic symptom or illness anxiety disorders. Pain complaints associated with psychological distress and suffering may emanate from complex factors in the patient's developmental life history. A clinical correlation of somatic suffering may take time to uncover yet may not be possible due to the complexity of the patient's mental structure. Patients with a continued somatization habit may use this non-symbolic form of communication about stress and distress as a result of an immature personality.

Studies of the psychology of patients with pain have found that alexithymia is a common finding. Alexithymia is the inability to identify and use verbal language to describe feelings, a lack of symbolic (imaginative) capacity and an inordinate focus upon physical experiences and external occurrences. Patients with this type of mental organization are prone to amplify somatic stimuli. It has also been noted that alexithymia may occur as a secondary complication of the suffering inherent in prolonged chronic illness and pain.

Cognitive impairment is common in pain patients. Depression, pharmacotherapy regimens consisting of multiple medications which have central nervous system side effects, and the loss of cortical volume which has been demonstrated due to pain-related central sensitization are the most common causes. As well, diminished functionality can cause impairments in attention, memory, and processing.

Addiction to opiates and benzodiazepines, self-soothing with compulsive overeating, and the development of other compulsive behaviors (shopping, gambling, and video games) can occur with chronic pain. Sexual functioning is commonly affected due to medications, weight gain, lack of vitality, and decreased self-esteem. Sleep cycle disorders are endemic to the chronic pain condition and difficult to manage due to neurobiological alterations associated with sensitization, medications, and inactivity. Delusional disorders and psychosis are rare but can occur if stress levels are unmanageable in a patient with significant vulnerability. Personality changes are also frequent – underlying tendencies such as dependency or loss of emotional control can be accentuated with lowered coping and self-regulation.

Evidence for Efficacy

The efficacy of psychological interventions to improve outcomes in chronic pain has been unequivocally established. These include psychotherapy, behavioral therapy, and psychiatric medication management. The refinement of protocols for interventional pain therapies has led to the requirement that patients being considered for neuromodulation, spinal surgery, and infusions with possible brain-related side effects undergo a screening psychological evaluation.

With regard to psychotherapy, there are many treatment options. An assessment of the patient's needs, goals, and capacities as well as resources prior to settling on the choice of psychotherapy will improve the outcome. Patients should agree to psychotherapy and not be forced into it.

For patients who require training in stress management and conscious control of negative symptoms, cognitive behavioral therapy (CBT), acceptance commitment therapy (ACT), and dialectical behavioral therapy (DBT) are optimal choices. These modalities are generally oriented to the improvement of coping skills and are provided on a short-term basis with goals directed at changes in emotional processing, thinking, and behavior.

Psychodynamic psychotherapy is indicated for those for whom attention paid to the deeper causes and consequences of distress, improvement in relationships, and an understanding of the meaning of traumatic experiences are sought after and for somatoform disorders. This type of therapy is directed at transformation of emotional experience and is usually long term in duration. There is less specific evidence for psychodynamic psychotherapy with pain patients (most of the medical data is with somatization disorders), yet clinical observation by clinicians providing this care has indicated positive gains.

Many providers of psychotherapy apply a multimodal approach. As such, elements of different psychotherapy orientations are combined. This strategy is practical and potentially serves the complex needs of patients with chronic pain who may not find full benefit from one technique.

Couples therapy, family therapy, and group therapy are other psychotherapy modalities which are indicated based upon the problems which pain has created for the individual patient.

Behavioral therapies can promote self-regulation and initiate a self-efficacy with distress.

Referral to a psychiatrist for psychotropic medication management may be indicated for select pain patients. However, uncomplicated psychological symptoms can be managed by the pain medicine physician. This is especially so as there is an overlap between pain and psychic distress which is covered by many pharmacotherapy agents used in pain medicine.

Main Points

1. The biopsychosocial model is the standard of care for patients with pain, and recent advances have enlarged this model.
2. Patients with chronic pain have high levels of psychiatric comorbidity.
3. Depression and anxiety are the most prevalent disorders in pain patients, but the full range of psychiatric disorders can occur.
4. There are varied criteria for evaluation of psychological symptoms comorbid to illness.
5. There is no one psychotherapy for pain patients – the choice depends upon the patient, and a combination of approaches may be the most effective (multimodal therapy).

Recommended Reading

1. Block AR, Sarwer DB. Presurgical psychological screening: understanding patients, improving outcomes. Washington, DC: American Psychological Association; 2013.
2. Borrell-Carrio F, Suchman AL, Epstein RM. The biopsychosocial model 25 years later: principles, practice and scientific inquiry. Ann Fam Med. 2004;2(6):576–82.
3. Ehde DM, Dillworth TM, Turner JA. Cognitive-behavioral therapy for individuals with chronic pain: efficacy, innovations and directions for research. Am Psychol. 2014;69(2):153–66.
4. Fava GA, Sonino N, Wise TN. The psychosomatic assessment: strategies to improve clinical practice. Basel: S. Karger A.G; 2012.
5. Hann KEJ, McCracken LM. A systematic review of randomized controlled trials of Acceptance and Commitment Therapy for adults with chronic pain: outcome domains, design quality, and efficacy. J Contextual Behav Sci. 2014;3:217–27.
6. Hodgkiss A. From lesion to metaphor: chronic pain in British, French and German medical writings, 1800-1914. Amsterdam: Brill Rodopi; 2000.
7. Knaster P, Karlsson H, Estlander AM, Kalso E. Psychiatric disorders as assessed with SCID in chronic pain patients: the anxiety disorders precede the onset of pain. Gen Hosp Psychiatry. 2012;34:46–52.
8. Roy R. Abuse, chronic pain and psychodynamic psychotherapy. In: Psychosocial interventions for chronic pain: in search of evidence. New York: Springer; 2008.

17 Psychological Evaluation for Those Receiving Devices for the Treatment of Pain

Ioannis M. Skaribas and Kevin Smith

Introduction

To date, spinal cord stimulators and intrathecal pump delivery systems represent the most common implantable devices in pain medicine. Pre-surgical psychological evaluations have been recommended since the very first use of the technology in 1967. Reasons for these evaluations are frequently unclear to patients and physicians alike. Evidence-based treatment guidelines have made psychological evaluation a prerequisite for implantable devices including implantable intrathecal drug delivery systems (IT), because there is considerable literature on the predictive value of biopsychosocial risk factors that impact surgical outcome. A pain management specialist must be able to appreciate the necessity of utilizing these psychological evaluations as part of the patient selection process and understand how this biopsychological assessment can predict treatment outcomes.

Background and Historical Perspectives

It is commonly accepted in the medical community that the psychological status of the patient is important in determining the success or failure of spinal cord stimulators and implantable pumps, but many pain physicians, and consequently their patients, remain unclear about why the psychological status of the patient is so important. The theoretical basis for spinal cord stimulation is the gate control theory of pain that included a role for psychological factors (affective, cognitive) in the modulation of pain. Although the exact mechanism is not well understood, the basic theory is that specific fibers of the dorsal horn that are responsible for touch, pressure, and vibration and not involved in pain transmission, can modulate fibers that transmit pain signals if stimulated. The gate control theory of pain states that non-noxious stimuli can close the "gate" of pain transmission to the brain, but psychological factors can then impact how any given stimuli is interpreted by the patient. For example, not all patients interpret the "non-noxious" stimuli of spinal cord stimulation as benign. The original recommendation for selecting a patient for spinal cord stimulation was to ensure emotional stability, absence of depression, and cooperation with a rehabilitation program.

Uses and Indications

Outcomes for spinal cord stimulation have historically been estimated to be about 50%, and some have speculated that the reasons that the long-term results are not higher are largely due to technical factors (e.g., lead migration, lead position, complications, malfunctioning units). Other authors have suggested that psychological factors likely play a role in the efficacy of these devices because pain is multidimensional in nature. The presence of psychiatric comorbidities including substance abuse, high levels of distress, and extreme psychopathology has been associated with poor responses to treatment. Pre-surgical psychological evaluations are meant to improve outcomes by helping to select the best candidates for spinal cord stimulators (SCS) or intrathecal pumps (ITP). Both types of implantable devices represent a tertiary form of treatment that are offered to patients who have already exhausted other forms of treatment, including both conservative (medication management, physical therapy) and interventional/surgical interventions. Thus, these patients have usually failed nearly every other form of intervention. One psychological factor that has been shown to consistently predict treatment failure has been depression; however, depression is not the only predictor of surgical success that has been identified.

I. M. Skaribas (✉)
Expert Pain P.A., Department of Anesthesiology, McGovern Medical School, The University of Texas Health Science Center at Houston, Houston, TX, USA
e-mail: skaribasmd@expertpaincare.com

K. Smith
Kevin G. Smith, Ph.D. and Associates, P.C., Houston, TX, USA
e-mail: kevin@kevinsmithphd.com

T. R. Deer et al. (eds.), *Deer's Treatment of Pain*, https://doi.org/10.1007/978-3-030-12281-2_17

Cognitive capacity, pain perception, beliefs about pain, treatment expectations, pain acceptance, and coping skills are widely seen as important factors for predicting positive treatment outcomes with implantable devices. Untreated and unresolved psychological problems, such as active psychosis, suicidal ideation, major untreated mood disorders, somatization disorders, and substance abuse, including alcohol abuse have been exclusionary contraindications for implantable. Some studies have found that higher levels of anxiety, "catastrophizing," paranoia, and psychopathic deviation are associated with lower treatment outcomes. Patients with histories of physical/sexual abuse were found to be more likely to develop chronic pain following an injury.

There have been several authors that have proposed a variety of exclusionary and cautionary criteria which have been included in this chapter (see Table 17.1). This summary of the criteria is by no means a definitive explanation of the subject, but rather is meant to provide the reader with an overall perspective of the common criteria used to emphasize the complexity of the decision made by a psychologist.

Although there appears to be wide agreement that psychological factors including depression are important in predicting surgical outcome for implantable devices, there is no algorithm nor any exact method used to weigh or calculate the total of psychological influence in a consistent manner. Much is left to the subjective judgment of the psychologist. To date available methods for pre-surgical psychological evaluation provide for a method of determining what constitutes a high score, and demonstrates the utility of this method in the decision-making process for implantable devices. Using this method, a psychologist would make recommendations to the physician in five categories:

- (Green) Proceed with Surgery
- (Yellow I) Proceed with Surgery with Postoperative Psychological Sessions
- (Yellow II) Preoperative Psychological Sessions
- (Red I) Noninvasive Therapy Recommended
- (Red II) No Treatment of Any Kind (XXX)

In practice, many psychologists are likely to recommend:

1. Proceed with surgery with or without recommendations for follow-up care.
2. Recommend against surgery at this time pending psychological intervention.
3. Recommend against surgery as this patient is unlikely to meet the guidelines.

There are a variety of psychological tests that are used by psychologists as tools to improve decision-making. Psychologists typically include an overall measure of psychological adjustment and personality, such as the MMPI-2 in their battery. The MMPI-2, as well as the Depression Scale, has been widely used to establish which patients are good candidates for implantable therapies. There are other measures of coping skills (Coping Skills Questionnaire), attitudes and beliefs about health (Behavioral Health Inventory, Millon Behavioral Medicine), pain specific measures (e.g., McGill Pain Questionnaire, Survey of Pain Attitudes), and numerous symptom specific measures (e.g., Beck Depression Inventory, Spielberg State Trait Anxiety, Hamilton Depression Scale) that are used. We mention just a few of these measures, because an exhaustive review of the many psychological measures is beyond the scope of this chapter. The utilization of these instruments in the psychological and overall biopsychosocial assessment of the patient is substantial, but these instruments are not infallible, and they require a psychologist with appropriate training and clinical experience to conduct these types of assessments, to interpret these tests accurately and to make appropriate recommendations to the physician. Many of these tests will show scale elevations, such as false positives, that are not an accurate reflection of the patient's psychological functioning, and the psychologist must decide whether any given elevation is accurate or not. Reading comprehension ability, exaggeration, and idiosyncratic responses are frequent occurrences that can impact psychological test interpretation.

In addition to psychological testing, the evaluation includes a clinical interview to discuss the location, severity, and chronicity of the patient's pain condition. The interviewer asks questions such as the following: Does the pain

Table 17.1 Psychological exclusionary and cautionary criteria

Exclusionary criteria	Cautionary criteria
Active psychosis	Somatization with explainable pain
Active suicidality or homicidality	Nonorganic signs (e.g., Wadel's)
Severe depression, anxiety untreated	Mild to moderate depression or anxiety
Severe cognitive impairment	Mild cognitive impairment with support
Severe sleep disturbance	Severe doctor-patient conflict
Severe mood instability/ impulsiveness	Poor coping, pessimism, catastrophizing
Active alcohol/drug addiction	Past history of substance/tobacco abuse
Litigation/compensation questions	Job dissatisfaction
Unrealistic expectations for pain relief	Incorrect beliefs about pain
Personality disorder	Multiple medical problems/ obesity
Poor/inadequate family/social support	Unusual pain ratings/exaggeration
Defiant and poor compliance	Excessive perception of disability
Malingering/factitious disorder	History of sexual/physical abuse

follow a known dermatome distribution or is it more global? Does the patient accept their pain as likely chronic or do they expect to be cured? What meaning does the patient assign to pain? Does the patient believe that pain is a sign of on-going physical harm? Furthermore, the psychologist asks about healthcare utilization, medical/surgical history, current medications, opioid use/abuse, psychological distress, symptoms of psychiatric illness, history of psychiatric treatment, history of physical/sexual abuse or trauma, nicotine use, substance abuse history, adequacy of social support, and the presence of any cognitive deficits, including a neurocognitive mental status exam. The patient's educational background and work history is used to better understand their attitudes and perceptions of disability. The psychologist will also likely probe for patient expectations about the procedure, and ascertain whether the patient fully understands the procedure, as well as answer any remaining questions. What does the patient expect from the procedure? Do they have goals to reduce their reliance on pain medications and increase their activity level? If successful, how would an implantable device impact their lives generally? Could the patient return to work or school?

While it is unlikely that one psychological test can serve as the gold standard for these assessments, there is a greater chance for agreement on what types of psychological tests are needed to make these decisions and the types of questions used. We advocate the use of semi-structured clinical interviews for patient selection. As further research develops, there will likely be greater agreement on the exact criteria and methods for conducting these assessments, and it is likely that other objective measures, such as quantitative sensory testing and other psychophysiological measures, will be developed.

Evidence of Efficacy

It is increasingly recognized that psychosocial variables can predict medical treatment outcomes. One review of the literature showed that psychological factors correctly predicted the treatment outcome of spinal cord stimulation over 80% of the time, and another systematic review of the literature found a strong association between psychological factors and treatment outcome 92% of the time.

Some authors have found that certain psychological traits could predict variation in pain relief between post-implantation and 3 months following the procedure. For example, some patients initially had a positive response to a SCS trial post-implantation but later reported at a 3-month evaluation that there was no pain relief. One review of the literature found that the patient's ability to cope with pain and the emotional impact of coping was a major determinant of SCS outcomes and suggested that improved education/preparation and cognitive behavioral therapy (CBT) for patients prior to undergoing SCS may improve outcomes by combining psychosocial intervention with implantable devices.

It is commonly accepted that depression and chronic pain are often correlated with one another, and there is data that show that high percentages of patients suffering from major depression (42%) are likely to develop low back pain. There is data that shows that high percentages (50–80%) of patients seen in pain centers suffer from some form of psychopathology. Patients with depression and low back pain tend to have poorer responses to treatment in general and greater chronicity of pain over time.

In clinical settings, it is not uncommon for many patients to say to a pain management physician, "I am depressed merely because of my pain, and getting me out of pain would resolve my underlying depression." There is some objective truth to that statement, but it is not always that simple. These patients are trying to define their problem narrowly and may refuse to recognize the role that depression and other psychosocial factors may play in determining their response to pain treatments. Patients and providers who try to ignore the psychosocial aspects of chronic pain will often do so at the expense of satisfactory treatment outcome. Some patients have psychological traumas or psychiatric conditions that predate their injuries that will influence their perception of their pain and will also influence how well they cope with pain (before and after an implantable device). After being injured, some patients face decidedly different prospects for their future. Patients are injured in a context. For those who may have many transferable job skills and an advanced degree, a back injury is often more of an inconvenience and not disabling, but for someone who may have a lower level of education, a learning disability, or a labor-intensive job, a back injury can be life-changing and hard for patients to come to terms with. Perceptions of disability, pending litigation, expectations for pain relief from the device, and current health status are all potentially cautionary things to consider when evaluating a patient with pain for a device. A patient's knowledge about the device can influence how they perceive the outcome of the initial trial. If a patient can experience a greater sense of mastery and control over their pain and their life, then they are more likely to view the implantable device as a successful long-term outcome.

Pearls and Pitfalls

While there appears to be a growing body of evidence that psychosocial factors play an important role in predicting medical treatment outcomes, there is no wide agreement on the precise method to determine who might be a candidate for implantable devices, nor a clear agreement about which psychological tests or cutoff scores should be used to make these decisions. There is no well-defined algorithm; therefore, a decision about a patient's candidacy for an implantable device is complex and is typically based on the combined clinical judgments of a psychologist and a physician. There have even been some retrospective studies that have questioned the effectiveness of psychological factors in predicting SCS outcomes.

While depression appears to be the factor that is most strongly linked to reducing efficacy in SCS, depression and quality of life can improve after SCS implantation. Although alcohol and substance abuse may be a valid exclusion criteria, there has been recent data that shows that patients with a history of alcohol abuse may show superior results from high-frequency spinal cord stimulation. The next generation of implantable devices has not been in use long enough for us to determine its long-term outcome.

Most of what we know about the psychological predictors for successful surgical outcome is based on data available as of the date of this publication, which represents older technology. While it is reasonable to think that psychological predictors are unlikely to change, it is not a foregone conclusion. New generations of spinal cord stimulation technology (Burst, HF-10, DRG) may have different results. Future studies are needed to further explore the best psychosocial predictors for this next generation of implantable devices.

Recommended Reading

1. American College of Occupational, Environmental Medicine. Chronic pain treatment guidelines. In: Hegmann K, editor. Occupational medicine practices. 2nd ed. Beverly Farms: OEM Press; 2008.
2. Atkinson JH, et al. Prevalence, onset and risk of psychiatric disorders in chronic pain patients: a controlled study. Pain. 1991;45:111–21.
3. Block AR. Psychological screening of spine surgery candidates. In: Hochshuler SH, Cotler HB, Guyer RD, editors. Rehabilitation of the spine: science and practice. St. Louis: Mosby; 1992. p. 617–25.
4. Block AR, Ahnmeiss DO, Guyer RD, Rashbaum RF, Hochschuler SH. The use of presurgical psychological screening to predict the outcome of spine surgery. Spine J. 2001;1:274–82.
5. Block AR, Gatchel RJ, Deardorff W, Guyer RD. The psychology of spine surgery. Washington D.C.: American Psychological Association; 2003.
6. Brandwin MA, Kewman DG. MMPI indicators of treatment response to spinal epidural stimulation in patients with chronic pain and patients with movement disorders. Psychol Reports. 1982;51:1059–64.
7. Bruns D, Disorbio JM. Assessment of biopsychosocial risk factors for medical treatment: a collaborative approach. J Clin Psychol Med Settings. 2009;16(2):127–47.
8. Burchiel KJ, Anderson VC, Wilson BJ, Denison DB, Olson KA, Shatin D. Prognostic factors in of spinal cord stimulation for chronic back and leg pain. Neurosurgery. 1995;36:1101–10.
9. Campbell CM, Jamison RN, Edward R. Psychological screening/phenotyping as predictors for spinal cord stimulation. Curr Pain Headache Rep. 2013;17(1):307.
10. Celestin J, Edwards RR, Jamison RN. Pretreatment psychosocial variables as predictors of outcomes following lumbar surgery and spinal cord stimulation: a systematic review and literature synthesis. Pain Med. 2009;10:659–3.
11. Colorado Division of Worker Compensation. Chronic Pain Task Force. (2007). Rule 17, Exhibit 9: Chronic pain disorder medical treatment guidelines. https://www.google.com/search?q=colorodo+division+of+worker+compensiation+chronic+pain+task+force+rule+17&oq=colorodo+division+of+worker+compensiation+chronic+pain+task+force+rule+17&aqs=chrome..69i57.25063j0j8&sourceid=chrome&ie=UTF-8. Retrieved from June 10, 2017.
12. Doleys DM. Psychological factors in spinal cord stimulation therapy: brief review and discussion. Neurosurg Focus. 2006;21(6):E1.
13. Evers AW, Kraaimaat FW, van Riel PL, Bijlsma JW. Cognitive, behavioral and physiological reactivity to pain as a predictor of long-term pain in rheumatoid arthritis patients. Pain. 2001;93:139–46.
14. Fishbain DA. Approaches to treatment decisions for psychiatric comorbidity in the management of the chronic pain patient. Med Clin North Am. 1999;83:737–60.
15. Giordan N, Lofland K. A literature review of psychological predictors of spinal cord stimulator outcomes. J Pain. 2005;6(3 Suppl):S67.
16. Giordano N, Lofland K, Guay J, Ghelminski S, Blonsky E, Katz J, et al. Utilization of and beliefs about presurgical psychological screening: a national survey of anesthesiologists. J Pain. 2005; 6(3 Suppl):S67.
17. Jamison RN, Washington TA, Fanciullo GJ, Ross EL, McHugo GJ, Baird JC. Do implantable devices improve mood? Comparisons of chronic pain patients with or without an implantable device. Neuromodulation. 2008;11:260–6.
18. Jamison RN, Edwards RR, Liu X, Ross EL, Michna E, Warnick M, et al. Relationship of negative affect and outcome of an opioid therapy trial amoun low back pain patients. Pain Pract. 2013;13(3):173–81.
19. Kalso E, Edwards JE, Moor RA, McQuay HF. Opioids in chronic non-cancer pain: systematic review of efficacy and safety. Pain. 2004;112:372–80.
20. Kemler MA, Barendse GA, van Kleef M, de Vet HC, Rijks CP, Furnee CA, et al. Spinal cord stimulation in patients with chronic reflex sympathetic dystrophy. N Engl J Med. 2000;343:618–24.
21. Melzack R, Wall PD. Pain mechanisms: a new theory. Science. 150:971–9.
22. North RB, Kidd DH, Wimberly RL, Edwin D. Prognostic value of psychological testing in patient undergoing spinal cord stimulation: a prospective study. Neurosurgery. 1996;39:301–10.
23. Rome HD Jr, Rome JD. Limbically augmented pain syndrome (LAPS): kindling, corticolimbic sensitization, and the convergence of affective and sensory symptoms in chronic pain disorders. Pain Med. 2000;1:7–23.
24. Schofferman J, Anderson D, Hines R, Smith G, White A. Childhood psychological trauma correlates with unsuccessful lumbar spine surgery. Spine. 1992;17(6 Suppl):S138–44.
25. Schofferman J, Anderson D, Hines R, Smith G, Keane G. Childhood psychological trauma and chronic refractory low back pain. Clin J Pain. 1993;9:260–5.
26. Shaw WS, Means-Christensen AJ, Slater MA, Webster JS, Patterson GI, Garfin SR, Wahlgren DR, Patel S, Atkinson JH. Psychiatric disorders and risk of transition to chronicity with first onset low back pain. Pain Med. 2010;11:1391–400.

27. Shealy CN, Taslitz N, Morimer JT, Reswick JB. Electrical inhibition of pain by stimulation of the dorsal columns: preliminary report. Anesth Analg. 1967;46:489–91.
28. Shealy CN, Taslitz N, Morimer JT, Becker DP. Electrical inhibition of pain: experimental evaluation. Anesth Analg. 1967;46:299–305.
29. Shocket KG, Gatchel RJ, Stoewll AW, Deschner M, Robinson R, Lou L, Whitworth T, Bernstein D. A demonstration of a pre-surgical behavioral medicine evaluation for categorizing patients for implantable therapies. A preliminary study. Neuromodulation. 2008;11:237–48.
30. Sparkes E, Raphael JH, Duarte RV, Lemarchand K, Jackson C, Ashford RL. A systematic literature review of psychological characteristics as determinants of outcome for spinal cord stimulation therapy. Pain. 2010;150:284–9. This is comprehensive, systematic review of the literature focused on psychological characteristics determining SCS outcome
31. Sparkes E, Duarte RV, Raphael JH, Denny E, Ashford RL. Qualitative exploration of psychological factors associated with spinal cord stimulation outcome. Chronic Illn. 2012;8(4):239–51.
32. Wolter T, Fauler I, Kieselbach K. The impact of psychological factors on outcomes for spinal cord stimulation: an analysis with long-term follow-up. Pain Physician. 2013;16:265–75.
33. Work Loss Data Institute. Official disability guidelines. Encinitas: Work Loss Data Institute; 2016.
34. Worker's Compensation Medical Treatment Guidelines in Texas (1999). https://www.tdi.texas.gov/reports/wcreg/documents/medtreat-guides.pdf. Accessed 10 June 2017.

Part IV

Pharmacological Treatment of Pain

Acetaminophen and Nonsteroidal Anti-inflammatory Drugs

18

Rishi Raj Agarwal, Rishi Gaiha, and Geeta Nagpal

Introduction

Nonsteroidal anti-inflammatory drugs are the most widely used non-opioid analgesics in the world and have been used to treat a wide variety of pain conditions for thousands of years. Today, annual use of NSAIDs by millions of Americans accounts for billions of dollars in sales, as they treat conditions ranging in severity from headaches to metastatic cancer. Though extremely disparate in chemical structure (Fig. 18.1), the NSAIDs are allied by an ability to inhibit cyclooxygenase (COX), the enzyme responsible for the formation of prostaglandins. COX inhibition enables the antipyretic, anti-inflammatory, and analgesic properties of NSAIDs. Acetaminophen, which is commonly included in discussions involving NSAIDs only because it is another commonly used non-opioid analgesic, has no clinically relevant COX inhibition and does not have adverse effects on platelet function and gastric mucosa. In fact, the mechanism by which acetaminophen works remains unknown.

Background and Historical Perspective

Documented use of natural sources of salicylates such as myrtus and willow bark to treat numerous pain conditions dates as far back as 1500 B.C. Between 1827 and 1899, salicylic acid (Salacin) was synthesized and used for the treatment of pain. However, it had terrible gastrointestinal side effects as well as foul taste and could only be tolerated for a few days. Now, medications such as acetylsalicylic acid (circa 1899), ibuprofen (circa 1969), and acetaminophen (circa 1877) are among the most widely used medications globally and are on the World Health Organization (WHO) Model List of Essential Medicines, which designates medications considered to be most effective and safe to meet the most important needs in a health system.

There are more than 20 commonly used NSAIDs today (Table 18.1), most of which fall into one of the following chemical classes: salicylates, propionic acid, acetic acid, anthranilic acid, oxicam, COX-2 inhibitors, and aniline derivatives. Each drug has a unique dosing pattern, half-life, and safety profile. Although there is complete lack of chemical similarity between the different NSAID medications, they all decrease inflammation by acting as COX inhibitors, which results in the inhibition of arachidonic acid synthesis and conversion into prostaglandins. The term *prostaglandin* was coined in the 1930s to describe and extract from semen that contracted uterine smooth muscle. It was later realized that prostaglandins are found in many parts of the body, and they play a key part in the inflammatory pathway and the pyretic response. Unlike hormones, prostaglandins cannot be stored and are released as soon as they are synthesized.

In inflammation or in injury states, prostaglandin formation is upregulated, either in the periphery or in the central nervous system (CNS) or both. In the event of cellular injury, phospholipids are released and converted to arachidonic acid. Cyclooxygenase then converts arachidonic acid to prostaglandin H2, which is in turn converted to tissue-specific prostaglandins (Fig. 18.2). In the periphery, there is an increase in the production of prostaglandin E (PGE). It is believed that the primary method of causing pain is the binding of PGE to nociceptive nerve endings whose cell bodies reside in the dorsal root ganglia, causing them to lower their firing thresholds, resulting in increased transduction of nociceptive signals to second-order neurons in the dorsal horn of the spinal cord.

These prostaglandins also contribute to the redness and swelling in the injured area. However, this is not the only method by which prostaglandins can contribute to pain. Following injury, even a surgical incision, the central nervous system upregulates prostaglandin formation causing a series of changes in pain transmission, making it far easier for the CNS to not only transmit but also to modulate and

R. R. Agarwal · R. Gaiha · G. Nagpal (✉)
Department of Anesthesiology, Northwestern University, Feinberg School of Medicine, Chicago, IL, USA
e-mail: rishi.gaiha@northwestern.edu; geeta.nagpal@nm.org

T. R. Deer et al. (eds.), *Deer's Treatment of Pain*, https://doi.org/10.1007/978-3-030-12281-2_18

Fig. 18.1 Chemical structures of select NSAIDs

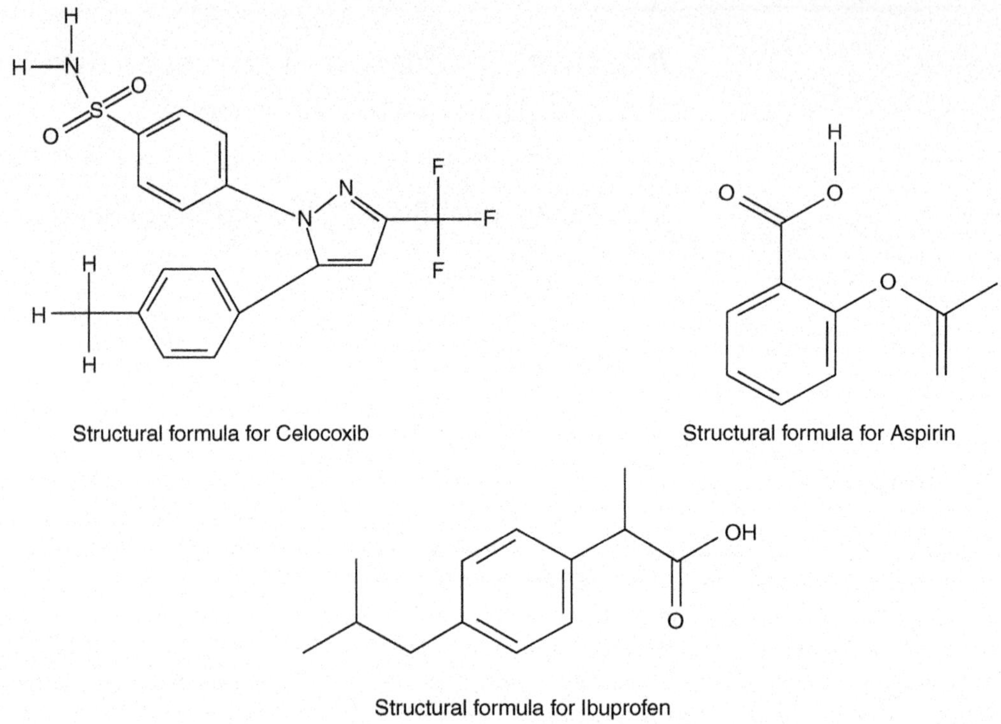

Table 18.1 Commonly prescribed NSAIDs

Medication (generic) name	Trade name	Half-life (hours)	Max daily dose	Adult daily dose	Dosage schedule	Comments
Salicylates						
Aspirin	Multiple names	2–3	4 g	600–1500 mg	QID	Irreversible inhibitor of cyclooxygenase
COX2-selective inhibitors						
Celecoxib	Celebrex	8–12	400 mg	200 mg	BID	Increased risk for CV events but decreased risk for GI side effects
Propionic acid derivatives						
Ibuprofen	Advil, Motrin	6	3200 mg	200–800 mg	QID	Nonselective COX 1 and COX 2
Naproxen	Naprosyn	14	1500 mg	250,375,500 mg	BID	Nonselective COX 1 and COX 2
Naproxen sodium	Aleve, Anaprox	14	1500 mg	275–550 mg	BID	
Ketoprofen	Orudis	2–4	300 mg	50–75 mg	TID	
Oxaprozin	Daypro	40–60	1800 mg	1.2	Daily	
Acetic acid derivatives						
Diclofenac	Voltaren	1–2	200 mg	50 mg, 75 mg	BID-QID	Preferential COX-2 inhibitor
Diclofenac gel	Voltaren Gel (1%)			2–4 g	BID-QID	Decreased systemic absorption
Diclofenac patch	Flector Patch (1.3%)	12		1 patch (180 mg)	BID	Decreased systemic absorption
Indomethacin	Indocin	~4	200 mg	25–50 mg, SR 75 mg	BID	Preferential COX-2 inhibitor
Ketorolac	Toradol	5–6	40 mg (max 4 days)	Oral: 10 mg	QID	Limited use <5 days, risk of acute kidney injury
Nabumetone	Relafen	20–24	2000 mg	500–700 mg	BID	Gastroprotective prodrug that is converted to the active molecule
Oxicam						
Meloxicam	Mobic	15–20	15 mg	7.5 mg (OA) 15 mg (RA)	Daily	COX-2 selective at 7.5 mg dose

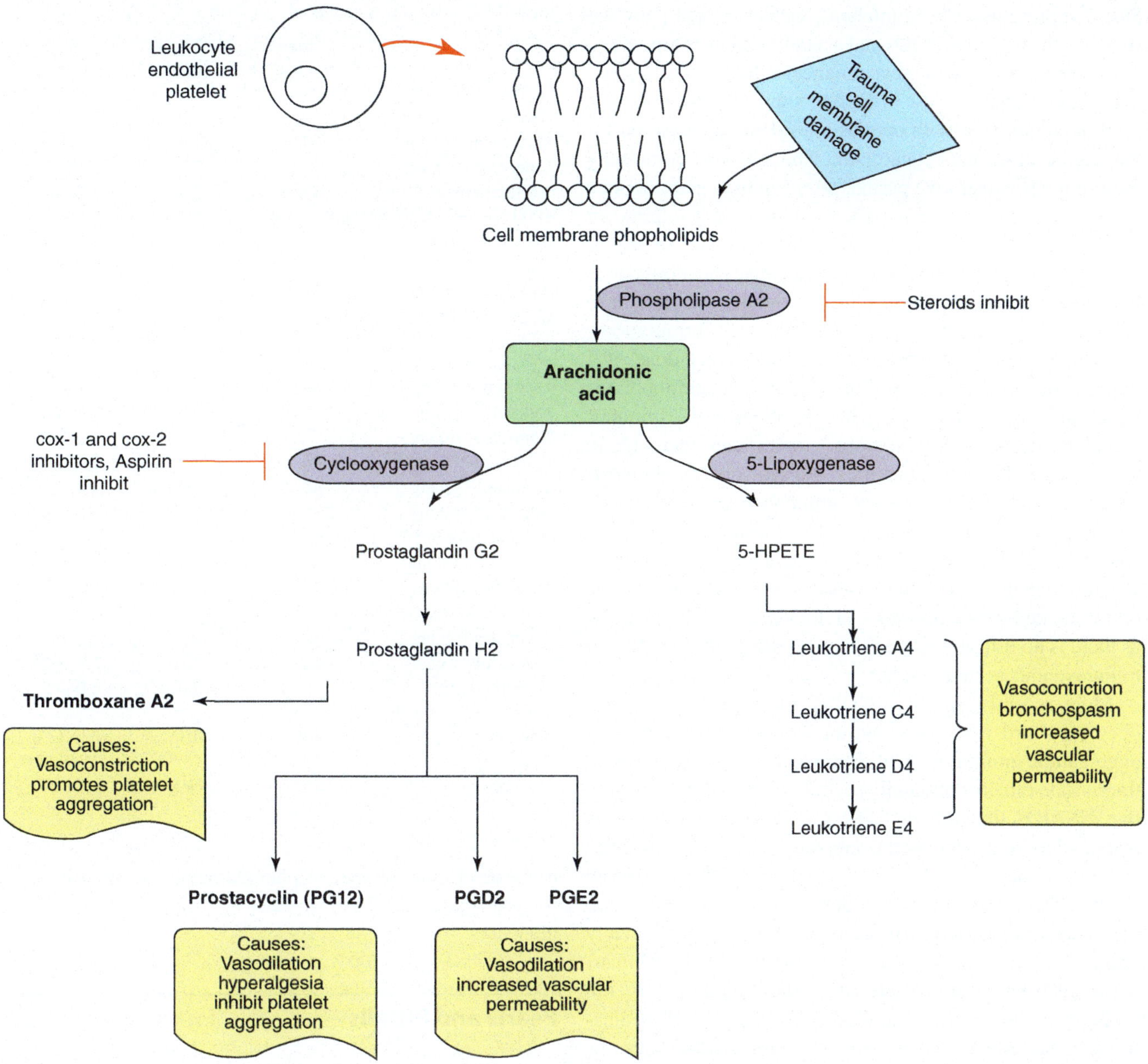

Fig. 18.2 Inflammatory pathway and the mechanism of action of NSAIDs

amplify pain transmission. This explains why NSAIDs can relieve pain even when the four hallmarks of inflammation (rubor/tumor/calor/dolor) are not present, such as in headache pain.

Uses and Indications

Whether used for acute or chronic pain conditions, and whether used alone or in combination with other analgesics such as opioids, NSAIDs and acetaminophen are proven to provide significant pain relief to patients of all demographics. NSAIDs can be divided into short acting (less than 6 hours: ibuprofen, diclofenac, ketoprofen, indomethacin, ketorolac) and long acting (more than 6 hours: naproxen, celecoxib, meloxicam, nabumetone, piroxicam) depending on their half-lives (Table 18.1), and thus the choice of NSAIDs can be tailored not only based on side effect and safety profiles but the acuity or chronicity of the type of pain being treated. Furthermore, NSAIDs can be administered by numerous routes: orally, rectally, topically, intramuscularly, and intravenously. This versatility facilitates pain control in patients who may have contraindications to certain drug administration routes.

Though not evidence-based, the WHO "analgesic ladder" approach to the treatment of cancer pain involves three steps:

Step 1 represents mild to moderate cancer-related pain and suggests the use of NSAIDs and acetaminophen; Steps 2 and 3 represent moderate to severe cancer-related pain, respectively, and suggest the use of NSAIDs and acetaminophen be used in conjunction with opioids considered appropriate for the degree of cancer-related pain. Though most commonly used in the perioperative period, intravenous acetaminophen is an excellent option for patients who cannot tolerate or have contraindications to drug administration via the oral or rectal routes, such as certain cancer patients. The intravenous formulation of acetaminophen has essentially the same dose and frequency guidelines as the oral and rectal formulations: max single dosage of 650–1000 mg, max daily dose of 4 grams. The onset of action of intravenous acetaminophen is rapid and predictable, occurring in about 5–10 minutes, compared to oral formulations, which can take 10 to >60 minutes. However, one must always consider the cost-effectiveness of intravenous acetaminophen, as the price difference is significant (a single tablet of oral acetaminophen costs less than 10 cents, whereas a single vial of intravenous acetaminophen costs about $35–45). Whenever possible, the oral or rectal formulations of acetaminophen should be used, as there is no difference in efficacy of pain control compared to intravenous acetaminophen.

More recently, selective COX-2 inhibitors were developed to afford patients analgesia without causing platelet aggregation inhibition or ulceration of the gastrointestinal tract – side effects commonly seen with the use of nonselective NSAIDs that inhibit COX-1. The COX-1 enzyme is responsible for producing thromboxane A2 (TXA2) in platelets, which facilitates platelet aggregation, and prostaglandin E2 (PGE2) in the stomach, which decreases acid secretion and increases gastric mucus secretion. However, the widely publicized withdrawal of rofecoxib (Vioxx™) from the market in 2004 revealed that selective COX-2 inhibitors are not without significant risk of morbidity, as this class of medication can increase the risk of heart attack and stroke. Selective COX-2 inhibitors should be used with caution, or not at all, in patients with cardiovascular disease, or with stage 4 or 5 chronic kidney disease, as these conditions can become worsened with the use of these medications. Nonetheless, selective COX-2 inhibitors such as celecoxib are an excellent analgesic choice in patients who are otherwise considered at high risk for gastrointestinal disease or who are on other anticoagulants.

Evidence for Efficacy

Statistical analysis of the efficacy of medications utilizes the concept of "number needed to treat," which compares the efficacy of an active treatment to placebo (Table 18.2). For the purpose of analgesic medications such as NSAIDs, this translates to the number of patients needed to treat in order for one patient to have at least a 50% reduction in pain intensity.

Table 18.2 Efficacy of commonly prescribed NSAIDs

Analgesic and dose	Percent with at least 50% pain relief	Number needed to treat	Confidence interval
Etoricoxib 120 mg	70	1.6	1.5–1.8
Diclofenac 100 mg	69	1.8	1.6–2.1
Celecoxib 400 mg	52	2.1	1.8–2.5
Acetaminophen 1000 mg + Codeine 60 mg	57	2.2	1.7–2.9
Rofecoxib 50 mg	54	2.3	2.0–2.6
Aspirin 1200 mg	61	2.4	1.9–3.2
Ibuprofen 400 mg	55	2.5	2.4–2.7
Oxycodone IR 10 mg + Acetaminophen 650 mg	66	2.6	2.0–3.5
Diclofenac 25 mg	53	2.6	2.2–3.3
Ketorolac 10 mg	50	2.6	2.3–3.1
Naproxen 500 mg	52	2.7	2.3–3.3
Ibuprofen 200 mg	48	2.7	2.5–2.9
Tramadol 150 mg	48	2.9	2.4–3.6
Naproxen 200 mg	45	3.4	2.5–4.9
Acetaminophen 500 mg	61	3.5	2.2–13.3
Celecoxib 200 mg	40	3.5	2.9–4.4
Ibuprofen 100 mg	46	3.8	3.4–4.4
Aspirin 600 mg	38	4.4	4.0–4.9
Tramadol 100 mg	30	4.8	3.8–6.1
Tramadol 75 mg	32	5.3	3.9–8.2
Acetaminophen 300 mg + Codeine 60 mg	26	5.7	4.0–9.8
Tramadol 50 mg	19	8.3	6.0–13.0
Codeine 60 mg	15	16.7	11.0–48.0
Placebo	18	N/A	N/A

Pearls and Pitfalls

- The risk of acute renal failure is increased in patients with preexisting glomerular disease, renal insufficiency, hypercalcemia, and various states of effective or actual volume depletion (cirrhosis, heart failure, gastrointestinal or renal salt and water losses).
- Inhibition of COX-1 by nonselective NSAIDs reduces production of prostaglandin E2 (PGE2), which decreases gastric acid production and increases gastric mucus secretion, thereby predisposing patients to gastrointestinal toxicity.
- The risk of gastrointestinal toxicity is increased in patients with a history of GI ulcer or hemorrhage, age > 60, high dose of NSAID, chronic use of NSAID, concurrent use of glucocorticoids, concurrent use of anticoagulants (e.g., aspirin, warfarin, clopidogrel), untreated *H. pylori* infection, and the use of SSRI antidepressants.

- The risk of adverse cardiovascular effects (i.e., hypertension, myocardial infarction, stroke, heart failure, atrial fibrillation, cardiovascular death) is increased with the use of nonselective NSAIDs in patients with or without baseline cardiovascular disease and depends primarily on dosage and duration of NSAID therapy, though patients with baseline cardiovascular disease are at increased risk.
- NSAIDs can cause a transient elevation of transaminase, and though the incidence of acute liver injury in extremely low, acute liver toxicity should be suspected in patients who have transaminase levels three times the upper limit of normal, decreased albumin, or prolonged INR.
- Aspirin-exacerbated respiratory disease (AERD) or NSAID-exacerbated respiratory disease (NERD) is a condition whereby COX-1 inhibition by nonselective NSAIDs precipitates acute exacerbations of airway inflammation that presents as bronchospasm in patients with underlying asthma, chronic rhinosinusitis, or nasal polyposis.
- The antiplatelet effects of NSAIDs are due to the inhibition of COX-1 in platelets which leads to decreased production of thromboxane A2 (TXA2), an integral molecule required for proper platelet aggregation.
- Platelet function normalizes in about 3 days for most NSAIDs, which reversibly bind to platelet cyclooxygenase, but normalizes in about 1 week for aspirin, which irreversibly binds to platelet cyclooxygenase.
- Selective COX-2 inhibitors such as celecoxib should not be used in patients with cardiovascular disease or renal disease.
- The recommended max single dose of acetaminophen is 650 milligrams, and the max daily dose of acetaminophen is 4 grams in healthy patients, or 3 grams in patients with preexisting liver disease.
- Since 2014, the FDA has mandated that any drug made in combination with acetaminophen contains no more than 325 mg of acetaminophen in order to reduce the risk of overdose.
- Acetaminophen toxicity presents in four distinct phases: Stage I (0.5–24 hours), nausea, vomiting, diaphoresis, pallor, lethargy, and malaise; Stage II (24–72 hours), elevated AST/ALT, right upper quadrant pain, liver enlargement, and elevated PT; Stage III (72–96 hours), liver function abnormalities peak, jaundice, hepatic encephalopathy, and bleeding diathesis; Stage IV (4 days to 2 weeks), recovery, if patient survived Stage III.
- Ketorolac is indicated only for moderate-severe acute pain and should be used for no more than 5 days consecutively, whether administered intramuscularly (30 mg every 6 hours, max daily dose 120 mg) or intravenously (30 mg every 6 hours, max daily dose 120 mg); oral administration (10 mg every 6 hours, max daily dose 40 mg) can be used as a continuation of IM or IV therapy.

Recommended Reading

1. Buckley MM, Brogden RN. Ketorolac. A review of its pharmacodynamics and pharmacokinetic properties, and therapeutic potential. Drugs. 1990;39:86–109.
2. Buvanendran A, Kroin JS, Berger RA, et al. Upregulation of prostaglandin E2 and interleukins in the central nervous system and peripheral tissue during and after surgery in humans. Anesthesiology. 2006;104:403–10.
3. Cashman JN. The mechanisms of action of NSAIDs in analgesia. Drugs. 1996;52(suppl 5):13–23.
4. Derry C, Derry S, Moore RA, McQuay HJ. Single dose oral ibuprofen for acute postoperative pain in adults. Cochrane Database Syst Rev. 2009;3:CD001548.
5. Derry C, Derry S, Moore RA, McQuay HJ. Single dose oral naproxen and naproxen sodium for acute postoperative pain in adults. Cochrane Database Syst Rev. 2009;1:CD004234.
6. Derry C, Derry S, Moore RA, McQuay HJ. Single dose oral etoricoxib for acute postoperative pain in adults. Cochrane Database Syst Rev. 2012;4:CD004309.
7. Derry C, Derry S, Moore RA, McQuay HJ. Single dose oral celecoxib for acute postoperative pain in adults. Cochrane Database Syst Rev. 2012;3:CD004233.
8. Derry C, Derry S, Moore RA, McQuay HJ. Single dose oral ibuprofen plus paracetamol for acute postoperative pain in adults. Cochrane Database Syst Rev. 2013;6:CD010210.
9. Godal HC, Eika C, Dybdahl JH, et al. Aspirin and bleeding-time. Lancet. 1979;1:1236.
10. Jouzeau JY, Terlain B, Abid A, et al. Cyclo-oxygenase isoenzymes. How recent findings affect thinking about nonsteroidal anti-inflammatory drugs. Drugs. 1997;53:563–82.
11. Laine L. Approaches to nonsteroidal anti-inflammatory drug use in the high-risk patient. Gastroenterology. 2001;120:594–606.
12. McGettigan P, Henry D. Cardiovascular risk and inhibition of cyclooxygenase: a systematic review of the observational studies of selective and nonselective inhibitors of cyclooxygenase 2. JAMA. 2006;296:1633–44.
13. Sinatra RS, Jahr JS, Reynolds LW, et al. Efficacy and safety of single and repeated administration of 1 gram intravenous acetaminophen injection (paracetamol) for pain management after orthopedic surgery. Anesthesiology. 2005;102:822–31.
14. Toms L, Derry S, Moore RA, McQuay HJ. Single dose oral paracetamol with codeine for postoperative pain in adults. Cochrane Database Syst Rev. 2009;1:CD001547.
15. Wallace JL. Nonsteroidal anti-inflammatory drugs and gastroenteropathy: the second hundred years. Gastroenterology. 1997;112:1000–16.

Anticonvulsants in the Treatment of Pain

19

Clarence T. Li and James C. Watson

Introduction

Anticonvulsants are commonly used in the management of neuropathic pain, alone or as adjuncts to other treatments. Anticonvulsants have also shown efficacy in the treatment of fibromyalgia (pregabalin) and in some headache disorders. These agents offer the advantages of being non-habit forming as well as often having a more favorable side effect profile compared to other pharmacologic agents used for neuropathic pain. This chapter will focus on the role of anticonvulsants for neuropathic pain as this is where the bulk of the literature rests; however, evidence-based roles of anticonvulsants for other pain indications will also be noted where appropriate.

Neuropathic pain is defined by the International Association for the Study of Pain as pain that arises as a direct consequence of a lesion or disease affecting the somatosensory system. It can stem from either damage to the peripheral nervous system or to the central nervous system.

Common descriptors of neuropathic pain are listed in Table 19.1. These symptoms alone or in combination are limited in both sensitivity and specificity for neuropathic pain (70–85% compared to formal clinical evaluation). Stimulus-evoked responses including allodynia (pain from non-painful stimuli) and hyperalgesia (excessive pain from a painful stimulus) are highly specific indicators of neuropathic pain.

The mechanisms behind neuropathic pain are complex and incompletely understood. Relative to treating pain, anticonvulsants may act at the site of peripheral nociceptor injury, in the modulation of nociceptive transmission (peripheral and central nervous system), or in the modulation of sensitized central nociceptive centers. The former are particularly relevant to peripheral neuropathic pain types, the latter to central neuropathic pain syndromes and in central sensitization disorders (including fibromyalgia).

Table 19.1 Common descriptors used for neuropathic pain

Less specific	Highly specific
Burning Freezing Tingling Lancinating, electric shock-like Shooting Stabbing Itching	Allodynia – pain from non-noxious stimulus Hyperalgesia – exaggerated pain response to a painful stimulus

Common etiologies of peripherally mediated neuropathic pain include peripheral neuropathy, postherpetic neuralgia (PHN), trigeminal neuralgia, complex regional pain syndrome (CPRS), and neuronal trauma. In the central nervous system, the most well-studied subtypes of neuropathic pain include central poststroke pain, multiple sclerosis-related pain, and spinal cord injury-related pain, both at the level and below the level of injury.

Pharmacologic treatment of neuropathic pain is multimodal and includes anticonvulsants, antidepressants in the serotonin-norepinephrine reuptake inhibitor (SNRI) and tricyclic (TCA) classes, and topical agents treating other underlying comorbidities (see Fig. 19.1 – an evidence-based medicine neuropathic pain treatment ladder). Relative to anticonvulsants, data supports the use of gabapentin and pregabalin as first-line agents for neuropathic pain, while other agents such as lamotrigine, topiramate, and lacosamide have more limited data available to support their use. Other anticonvulsants such as carbamazepine and oxcarbazepine are used as first-line agents in specific neuropathic pain syndromes, namely, trigeminal neuralgia, but have more limited efficacy in other neuropathic pain syndromes.

C. T. Li
Departments of Neurology, Mayo Clinic, Rochester, MN, USA
e-mail: Li.Clarence@mayo.edu

J. C. Watson (✉)
Departments of Neurology, Mayo Clinic, Rochester, MN, USA

Departments of Anesthesiology, Pain Medicine, Mayo Clinic, Rochester, MN, USA
e-mail: Watson.james@mayo.edu

T. R. Deer et al. (eds.), *Deer's Treatment of Pain*, https://doi.org/10.1007/978-3-030-12281-2_19

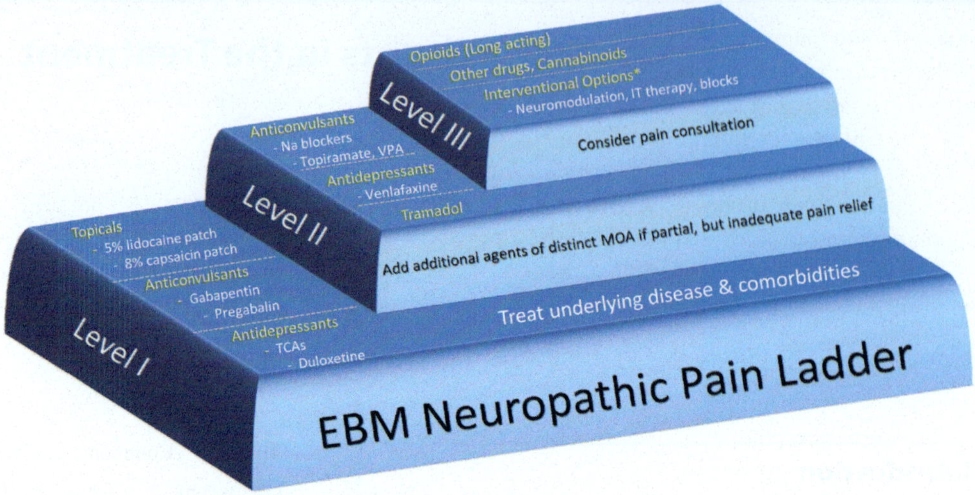

Fig. 19.1 An evidence-based medicine neuropathic pain treatment ladder. *For some neuropathic pain conditions, interventional options will be used earlier in the treatment algorithm

Background and Historical Perspective

Anticonvulsants were first used as analgesics in the 1960s, with clinical trials supporting the use of carbamazepine for trigeminal neuralgia. Subsequent clinical trials involving the use of anticonvulsants for pain were sparse. Phenytoin was trialed given its mechanistic similarities to carbamazepine and showed mixed results as an analgesic, but with an intolerable side effect profile.

Gabapentin was developed in the mid-1990s and initially showed promise in case reports and animal studies in the treatment of neuropathic pain. In 1998, two randomized control trials were published showing significant improvement in pain scores of patients with pain associated with diabetic neuropathy and PHN. Gabapentin was approved by the FDA as a primary agent in the treatment of PHN in 2004. Since then, various studies have been conducted evaluating the use of anticonvulsants as agents for the treatment of neuropathic pain with mixed results.

There is significant overlap between the targets of anticonvulsants and the pathophysiologic mechanisms underlying chronic neuropathic pain generation. Ultimately, chronic neuropathic pain involves morphologic changes at the nociceptor level, leading to chronic nociceptive afferent input into the central nervous system (nociceptor irritability) which perpetuates the pain process and induces central sensitization. Mechanisms that have been well established include ectopic activity, peripheral sensitization, central sensitization, impaired inhibitory modulation, and microglial activation. These mechanisms frequently involve phenotypic changes in the expression of ion channels or neurotransmitters in the neuron, which are felt to be the basis of the analgesic effect of anticonvulsants.

Following initial nerve injury, there is an increase in voltage-gated sodium channels and aberrant nodes. These generate hyperexcitability in the primary afferent neurons and send ectopic action potentials from the periphery to the central nervous system. Specific voltage-gated sodium channels shown to be altered and overexpressed in this process include $Na_v1.3$, $Na_v1.6$, and $Na_v1.9$. Other channels such as voltage-gated calcium channels, voltage-gated potassium channels such as KCNQ K_v7, and hyperpolarization-activated cyclic nucleotide-gated channels have also demonstrated alteration following nerve injury.

In addition to ectopic action potentials, the physiologic channels of the primary afferent neurons in the peripheral nervous system also show evidence of hyperexcitability and reduced activation threshold potential following injury. Specifically, the fibers responsible for pain transmission, Aδ- and C-fibers, have their activation threshold reduced.

The central nervous system contains second-order nociceptive neurons in the outer margins of the dorsal horn of the spinal cord, in regions referred to as Rexed laminae I–II, or the marginal nucleus and substantia gelatinosa. The axons of these neurons then transmit information to the nucleus proprius (Rexed laminae IV–VI), which projects ascending fibers to the contralateral thalamus as the spinothalamic tract, which relays pain and temperature sensation. This is mediated through the release of neuropeptides such as calcitonin gene-related peptide (CGRP) and substance P as well as the excitatory neurotransmitter glutamate and activation of the NMDA receptor. In addition, the Aβ-fibers themselves undergo phenotypic changes that increase their expression of CGRP, substance P, and glutamate. There is an intersection of pathways in wide dynamic range neurons of the dorsal horn. Under physiologic conditions, nociceptive neurons in the dorsal horn selectively respond to noxious stimuli transmitted by Aδ-fibers and C-fibers. Following nerve damage, however, the background activity in these nociceptive neurons increases, and their response to all afferent stimuli, including non-painful stimuli, increases. This in turn allows for even non-painful stimuli carried by large myelinated Aβ-fibers to activate the pain-signaling pathway through sensitized dorsal horn wide dynamic range neurons (the clinical phenomenon of allodynia and an indicator of central sensitization).

While nerve damage upregulates excitatory transmission, there is also a downregulation of inhibitory GABAergic inhibitory neurons which further contributes to the chronic neuropathic pain process. Additionally, non-neuronal glial cells undergo changes that enhance the release of substance P and glutamate from neuronal terminals.

Mechanistically, anticonvulsants suppress the hyperexcitability and excessive depolarization in the central nervous system by targeting a wide array of ion channels, ligand receptors, and neurotransmitters (Fig. 19.2). Of particular interest to neuropathic pain therapy are the presynaptic voltage-gated sodium channels and L-type calcium channels, the postsynaptic chloride channels, as well as NMDA and GABA receptors. Anticonvulsants that have been studied in pain modulation are typically associated with one or more of these mechanisms (Fig. 19.2).

Uses, Indications, Dosing, and Notable Side Effects

General Principles

The treatment of neuropathic pain is difficult, and one should take a stepwise approach to treating based on the level of evidence supporting the efficacy of a particular drug (Fig. 19.2). Of the anticonvulsants, gabapentin and pregabalin have the most evidence, with their usage as a first-line neuropathic pain agent supported in multiple published meta-analyses.

Generally, doses should be started low to minimize side effects and titrated every 4–7 days. The initial goal should be the lowest dose proven to be useful for neuropathic pain in the literature (Table 19.2). The titration may be stopped at the lowest efficacious dosage even prior to reaching the goal dose. If a patient's pain persists but they are tolerating the medication, then it may be titrated upward to the maximum

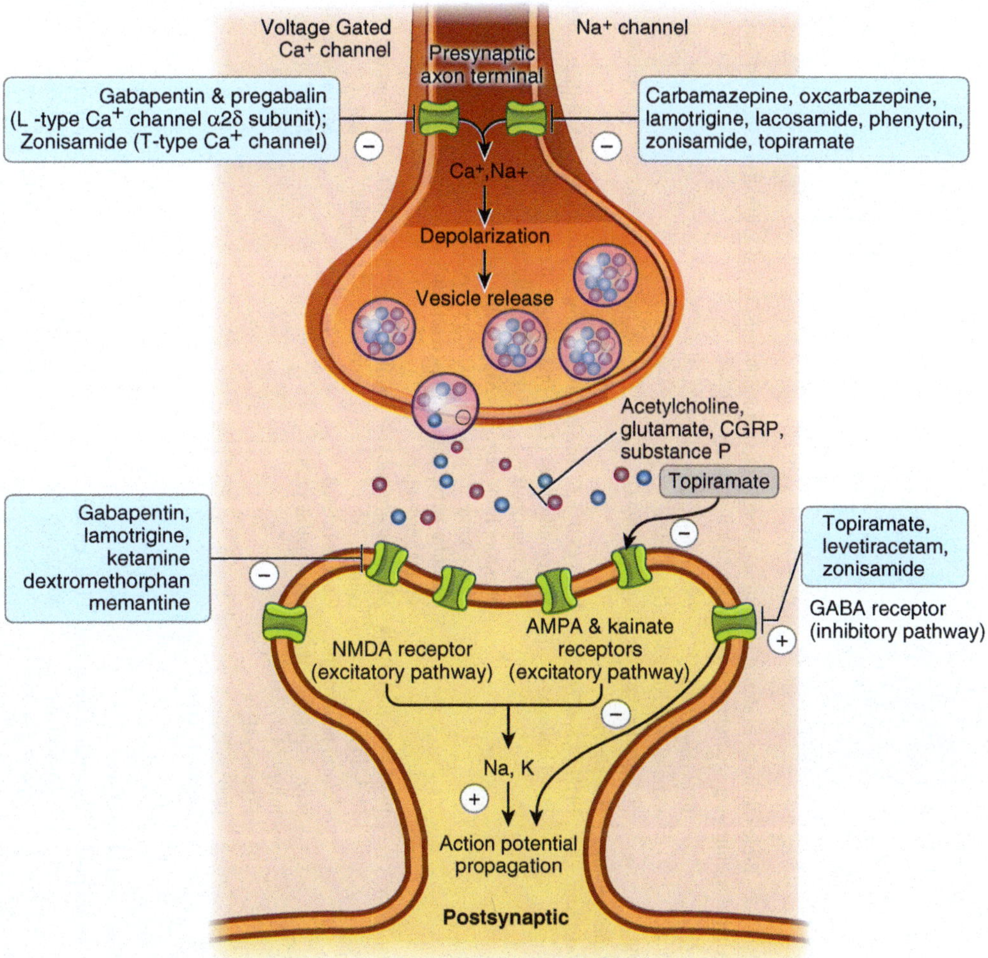

Fig. 19.2 Stepwise approach to the evidence-based treatment of neuropathic pain. TCAs, tricyclic antidepressants. Other drugs: mexiletine, dextromethorphan, ketamine, memantine, cannabinoids (central pain), IVIG, IV steroids

Table 19.2 Table outlining evidence for efficacy, dosing recommendations, and side effects of selected anticonvulsants in the treatment of neuropathic pain. All anticonvulsants should be tapered off when discontinuing secondary to risk of seizure if abruptly stopped

Drug	FDA-approved indications (NNT 30% improvement)	Other pain indications (NNT 30% improvement)	Dosing recommendations	Goal dosing	Precautions	Common side effects	Comments
Calcium channel – α2δ ligands							
Gabapentin	PHN (4.8–6.7) Focal epilepsy	PDN (5.9–6.6), mixed neuropathic pain (7.2) HIV neuropathy, phantom limb pain, direct nerve injury, radicular nerve pain, spinal cord injury	Initial dose: 300 mg QHS. Increase by 300 mg every 4 days to TID dosing. May further increase by 300 mg every 4 days based on clinical response	Minimum: 600 mg TID Maximum: 1200 mg TID	Dose adjustment for renal impairment Caution in elderly and patients with gait instability	Cognitive impairment, somnolence, dizziness, ataxia, visual disturbance, mood lability, tremor, and peripheral edema	Few drug interactions 100 mg increments available for slower titration Reduced bioavailability at higher doses
Pregabalin	PHN (5.1–6.9), PDN (6.3–11) Central neuropathic pain – spinal cord injury (4.0–7.0) Fibromyalgia (6.6–9.2) Focal epilepsy	Mixed neuropathic pain (7.7) Cancer-related neuropathic pain	Initial dose: 75 mg BID Increase by 75 mg BID every 4–7 days	Minimum: 150 mg BID Maximum: 300 mg BID	Dose adjustment for renal impairment Caution in elderly and patients with gait instability Psychiatric disease or addiction history (euphoria risk)	Cognitive impairment, somnolence, dizziness, ataxia, visual disturbance, mood lability, tremor, and peripheral edema	May convert directly from gabapentin (6:1 dosing ratio) 25 and 50 mg dosing available for slower titration Few drug interactions
Sodium channel blockers							
Carbamazepine	Trigeminal neuralgia Focal epilepsy Bipolar disorder	PDN, central poststroke pain	Initial dose: 200 mg XR once daily Increased by 200 mg after 1 week and may be further increased by 200–400 mg the following week	Minimum: 400 mg Maximum: 1200 mg	Hepatic cytochrome inducer, multiple drug interactions Dose adjust with renal and hepatic impairment	Hyponatremia, rash (Stevens-Johnson syndrome), blood dyscrasias, hepatic dysfunction, somnolence, dizziness, diplopia, nausea, vomiting	Higher risk of developing SJS in Han Chinese patients or patients with expression of HLA-B*1502 Must monitor CBC and LFTs
Oxcarbazepine	Focal epilepsy	Trigeminal neuralgia (similar efficacy to carbamazepine), PDN	Initial dose: 300 mg once daily Increase to 300 mg BID after 4–7 days. Titrate by 300 mg increments based on clinical response	Minimum: 300 mg BID Maximum: 1200 mg BID (neuropathic syndromes usually 600–900 mg BID)	High rate of hypersensitive cross-reactivity to carbamazepine reactions Dose adjust with renal and hepatic impairment	Hyponatremia, rash (Stevens-Johnson syndrome), dizziness, somnolence, diplopia, nausea, vomiting	More favorable side effect profile than carbamazepine and fewer drug interactions Routine CBC and LFT monitoring not necessary

Lamotrigine	Generalized and focal epilepsy Bipolar disorder	PDN, trigeminal neuralgia, HIV neuropathy, central poststroke pain	Initial dose: 25 mg once daily for 2 weeks Increase to 25 mg BID for 2 weeks, then 50 mg BID for 1 week, then 75 mg BID for 1 week, and then 100 mg BID; may increase further by 50–100 mg in weekly intervals	Minimum: 100 mg BID Maximum: 200 mg BID	SJS more likely with rapid titration and in young patients Dose adjust with renal or hepatic impairment	Rash (Stevens-Johnson syndrome), abdominal pain, diplopia, diarrhea, headache, dizziness	Affected by hepatic CYP450 metabolism. Patients receiving medications, such as valproic acid, which inhibit hepatic p450 system require slower titration calendar and patients receiving medications, such as carbamazepine, which induce hepatic p450 system require faster titration
Lacosamide	Focal epilepsy	PDN (10.0–12.0)	Initial dose: 50 mg BID Increase weekly by 50 mg BID	Target dose: 200 mg BID	Obtain ECG prior to starting treatment Dose adjust with renal impairment	First-degree AV block, nausea, vomiting, dizziness, sedation	Favorable side effect profile (particularly low sedation and cognitive effects) with few drug interactions
Multiple receptor effects[a]							
Topiramate	Focal and generalized epilepsy Migraine	DPN	Initial dose: 50 mg BID Increase by 50–100 mg weekly	Minimum: 50 mg BID Maximum: 200 mg BID For migraine 50–100 mg BID effective For neuropathic pain, 100–200 mg BID effective	Check baseline renal function (if risk insufficiency) and bicarbonate Dose adjust with renal impairment	Prominent side effects: weight loss, renal stones, cognitive side effects, paresthesias (dose dependent)	Contraindicated in patients with history of renal stones

NNT number needed to treat, *PDN* painful diabetic neuropathy, *PHN* postherpetic neuralgia, *SJS* Stevens-Johnson syndrome, *BID* twice daily, *TID* thrice daily, *CBC* complete blood count, *LFTs* liver function tests, *ECG* electrocardiogram

[a]Topiramate mechanisms of action: sodium channel blocker, augmentation of inhibitory activity via chloride channels at some GABA receptor subtypes, antagonism of AMPA/kainate subtype of the glutamate receptor, inhibition of the carbonic anhydrase enzyme (also induces risk of nephrolithiasis)

dose. The patient should be maintained at a goal dose for several weeks to assess for efficacy.

Expectation management is paramount when treating patients with neuropathic pain. The benefits of all medications (including anticonvulsants) used to treat neuropathic pain are usually incomplete, and results of studies evaluating the efficacy of anticonvulsants in neuropathic pain treatment are generally reported as a number needed to treat (NNT) to achieve a 30–50% reduction in pain. It has been demonstrated that a 30% reduction in pain level (or 2 points on a 0–10 Numeric Pain Rating Scale) correlate with a patient's impression of a clinically significant improvement.

Because of incomplete pain control with monotherapy, even when efficacious, chronic neuropathic pain treatment frequently requires rationale polypharmacy using more than one agent with distinct mechanisms of action (e.g., anticonvulsant and antidepressant class neuropathic pain adjuvant). Nearly all studies that have examined this have shown combination therapy to be superior to monotherapy (even when both of those monotherapies were superior to placebo). The benefits and tolerance of polypharmacy regiments should be reassessed regularly.

Additionally, all agents have side effects. Patients with a lesion in the nervous system that causes cognitive, behavioral, balance, or sensorimotor deficits in addition to their pain may be more vulnerable to these side effects. Caution should be used in the elderly, who are particularly intolerant of medication side effects.

Depression, anxiety, and sleep issues are common comorbidities with chronic neuropathic pain, and failure to address these issues will sabotage the likelihood of an efficacious trial of any neuropathic pain agent (including anticonvulsants).

Gabapentin

Indications

Gabapentin is an anticonvulsant initially developed for the treatment of focal seizures. It currently has FDA approval in the treatment of PHN. However, the clinical use of gabapentin extends far beyond its FDA-approved applications given its favorable side effect profile and minimal drug-drug interactions. Common off-label uses for gabapentin include painful diabetic neuropathy, CPRS, nonspecific neuropathic pain, migraine (for both prophylaxis of acute migraine and the treatment of chronic migraine), restless leg syndrome (RLS), trigeminal neuralgia, and a variety of psychiatric mood disorders.

Mechanism of Action (MOA)

The mechanism of gabapentin is incompletely described. The chemical structure is similar to the endogenous neurotransmitter GABA, but the drug has not been shown to bind to or directly interact with GABA receptors. Its binding to the α2δ-1 subunit of the presynaptic L-type calcium channel is of particular interest as a mechanism of its role in pain attenuation. In the nervous system, α2δ subunits are expressed in high concentrations in the dorsal horn, particularly in the marginal zone and substantia gelatinosa as well as in the unmyelinated C-fibers responsible for carrying pain and temperature input. Areas of the brain associated with nociceptive processing also have been found to express high levels of α2δ subunits. Numerous studies have shown upregulation of α2δ-1 subunits in the dorsal root ganglia and spinal cord following nerve injury, leading to afferent hyperexcitability and an exaggerated pain response. Gabapentin has been shown to reverse this upregulation and inhibit upstream propagation of the pain cascade. In transgenic mice, ablation of the α2δ-1 subunit completely abolishes the antinociceptive effect of gabapentin.

Dosing and Considerations (See Table 19.2)

Gabapentin is currently only available in oral formulations. It is rapidly absorbed from the small intestine rapidly via a very specific but unidentified transport mechanism. This mechanism is saturated at higher doses, resulting in decreased bioavailability at higher doses. Gabapentin has an oral bioavailability of 60% at a total daily dose of 900 mg/day divided into three times a day dosing. This decreases to 34% at 2400 mg/day. The half-life of gabapentin requires three times a day dosing. Gabapentin is not metabolized in the body and is excreted renally. Dosage adjustments may be needed in patients with renal impairment. It does not induce or inhibit hepatic enzymes, and interactions with other medications are minimal.

Gabapentin is available in an extended-release formulation, with FDA approval for treatment of PHN and some evidence supporting its use in the treatment of painful diabetic neuropathy. Its release mechanism is a polymer-based Acuform technology, which swells and is retained in the stomach. This overcomes the saturable gabapentin transport mechanisms, resulting in increased bioavailability. Initial dosing is once daily at 300 mg and titrated upward to a daily dose of 1800 mg over 15 days. Dosing is not interchangeable with immediate-release gabapentin, and it is not appropriate for epilepsy treatment.

Gabapentin enacarbil (GEn), which is the prodrug of gabapentin, is another available formulation and is approved for treatment of PHN and RLS. GEn is absorbed by high capacity, non-saturable transporters throughout the GI tract and is hydrolyzed by enterocytes into gabapentin. It offers the advantage of predictable bioavailability and sustained systemic exposure. Dosing for PHN is 600 mg daily for 3 days, followed by 600 mg twice daily as a goal dose. Dosing for RLS is 600 mg at 5 pm. GEn has a black box warning regarding possible impairment in driving ability, and patients should not drive while on the medication until they have fully assessed their tolerance of the drug.

Pregabalin

Indications

Indications for pregabalin in the treatment of pain are similar to gabapentin. It has FDA approval for the treatment of PHN and painful peripheral diabetic neuropathy. Unlike gabapentin, it has additional FDA approval for the treatment of central neuropathic pain from spinal cord injury and fibromyalgia.

MOA

Pregabalin has a similar mechanism of action to gabapentin. It binds to the $\alpha 2\delta$-1 subunit of the presynaptic voltage-gated calcium channels, resulting in downregulation and a decrease in substance P, glutamate, CGRP, and other pain potentiating neurotransmitters. Compared to gabapentin, it has a higher binding affinity for this site. Pregabalin does not have meaningful interaction with the GABA receptor.

Dosing and Considerations (See Table 19.2)

Pregabalin is only available as an oral formulation. When compared to gabapentin, pregabalin has a more predictable absorption (not saturable) and bioavailability profile (90% bioavailability even at higher dosages). Like gabapentin, pregabalin is excreted renally (requiring dosage adjustment with renal insufficiency) without significant metabolism, no effect on hepatic metabolism, and few drug-drug interactions.

Pregabalin was initially approved for three times a day dosing. Further studies have evaluated all of its approved uses for twice daily dosing, showing equal efficacy along with better tolerability and patient compliance. Typical dosing regimens are reported in Table 19.2. While goal dosing for neuropathic pain is 300–600 mg/day (split twice daily), studies for fibromyalgia used 450 mg/day as the maximal dosage. Patients can get to a potentially efficacious dosage (300 mg/day) very quickly with pregabalin (potentially starting at that dosage), whereas gabapentin requires a slower titration to goal dosing of at least 1800 mg/day.

There are no good head to head trials of gabapentin to pregabalin. Some patients who have inadequate responses or limiting side effects to one may find better tolerance and efficacy from the other. Given similar mechanisms of action, they are not typically used in combination. Cross titration from gabapentin to pregabalin is relatively straightforward. The ratio of dosing for gabapentin to pregabalin is 6:1 (pregabalin binds six times more potently to the receptor). The morning dose of gabapentin may be switched for the equivalent dose of pregabalin, and the patient can continue on a twice daily dosing schedule of pregabalin in substitution for the gabapentin. Another strategy is to taper the dose of gabapentin to half of the patient's maintenance dose and then to titrate the pregabalin dose up.

Carbamazepine and Oxcarbazepine

Indications

Carbamazepine is an antiepileptic primarily used in the treatment of focal epilepsy. In pain management, it is a gold standard agent for the treatment of trigeminal neuralgia and has FDA approval for this use. While oxcarbazepine does not have formal FDA approval for the treatment of trigeminal neuralgia, the current body of evidence shows essentially equivalent efficacy when compared to carbamazepine. The data is mixed (and particularly limited for carbamazepine) for the use of these agents in other neuropathic pain conditions.

MOA

The binding site for carbamazepine is the presynaptic voltage-gated sodium channel. Carbamazepine binds to the sodium channel, decreasing the availability of the channels and resulting in a net decrease in the firing of ectopic action potentials. Additionally, carbamazepine has been shown to potentiate GABA receptor expression, further decreasing nervous system hyperexcitability. Oxcarbazepine is a structural derivative of carbamazepine with a similar MOA.

Dosing and Considerations (See Table 19.2)

Carbamazepine is extensively metabolized by the liver by the cytochrome P-450 system. It is an inducer of the cytochrome P-450 system and has numerous drug interactions as a result, including reducing the effectiveness of oral contraceptives, warfarin, and other anticonvulsants including itself, as carbamazepine undergoes auto-induction at higher doses. Of note, grapefruit juice has been shown to decrease carbamazepine bioavailability via inhibition of CYP3A4 enzymes in the liver and gut wall. Oxcarbazepine is purported to have fewer drug interactions but still has several and can specifically still lower contraceptive and immunosuppressant serum levels (decreasing their efficacy).

As a first-generation anticonvulsant, carbamazepine has a myriad of side effects that may limit its long-term use in patients. Less frequent but serious documented side effects include blood dyscrasias including aplastic anemia, drug-induced lupus erythematosus, hepatotoxicity, and Stevens-Johnson syndrome (SJS). Patients of Han Chinese ethnicity are at significantly higher risk of developing SJS or toxic epidermal necrolysis (TEN) with carbamazepine due to more frequent expression of the human leukocyte antigen allele, HLA-B*1502, and care is frequently taken in considering for individuals of non-Japanese Asian descent. Serum blood counts, liver enzymes, and sodium levels should be periodically monitored while a patient is on carbamazepine. Oxcarbazepine has fewer serious adverse side effects than carbamazepine, with a lower incidence of blood dyscrasias and hepatic dysfunction (and no need for routine blood count or liver function monitoring). Cross-reactivity with carbamazepine is common and occurs in about 25% of patients, so oxcarbazepine should be avoided in patients with serious adverse reactions to carbamazepine. Side effects common to both drugs include somnolence, dizziness, diplopia, and hyponatremia.

Lamotrigine

Indications

Lamotrigine is an anticonvulsant with FDA approval for the treatment of generalized and focal epilepsy and bipolar disorder. Data regarding its efficacy in treating neuropathic pain is mixed. It is used as a second-line agent for the treatment of neuropathic pain conditions including painful diabetic neuropathy, trigeminal neuralgia, HIV neuropathy, and central neuropathic pain.

MOA

The primary mechanism of action for lamotrigine is stabilization of the inactivated state of the presynaptic voltage-gated sodium channel. Other effects include GABAergic activity and minor inhibition of presynaptic calcium channels. It is chemically distinct from other antiepileptics that bind to the sodium channel.

Dosing and Considerations (See Table 19.2)

Notable drug interactions include valproic acid, which inhibits lamotrigine metabolism, and oral contraceptives, which induce lamotrigine metabolism.

The main side effect of lamotrigine is rash and risk of SJS and TEN. About 10% of patients develop a rash with lamotrigine, although the risk of developing a SJS or TEN is much lower. Risk factors for the development of SJS or TEN include young age, a high initial dose, titration of the dosage too quickly, or concomitant use of valproic acid. Almost all documented cases of serious rash occurred in the first 2–8 weeks of treatment. Other notable side effects include diplopia, dizziness, and somnolence.

To minimize the risk of SJS or TEN, lamotrigine should be titrated slowly over the course of at least 6 weeks (see Table 19.2). Lamotrigine should be discontinued if there is development of a rash and urgent dermatologic evaluation if it is exfoliating.

Lacosamide

Indications

Lacosamide is a newer novel-type voltage-gated sodium channel blocker anticonvulsant primarily used in the treatment of partial epilepsy. Several studies suggested lacosamide is effective for neuropathic pain, but concerns were expressed as to these studies' intention to treat analyses, and this effect is therefore uncertain.

MOA

Unlike other sodium channel blockers such as carbamazepine, which act primarily on the fast inactivation of voltage-gated sodium channels, lacosamide acts through a different mechanism and enhances the slow inactivation of these channels.

Dosing and Considerations (See Table 19.2)

Lacosamide is excreted renally and should be dose adjusted in patients with renal dysfunction. Drug-drug interactions are minimal.

The side effect profile for lacosamide is favorable, and the drug is generally well tolerated with notably low incidences of sedation or confusion and may be considered in patients who have struggled with side effects from other neuropathic pain adjuvants. First-degree AV block has been documented in about 0.5% of patients, and ECG should be considered prior to use in older patients or if there is prior cardiac disease. Other side effects include dizziness, nausea, and sedation.

Topiramate

Indications

Topiramate is an anticonvulsant with FDA approval for the treatment of epilepsy and migraine headache. There is limited data supporting its use in the treatment of painful diabetic neuropathy, but it may be trialed when patients have comorbid migraine or wish a medication more likely to cause weight loss than gain.

MOA

The mechanism of topiramate is incompletely understood, and it has a variety of targets within the body. It inhibits presynaptic voltage-gated sodium channels and also has postsynaptic effects through augmentation of inhibitory effects through chloride channels via some GABAergic receptors and antagonism of AMPA/kainate subtypes of the glutamate receptor. Topiramate also weakly inhibits endogenous carbonic anhydrase activity, which is felt to contribute to its side effect profile (risk of nephrolithiasis) but has unclear significance in its pharmacologic efficacy.

Dosing and Considerations (See Table 19.2)

The most notable side effects of topiramate are the development of urolithiasis, paresthesias, weight loss, and cognitive side effects. Urolithiasis occurs in about 2% of patients taking topiramate, and topiramate is contraindicated in patients with a history of urolithiasis. Weight loss of 2.5 kg or more has been reported in over 75% of patients taking topiramate. Adverse effects on cognition ("dope-a-max") occur in about 10% of patients and seem to be dose dependent. As such low dosages used for migraine (100–200 mg/day) are usually well tolerated, whereas higher dosages used for epilepsy and neuropathic pain (200–400 mg/day) are frequently poorly tolerated.

Other AEDs

Phenytoin is a first-generation voltage-gated sodium channel inhibitor with some evidence supporting its efficacy in treating neuropathic pain. However, its side effect profile is very unfavorable, and the pharmacodynamics of the medication results in an extremely narrow therapeutic window, especially in the elderly. Potential side effects include nystagmus, ataxia, cerebellar atrophy, aplastic anemia, SJS, gingival hyperplasia, and decreased bone density.

Other commonly used anticonvulsants such as levetiracetam, valproic acid, and zonisamide have not demonstrated clear efficacy in treating neuropathic pain.

Agents which work on the NMDA receptor will be covered separately in Chap. 25.

Evidence for Efficacy and Limitations of Available Evidence

The majority of randomized controlled studies evaluating anticonvulsants for neuropathic pain have studied painful diabetic neuropathy or postherpetic neuralgia given their prevalence and ability to define a homogeneous population of patients. Evidence outside of these conditions is much more limited. We commonly extrapolate proven efficacy of an agent for one neuropathic condition to another condition given these holes in evidence. This is rationale, but imperfect. For example, while sodium channel blockers like carbamazepine or oxcarbazepine are highly efficacious for the paroxysmal pain of trigeminal neuralgia, their effect for the burning dysesthetic pain of diabetic neuropathy is limited. Similarly while gabapentin, lamotrigine (to a lesser extent), and the tricyclic antidepressants amitriptyline and nortriptyline have good evidence for the treatment of painful diabetic neuropathy, well-designed trials for some forms of chemotherapy-induced peripheral neuropathy failed to demonstrate efficacy.

Despite most neuropathic pain conditions being chronic, most trials are of short duration (8 weeks or less). Additionally, there are few head to head trials comparing the efficacy of different anticonvulsants against each other or other medications (antidepressants, analgesics) used for neuropathic pain treatment.

Gabapentin

Gabapentin has shown clear efficacy in the treatment of PHN (FDA approved) and painful diabetic neuropathy. Data regarding its efficacy in the treatment of other neuropathic pain etiologies such as central neuropathic pain, mixed neuropathic pain, or chemotherapy-associated peripheral neuropathy is less robust and shows mixed results.

A 2017 Cochrane review meta-analysis of gabapentin in the treatment of neuropathic pain includes 37 randomized controlled trials with total daily doses ranging from 1200 to 3600 mg. Included in the analysis were trials that used the extended-release formulation of gabapentin or gabapentin enacarbil. For treatment of postherpetic neuralgia, 32% of patients experienced substantial (50% or greater) pain relief compared to 17% of patients treated with placebo, and 46% of the studied patients experienced moderate (25% or greater) pain relief compared to 29% with placebo. The NNT for substantial benefit was 6.7 and 4.8 for moderate benefit. For treatment of painful diabetic neuropathy, 38% of patients experienced substantial pain relief compared to 21% of patients treated with placebo, and 52% of the studied patients experienced moderate pain relief compared to 37% with placebo. The NNT for substantial benefit was 5.9 and 6.6 for moderate benefit. Gabapentin studies done with heterogeneous neuropathic pain types showed mixed results.

A separate meta-analysis of 14 placebo-controlled studies evaluating gabapentin in the treatment of neuropathic pain showed 35% of patients having at least a 30% improvement in pain with gabapentin compared to 20% with placebo, with a NNT of 7.2. The majority of studies included in this analysis were for PHN and painful diabetic neuropathy, but neuropathic pain from nerve injury, spinal cord injury, and mixed causes was also included.

Trials of gabapentin in the treatment of other causes of neuropathic pain such as radicular leg pain, HIV neuropathy, phantom limb pain, direct nerve injury, and spinal cord injury are limited due to few available studies and low statistical power from a small number of patients. Trends in the studies evaluating efficacy for HIV neuropathy, phantom limb pain, and direct nerve injury were favorable for gabapentin, but did not reach statistical significance. The results for spinal cord injury and radicular leg pain were mixed. Studies of gabapentin for the treatment of chemotherapy-related neuropathic pain have failed to show benefit, though baseline pain scores were low limiting the sensitivity of detecting a demonstrable benefit.

Pregabalin

The most robust evidence supporting the use of pregabalin is in the treatment of painful diabetic neuropathy, PHN, central neuropathic pain, and fibromyalgia (all of which are FDA-approved indications). Response to pregabalin shows a gradient effect, with a lower NNT needed at higher doses.

Pooled data of all types of neuropathic pain from 25 studies showed 38% of patients achieving at least 30% pain reduction with pregabalin at daily doses of 300–600 mg compared to 24% with placebo with a NNT of 7.7.

For the treatment of PHN, a pooled analysis of five studies showed that 39%, 49%, and 62% of patients achieved 30% pain improvement with pregabalin at daily doses of 150, 300, and 600 mg, respectively, compared to 17%, 17%, and 24% of patients receiving placebo. Corresponding NNT were 4.6, 4.0, and 2.7. The proportion of patients to achieve 50% pain reduction were 25%, 32%, 41% for 150, 300, and 600 mg compared to 11%, 11%, and 15% for placebo, with NNT of 6.9, 5.1, and 3.9.

Analysis of seven studies evaluating pregabalin efficacy painful diabetic neuropathy showed 50% or more pain reduction in 38% and 46% of patients receiving pregabalin in daily doses of 300 mg and 600 mg, respectively, compared to 29% and 30% with placebo, with a NNT of 11 and 6.3. Only the 600 mg dosing of pregabalin showed efficacy over placebo for patients experiencing a 30% reduction in pain, with 62% of patients achieving this outcome versus 48% for placebo, with a NNT of 6.8.

Four placebo-controlled randomized control studies have been conducted evaluating the efficacy of pregabalin in central neuropathic pain. Two of these studies evaluated patients with central neuropathic pain from spinal cord injury, one study included central neuropathic pain etiologies of all types, and one study included only poststroke central neuropathic pain. Results were favorable for pregabalin in the spinal cord and mixed central pain studies, with 42–48% of patients achieving pain improvement of 30% or more compared to 13–38% with placebo, with a NNT ranging from 4.0 to 7.0. Outcomes were less favorable in the study solely evaluating poststroke central neuropathic pain, where pregabalin did not demonstrate efficacy over placebo.

For the treatment of fibromyalgia, pregabalin showed favorable efficacy over placebo, but the gradient effect seen with treatment of other forms of neuropathic pain was not present. Data suggests that a daily dose of 450 mg has the greatest efficacy in this subgroup of patients. In a pooled analysis of five studies, pregabalin was found to have a 30% reduction in pain intensity in 39%, 43%, and 39% of patients compared to 28% in placebo, with a NNT of 9.2, 6.6, and 9.1 for doses of 300 mg, 450 mg, and 600 mg, respectively. Corresponding results for 50% pain reduction were 21%, 25%, and 24% compared to 14%, 15%, and 14% in placebo with NNT of 14.0, 9.8, and 11.0.

Data is limited regarding pregabalin efficacy in cancer-related neuropathic pain, but it does appear to decrease the need for rescue doses of morphine. Two randomized controlled trials for HIV neuropathy failed to demonstrate pregabalin efficacy.

Carbamazepine and Oxcarbazepine

Many studies evaluating carbamazepine efficacy in the treatment of neuropathic pain are older and limited by small sample size, lack of placebo control, and short study duration. However, in the studies available, carbamazepine has shown efficacy in the treatment of trigeminal neuralgia, as well as more limited data supporting efficacy in the treatment of painful diabetic neuropathy and central poststroke pain.

Although carbamazepine is considered the gold standard medical treatment for trigeminal neuralgia, the body of evidence supporting its use in the condition mostly consists of older studies with a relatively small sample size. Three placebo-controlled randomized controlled trials are available for analysis, with daily doses ranging from 400 to 2400 mg. Patients showed a 32–70% improvement in pain after treatment ranging from 5 days to 2 weeks. NNT was not calculated in these studies, and sample size was fewer than 60 patients in each study. No placebo-controlled trials exist for evaluating the efficacy of oxcarbazepine in trigeminal neuralgia. One study evaluated the use of oxcarbazepine in patients with trigeminal neuralgia refractory to carbamazepine and found a reduction in paroxysmal pain occurrence from 12.26 days per month to 5.6 after treatment with a daily dose of 800 mg for 12 weeks. Another study compared the efficacy of carbamazepine and oxcarbazepine and found similar efficacy between the two drugs, with 98% of patients improving with carbamazepine and 94% of patients improving with oxcarbazepine.

Data is generally supportive for the use of carbamazepine in the treatment of diabetic neuropathy, although the clinical implications of the studies are difficult to interpret due to limitations in methodology. One trial reported that 60% of patients treated for pain preferred carbamazepine after 1 week of treatment compared to 35% preferring placebo. Another trial reported 56% of patients experiencing improvement in pain with carbamazepine after 2 weeks compared to 7% with placebo. Other trials have shown comparable efficacy of carbamazepine with SNRIs such as nortriptyline and venlafaxine. Data is mixed regarding efficacy of oxcarbazepine. Only one placebo controlled trial was positive and showed a 50% reduction in pain after 16 weeks in 35% of the oxcarbazepine group compared to 18% of the placebo group, with a NNT of 6.0. However, this was only for a daily dose of 1800 mg, and lower doses did not show a significant difference. Other trials did not show a significant benefit over placebo, even at higher doses.

Poststroke pain treatment data is limited to one crossover trial showing an improvement in pain after 4 weeks in 5 of 15 patients with carbamazepine, compared to 10 of 15 with amitriptyline and 1 of 15 with placebo. Trials for carbamazepine in the treatment of radiculopathy have been negative.

Lamotrigine

Data regarding the efficacy of lamotrigine in treating neuropathic pain is mixed. There is limited evidence supporting the use of lamotrigine in the treatment of painful diabetic neuropathy, trigeminal neuralgia, HIV painful neuropathy, and central neuropathic pain.

One crossover study compared efficacy of lamotrigine compared to amitriptyline in patients with painful diabetic neuropathy. Good, moderate, and mild pain relief were reported in 41%, 13%, and 15% compared to 28%, 11%, and 33% of patients in the amitriptyline group. Notably, side effects for lamotrigine (25% experiencing) were lower than for amitriptyline (75% experiencing). Rash was experienced by 7% of patients, none of whom developed SJS. Another study of 53 patients showed 50% pain reduction in 44% of the lamotrigine group at a daily dose of 400 mg compared to 19% on placebo. However, subsequent larger placebo controlled trials were negative.

One small study of 20 patients showed an improvement in pain of patients with poststroke central pain after taking lamotrigine at 200 mg after 8 weeks, with 60% of patients experiencing pain improvement versus 15% with placebo. Studies evaluating lamotrigine use in neuropathic pain from spinal cord injury have been negative.

The use of lamotrigine for HIV neuropathy was evaluated in a study of 92 patients and showed that in patients receiving antiretroviral therapy, 57% of patients had significant pain improvement compared to 23% of placebo.

As combination therapy, lamotrigine at a daily dose of 400 mg showed improvements in patients with trigeminal neuralgia refractory to phenytoin or carbamazepine.

Lacosamide

Several large, placebo-controlled trials modestly supported the efficacy of lacosamide for treating painful diabetic neuropathy with a goal dosage of 400 mg/day (30% improvement in 58% of lacosamide cohort vs. 46% with placebo in one trial). NNT for these studies was modest and ranged from 10 to 12.

Topiramate

Like lacosamide, studies evaluating the efficacy of topiramate have primarily evaluated its use in the treatment of painful diabetic neuropathy. One study of 208 patients showed that 36% of patients in the topiramate group (goal dosage of 400 mg, mean of 320 mg) experienced greater than 50% pain relief (vs. 21% of placebo cohort) and 50% of patients experienced greater than 30% pain (34% with placebo). However, several other placebo controlled trials failed to show topiramate efficacy. Of note, patient withdrawal from these studies is significant at higher doses, with greater than 50% of patients withdrawing from the study due to side effects at a daily dose of 400 mg.

Topiramate has also been evaluated in a small randomized crossover trial of 41 patients evaluating its use in lumbar radiculopathy, with 37% of patients in the topiramate group (mean dosage 200 mg) experiencing moderate pain relief compared to 17% of the placebo group.

Pearls and Pitfalls

- Gabapentin and pregabalin are first-line neuropathic pain agents.
- Carbamazepine and oxcarbazepine are first-line agents in the treatment of trigeminal neuralgia and are useful in other neuropathic pain syndromes with paroxysmal pains.
- Combination therapy (utilizing neuropathic pain adjuvants of distinct mechanisms of action) is more efficacious than monotherapy (e.g., anticonvulsant + antidepressant).
- Polypharmacy should be rational and done with drugs of different mechanisms of action.
- Anticonvulsants should not be discontinued abruptly as precipitous withdraw could precipitate a seizure.
- Neuropathic pain adjuvants (including anticonvulsants and antidepressants) are underutilized in patients with painful neuropathy. Only 55–60% of those utilizing chronic opioid therapy for their neuropathic pain have been trialed on a neuropathic pain adjuvant.
- As with antidepressants, there is a small but important risk with anticonvulsants of emerging suicidality. Based on a meta-analysis of anticonvulsants as a drug class, anticonvulsants have a suicide risk to 0.43% (compared to 0.22% with placebo).
- Many anticonvulsants are teratogenic. Discussion regarding risks, benefits, and need to use contraception (barrier method preferable) should be held with any female patient of childbearing age prior to starting the medication. The medication should be weaned if possible prior to trying to get pregnant, and folic acid supplementation should be encouraged.
- Anticonvulsants that inhibit the cytochrome P450 system in the liver reduce the efficacy of oral contraceptives.
- Treatment of comorbid medical and psychiatric conditions in patients is critical, and a multidisciplinary approach is often needed to adequately address neuropathic pain.

Recommended Reading (Highlight references are marked in *)

1. Al-Quliti KW. Update on neuropathic pain treatment for trigeminal neuralgia: the pharmacological and surgical options. Neurosciences (Riyadh). 2015;20(2):107–14. https://doi.org/10.17712/nsj.2015.2.20140501.
2. Backonja M, Beydoun A, Edwards KR, Schwartz SL, Fonseca V, Hes M, et al. Gabapentin for the symptomatic treatment of painful neuropathy in patients with diabetes mellitus: a randomized controlled trial. JAMA. 1998;280(21):1831–6.
3. Backonja MM, Canafax DM, Cundy KC. Efficacy of gabapentin enacarbil vs placebo in patients with postherpetic neuralgia and a pharmacokinetic comparison with oral gabapentin. Pain Med. 2011;12(7):1098–108. https://doi.org/10.1111/j.1526-4637.2011.01139.x.
4. Bennett M. The LANSS Pain Scale: the Leeds assessment of neuropathic symptoms and signs. Pain. 2001;92(1–2):147–57.
5. Blom S. Trigeminal neuralgia: its treatment with a new anticonvulsant drug (G-32883). Lancet. 1962;1(7234):839–40.
6. Campbell JN, Meyer RA. Mechanisms of neuropathic pain. Neuron. 2006;52(1):77–92. https://doi.org/10.1016/j.neuron.2006.09.021.
7. Cardenas DD, Nieshoff EC, Suda K, Goto S, Sanin L, Kaneko T, et al. A randomized trial of pregabalin in patients with neuropathic pain due to spinal cord injury. Neurology. 2013;80(6):533–9. https://doi.org/10.1212/WNL.0b013e318281546b.
8. Costigan M, Scholz J, Woolf CJ. Neuropathic pain: a maladaptive response of the nervous system to damage. Annu Rev Neurosci. 2009;32:1–32. https://doi.org/10.1146/annurev.neuro.051508.135531.
9. Dogra S, Beydoun S, Mazzola J, Hopwood M, Wan Y. Oxcarbazepine in painful diabetic neuropathy: a randomized, placebo-controlled study. Eur J Pain. 2005;9(5):543–54. https://doi.org/10.1016/j.ejpain.2004.11.006.
10. *Finnerup NB, Attal N, Haroutounian S, McNicol E, Baron R, Dworkin RH, et al. Pharmacotherapy for neuropathic pain in adults: a systematic review and meta-analysis. Lancet Neurol. 2015;14(2):162–173. https://doi.org/10.1016/s1474-4422(14)70251-0.
11. Fukada C, Kohler JC, Boon H, Austin Z, Krahn M. Prescribing gabapentin off label: perspectives from psychiatry, pain and neurology specialists. Can Pharm J (Ott). 2012;145(6):280–284.e281. https://doi.org/10.3821/145.6.cpj280.
12. Gilron I, Bailey JM, Tu D, Holden RR, Weaver DF, Houlden RL. Morphine, gabapentin, or their combination for neuropathic pain. N Engl J Med. 2005;352(13):1324–34. https://doi.org/10.1056/NEJMoa042580.
13. Gilron I, Bailey JM, Tu D, Holden RR, Jackson AC, Houlden RL. Nortriptyline and gabapentin, alone and in combination for neuropathic pain: a double-blind, randomised controlled crossover trial. Lancet. 2009;374(9697):1252–61. https://doi.org/10.1016/s0140-6736(09)61081-3.
14. *Gilron I, Baron R, Jensen T. Neuropathic pain: principles of diagnosis and treatment. Mayo Clin Proc. 2015;90(4):532–545. https://doi.org/10.1016/j.mayocp.2015.01.018.
15. Gomez-Arguelles JM, Dorado R, Sepulveda JM, Herrera A, Arrojo FG, Aragon E, et al. Oxcarbazepine monotherapy in carbamazepine-unresponsive trigeminal neuralgia. J Clin Neurosci. 2008;15(5):516–9. https://doi.org/10.1016/j.jocn.2007.04.010.
16. Gronseth G, Cruccu G, Alksne J, Argoff C, Brainin M, Burchiel K, et al. Practice parameter: the diagnostic evaluation and treatment of trigeminal neuralgia (an evidence-based review): report of the Quality Standards Subcommittee of the American Academy of Neurology and the European Federation of Neurological Societies. Neurology. 2008;71(15):1183–90. https://doi.org/10.1212/01.wnl.0000326598.83183.04.
17. Guy S, Mehta S, Leff L, Teasell R, Loh E. Anticonvulsant medication use for the management of pain following spinal cord injury: systematic review and effectiveness analysis. Spinal Cord. 2014;52(2):89–96. https://doi.org/10.1038/sc.2013.146.
18. Hahn K, Arendt G, Braun JS, von Giesen HJ, Husstedt IW, Maschke M, et al. A placebo-controlled trial of gabapentin for painful HIV-associated sensory neuropathies. J Neurol. 2004;251(10):1260–6. https://doi.org/10.1007/s00415-004-0529-6.
19. Hearn L, Derry S, Moore RA. Lacosamide for neuropathic pain and fibromyalgia in adults. Cochrane Database Syst Rev. 2012;2:Cd009318. https://doi.org/10.1002/14651858.CD009318.pub2.
20. Jensen TS. Anticonvulsants in neuropathic pain: rationale and clinical evidence. Eur J Pain. 2002;6(Suppl A):61–8. https://doi.org/10.1053/eujp.2001.0324.
21. Jose VM, Bhansali A, Hota D, Pandhi P. Randomized double-blind study comparing the efficacy and safety of lamotrigine and amitrip-

tyline in painful diabetic neuropathy. Diabet Med. 2007;24(4):377–83. https://doi.org/10.1111/j.1464-5491.2007.02093.x.

22. Kim JS, Bashford G, Murphy TK, Martin A, Dror V, Cheung R. Safety and efficacy of pregabalin in patients with central post-stroke pain. Pain. 2011;152(5):1018–23. https://doi.org/10.1016/j.pain.2010.12.023.
23. Kukkar A, Bali A, Singh N, Jaggi AS. Implications and mechanism of action of gabapentin in neuropathic pain. Arch Pharm Res. 2013;36(3):237–51. https://doi.org/10.1007/s12272-013-0057-y.
24. Lee DO, Ziman RB, Perkins AT, Poceta JS, Walters AS, Barrett RW. A randomized, double-blind, placebo-controlled study to assess the efficacy and tolerability of gabapentin enacarbil in subjects with restless legs syndrome. J Clin Sleep Med. 2011;7(3):282–92. https://doi.org/10.5664/jcsm.1074.
25. Levendoglu F, Ogun CO, Ozerbil O, Ogun TC, Ugurlu H. Gabapentin is a first line drug for the treatment of neuropathic pain in spinal cord injury. Spine (Phila Pa 1976). 2004;29(7):743–51.
26. Levinson SR, Luo S, Henry MA. The role of sodium channels in chronic pain. Muscle Nerve. 2012;46(2):155–65. https://doi.org/10.1002/mus.23314.
27. Minton GC, Miller AD, Bookstaver PB, Love BL. Topiramate: safety and efficacy of its use in the prevention and treatment of migraine. J Cent Nerv Syst Dis. 2011;3:155–68. https://doi.org/10.4137/jcnsd.s4365.
28. Mishra S, Bhatnagar S, Goyal GN, Rana SP, Upadhya SP. A comparative efficacy of amitriptyline, gabapentin, and pregabalin in neuropathic cancer pain: a prospective randomized double-blind placebo-controlled study. Am J Hosp Palliat Care. 2012;29(3):177–82. https://doi.org/10.1177/1049909111412539.
29. Moore RA, Straube S, Wiffen PJ, Derry S, McQuay HJ. Pregabalin for acute and chronic pain in adults. Cochrane Database Syst Rev. 2009;3:Cd007076. https://doi.org/10.1002/14651858.CD007076.pub2.
30. Moore RA, Wiffen PJ, Derry S, Toelle T, Rice AS. Gabapentin for chronic neuropathic pain and fibromyalgia in adults. Cochrane Database Syst Rev. 2014;4:Cd007938. https://doi.org/10.1002/14651858.CD007938.pub3.
31. Moore RA, Wiffen PJ, Derry S, Lunn MP. Zonisamide for neuropathic pain in adults. Cochrane Database Syst Rev. 2015;1:Cd011241. https://doi.org/10.1002/14651858.CD011241.pub2.
32. *Moulin D, Boulanger A, Clark AJ, Clarke H, Dao T, Finley GA, et al. Pharmacological management of chronic neuropathic pain: revised consensus statement from the Canadian Pain Society. Pain Res Manag. 2014;19(6):328–335.
33. Patel R, Dickenson AH. Mechanisms of the gabapentinoids and α. Pharmacol Res Perspect. 2016;4(2):e00205. https://doi.org/10.1002/prp2.205.
34. Patel R, Bauer CS, Nieto-Rostro M, Margas W, Ferron L, Chaggar K, et al. alpha2delta-1 gene deletion affects somatosensory neuron function and delays mechanical hypersensitivity in response to peripheral nerve damage. J Neurosci. 2013;33(42):16412–26. https://doi.org/10.1523/jneurosci.1026-13.2013.
35. Petersen KL, Fields HL, Brennum J, Sandroni P, Rowbotham MC. Capsaicin evoked pain and allodynia in post-herpetic neuralgia. Pain. 2000;88(2):125–33.
36. Rauck RL, Shaibani A, Biton V, Simpson J, Koch B. Lacosamide in painful diabetic peripheral neuropathy: a phase 2 double-blind placebo-controlled study. Clin J Pain. 2007;23(2):150–8. https://doi.org/10.1097/01.ajp.0000210957.39621.b2.
37. Rintala DH, Holmes SA, Courtade D, Fiess RN, Tastard LV, Loubser PG. Comparison of the effectiveness of amitriptyline and gabapentin on chronic neuropathic pain in persons with spinal cord injury. Arch Phys Med Rehabil. 2007;88(12):1547–60. https://doi.org/10.1016/j.apmr.2007.07.038.
38. Rogawski MA, Loscher W. The neurobiology of antiepileptic drugs for the treatment of nonepileptic conditions. Nat Med. 2004;10(7):685–92. https://doi.org/10.1038/nm1074.
39. Serpell MG. Gabapentin in neuropathic pain syndromes: a randomised, double-blind, placebo-controlled trial. Pain. 2002;99(3):557–66.
40. Shaibani AI, Pope LE, Thisted R, Hepner A. Efficacy and safety of dextromethorphan/quinidine at two dosage levels for diabetic neuropathic pain: a double-blind, placebo-controlled, multicenter study. Pain Med. 2012;13(2):243–54. https://doi.org/10.1111/j.1526-4637.2011.01316.x.
41. Sills GJ. The mechanisms of action of gabapentin and pregabalin. Curr Opin Pharmacol. 2006;6(1):108–13. https://doi.org/10.1016/j.coph.2005.11.003.
42. Simpson DA. Gabapentin and venlafaxine for the treatment of painful diabetic neuropathy. J Clin Neuromuscul Dis. 2001;3(2):53–62.
43. Tolou-Ghamari Z, Zare M, Habibabadi JM, Najafi MR. A quick review of carbamazepine pharmacokinetics in epilepsy from 1953 to 2012. J Res Med Sci. 2013;18(Suppl 1):S81–5.
44. Vargas-Espinosa ML, Sanmartí-García G, Vázquez-Delgado E, Gay-Escoda C. Antiepileptic drugs for the treatment of neuropathic pain. Med Oral Patol Oral Cir Bucal. 2012;17(5):e786–93. https://doi.org/10.4317/medoral.18001.
45. Verma V, Singh N, Singh Jaggi A. Pregabalin in neuropathic pain: evidences and possible mechanisms. Curr Neuropharmacol. 2014;12(1):44–56. https://doi.org/10.2174/1570159x1201140117162802.
46. Vranken JH, Dijkgraaf MG, Kruis MR, van der Vegt MH, Hollmann MW, Heesen M. Pregabalin in patients with central neuropathic pain: a randomized, double-blind, placebo-controlled trial of a flexible-dose regimen. Pain. 2008;136(1–2):150–7. https://doi.org/10.1016/j.pain.2007.06.033.
47. Watson JC, Dyck PJ. Peripheral neuropathy: a practical approach to diagnosis and symptom management. Mayo Clin Proc. 2015;90(7):940–51. https://doi.org/10.1016/j.mayocp.2015.05.004.
48. Watson JC, Sandroni P. Central neuropathic pain syndromes. Mayo Clin Proc. 2016;91(3):372–85. https://doi.org/10.1016/j.mayocp.2016.01.017.
49. Weingarten TN, Watson JC, Hooten WM, Wollan PC, Melton LJ 3rd, Locketz AJ, et al. Validation of the S-LANSS in the community setting. Pain. 2007;132(1–2):189–94. https://doi.org/10.1016/j.pain.2007.07.030.
50. Wiffen PJ, Derry S, Lunn MP, Moore RA. Topiramate for neuropathic pain and fibromyalgia in adults. Cochrane Database Syst Rev. 2013;8:Cd008314. https://doi.org/10.1002/14651858.CD008314.pub3.
51. Wiffen PJ, Derry S, Moore RA. Lamotrigine for chronic neuropathic pain and fibromyalgia in adults. Cochrane Database Syst Rev. 2013;12:Cd006044. https://doi.org/10.1002/14651858.CD006044.pub4.
52. Wiffen PJ, Derry S, Moore RA, Aldington D, Cole P, Rice AS, et al. Antiepileptic drugs for neuropathic pain and fibromyalgia - an overview of Cochrane reviews. Cochrane Database Syst Rev. 2013;11:Cd010567. https://doi.org/10.1002/14651858.CD010567.pub2.
53. Wymer JP, Simpson J, Sen D, Bongardt S. Efficacy and safety of lacosamide in diabetic neuropathic pain: an 18-week double-blind placebo-controlled trial of fixed-dose regimens. Clin J Pain. 2009;25(5):376–85. https://doi.org/10.1097/AJP.0b013e318196d2b6.
54. Zhou M, Chen N, He L, Yang M, Zhu C, Wu F. Oxcarbazepine for neuropathic pain. Cochrane Database Syst Rev. 2013;3:Cd007963. https://doi.org/10.1002/14651858.CD007963.pub2.

20 Botulinum Toxin

Kris Ferguson and Nicole Wolfgram

Introduction

The World Health Organization ranks migraines as the sixth highest cause of disability when considered alone and third highest when medication-overuse headache is included. Medication-overuse headache is a common and disabling condition which further complicates the underlying pain. The social and economic burden is staggering resulting in missed days of work, economic loss, pain, and sufferance which can cause and potentiate depression.

Most patients with primary headache do not receive satisfactory treatment. A European study showed that between 43% and 81% of people with chronic headaches were not satisfied with the headache management. The main reason for the lack of satisfaction is the lack of efficacy and side effect profile of existing oral medications.

Background/History

Botulinum toxin is a neurotoxin protein produced by the bacterium *Clostridium botulinum* and related species. There are seven types of botulinum toxin, types A–G, but only types A and B are FDA approved to be used in humans. Only vertebrate animals are sensitive to the botulinum neurotoxin. The neurotoxin affects the peripheral cholinergic nerve terminals of skeletal muscle and cholinergic nerve terminals of autonomic ganglia. By inhibiting the soluble N-ethylmaleimide-sensitive factor attachment protein receptor (SNARE complex), botulinum toxin causes flaccid paralysis and inactivity of the cholinergic neurons (see Fig. 20.1).

Mechanism of Action

The botulinum toxin is composed of a heavy chain and a light chain held together by a disulfide bond. This structure allows the botulinum toxin to interact with two independent receptors on the presynaptic membrane that allows internalization into a vesicle. Of note, neuronal activity enhances botulinum uptake. This is clinically relevant because when treating syndromes characterized by hyperactive nerve terminals, the hyperactive nerve terminals will preferentially uptake the botulinum toxin.

The endocytosis process may seem esoteric but it does have clinical implications. After binding to the membrane protein, the botulinum toxin resides in the lumen of the synaptic vesicle. Of note, there are only one or two botulinum toxin molecules per vesicle. On the presynaptic membrane, there are specialized active sites with proteins involved in endocytosis and the formation of the synaptic vesicle. Prior to the formation of the synaptic vesicle, the membrane proteins are similar. Once the synaptic vesicle is formed and endocytosed, there are various membrane profiles the vesicle can take which impact future pathways. For example, a synaptic vesicle can be immediately recycled, it can be acidified by an ATPase proton pump which creates a gradient allowing for accumulation of specific neurotransmitters, or it can fuse with endosomal compartments. These various pathways allow for the trafficking of the synaptic vesicle allowing for mobility of the botulinum toxin.

The consequence of local botulinum toxin is either muscle paralysis or inactivity of cholinergic glands. There is evidence of retrograde transport of botulinum toxin in the spinal cord via the motor and sensory nerves. Currently, there is no

K. Ferguson (✉) · N. Wolfgram
Aspirus Hospital, Wausau, WI, USA

T. R. Deer et al. (eds.), *Deer's Treatment of Pain*, https://doi.org/10.1007/978-3-030-12281-2_20

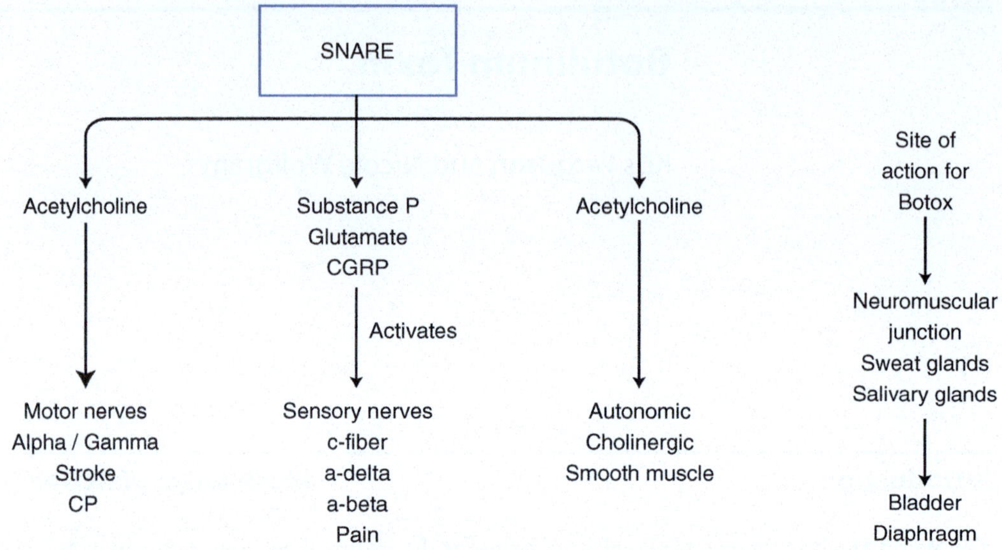

SNARE complex. Single site of action = SNARE protein via SNAP-25.

Fig. 20.1 SNARE complex. Single site of action, SNARE protein via SNAP-25

evidence of pathologic signs or symptoms resulting from the retrograde transport of the botulinum toxin into the CNS (see Fig. 20.2). However, this retrograde transport suggests a possible pathway by which botulinum toxin can help with central pain syndromes.

Botulinum toxin can enter the body via several routes: oral ingestion, anaerobic wounds, inhalation, and intramuscular injection of excessive doses. Botulinum poisoning is rare with improved food processing techniques that prevent anaerobic bacterial growth. The main pathologic symptom of systemic botulinum toxin is flaccid paralysis. The effects start with the ocular muscles and then spread systemically causing respiratory failure. If the patient can be mechanically ventilated and appropriately supported, the recovery is typically complete. Of significance, if botulinum toxicity is being treated with ventilatory support, they likely will not be able to move and will appear asleep. However, they will be fully conscious of the event and should be sedated or the patient will be at risk for psychological trauma.

Unique among many nerve toxins, botulinum toxin is reversible. There are reports of severe botulinum intoxication resulting in total paralysis and the patients making a virtually complete recovery with the aid of supportive care. This is because botulinum toxin is not neurotoxic and cytotoxic or causes axonal degeneration. In vitro studies may show cytotoxicity, but that is because the concentration and amount of botulinum toxin used is orders of magnitude higher that can be reasonably expected in vivo. Clinical experience with botulinum for therapeutic and cosmetic indications has not demonstrated any neurotoxicity or side effects, even after continuous repeated treatments. The caveat is that only botulinum toxin type A and B are FDA approved, and there may be toxicity associated with the other isoforms.

Onabotulinum toxin A is the primary commercially prepared type of Botox. It is marketed for cosmetic use as in Botox Cosmetic and for medical use at Botox. While rimabotulinum toxin B (Myobloc) is FDA approved for use, it is not used as readily in the United States.

Clinical applications for type A in both FDA (bolded) and off-label uses:

- *Limb spasticity*
- *Overactive bladder*
- *Cervical dystonia*
- *Primary axillary hyperhidrosis*
- *Blepharospasm and strabismus*
- Postherpetic neuralgia
- Trigeminal neuralgia
- Posttraumatic/postsurgical neuralgia
- Diabetic neuropathy
- Occipital neuralgia
- *Chronic migraines*
- Residual limb pain/phantom limb pain
- Myofascial trigger points
- Anterior knee pain

Clinical applications for type B in both FDA (bolded) and off-label uses:

- *Cervical dystonia*
- Spasmodic torticollis
- Hemifacial spasm
- Spasmodic dysphonia

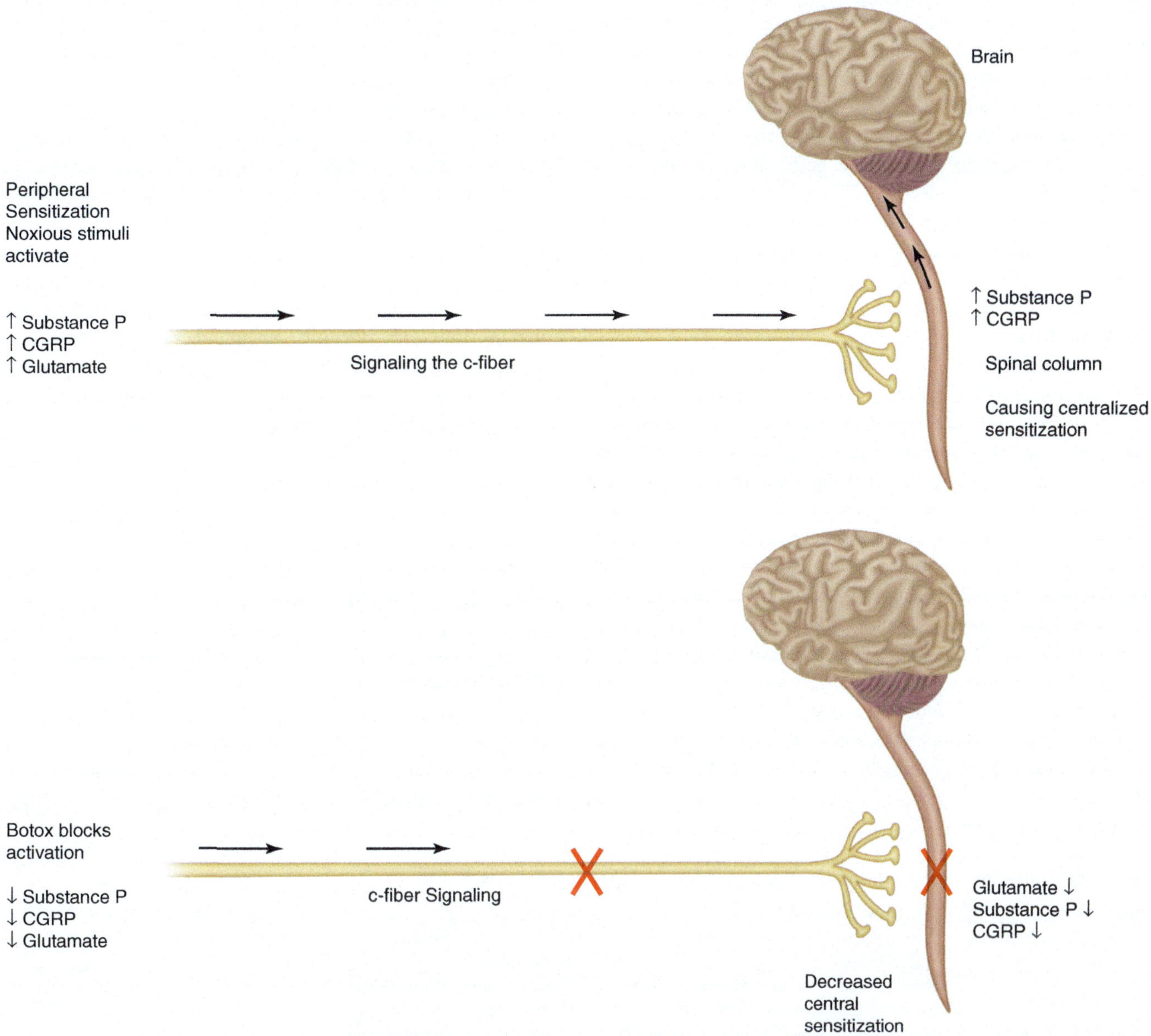

Fig. 20.2 The consequence of local botulinum toxin is either muscle paralysis or inactivity of cholinergic glands. There is evidence of retrograde transport of botulinum toxin in the spinal cord via the motor and sensory nerves. Currently, there is no evidence of pathologic signs or symptoms resulting from the retrograde transport of the botulinum toxin into the CNS

- Primary axillary hyperhidrosis
- Blepharospasm and strabismus
- Neuropathic pains
- Headaches
- Myofascial pain
- Stroke-related spasticity

FDA black box warning Potential for distal spread of the medication which can lead to life-threatening issues with breathing and swallowing.

Special Considerations

Use cautiously in patients with pre-existing neuromuscular disorders or respiratory disorders.

Contraindications

Infection, pregnancy, breastfeeding, and urinary tract infection (intradetrusor injections)

Dosing

Dosing is variable based on the type used and the area being injected. There are no clear guidelines established for appropriate dosing. Prior to injection the Botox needs to be reconstituted with sterile, preservative free, 0.9% saline. In general, the smaller the muscle being injected, the more dilute the solution needs to be. The package insert gives specific dilution instructions. Sterile technique should be used when administering the injections.

Headaches

For headaches, there are several different protocols that can be used. These include a fixed-site approach, the follow-the-pain approach, and a combination approach. The fixed-site approach uses symmetric injection sites in predetermined doses. The follow-the-pain approach uses asymmetric injection site, and the dose varies based on pain response to palpation. The combination approach supplements the fixed sites utilizing a follow-the-pain response in which painful areas outside of the fixed sites are injected. Based on the results of the PREEMPT (Phase III Research Evaluating Migraine Prophylaxis Therapy) trial study, the areas that are recommended to inject include the corrugator, the procerus, the frontalis, the occipitalis, the temporalis, cervical paraspinal muscles, and the trapezius muscles (see Table 20.1 and Fig. 20.3).

Cervical Dystonia

Cervical dystonia is treated with Botox based on the affected muscles involved. There may be benefit to having EMG testing to help identify which muscles are causing the spasticity. The muscles can be tonic or in a prolonged contracture or spasm or clonic where there is more "jerky" type movement or a combination of the two. Dosing for dystonia is based on the location being treated. Posterior injection sites include the semispinalis muscles (30–100 units), longissimus (30–100 units), trapezius (20–100 units), and levator scapulae (20–100 units). Anterior/lateral injection sites include the splenius capitis (15–100 units), splenius cervicis (20–60 units), scalene complex (15–50 units), and sternocleidomastoid (15–100 units). Caution should be taken with injections into the sternocleidomastoids as dysphagia can occur.

Others

The dose range for other types of injections is generally 5–200 units. For joint injections, the average amount is 100 units.

Efficacy/Duration

The duration of action of botulinum toxin is dependent on the type of botulinum used A vs. B, dose, method of administration, and the type of synapse affected (muscle vs. cholinergic

Table 20.1 PREEMPT (Phase III Research Evaluating Migraine Prophylaxis Therapy) trials

Area to inject	Anatomic location	Dosing	Additional dosing
Corrugator (bilateral)	Above the medial superior edge of the orbital ridge	0.1 mL (5 units) per injection 10 units/2 sites	
Procerus	Superior and midline to the medial superior aspect of the orbital ridge of each eye	0.1 mL (5 units) per injection 5 units/1 site	
Frontalis (bilateral)	Central and forehead region just beneath the surface of the skin Total of four injections	0.1 mL (5 units) per injection 20 units/4 sites	
Occipitalis (bilateral)	Six sites superior to the supranuchal ridge bilaterally from the occipital protuberance	0.1 mL (5 units) per injection Up to additional 0.4 mL (40 units) can be injected 30 units/6 sites	*In areas of tenderness can inject up to two additional sites across the right and left occipitalis muscles
Temporalis (bilateral)	1st: anterior temporalis muscle 2nd and 4th: medial aspect temporalis muscle 3rd: posterior temporalis muscle repeat contralaterally for a total of 8 + any additional for areas of tenderness	0.1 mL (5 units) per injection Up to additional 0.4 mL (40 units) can be injected 40 units/8 sites	*In areas of tenderness can do additional injections
Cervical paraspinal (bilateral)	1st: lateral midline/inferior occipital protuberance 2nd: lateral/superior to 1st Repeat contralaterally for a total of four injections	0.1 mL (5 units) per injection Up to additional 0.4 mL (40 units) can be injected 20 units/4 sites	*In areas of tenderness can do additional injections

*Allows for additional dosing above standard protocal

Total dosing for 31 sites is 155 units (with no additional follow-the-pain injections)

Total maximum dosing for all 39 site is 195 units

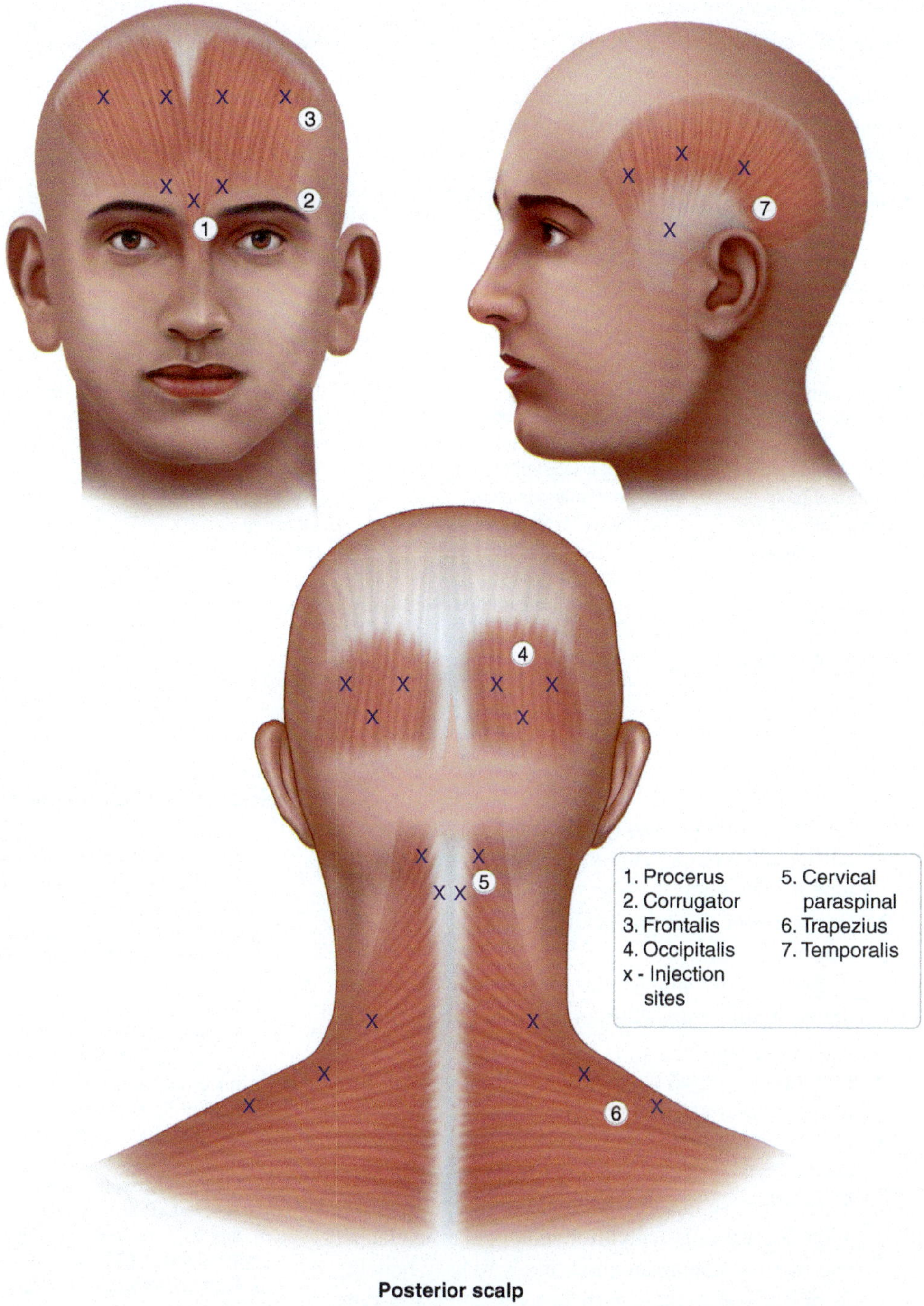

Fig. 20.3 The combination approach supplements the fixed sites with follow-the-pain response. Based on the results of the PREEMPT (Phase III Research Evaluating Migraine Prophylaxis Therapy) trial study, the areas that are recommended to inject include the corrugator, the procerus, the frontalis, the occipitalis, the temporalis, and the cervical paraspinal

synapse). Botulinum A works longer than B, and skeletal muscle recovers three times faster than the autonomic cholinergic nerves. In general, onset is 1–3 days with peak efficacy achieved around 2 weeks. The duration of action for skeletal muscle is 3–4 months, while for autonomic cholinergic nerves, it is approximately 1 year (see Table 20.1). For a summary of efficacy studies for various pain conditions, see Table 20.2.

Side Effects

Common side effects include injection site infection or bleeding, itching, fever, headaches, generalized muscular weakness, dysphagia, dysphonia, dysarthria, diplopia, ptosis, urinary incontinence, and breathing difficulties. Breathing difficulties and trouble swallowing are very rare.

Table 20.2 Evidence of efficacy

Condition	Studies	Results	Level of efficacy
Postherpetic neuralgia	(2) Class I	Both showed effectiveness	Effective
Trigeminal neuralgia	(1) Class I (multiple) Class IV	All showed effectiveness	Likely effective, more Class I research needed
Posttraumatic/postsurgical neuralgia	(1) Class I (1) Class IV	All showed effectiveness	Likely effective, more research needed
Diabetic neuropathy	(1) Class I (1) Class II	All showed effectiveness	Likely effective, more research needed
Occipital neuralgia	(2) Class IV	Mixed results	Insufficient evidence
Carpal tunnel	(1) Class I (1) Class IV	Mixed results	Insufficient evidence
Complex regional pain syndrome (CRPS)	(2) Class III (3) Class IV	Mixed results	Insufficient evidence
Residual limb pain/phantom limb pain	Case reports Prospective, randomized double-blind pilot study	Improved residual limb pain, no change in phantom limb pain	Insufficient evidence
Anterior knee pain	Open-label pilot study	Effective	Insufficient evidence
Myofascial pain	Systematic reviews	Mixed results	Insufficient evidence
Migraine headaches	Phase III PREEMPT	Effective	Effective
Cervical dystonia	(2) Cochrane reviews, meta-analysis	Effective	Effective
Low back pain	Randomized, double-blind study (3) Trials	Mixed results	Insufficient evidence
Chronic pelvic pain	Case reports (3) Prospective studies	Effective	Likely effective, more research needed

Clinical Pearls

- Dosing from type A to type B is not a 1:1 ratio.
- Dosing of type A "Botox" is not a 1:1 ratio with type A "Dysport."
- Dysport type A seems to disperse to a larger area than Botox type A.
- In general, the smaller the muscle being injected, the more dilute the solution needs to be (such as in ocular injections).
- Injection of a high concentration in a small volume results in a more localized effect.
- Using EMG when treating complex dystonia can be useful.
- Most effective in focal dystonia.
- Migraine patients with allodynia, ocular headache, and imploding pain are more likely to have benefits from Botox than those with episodic or tension-type headaches.

Recommended Reading

1. Beal B, Wallace M. An overview of pharmacologic management of chronic pain. Med Clin N Am. 2016;100(1):65–79.
2. Bomba-Warczak E, Vevea J, Brittain J, Figueroa-Bernier A, Tepp W, Johnson E, et al. Interneuronal transfer and distal action of tetanus toxin and botulinum neurotoxins A and D in central neurons. Cell Rep. 2016;16(7):1974–87.
3. Broide R, Cai B, Francis J, Brin M. Botulinum neurotoxin type A–cleaved SNAP25 is confined to primary motor neurons and expressed on the plasma membrane following intramuscular toxin injection. Toxicon. 2016;123:S8.
4. Godoy I, Donahue D, Torriani M. Botulinum toxin injections in musculoskeletal disorders. Semin Musculoskelet Radiol. 2016;20(05):441–52.
5. Halder G, Scott L, Wyman A, Mora N, Miladinovic B, Bassaly R, et al. Botox combined with myofascial release physical therapy as a treatment for myofascial pelvic pain. Investig Clin Urol. 2017;58(2):134.
6. Hong B, Yao L, Ni L, Wang L, Hu X. Antinociceptive effect of botulinum toxin A involves alterations in AMPA receptor expression and glutamate release in spinal dorsal horn neurons. Neuroscience. 2017;357:197–207.

7. Kermen R. Botulinum toxin for chronic pain conditions. Dis Mon. 2016;62(9):353–7.
8. Matak I, Riederer P, Lackovic Z. Botulinum toxin's axonal transport from periphery to the spinal cord. Neurochem Int. 2012;61(2):236–9.
9. Mittal S, Safarpour D, Jabbari B. Botulinum toxin treatment of neuropathic pain. Semin Neurol. 2016;36(01):073–83.
10. Moon Y, Choi J, Park H, Park J, Kim J. Ultrasound-guided nerve block with botulinum toxin type a for intractable neuropathic pain. Toxins. 2016;8(1):18.
11. Morra M, Elgebaly A, Elmaraezy A, Khalil A, Altibi A, Vu T, et al. Therapeutic efficacy and safety of botulinum toxin A therapy in trigeminal neuralgia: a systematic review and meta-analysis of randomized controlled trials. J Headache Pain. 2016; 17(1):63.
12. Oh H, Chung M. Botulinum toxin for neuropathic pain: a review of the literature. Toxins. 2015;7(8):3127–54.
13. Pirazzini M, Rossetto O, Eleopra R, Montecucco C. Botulinum neurotoxins: biology, pharmacology, and toxicology. Pharmacol Rev. 2017;69(2):200–35.
14. Silberstein S. The use of botulinum toxin in the management of headache disorders. Semin Neurol. 2016;36(01):092–8.
15. Singer B, Silbert B, Silbert P, Singer K. The role of botulinum toxin type A in the clinical management of refractory anterior knee pain. Toxins. 2015;7(9):3388–404.
16. Wheeler A, Smith H. Botulinum toxins: mechanisms of action, antinociception and clinical applications. Toxicology. 2013;306:124–46.
17. Wissel J, Bensmail D, Ferreira J, Molteni F, Satkunam L, Moraleda S, et al. Safety and efficacy of incobotulinumtoxinA doses up to 800 U in limb spasticity. Neurology. 2017;88(14):1321–8.

Sodium Channel Antagonists

21

Katherine D. Travnicek

Introduction

Voltage-gated sodium channels (Na_v) have been analgesic targets for over 100 years. They have been studied extensively since the 1950s with significant strides made in understanding their mechanisms in the past decade. Voltage-gated sodium channels regulate signals by generating and conducting neuropathic and inflammatory pain electrical signals along predominantly peripheral sensory nerves to the central nervous system where the signals can be chronically maintained. These chronic and pathological pain sensations arise as a result of changes in peripheral sensory neuron excitation in common conditions such as painful diabetic neuropathy and postherpetic neuralgia (see Fig. 21.1).

There are nine known sodium channels, all with a similar overall structure but with different amino acid sequences, and different physiological properties, and functions, and four of these channels (Na_v1.3, Na_v1.7, Na_v1.8, and Na_v1.9) are potential analgesic targets. There are ten different α subunits, Na_v1.1–Na_v1.9 and Na_x, which are encoded by genes SCN1A–SCN11A, and four β subunits, Na_v β1–Na_v β4, encoded by genes SCN1B–SCN4B. Voltage-gated sodium channels are large, dynamic transmembrane proteins consisting of a pore-forming α subunit that regulates sodium passage and β subunits that modulate channel gating, expression, and localization. The ten different α subunits have four homologous domains (I–IV), each consisting of six transmembrane α helices labeled S1–S6. The outer part of the channel's pore has additional loops to join the S5–S6 segments, while the S6 segment forms the inner part of the pore. The S1–S4 segments are voltage sensors with the translocation of positively charged S4 residues initiating channel activation in response to membrane potential changes. The majority of all sodium channels are closed at resting membrane potentials and then, when depolarized, go through multiple activation states as S4 segment translocation allows sodium influx. The channel is inactivated by two α subunit domains III and IV that become covered by another looped structure. Inactivation lasts throughout depolarization, which is the reason for the refractory period. The channel recovers from inactivation to the resting, closed state and is then reprimed to for the next activation period.

The Na_v1.7, Na_v1.8, and Na_v1.9 channels have evolved relatively recently and are only found in mammals. These isoforms are expressed selectively in the PNS pain-conducting pathways. At present, the clinically available sodium channel antagonists are nonselective. Adverse side effects include cardiac toxicity, motor impairments, and multiple central nervous system effects such as sedation. The future of selective sodium channel antagonists may change current practice as more is learned about the different Na_v roles in pain management in various types of acute and chronic pain pathology.

Background and History Perspective

Sodium channel antagonists are used mainly for neuropathic pain, which can arise following increases in intrinsic nerve hyperexcitability and perhaps dysfunction in the surrounding milieu. Sodium channels are critical determinants of electrical excitability and play key role by controlling afferent impulse discharges. Peripheral nerve injury can induce axonopathy and demyelination, and these changes induce membrane remodeling, which results in neuronal hyperexcitability. In addition, nerve injury has been shown to result in changes in sodium channel gene expression, channel kinetics, and trafficking. Hyperexcitable neurons and excess discharges trigger and maintain central sensitization. Membrane-stabilizing sodium channel blockers suppress these discharges. Thus, sodium channel antagonists stabilize neuronal membranes and suppress membrane excitability.

Na_v1.7 expression was first discovered in peripheral neurons including somatosensory and sympathetic neurons but

K. D. Travnicek (✉)
Pain Institute of Nevada, Las Vegas, NV, USA
e-mail: kdt@paininstitute.com

T. R. Deer et al. (eds.), *Deer's Treatment of Pain*, https://doi.org/10.1007/978-3-030-12281-2_21

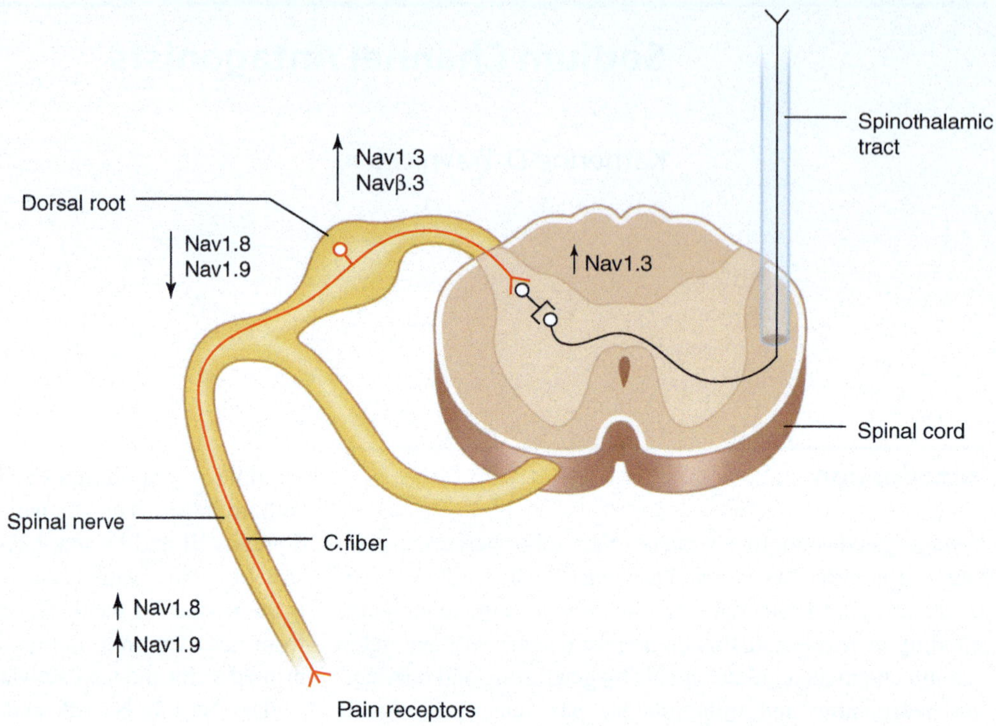

Fig. 21.1 The spinal cord and peripheral afferent pain pathway changes in Na_v channels after chronic nerve injury associated with chronic pain

now includes myenteric and visceral sensory neurons. This sodium channel is expressed in small (C fibers and A-delta)- and large (Aß)-diameter DRG neurons. It has attracted significant interest following two intriguing genetic discoveries both based on the *SCN9A* gene which encodes $Na_v1.7$. Waxman et al. found that in patients with the chronic familial pain disorder primary erythermalgia, $Na_v1.7$ is hyperexcitable due to a gain-of-function mutation in the *SCN9A* gene. Woods et al. found that $Na_v1.7$ is nonfunctional in those who cannot feel pain due to a loss-of-function gene mutation. Despite these genetic findings, not all of the $Na_v1.7$ mechanisms are fully understood. However, there is clear involvement in human pain and lack of serious cognitive, cardiac, and motor effects with total loss of $Na_v1.7$.

$Na_v1.8$ is expressed in DRG neurons and trigeminal ganglia, peripheral axon shafts, and free terminal nerve endings in the skin. $Na_v1.9$ is expressed in small-diameter, nonpeptidergic dorsal root ganglia, trigeminal ganglia, myenteric neurons, and free nerve terminals in the skin and cornea. Their role in neuropathic pain is unknown but in inflammatory pain states it is well documented in animal studies for $Na_v1.8$ and is convincing for $Na_v1.9$. There is recent evidence linking gain-of-function mutations of $Na_v1.8$ and $Na_v1.9$ to painful peripheral neuropathies. $Na_v1.3$ is normally expressed during embryogenesis, continues to be expressed in sympathetic neurons in adults, and is upregulated after a nerve injury in rodents. Recently it was discovered that $Na_v1.3$ mutations are linked to human childhood epilepsy and have been localized in human neuromas. Moreover, gene therapy experiments in rodents indicate that knockdown of $Na_v1.3$ can ameliorate neuropathic pain. This suggests it may play a larger role in human nociception than previously thought, but current data is conflicting. Until more is learned about the specifics of each sodium channel and their involvement in pain pathways, solely nonselective sodium channel blockers will be utilized.

Sodium channel antagonists fall into four different classes of medications: antidepressants (discussed elsewhere), local anesthetics, anticonvulsants, and anti-arrhythmic. In the late 1800s, cocaine was the first sodium channel antagonist used clinically for surgical anesthesia but due to toxicity was mostly abandoned. Long before the arrival of European explorers, the *coca* plant was used by the indigenous people of South America as a remedy for wide range of health conditions. The development of modern organic chemistry led to the synthesis of pure cocaine in late nineteenth century. Cocaine is the principal alkaloid found in cultivated coca leaves. Coca leaves were brought back to Europe after editorials on coca were published in *The British Medical Journal*. Albert Niemann, a German chemist, isolated cocaine from the imported coca leaves. A few years later, Dr. Karl Koller, a German ophthalmologist, announced his successful use of cocaine as a topical anesthetic for eye surgery. In Europe and the United States, there was an immediate surge of experimentation with cocaine, leading to revolutionary developments in regional anesthesia as well as new surgical procedures. However, the toxic effects of cocaine were soon identified as there were many deaths among both patients and addicted medical staff.

In 1905, procaine (Novocaine) was developed, and because it was not addictive and safer than cocaine, it became a popular local anesthetic. However, procaine could trigger severe allergic reactions, and it was quickly replaced with the first amide local anesthetic, lidocaine (Xylocaine), introduced in 1946. Lidocaine revolutionized pain control in medicine and surgery. It is on the World Health Organization's List of Essential Medicines, which is a list of the most effective and safest medicines needed in a health system. In succeeding years other amide local anesthetics were introduced and include mepivacaine, prilocaine, bupivacaine, ropivacaine, and levobupivacaine. The amides give the analgesia for periods from 20 minutes to as long as 3 hours, proved to be more rapid acting than the older ester-type drug, and were also safer from an allergic reaction perspective.

Mexiletine hydrochloride is an orally active sodium channel antagonist, Class 1B anti-arrhythmic agent, and structurally similar to lidocaine. Although it was primarily studied for the treatment of ventricular arrhythmias, it has been demonstrated to be useful also for the treatment of chronic painful diabetic neuropathy, neuropathic pain, skeletal muscle channelopathies, and recently muscle spasms in amyotrophic lateral sclerosis. It is a substrate for the metabolic pathways involving CYP2D6 and CYP1A2 enzymes, and inhibition or induction of either of these enzymes can alter mexiletine plasma concentrations. Due to its pro-arrthymic nature and multiple drug interactions, it is not commonly used.

The final class of sodium channel antagonists is anti-epileptic drugs (AEDs), which are prescribed for migraines, psychiatric conditions, epilepsy, and chronic neuropathic pain, and all likely have common pathophysiological mechanisms. Anti-epileptic medications are most effective at blocking high-frequency action potentials firing from sodium channels, or they can activate slow inactivation phase of sodium channels. They are not as effective in low-frequency action potential firing. The fast-firing-type sodium channel blockers include phenytoin, carbamazepine, oxcarbazepine, lamotrigine, felbamate, topiramate, valproic acid, zonisamide, rufinamide, and eslicarbazepine. Lacosamide is unique in that it selectively enhances the slow inactivation component of sodium channels. The only AED that is FDA approved for any neuropathic pain condition is carbamazepine (trigeminal neuralgia).

Uses and Indications

Local Anesthetics

Central and regional nerve block procedures with local anesthetics have a well-defined role as safe and effective for well over 100 years. Local anesthetics are used solo or in combination with other agents during surgery, dental procedures, and for diagnosis and management of various acute and chronic pain conditions. These nonselective sodium channel antagonists are available by various routes – topical, oral, rectal, intravenous, intramuscular, peripheral perineural blocks, epidural, and intrathecal in pumps.

Understanding local anesthetics structure helps explain their chemical activity. All local anesthetics have the same basic structure which includes four separate components. There is an intermediate chain of between 3 and 7 carbon equivalents, an ester or amide bond, a hydrophilic amine on one end, and a lipophilic aromatic ring on the other end. Variation of the amine or aromatic ends will change the chemical activity. The two classes of local anesthetics are named after the bond, the amino amides have an amide bond between the intermediate chain and the aromatic end, whereas amino esters have an ester link at the same position. Esters include cocaine, procaine, tetracaine, chloroprocaine, and benzocaine, and amides include lidocaine, mepivacaine, prilocaine, bupivacaine, and ropivacaine. Lidocaine and bupivacaine are the most commonly used in all stages of pain management and only ones discussed in detail in this chapter (see Table 21.1).

Table 21.1 Commonly used local anesthetics for pain

Local anesthetic	Dose ceiling	Onset	Duration of action	Properties
Lidocaine	4.5 mg/kg without EPI	PNB[a] ~ 30 seconds	Up to 120 minutes without EPI	pKa = 7.9
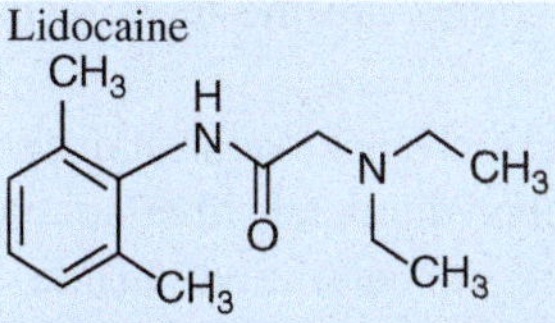	Not to exceed 300 mg at once			64% protein bound
			Up to 360 minutes with EPI	No chirality
	7 mg/kg with EPI			Sensory and motor blockade
	Not to exceed 500 mg			
Bupivacaine	2.5 mg/kg without EPI	PNB[a] ~ 30 seconds	About 4 hours without EPI	pKa = 8.1
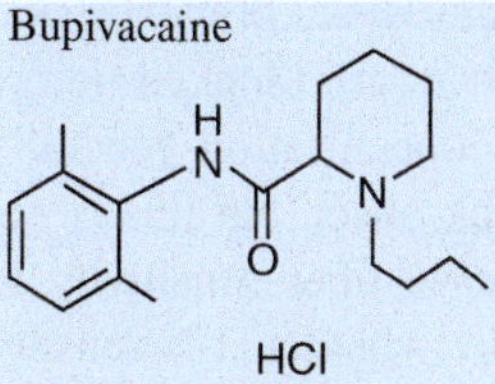	Not to exceed 175 mg at once			95% protein bound
	3 mg/kg with EPI	IT[b] ~ 30 seconds	About 8 hours with EPI	Sensory ≫ motor blockade
	Not to exceed 225 mg			

[a]*PNB* peripheral nerve block
[b]*IT* intrathecal

The most important chemical properties that determine local anesthetic pharmacology are the ionization (pKa), lipid solubility, and protein binding. These three properties determine local anesthetic clinical behaviors which are onset, potency, duration, and toxicity. The ionization constant (pKa) determines the proportion of ionized and non-ionized forms of anesthetic in solution. Local anesthetics with lower pKa have a more rapid onset of action. Lipid solubility determines local anesthetic potency, plasma protein binding, and duration of action. The lipid solubility is determined by chemical structure and increases with an increase in number of carbon substitution on aromatic ring or on the amino group.

A major determinant of local anesthetics' conduction blockade onset is the pKa, and the closer the pKa is to the body's pH, the faster the onset. The pKa is the pH at which 50% of the drug exists in the ionic and the other 50% in nonionic, base form. The pKa of most local anesthetics is alkaline with pKa's ranging from 7.7 to 9.0, which is higher than physiologic pH. Both neutral base and ionized cation forms of local anesthetics are necessary for activity. Local anesthetics are prepared at a pH of 5–6 so that a majority exists in the cation state. However, they enter nerve fibers faster if they are in nonionic, base form. Once injected, the extracellular surroundings buffer the local anesthetic to physiologic pH, and it moves down its concentration gradient into the nerve cell. After passing through the membrane into the axoplasm of the nerve, the drug equilibrates by accepting a hydrogen ion to the active, ionic form. For most local anesthetics, the cationic form blocks conduction. However, benzocaine is always neutral, which shows that the ionized form is not completely necessary for the block to occur.

Lipid solubility appears to be the most significant property of local anesthetic molecules in determining anesthetic potency and duration of action. The aromatic ring improves the lipid solubility, and this property can be enhanced further by aliphatic substitutions on the ring or at the amine end. Local anesthetic molecules which are highly lipophilic easily penetrate the nerve cell membrane and can bind to sodium channels with more affinity. Bupivacaine is considerably more lipid soluble and more potent than lidocaine by about ten times. Increasing the lipid solubility can decrease speed of onset but not significantly.

The protein-binding capacity, which is related to lipid solubility, of a local anesthetic also determines the duration of conduction block. In general, agents with greater protein binding have a greater attraction for receptors and remain within sodium channels for a longer period of time. This means that agents with higher protein-binding capacity are associated with a longer duration of action. Poorly protein bound agents, such as procaine, are easily washed out, and duration of local anesthetic blockade can be extremely short, whereas those which are highly protein bound, such as bupivacaine, are much more difficult to wash out in similar type in vitro experiments. In addition, the degree of protein binding is concentration dependent and influenced by the local pH. The percentage of drug bound decreases as the pH decreases. This is important because with the development of acidosis or infection, the amount of free drug increases. The magnitude of this phenomenon varies among each local anesthetic.

Despite their common clinical use, the mechanism of action at the sodium channel is not fully understood. In general, all local anesthetics bind to the alpha subunit on sodium channels and prevent sodium influx into the cell resulting in a reversible conduction block. They have the highest affinity for open and inactivated depolarized sodium channels and the lowest for closed, resting state sodium channels. The more often a nerve is stimulated, the greater the time its sodium channels are open and the more susceptible the nerve is to the local anesthetic.

In addition to the degree of ionization, the rate of local anesthetic diffusion rate into the nerve is determined by the drug's concentration, hydrophobicity, and the surrounding tissue characteristics. In general, faster rates of diffusion are associated with higher local anesthetic concentrations as they flow down a concentration gradient. However, the more lipophilic, hydrophobic local has a larger amount of nonionized drug that is bound to plasma proteins, thus a slower diffusion rate. The more acidic the area will slow down diffusion rate as well. Infected tissue is acidic, and this acidity reduces LA diffusion because the LA form is forced into an ionized state.

In terms of absorption, anatomical considerations that affect the rate of local anesthetic absorption include how cephalad the LA is placed, the vascularity of the area, and nerve fiber type and size. The more cephalic the injection (cervical epidurals) has a faster rate of LA absorption compared to caudal injections. All LAs are vasodilators except cocaine, and the higher vascularity of the area generally allows faster LA uptake. Smaller fibers are preferentially blocked before larger nerve fibers, and myelinated fibers are more easily blocked than nonmyelinated. As a result, the nonmyelinated, small-diameter C-fibers are the most resistant fibers to blockade.

Various elements of the conduction block occur at different times, and this is related to fiber diameter, fiber spatial relationships, and local anesthetic concentration. Inside a peripheral nerve, nerve fibers are arranged with proximal branches near the surface or mantle and distal branches near the center core. Thus, the mantle fibers are blocked before the core fibers. The higher the LA concentration generally means the faster the conduction block onset, but this is not always the case. In addition, the nerve fiber sensitivity to local anesthetics is not determined by whether it is sensory or motor but more related to size. A-gamma fibers that supply the muscle spindles are blocked first as they are smaller than muscle proprioceptive afferent (A-beta) and motor efferent fibers (A-alpha). The latter two types are equally sensitive as they have the same diameter.

The duration of the block depends on the local anesthetic lipid solubility, protein-binding strength, and vasodilation properties as well as the presence of any vasoconstrictors with the most important property being lipid solubility. Greater lipid solubility increases the potency and duration of action as lipophilic medications have greater affinity for the lipid membrane of the nerve. The longer the drug stays present or in the vicinity of the lipid membrane, the more likely it will have a longer effect. Lipophilic substances also increase toxicity risk for the same reason.

Local anesthetics toxicity and central nervous system effects occur in a dose-dependent manner. Toxicity first produces central nervous system stimulation and causes restlessness, disorientation, and tremor. As the plasma concentration increases, seizures occur, and the more potent the local anesthetic, the more readily convulsions may be produced. With even higher plasma concentration, the central nervous system becomes depressed resulting in respiratory failure and coma.

The initial focus of local anesthetic toxicity is airway management and seizure suppression with benzodiazepines. Propofol should be avoided in patients having signs of cardiovascular instability. It is possible that ACLS will be instituted and it will require adjustment of medications and perhaps prolonged effort. ASRA guidelines recommend avoiding vasopressin, calcium channel blockers, beta-blockers, and any further local anesthetic. In addition, reducing epinephrine doses to <1 mcg/kg is important as well as lipid emulsion (20%) therapy. Cardiac arrest due to local anesthetic toxicity is a rare but well-recognized complication that must be recognized.

Lidocaine

Lidocaine was introduced in 1948 by the Swedish company Astra, and it remains one of the most versatile and widely used local anesthetics on the market today. It is a Class 1b anti-arrhythmic and prototype of the amide local anesthetics. It is commonly used topically, in peripheral nerve blocks, epidural injections, and rarely intravenously. Topical drug delivery is an attractive alternative to other intravenous or oral as it generally allows a lower total systemic daily dose, local delivery, avoidance of first-pass metabolism, major drug interactions, and systemic side effects. Topical lidocaine comes in creams, ointments, and patches. It not only inhibits sodium channels but also has various effects on acid-sensing ion channels (ASIC), potassium and calcium channels, glutamate, γ-aminobutyric acid, glycine, and vanilloid receptors. Hepatic oxidative metabolism of lidocaine is carried out by CYP1A2 and CYP3A4 enzymes, and then metabolites are renally excreted. Lidocaine can be used in almost any peripheral nerve block in which anesthesia of intermediate duration is needed.

Bupivacaine

Since its introduction in 1963, bupivacaine has been one of the most commonly used local anesthetics. Its structure is similar to that of lidocaine, except that the amine-containing group is a butylpiperidine. Bupivacaine is also used in topical compounded creams, peripheral nerve blocks, epidurals, and intrathecal pumps. It is used in intrathecal pumps over lidocaine as it causes less motor blockade. Bupivacaine is metabolized in the liver via conjugation with glucuronic acid and is renally excreted. However, it is substantially more cardiotoxic than lidocaine; hence the IV route is not used. The cardiotoxicity of bupivacaine is cumulative and substantially greater than would be predicted by its potency. Bupivacaine-induced cardiotoxicity can be difficult to treat. Because of its toxicity profile, bupivacaine in large dosages should be avoided.

Oral Anti-arrthymic

Mexiletine

Case reports from the 1950s and 1960s suggested that intravenous lidocaine could provide pain relief in patients with postoperative pain and cancer pain. Subsequent reports in the 1980s suggested a similar benefit for mexiletine, which is a structural oral analogue of lidocaine. Mexiletine is a class 1b anti-arrhythmic agent and is administered orally with 90% bioavailability. The peak effect takes place in 1.5–4 hours, and it is 90% metabolized in the liver by CYP2D6 and less so by CYP1A2. Mexiletine has been used in the treatment of peripheral neuropathy after nerve injury, diabetic neuropathic pain, cancer-related neuropathic pain, phantom limb pain, complex regional pain syndromes, spinal cord injury, trigeminal neuralgia, and fibromyalgia. In the few studies completed, mexiletine doses ranged from 400 to 1200 mg per day, and the mean plasma level was 0.76 mg/ml in this dosing range. Gastrointestinal complaints, of which nausea was the most frequent, were the most common adverse events. Serious cardiac arrhythmias have not been reported in patients receiving mexiletine for painful diabetic neuropathy; however, transient tachycardia and palpitations have been reported. Mexiletine is contraindicated in patients with heart block and uncompensated heart failure. There are many drug interactions related to mexiletine. It inhibits CYP2D6-mediated metabolism of common medications such as metoprolol and others metabolized by cytochrome CYP1A2. Clearance of mexiletine is impaired in patients with hepatic dysfunction. Hence, dosage adjustments are necessary in patients with liver disease. Mexiletine can be an alternative agent for the treatment for neuropathic pain in carefully selected patients. However, safety data are limited because most studies were of relatively short duration and have a small number of patients. Finally, there are no well-controlled clinical trials completed to date.

Anticonvulsants

Carbamazepine

Carbamazepine is effective in neuropathic pain states due to its sodium channel blocking action, which is blocking high-frequency action potential neuronal firing. Its complete mode of action is not fully understood. Pain relief is believed to be associated with blockade of synaptic transmission in the trigeminal nucleus. Carbamazepine also has anticholinergic, central antidiuretic, anti-arrhythmic, muscle relaxant, antidepressant (possibly through blockade of norepinephrine release), sedative, and neuromuscular-blocking properties. It is the only FDA-approved medication for trigeminal neuralgia, and the response to carbamazepine is variable. In general, pain control can be maintained in most patients with 400–800 mg daily; however, as little as 200 mg up to 1200 mg daily have been effective. The CYP3A4 enzyme is the primary isoform responsible for the formation of its active metabolite, which is equipotent to carbamazepine with regard to its anticonvulsant activity. About 70% of the drug is excreted in the urine while the rest is in the feces. Due to CYP3A4 metabolism, the potential exists for interaction between carbamazepine and any agent that induces CYP3A4. Serious adverse side effects with carbamazepine include Stevens-Johnson syndrome, toxic epidermal necrolysis, aplastic anemia, and agranulocytosis. Retrospective case-control studies have found that patients with Chinese ancestry have a ten times higher risk of developing these serious skin rashes with carbamazepine treatment. In addition, this will occur in the first few months of therapy in 90% of patients. It is recommended to get baseline hematological lab work and monitor throughout treatment.

Oxcarbazepine

Oxcarbazepine is a structure derivative of carbamazepine, and it was made to reduce the impact on hepatic metabolism and prevent serious forms of anemia occasionally associated with carbamazepine. It is thought to have the same mechanism as carbamazepine, sodium channel antagonism; however, the exact mechanism is unknown. In research trials, oxcarbazepine is gradually increased from 300 mg to 2400 mg daily over 3 weeks and kept on for only 3 weeks. It is completely absorbed following oral administration. Oxcarbazepine is then extensively metabolized to its pharmacologically active 10-monohydroxy metabolite, which is further metabolized by conjugation with glucuronic acid. Oxcarbazepine is cleared from the body mostly in the form of metabolites which are predominantly excreted by the kidneys. At high dosages, oxcarbazepine can inhibit CYP2C19 and induce CYP3A4 and CYP3A5 with potentially important effects on plasma concentrations of other drugs in vitro. The clinical significance of this is unknown.

Lacosamide

Approved by the FDA in 2008 as an adjunctive treatment for partial onset seizures, lacosamide has dual mechanisms of action that may be useful in neuropathic pain. Lacosamide selectively enhances slow inactivation of sodium channels without any effect on fast inactivation. It also modulates the collapsin response mediator protein-2 (CRMP-2), which is part of neuronal signal transduction pathways mediating neuron plasticity. Lacosamide is a CYP2C19 substrate, and any other isoform contribution is unknown. Its metabolite has no known pharmacological activity and is renally excreted.

Phenytoin

Phenytoin is structurally related to barbiturates and FDA approved for a wide variety of seizures but has anti-arrhythmic and muscle relaxant properties. The mechanism of action is not clear, although several cellular actions have been described including effects on sodium channels, active transport, and neuronal membrane stabilization. Phenytoin has been proposed for several other therapeutic uses such as mood disorders and neuropathic pain, but its use is limited by adverse effects and interactions with other drugs. Phenytoin is primarily metabolized by CYP2C9. Most of the drug is excreted in the bile as inactive metabolites which are then reabsorbed from the intestinal tract and excreted in the urine.

Topiramate

Topiramate is a sulfamate that inhibits voltage-dependent sodium channels and non-NMDA glutamate receptors. Topiramate is FDA approved and prescribed for migraine prevention at dosages of 200–600 mg daily. Topiramate acts through inhibiting sodium channels and has been shown to be effective at reducing the frequency of migraine attacks. However, it acts on other targets as well, and therefore the therapeutic effect may be unrelated to sodium channel antagonism. Topiramate is rapidly absorbed, with a high bioavailability, and is not extensively metabolized. It is primarily eliminated unchanged in the urine.

Valproic Acid

Valproate is effective in reducing headache frequency and is reasonably well tolerated in adult patients with episodic migraine. It was FDA approved for this indication in 2008. Valproic acid dissociates to the valproate ion in the gastrointestinal tract and then binds to and inhibits GABA transaminase. Its anticonvulsant activity may be related to increased brain concentrations of gamma-aminobutyric acid by inhibiting enzymes that catabolize it or block its reuptake into glia and nerve endings. Valproic acid may also work by suppressing repetitive neuronal firing through inhibition of voltage-sensitive sodium channels. It is also been shown to be an inhibitor of an enzyme called histone deacetylase 1 (HDAC1), which is needed for HIV to remain in infected cells. A study published in August 2005 revealed that patients treated with valproic acid in addition to highly active antiretroviral therapy (HAART) showed a 75% reduction in latent HIV infection. It has a high oral bioavailability and is metabolized almost entirely by the liver. Due to its complex mechanisms, it's difficult to know how much sodium antagonism plays a role in migraine prevention.

Lamotrigine, Eslicarbazepine, and Rufinamide

All three are FDA approved for epilepsy; however, the mechanisms of action are still unclear. Lamotrigine has shown binding to sodium channels similar to local anesthetics. For rufinamide, in vitro studies suggest sodium channel modulation as it appears to prolong the inactive state of Na_v by slowing the recovery of these channels from inactivation. Eslicarbazepine is structurally related to carbamazepine and oxcarbazepine but with a more favorable metabolic profile. Whether these medications will be used for neuropathic pain in the future is unknown, and research is ongoing.

Evidence for Efficacy

Lidocaine and bupivacaine have a well-established role in regional anesthesia for peripheral nerve blocks and epidurals. There are other routes used for local anesthetics and other oral sodium channel antagonists which are widely used for various pain conditions; however, most trials evaluated and focused on postherpetic neuralgia or painful diabetic neuropathies. It is unknown if the results of these studies can be extrapolated to other neuropathic pain conditions. Long-term benefits and risks are unknown as the published studies looked at individuals for 3 months or less. Previous research trial methodology and outcome reporting have now changed over time, with more recent studies having more comprehensive protocols. The limitations of existing research for these medications and the pain states they are used to treat cannot be understated. Providers should always assess potential adverse outcomes or side effects, drug interactions, lab abnormalities, comorbidities, costs, abuse risk, and risk of unintentional overdose. Each individual's response will vary and is unpredictable.

Every few years the International Association for the Study of Pain has a neuropathic pain interest group (NeuPSIP) that publishes systematic reviews and guidelines for the pharmacological treatment of neuropathic pain. This interest group has only reviewed randomized double-blind studies, unpublished trials from clinicaltrials.gov, and pharmaceutical websites for oral and topical pharmacotherapy. The group has excluded the following routes of drug administration: IM, IV, epidural, and IT. All of these routes are used in many clinical situations, but literature on intrathecal bupivacaine is limited to small case studies, small retrospective studies, and anecdotal reports. The only first-line agent that is also a sodium channel blocker is topical lidocaine transdermal patches.

Topical lidocaine 5% transdermal patches were FDA approved in 1999 for postherpetic neuralgia. Topical lidocaine is preferred due to its lack of systemic side effects and favorable therapeutic index. Efficacy in placebo-controlled, small RTCs has been shown in patients with allodynia due to various neuropathic pain conditions and postherpetic neuralgia. There is one multicenter, noninferiority study that compared lidocaine 5% patch to standard of care pregabalin for patients with postherpetic neuralgia or painful diabetic neuropathy. Noninferiority was not found for lidocaine patches at the 4-week end point, and there was a higher response rate in patients with postherpetic neuralgia. The paucity of double-blind RTCs evaluating topical lidocaine for treatment of peripheral neuropathic pain was illustrated in a Cochrane review in 2014. They noted that all evidence was of very low quality but that there was some indication lidocaine is beneficial. It is recommended as first line mostly due to its tolerability and safety compared to other treatment options.

The clinical use of systemic (IV) lidocaine was introduced in 1961 for postoperative acute pain control, but its use is complicated by its cardiac and central nervous system side effects. Published studies since 1982 on intravenous lidocaine have shown it to be effective in reducing peripheral and central neuropathic pain, including thalamic pain, trigeminal neuralgia, and phantom limb pain. In a study by Boas in 1982, IV lidocaine dosed at 3 mg/kg over 3 minutes followed by a continuous infusion of 4 mg/kg for 60 minutes relieved central pain but did not provide any beneficial effect on peripherally induced nociception. Similar results were reported in a review of 211 chronic pain cases in which a bolus dose of lidocaine was given with or without continuous infusion by Edwards in 1985. Ferrante gave subjects with neuropathic pain lidocaine IV 500 mg at a rate of 8.35 mg/min for 60 minutes in order to determine a dose-response and plasma concentration-response relationship. He found that the lidocaine infusion resulted in complete pain relief in 10 out of 13 patients. Small changes in the lidocaine dose caused a significant reduction in pain scores once the plasma lidocaine concentration reached 0.62 mg/ml. In a randomized, double-blind, placebo, crossover study of IV lidocaine, a dosage of 5 mg/kg over 30 minutes reduced diabetic neuropathic pain symptoms for up to 3 weeks (Bath 1990). Later in a 1991 Rowbotham study, the IV lidocaine dose was targeted to 5 mg/kg (maximal 450 mg), and this significantly decreased postherpetic neuralgia pain scores compared to saline controls. Interestingly, subcutaneous 10% lidocaine also has been shown to be effective in treating neuropathic pain in cancer patients who failed to respond to opioids. In successful cases, the plasma concentration of subcutaneous lidocaine was comparable to that of lidocaine infusion. It is possible that it is the plasma level of lidocaine rather than the route of administration that determines the effectiveness of systemic lidocaine. A 2005 meta-analysis done by Tremont-Lukats analyzed randomized double-blind controlled trials from 1987 to 2002. They felt that lidocaine IV was superior to placebo in chronic neuropathic pain. However the studies analyzed had a variation of lidocaine doses and durations, each trial had 30 patients or less, and there was a large heterogeneity in diagnoses. From the current data published, there seems to be an effective dose range of systemic lidocaine (1.5 ± 5.0 mg/kg) and effective plasma level (0.62–5.0 ug/ml), but it's unclear if the same dose is comparable among different neuropathic pain conditions.

Unfortunately, lidocaine infusions rarely provide pain relief that persists beyond the duration of the infusion (at most 3–4 weeks has been reported), and it cannot be used continuously long term in its current IV form. Diagnostically, systemic lidocaine may help establish the presence of neuropathic pain and responsiveness to oral sodium channel antagonism. However, the data supporting diagnostic infusions remain sparse. Intravenous infusion of all local anesthetics for the treatment of chronic pain, including, but not limited to, chronic neuropathic pain and fibromyalgia, is considered investigational at this time.

All types of pharmacotherapy for neuropathic pain in adults were reviewed in a 2015 meta-analysis published in *The Lancet*. Finnerup et al. analyzed 229 published studies, and the primary outcomes were one of the two: greater than 30% pain relief and/or the numbers needed to treat (NNT) of 50% pain relief. They also assessed publication bias, which was estimated that there is a 10% overstatement of treatment effects. Trial outcomes were generally modest even for effective drugs, and they noted the NNT was undetermined for lidocaine patches, which also had low-quality evidence. The data for drug combinations, anti-epileptics, and topical drugs were inconclusive. For the medications analyzed, the reported impression was that there is limited efficacy, large placebo responses, inadequate diagnostic criteria, and poor phenotypic profiling that probably account for modest trial outcomes. Most studies using anti-epileptic drugs (carbamazepine, topiramate, oxcarbazepine) were negative for efficacy of pain relief, and they have the lowest safety profile.

A majority of reviews and guidelines note that anti-epileptic medications used for neuropathic pain and mexiletine have shown mixed results in single random controlled trials or inconsistent results in multiple random controlled trials for neuropathic pain conditions. The most commonly studied neuropathic pain conditions with anti-epileptics are painful DNP, PHN, and HIV neuropathy. The most common off-label use is for diagnoses such as neuropathic pain, back pain, cancer pain, complex regional pain syndrome, postoperative pain, and lumbar radicular pain.

Mexiletine has been studied in patients with painful diabetic neuropathy and other types of neuropathic pain. The studies show modest to no difference compared to placebo. In addition, it was mostly effective at higher dosages, which is poorly tolerated by patients.

Carbamazepine is first-line therapy for trigeminal neuralgia (TN) as it has established efficacy since the 1960s. The newer oxcarbazepine is probably effective for TN and has a better safety profile. For both of these medications, random control trials (RCTs) for all other neuropathic pain conditions have been inconsistent, but the research methods have been limited. In a recent well done 2008 randomized, double-blind, placebo-controlled, multicenter trial, Silberstein et al. explored the efficacy, safety, and tolerability of oxcarbazepine at 1200 mg/day versus placebo for the prevention of migraine. There was no statistically significant difference in pain relief between oxcarbazepine and the placebo group. Another important 2014 RTC, double-blind, placebo-controlled study found that the effect of oxcarbazepine in peripheral neuropathic pain depends on pain phenotype determined by detailed quantitative sensory testing. This finding underscores how little is known about these agents and the pain pathology they treat.

Lacosamide has been studied for painful diabetic neuropathy but was not FDA approved for this condition due to unknown reasons. A 2012 Cochrane review on lacosamide for neuropathic pain and fibromyalgia included five studies on painful diabetic neuropathy and one on fibromyalgia. Lacosamide was concluded to have limited efficacy in painful DN and an unclear benefit in fibromyalgia. Similar conclusions of lack of efficacy for pain have been made on valproic acid and phenytoin for neuropathic pain. For valproic acid, there are three positive trials in painful DPN reported by a single center and one negative RCT for painful polyneuropathies by a separate group. While Phenytoin has been studied, there appears to be no good-quality studies to date. Topiramate is mostly used for migraine prevention, and study results for other neuropathic pain conditions, such as radiculopathy and painful DPN, have been negative or shown no difference with placebo for pain relief.

Conclusion

Voltage sodium channel antagonists are clinically useful for treating pain, but they often provide only partial relief, and adverse effects can limit their use. Electrophysiological and pharmacological studies have revealed that specific sodium channel subtypes particularly $Na_v1.3$, $Na_v1.7$, $Na_v1.8$, and $Na_v1.9$ are predominantly expressed and involved in the peripheral nociceptive neurons. In the future, it should be possible to develop specific sodium channel blockers with lower toxicity and enhanced efficacy for treating neuropathic pain.

Pearls and Pitfalls

- Nav1.3, Nav1.7, Nav1.8, and Nav1.9 play key roles in neurobiology of pain.
- All current sodium channel antagonist medications are nonselective.
- The higher the LA concentration, the more potent but no change in duration of action.
- The more lipid soluble an LA is, the more potent and longer duration of action.
- Mixing local anesthetics makes characteristics of each LA unpredictable – if long duration is desired, use long acting alone.
- Always check drug interactions for AEDs and Mexiletine.

Recommended Reading

1. Akopian AN, et al. A tetrodotoxin-resistant voltage-gated sodium channel expressed by sensory neurons. Nature. 1996;379:257–62.
2. Akopian AN, Souslova V, England S, Okuse K, Ogata N, Ure J, et al. The tetrodotoxin resistant sodium channel SNS has a specialized function in pain pathways. Nat Neurosci. 1999;2:541–8.
3. Cao L, Nitzsche N, McDonnell A, Alexandrou A, Saintot P-P, Loucif AJC, Brown AR, Young G, Mis M, Randall A, Waxman SG, Stanley P, Kirby S, Tarabar S, Gutteridge A, Butt R, McKernan RM, Whiting R, Ali Z, Bilsland J, Stevens EB. Pharmacological reversal of pain phenotype in iPSC-derived sensory neurons and human subjects with inherited erythromelalgia. Sci Transl Med. 2016;8(335):335ra56. PMID: 27099175 (first demonstration of proof-of-principle that Nav1.7 blocker can attenuate pain in humans).
4. Cummins TR, Waxman SG. Down regulation of tetrodotoxin-resistant sodium currents and up-regulation of a rapidly repriming tetrodotoxin-sensitive sodium current in small spinal sensory neurons after nerve injury. iJ Neurosci. 1997;17:3503–14.
5. Cummins TR, Dib-Hajj SD, Black JA, Akopian AN, Wood JN, Waxman SG. A novel persistent tetrodotoxin-resistant sodium current in small primary sensory neurons. J Neurosci. 1999;19:RC43.
6. de León-Casasola OA, Mayoral V. The topical 5% lidocaine medicated plaster in localized neuropathic pain: a reappraisal of the clinical evidence. J Pain Res. 2016;12(9):67–79. https://doi.org/10.2147/JPR.S99231. eCollection 2016.
7. Devor M. Sodium channels and mechanisms of neuropathic pain. J Pain. 2006;7(Suppl 1):S3–S12.
8. Dib-Hajj SD, Cummins TR, Black JA, Waxman SG. Sodium channels in normal and pathological pain. Ann Rev Neurosci. 2010;33:325–47. PMID: 20367448 (Overview of Na channels in pain).
9. Dib-Hajj SD, Yang Y, Black JA, Waxman SG. The NaV1.7 sodium channel: from molecule to man. Nat Rev Neurosci. 2013;14(1):49–62. PMID: 23232607 (the most complete review on Nav1.7 and pain).
10. Dib-Hajj SD, Black JA, Waxman SG. NaV1.9: a sodium channel linked to human pain. Nat Rev Neurosci. 2015;16:511–9. PMID 26243570 (the most complete review on Nav1.9 and pain).
11. Faber CG, Lauria G, Merkies ISJ, Cheng X, Han C, Ahn H-S, Persson A-K, Hoeijmakers JGJ, Gerrits MM, Pierro T, Lombardi R, Kapetis D, Dib-Hajj SD, Waxman SG. Gain-of-function $Na_V1.8$ mutations in painful neuropathy. Proc Natl Acad Sci. 2012;109:19444–9. PMID: 23115331.
12. Finnerup NB, et al. Pharmacotherapy for neuropathic pain in adults: a systematic review and meta-analysis. Lancet Neurol. 2015;14(2):162–73.
13. Geha P, Yang Y, Estacion M, Schulman BR, Tokuno H, Apkarian AV, Dib-Hajj SD, Waxman SG. Pharmacotherapy for pain in a family with inherited erythromelalgia guided by genomic analysis and functional profiling. JAMA Neurol. 2016;73(6):659–767. https://doi.org/10.1001/jamaneurol.2016.0389. PMID: 27088781. (first study using pharmacogenomics to treat patients in a personalized, "precidion": manner with a Na channel blocker).
14. Han C, Huang J, Waxman SG. Sodium channel $Na_V1.8$: emerging links to human disease. Neurology. 2016;86:473–83. PMID 26747884.
15. Levinson SR, et al. The role of sodium channels in chronic pain. Muscle Nerve. 2012;46(2):155–65.
16. Mao J, Chen LL. Systemic lidocaine for neuropathic pain relief. Pain. 2000;87(1):7–17.
17. Rogawski MA, Loscher W. The neurobiology of antiepileptic drugs for the treatment of nonepileptic conditions. Nat Med. 2004;10(7):685–92.
18. Sidhu HS, Sadhotra A. Current status of the new antiepileptic drugs in chronic pain. Front Pharmacol. 2016;7:276. https://doi.org/10.3389/fphar.2016.00276. Published online 2016 Aug 25. PMCID: PMC4996999.
19. Sommer C, Cruccu G. Topical treatment of peripheral neuropathic pain: applying the evidence. J Pain Symptom Manag. 2017;53:614–29.
20. Tan A, Samad O, Dib-Hajj SD, Waxman SG. Virus-mediated knockdown of Nav1.3 in dorsal root ganglia of STZ-induced diabetic rats alleviates tactile allodynia. Mol Med. 2015;21:544–52. PMID 26101954.
21. Tremont-Lukats IW, Challapalli V, McNicol ED, et al. Systemic administration of local anesthetics to relieve neuropathic pain: a systematic review and meta-analysis. Anesth Analg. 2005;101:1738–49.
22. Wood JN, et al. Voltage-gated sodium channels and pain pathways. J Neurobiol. 2004;61(1):55–71.

Antispasmodics and Muscle Relaxants

22

Katherine D. Travnicek

Introduction

Musculoskeletal pain is a common clinical complaint in the healthcare setting. The pathophysiology of musculoskeletal pain is not well understood, and possible causes include inflammation, tissue break down, fibrosis, and abnormal neurotransmitter levels. It has been shown that substance P and calcitonin-related peptide can be elevated in injured tissue, the dorsal root ganglia, and the spinal cord dorsal horn, which then can lead to centralization of pain from peripheral nociceptor sensitization. Low back pain is the most common example of chronic musculoskeletal pain. In the United States, acute low back pain is the second most common cause for physician visits, and low back pain with or without radiculopathy is the leading cause of years lived with disability. Approximately 50% of working-age adults report having symptoms, and low back pain has been reported to affect 80–85% of the population over their lifetime. The economic burden of musculoskeletal pain is second only to that of cardiovascular disease with total medical costs for low back pain alone totaling more than $100 billion yearly. Two-thirds of these costs are indirect and attributable to lost wages and reduced productivity. The exact etiology of acute low back pain can be difficult to define. In addition, there is little data showing how many patients recover fully, experience recurrent pain, or progress to chronic low back pain. It is estimated that up to 20% of cases will develop chronic low back pain, which is responsible for high treatment costs, sick leave, and individual suffering.

The initial management of acute low back pain is conservative and multimodal including modalities (heat, ice, TENs unit), physical therapy with an exercise program (aerobic, strengthening, and stretching), medications, education in reducing or modifying workload, and stress management if needed. In general, prolonged bed rest should be discouraged as this can cause further deconditioning and exacerbate the symptoms long term. Treatment should focus on managing the patient's discomfort by reducing their pain and associated symptoms with pharmacologic options such as anti-inflammatory medications and muscle relaxants. Skeletal muscle relaxants are frequently prescribed to decrease muscle spasms associated with back pain. "Muscle relaxant" is a broad term that encompasses a class of medications that can decrease muscle excitability and pain, possibly improving disability and function. The goal of pharmacologic treatment is to reduce bothersome symptoms and encourage patients to return to their normal daily activities. In addition to acetaminophen and anti-inflammatory medications, skeletal muscle relaxants are prescribed frequently. In 2004 Dillon et al. found that approximately two million US adults used skeletal muscle relaxants using data from the third National Health and Nutrition Examination Survey, which captures information from 1988 to 1994. He also showed that 44.5% took muscle relaxants for more than 1 year. This finding is concerning because clinical efficacy is lacking past the acute period and has not been studied in chronic pain.

Background and Historical Perspective

Currently, no clinical practice guidelines recommend the use of muscle relaxants as the first-line treatment for musculoskeletal pain. In 1994, the Agency for Health Care Policy and Research (AHCPR) published guidelines with the recommendation for the use of acetaminophen as a first-line treatment. Nonsteroidal anti-inflammatory drugs (NSAIDs) were less preferred than acetaminophen as these may cause significant adverse effects such as gastrointestinal ulceration and renal impairment. The AHCPR panel also evaluated the use of cyclobenzaprine and did not recommend the use of skeletal muscle relaxants due to limited efficacy in comparison to NSAIDs. Furthermore, muscle relaxants are commonly associated with drowsiness and sedation.

K. D. Travnicek (✉)
Pain Institute of Nevada, Las Vegas, NV, USA
e-mail: kdt@paininstitute.com

T. R. Deer et al. (eds.), *Deer's Treatment of Pain*, https://doi.org/10.1007/978-3-030-12281-2_22

In 2007, a joint clinical practice guideline published by the American College of Physicians and the American Pain Society recommended acetaminophen and nonsteroidal anti-inflammatories as the first-line treatment, while reserving skeletal muscle relaxants as adjunct or alternative therapy after the first-line therapies have failed. These guidelines were then updated in 2017 as new evidence and medications became available. Chou et al. evaluated new randomized trials that compared placebo or another treatment to specific outcomes such as pain reduction, change in function, or adverse effects of muscle relaxants. Skeletal muscle relaxants give small to moderate pain reductions in acute low back pain in the short term. The functional outcomes were even less substantial, and these medications cause drowsiness and dizziness in comparison to placebo.

Based on current literature, muscle relaxants appear to have a favorable role in short-term use for acute management of low back pain; however the effectiveness is unclear for chronic low back pain. The role of skeletal muscle relaxants in managing low back pain remains controversial, and major adverse effects associated with muscle relaxants should be considered before initiating these medications.

There are two settings in which skeletal muscle relaxants can be utilized as pharmacologic treatments – spasticity and musculoskeletal pain conditions. The main distinction is that muscle relaxants as a group can either be anti-spasticity or antispasmodic agents. The primary goal of using anti-spasticity agents is to decrease spasticity, whereas the goal of antispasmodic agents is to reduce musculoskeletal pain and spasms.

Spasticity is an involuntary, velocity-dependent increase in muscle tone that causes resistance to movement. Spasticity is the result of dysfunction within the central nervous system, producing an upper motor neuron syndrome that is associated with an elevated reflex activity and hypertonia. Spasticity is most commonly associated with stroke, traumatic brain injury, spinal cord injury, multiple sclerosis, and cerebral palsy. In the United States, the Food and Drug Administration (FDA) has approved three skeletal muscle relaxants for the treatment of spasticity-related disorders, and they include baclofen, dantrolene, and tizanidine.

Musculoskeletal conditions, on the other hand, are ubiquitous and can comprise of a myriad of common complaints such as neck pain, back pain, shoulder, hip, and extremity pain. Musculoskeletal pain affects the muscles, ligaments, tendons, and bones. This pain is caused by overuse injuries, poor ergonomics, and trauma such as car accidents or falls. Muscle spasms are a common symptom of these injuries.

Muscle spasms can cause persistent and painful activation of muscle groups, which are typically localized to an area and can result in chronic pain. Several psychogenic factors such as anxiety and stress can further exacerbate these symptoms. It has been proposed that muscle spasms can perpetuate a cycle of spasm-pain-spasm, in which muscle spasms worsen the pain by stimulating nociceptive receptors in peripheral tissues. Thus, skeletal muscle relaxants could counteract the additional muscle spasms and interrupt this cycle. Muscle relaxants have the possibility of improving range of motion and subsequently improving function. Most skeletal muscle relaxants depress the central nervous system and do not act directly on muscles or synaptic pathways. In animal model research, it is believed that these agents display a muscle relaxation effect by exerting an inhibitory response on brain's descending reticular formation as well as the polysynaptic neurons of the spinal cord. In humans, it is unclear if improvements in pain symptoms with skeletal muscle relaxants are related to muscle relaxation or the sedative effect from CNS depression.

While there is some overlap in clinical usage of muscle relaxants, each can be used for either spasticity or musculoskeletal pain conditions. In the United States, carisoprodol, chlorzoxazone, cyclobenzaprine, metaxalone, methocarbamol, and orphenadrine have been approved by the US Food and Drug Administration (FDA) for the treatment of acute musculoskeletal conditions. Other muscle relaxants, such as baclofen, tizanidine, and dantrolene, are FDA approved for spasticity. Oral baclofen and tizanidine are prescribed by clinicians for low back pain, despite the lack of approved indication by the FDA. Additionally, benzodiazepines, such as diazepam, are frequently utilized for musculoskeletal conditions. While all of these agents may be prescribed for the acute phase of low back pain, none of them have been studied for chronic low back pain.

Uses and Indications

Carisoprodol

Carisoprodol was approved by the Food and Drug Administration (FDA) in 1959 for the short-term management of acute, painful musculoskeletal conditions in adult as an adjunctive treatment to the standard regimen of rest and physical therapy. It is a central nervous system depressant and does not directly interact with human skeletal muscle. It is metabolized in the liver by cytochrome P450 2C19 with onset of action within 30 minutes, and the duration of action is 4–6 hours. Once metabolized, carisoprodol is converted to hydroxycarisoprodol, hydroxymeprobamate, and meprobamate, and these metabolites are all excreted by the kidney (see Fig. 22.1 and Table 22.1).

Meprobamate specifically modulates and activates gamma-aminobutyric acid A ($GABA_A$) receptors. Due to this, it is a schedule IV controlled substance of the Controlled Substances Act (CSA) with a well-established abuse potential similar to benzodiazepines. Carisoprodol usage can

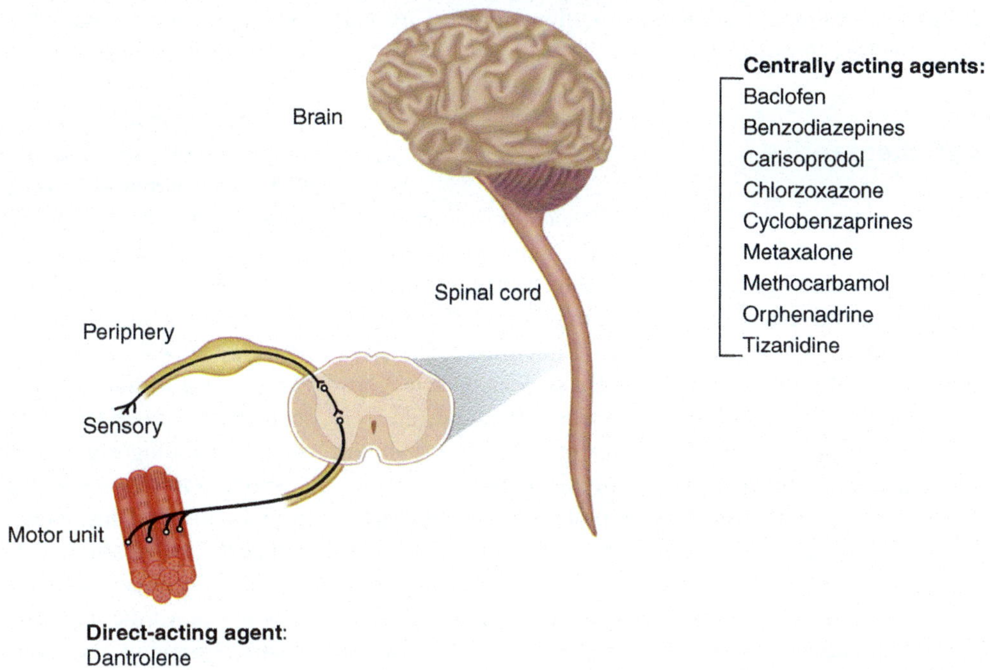

Fig. 22.1 Skeletal muscle relaxants and site of action

Table 22.1 Skeletal muscle relaxants: mechanism of action

	Classification	Medications
Centrally acting agents	Anticholinergic and antihistamine	Orphenadrine
	CNS depressants	Carisoprodol Chlorzoxazone Metaxalone Methocarbamol
	Centrally acting α_2-adrenergic agonist	Tizanidine
	Gamma-aminobutyric acid (GABA) agonists	Baclofen Benzodiazepines
	Tricyclic antidepressants	Cyclobenzaprine
Direct-acting agents	Postsynaptic muscle relaxant	Dantrolene

result in physical and psychological dependence. Furthermore, it has a narrow therapeutic window with common adverse effects including drowsiness, dizziness, and headache. More severe adverse effects can occur such as tachycardia, hypotension, respiratory depression, increased muscle tone, sedation, coma, and even death.

When taken in higher than therapeutic dosages, there is an increased risk of developing hallucinations, euphoria, and irritability. This can create significant abuse potential as carisoprodol could be utilized to produce psychotropic effects or enhance illicit drugs. In 2008, carisoprodol was 1 of the top 25 drugs frequently associated with drug abuse cases in the United States. Due to increasing rates of intoxication, carisoprodol was withdrawn from Norway and the European Union in 2008. According to the 2012 National Survey on Drug Use and Health, over three million people in the United States have reported recreational use of Soma at some point in their lives. Effective on January 11, 2012, carisoprodol became classified as a schedule IV controlled substance. Finally, if patients on large doses of carisoprodol abruptly stop, they can suffer from withdrawal symptoms such as anxiety, tremors, and seizures. This medication should be slowly tapered, which can take days to weeks.

Chlorzoxazone

Chlorzoxazone came onto the market in 1958, and while the exact mechanism of action is unclear, it is believed that it inhibits multiple synaptic reflex arcs in the spinal cord and subcortical areas of the brain, resulting in decreased muscle spasms and sedative effects. Chlorzoxazone is metabolized in the liver by cytochrome P450 2E1 with onset of action within 1 hour, and the duration of action is 3–5 hours. It is excreted by the kidneys and does not appear to have significant drug-drug interactions. As with other muscle relaxants, the most common adverse effects include drowsiness and dizziness. In patients with concomitant chronic alcohol abuse or cardiovascular disease, there is a rare risk of hepatocellular toxicity. Patients with hepatic impairment need serial monitoring of liver enzymes. Patients may also experience sensitivity such as pruritis, angioedema, and erythema. The majority of chlorzoxazone research shows inadequate evidence for efficacy. However, these studies were conducted prior to 1980 with very small sample sizes and poor scientific quality. Overall, the role of chlorzoxazone in the management of acute musculoskeletal conditions remains unclear given the lack of proven efficacy.

Cyclobenzaprine

Cyclobenzaprine was initially marketed for human use in 1977 and is widely prescribed for the treatment of muscle spasms and acute musculoskeletal pain. It is FDA indicated as an adjunct to rest and physical therapy for relief of muscle spasms associated with acute, painful musculoskeletal conditions. It is also the most well-studied skeletal muscle relaxant agent in terms of efficacy and adverse effect profile.

Cyclobenzaprine is a tricyclic agent that differs from the antidepressant amitriptyline by only a single double bond. Cyclobenzaprine has very limited potency as an antidepressant and has better muscle-relaxing properties. Similar to other muscle relaxants, it does not directly affect the muscle fibers. The mechanism of action has been largely studied in animal models, and it is believed cyclobenzaprine exerts an effect on the central nervous system while sparing the neuromuscular junctions and skeletal muscle. Cyclobenzaprine appears to act first on brainstem functions, followed by the spinal cord interneurons involved in muscle reflex, and then eventually decreases in muscle tone and spasms. It also augments norepinephrine and antihistamine receptors. It has been proposed that cyclobenzaprine acts on both α motor and γ motor pathways on the descending noradrenergic neurons. Furthermore, it appears to inhibit serotonergic pathways since it is also a 5-HT_2 receptor antagonist.

Some studies indicate cyclobenzaprine given as 10 mg three times daily provides superiority over placebo for the improvement of muscle spasms and pain. However, there is an increased incidence in adverse effects associated with this dosing schedule, and 5 mg dose may be effective for acute musculoskeletal conditions and with less sedation. Cyclobenzaprine is metabolized by the cytochrome P450 system, mainly the PA2, 2D6, and CYP3A4 isoforms, and excreted by the kidney and by the GI tract. The onset of action is less than 1 hour with duration of action for 12–24 hours.

Due to its resemblance to TCAs, cyclobenzaprine has anticholinergic properties and can produce undesired adverse effects such as tachycardia, dysrhythmias, drowsiness, dizziness, dry mouth, nausea, and hypotension. Risk of adverse effects increases with higher (more than 5 mg) or more frequent dosing. Cyclobenzaprine should be avoided in hepatic insufficiency, congestive heart failure, recent myocardial infarction, and acute glaucoma. It should be used with caution in the elderly due to the increased risk of confusion and hallucinations.

Furthermore, there is a possible increased risk of seizure with concomitant tramadol use. Infrequently, serotonin syndrome has been observed with concurrent cyclobenzaprine usage in patients who are receiving pro-serotoninergic medications (monoamine oxidase inhibitors, MAOI; selective serotonin reuptake inhibitors, SSRI). Due to this potential risk of serotonin syndrome, cyclobenzaprine should not be prescribed if the patient is taking concomitant MAOIs or has taken an MAOI within the last 14 days.

Doses of 20–80 mg have been reported for recreational use due to the mood-altering properties, but cyclobenzaprine does not appear to have significant abuse potential despite its widespread availability. Although fatal overdoses of cyclobenzaprine have been published, fatalities are usually associated with co-ingestion of other drugs. In the case of 400 pure cyclobenzaprine ingestions, there were no deaths. Clinical toxicity often manifests in anticholinergic activities, such as agitation, tachycardia, and QT prolongation. In general, no serious side effects were observed with ingestion of less than 100 mg at a time. Otherwise, supportive strategies such as gastric emptying, mechanical ventilation, fluids, and physostigmine can be utilized for suspected cases of significant cyclobenzaprine ingestion.

Metaxalone

Metaxalone was approved by the FDA in 1964 for the relief of muscle pain and spasms associated with acute, painful musculoskeletal conditions. It is another centrally acting muscle relaxant agent that does not exert direct effect on skeletal muscles. The exact mechanism of action has not been established in humans, but most likely it causes central nervous depression. One advantage of metaxalone is that it generally has less sedating properties than the other muscle relaxants. The drug is metabolized in the liver with initial onset within 1 hour, with duration of 4–6 hours, and is excreted in urine. It does not have significant drug-drug interactions.

Metaxalone should be avoided in patients with hepatic or renal impairment. Patients on long-term metaxalone should have serial monitoring of their liver function as impaired liver function can occur, even though this is rare. Most of the adverse side effects are neurological and include dizziness, headache, and drowsiness. Hypersensitivity reactions resulting in jaundice, leukopenia, hemolytic anemia, and rare cases of deaths have been associated with metaxalone overdose. More serious adverse events occurred with moderate effects after ingestion of >2400 mg, and for patients with drug-induced anemia, metaxalone should be avoided. This medication is not associated with abuse potential. A small number of patients reported gastrointestinal upset, including nausea, emesis, as well as nervousness. Interestingly, another potential adverse effect is paradoxical muscle cramps. There are a limited number of studies evaluating the efficacy and safety of metaxalone, which seems to have a limited utility for acute musculoskeletal conditions.

Methocarbamol

Methocarbamol is also a central nervous system depressant with sedative and musculoskeletal relaxant properties. It is a carbamate derivative of guaifenesin with an unclear mechanism of action. Methocarbamol has been available since the 1980s as either oral tablets or parenteral formulation. Several adverse effects have been observed with the intravenous or intramuscular form, such as sloughing of the skin or thrombophlebitis. Although it was designed to be longer acting, the onset of action occurs within the first 30 minutes with duration lasting only 4–6 hours. Methocarbamol is metabolized by dealkylation and hydroxylation in the liver, and essentially all methocarbamol metabolites are eliminated in the urine. As with other muscle relaxants, common adverse effects include dizziness, headache, and drowsiness. There are reports of potential fetal abnormalities; however, this is rare.

There is abuse potential similar to other sedative/hypnotic drugs at higher than therapeutic doses of methocarbamol at 2.25 grams or higher. There is an increased incidence of dysphoria, impaired psychomotor, and cognitive performance. These undesired adverse effects lower the abuse potential of methocarbamol in comparison to benzodiazepines. Overall, there are relatively few well-designed studies to thoroughly evaluate the effectiveness of methocarbamol versus placebo in managing acute musculoskeletal conditions.

Orphenadrine

Orphenadrine is a derivative of diphenhydramine that was developed in the 1940s for the treatment of Parkinson's disease as it is particularly useful for involuntary resting tremors. Additionally, randomized clinical trials have demonstrated orphenadrine's muscle relaxation properties as well as analgesia. There is also evidence of its effectiveness versus placebo in painful musculoskeletal conditions. Orphenadrine is available in either oral or parenteral forms, and it is readily absorbed from the GI tract. Unfortunately, the parenteral formulation carries the risk of severe anaphylactic reactions. The onset of action is less than 1 hour with duration of action for 2–4 hours. This medication targets muscarinic receptors, histaminic receptors, N-methyl-D-aspartate (NMDA) receptors, and the noradrenalin reuptake system. The drug also has mostly anticholinergic with mild antihistamine activity, and it does exhibit local anesthetic properties in animal models. The exact mechanism for its antinociceptive properties remains unknown, but current research indicates that orphenadrine can cause inhibition of voltage-gated sodium channels similar to other local anesthetics. Typical adverse effects at therapeutic level include nausea, headache, drowsiness, dizziness, dry mouth, and urinary retention. There are also rare cases of aplastic anemia reported, and at higher doses, patients may experience tachycardia, skin rash, hallucination, and agitation. Due to its anticholinergic activity, it should be avoided in patients with glaucoma, pyloric or duodenal obstruction, urinary obstruction, enlarged prostate, myasthenia gravis, and in the elderly.

Anti-spasticity Agents

Medications with muscle relaxation properties and that are FDA indicated for spasticity include baclofen, tizanidine, and dantrolene. Spasticity is a common problem in patients with neurological disease and only occurs with central nervous system pathology. It is highly likely that multiple mechanisms are responsible for spasticity, many of which still remain to be fully elucidated. Muscle spasticity often interferes with motor function or causes distressing symptoms, such as painful muscle spasms. If untreated, spasticity may also lead to fixed contractures. However, spasticity can also be beneficial to patients. The best treatment outcomes for spasticity are usually achieved when pharmacological and non-pharmacological treatment modalities are used in tandem.

Baclofen

Baclofen was introduced in 1988 as a first-line treatment of spasticity due to central nervous system disorders such as spinal cord injury and multiple sclerosis. Baclofen is an analog of GABA-type B receptors and inhibits both monosynaptic and polysynaptic reflexes at the spinal cord level to reduce muscle spasticity. This results in systemic muscle relaxation but can also cause sedation and fatigue. The onset time is 2–3 hours with onset duration of 3–4 days. Baclofen is excreted by the kidneys and should be avoided in patients with renal impairment. The oral form is available as either 10 or 20 mg tablets with limited efficacy in lower doses (5 mg) due to inefficient penetration of the blood-brain barrier. Typical dosing for spasticity treatment is up to 80 mg per day in divided daily dosing. Intrathecal baclofen is also available for severe spasticity or intolerance to the oral formulation. Baclofen should not be abruptly stopped due to risk of withdrawal symptoms including seizures, hyperthermia, altered mental status, and death. It should be tapered slowly. Common adverse reactions include headache, weakness, dizziness, drowsiness, and hypotension. Due to its adverse effect profile, it should be avoided in the elderly and patients with renal impairment. It is also used in musculoskeletal pain disorders also at lower dosages.

Tizanidine

Tizanidine arrived on the market in 1997 for the management of spasticity from central nervous system disorders. It is a centrally acting α_2-adrenergic receptor agonist that is closely related to clonidine, although tizanidine's potency in reducing blood pressure is only 1/10th–1/50th of clonidine. Tizanidine is short-acting and metabolized by the liver enzymes CYP450 1A2 with renal excretion. A proposed mechanism for tizanidine is the inhibition of neurotransmitter release with subsequent presynaptic inhibition of spinal motor neurons. There is no direct effect on the skeletal muscle fibers. The onset of action occurs within the first hour with duration lasting 3–6 hours. Given the short onset and duration of action, tizanidine should be utilized for time-dependent activities.

Patients may experience somnolence, hypotension, hallucination, and dry mouth, and tizanidine should be avoided in patients on hypertension medication due to risk of developing hypotension. QT interval prolongation is also another rare risk described in the literature. Caution should be used in patients with renal impairment or concomitant use of fluvoxamine and ciprofloxacin as these medications can significantly increase serum level of tizanidine. This is mainly due to their interactions with the CYP450 system. Similarly, there are documented cases of hepatic injury with tizanidine use, and patients with impaired liver function should have liver enzymes monitored during the first 6 months of treatment. Although tizanidine is indicated for the treatment of spasticity, it also appears to demonstrate antinociceptive effect in animal models indicating possible benefit for those with musculoskeletal conditions.

Dantrolene

Dantrolene had been in use since 1979 with both intravenous and oral forms. The indication for IV dantrolene is malignant hyperthermia, whereas the oral form is primarily used for spasticity management. It is a direct muscle relaxant by interfering the release of intracellular calcium from the sarcoplasmic reticulum, dissociating the excitation and contraction of the muscle. Oral dantrolene has an onset within 1 week and duration of action from 6 to 12 hours. It is metabolized entirely by the liver, and caution should be exercised in patients with hepatic impairment due to potential risk of hepatotoxicity associated with doses exceeding 800 mg/day. A baseline liver function test should be ordered prior to starting dantrolene, and periodic LFT monitoring is recommended.

Dantrolene can also cause central nervous system adverse effects, including drowsiness, confusion, dizziness, and headache. In some instances, it can cause generalized muscle weakness. Dantrolene should not be used in patients with cardiac or pulmonary disease since other potential serious adverse effects such as pleural effusion, pericarditis, and heart failure can occur. While dantrolene can be used for painful musculoskeletal conditions, such as severe muscle spasms after teeth extraction, the best evidence for this medication involves painful muscle contractures in spasticity. It generally is recommended as a second-line agent.

Diazepam

Diazepam is a benzodiazepine introduced in 1963 with anxiolytic, anticonvulsant, and muscle-relaxing properties. It was one of the first agents used to treat spasticity. This medication potentiates the action of $GABA_A$ receptors in the central nervous system, resulting in neuronal inhibition of polysynaptic pathways at the level of the spinal cord. The onset of action depends on if the patient has consumed a meal (up to 45 minutes) or is fasting (15 minutes), and duration of action varies as the half-life ranges from 20 to 100 hours. Diazepam and its metabolites are highly protein bound and cross the blood-brain barrier. It is metabolized by CYP3A4 and 2C19 isoforms to N-desmethyldiazepam, which is then hydroxylated to temazepam and oxazepam. It is eliminated in urine.

In the past, diazepam was commonly prescribed for muscle spasms. However, due to its sedative and hypnotic effects, it has significant abuse potential, and it is a schedule IV medication in the United States. Concomitant use of benzodiazepine and opioids can significantly increase the risk of adverse effects such as mortality due to respiratory depression. Given its adverse effect profile and abuse potential, diazepam should not be prescribed as a first-line agent for the treatment of acute musculoskeletal conditions. Upon discontinuing diazepam, it should be tapered down slowly over time and not abruptly stopped due to withdrawal symptoms such as anxiety, tremors, panic attacks, confusion, insomnia, and irritability.

Evidence of Efficacy

Despite lack of supportive data, long-term use of muscle relaxants and anti-spasticity agents is widespread and common. The FDA advises short-term use of about 2–3 weeks because adequate evidence of effectiveness for longer use is not available. Current review of the medical literature does not show superiority of one muscle relaxant over another, and available evidence is rated poor to fair quality. Adverse event rates cannot reliably be established on current evidence, and there are no studies lasting longer than 12 weeks.

Cyclobenzaprine has the most data behind its short-term use and has been shown to have superiority over placebo but not other muscle relaxants. In the Canadian Agency for Drugs and Technologies in Health meta-analysis, the long-term use of cyclobenzaprine for pain was assessed in 2015. The authors evaluated seven reviews published from 2001 to 2011 and three random controlled trials. There has since been a JAMA published RTC in 2015 in patients who presented to the ER with acute low back pain. The authors found no difference in giving Naprosyn with placebo versus Naprosyn with cyclobenzaprine for acute low back pain at 21 days. All trials evaluated between 20 and 200 patients, all were 12 weeks or less in duration, and the review results were mixed. No trials showed a statistical difference between cyclobenzaprine doses, no differences compared to placebo, and no differences between short-acting and extended release cyclobenzaprine. It has not been found effective in the treatment of spasticity associated with central nervous disorders.

There are three Cochrane reviews on muscle relaxants to date. A 2003 Cochrane review noted that muscle relaxants are effective in the short term and similar in performance for the management of non-specific low back pain. In 2009 a Cochrane review of cyclobenzaprine use in myofascial pain noted there is insufficient evidence to support the use of cyclobenzaprine. However, there were only two small studies in which a total of 35 participants were given cyclobenzaprine. In 2012 another Cochrane review noted that muscle relaxants in general are not effective in inflammatory or rheumatoid arthritis.

Combining reviews for spasticity due to any upper motor neuron cause, the data is comparable. A recent 2016 review in the *MS Journal* on spasticity management in multiple sclerosis has similar conclusions to past systematic reviews and guidelines. For spasticity management, evidence supports baclofen or tizanidine as first-line agents, while dantrolene and diazepam are second line. Unfortunately, the available studies on spasticity treatment are also of variable methodological quality. Another recently done review in the *Journal of Rehab Medicine* is consistent with the *MS Journal* findings in that oral baclofen was determined to be effective at relieving spasticity with no significant differences in efficacy compared to tizanidine. Weakness and other adverse effects are common with oral baclofen; however, the range of adverse effects was quite large from 10% up to 75% having symptoms. The largest review of 30 trials found no significant treatment differences with oral baclofen compared with tizanidine. Adverse effects in all studies were dose related and tended to disappear when doses were reduced.

The systematic reviews generally have been well done and helpful in assessing all of the data; however, the ability to draw clear conclusions is limited. This is due to the quality of evidence, which was poor to fair quality. The lack of quality with low numbers of patients, short duration, heterogeneity of patients, and variable outcome measures all lead to inconclusive results. Many studies were done before the 2000s, and today research methods are better defined and more robust. Finally, methods to measure positive outcomes have also been a point of contention and debate. For example, spasticity can be measured using the Modified Ashworth Scale (MAS), the Tardieu Scale, the Modified Tardieu Scale, the Triple Spasticity Scale (TSS), and/or laboratory measures such as the stretch-induced electromyography (EMG) activity. Various published reviews have found that none of these scales are reliable or valid. Better clinical tools that are easily interpreted and reproduced and clinically feasible need to be developed.

Conclusion

Deciding the most sensible muscle relaxant medication to prescribe is up to the clinician's best judgment. The majority of studies on muscle relaxants were performed from the 1960s to 1980s with dated methodologies and inconsistent quantification of back pain outcomes. From the limited available data, there appears to be some benefit to using skeletal muscle relaxants in the acute phase (<1–2 weeks) to help patients with discomfort and assist in their recovery during this phase. The majority of patients with acute musculoskeletal conditions will likely have improvements within 2–3 months. Current studies show no superiority of one muscle relaxant over another, no clear differences in adverse effects, and no evidence to support prolonged use of these agents in treating chronic musculoskeletal conditions. Due to increased risk of abuse and addiction to carisoprodol and diazepam, these agents should be avoided in patients on opioids or with a substance use disorder. The physician should evaluate each patient individually and prescribe the most appropriate skeletal muscle relaxant if appropriate.

Table 22.2 Common antispasmodic dosing

Medication	Dosage	Additional consideration
Baclofen	5–10 mg PO three times daily	Avoid in elderly and renal impairment Should be tapered off slowly
Carisoprodol	250–350 mg PO three times daily and nighttime	Schedule IV controlled substance with habit-forming potential Taper off gradually Should not be prescribed as first-line agent
Chlorzoxazone	250–500 mg PO three to four times daily	Lack of efficacy Common adverse effects include drowsiness and sedation Possible risk of idiosyncratic hepatocellular toxicity
Cyclobenzaprine	5–10 mg PO three times daily	Anticholinergic properties Avoid if the patient is taking concomitant MAOI or took an MAOI within the last 14 days
Diazepam	2–10 mg PO four times daily	Sedative and hypnotic High abuse potential Should not be prescribed as first-line agent
Metaxalone	800 mg PO three to four times daily	Avoid in hepatic or renal impairment Possible hypersensitivity reactions
Methocarbamol	750–1500 mg PO four times daily	Consider initial dose of 8 grams per day for first 48 to 72 hours if having severe pain Low abuse potential
Orphenadrine	100 mg PO two times daily	Mostly anticholinergic activity Avoid in elderly
Tizanidine	4–8 mg PO four times daily	Concomitant use of fluvoxamine and ciprofloxacin can cause increased serum level of tizanidine Avoid in liver impairment, and consider LFT monitoring in first 6 months of treatment

The emphasis should be to relieve pain and return the patient to a normal level of function while minimizing adverse side effects (Table 22.2).

Pearls and Pitfalls

- Skeletal muscle relaxants may be beneficial in the acute phase of musculoskeletal injuries.
- No evidence for long-term use of these medications exists.
- Due to high abuse potential, avoid prescribing carisoprodol or diazepam for acute musculoskeletal conditions.
- Cyclobenzaprine has the most supportive evidence for short-term use.
- First-line agents for spasticity are baclofen and tizanidine. Second line is dantrolene.

Recommended Reading

1. Alencar FG Jr, Viana PG, Zamperini C, Becker A. Patient education and self-care for the management of jaw pain upon awakening: a randomized controlled clinical trial comparing the effectiveness of adding pharmacologic treatment with cyclobenzaprine or tizanidine. J Oral Facial Pain Headache. 2014;28(2):119–27.
2. Alpaslan C, Kahraman SA, Durmuslar C, Cula S. Comparative efficacy of four muscle relaxants on signs and symptoms of the myofascial pain syndrome associated with temporomandibular disorders: a randomized clinical trial. J Musculoskelet Pain. 2012;20(4):310–6.
3. American Geriatrics Society 2012 Beers Criteria Update Expert Panel. American Geriatrics Society updated Beers Criteria for potentially inappropriate medication use in older adults. J Am Geriatr Soc. 2012;60(4):616–31.
4. Beebe FA, Barkin RL, Barkin S. A clinical and pharmacologic review of skeletal muscle relaxants for musculoskeletal conditions. Am J Ther. 2005;12(2):151–71.
5. Borenstein DG, Lacks S, Wiesel SW. Cyclobenzaprine and naproxen versus naproxen alone in the treatment of acute low back pain and muscle spasm. Clin Ther. 1990;12(2):125–31.
6. Browning R, Jackson JL, O'malley PG. Cyclobenzaprine and back pain: a meta-analysis. Arch Intern Med. 2001;161(13):1613–20.
7. Chou R, Peterson K, Helfand M. Comparative efficacy and safety of skeletal muscle relaxants for spasticity and musculoskeletal conditions: a systematic review. J Pain Symptom Manag. 2004;28(2):140–75.
8. Chou R, et al. Diagnosis and treatment of low back pain: a joint clinical practice guideline from the American College of Physicians and the American Pain Society. Ann Intern Med. 2007;147(7):478–91.
9. Chou R, Huffman LH, American Pain Society, American College of Physicians. Medications for acute and chronic low back pain: a review of the evidence for an American Pain Society/American College of Physicians clinical practice guideline [published correction appears in Ann Intern Med. 2008;148(3):247–248]. Ann Intern Med. 2007;147(7):505–514.
10. Chou R, Deyo R, Friedly J, Skelly A, Weimer M, Fu R, Dana T, Kraegel P, Griffin J, Grusing S. Systemic pharmacologic therapies for low back pain: a systematic review for an American College of Physicians Clinical Practice Guideline. Ann Intern Med. 2017;166:480–92.
11. Cimolai N. Cyclobenzaprine: a new look at an old pharmacological agent. Expert Rev Clin Pharmacol. 2009;2(3):255–63.
12. Dillon C, et al. Skeletal muscle relaxant use in the United States: data from the Third National Health and Nutrition Examination Survey (NHANES III). Spine. 2004;29(8):892–6.
13. Ertzgaard P, Campo C, Calabrese A. Efficacy and safety of oral baclofen in the management of spasticity: a rationale for intrathecal baclofen. J Rehabil Med. 2017;49:193–203.
14. Fass JA. Carisoprodol legal status and patterns of abuse. Ann Pharmacother. 2010;44(12):1962–7.
15. Fitzcharles MA, Ste-Marie PA, Goldenberg DL, Pereira JX, Abbey S, Choiniere M. 2012 Canadian guidelines for the diagnosis and management of fibromyalgia syndrome [Internet] The Canadian Fibromyalgia Guidelines Committee. Management. 2012;2012:1–6.
16. Fleuren JF, Voerman GE, Erren-Wolters CV, Snoek GJ, Rietman JS, Hermens HJ, Nene AV. Stop using the Ashworth Scale for the assessment of spasticity. J Neurol Neurosurg Psychiatry. 2010;81(1):46–52.
17. Forrester MB. Adult metaxalone ingestions reported to Texas poison control centers, 2000-2006. Hum Exp Toxicol. 2010;29(1):55–62.
18. Friedman BW, Dym AA, Davitt M, et al. Naproxen with cyclobenzaprine, oxycodone/acetaminophen, or placebo for treating acute low back pain: a randomized clinical trial. JAMA. 2015;314(15):1572–80.

19. Jackson J, Anania FA. Chlorzoxazone as a cause of acute liver failure requiring liver transplantation. Dig Dis Sci. 2007;52(12):3389–91.
20. Johansson H, et al. Pathophysiological mechanisms involved in genesis and spread of muscular tension in occupational muscle pain and in chronic musculoskeletal syndromes: a hypothesis. Med Hypotheses. 1991;35:196–203.
21. Kamen L, Henney HR III, Runyan JD. A practical overview of tizanidine use for spasticity secondary to multiple sclerosis, stroke, and spinal cord injury. Curr Med Res Opin. 2008;24:425–39.
22. Khwaja SM, Minnerop M, Singer AJ. Comparison of ibuprofen, cyclobenzaprine or both in patients with acute cervical strain: a randomized controlled trial. CJEM. 2010;12(1):39–44.
23. Leite FM, Atallah AN, El Dib R, Grossmann E, Januzzi E, Andriolo RB, et al. Cyclobenzaprine for the treatment of myofascial pain in adults. Cochrane Database Syst Rev. 2009;8(3):CD006830.
24. Malanga GA, Gwynn MW, Smith R, Miller D. Tizanidine is effective in the treatment of myofascial pain syndrome. Pain Physician. 2002;5(4):422–32.
25. Malanga G, Reiter RD, Garay E. Update on tizanidine for muscle spasticity and emerging indications. Expert Opin Pharmacother. 2008;9(12):2209–15.
26. Malanga GA, Ruoff GE, Weil AJ, Altman CA, Xie F, Borenstein DG. Cyclobenzaprine ER for muscle spasm associated with low back and neck pain: two randomized, double-blind, placebo-controlled studies of identical design. Curr Med Res Opin. 2009;25(5):1179–96.
27. Melloh M, Röder C, Elfering A, Theis JC, Müller U, Staub LP, et al. Differences across health care systems in outcome and cost-utility of surgical and conservative treatment of chronic low back pain: a study protocol. BMC Musculoskelet Disord. 2008;9:81. https://doi.org/10.1186/1471-2474-9-81.
28. Otero-Romero S, Sastre-Garriga J, Comi G, Hartung H-P, Soelberg Sørensen P, Thompson AJ, Vermersch P, Gold R, Montalban X. Pharmacological management of spasticity in multiple sclerosis: Systematic review and consensus paper. Mult Scler J. 2016;22(11):1386–96.
29. Peloso P, Gross A, Haines T, Trinh K, Goldsmith CH, Burnie S, et al. Medicinal and injection therapies for mechanical neck disorders. Cochrane Database Syst Rev. 2007;18(3):CD000319.
30. Preston KL, Guarino JJ, Kirk WT, Griffiths RR. Evaluation of the abuse potential of methocarbamol. J Pharmacol Exp Ther. 1989;248(3):1146–57.
31. See S, Ginzburg R. Choosing a skeletal muscle relaxant. Am Fam Physician. 2008;78(3):365–70.
32. See S, Ginzburg R. Skeletal muscle relaxants. Pharmacotherapy. 2008;28(2):207–21.
33. Shea BJ, Grimshaw JM, Wells GA, Boers M, Andersson N, Hamel C, et al. Development of AMSTAR: a measurement tool to assess the methodological quality of systematic reviews. BMC Med Res Methodol. 2007;7:10.
34. Smith B, Peterson K, Fu R, McDonagh M, Thakurta S. Drug class review: drugs for fibromyalgia: final original report [Internet]. Portland: Oregon Health & Science University; 2011. [cited 2015 Jan 29]. (Drug Class Reviews). Available from: http://www.ncbi.nlm.nih.gov/pubmedhealth/PMH0010224/pdf/TOC.pdf.
35. Tofferi JK, Jackson JL, O'Malley PG. Treatment of fibromyalgia with cyclobenzaprine: a meta-analysis. Arthritis Rheum [Internet]. 2004;51(1):9–13.
36. van Tulder MW, Touray T, Furlan AD, Solway S, Bouter LM. Muscle relaxants for non-specific low back pain. Cochrane Database Syst Rev. 2003;2:CD004252.
37. Van Tulder MW, Touray T, Furlan AD, Solway S, Bouter LM, Cochrane Back Review Group. Muscle relaxants for nonspecific low back pain: a systematic review within the framework of the Cochrane Collaboration. Spine. 2003;28(17):1978–92.
38. Van Tulder MW, Koes B, Malmivaara A. Outcome of non-invasive treatment modalities on back pain: an evidence-based review. Eur Spine J. 2006;15(Suppl 1):S64–81.
39. Witenko C, Moorman-Li R, Motycka C, Duane K, Hincapie-Castillo J, Leonard P, Valaer C. Considerations for the appropriate use of skeletal muscle relaxants for the management of acute low back pain. P T. 2014;39(6):427–35.

Antidepressants in Pain Management

23

Kris Ferguson and Nicole Wolfgram

Introduction

Patients with chronic pain often have several pain generators, and therefore, the treatment of their pain requires a multifaceted approach. One resource used by providers is the use of antidepressant medications. Historically, the use of the tricyclic antidepressants has been the mainstay as adjunctive therapy in pain management, particularly for neuropathic conditions. More recently, the use of selective norepinephrine reuptake inhibitors has become more widespread due to decreased risk of side effects. While it is generally accepted that it is the reuptake of serotonin and norepinephrine that allows for analgesia, their mechanism of action in pain management is not well understood.

Background/History

Antidepressants entered the arsenal of medicine in the 1950s. The first drug, iproniazid, was introduced in 1958. It had been developed as a cousin drug to isoniazid, an antitubercular treatment, after it was noted to have a euphoric effect on patients. Iproniazid became the first antidepressant to be marketed. This discovery led to the development of monoamine oxidase inhibitors (MAOIs). Concurrently, the tricyclic antidepressants (TCAs) were also being developed. Imipramine was released in 1957. The MAOIs and the TCAs are considered to be the first generation of antidepressants. The effect of these initial medications in the world of psychiatry and our social understanding of depression are immeasurable. It was not until the late 1980s that fluoxetine (Prozac) a selective serotonin reuptake inhibitor (SSRI) was introduced. The SSRIs are the second generation of antidepressants. The 1990s brought the third generation of medications in the serotonin-norepinephrine reuptake inhibitors (SNRI).

K. Ferguson (✉) · N. Wolfgram
Aspirus Hospital, Wausau, WI, USA

The use of antidepressant medications in the use of pain was serendipitous. Their use in pain management historically had primarily been grounded in the idea that most pain patients are depressed, and treating their depression will help improve their pain. It was not until the 1970s that the use of antidepressants in pain was studied. Merskey and Hester along with other researchers theorized and later proved that these medications could give analgesia apart from their principal function in altering mood (see Table 23.1).

Tricyclic (Heterocyclic) Antidepressants

TCAs as a class of medications have been extensively studied in multiple pain conditions and found to be multipurpose, nonspecific analgesic adjuncts. Analgesic effects from the TCAs occur at doses lower than those used for treatment of depression. Pain-relieving efficacy typically starts a week or less after starting therapy. The TCA medications most commonly prescribed for adjunctive pain management are dependent on the pain condition being treated because of the variation in the mechanism of action of each drug. Prescribing patterns should reflect the symptoms being targeted.

Mechanism of Action

As a class, the TCAs affect many pain receptors. They alter the monoamine transmitter activity at the synapse by blocking presynaptic norepinephrine and serotonin reuptake. The opioidergic effect is achieved through modification of the opioid receptor densities and by increasing opioid levels in areas of the brain. Furthermore, TCAs bind to the N-methyl-D-aspartate (NMDA) receptor complexes and alter their binding capacity. The reuptake of adenosine is inhibited, and sodium channels are blocked. There is also an increase in the densities of L-type calcium channels, and nonselectively, there is blocking of the postsynaptic histamine, the postsynaptic acetylcholine, and muscarinic and nicotinic receptors.

T. R. Deer et al. (eds.), *Deer's Treatment of Pain*, https://doi.org/10.1007/978-3-030-12281-2_23

Table 23.1 Classification of antidepressants

Monoamine oxidase inhibitors (MAOIs) *(That are still on the market)* Isocarboxazid (Marplan) Moclobemide (Aurorix/Manerix) Phenelzine (Nardil) Pirlindole (Pirazidol) Selegiline (Deprenyl/Eldepryl/Emsam) Tranylcypromine (Parnate) Toloxatone (Humoryl)	Tetracyclic antidepressants (TeCA) Amoxapine (Asendin/Demolox) Maprotiline (Deprilept/Ludiomil) Mianserin[a] (Many) Mirtazapine (Remeron) Trazodone (Oleptro)
Dopamine reuptake inhibitors Amineptine[b] (Survector/Maneon) Bupropion (Wellbutrin) Serotonin-norepinephrine reuptake inhibitors (SNRIs) Duloxetine (Cymbalta) Milnicipran (Savella) Venlafaxine (Effexor) Selective serotonin reuptake enhancer Tianeptine[b](Coaxil/Stablon)	Tricyclic antidepressants (TCA) Amitriptyline (Elavil) Clomipramine (Anafranil) Desipramine (Norpramin) Dothiepin[a] (Dosulepin/Prothiaden) Doxepin (Silendor/Zonalon) Imipramine (Tofranil) Iprindole[a] (Pramindole/Prondol) Lofepramine[a] (Lomont/Emdalen) Nortriptyline (Pamelor/Norpress) Opipramol[a] (Insidon/Pramolan) Protriptyline (Vivactil) Trimipramine (Surmontil)
Selective serotonin reuptake inhibitors (SSRIs) Citalopram (Celexa) Escitalopram (Lexapro) Fluoxetine (Prozac) Fluvoxamine (Luvox) Paroxetine (Paxil) Sertraline (Zoloft)	

[a]Not approved in the US
[b]Also chemically a TCA

Because of their effect on the neurotransmitters, it is recommended that an EKG be obtained prior to initiation of TCAs, particularly in patients with a preexisting cardiac condition.

General Contraindications

- In conjunction with any anti-arrhythmic medications that prolong the QTc interval
- Concurrent use with MAOIs (must wait 14+ days after discontinuation to start)
- Uncompensated heart failure or recent MI
- Proven hypersensitivity to other TCAs
- In conjunction with medications that inhibit CYP2D6 (i.e., duloxetine, paroxetine, cimetidine, valproic acid as the plasma concentration will be increased).
- Closed angle glaucoma
- Pregnancy
- Breastfeeding

Special Considerations

Use with caution in patients with known renal or hepatic impairment. The TCAs should be used cautiously in the elderly, and one may need to use a lower than normal dose. Avoid use in those with history of psychotic or bipolar disorder.

All TCAs carry an FDA Black Box Warning regarding the increased risk of suicide.

Severe/Life-Threatening Side Effects

Orthostatic hypotension, tachycardia, QTc prolongation, increased intraocular pressure, paralytic ileus, and hyperthermia. Rare: death, activation of mania, suicidal ideation, and worsening of existing seizure disorder.

Overdose

Causes cardiac arrhythmias, severe hypotension, CNS depression, seizures, and coma. Sodium bicarbonate beneficial for arrhythmia management. Vasopressors, oxygen, and steroids beneficial for shock-type symptoms.

Amitriptyline (Elavil)

Pharmacokinetics Generally, well absorbed orally. Peak plasma concentrations in 4–8 hours. Metabolized extensively in the liver (CYP450 system) to nortriptyline. Highly lipophilic. Bioavailability 33–62% with oral dosing. 1/3–1/2 of the drug is excreted within 24 hours. Plasma half-life 10–28 hours for the active amitriptyline. Plasma half-life for the metabolite nortriptyline is 16–80 hours.

Common uses both FDA approved (bolded) and off label:

- **Depression**
- Anxiety
- Bulimia nervosa
- Fibromyalgia
- Headache (migraine, tension type) prophylaxis: *Goal to have 50+% reduction in frequency and severity*
- Insomnia

- Neuropathy/neuralgia (diabetic, peripheral with pain, postherpetic, phantom limb). *Goal to give reduction in intensity/symptoms; will not produce total symptom remission*
- Nocturnal enuresis
- Pseudobulbar affect

Dosing Start low and titrate every few days as tolerated. Initial dose 10–25 mg/day taken 1 hour before bed. Dose range 10–400 mg/day but usually less than 150 mg/day. Extreme caution with titration above 150 mg/day.

Available tablet sizes: 10, 25, 50, 75, 100, and 150 mg

Time to Efficacy
- **Migraines:** 2 weeks to 3 months.
- **Neuropathic pain:** up to 4 weeks.
- **Insomnia/anxiety/depression:** immediately to 4 weeks.

Common Side Effects (Most Common Bold)
Sedation, dry mouth, **constipation**, diarrhea, nausea, heartburn, increased appetite, **weight gain**, blurred vision, urinary retention, sweating, itching, rash, fatigue, weakness, and sexual dysfunction.

Clinical Pearls
- Check EKG for QTc prolongation prior to initiating therapy and periodically afterward.
- If patient is on diuretic, check baseline magnesium and potassium prior to starting therapy and periodically afterward.
- If fatigue is problematic, consider switching to nortriptyline.
- For more severe side effects, lower dosage or stop.
- Magnesium supplementation is often helpful in managing constipation.
- If using for headaches, consider concurrent use with topiramate to offset weight gain.
- Concurrent use with tramadol increases risk of seizures.
- If not effective, wean off slowly to avoid withdrawal symptoms. Most tolerate a 50% reduction every 3 days with total discontinuation at Day 6.

Nortriptyline (Pamelor)

Pharmacokinetics Generally well absorbed orally. Peak plasma concentrations in 5 hours. Metabolized extensively in the liver (CYP450 system). Bioavailability 51% with oral dosing. Plasma half-life is 16–80 hours. Excreted by the kidneys. Elimination half-life 26 hours.

Common uses both FDA approved (bolded) and off label:

- **Major depression**: *Goal of treatment is complete remission of symptoms, prevent relapses*
- Anxiety
- Insomnia
- Neuropathy/neuralgia (diabetic, peripheral with pain, postherpetic, phantom limb). *Goal to give reduction in intensity/symptoms, will not produce total symptom remission*
- Treatment-resistant depression

Dosing Start low and titrate every 3–7 days as tolerated by 25 mg. Initial dose 10–25 mg/day taken at bedtime. Dose range 10–300 mg/day though generally 150 mg/day in pain. Titration can be done above this with caution, particularly in those with heart disease or with concomitant use of tramadol.

Available capsules: 10, 25, 50, and 75 mg
Liquid: 10 mg/5 mL

Time to Efficacy
- **Neuropathic pain:** ~6–8 weeks.
- **Insomnia/anxiety/depression:** immediately to 4 weeks for insomnia, anxiety; 2–4 weeks for depression.

Common Side Effects (Most Common Bold)
Sedation, dry mouth, constipation, diarrhea, nausea, heartburn, unusual taste in the mouth, **weight gain**, blurred vision, urinary retention, sweating, itching, rash, dizziness, fatigue, weakness, and sexual dysfunction.

Clinical Pearls
- Check EKG for QTc prolongation prior to initiating therapy and periodically afterward.
- If patient is on diuretic, check baseline magnesium and potassium prior to starting therapy and periodically afterward.
- Monitor weight and BMI.
- For more severe side effects, lower dosage or stop.
- Concurrent use with tramadol increases risk of seizures.
- If patient experiences nightmare, split dose and do not give large bedtime dose.
- Underweight patients are more likely to experience side effects.
- Can be used for smoking cessation.
- Can cause photosensitivity and/or blue-green urine.

Desipramine (Norpramin)

Pharmacokinetics Generally, well absorbed orally. Peak plasma concentrations in 2–6 hours. Metabolized extensively in the liver (CYP450 system). Bioavailability 40% with oral dosing. Plasma half-life is 12–54 hours. Approximately 70% excreted by the kidneys. Elimination half-life 24 hours.

Common uses both FDA approved (bolded) and off label:

- **Depression**: *Goal of treatment is complete remission, prevention of relapses*
- Anxiety
- Insomnia
- Neuropathy/neuralgia (diabetic, peripheral with pain, postherpetic, phantom limb. *Goal to give reduction in intensity/symptoms, will not produce total symptom remission*
- Treatment-resistant depression

Dosing Start low and titrate every 3–7 days as tolerated by 25 mg. Initial dose 25 mg/day taken at bedtime. Dose range 25–300 mg/day though again generally maximum of 150 mg/day for pain.

Available tablets: 10, 25, 50, 75, 100, and 150 mg

Time to Efficacy
- **Neuropathic pain:** ~6–8 weeks.
- **Insomnia/anxiety/depression:** immediately to 4 weeks for insomnia, anxiety; 2–4 weeks for depression.

Common Side Effects (Most Common in Bold)
Sedation, dry mouth, constipation, diarrhea, nausea, heartburn, unusual taste in the mouth, **weight gain**, blurred vision, urinary retention, sweating, itching, rash, dizziness, fatigue, weakness, and sexual dysfunction.

Clinical Pearls
- Check EKG for QTc prolongation prior to starting therapy and periodically afterward.
- If patient is on diuretic, check baseline magnesium and potassium prior to starting therapy and periodically afterward.
- Monitor weight and BMI.
- For more severe side effects, lower dosage or stop.
- Using adjunctively with gabapentin for neuropathic pain may be beneficial.
- Concurrent use with tramadol increases risk of seizures.
- If patient experiences nightmare, split dose and do not give large bedtime dose.
- Typically has fewer side effects than other TCAs.

Trazodone (Desyrel, Oleptro)

FDA Black Box Warning: Increased Risk of Suicide

Pharmacokinetics Generally well absorbed orally. Peak plasma concentrations in 2–6 hours. Metabolized extensively in the liver (CYP450 system). Bioavailability 40% with oral dosing. Approximately 70–75% excreted by the kidneys. Elimination half-life 3–9 hours.

Common uses both FDA approved (bolded) and off label:

- **Depression**: *Goal of treatment is complete remission, prevention of relapses*
- Anxiety
- Insomnia
- Diabetic neuropathy/complex regional pain syndrome: *Goal to give reduction in intensity/symptoms, will not produce total symptom remission*
- Fibromyalgia
- Bulimia nervosa

Dosing Start low and titrate every 3–4 days as tolerated by 50 mg. Initial dose 150 mg/day in divided doses. Dose range 50–400 mg/day.

Available tablets: 50, 100, and 150 mg

Time to Efficacy
- **Neuropathic pain:** ~1 week.
- **Insomnia/anxiety/depression:** immediately to 4 weeks for insomnia, anxiety; 4 weeks for depression.

Common Side Effects (Most Common Bold)
Sedation, headache, nausea, unusual taste in the mouth, dry mouth, diarrhea, constipation, weakness, fatigue, memory or concentration issues, blurred vision, and sexual dysfunction.

Clinical Pearls
- May increase digoxin, phenytoin levels.
- Grapefruit can interfere with trazodone metabolism.
- Good choice for patients with sleeping difficulties.
- May be a better choice in the elderly due to minimal anticholinergic activity.

Selective Serotonin Reuptake Inhibitors (SSRIs)

Selective serotonin reuptake inhibitors (SSRIs) are the second generation of antidepressants. They came on the market in the 1980s with the introduction of fluoxetine (Prozac). As a group, the efficacy of SSRIs for pain management is less than that of TCAs. Despite this, their use can be beneficial, particularly in cases where the use of TCAs is contraindicated or not well tolerated due to side effects. Within the class, the two that have found the most evidential support for use in pain are paroxetine (Paxil) and fluoxetine (Prozac). Unfortunately, the support is modest at best. As with the TCAs, the SSRIs carry the FDA Black Box warning regarding the increased risk of suicide.

Mechanism of Action

Selectively blocks the reuptake of serotonin by blocking the sodium/potassium adenosine triphosphate pump.

Paroxetine (Paxil)

Pharmacokinetics Generally, well absorbed orally. Peak plasma concentrations in 5–7 hours. Metabolized extensively in the liver (CYP2D6). Approximately 60–65% excreted by the kidneys. Elimination half-life 21–24 hours.

Common uses both FDA approved (bolded) and off label:

- **Depression**: *Goal of treatment is complete remission, prevention of relapses*
- **Generalized/social anxiety**
- **Obsessive compulsive disorder (OCD)**
- **Panic disorder**
- Insomnia
- **Post-traumatic stress disorder (PTSD)**
- Headache prophylaxis
- Diabetic neuropathy: *Goal of treatment is reduction in symptoms, not total remission*

Dosing Start low and titrate every 7–14 days as tolerated by 10 mg. Initial dose 20 mg/day. Dose range 20–50 mg/day.

Available tablets: 10, 20, 30, and 40 mg
Available controlled release: 12.5, 25 mg
Liquid: 10 mg/mL–250 mL bottle

Time to Efficacy
- **Neuropathic pain:** *anecdotally* 2–4 weeks but generally 6–8 weeks.
- **Insomnia/anxiety/depression:** immediately to 4 weeks for insomnia, anxiety; 2–4 weeks for depression.

Special Considerations

Use with caution in patients with known renal or hepatic impairment. Should also be used cautiously in the elderly. You may need to use a lower than normal dose. Avoid use in those with history of psychoses or bipolar disorder.

Contraindications

- Multiple potential medication interactions including thioridazine, pimozide, tamoxifen, codeine, and triptans
- Should not be used with Coumadin (warfarin)
- MAOI concurrent use. Must have a minimum of a 14-day break between ending the MAOI and starting paroxetine
- Narrow angle closure glaucoma
- Pregnancy
- Breastfeeding

Common Side Effects (Most Common Bold)
Weight gain, decreased appetite, nausea, diarrhea, constipation, dry mouth, dry mouth, insomnia, **sedation**, agitation, tremors, headaches, blurred vision, dizziness, sweating, and sexual dysfunction.

Severe/Life-Threatening Side Effects

Mania, suicidal ideation, worsening of seizure disorder, serotonin syndrome, and neuroleptic malignant syndrome.

Overdose

Causes nausea, vomiting, ataxia, tachycardia, and seizures. Considered to be relatively low risk in overdose.

Clinical Pearls
- Side effects are typically dose dependent.
- Simultaneous dosing with bupropion may offset mental flattening, cognitive slowing, and sexual dysfunction.
- Higher than normal plasma levels of Coumadin or benzodiazepines will occur with concurrent dosing.

Serotonin-Norepinephrine Reuptake Inhibitors (SNRIs)

Serotonin-norepinephrine reuptake inhibitors (SNRIs) came on the market in the 1990s and are considered to be the third generation of antidepressants. Within the class is duloxetine (Cymbalta) which is the first antidepressant in the USA to have a specific pain indication. The SNRIs act on the 5-HT receptors which are the serotonin receptors in the peripheral and central nervous system. Their function is modulation of neurotransmitters and hormones including several that are implicated in pain modulation. These include dopamine, acetylcholine, norepinephrine, glutamate, GABA, and acetylcholine.

Mechanism of Action

Selectively blocks the reuptake of norepinephrine and serotonin.

General Contraindications

- Concurrent use with MAOIs (must wait 14+ days after discontinuation to start).
- Proven hypersensitivity to other SNRIs.
- With duloxetine, avoid use with medications that inhibit CYP1A2 (i.e., fluvoxamine, cimetidine, quinolones, antimicrobials [e.g., Cipro], valproic acid) as this can cause elevated plasma levels.
- With venlafaxine, avoid use with medications that inhibit CYP2D6 (i.e., fluoxetine, paroxetine, bupropion), cimetidine, valproic acid, and CYP3A4 inhibitors (clarithromycin, ketoconazole, itraconazole) as they can cause elevated plasma levels.
- Hepatic impairment.
- End-stage renal disease (creatinine clearance <30 mL/minute).
- Pregnancy.
- Breastfeeding.

Special Considerations

Use with caution in patients with known renal impairment. The SNRIs should not be used in patients with hepatic impairment. Avoid use in those with history of psychotic or bipolar disorder. Venlafaxine should be used with caution in the elderly as a lower than normal dose may be needed.

Severe/Life-Threatening Side Effects

Serotonin syndrome, hepatotoxicity, hepatitis, increased intraocular pressure, paralytic ileus, hyperthermia, worsening of seizure disorder, activation of mania, depression, and suicidal ideation. With venlafaxine, tachycardia, cardiac arrhythmias, extrapyramidal effects, bowel perforation, and rhabdomyolysis may occur.

Overdose

At doses as low as 1000 mg with duloxetine – somnolence, coma, serotonin syndrome, seizures, syncope, tachycardia, hypotension, hypertension, vomiting, and death. Venlafaxine may cause hyponatremia, tachycardia, cardiac arrhythmias, and CNS depression. No specific antidote.

Duloxetine (Cymbalta)

Available as a generic? Yes

FDA Black Box Warning: Increased Risk of Suicide

Pharmacokinetics Generally, well absorbed orally. Peak plasma concentrations in 6–10 hours. There is a 3-hour delay in absorption and a one-third increase in clearance of duloxetine after an evening dose as compared to a morning dose. Metabolized extensively in the liver (CYP450 system). Bioavailability 50% with oral dosing. Elimination half-life 8–17 hours.

Common uses both FDA approved (bolded) and off label:
- **Major depression**
- **Generalized anxiety**
- **Fibromyalgia**: *Goal is to reduce pain intensity, symptoms, reduce analgesic use, improve quality of life*
- **Diabetic peripheral neuropathy pain**: *Goal reduce pain intensity, will not cause remission*
- **Chronic musculoskeletal pain**
- Headache (migraine/tension type) prophylaxis
- Other painful peripheral neuropathies
- Neuropathic cancer pain
- Stress urinary incontinence

Dosing Start low and titrate every few days as tolerated. Initial dose 20–30 mg/day. Dose range 20–120 mg/day but usually no added benefit for pain management above 60 mg/day. Can be given as single or divided dose.

Available capsule sizes: 20, 30, and 60 mg

Time to Efficacy
- **Headaches:** Migraines 2–10 weeks, tension type 4–8 weeks.
- **Neuropathic pain:** up to 4 weeks.
- **Diabetic neuropathy:** significant improvement with high doses at 6 weeks.
- **Depression:** 2 weeks, full effect up to 2 months.

Common Side Effects (Most Common Bold)
Orthostatic hypotension, syncope, hypertension, dizziness, fatigue, asthenia, **weight loss or gain**, diarrhea, constipation, dry mouth, sweating, headaches, insomnia, and **somnolence**.

Clinical Pearls
- Use with rifamycin, nicotine, phenobarbital or other CYP2D6, or CYP1A2 inhibitors can reduce plasma levels.

- Monitor blood pressure before starting to establish baseline and then periodically thereafter.
- Prior to initiating therapy, check liver function to establish baseline. This should be checked periodically thereafter.
- Orthostatic hypotension and syncope usually occur within the first week of therapy.
- Magnesium may be beneficial for constipation.
- If not effective, wean off slowly to avoid withdrawal symptoms. Most tolerate a 50% reduction every 3–4 days.

Venlafaxine (Effexor)

Pharmacokinetics Generally, well absorbed orally. Peak plasma concentrations in 2–3 hours. Metabolized extensively in the liver (CYP450 system) to desvenlafaxine. Bioavailability 40–45% with oral dosing. Plasma half-life for the immediate release venlafaxine is 5 hours. 87% excreted in the urine within 48 hours of dosing.

Common uses both FDA approved (bolded) and off label:

- **Depression**
- **Generalized anxiety**
- **Panic disorder**
- **Social phobia**
- Headache (migraine, tension type) prophylaxis: *Goal to have 50+% reduction in frequency and severity.*
- Fibromyalgia
- Neuropathy/neuralgia (diabetic, peripheral with pain): *Goal to give reduction in intensity/symptoms, will not produce symptom remission*
- Depression secondary to stroke
- Insomnia
- Stress urinary incontinence
- Post-traumatic stress disorder

Dosing Start low and titrate as tolerated. Initial dose 37.5–75 mg/day. Dose range 37.5–375 mg/day. Dose range for pain is usually 150–375 mg/day.

Available tablet sizes: 25, 37.5, 50, 75, and 100 mg
Extended release: 37.5, 75, and 150 mg

Time to Efficacy

- **Migraines:** 2 to 10 weeks.
- **Neuropathic pain:** up to 4 weeks.
- **Diabetic neuropathy:** significant improvement with high doses at 6 weeks.
- **Depression:** 2 weeks, full effect up to 2 months.

Common Side Effects (Most Common Bold)
Constipation, dry mouth, loss of appetite, weight loss or gain, blurred vision, sweating, headache, hypertension, dizziness, tremor, insomnia, somnolence, itching, rash, fatigue, weakness, and sexual dysfunction.

Clinical Pearls

- Efficacy and side effects are dose dependent.
- Check blood pressure at initiation for baseline measurement and then periodically after as medication may worsen hypertension.
- At lower doses, venlafaxine acts more like an SSRI (<150 mg/day).
- If not effective, wean off slowly to avoid withdrawal symptoms.

Milnacipran (Savella)

Pharmacokinetics Generally, well absorbed orally. Peak plasma concentrations in 2–4 hours. Metabolized via the glucuronidation pathways. Bioavailability 85% with oral dosing. Plasma half-life is 6–8 hours. 90% eliminated in urine.

Common Uses

- Fibromyalgia
- Major depression
- Neuropathic pain/chronic pain

Dosing Start low and titrate every few days as tolerated. Initial dose 12.5 mg day 1; 12.5 mg twice daily on days 2 and 3; 25 mg twice daily on days 4, 5, and 6, 50 mg twice daily on day 7.

Available capsule sizes: 25, 50 mg
Available tablet sizes: 12.5, 25, 50, and 100 mg

Time to Efficacy
2–4 weeks

Common Side Effects (Most Common Bold)
Sedation, dry mouth, **constipation**, diarrhea, nausea, heartburn, increased appetite, **weight gain**, blurred vision, urinary retention, sweating, itching, rash, fatigue, weakness, and sexual dysfunction.

Clinical Pearls

- Check EKG for QTc prolongation prior to initiating therapy and periodically afterward.

- If patient is on diuretic, check baseline magnesium and potassium prior to starting therapy and periodically afterward.
- If fatigue is problematic, consider switching to nortriptyline.
- For more severe side effects, lower dosage or stop.
- Magnesium supplementation is often helpful in managing constipation.
- If using for headaches, consider concurrent use with topiramate to offset weight gain.
- Concurrent use with tramadol increases risk of seizures.
- If not effective, wean off slowly to avoid withdrawal symptoms. Most tolerate a 50% reduction every 3 days with total discontinuation at day 6 (see Table 23.2).

Table 23.2 Medication Range

Medication	Starting dosage	Timing
Amitriptyline	10–25 mg daily	Typically 1 hour before bedtime
Nortriptyline	10–25 mg daily	Typically 1 hour before bedtime
Desipramine	25 mg daily	Typically at bedtime
Trazodone	150 mg daily in divided doses	AM/PM or three times daily
Paroxetine	20 mg daily	AM or PM
Duloxetine	20–30 mg daily	AM or PM
Venlafaxine	37.5–75 mg daily	AM or PM
Milnacipran	12.5 mg titration to 100 mg by day 7	Twice daily

Recommended Reading

1. Argoff C, McCleane G. Pain management secrets. Philadelphia: Mosby/Elsevier; 2009.
2. Argoff C, Albrecht P, Irving G, Rice F. Multimodal analgesia for chronic pain: rationale and future directions. Pain Med. 2009;10(suppl 2):S53–66.
3. Attal N, Bouhassira D. Pharmacotherapy of neuropathic pain. Pain. 2015;156:S104–14.
4. Finnerup N, Attal N, Haroutounian S. Pharmacotherapy for neuropathic pain in adults: a systematic review and meta-analysis. Lancet. 2015;14(2):162–73.
5. Griebeler M, Morey-Vargas O, Brito J, Tsapas A, Wang Z, Carranza Leon B, et al. Pharmacologic interventions for painful diabetic neuropathy. Ann Intern Med. 2014;161(9):639.
6. Hearn L, Derry S, Phillips T, Moore R, Wiffen P. Imipramine for neuropathic pain in adults. Cochrane Database Syst Rev. 2014;5:CD010769.
7. Julien R. A primer of drug action. New York: Henry Holt and Company; 2013.
8. Lipkovich I, Choy E, Van Wambeke P, Deberdt W, Sagman D. Typology of patients with fibromyalgia: cluster analysis of duloxetine study patients. BMC Musculoskelet Disord. 2014;15(1):450.
9. Lunn M, Hughes R, Wiffen P. P68 Duloxetine for treating painful neuropathy or chronic pain; a Cochrane systematic review. Neuromuscul Disord. 2010;20:S23.
10. O'Connor A, Dworkin R. Treatment of neuropathic pain: an overview of recent guidelines. Am J Med. 2009;122(10A):S22–32.
11. Tanenberg R, Clemow D, Giaconia J, Risser R. Duloxetine compared with pregabalin for diabetic peripheral neuropathic pain management in patients with suboptimal pain response to gabapentin and treated with or without antidepressants: a post hoc analysis. Pain Pract. 2013;14(7):640–8.
12. Waldfogel J, Nesbit S, Dy S, Sharma R, Zhang A, Wilson L, et al. Pharmacotherapy for diabetic peripheral neuropathy pain and quality of life. Neurology. 2017;88(20):1958–67.
13. Zilliox L. Neuropathic pain. Continuum. 2017;23:512–32.

Ketamine and NMDA-Receptor Antagonists

24

Mihir M. Kamdar

Introduction

The *N*-methyl-*D*-aspartate (NMDA) pathway plays an important role in the development, maintenance, and amplification of pain. Both acute and chronic pain states are associated with increased expression and activation of the NMDA pathway.

The NMDA receptor is an ionotropic receptor that is activated by ubiquitous excitatory neurotransmitter glutamate (see Fig. 24.1). In its resting state, the NMDA receptor is blocked by magnesium and remains inactive. When activated by glutamate, the channel is opened, and an influx of extracellular calcium occurs. This results in neuronal activation and propagation of pain signals.

The dorsal horn of the spinal cord is a major site of NMDA-receptor activation and contributes to neuroplastic changes that mediate central sensitization. Activation of NMDA pathways in the dorsal horn results in neuronal hyperexcitability, thereby causing increased pain signaling via ascending spinal pathways. The NMDA receptor has also been associated with reduction in opioid responsiveness, as activation of the opioid pathway leads to activation of the NMDA receptor, which in turn results in downregulation of the opioid receptor.

Clinically, upregulation and activation of the NMDA receptor in the dorsal horn have been associated with the development of chronic pain states, hyperalgesia, decreased opioid responsiveness, and neuropathic pain. Hence the NMDA pathway presents an attractive non-opioid analgesic target for a variety of clinical pain states.

This chapter will focus heavily on ketamine, as it is the most widely used and well-studied non-opioid NMDA-receptor antagonist used in the treatment of pain. As will be discussed, there is limited data for the use of the remaining non-opioid NMDA-receptor antagonists. Opioids that possess NMDA-receptor antagonism properties will be touched on in this chapter but will be discussed in greater detail in other sections of this text.

M. M. Kamdar (✉)
Divisions of Palliative Care and Anesthesia Pain Medicine, Massachusetts General Hospital, Boston, MA, USA
e-mail: mmkamdar@mgh.harvard.edu

Background, Uses, and Indications

Ketamine

Introduction and History

Ketamine is the one best studied and most widely used NMDA antagonists. First developed in the early 1960s, it was approved for clinical use in the United States in 1970. It was initially used as a surgical anesthetic and was not used specifically as an analgesic therapy until the late 1980s. Ketamine has since been used to treat a host of acute and chronic pain conditions.

Mechanism of Action

Structurally, ketamine is a phencyclidine (PCP) analog. It is a high-affinity NMDA-receptor antagonist. Ketamine also exerts effects on calcium channels, as well as cholinergic, dopaminergic, noradrenergic, and descending inhibitory pathways. Interestingly, ketamine may also a play a role in regulating immune responses involved in pain signaling. For example, ketamine interacts with toll-like receptors on immune cells to reduce expression of inflammatory cytokines. The clinical significance of this immunoregulatory feature is not clear in humans but theoretically may result in reduction of both acute and chronic pain.

Ketamine is present in both *S* and *R* isomers, though the *S* isomer has significantly greater affinity for the NMDA pathway and may be more clinically relevant. In the United States, only the racemic mixture is commercially available.

Pharmacokinetics and Routes of Delivery

In humans, ketamine is metabolized by the hepatic p450 CYP3A4 and CYP2B6 pathways. Its metabolites, including its primary metabolite norketamine, are primarily renally

T. R. Deer et al. (eds.), *Deer's Treatment of Pain*, https://doi.org/10.1007/978-3-030-12281-2_24

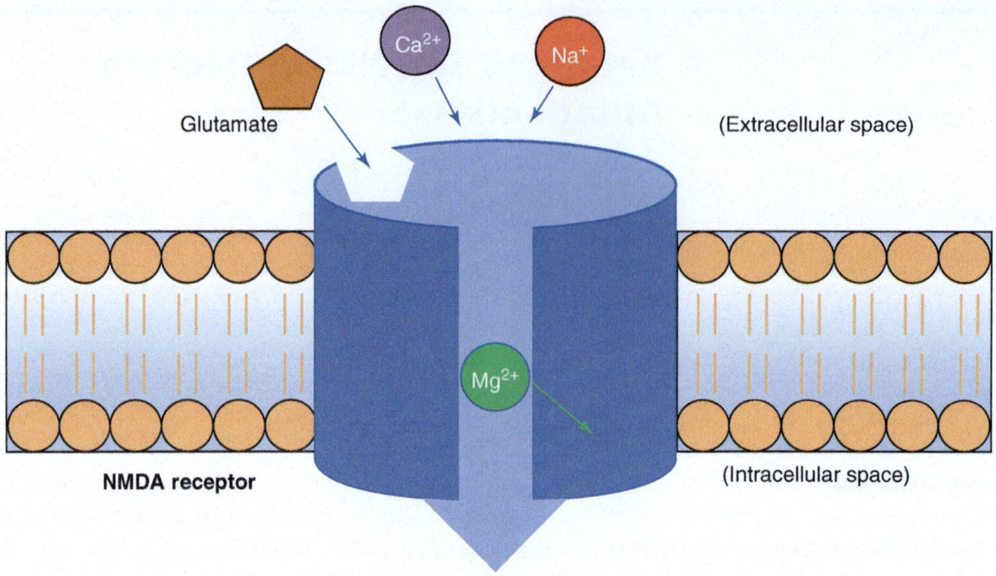

Fig. 24.1 Schematic of NMDA receptor. Binding of the glutamate to the NMDA receptor results in disassociation of magnesium, influx of positive ions, and neuronal activation

excreted. Less than 5% of ketamine is excreted unmetabolized via feces and urine. Ketamine is lipid-soluble, which results in a large volume of distribution and yields several available routes of delivery.

Ketamine can be administered via intravenous, subcutaneous, intramuscular, intranasal, oral, sublingual, and topical routes. Oral bioavailability of ketamine is poor because of significant first-pass metabolism, though surprisingly oral dosing seems roughly equianalgesic to intravenous dosing. This may be related to analgesic activity of norketamine, which is present in high concentration following oral administration, though this has not been demonstrated in humans.

Elimination half-life following single bolus dose infusion of ketamine is 2–3 hours. However, prolonged infusions of ketamine are associated with significantly longer analgesic effects, which may be due to elevated levels of norketamine that occur with continued administration. Presently there is no commercially available oral formulation, but an oral solution can be prepared from the intravenous solution by local pharmacies. Spinal use of ketamine may be limited by neurotoxicity.

Onset of action of intravenous and intramuscular ketamine is approximately 5 minutes, versus 15–30 minutes for subcutaneous administration and 30 minutes for the oral route. Time to peak plasma concentration is 30 minutes for the subcutaneous route, while the oral route takes approximately 60 minutes to reach peak plasma levels. Plasma half-life of intravenous and intramuscular ketamine is 1–3 hours, while the plasma half-life of oral ketamine is approximately 3 hours. Duration of action of intravenous and intramuscular ketamine is 30 minutes to 2 hours following bolus administration, while the duration of action for oral ketamine is approximately 4–6 hours.

Anesthetic Versus Subanesthetic Dosing

At higher doses (generally greater than 1 mg/kg), ketamine functions as a disassociative anesthetic. For pain indications, ketamine is used at "subanesthetic doses," which are typically 10–20% of those used for anesthesia. Subanesthetic doses of ketamine generally range from 0.1 to 0.5 mg/kg in oral or intravenous bolus doses, or in continuous infusions of 0.1–0.5 mg/kg/hour via intravenous or subcutaneous administration.

Uses and Indications

Ketamine is used as an analgesic in a wide array of clinical scenarios. In the acute pain setting, ketamine is used as a perioperative adjunct, as an opioid-sparing analgesic in the emergency department, and as a sedative analgesic for wound dressing changes. In the chronic pain setting, ketamine has been used for nonmalignant neuropathic pain such as complex regional pain syndrome and phantom limb syndrome. Ketamine has also been used as an analgesic to treat opioid nonresponsive pain in the cancer population.

Interestingly there has been a recent body of growing literature examining non-pain benefits of ketamine on mood disorders. For example, ketamine has gained significant attention for the acute treatment of refractory depression and suicidality.

Memantine, Amantadine, and Dextromethorphan

Memantine, amantadine, and dextromethorphan are NMDA-receptor antagonists that are generally used to treat non-pain conditions. Memantine is a partial NMDA antagonist that is commonly used to treat Alzheimer's disease. Amantadine is a NMDA-receptor antagonist that is used in the treatment of Parkinson's disease and as antiviral therapeutic. Its NMDA-receptor antagonism is unique in that it likely accelerates calcium channel closure rather than blocking channels. Dextromethorphan is commonly used a cough suppressant at low doses. At higher doses, however, dextromethorphan causes antagonism of the NMDA receptor similar to disassociative anesthetics.

Opioids with NMDA Antagonism: Methadone and Levorphanol

Methadone and levorphanol are unique long-acting opioids that antagonize the NMDA receptor in addition to activating the mu-opioid pathway. Methadone was initially developed in Germany and used in World War II in the setting of a morphine shortage. Methadone was first introduced in the United States in 1947 as a pain medication. In the 1970s, methadone began to be used for the treatment of opioid addiction, which is now its most common indication. Nonetheless, methadone remains an effective medication for pain. Levorphanol was also developed in Germany in the 1940s as a morphine substitute. Levorphanol is used solely for pain and not addiction. It is less utilized and well-studied than methadone.

Evidence for Efficacy

Ketamine

Acute Pain

Perioperative Pain Management

Low-dose intravenous ketamine administered both intra- and postoperatively has demonstrated multiple benefits including improved pain control, less postoperative nausea and vomiting, and a reduction in postoperative opioid use. Perioperative benefits of ketamine have been demonstrated in spinal, thoracic, orthopedic, major abdominal, and pediatric surgeries. As compared to other intravenous anesthetics, ketamine does not impair cardiac output and hence may an excellent option for hemodynamically unstable patients. Furthermore, addition of ketamine to hydromorphone or morphine PCA in the postoperative setting has been shown to improve pain control with opioid-sparing effects, as well as less postoperative nausea and vomiting. A review of perioperative ketamine demonstrated that 78% of ketamine treatment groups required less postoperative analgesia and reported less postoperative pain. Another review also demonstrated similar results. Based on this large volume of data, ketamine is a useful and effective adjunct in the management of perioperative pain.

Use of Ketamine in the Emergency Department (ED)

A meta-analysis of low-dose ketamine in the emergency department demonstrated that it may be a beneficial adjunct for acute pain in the emergency setting with less cardiopulmonary side effects than opioids. Benefits may apply to a host of acute pain conditions commonly seen in the ED including orthopedic fracture, sickle cell crises, abdominal, and back pain. Some studies suggest that ketamine may have opioid-sparing effects and benefits in opioid-tolerant patients, both of which are key considerations in the treatment of pain in the emergency department.

Chronic Non-cancer Pain

Complex Regional Pain Syndrome (CRPS)

Several studies have examined the effects of inpatient and outpatient intravenous infusions of ketamine on CRPS with most studies demonstrating analgesic benefit. The degree and duration of pain relief were varied, with improvements typically lasting several weeks. However, the quality of most of these studies was suboptimal, and a recent systematic review concluded there was only weak evidence for the use of ketamine for CRPS. The authors did note the benefits seen in the existing low-quality studies did make a compelling argument for higher-quality randomized controlled trials. Interestingly there has been suggestion that anesthetic doses of ketamine may have greater efficacy, though this assumes a greater degree of risk, requires more intensive monitoring, and has not been directly compared to subanesthetic dosing.

Phantom Limb Pain

Studies examining the role of ketamine in the treatment of phantom limb pain are limited. Two small studies demonstrated benefits of ketamine infusions in patients with phantom limb pain. A recent Cochrane database review of treatments for phantom limb pain suggested the exact role of ketamine in management of phantom limb pain is unclear and that larger, more rigorous randomized controlled trials are needed.

Fibromyalgia

Ketamine has been studied in three trials utilizing intravenous infusions for patients with fibromyalgia. While two studies showed an initial response, the benefits were short-lived and did not last longer than a few hours post-infusion. Larger, well-designed studies exploring both dosing and duration of ketamine may be of benefit in determining the role of ketamine in fibromyalgia pain.

Prevention of Chronic Postoperative Pain

Because of the potential role that the NMDA pathway may play in the transition from acute to chronic pain, ketamine has positioned as a possible agent to prevent chronic postoperative pain. Systematic reviews have failed to demonstrate the prevention of chronic pain with both epidural and intravenous ketamine. Subgroup analysis of patients who received only intravenous ketamine did in fact demonstrate a reduction in chronic pain up to 6 months following surgery. The variety of surgical types in addition to differences in the timing and dossing of ketamine complicates the ability to draw clinical conclusions about its role in preventing chronic postoperative pain. Further well-structured and controlled studies are warranted.

Cancer Pain

Case reports and small prospective studies have demonstrated benefits of ketamine in patients with refractory cancer pain. Initial beneficial studies often used "burst" protocols that involved short-term infusions (48 hours or less) which yielded analgesic benefits that lasted well beyond the half-life of the drug (days to weeks).

However, a large randomized controlled trial of subcutaneous ketamine that utilized a rapid titration, high-dose protocol failed to demonstrate improvement in analgesia in patients with opioid-refractory cancer pain. The drop-out rate in the treatment arm, significantly higher compared to the control arm, primarily related to cognitive disturbance and skin site irritation from subcutaneous administration. A subsequent Cochrane review concluded that more randomized controlled trials are necessary to fully assess the benefits and risks of ketamine in opioid-refractory cancer pain.

Reversal of Opioid-Induced Hyperalgesia

Opioid-induced hyperalgesia (OIH) is a clinical phenomenon by which exposure to opioids paradoxically lowers the threshold to experience pain. Numerous case reports have suggested that addition of ketamine to opioid-tolerant with refractory acute and chronic pain results in improved analgesia and reduction in opioid use. Several case reports have described clinical scenarios consistent with possible opioid-induced hyperalgesia (severe pain, diffuse allodynia, neurotoxicity) that improved with ketamine treatment. While these reports suggest that ketamine may have a role in the reversal of opioid-induced hyperalgesia, structured clinical trials are warranted to more clearly elucidate the role of ketamine in the treatment of OIH. The diagnosis of OIH remains a clinical diagnosis which adds to the complexity of designing studies to examine this phenomenon in a prospective manner.

Topical Ketamine

The recognition of the presence of NMDA receptors on afferent endings of peripheral sensory neurons has resulted in an interest in the use of topical ketamine. Furthermore, ketamine's activity of sodium and calcium channels in addition to its immunomodulatory effects provides further rationale for topical use of ketamine. Lastly, the potential for a reduction of systemic side effects makes topical application of ketamine an attractive modality.

Data for use of topical ketamine monotherapy is mixed. Initial case reports demonstrated benefits of topical ketamine for neuropathic pain. A subsequent phase II study of patients with cancer-related mucositis pain demonstrated benefit with the use of oral ketamine rinses. However, randomized controlled trials exploring the use of topical ketamine monotherapy for non-cancer pain, including one examining CRPS, have not yet demonstrated such benefits.

Conversely, studies examining the use of ketamine in combination with other topical analgesics have demonstrated benefit. Retrospective case reports and case series examining the role of topical ketamine combinations have demonstrated response rates of up to 75%. Randomized controlled trials of topical combination ketamine compounds have suggested benefit, but doses, ratios, and optimal agent selection have not been delineated. Topical ketamine appears to be a safe treatment modality, but further randomized controlled trials examining the role of topical ketamine either as a monotherapy or in combination with other topical analgesics are needed.

Ketamine for Mood

The use of ketamine for refractory mood issues has become an exciting area of research. Burst dosing of intravenous ketamine has demonstrated a rapid benefit in patients with refractory major depression, bipolar disorder, and actively suicidal patients. Similar to pain, the benefits of ketamine administration seem to far outlive the half-life of the drug. A detailed review of this indication is beyond the scope of this chapter, but the results are interesting particularly given the concomitant incidence of mood issues in patients dealing with chronic pain. The utility of other NMDA antagonists besides ketamine is also being explored for depression.

Memantine

Memantine has been used for decades for the treatment of Parkinson's disease. Memantine blocks the NMDA receptor, though its potency is weaker than other NMDA-receptor antagonists. A study examining the effects of memantine in patients with fibromyalgia patients demonstrated increased cerebral metabolism on magnetic resonance spectroscopy as compared to controls. Likewise, functional MRI imaging of patients with CRPS given morphine with or without memantine demonstrated changes in cerebral processing as compared to morphine alone.

Unfortunately, most trials exploring the use of memantine for chronic pain have been negative. Several studies of neuropathic pain have not shown benefit as compared to placebo. Memantine was also not found to be helpful in the prophylaxis of tension-type chronic headache in a double-blind randomized controlled trial. More recent studies have shown some promise. A randomized controlled trial of memantine for the prevention of postmastectomy pain showed reduced pain scores and less analgesic use at 3 months. A double-blind randomized controlled trial of patients with fibromyalgia also demonstrated reduction in pain scores up to 6 months from initiation of memantine. Further larger studies are warranted to better determine the analgesic role of memantine in both acute and chronic pain states.

Amantadine

Amantadine is approved by the US Food and Drug Administration (FDA) as both an antiparkinsonian and antiviral agent. Studies examining the use of amantadine for pain are limited. An early study of amantadine for pain demonstrated reduced sensitization in patients with chronic low back pain. Small studies have demonstrated some possible benefit for postoperative and neuropathic pain. However, the largest study examining the use of intravenous amantadine for neuropathic pain in patients with sciatica failed to show benefit compared to intravenous lidocaine or placebo. A double-blind study also failed to show benefit of perioperative amantadine in patients undergoing mandibular fracture surgery. Larger studies are needed to delineate the role of amantadine for both acute and chronic pain.

Dextromethorphan

Dextromethorphan is a dose-dependent NMDA-receptor antagonist that is most commonly used for the treatment of cough. It is also FDA-approved for the treatment of pseudobulbar affect (emotional lability). A review of six studies of dextromethorphan for the treatment of pain demonstrated benefit in four of the studies. Two trials examined the benefits of dextromethorphan in patients with diabetic neuropathy and postherpetic neuralgia. Both studies showed significant benefits in the diabetic neuropathy group but not in patients with postherpetic neuralgia. A small study of dextromethorphan for phantom limb pain did show benefit. Larger, well-designed controlled studies are needed to elucidate the analgesic role of dextromethorphan.

Methadone and Levorphanol

Methadone is a well-studied opioid with benefits in acute, chronic non-cancer, and cancer pain. A full review of the opioid benefits of methadone is beyond the scope of this chapter. The specific clinical significance of methadone's NMDA antagonism effect is less clear. Animal studies and small human studies suggest that methadone may have greater effects on neuropathic pain. However, large studies demonstrating the NMDA-specific benefits of methadone in humans are lacking. Levorphanol is less well studied but has demonstrated benefit in a few studies of patients with chronic non-cancer pain (including a variety of neuropathic pain states) and cancer pain.

Pearls and Pitfalls

Ketamine

- Side effects of ketamine can include psychomimetic effects (including delirium, psychosis, vivid dreams, and disassociation), tachycardia, intracranial hypertension, bladder toxicity, hepatic toxicity, and sialorrhea.
- Patient selection is very important when deciding whether to administer ketamine. Ketamine should be avoided in patients with a history or risk of psychosis or delirium. Ketamine should be used cautiously in patients with hepatic dysfunction or with elevated intracranial pressures (though systematic reviews suggest effects on intracranial pressure may be less of a concern than initially reported). Because of its use as a street drug, caution should be given when considering administration to a patient with a history of substance use disorder in a noncontrolled setting.
- The psychomimetic effects of ketamine (delirium, agitation, disassociation) can often be prevented or treated by either neuroleptics or benzodiazepines. Many clinicians prefer use of a neuroleptic such as haloperidol as benzodiazepines may cause paradoxical agitation or delirium.
- Despite its poor bioavailability, oral ketamine appears to have near equianalgesic potency to intravenous ketamine. Hence, the subanesthetic oral and intravenous bolus dose range is generally between 0.2 and 0.5 mg/kg. Subanesthetic continuous administration via the intravenous or subcutaneous routes is often dosed at 0.1–0.5 mg/kg/hour. Subcutaneous infusion is associated with painful skin irritation, so the intravenous route is often preferred for continuous infusions.
- Because of its short half-life, bolus doses are generally administered every 6–8 hours. Length of continuous infusions can range from 1 hour to several days. Ketamine can be titrated daily if needed as plasma levels should reach steady state within 24 hours.
- There is no commercially available oral version of ketamine available in the United States presently. Hence the intravenous solution is generally used when administered orally and is associated with a bitter taste. Patients can mix the solution in orange juice, and local pharmacies may be able to formulate the solution in flavored syrups or tablets to avoid the noxious taste.

- A subset of opioid-tolerant patients may experience sedation due to the effects of ketamine on opioid tolerance. If mild sedation is noted following ketamine administration, clinicians may consider reducing the opioids by 20–25%.
- No physiologic withdrawal has been associated with cessation of ketamine, but psychologic cravings can occur. Diffuse hyperalgesia and allodynia have been reported in patients who have abruptly ceased ketamine after weeks of use.

Memantine

- Optimal dosing of memantine for pain is not well established. Studies examining the use of memantine for pain generally used doses of 5–20 mg orally per day.
- Memantine is generally well tolerated. Side effects occurring at an incidence of >5% include dizziness, headache, confusion, constipation, and diarrhea.

Amantadine

- Optimal dosing of amantadine for pain indications is not well established. Oral amantadine is generally dosed at 100–200 mg daily.
- Amantadine is generally well tolerated. Nausea, insomnia, and dizziness occur at an incidence of 5–10%. Less common side effects include blurry vision, confusion, depression, anxiety, peripheral edema, orthostatic hypotension, and fatigue. Caution should be used in patients with seizures.

Dextromethorphan

- Optimal dosing of dextromethorphan for pain is not well established. In studies examining its use for pain, doses generally between 30 and 180 mg orally per day were used.
- Dextromethorphan is usually well tolerated. Side effects can include gastrointestinal issues such as diarrhea and upset stomach.

Methadone

- Methadone is a nuanced opioid whose clinical use comes with greater complexity than typical opioids. Detailed advice on the use of methadone for pain is beyond the scope of this chapter and can be found elsewhere. Clinicians should familiarize themselves with the unique pharmacokinetics, equianalgesic conversions, and cardiac effects of methadone to use the drug safely and effectively.

Recommended Reading

1. Aiyer R, Mehta N, Gungor S, Gulati A. A systematic review of NMDA receptor antagonists for treatment of neuropathic pain in clinical practice. Clin J Pain. 2018;34(5):450–67.
2. Badiola IJ. Can chronic pain be prevented? Anesthesiol Clin. 2016;34(2):303–15.
3. Bell RF, Eccleston C, Kalso EA. Ketamine as an adjuvant to opioids for cancer pain. Cochrane Database Syst Rev. 2017;6:CD003351.
4. Connolly SB, Prager JP, Harden RN. A systematic review of ketamine for complex regional pain syndrome. Pain Med. 2015;16(5):943–69.
5. Maher DP, Chen L, Mao J. Intravenous ketamine infusions for neuropathic pain management: a promising therapy in need of optimization. Anesth Analg. 2017;124(2):661–74.
6. Peltoniemi MA, Hagelberg NM, Olkkola KT, Saari TI. Ketamine: a review of clinical pharmacokinetics and pharmacodynamics in anesthesia and pain therapy. Clin Pharmacokinet. 2016;55(9):1059–77.
7. Pourmand A, Mazer-Amirshahi M, Royall C, Alhawas R, Shesser R. Low dose ketamine use in the emergency department, a new direction in pain management. Am J Emerg Med. 2017;35(6):918–21.
8. Quibell R, Fallon M, Mihalyo M, Twycross R, Wilcock A. Ketamine. J Pain Symptom Manag. 2015;50(2):268–78.
9. Sawynok J. Topical and peripheral ketamine as an analgesic. Anesth Analg. 2014;119(1):170–8.

Novel Analgesics

25

Vitaly Gordin, Daniel Morgan, Michael Mueller, Alba Guevara, and Yuri Gordin

Introduction

The most common reason patients seek medical care is pain. With the advances of medicine the US population is living, longer and chronic pain conditions associated with advanced age such as osteoarthritis, osteoporosis commonly associated with compression fractures, and diabetic neuropathy are becoming more prevalent. Successes in cancer treatments have resulted in cancer-related illness turning into chronic disease with a significant number of patients suffering from the side effects related to cancer treatments such as chemotherapy-induced peripheral neuropathy, postradiation pain, and pain associated with the residual effects of surgery for cancer. All these conditions can lead to chronic pain and poor quality of life. According to the Institute of Medicine, approximately 100 million North Americans suffer from chronic noncancer pain with associated direct and indirect costs over $600 billion which continues to climb. Currently available analgesics and adjuvant medications provide only modest improvement of pain and have significant side effects. The most commonly used medications include nonsteroidal anti-inflammatory agents, acetaminophen, antiepileptic medications, antidepressants possessing norepinephrine reuptake inhibition, and opioids. The notion prevailing in the 1990s that opioids do not have a ceiling effect and should be titrated to complete or almost complete analgesic state led to overprescribing of opioids. This in turn caused many patients on chronic opioids to turn to heroin. According to the literature, three out of four new heroin users admit to abusing prescription opioids before turning to heroin. According to the CDC in 2015, more than 33,000 people died from overdosing on opioids, and the number of opioid-related deaths continues to climb. The economic cost of the opioid epidemic is estimated to be $95 billion for 2016. In the light of these factors, and with the number of patients with chronic pain increasing, it is important to develop new classes of analgesic medications that would have less side effects, that their action would be targeting the underlying mechanisms that are causing pain, and that would have low abuse potential.

Clinical manifestations of pain syndromes depend on the anatomical structures that are involved in the pathological process. Depending on the affected tissue, pain can be somatic, neuropathic, or mixed. Under certain conditions when the pathological process involves neural structures, widespread pain can arise caused by central sensitization and amplification. This amplified state of the central nervous system is manifested by such phenomena as allodynia and hyperesthesia, which are the hallmarks of neuropathic pain. Based on the above reasons, it is impossible to have a single agent that would treat the broad range of conditions associated with acute and especially chronic pain.

While there are many agents that have shown promise in preclinical studies in pain models, many of them have been either marginally effective in clinical trials or their use has been associated with unacceptable side effects. New agents that are targeting various ion channels, enzymes, and G protein-coupled receptors (GPCRs) have shown promising results in the lab and are being studied in human subjects.

In this chapter, we review some of the new agents that have become recently available or have shown a significant potential in treating pain in lab models.

V. Gordin (✉) · D. Morgan · M. Mueller · A. Guevara
Department of Anesthesiology and Perioperative Medicine, Pennsylvania State University, Hershey, PA, USA
e-mail: vgordin@pennstatehealth.psu.edu; dmorgan1@pennstatehealth.psu.edu; mmueller@pennstatehealth.psu.edu; aguevara@pennstatehealth.psu.edu

Y. Gordin
Department of Physical Medicine and Rehabilitation, Pennsylvania State University, Hershey, PA, USA
e-mail: ygordin@pennstatehealth.psu.edu

T. R. Deer et al. (eds.), *Deer's Treatment of Pain*, https://doi.org/10.1007/978-3-030-12281-2_25

Neurobiology of Pain

One cannot review pharmacologic agents without an understanding of pain mechanisms and pathways and where these agents exert their action. Under physiologic conditions, pain is essential for survival of species by providing a warning signal which is eliciting a protective response. However, under certain conditions, which can be due to the injury of the nervous system, persistent inflammation, psychological composition, and genetic factors of the affected individual, pain becomes chronic and is no longer serving a protective function. It becomes a disease state leading to maladaptive behavior and decreased function resulting in poor quality of life.

One of the features of chronic neuropathic pain is its spontaneous nature due in part to the ectopic activity of primary sensory neurons which no longer require external stimulation. This ectopic activity is modulated by several voltage-gated channels, such as Nav1.7, Nav1.8, calcium channels Cav2.2, and potassium channels KCNQ among others. Their role becomes especially prominent after peripheral nerve injury. There has been a lack of reliable animal models of ectopic spontaneous pain, making development of new agents difficult. The persistent inflammation involving peripheral sensory neurons results in windup which in turn leads to the decreased threshold necessary for activation of these neurons. Such well-described phenomena as allodynia, hyperesthesia, and involvement of the surrounding tissue (secondary hyperalgesia) are the clinical hallmarks of chronic neuropathic pain. These phenomena develop due to peripheral mechanisms as well as central sensitization. In addition to the spontaneous ectopic excitatory activity, there is also a decreased influence of the inhibitory pathways regulated by norepinephrine, gamma-aminobutyric acid (GABA), endogenous opioid peptides, as well as endocannabinoids. It appears that central sensitization mechanisms are dominant in such conditions as chronic low back pain, whiplash injuries, chronic tension headaches, endometriosis, fibromyalgia, and irritable bowel syndrome.

Under physiologic conditions, endogenous opioid peptides and endocannabinoids provide analgesia by blocking transmission of pain signals. The endogenous cannabinoid system and its ligands have been extensively studied over the past two decades. Clinical applications of this system and its ligands are discussed separately in this chapter. Cannabinoids bind to two distinct G-protein-coupled receptors, CB1 and CB2. CB1 receptors are predominantly found in the CNS and along the pain pathways, while the CB2 are predominantly expressed outside the CNS in the peripheral tissues and play an important role in immune responses. Activation of the CB1 receptors reduces the stress response via inhibition of noradrenaline release from presynaptic terminals. Cannabinoids directly stimulate glycine receptors which modulate NMDA receptor activity. Additionally, by activating CB2 receptors, cannabinoids increase the release of endogenous opioids from keratinocytes in the epidermis thus reducing nociceptor activation. Recent studies in preclinical models have discovered that cannabinoids can produce antinociception and anti-hyperalgesia by inhibiting degranulation of mast cells, decreasing activity and responses to noxious stimuli of nociceptive neurons at peripheral, spinal, and supraspinal sites. It has been noticed that peripherally acting cannabinoids can potentiate the antinociceptive effect of opioids. Additionally, there have been observations that cannabinoids are involved in deletion of negative memories associated with noxious stimuli. This effect is executed by inhibition of GABAergic circuits and glutamatergic synapses in the amygdala.

Multiple pre- and postsynaptic mechanisms in the periphery as well as along the pain pathways and in the brain have been implicated in the development of chronic pain states, which makes treatment of chronic neuropathic pain challenging. In addition to the role played by these peripheral and central mechanisms, there is a well-described influence of negative emotions, anxiety, and depression on the development and persistence of chronic pain. On the other hand, pain relief is associated with a strong reward encoded in the mesolimbic system, and motivation to obtain pain relief can be also very strong.

The Opioid System

The first opioid ligands were isolated from *Papaver somniferum* more than 3000 years ago and have been used ever since. Until recently, three major families of receptors were identified, μ (MOR), δ (DOR), and κ (KOR). Recently, another family of opioid receptors activated by neuropeptide nociceptin (NOR) has been identified. Activation of the latter receptors is not reversed by naloxone. Opioid receptor agonists utilize GPCR signaling. They cause hyperpolarization of the cellular membrane by increasing potassium conductance. Opioid receptors are ubiquitous throughout the peripheral and central nervous system with the highest density in the substantia gelatinosa, amygdala, hippocampus, hypothalamus, thalamus, periaqueductal gray, and other structures. Depending on which particular receptor is activated, their stimulation is associated with a broad range of physiologic reactions such as analgesia, respiratory depression, miosis, euphoria, dysphoria, sedation, and decreased GI tract motility among others. While opioid analgesics provide superior pain control in the acute setting and in terminally ill patients who suffer from pain, their chronic use is associated with tolerance and physical and psychological dependence and can lead to addiction. There has been a lack of high-quality data on the benefits vs harms of long-term use of opioids for chronic musculoskeletal pain. In a recent pragmatic randomized trial in 240 patients with moderate to severe low back pain or pain related to hip or knee osteoarthritis, the use of opioid analgesics vs nonopioid medications did not result in improved pain-related function over the 12-month period. Pain intensity decreased more in the nonopioid group (3.5 vs 4.0), while adverse medication-related effects were significantly common in the opioid group.

Carefully selected patients with anatomically based pain can benefit from chronic opioid use while being closely monitored for pain relief, side effects, effect on the quality of life, compliance, and aberrant drug-taking behaviors.

Abuse-Deterrent Formulations

Tremendous strides have been made by the pharmaceutical industry to create abuse-deterrent formulations (ADFs). Since these formulations are utilizing μ-receptor agonists that have been used for many decades, they will not be discussed in any detail in this chapter.

The premise of extended release (ER) opioids is that the slow-release mechanism does not facilitate euphoric reactions to the same degree as the short-acting opioids which cause a rapid increase and decline in plasma concentration which can precipitate craving and withdrawal both of which can lead to the development of addiction. However, it has been shown that ER formulations are more desirable to abusers as they typically contain a higher dose that can be extracted. ADFs are designed to make it rather difficult to extract the opioid, thus limiting the likelihood of abusing these formulations. Several mechanisms have been developed to prevent abuse of opioids. Some formulations use chemical and physical barriers that prevent extraction of opioids with crushing, grinding, chewing, or using solvents. Examples include crush-resistant pills and tablets, capsules that contain high-viscosity gelatin, and extruded pellets among others. Another approach is the addition of an opioid antagonist, such as naloxone or naltrexone, which is only released when an individual is tampering with the pill. Depending on the specific antagonist, one (naltrexone) decreases the euphoric effect while the other (naloxone) precipitates withdrawal. It should be emphasized that utilizing ADFs is only one of the several approaches aimed at decreasing abuse of opioids. In spite of sophisticated abuse-deterrent mechanisms, these formulations can still be abused by taking them more frequently than prescribed which is the most frequent way of abuse. It has been noted that when the reformulated ADF of oxycodone ER was introduced, heroin abuse increased by 23%. On the other hand, the beginning of the rise of heroin abuse preceded introduction of ADFs to the market. It should be emphasized that ADFs are not the treatment of choice of addiction, and individuals with substance use disorder should be referred to an addiction treatment program.

Novel Opioid Agonists

Research in developing new opioid agonists is booming with several promising agents undergoing phase II and phase III studies. There have been efforts to develop new selective ligands to target κ- or δ-receptors as it has been postulated that these ligands cause very little if any predisposition for developing physical dependence and abuse. On the contrary, their centrally mediated effects may cause adverse reactions. The peripherally restricted κ-receptor agonist difelikefalin, (formerly CR845) developed by Cara Therapeutics, can be administered either intravenously or orally and was effective, safe, and well tolerated in phase II trials studying postoperative abdominal pain. The oral formulation of difelikefalin is undergoing separate phase II trials for chronic knee pain and uremic pruritus in patients undergoing chronic hemodialysis.

Another direction in drug development in this area is the emergence of biased ligands. Analgesia produced by conventional opioids is mediated by G-proteins. Conventional opioids also cause recruitment of β-arrestin which is responsible for desensitization of opioid receptors and their internalization as well as common side effects associated with opioids such as constipation and respiratory depression. Studies of the analgesic effect of morphine in knockout mice which are lacking β-arrestin showed increased analgesic effect while significantly less GI and respiratory side effects. A new G-protein-biased ligand of the μ-receptor oliceridine (formerly TRV130) caused G-protein activation with only a minor β-arrestin activation. After showing a strong analgesic effect with simultaneously decreased incidence of side effects in preclinical studies, it has been studied in volunteers. When compared to 10 mg of morphine, oliceridine showed equianalgesic or greater analgesic effect in well-established experimental pain models while having a lesser impact on respiratory drive and causing less nausea in volunteers. In a randomized, double-blind, adaptive design study in patients undergoing bunionectomy, oliceridine in four different doses ranging from 0.5 mg to 3 mg was compared to morphine and placebo. Oliceridine 3 mg produced a 6-point group mean decrease in NRS pain intensity 10 minutes after administration in the absence of serious side effects. At this dose, the peak effect occurred faster than with 4 mg morphine.

It has been shown with the help of positron emission tomography that fast penetration of blood-brain barrier is promoting addictive behavior in susceptible individuals and is responsible for respiratory depression and sedation. A new μ-receptor agonist NKTR-181 with inherently slow rate of entry into the CNS independent of dose level and route of administration has been developed. When compared to oxycodone in a randomized, double-blind, active- and placebo-controlled crossover study in recreational opioid users, NKTR-181 demonstrated lower abuse potential determined by Drug Liking VAS and Drug High VAS.

Ion Channel Blockers

Ion channels possess a voltage-sensing domain that interprets and responds to the electric current of the cell by initiating a conformational change in the channel structure. Current analgesics that bind to ion channels involved in the pain pathway are neither specific nor selective to ion channels or their subtypes. Future analgesics targeting ion channels will be as specific as possible – not just to channel subtypes, but, more selectively still, to the pathological state the channel maintains during the transmission of pain. Targeting pathologic ion channels which have become upregulated in pain states and cycle through these states at an increased frequency allows for increased drug efficacy while minimizing adverse reactions. The proposed effect of this is as follows: (a) to inhibit the further spread of upregulated/pathological ion channel action, (b) to reverse channel upregulation, and (c) to increase the therapeutic index of the drug as it would target channels that are functioning pathologically. This hypothesis is potentially mitigated by the fact that channel state selectivity depends upon multiple drug and ion channel factors.

Due to the multitude of novel compounds in preclinical development and the lack of successful transition from positive preclinical to clinical trials we will focus on drugs that have had success in clinical trials. We will also briefly discuss some highly promising agents.

Voltage-gated calcium channels (VGCCs) are found throughout the body, and their activation results in broad physiologic effects. This ubiquity makes pharmacological development difficult due to the specificity required to avoid overly broad drug effects. Conversely, the cascade of calcium channel effects provides several points for targeted drug development. This cascade of effects is due to the VGCC's location, unique subunit composition, neurotransmitter release, effect on transcription, and cellular adaptation.

The specific subtypes of VGCCs are based upon which proteins form the CaVα1 subunit of the ion channel pore: L-(CaV1.1–4), P/Q-(CaV2.1), N-(CaV2.2), R-(CaV2.3), and T-type (CaV3.1–3). All VGCC subtypes are found in the central and peripheral nervous systems in varying location, density, and proximity to other receptors.

P/Q-Type Calcium Channels (P/QTCC): (Cav2.1)

Pain-modulating P/Q-(CaV2.1) and N-(CaV2.2) channels are found on presynaptic primary afferent neurons. They inhibit the release of pain-modulating and inflammatory peptides such as substance P, glutamate, and CGRP in the Rexed laminae of the dorsal horn in the spinal cord. Current research focuses on the role of these channels in migraines. While the conopeptide ziconotide does bind to P/QTCCs, it has much greater affinity to N-type calcium channels (NTCC).

N-Type Calcium Channels (NTCC): (Cav2.2)

NTCCs are found throughout the central and peripheral nervous system. Their activation can cause neuropathic pain due to release of pain-modulating and inflammatory substances such as substance P, glutamate, and CGRP at presynaptic terminals of primary afferent neurons in the dorsal horn and dorsal root ganglia. Peripheral nerve injury can cause upregulation of this channel.

Research on novel analgesics specific to NTCCs has focused largely on conopeptides, which are derived from the venom of several species of snakes, spiders, and marine cone snails.

While animal experiments demonstrated the effect of conotoxins in the 1980s, only one drug targeting NTCC receptors is clinically available. Ziconotide (Prialt), synthesized from cone snail toxin, is administered intrathecally and approved for refractory chronic pain by acting primarily on the NTCC, via irreversible binding. An advantage of ziconotide over intrathecal morphine is that it does not produce tolerance, dependence, or respiratory depression. However, it can cause a variety of adverse effects through activation of the NTCCs found outside of the dorsal horn, primarily CNS impairment including hallucinations. While ziconotide's adverse effects and the requirement for intrathecal administration limit its use, the drugs potent analgesic effects and lack of tolerance and euphoria have prompted further research into conopeptides.

Current drug development of conotoxin derivatives has focused on simplifying the peptide structure in an attempt to reduce the molecular size which limits ziconotide from crossing the blood-brain barrier. Because of this, ziconotide requires intrathecal route of administration. It is trialed via single bolus efficacy trials and, if the trial is successful, is delivered with the help of a surgically implanted intrathecal pain pump. Studies are underway to develop drugs with a smaller molecular size which would allow for transport across the blood-brain barrier and eliminate the need for intrathecal administration, reduce the manufacturing cost, and enhance receptor specificity, which is likely to reduce adverse effects.

ZC88, CNV2197944, and A-1264087 are all state-dependent antagonists at the NTCC in development. While selective NTCC antagonists have been shown to be safe and do not share the broad adverse effect profile of ziconotide, they, for an unknown reason, have not shown analgesic efficacy.

Of the molecules listed, only ZC88 and CNV2197944 act solely as NTCC antagonists. In animal models, ZC88 was found to reverse morphine tolerance, likely by interacting with G-protein activation on mu-opioid receptors and causing inhibition of NTCC with oral administration.

Two phase II studies of CNV2197944 have been completed, one on its effect on postherpetic neuralgia and the other one on diabetic peripheral neuropathy. No results have been published in part due to multiple pharmaceutical company acquisitions.

Leconotide, which is also known as ω-conotoxin CVID, is significantly less toxic than ziconotide and is suitable for intravenous administration. Leconotide binds preferentially to Cav2.2 over Cav2.1 (100:1) and inhibits neurotransmitter release from preganglionic cholinergic neurons in animal studies. It also has an improved therapeutic index and avoids the cardiovascular adverse effects of ziconotide.

R-Type Calcium Channels (RTCCs): (Cav2.3)

RTCCs, also known as CaV2.3, are found on primary afferent neuronal body and dendrites.

Studies of RTCCs thus far have found limited evidence of their role in pain pathways, but their location on the dorsal root ganglion suggests a role in the ascending pain pathway. Clinical trials using a tarantula toxin, SNX-482, have demonstrated pain modulation with preference for the RTCCs.

T-Type Calcium Channels (TTCC): (CaV3.1–3)

While TTCCs are associated with pain, there has not been much success in finding specific analgesics for this channel subtype.

Z944 is the first TTCC-specific drug shown to have clinical efficacy in human trials. Effective in both neuropathic and inflammatory pain caused by capsaicin and UV light and monitored by laser-evoked potentials, these positive results have prompted development of a long-acting formulation for future trials.

Ethosuximide is a non-specific TTCC modulator and has shown modest inhibition of both inflammatory and neuropathic pain in animal models.

Nonselective Voltage-Gated Calcium Channels (VGCC) Antagonists and State-Dependent Antagonists

A group of molecules called state-dependent antagonists are thought to have potential in chronic pain states. These molecules are designed to have higher affinity for VGCC when they are in specific states, such as resting vs. open, or firing at high frequency. The hypothesis is that chronic pain induces unique changes in VGCC that could be more selectively targeted. However, no state-dependent antagonists have thus far demonstrated clinical efficacy.

A-1264087 is a state-dependent antagonist of T-(CaV3), P/Q-(CaV2.1), and N-(CaV2.2) channels which shows the ability to reduce neuropathic pain and hypersensitive response to mechanical stimuli. In separate studies, rats with induced neuropathy and osteoarthritis showed a reduced response to mechanical stimulus.

α2δ Ligands

Due to the high affinity of gabapentinoids for the α2δ subunit in the VGCC pore, this ligand has been the target of research in regard to its role in pain transmission. It is proposed that gabapentinoids reduce trafficking of α2δ without affecting its endocytosis. However, the exact mechanism of action of gabapentin and pregabalin remains unclear as they bind to both the α2δ1 and α2δ2 subunits which may have differences in analgesic effect when tested individually.

While the development of novel compounds that bind specifically to these α2δ subunits remains elusive, continued improvement of the gabapentinoids pharmacokinetic profile has resulted in several new formulations of the drug including an extended release formulation (gabapentin enacarbil or Horizant), improved CNS penetration (4-methylpregabalin), and greater potency (mirogabalin).

Mirogabalin (DS-5565) has positive results from two phase II trials in diabetic neuropathy, and phase III trials in fibromyalgia and diabetic neuropathy are underway.

Voltage-Gated Sodium Channel Blockers

There are currently nine subtypes of voltage-gated sodium channels found primarily in the central and peripheral nervous systems on neurons and glial cells named by their pore-forming α-subunit – NaV1.1–1.9 all of which have multiple neurophysiologic effects. While NaV1.4 and NaV1.5 are found primarily in skeletal and cardiac myocytes, the other sodium channels are found both in the brain and dorsal root ganglion and are involved in the transmission and processing of pain. Most notable of these are V1.3, found in the CNS in developmental stages, and 1.7, 1.8, and 1.9 all found in the dorsal root ganglion. However, preclinical data is often mixed or nonexistent for most of the channels. We will discuss only those with successful clinical data.

It has been long known that sodium channels play a role in pain transmission. Local anesthetics, tricyclic antidepressants, and anticonvulsants, such as lamotrigine, have shown modest effect in reducing chronic neuropathic pain while having a relatively narrow therapeutic index.

Current research involves numerous peptide toxins isolated from several different invertebrates. Thus far, a lack of receptor specificity has kept these agents from coming to market. A further pharmacokinetic goal in sodium channel chemistry is the theorized superiority of creating a molecule that can stabilize the channel after depolarization while it is inactivated, instead of blocking the open channel. Many of the compounds in development have effects at multiple sodium channels, often in conjunction with additional receptors as well.

Nonselective Antagonists

Ralfinamide acts on NaV1.3, NaV1.7, NaV1.8, as well as voltage-gated calcium channel CaV2.2 and NMDA antagonism. Despite early clinical promise in animal-based models, ralfinamide was no better than placebo in treating neuropathic low back pain.

NaV1.7

This sodium channel is the most likely target for pharmacologic intervention due to its unique location and alterations in electrophysiology. Due to the fact that it is found solely within sympathetic and nociceptive neurons, its targeting may minimize the adverse effects associated with targeting of the channels expressed in both the nervous tissue and cardiac myocytes. Channelopathies of NaV1.7 result in several pain pathologies. Mutations of the gene coding for NaV1.7 results in erythromelalgia and the absence of the channel results in congenital insensitivity to pain.

Vixotrigine (previously known as raxatrigine or CNV1014802) is purported to be a selective NaV1.7 antagonist with a preference for the open/inactivated state. While its selectivity is not fully proven, it has shown efficacy in two separate phase II clinical trials in patients with low back pain and trigeminal neuralgia, respectively. Phase III trials in both of these patient populations have been initiated.

NaV1.8

There have been multiple studies utilizing animal models which indicated a role played by NaV1.8 in both inflammatory and neuropathic pain. While several novel compounds have shown promise in animal models, none have progressed beyond phase I of clinical trials.

NMDA Receptor Antagonists

Overview

N-methyl-d-aspartate (NMDA) is a receptor for glutamate, an excitatory neurotransmitter. Glutamate is released with noxious peripheral stimulation and goes on to activate the NMDA receptors. Research has demonstrated an association between the activation of NMDA receptors and hyperalgesia, neuropathic pain, and the decreased functionality of opioid receptors. The hyperalgesia and/or neuropathic pain often noted in chronic pain is in part a result of increased sensitization at the level of the spinal neuron which consequently leads to a heightened level of pain. Due to the growing prevalence of chronic pain coupled with increasing opioid tolerance, NMDA receptor antagonists may play an important role in pain management, especially for those conditions that have proven refractory to other treatment modalities.

NMDA receptor antagonists include ketamine, dextromethorphan, memantine, and amantadine. The opioid methadone is also an antagonist at the NMDA receptor site. They each differ in their level of activity at the NMDA receptor site.

Ketamine

Ketamine is a noncompetitive NMDA receptor antagonist and analgesic with anti-hyperalgesia and anti-allodynia properties in multiple pain settings. When used for chronic pain conditions, doses substantially lower than those used in anesthesia are utilized. When administered with opioids, ketamine has demonstrated a synergistic effect resulting in superior pain control and reduced opioid use versus opioid administration alone. Additionally, at analgesic doses, ketamine has significantly less risk of respiratory depression, less sedation, and diminished risk of developing tolerance to the drug. Ketamine is the most studied NMDA receptor antagonist for the treatment of neuropathic pain and has been shown to be a high-affinity antagonist, which results in long-term blocking of the receptor site thus inhibiting the neuronal hyperexcitability that occurs in neuropathic pain syndromes. Thus far ketamine has been used primarily in inpatient settings, and further studies are required to make outpatient treatment safe and successful in the treatment of chronic pain.

Dextromethorphan

Dextromethorphan (DMX) is a noncompetitive NMDA receptor antagonist that acts by decreasing the excitatory transmission of the primary afferent pathway. Recent studies have demonstrated that DMX is effective in controlling neuropathic pain in patients that are unable to receive ketamine. Like ketamine, DMX works synergistically when administered with opioids and has shown little psychomimetic effects at clinically administered doses. DMX has a reduced affinity for the NMDA receptor when compared to ketamine. Additionally, DMX has a significant first-pass effect in the liver via CYP2D6 and might have a better efficacy when coadministered with a

CYP2D6 inhibitor like quinidine. In a study, patients who were known to be extensive metabolizers of DMX experienced superior pain relief versus poor metabolizers of DMX; however, more studies need to be performed for further validation.

Methadone

Methadone is a synthetic opioid that was initially introduced in the 1940s as an analgesic, and it later became widely used as supportive treatment for opioid addiction. Methadone is a racemic mixture with a high affinity for the opioid receptor and inhibition of NMDA receptor. It has proven an efficacious option for those patients that experience dose-limiting adverse effects while on other opioids, for example, patients with cancer-related pain and patients with refractory neuropathic pain. Unfortunately, methadone exhibits variability in both bioavailability and elimination half-life, and accumulation of methadone due to prolonged elimination may increase the risk of respiratory depression. It is also metabolized by a number of P450 (CYP) enzymes, and physicians need to be cautious in managing drug interactions.

More research is needed regarding NMDA receptor antagonists; however, they have demonstrated promise regarding the treatment of neuropathic and opioid-resistant pain. Thus far, clinical trials regarding ketamine and methadone have been mostly positive in reducing pain; however, the adverse CNS effects have limited their use.

Endocannabinoid Signaling System

The endocannabinoid signaling system (ECS) consists of endogenous endocannabinoid ligands, two known cannabinoid receptors, and the enzymes responsible for the production and breakdown of endocannabinoid agonists. The cannabinoid receptor subtype 1 (CB_1) is widely expressed throughout the nervous system including in primary afferent sensory neurons, neurons in the cortex, limbic system, and periaqueductal gray that modulate cognitive and affective components of pain. As a consequence, CB_1 can modulate many aspects of physiology including pain. CB_1 is responsible for the psychoactive effects of cannabinoid drugs including delta-9-tetrahydrocannabinol (Δ^9-THC), the principal psychoactive cannabinoid in the cannabis plant. However, the analgesic effects of cannabinoids are mediated by CB_1 and also CB_2, the other cannabinoid receptor that was first cloned from a human promyelocytic leukemia cell line (HL60). CB2 is most abundant in immune cells although low neuronal CB_2 expression has been reported in the brain. Two main endocannabinoids have been identified, N-arachidonoylethanolamine (AEA; anandamide) and 2-arachidonoyl-glycerol (2-AG).

Currently Approved Uses for Cannabinoid Drugs

Dronabinol

Dronabinol consists of isomerically pure, synthetic Δ^9-THC and is marketed under the trade name, Marinol. Dronabinol is approved in the United States and Europe for the treatment of anorexia in patients with human immunodeficiency virus (HIV) and refractory nausea and vomiting associated with cancer chemotherapy. In the United States, dronabinol is a Schedule III compound under the Controlled Substance Act. Dronabinol (Δ^9-THC) exerts pharmacodynamic effects on appetite and emesis through the activation of CB_1, while the effects on analgesia are mediated through action at both CB_1 and CB_2.

Nabiximols

Nabiximols is an extract of cannabis containing a 1:1 ratio of Δ^9-THC and cannabidiol (CBD) that is also known by the trade name Sativex. Sativex was developed by GW Pharmaceuticals and is administered as oromucosal spray that delivers 2.7 mg of Δ^9-THC and 2.5 mg of CBD per actuation. The presence of Δ^9-THC produces analgesia through the activation of both CB_1 and CB_2, while the presence of CBD may reduce adverse side effects of Δ^9-THC including psychoactivity. The mechanism of action through which CBD dampens side effects is not completely understood but may involve the ability of CBD to act as a negative allosteric modulator at CB_1. In the United States, Sativex is restricted as a Class I controlled substance. Sativex is approved for the treatment of muscle spasticity associated with multiple sclerosis (MS) in the United Kingdom (UK), Canada, and most countries of the European Union (EU). It is also approved in Canada for the treatment of cancer pain and neuropathic pain associated with MS.

Nabilone

Nabilone is a synthetic cannabinoid, marketed under the trade name Cesamet, that is a structurally and chemically similar to Δ^9-THC. Nabilone is scheduled as a Class II controlled substance in the United States where it has been approved by the FDA for the treatment of refractory nausea and vomiting caused by cancer chemotherapy. Similar to dronabinol, the pharmacodynamics effects of nabilone on emesis are likely mediated through the CB_1 receptor while off-label effects on analgesia are mediated through both CB_1 and CB_2.

Medical Marijuana

Medical marijuana, also known as cannabis, is the psychoactive, organic material derived from the *Cannabis sativa* plant. Medical marijuana is typically administered through the inhalation of combusted plant material as a cigarette or using an inhalation device such as a pipe. This mixture of inhaled compounds consists of terpenes and more than 60 cannabinoid drugs including psychoactive compounds such as Δ^9-THC, Δ^8-THC, and 11-hydroxy-tetrahydrocannabinol (11-OH-THC) and non-psychoactive cannabinoids such as CBD. Thus, this complex chemical composition of inhaled cannabis raises the possibility of an "entourage effect" for medical marijuana that is pharmacologically different than that of Δ^9-THC or CBD alone. In the United States, medical marijuana is heavily restricted as a Schedule I compound by the Controlled Substances Act. Although the distribution and possession of marijuana are illegal under federal law in the United States, it has been legalized by 29 states for a range of medical uses including, but not limited to, cancer, glaucoma, HIV, chronic pain, multiple sclerosis, seizures, inflammatory bowel disease, Crohn's disease, sickle cell anemia, cachexia or wasting syndrome, nausea, Parkinson's disease, and Alzheimer's disease. Due to the complicated mixture of compounds in inhaled cannabis, a complete understanding of its pharmacodynamic mechanism/s of action is difficult to fully assess. It is well known that most of the psychoactive effects of marijuana occur through the action of Δ^9-THC at CB_1. However, the analgesic effects of marijuana are likely mediated through the action of Δ^9-THC and/or other cannabinoids such as CBD at both cannabinoid receptors.

Efficacy of Cannabinoid Drugs for the Treatment of Chronic Pain

A recent meta-analysis examined the level of support from 79 clinical trials for a range of medical uses for different cannabinoid drugs including dronabinol (Δ^9-THC), Sativex, nabilone, and medical marijuana. This meta-analysis provided additional confirmation that cannabinoids are effective in the treatment of nausea and vomiting associated with cancer chemotherapy and wasting syndrome due to HIV. For chronic pain, meta-analysis found that the 37% of patients that exhibited a clinically relevant 30% or greater reduction in pain scores for the cannabinoid group was higher compared to 31% of patients in the placebo group (odds ratio of 1.41) (16). Meta-analysis also indicated an overall reduction in pain scores of −0.46 on a 0–10 point numerical rating scale for patients that were treated with cannabinoids versus placebo. This meta-analysis incorporated the results of eight randomized, placebo-controlled clinical trials, of which six of the eight trials were also double-blind. The clinical trials included in this meta-analysis evaluated the effect of Sativex (seven trials) and smoked medical marijuana (one trial) on several types of chronic pain including neuropathic pain, cancer pain, diabetic neuropathy, and HIV-associated neuropathy.

Adverse Effects Associated with Cannabinoid Drugs

A large number of randomized, double-blind, placebo-controlled clinical trials have investigated the efficacy of cannabinoid drugs for a range of medical conditions including different types of pain. Overall, these studies demonstrate a significant increase in the number of adverse events for patients treated with cannabinoids versus placebo. The percentage of patients that reported adverse events from 29 clinical trials was meta-analyzed by Whiting and colleagues. Overall, 81% of patients treated with cannabinoids reported an adverse event compared to 62% of patients in the placebo group (odds ratio 3.03). However, these adverse events were generally well tolerated and mild-moderate in severity with dizziness, intoxication, dry mouth, nausea, fatigue, somnolence, and gastrointestinal issues being the most commonly reported.

Biologics in the Treatment of Chronic Pain

Introduction

Over the last several decades, investigators have increasingly pointed to the activation of glial cells and the pro-inflammatory signaling cascades they initiate following nerve injury, rather than direct mechanical irritation or injury to the nerve itself, as the major precipitants of neuropathic pain. These processes are especially effective at ensuring the acute inflammatory response, thanks to redundant signaling pathways and positive feedback that collectively further perpetuate neuropathic and inflammatory pain. Given the complexity of these processes and the multitude of prospective targets for pain modulation, monoclonal antibodies have evolved as promising agents able to target mechanism-specific pathways. Among the molecular targets are (1) the pro-inflammatory signaling molecules, (2) their complementary cell surface receptors, and (3) a wide variety of downstream signaling pathways that mediate cell activation and the inflammatory response. The cost associated with development of biologics and administration of these regimens remains a barrier to clinical investigations and has made it difficult to justify prescribing such agents over conventional pain therapies.

Within the local microenvironment surrounding the site of injury, a number of signaling mediators are released. Pronociceptive factors including reactive oxygen species, potassium and hydrogen ions, adenosine triphosphate (ATP), and glutamate are released from the cytosol of the injured neuron, as well as from adjacent afferent nerves. These molecular mediators increase nearby afferent neurons' excitability, initiate glial cell activation, and propagate signaling cascades that cause pain sensitization. Sufficient repetitive noxious stimulation, as is experienced by patients with chronic pain conditions, reinforces long-term potentiation and hyperalgesia. Factors released by glial support cells can promote or decrease expression of receptors with pain-related pathways. Activated microglia can modulate spinal cord synaptic transmission by increasing the excitability of neurons and suppressing inhibitory synaptic transmission, leading to sensitization to pain signaling. Astrocytes regulate neuronal growth and synaptogenesis in developing nervous tissue and can augment long-term potentiation of pain.

TNF-α

Tumor necrosis factor-alpha (TNF-α) is produced de novo mainly by Schwann cells in peripheral nerves, satellite glial cells in the DRG, and microglia in the dorsal horn. This cytokine directly mediates the acute inflammatory response and has been isolated from peripheral nerves in patients with peripheral neuropathy. TNF-α enhances expression of voltage-gated sodium channels in nociceptive DRG neurons and can modulate synaptic plasticity by increasing expression of AMPA receptors. Several anti-TNF-α monoclonal antibodies (mAb) have been studied in phase II clinical studies; one open-label study with infliximab revealed promising results in treating sciatica, but subsequent randomized controlled trials failed to show benefits of systemic anti-TNF-α treatment for sciatica or discopathy. Another agent, etanercept, was shown to reduce pain in the treatment of sciatica, both via epidural and subcutaneous administration. When compared to intravenous infliximab in a study of rats with discopathy, epidural administration of etanercept led to earlier recovery from radiculopathy-related allodynia. A recent meta-analysis of efficacy and safety of etanercept for treating sciatica found this mAb to be superior to placebo at improving leg pain scores, and possibly better than steroids; however, etanercept was not found to be superior to placebo nor steroid treatment of back pain.

In spite of mixed results for pain control, the TNF-α/TNFR ligand/receptor superfamily remains a promising target for monoclonal antibodies since it has been implicated in somatic and neuropathic pain in animal models and human subjects. TNFR1 and TNFR2 are expressed in both peripheral nerves and DRG, and that expression was found to be upregulated in murine studies of Wallerian degeneration. TNFR1 predisposes neurons to excitotoxicity via glutamate release secondary to the activation of voltage-gated channels on microglia, ultimately promoting apoptosis via caspase signaling. On the contrary, TNFR2 was shown to play a neuroprotective role. An intra-sciatic injection of TNF-α in rats produced pain hypersensitivity that can be reversed with anti-TNFR1 antibodies. Recent work by Zeng et al. [28] found that both receptors are equally essential for development of neuropathic pain and its maintenance in an investigation of the impact of spare nerve injury on their expression in the red nucleus in rats. Both anti-TNFR1 and anti-TNFR2 monoclonal antibodies successfully produced an analgesic effect and have generated interest for future pain pathway-targeting biologics under development.

Nerve Growth Factor (NGF)

Nerve growth factor (NGF) is a neurotrophin expressed in developing an adult nervous tissue and has emerged as the most promising candidate for targeting by biologics. NGF promotes growth, differentiation, and survival of neurons during embryonic development, while in adults this factor promotes the survival and maintenance of sympathetic and sensory neurons. NGF is released in peripheral tissue in response to noxious stimuli stemming from the signaling cascades set in motion by pro-inflammatory cytokines and has been shown to play a role in both activation and sensitization of nociceptors. Not only does tissue injury cause NGF release but it also increases NGF synthesis. NGF binds to two classes of receptors: tropomyosin receptor kinase A (trkA) and the p75 neurotrophin receptor (p75NTR). Binding between NGF and the trkA receptor causes dimerization and autophosphorylation of the tyrosine residue of the cytoplasmic tail by adjacent trk receptors. The NGF-trkA complex is internalized and transported by the afferent neuron in retrograde fashion to the dorsal root ganglion. In the DRG, the NGF-trkA complex causes activation of downstream signaling pathways, including PI 3-kinase, Ras protein family, and phospholipase C. Depending on whether NGF and its precursor molecule proNGF bind the target receptor with high or low affinity, either axonal survival and growth or apoptosis will be promoted. High-affinity binding between proNGF, a membrane glycoprotein sortilin, and NGF receptor p75NTR can result in either survival or programmed cell death. NGF-trkA signaling also leads to transcriptional changes and central sensitization in the posterior horns. Binding trkA receptors on mast cells adjacent to the nociceptive neurons also causes the release of pro-inflammatory mediators such as histamine, 5-HT, and more of NGF, thus further amplifying inflammatory pain. TrkA receptors are selectively expressed by unmyelinated C-fibers. NGF-trkA signaling also leads to increased expression of the pronociceptive neurotransmitters substance P (SP), calcitonin gene-related peptide (CGRP), and BDNF, further predisposing to central sensitization.

Systemic injection of anti-NGF mAbs has been shown to reduce tactile allodynia and hyperalgesia in rodents. Clinical studies have shown significant dose-dependent hyperalgesia at the site of NGF injection. NGF levels are elevated in several forms of chronic pain, including neuropathic pain, cancer-related pain, and visceral pain. NGF levels and pain severity in patients with chemotherapy-induced peripheral neuropathy were found to be inversely correlated. A 2015 meta-analysis conducted by Schnitzer and Marks assessing several anti-NGF mAbs found these agents were superior to nonsteroidal anti-inflammatory or opioid regimens for pain control, and the three studies comparing tanezumab monotherapy to an active control (NSAID or opioid) also demonstrated superior efficacy. Although anti-NGF antibodies tanezumab and fulranumab effectively reduce pain, specifically in osteoarthritis and neuropathic pain, a scientometric assessment by Kissin [10] of pain-related molecular targets suggested that the cost of administering these agents was greater by an order of magnitude than that of conventional pain treatments.

Tanezumab is an anti-NGF monoclonal antibody developed by Pfizer. In 2010, the FDA halted all such agents' clinical trials as a result of reports of adverse events including joint degeneration and osteonecrosis requiring knee replacement surgery. Treatment-related adverse events were similar for all anti-NGF therapies, suggestive of a class-specific effect. More common side effects of anti-NGF therapy include peripheral edema, arthralgia, extremity pain, and peripheral neuropathy. Further work on tanezumab and fasinumab resumed after the FDA lifted its hold in March 2015, but development of other anti-NGF mAbs was halted by other manufacturers. Several placebo-controlled phase III studies involving tanezumab in patients with hip and/or knee OA show a reduction in pain at a variety of single doses ranging from 2.5 to 10 mg administered at 8-week intervals, although the likelihood of adverse events was lower in those patients given lower doses. Investigators concluded that tanezumab may have therapeutic utility in patients with OA who experience inadequate analgesia with NSAIDs. A multicenter investigation of knee and hip OA in 2700 subjects experiencing inadequate pain relief on a stable oral NSAID regimen received IV tanezumab 5 or 10 mg as monotherapy or in combination with NSAID compared to NSAID monotherapy. Tanezumab provided significant improvement in pain and function either as monotherapy or when combined with an NSAID vs NSAID monotherapy. As shown by Schnitzer and Marks [20], the frequency of adverse effects was higher in patients receiving tanezumab when compared to NSAIDs when these two medications were administered alone and was the highest in the combination therapy group. Importantly, incidence of OA requiring total joint replacement was similar in monotherapy with either tanezumab or an NSAID but was doubled when these medications were combined. A study by Sopata et al. [23] of 8-week interval administration of 10 mg IV tanezumab in patients with pain secondary to metastatic bone cancer showed that patients in a 40-week extension of the study had significantly decreased pain scores compared to baseline. A one-time 20 mg IV dose of tanezumab significantly reduced average pain scores at 4 weeks and 8 weeks after treatment in patients with diabetic neuropathy, according to Bramson et al. [1]. Miyagi et al. [18] showed improvement on gait analysis and suppression of CGRP expression in DRG of mice in response to intraperitoneal injection of anti-NGF antibody, suggesting decreasing pain signaling via this blockade could be achieved. Tanezumab has also shown promise in treatment of visceral pain; Evans et al. [5] showed that a single dose of tanezumab reduced chronic visceral pain in patients with interstitial cystitis, with significant reduction in pain scores assessed daily over a 6-week period. In contrast, a study of patients suffering from chronic prostatitis and pelvic pain syndrome performed by Nickel et al. [17] suggested this mAb elicited no significant pain reduction compared to placebo.

Several studies of patients with chronic low back pain administered a single dose of IV tanezumab have shown superior pain relief compared with naproxen and placebo. Phase II studies in patients with chronic mechanical low back pain receiving extended IV tanezumab therapy at 8-week intervals found that both 10 mg and 20 mg dosages exhibited efficacy in pain and physical function at 16 weeks, superior to both placebo and naproxen; at multiple intervals, patients reported improvements in pain from baseline, with slightly greater efficacy in the 20 mg group vs the 10 mg treatment group. Other anti-NGF mAbs such as fulranumab and fasinumab have demonstrated significant analgesia compared to placebo, with a low incidence of adverse effects, in patients with chronic knee and hip OA; however, few phase II studies in patients with chronic LBP have been undertaken with the antibodies fulranumab and fasinumab, and as such less data on adverse events is available.

Although most patients tolerated anti-NGF agents well, neurosensory symptoms occurred frequently, and some patients developed new or worsened peripheral neuropathies. However, the most problematic safety issue was rapidly destructive arthropathies, leading to joint replacement surgery. Some risk factors include receiving higher doses of anti-NGF mAbs, longer drug exposure, nonsteroidal anti-inflammatory drug (NSAID) use, and pre-existing subchondral insufficiency fractures. Low-dose anti-NGF mABs may exhibit a favorable risk-benefit ratio in selected patients with certain chronic pain conditions, especially symptomatic osteoarthritis.

Interleukins (IL)

Interleukins may facilitate pain transmission through coupling to neuronal glutamate receptors, but relatively few investigations of pain modulation have been completed to date. Canakinumab is an anti-IL1Beta-specific human monoclonal antibody approved by the FDA in 2009, at which time Novartis began to manufacture Ilaris® initially for a number of rare autoinflammatory conditions, and in May 2013 was approved for treatment of systemic juvenile idiopathic arthritis. In a 2014 Cochrane review of interleukin-1 inhibitors in treatment of acute gout, canakinumab was found to be superior to low-dose steroid but costs approximately 5000 times more. As with other biologics, this cost hurdle stifles development of this important subset of such agents.

Calcitonin Gene-Related Peptide (CGRP)

To date, no clinical studies to assess the effectiveness of biologics targeting calcitonin gene-related peptide (CGRP) for pain conditions have been completed, aside from preventive treatment of episodic migraine headaches [6]. CGRP is released from trigeminal nerve endings, trigeminal ganglia cells, and higher order neurons and promotes cerebrovascular and dural vasodilation. Moreover, CGRP affects nociceptive transmission by modulating the function of other neurotransmitters and, in the trigeminal ganglion, is often co-expressed with substance P and serotonin receptors. According to a 2017 meta-analysis including four studies of anti-CGRP mAbs conducted by Hong et al., these agents were found to be effective in preventive treatment of episodic migraine compared to baseline up to 9–12 weeks postinjection. The a-isoform of CGRP is more prevalent throughout the central and peripheral nervous systems and acts on calcitonin receptor-like receptor (CALCRL) linked to receptor activity-modifying protein 1 (RAMP1) receptors. CGRP is elevated in plasma, synovial fluid, and CSF in patients with musculoskeletal pain. A 2017 systematic review by Schou et al. revealed an association between measured CGRP levels and somatic, visceral, neuropathic, and inflammatory pain, in spite of a paucity of studies of the efficacy of monoclonal antibodies against CGRP receptor in non-headache pain conditions. Despite early evidence of efficacy of galcanezumab in several models of osteoarthritis-related pain, this high-affinity anti-CGRP monoclonal antibody failed to improve pain compared with placebo in a randomized clinical trial of galcanezumab in patients with osteoarthritis knee pain. CGRP mediates the release of inflammatory mediators from mast cells and as such may promote inflammatory pain in conditions including OA and chronic low back pain, although no consensus has been reached regarding its role in neuropathic pain.

Anti-epidermal Growth Factor Receptor Monoclonal Antibodies

Epidermal growth factor receptor (EGFR) is a member of the ErbB family of tyrosine kinase receptors. Given the role of this growth factor in promoting carcinoma progression and tumor growth, anti-EGFR antibodies' potential as analgesics was discovered in patients with chemotherapy-induced peripheral neuropathy, which improved with cetuximab treatment. In an open-label study of patients with neuropathic pain who were taking cetuximab, panitumumab, gefitinib, or erlotinib, Kersten et al. found pain relief was significant and rapid in onset with only mild hypersensitivity reactions such as skin rash seen. EGFR influences mitogen-activated protein kinase (MAPK) expression on the cell surface on astrocytes following nerve damage, as shown by Liu and Neufeld in 2007. A separate mechanism by which EGFR may produce pain is upregulation of expression of voltage-gated sodium channels, including Nav1.7. While EGFR can be targeted and thus prevent $Na_v1.7$ channel activation, direct targeting of voltage-gated channels has also been explored.

Conclusion

In the past decade, a number of exciting discoveries of new agents for the treatment of pain have been made. The tremendous toll on the US population by the opioid epidemic necessitates the need for agents that are lacking abuse potential or have a substantially smaller propensity for abuse. New agents acting on voltage-gated ion channels are undergoing phase II and III studies and hold a considerable promise. Advances in pain research have led to a better understanding of the role of inflammatory mediators, glial cells, and cytokines and neurotrophic factors in the development of chronic pain, which in turn resulted in discovery of target-specific monoclonal antibodies. With the dramatic changes caused by legalization of marijuana for medical use by the majority of states, thousands of patients gained access to THC and CBD preparations. However, the role of these substances in the treatment of pain conditions and their interaction with opioid and nonopioid analgesic are still emerging. One can be cautiously optimistic that in the next decade, the medical community will see new agents being added to the armamentarium for the treatment of pain. This is going to happen only if the "war on drugs" is accompanied by a simultaneous adequate funding by the government of research and development of new agents for the treatment of pain.

Recommended Reading

1. Bramson C, Herrmann DN, Carey W, Keller D, Brown MT, West CR, Verburg KM, Dyck PJ. Exploring the role of tanezumab as a novel treatment for the relief of neuropathic pain. Pain Med. 2015;16(6):1163–76.
2. Bullock CM, Kelly S. Calcitonin gene-related peptide receptor antagonists: beyond migraine pain--a possible analgesic strategy for osteoarthritis? Curr Pain Headache Rep. 2013;17(11):375. https://doi.org/10.1007/s11916-013-0375-2.
3. Chang DS, Hsu E, Hottinger DG, Cohen SP. Anti-nerve growth factor in pain management: current evidence. J Pain Res. 2016;9:373–83.
4. Empl M, Renaud S, Erne B, Fuhr P, Straube A, Schaeren-Wiemers N, Steck AJ. TNF-alpha expression in painful and nonpainful neuropathies. Neurology. 2001;56:1371–7.
5. Evans RJ, Moldwin RM, Cossons N, Darekar A, Mills IW, Scholfield D. Proof of concept trial of tanezumab for the treatment of symptoms associated with interstitial cystitis. J Urol. 2011;185(5):1716–21.
6. Gimbel JS, Kivitz AJ, Bramson C, et al. Long-term safety and effectiveness of tanezumab as treatment for chronic low back pain. Pain. 2014;155(9):1793–801.
7. Iyengar S, Ossipov MH, Johnson KW. The role of calcitonin gene-related peptide in peripheral and central pain mechanisms including migraine. Pain. 2017;158(4):543–59.
8. Jing S, Yang C, Zhang X, Wen S, Yuankui L. Efficacy and safety of etanercept in the treatment of sciatica: a systematic review and meta-analysis. J Clin Neurosci. 2017;44:69–74.
9. Kapural L, Kapural M, Bensitel T, et al. Opioid-sparing effect of intravenous outpatient ketamine infusions appears short-lived in chronic-pain patients with high opioid requirements. Pain Physician. 2010;13:389–94.
10. Kissin I. Scientometrics of drug discovery efforts: pain-related molecular targets. Drug Des Devel Ther. 2015;9:3393–404.
11. Knezevic NN, Yekkirala A, Yaksh TL. Basic/translational development of forthcoming opioid- and nonopioid-targeted pain therapeutics. Anesth Analg. 2017;125(5):1714–32. https://doi.org/10.1213/ANE.0000000000002442.
12. Langford RM, Mares J, Novotna A, Vachova M, Novakova I, Notcutt W, et al. A double-blind, randomized, placebo-controlled, parallel-group study of THC/CBD oromucosal spray in combination with the existing treatment regimen, in the relief of central neuropathic pain in patients with multiple sclerosis. J Neurol. 2013;260(4):984–97.
13. Leppert W. The role of methadone in cancer pain treatment—a review. Int J Clin Pract. 2009;63(7):1095–109.
14. Leung L, Cahill CM. TNF-alpha and neuropathic pain--a review. J Neuroinflammation. 2010;7:27.
15. Madariaga-Mazón A, Marmolejo-Valencia AF, Li Y, Toll L, Houghten RA, Martinez-Mayorga K. Mu-opioid receptor biased ligands: a safer and painless discovery of analgesics? Drug Discov Today. 2017;22(11):1719–29.
16. Mercadante S, Arcuri E, Tirelli W, Casuccio A. Analgesic effect of intravenous ketamine in cancer patients on morphine therapy: a randomized, controlled, double-blind, crossover, double-dose study. J Pain Symptom Manage. 2000;20:246–52.
17. Miyagi M, Ishikawa T, Kamoda H, Suzuki M, Inoue G, Sakuma Y, Oikawa Y, Orita S, Uchida K, Takahashi K, Takaso M, Ohtori S. Efficacy of nerve growth factor antibody in a knee osteoarthritis pain model in mice. BMC Musculoskelet Disord. 2017;18(1):428.
18. Nickel JC, Atkinson G, Krieger JN, et al. Preliminary assessment of safety and efficacy in proof-of-concept, randomized clinical trial of tanezumab for chronic prostatitis/chronic pelvic pain syndrome. Urology. 2012;80(5):1105–10.
19. Niesters M, Martini C, Dahan A. Ketamine for chronic pain: risks and benefits. Br J Clin Pharmacol. 2014;77:357–67.
20. Schnitzer TJ, Marks JA. A systematic review of the efficacy and general safety of antibodies to NGF in the treatment of OA of the hip or knee. Osteoarthr Cartil. 2015;23(Suppl 1):S8–S17.
21. Schou WS, Ashina S, Amin FM, Goadsby PJ, Ashina M. Calcitonin gene-related peptide and pain: a systematic review. J Headache Pain. 2017;18(1):34.
22. Selvarajah D, Gandhi R, Emery CJ, Tesfaye S. Randomized placebo-controlled double-blind clinical trial of cannabis-based medicinal product (Sativex) in painful diabetic neuropathy: depression is a major confounding factor. Diabetes Care. 2010;33(1):128–30.
23. Sopata M, Katz N, Carey W, et al. Efficacy and safety of tanezumab in the treatment of pain from bone metastases. Pain. 2015;156(9):1703–13.
24. Wen YR, Tan PH, Cheng JK, Liu YC, Ji RR. Microglia: a promising target for treating neuropathic and postoperative pain, and morphine tolerance. J Formos Med Assoc. 2011;110(8):487–94.
25. Whiting PF, Wolff RF, Deshpande S, Di Nisio M, Duffy S, Hernandez AV, et al. Cannabinoids for medical use: a systematic review and meta-analysis. JAMA. 2015;313(24):2456–73.
26. Yeh JF, Akinci A, Al Shaker M, Chang MH, Danilov A, Guileen R, Johnson K, Kim YC, El-Shafei A, Skljarevski V, Duenas H, Tassanawipas W. Monoclonal antibodies for chronic pain: a practical review of mechanisms and clinical applications. Mol Pain. 2017;13:174480691774023.
27. Zamponi GW, Striessnig J, Koschak A, Dolphin AC. The physiology, pathology, and pharmacology of voltage-gated calcium channels and their future therapeutic potential. Pharmacol Rev. 2015;67(4):821–70. https://doi.org/10.1124/pr.114.009654.
28. Zeng XY, Zhang Q, Wang J, Yu J, Han SP, Wang JY. Distinct role of tumor necrosis factor receptor subtypes 1 and 2 in the red nucleus in the development of neuropathic pain. Neurosci Lett. 2014;569:43–8.

Injectable Corticosteroids

26

Devang Padalia, Neal Shah, Jaspreet Singh, Navdeep Jassal, Corey Reeves, and Randall P. Brewer

Introduction

Corticosteroids are endogenous regulatory hormones produced in the adrenal glands that have achieved prominence in the treatment of many acute and chronic inflammatory conditions and endocrinologic disorders. The two main classes are mineralocorticoids (e.g., aldosterone) and glucocorticoids (e.g., cortisol), which are both regulated by the hypothalamic-pituitary-adrenal axis. Mineralocorticoids help regulate water and electrolyte balance, whereas glucocorticoids play a prominent role in the regulation of physiologic stress, metabolic homeostasis, and immunologic function. It is the anti-inflammatory and analgesic properties of glucocorticoids that are the focus of use in pain management.

Once glucocorticoids are injected into the body, they move to the cell cytoplasm and bind to specific receptors to form a steroid-receptor complex. This complex then interacts with DNA to alter the transcription of messenger RNA (mRNA). Ultimately this leads to an increased production of a specific glycoprotein called lipocortin I, also known as annexin A1 (AA1). AA1 blocks the release of arachidonic acid, the precursor of prostaglandins and leukotrienes, from phospholipids by inhibiting of the activity of phospholipase A2. In addition to blocking this inflammatory pathway, glucocorticoids also act at the level of the cyclooxygenase (COX) enzyme to further decrease prostaglandin production. Prostaglandins play a role in both sensitizing neurons to pain and being pro-inflammatory (Fig. 26.1). Furthermore, glucocorticoids enhance analgesia by dilution and dispersion of pro-inflammatory compounds, direct analgesic effects on pain fibers, and osmolality alterations which can benefit nerve function.

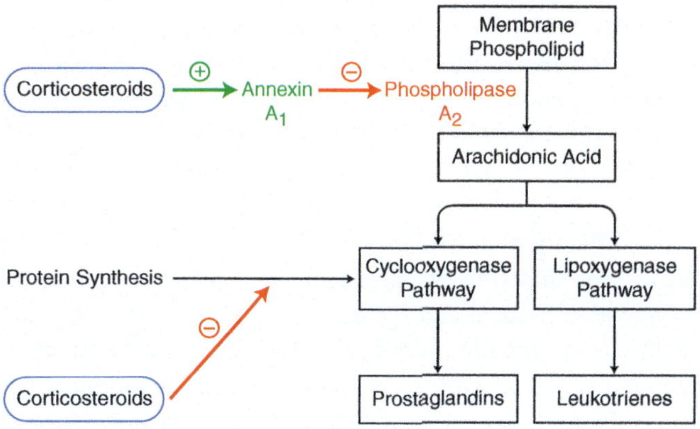

Fig. 26.1 Mechanism of action of corticosteroids

The adverse effects of corticosteroids must also be considered prior to their therapeutic use. The most common local adverse effect of corticosteroid injections is postinjection pain that develops within hours and can last 2 or 3 days. Other local adverse effects include subcutaneous fat atrophy, skin depigmentation, and soft tissue calcification. Systemic adverse events include the inhibition of bone healing, tendon rupture, hyperglycemic effects in diabetic patients, and articular hyaline cartilage damage. Suppression of the hypothalamic-pituitary-adrenal axis may occur, even following a single dose of injected corticosteroids. Repeated systemic exposure to corticosteroids can result in corticosteroid dependency, which, upon cessation of steroid administration, leads to corticosteroid withdrawal symptoms. Contraindications to injectable corticosteroids include significant hyperglycemia, poorly controlled hypertension, history of untoward psychiatric effects,

D. Padalia (✉) · N. Shah
Interventional Pain Department, Moffitt Cancer Center, University of South Florida, Tampa, FL, USA
e-mail: devang.padalia@moffitt.org; neal.a.shah@moffitt.org

J. Singh · N. Jassal
Department of Neurology, University of South Florida, Tampa, FL, USA

C. Reeves
Department of Physical Medicine and Rehabilitation, University of South Florida, Tampa, FL, USA

R. P. Brewer
Department of Neurology and Anesthesiology, Louisiana State University, Shreveport, LA, USA
e-mail: brewer.randall@duke.edu

T. R. Deer et al. (eds.), *Deer's Treatment of Pain*, https://doi.org/10.1007/978-3-030-12281-2_26

infection or fracture at the site of intended administration, and ligamentous instability.

Background and Historical Perspective

Cortisone was discovered in the 1940s by Mayo Clinic researchers, Edward Kendall, Ph.D., and Philip Hench, M.D. The drug was first used to treat rheumatoid arthritis, where it was hailed as a miracle drug. In 1950, the researchers were awarded the Nobel Prize in Medicine for the discovery. Over the ensuing decades, the observed potent anti-inflammatory effects in a variety of medical conditions resulted in the vast expansion of cortisone in the treatment of inflammatory conditions. As experience with the drug increased, the occurrence of severe systemic side effects became acknowledged as a result of chronic steroid treatment, with the ensuing utilization of shortened courses or "bursts" of steroid treatments. Local application of corticosteroids also emerged as a primary strategy to locally "control" inflammation while limiting systemic exposures to the drug. The injection of corticosteroids into joints, muscles, connective tissues, and the spinal structures for pain relief gained widespread acceptance as a means to treat both nociceptive and neuropathic spinal pain as well as joint and tissue inflammation. In particular, over the past few decades, there has been widespread use of steroid injections for the treatment of nociceptive articular and neuropathic radicular pain arising from the degenerative disorders of the zygapophysial joints and intervertebral discs. However, after repeated exposure to injectable corticosteroids, the occurrence of systemic side effects was also observed, prompting clinicians to carefully consider the frequency and accumulated dosing of injectable corticosteroids for painful conditions. More recently there have been questions raised as to both the safety and efficacy of injectable corticosteroids in inflammatory conditions. Factors which have directed increased attention to the relative value of injections include rises in healthcare costs and the rare occurrences of serious adverse events related to spinal injections, particularly the potentially fatal complications of brainstem and spinal ischemia and meningitis.

Prednisolone is a synthetic glucocorticoid from which the most commonly used injectable corticosteroids are derived. The six most commonly used steroids include methylprednisolone acetate (MA), triamcinolone acetonide (TA), triamcinolone hexacetonide (TH), betamethasone sodium phosphate (BSP), betamethasone acetate (BA), and dexamethasone sodium phosphate (DSP). Depending on the formulation, these medications can be either water soluble or insoluble. Those with acetate or acetonide formulations, such as TH, MA, TA and BA, have low solubility and therefore can form particles in solution. This causes a slower release time at the site of injection and is believed to result in prolonged anti-inflammatory effects. Those with a salt preparation, including BSP and DSP, are freely water-soluble compounds which allows for a rapid uptake into their site of action. DSP is considered the only widely used non-particulate steroid for injection. Each corticosteroid has a unique set of properties, with particles of differing size, water solubility, tendency to aggregate, and potency. (See Table 26.1, Fig. 26.2).

Lacking clear evidence to guide corticosteroid selection for therapeutic injections, providers generally base the decision of which corticosteroid to utilize on a combination of clinical experience and personal preference. Intra-articular corticosteroids reduce synovial blood flow, decrease joint fluid immune cells and modulators, and reduce collagen synthesis. Branched esterification further reduces solubility, allowing steroids to remain at the injection site longer. Clinically, insoluble steroids have a longer duration of action and a higher incidence of cutaneous side effects. TH is the least soluble of the commonly used injectable steroids, followed by TA.

Table 26.1 Properties of injectable corticosteroids

Corticosteroid	Dexamethasone sodium phosphate	Triamcinolone acetate and triamcinolone hexacetonide	Betamethasone sodium phosphate and betamethasone acetate compound	Methylprednisolone acetate
Particulate or non-particulate	Non-particulate	Particulate	Particulate/non-particulate	Particulate
Particles >10 μm (%)	0	29	39	40
Maximum particle size (μm)	0.5	>500	500	>500
Aggregation	None	Extensive	Some	Few
Anti-inflammatory Potency[a]	25	5	25	5
Injectable dose range (mg)	4–16	40–80	6–12	40–80

Comparisons of most commonly used injectable corticosteroids by physicochemical properties, potency, and dose equivalency
[a]Corticosteroid potency relative to the potency cortisol (standard of 1)

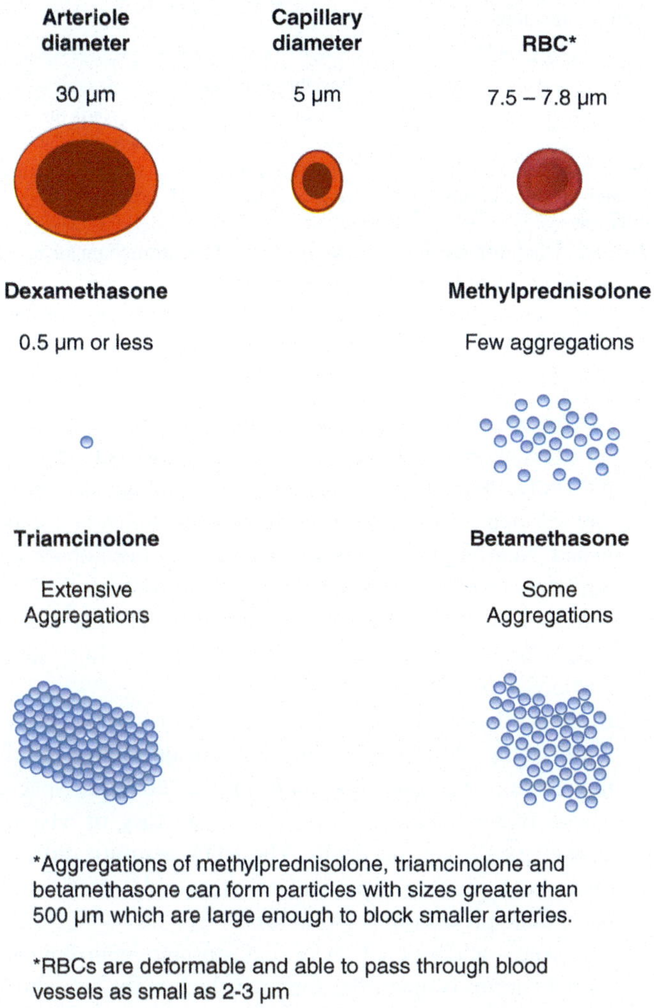

Fig. 26.2 Comparison of vessel size with corticosteroid particle size

For intra-articular injections, MA is the most commonly used steroid, followed by TH and TA. BA, with high solubility, shorter duration of action, fewer cutaneous side effects, is commonly utilized for soft tissue injections.

Most Common Uses of Injectable Corticosteroids in Pain Management:

1. Osteoarthritis (intra-articular: zygapophysial, shoulder, knee, sacroiliac, hip)
2. Inflammatory arthritides (rheumatoid arthritis, crystalline arthritis, spondyloarthritis syndromes)
3. Perineural spinal injections: caudal, interlaminar, and transforaminal epidural steroid injections
4. Peripheral nerve blockade and entrapment (occipital nerve block, carpal tunnel syndrome)
5. Sympathetic nerve blocks (cervical, thoracic, lumbar)
6. Connective tissue inflammation: tendinitis, synovitis, bursitis, and fasciitis
7. Muscle trigger points
8. Ganglion cysts and neuromas

Evidence for Efficacy

Readers are referred to chapters dedicated to specific conditions for a full review of the efficacy related to the wide variety of conditions in which the utilization of injectable corticosteroids exists. Here, we will briefly summarize the data regarding the utilization of injectable corticosteroids for epidural spinal injections, where the predominance of controversy exists over the selection and route of epidural administration, and review musculoskeletal indications.

Epidural injections. A recent systematic review of the efficacy of particulate versus non-particulate corticosteroids in epidural injections was completed. The results were as follows:

1. Systematic review of three different studies showed no statistical difference between the two preparations in cervical transforaminal epidural steroid injections (TFESI) in terms of pain reduction on visual analog scale (VAS). Particulate steroids could cause vascular obstruction, and therefore the authors recommended the use of non-particulate steroid for cervical TFESI (Table 26.2).
2. In patients with lumbar radiculopathy due to stenosis or disk herniation, systematic review of four different studies showed TFESI using particulate or non-particulate is equivocal in reducing pain and improving function. Particulate steroids could cause vascular obstruction, and therefore the authors recommended the use of non-particulate steroid for lumbar TFESI.
3. Because there is only one study comparing particulate versus non-particulate in lumbar interlaminar epidural steroid injection (ILESI), there is insufficient information to make a recommendation of one steroid over the other in lumbar ILESI.

A meta-analysis and systematic review showed the current evidence on optimal procedure-related variables as follows:

1. Steroid dosage: Individual randomized controlled trials found that increasing steroid doses for ESI did not show a correlation in benefits.
2. Number of ESI treatments: In systematic reviews, there was no evidence that a series of ESI was any more effective that just one injection.
3. Injection technique: A systematic review of caudal, interlaminar, and transforaminal ESI showed no specific injection technique improved back pain over another technique. There was a statistically significant short-term reduction in leg pain with caudal ESI as well as long-term leg pain with TFESI. There was also a statistically significant reduction in short-term disability with caudal ESI, but not for ILESI or TFESI.

Table 26.2 Recommendations on particulate vs non-particulate epidural steroid injections

Type of ESI studied	# of studies reviewed	Interventions	Results	Recommendations
Cervical TFESI	3	Dexamethasone vs triamcinolone	No statistical difference on VAS	Use of non-particulate steroids due to possible spinal cord ischemia
Lumbar TFESI	4	Dexamethasone vs betamethasone and/or dexamethasone vs triamcinolone	All were equivocal in reducing pain and improving function	Use of non-particulate steroids due to possible spinal cord ischemia
Lumbar ILESI	1	Dexamethasone vs methylprednisolone	No significant difference in mean pain between steroids	Not enough information to make a recommendation

Summary of studies of injectable corticosteroids for epidural administration. For illustrative purposes and not a complete representation of all data
TFESI transforaminal epidural steroid injection, *ILESI* interlaminar epidural steroid injection

4. Volume of injectate: There are currently no consensus guidelines on the ideal volume to administer during ESI.

Pearls and Pitfalls

- Unlike TA, BA, and MA injectable suspensions, DSP is considered a non-particulate medication. For this reason, DSP is less likely to cause arterial or capillary obstruction if inadvertently injected into a vertebral or radicular artery. (See Fig. 26.2).
- Due to the 19 reported cases of spinal cord infarction after the administration of particulate steroid in lumbar TFESI, the use of non-particulate steroid is recommended for these procedures.
- Since 2002, there have been at least 13 reported cases of spinal cord ischemia and posterior circulation infarction after cervical TFESI. Specifically, reports on spinal cord ischemia after transforaminal injections have raised concerns about the potential for embolization of particulate corticosteroids during the procedure. No serious complications have been cited that were caused by the injection of a non-particulate steroid.
- Safeguards, such as fluoroscopy with contrast and digital subtraction imaging, can be implemented to reduce intravascular complications from injectable corticosteroids.
- When performing a TFESI, one must consider the potential complication resulting from damage to the largest anterior segmental medullary artery, known as the artery of Adamkiewicz. This vessel enters the spinal canal through an intervertebral foramen and supplies the lower two-thirds of the spinal cord via the anterior spinal artery. It typically enters on the left from T8-L1 but can enter on either side from T5-L4. Damage or blockage of this structure can cause anterior spinal artery syndrome which can lead to impaired motor function, as well as urinary and fecal incontinence.
- Some commercially available corticosteroid formulations contain other compounds, including preservatives (benzyl alcohol) and a drug vehicle (polyethylene glycol). Neurotoxic effects such as demyelination, neural degeneration, and paraplegia have been associated with benzyl alcohol. Polyethylene glycol is considered biologically inert, and no neurotoxic effects have been definitively established. Neurologic complications have only been observed with the *intrathecal* administration of corticosteroids.
- Single-dose vials of DSP are currently the only available "preservative-free" preparations of injectable corticosteroids
- In 2014, the US Food and Drug Administration (FDA) required the addition of a warning to the drug labels of all injectable corticosteroids used in the epidural space. These include adverse events such as loss of vision, stroke, paralysis, and death. The FDA warning did not distinguish between particulate (insoluble) and non-particulate preparations (soluble).
- The true incidence of these catastrophic neurological complications is unknown due to the lack of the large prospective studies that would provide accurate numerator (all adverse events) and denominator (total epidural injections performed) data. The FDA also stated that the effectiveness and safety of epidural corticosteroid injections were not established in the treatment of spinal disorders. Because corticosteroids are not approved in epidural injections, their injection represents off-label use.

Musculoskeletal Injections: Review of Evidence for Efficacy

1. Trigger points are common musculoskeletal conditions that have been traditionally treated with injectable corticosteroids. Recent data suggests local anesthetic alone, or dry needling without an injectate may be equally effective methods of treating myofascial trigger points. Pain at the site of injection is highest with dry needling.
2. Moderate to strong evidence suggests short-term benefit of injectable corticosteroids in DeQuervain synovitis, adhesive capsulitis, carpal tunnel syndrome, greater trochanteric bursitis, lateral epicondylitis, trigger finger, and osteoarthritis of the knee and hip.

3. Evidence for long-term benefit is weak for most musculoskeletal conditions. The strongest evidence (fair to moderate) exists for osteoarthritis of the hip, greater trochanteric bursitis, and adhesive capsulitis.
4. Evidence is weak for benefits of corticosteroid injections for subacromial impingement and osteoarthritis of the wrist and hand.
5. Injections for osteoarthritis of the hip and knee suggest good evidence for short-term benefit.

Pearls and Pitfalls: Musculoskeletal Corticosteroid Injections

- Injections early in the course of treatment tend to have the most favorable results.
- Patients wishing to delay joint replacement surgery of the hip or knee may benefit from corticosteroid injections.
- Results of musculoskeletal injections are improved when combined with physical therapy measures aimed to simultaneously address musculoskeletal deficits, such as range of motion, stretching, joint manipulation, and targeted strengthening.
- Particulate or "depot" corticosteroids such as TA, TH, and MP may have improved efficacy, with lower relative vascular risk compared to perispinal injections, in intra-articular musculoskeletal injections.
- Steroid injections can weaken tendons and ligaments, so extreme caution must be utilized when deciding to start or repeat injections in high-risk locations.

Injectable Corticosteroids: Safety Concerns

The primary rationale for the utilization of injected corticosteroids is for the delivery of maximal anti-inflammatory effect to the area of inflammation and pain while minimizing systemic exposure to the drugs. Long-standing knowledge exists regarding the potential side effects associated with the systemic utilization of corticosteroids. In certain patient populations, or in normal individuals undergoing high-dose or frequent injections, significant systemic side effects may occur and result in serious medical complications. Table 26.3 summarizes the most common systemic steroid side effects and provides information regarding side effect prevention.

Table 26.3 Adverse events associated with corticosteroids

Adverse event	Risks	Preventive strategies
Hyperglycemia	Metabolic syndrome, diabetes mellitus	Lowest effective corticosteroid dose Dietary restrictions during steroid therapy Adjust diabetic medications following procedure
Infection	Immunocompromised status	Consider tuberculosis screening, antifungal therapy in predisposed individuals, vaccinations (influenza, pneumococcal)
Impaired tissue repair/wound healing	Recent trauma or surgery	Avoid corticosteroid injections for 4–6 weeks
Gastrointestinal mucosal ulceration	Peptic ulcer disease, nonsteroidal anti-inflammatory therapy, aspirin	Concomitant preventive therapy with antihistamine or proton pump inhibitor
Osteoporosis	Osteoporosis risk factors, deconditioning, debilitated status, metabolic bone disease	Bone densitometry monitoring, calcium, vitamin D, osteoporosis treatment, weight-bearing exercise
Weight gain	Obesity, concomitant obesogenic medications (antidepressants, anticonvulsants)	Dietary consultation for obese patients, limit doses and frequency of injections, exercise
Insomnia	History of insomnia, concomitant psychostimulant or caffeine use	Sleep hygiene counseling, avoid stimulants for 1–2 weeks following injection, sleep aids
Psychological adverse events	Psychotic disorders, anxiety, depression, bipolar disorder	Thorough psychological history, limit doses and frequency of injections, collaborative psychological/psychiatric care
Hypertension	Poorly controlled hypertension, latent essential hypertension	Dietary sodium management, antihypertensive dose adjustments for 1–2 weeks following injection
Fluid retention	Pre-existing edema, renal insufficiency, cardiac disease, chronic venous stasis	Dietary sodium management, consider diuretic dose adjustments for 1–2 weeks following injection
Ophthalmologic adverse events (glaucoma, cataracts)	Elderly, chronic steroid use	Regular ophthalmologic exams
Atherosclerosis	Hypertension, hyperlipidemia, smoking, diabetes	Risk factor management, smoking cessation, aerobic exercise
Osteonecrosis (avascular necrosis)	High dose or chronic steroid exposure, metabolic bone disease, debilitated status	Avoid high doses, prolonged exposure, high-level attention to new-onset groin pain
Steroid-induced myopathy (acute and chronic)	High dose or chronic steroid exposure, elderly, debilitated, cancer, concomitant myopathic medications (e.g., omeprazole, statins)	Avoid high dose, prolonged exposure, exercise, avoid concomitant myopathic medications during steroid treatment

Adverse events and systemic side effects associated with injectable corticosteroids

Pearls and Pitfalls: Safety of Injectable Corticosteroids

- Always ask patients regarding their prior personal history with corticosteroid exposure regarding adverse events.
- Corticosteroid "allergies" are exceptionally rare.
- Limit corticosteroid dosage to the minimal effective dose for each patient.
- Check serum blood glucose prior to injection in all diabetics.
- Consider alternative treatments in patients who are "pre-diabetic" and poorly controlled diabetics and ensure diabetic patients closely monitor glucose levels during any treatment with corticosteroids.
- Poor diabetic control worsens outcomes in chronic pain treatments; ensure that diabetic control is unaffected by injected corticosteroid treatment by collaborating with diabetes treatment provider.
- Always advise patients of potential corticosteroid side effects prior to injection.
- Review bone densitometry results in high-risk patient populations prior to injection.
- Avoid high-dose injections in patients with poorly controlled hypertension and decompensated congestive heart failure.
- Carefully record adverse events that occur related to the corticosteroid dose and duration of event.
- Avoid corticosteroid injections in patients with a recent or new infection that is not being treated with antimicrobial therapy.
- In patient with pre-existing psychotic and mood disorders, avoid corticosteroid injections if there is a history of severe, steroid-related psychiatric complications.
- Closely monitor body mass index in overweight and obese patients undergoing regular corticosteroid injections for chronic pain conditions.
- One in 300 patients will develop a serious adverse event following a corticosteroid injection severe enough to require hospitalization.
- A daily dose of more than 8 mg of systemic prednisone was associated with a dose-related, linear increase in all-cause and cardiovascular mortality in a long-term study of rheumatoid arthritis patients.

Recommended Reading

1. Bateman BT, Brenner GJ. An important step forward in the safe use of epidural steroid injections. Anesthesiology. 2015;122:964–6.
2. Benzon HT, et al. Comparison of the particle sizes of different steroids and the effect of dilution: a review of the relative neurotoxicities of the steroids. Anesthesiology. 2007;106(2):331–8.
3. Craig DB, Habib GG. Flaccid paraparesis following obstetrical epidural anesthesia: possible role of benzyl alcohol. Anesth Analg. 977(56):219–21.
4. Denis I, Claveau G, Filiatrault M. Randomized double-blind controlled trial comparing the effectiveness of lumbar transforaminal epidural injections of particulate and nonparticulate corticosteroids for lumbosacral radicular pain. Pain Med. 2015;16:1697–708.
5. Derby R, Lee SH, Date ES, Lee JH, Lee CH. Size and aggregation of corticosteroids used for epidural injections. Pain Med. 2008;9(2):227–34.
6. Dreyfuss P, Baker R, Bogduk N. Comparative effectiveness of cervical transforaminal injections with particulate and nonparticulate corticosteroid preparations for cervical radicular pain. Pain Med. 2006;7:237–42.
7. El-Yahchouchi CE, Geske J, Carter RE. The noninferiority of the nonparticulate steroid dexamethasone vs the particulate steroids betamethasone and triamcinolone in lumbar transforaminal epidural steroid injections. Pain Med. 2013;14:1650–7.
8. Foster Z, Voss T, Hatch J, Drimodig A. Corticosteroid injections for common musculoskeletal conditions. Am Fam Physician. 2015;92:694–9.
9. Freire V, Bureau NJ. Injectable corticosteroids: take precautions and use caution. Semin Musculoskelet Radiol. 2016;20:401–8.
10. Jüni P, Hari R, Rutjes AWS, Fischer R, Silletta MG, Reichenbach S, da Costa BR. Intra-articular corticosteroid for knee osteoarthritis. Cochrane Database Syst Rev. 2015;10:CD005328. https://doi.org/10.1002/14651858.CD005328.pub3.
11. Kennedy DJ, Plastaras C, Casey E. Comparative effectiveness of lumbar transforaminal epidural steroid injections with particulate versus nonparticulate corticosteroids for lumbar radicular pain due to intervertebral disc herniation: a prospective, randomized, double-blind trial. Pain Med. 2014;15:548–55.
12. Kim D, Brown J. Efficacy and safety of lumbar epidural dexamethasone versus methylprednisolone in the treatment of lumbar radiculopathy: a comparison of soluble versus particulate steroids. Clin J Pain. 2011;27:518–22.
13. Lee JW, Park KW, Chung SK. Cervical transforaminal epidural steroid injection for the management of cervical radiculopathy: a comparative study of particulate verse non-particulate steroids. Skelet Radiol. 2009;38:1077–82.
14. MacMahon PJ, Eustace SJ, Kavanagh EC. Injectable corticosteroid and local anesthetic preparations: a review for radiologists. Radiology. 2009;252(3):647–61.
15. MacMahon PJ, Huang AJ, Palmer WE. Spine injectables: what is the safest cocktail? AJR. 2016;207:526–33.
16. Manchikanti L. Role of neuraxial steroids in interventional pain management. Pain Physician. 2002;5:182–99.
17. Mehta P, Syrop I, Singh JR, Kirschner J. Systematic review of the efficacy of particulate versus nonparticulate corticosteroids in epidural injections. PMRJ. 2017;9(5):502–12. https://doi.org/10.1016/j.pmrj.2016.11.008.
18. Park CH, Lee SH, Kim B. Comparison of the effectiveness of lumbar transforaminal epidural injection with particulate and nonparticulate corticosteroids in lumbar radiating pain. Pain Med. 2010;11:1654–8.
19. Pinto RZ, Maher CG, Ferreira ML, et al. Epidural corticosteroid injections in the management of sciatica: a systematic review and meta-analysis. Ann Intern Med. 2012;157(12):865–77.
20. Rincon I, Battafarano D, Restrepo J, Erikson J, Escalante A. Glucocorticoid dose thresholds associated with all-cause and cardiovascular mortality in rheumatoid arthritis. Arthritis Rheumatol. 2014;66:264–72.
21. Shakir A, Ma V, Mehta B. Comparison of pain score reduction using triamcinolone vs. dexamethasone in cervical transforaminal epidural steroid injections. Am J Phys Med Rehabil. 2013;92:768–75.
22. Shamliyan TA, Bart Staal J, Goldmann D, Sands-Lincoln M. Epidural steroid injections for radicular lumbosacral pain: a systematic review. Phys Med Rehabil Clin N Am. 2014;25:471–89.
23. U.S. Food and Drug Administration (FDA). FDA drug safety communication: FDA requires label changes to warn of rare but serious neurologic problems after epidural corticosteroid injections for pain. FDA Website. www.fda.gov/Drugs/DrugSafety/ucm394280.htm. Published April 23, 2014. Accessed 13 May 2016.

Topical Therapies

27

Devang Padalia, Neal Shah, Jaspreet Singh, Samia Malik, Osama Hafez, and Randall P. Brewer

Introduction

Topical analgesics are an integral but often overlooked component of the multimodal approach to pain management. This diverse group of medications is used in the treatment of a variety of acute and chronic pain conditions. These agents are applied to the skin overlying a painful area and may exert their effects on receptors on nociceptive sensory nerve endings, regionally circulating immune cells and keratinocytes. The term "topical" analgesic must always be distinguished from the term "transdermal" which entails the systemic delivery of a drug utilizing a transdermal mechanism. The utilization of topical medications has benefits which include a reduction in adverse events associated with higher systemic levels of the drug and drug-drug interactions. However, there can be variability in the penetration and absorption of topical analgesics arising from the components of the topical formulation and the individual's variability in skin absorption. Conversely, depending upon the drug administered, dose, and individual characteristics, central nervous system and/or systemic effects are possible with the utilization of "topical analgesics." For ostensibly adequate concentrations of the drugs to reach target peripheral receptors, penetration of the outer layer of the skin requires lipophilic, hydrophilic, and low-molecular-weight properties, which is facilitated via various "vehicles" with an "oil-in-water" base to provide maximum skin penetration and target tissue delivery.

This therapy is most frequently used in the management of pain arising from acute soft tissue injuries, chronic musculoskeletal pain and peripheral neuropathic pain syndromes. The utilization of topical analgesics is limited to the pain syndromes with regional or limited somatic distribution, and the use of topical analgesics with large areas of involvement such as widespread musculoskeletal pain, diffuse myofascial pain, and central neuropathic pain is not warranted.

Background and Historical Perspective

Historical references to the use of naturally occurring substances applied topically to provide analgesia exist from some of the earliest recordings of human medicine. Menthol, a popular component of over-the-counter topical analgesics, was used to impart a cool sensation over irritated skin, and mandrake root extract was used to relieve joint and muscle pain. In modern medicine, the mode of action of some ancient remedies has been elucidated. Primary nociceptive sensory afferent neurons can be activated by a range of inflammatory mediators released during tissue injury or inflammation, which include substance P, prostaglandins, bradykinin, adenosine triphosphate (ATP), histamine, and serotonin. These neurons also express a variety of inhibitory receptors including opioid, alpha-adrenergic, cholinergic, and adenosine. These pathways of activation and inhibition represent the hypothetical mechanisms for effective clinical use of the drugs and are targets for future drug development. Figure 27.1 demonstrates the cellular and molecular targets most often cited in the utilization of molecular targets in the treatment of inflammatory and neuropathic pain.

D. Padalia (✉) · N. Shah
Interventional Pain Department, Moffitt Cancer Center, University of South Florida, Tampa, FL, USA
e-mail: devang.padalia@moffitt.org; neal.a.shah@moffitt.org

J. Singh · S. Malik
Department of Neurology, University of South Florida, Tampa, FL, USA

O. Hafez
Department of Anesthesiology, Moffitt Cancer Center, University of South Florida, Tampa, FL, USA
e-mail: osama.hafez@moffitt.org

R. P. Brewer
Department of Neurology and Anesthesiology, Louisiana State University, Shreveport, LA, USA
e-mail: brewer.randall@duke.edu

T. R. Deer et al. (eds.), *Deer's Treatment of Pain*, https://doi.org/10.1007/978-3-030-12281-2_27

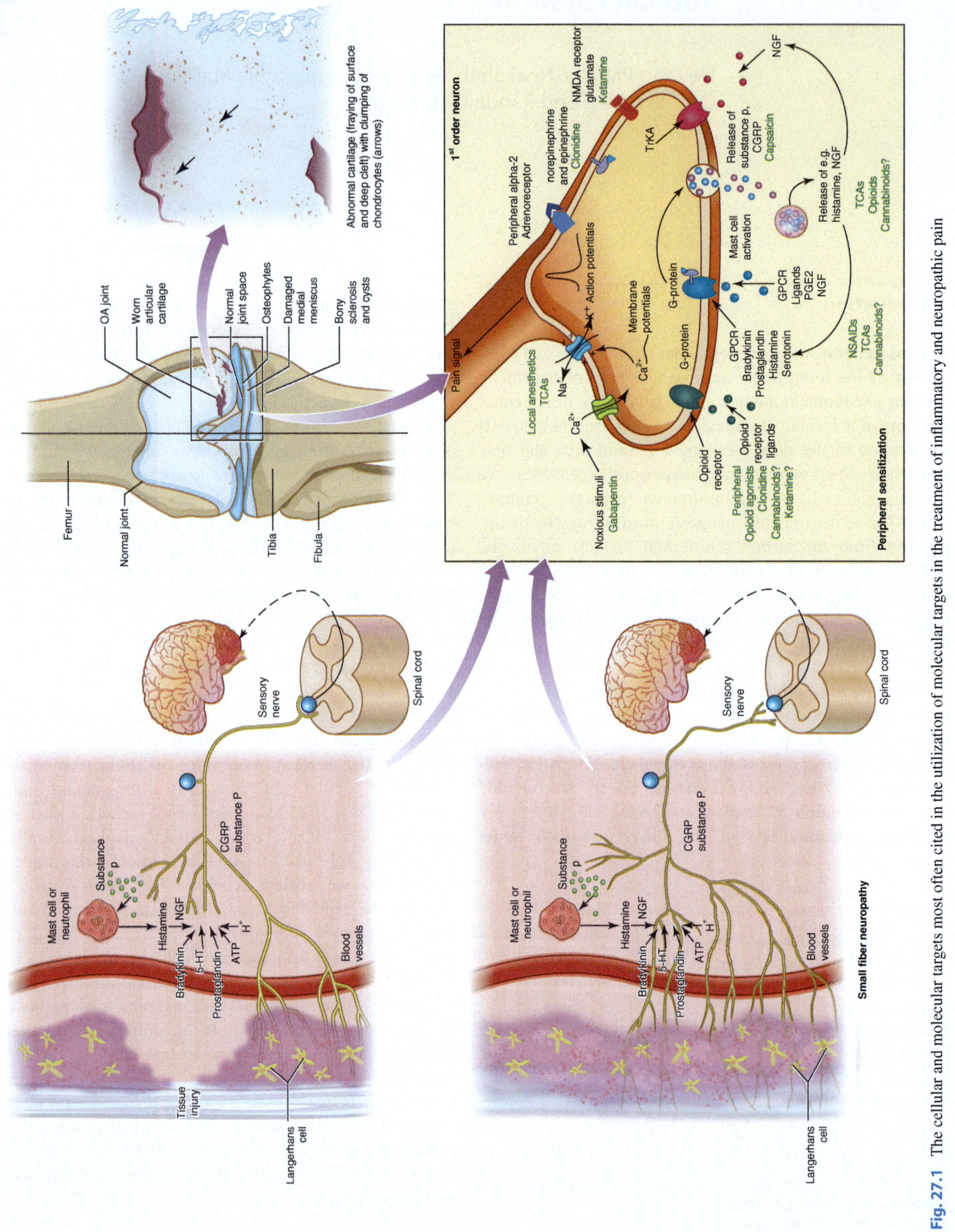

Fig. 27.1 The cellular and molecular targets most often cited in the utilization of molecular targets in the treatment of inflammatory and neuropathic pain

Uses of Topical Analgesics in Pain Management

1. Peripheral neuropathic pain (e.g., post-herpetic neuralgia, Morton's neuroma, diabetic peripheral neuropathy, scar-related pain)
2. Chronic musculoskeletal pain (osteoarthritis, rheumatoid arthritis)
3. Acute pain: soft tissue injuries (sprains, strains, and tendonitis)
4. Dermal anesthesia for venipuncture, lumbar puncture, intramuscular injection, and circumcision

Drugs Utilized as Topical Analgesics

Topical analgesics available to patients and providers can be broadly classified into one of the three following categories:

1. Over-the-counter topical analgesics – minimum standards of safety and efficacy must be met for consumer targeted symptom management, indicated for short-term symptomatic use with broad indications.
2. Prescription drugs – rigorous process of drug development demonstrating safety and efficacy to achieve FDA approval for specific indications.
3. Compounded pharmaceuticals – FDA-approved drugs repurposed through utilizing compounding pharmacy principles for manufacturing and delivering. As drugs have already gained FDA approval, the base chemicals are not required to undergo re-evaluation for new indications under the scope of compounding pharmacy practice.

Indicated above, the term "topical analgesic" can apply to a wide variety of drugs, each of which may enter into a pain management treatment regimen through vastly different pathways of development, approval, and marketing. Table 27.1 summarizes the evidence of various agents utilized as TA. The following section will describe the drugs, by class, that are available for utilization as topical analgesics.

Capsaicinoids

Capsaicin is a natural vanilloid derived from the capsicum plant and acts as a vanilloid receptor subtype 1 (*t*ransient *r*eceptor *p*otential cation channel subfamily *V* – TRPV1) receptor agonist. Topical capsaicin binds to TRPV1 receptors on the cutaneous fibers of sensory A-delta C neurons and causes release of substance P and calcitonin gene-related peptide (CGRP). Chronic exposure to capsaicin is hypothesized to result in the depletion of substance P in C fibers, reducing peripheral sensitization and long-term elevations in nociceptive thresholds. Reports of benefit for the utilization of capsaicin include the treatment of pain associated with diabetic peripheral neuropathy (DPN), post-herpetic neuralgia (PHN), and fibromyalgia. Positive results have been demonstrated in randomized studies with capsaicin cream in patients with osteoarthritis (OA), fibromyalgia, and chronic non-specific back pain; and some guidelines recommend 0.025% capsaicin as first-line therapy in the treatment of pain associated with OA. The concentration of capsaicin used in clinical studies has varied from 0.025% to an 8% patch (see Table 27.1). Topical capsaicin is present in a variety of over-the-counter topical analgesic preparations in

Table 27.1 Summary of studies using topical analgesics

Agent	Author	# Participants	Concentration	Type of pain	Duration	Results
Capsaicin	Derry et al. (2013) [10] (literature review)	1272 (Total)	8% patch (single dose)	PHN	12 weeks	NNT – 7 for much or very much improvement
	Casanueva et al. (2013) [8]	130	0.075%	Fibromyalgia	6 weeks	28% reduction in pain
	Kulkantrakor et al. (2013) [20]	33	0.025%	DN	8 weeks	No statistical difference
NSAIDs	Jousselin (2003) [17]	134	1.3% Diclofenac patch	Minor ankle sprain	7 days	Significant pain reduction
Lidocaine	Ho et al. (2008) [16]	35	5%	DN, PHN	1 week	Statistically reduced pain
	Katz et al. (2002) [18]	332	5% patch	PHN	1 week	66% of patients improved
Gabapentin	Boardman et al. (2008) [5]	51	2%–6%	Vulvodynia	8 weeks	65% reduction in pain
Ketamine	Quan, et al. (2003) [24]	23	0.5%	PHN	Varied	Significant pain reduction
	Maloney et al. (2012) [21]	17	5%	DN	4 weeks	No statistical difference
Amitriptyline	Ho et al. (2008) [16]	35	5%	PHN, DN	1 week	No statistical difference
Clonidine	Campbell et al. (2012) [6]	344	0.1%	DN	12 weeks	41% reduction
4% Amitriptyline, 1% baclofen, 2% ketamine	Barton et al. (2011) [4]	208	–	CIPN	4 weeks	Statistically reduced pain

NNT number needed to treat, *DN* diabetic neuropathy, *PHN* post-herpetic neuralgia, *CIPN* chemotherapy-induced peripheral neuropathy low concentrations (0.025–0.1%) for use in the "temporary relief" of a variety of painful musculoskeletal conditions. The 8% capsaicin patch is approved by the Food and Drug Administration (FDA) for the treatment of post-herpetic neuralgia. A phase IV open-label 52-week study of the 8% capsaicin patch in patients with peripheral neuropathic pain conditions such as HIV polyneuropathy, PHN, and post-traumatic/postsurgical nerve injury reported acceptable levels of tolerability, sustained albeit modest improvements in pain, and variable alterations of sensory function with long-term administration of the high-dose preparation. Adverse events are experienced in one-third of patients and include its known effects related to substance P release: erythema, itching, stinging, and burning upon application. Adverse events associated with high-dose capsaicin 8% included moderate transient burning, papules, swelling, and dryness. Rare, but serious, skin reactions have been reported. The number needed to treat (NNT), for a 50% reduction in pain scores, for capsaicin in musculoskeletal pain was 8.1, and for neuropathic pain, the NNT was 5.7. In summary, capsaicin has demonstrated efficacy in OA and PHN, and reports of benefit in other musculoskeletal and neuropathic conditions warrant consideration in treatment refractory chronic pain conditions associated with regional distributions.

Nonsteroidal Anti-inflammatory Drugs (NSAIDs)

NSAIDs are widely used for their analgesic and anti-inflammatory effects. Their primary mechanism of action is inhibition of the enzyme cyclooxygenase (COX)1 and 2, which leads to a decrease in prostaglandin production. This decrease leads to a reduction in tissue inflammation and reduced sensitization of peripheral nociceptive neurons. Plasma concentrations typically range only from 5% to 15% of that observed after systemic administration. Reduced systemic levels of the drugs are believed to result in lower risks of the major adverse events associated with systemic NSAIDs: gastrointestinal toxicity, elevated risks for cardiovascular events and stroke, and renal toxicity. Additionally, reduced systemic concentrations also have the potential to limit the antiplatelet effects of systemic NSAID administration and therefore clinically significant hemorrhagic events. Compared with oral administration, topical NSAID administration leads to higher drug concentrations in the dermis and, variably, equivalent or higher concentrations in muscle. Variable concentrations have been detected in cartilage, ligament, and tendon tissue. The synovium, which is highly vascular, and synovial fluid concentrations are less reliably elevated with topical administration versus systemic administration. It is likely that a number of factors unique to drug formulations and individual patient characteristics influence the concentration and distribution of NSAID and other topical analgesics in target tissue. Topical NSAID treatment is commonly used for joint pain (osteoarthritis and rheumatoid arthritis), soft tissue injuries (sprains, strains, and tendonitis), and peripheral neuropathic pain. Diclofenac is the most commonly used topical NSAID which is available in a compounded form as well as a topical 1.3% patch. This patch has shown efficacy in reducing acute musculoskeletal pain secondary to minor strains and sprains. The 1% topical diclofenac gel demonstrated efficacy in OA of small and medium joints, and the 1.5% and 2% topical diclofenac solution demonstrated efficacy in OA of the knee. The 1.5% and 2% solutions are noted to have the addition of the solvent dimethyl sulfoxide (DMSO), an antioxidant and anti-inflammatory agent, which enhances the delivery of diclofenac into tissue following topical administration. Trolamine salicylate 10%, an over-the-counter NSAID preparation, has a long history of availability and has shown efficacy in a randomized, placebo-controlled study of OA of the hands. Methyl salicylate, another over-the-counter ingredient that has both counterirritation and salicylate properties, has demonstrated benefit in randomized double-blind trials, particularly in acute pain. Adverse effects of topical NSAIDs are typically limited to local skin rashes and pruritus, although the prescribing information includes the warnings of adverse events associated with the NSAID drug class. It is important to note that long-term data pertaining to topical therapies, including NSAIDs, is limited, especially in the elderly and other patient populations with multiple co-morbidities, such that the safety, tolerability, and efficacy of therapy should be routinely assessed during the course of therapy.

Specific Conditions

1. Acute pain: Topical NSAIDs are recommended for acute soft tissue injuries for up to 2 weeks, with the advantage of limited risk of systemic adverse effects as compared to systemic NSAIDs, particularly gastrointestinal toxicity. Equivalent analgesic efficacy has been shown with topical diclofenac, ibuprofen, ketoprofen, and piroxicam. The NNT (50% pain reduction), for all topical NSAIDs combined vs. placebo was 4.5 for treatment periods of 6–14 days.
2. OA and tendinitis: Topical NSAIDs are recommended for up to 12 weeks in treatment of pain associated with OA and tendinitis, especially in treatment areas considered amenable to topical therapy. These areas include OA of the hands, elbows, wrists, ankles, and knee. In the long-term studies for OA of the low back, neck, hip, and shoulder, there is insufficient evidence to recommend topical NSAIDs.

Local Anesthetics (LA)

LA reversibly block nerve conduction by decreasing the permeability of the nerve cell membrane to sodium ions, also commonly described as "sodium channel blockers." LA bind to the intracellular "inactivation gate" within the cytoplasm of axons, prolonging the duration of sodium channel reactivation and action potential propagation. This results in a decreased depolarization rate and an increase in the excitability threshold of nociceptive sensory neurons. Neurons with hyperexcitability, with reduced thresholds to stimulation, such as following tissue injury or inflammation, have been shown to be preferentially blocked by LA. LA block small fibers that mediate pain and temperature sensation at lower concentrations than required for the blockade of "large" fibers, neurons that transmit joint and position sensation, muscle contraction, and proprioception. The primary goal in the use of LA in the management of a painful condition is to provide a sufficient "therapeutic" concentration of LA at the site of pain that will reduce pain and without functional impairment. These agents have been used to reduce pain prior to venipuncture, for myofascial trigger points, and to suppress abnormal nociceptor activity. The important distinction between the agents available topically which contain local anesthetic is the extent to which the formulation preserves, or suppresses, dermal sensitivity. The most commonly used local anesthetic is lidocaine which is available as an over-the-counter product in both cream and gel form. Other common prescription topical agents include compounded bupivacaine, a 5% lidocaine patch, a eutectic mixture of local anesthetics (EMLA) with a combination of prilocaine 2.5% and lidocaine 2.5%, and a patch containing equal amounts of lidocaine and tetracaine. Over-the-counter topical lidocaine is available in a 4% patch and various topical formulations.

The lidocaine 5% patch has shown benefit for patients suffering from post-herpetic neuralgia, and the lidocaine 5% gel has been used to reduce pain from HIV-associated distal symmetric polyneuropathy. EMLA has been successfully used for dermal analgesia for venipuncture, intramuscular injection, and circumcision, and the drug reduced acute and chronic pain in patients undergoing breast cancer surgery. Studies of EMLA in PHN have demonstrated favorable results in nonrandomized studies, whereas a randomized, controlled study failed to show efficacy over placebo. The mixture of local anesthetics in this agent decreases its melting point and is therefore well absorbed into the dermis. Its use in chronic pain is limited secondary to the risk of prilocaine-induced methemoglobinemia and effects upon skin sensation. There are ongoing studies with the use of a variety of topical local anesthetics in the treatment of myofascial pain as well as shoulder impingement syndrome.

NMDA Receptor Antagonists: Ketamine

The analgesic pathways of ketamine are not completely understood but seem to be through a variety of mechanisms. One major pathway is the prevention of central sensitization in the dorsal horn of the spinal cord via its noncompetitive N-methyl-D-aspartate (NMDA) receptor antagonism. It has also been shown to attenuate hyperalgesia by blocking calcium and sodium channels as well as inhibiting the production of nitric oxide, which is a neurotransmitter involved in pain perception. As a topical agent, ketamine has been evaluated in the peripheral neuropathic pain syndromes DPN, PHN, and complex regional pain syndrome (CRPS). Studies have utilized concentrations ranging from 0.5% to 10% ketamine with and without other agents. The lack of control subjects, routine serum testing, combination with other drugs, and small sample sizes contribute to the lack of consensus regarding the efficacy of topical ketamine.

Alpha-2 Agonists: Clonidine

Clonidine is an alpha-2 adrenergic receptor agonist which is mostly commonly used as an antihypertensive. It exerts its analgesic effects via receptors that are found throughout the central nervous system as well as on sensory neurons in the epidermis. Activation of these receptors leads to a downregulation of adenylate cyclase and the second messenger system which is involved in maintaining the abnormal excitability of nociceptors. The peripheral analgesic action of clonidine may be related to alpha-2 adrenoreceptor modulation of the peripheral opioid system. The therapeutic use of epidural and intrathecal clonidine administration, while effective as an analgesic, has been limited by side effects, predominantly hypotension. Topical 0.1% clonidine demonstrated analgesic benefit in patients with DPN in a placebo-controlled study. No significant absorption was noted and cardiovascular parameters remained unchanged with treatment. The drug has also demonstrated to relieve hyperalgesia in patients with sympathetically maintained pain.

Muscle Relaxants: Baclofen

The target of topical baclofen is specifically the gamma-amino butyric acid B ($GABA_B$) receptors found on peripheral C fibers and keratinocytes, through action on peripheral potassium channels. Baclofen monotherapy is rarely used but is more often applied as a compounded mixture with other topical medications and demonstrated benefit in combination with amitriptyline for vulvodynia. Compounded topical baclofen 5% showed benefit in neuropathic pain associated with chemotherapy. Although some results are favorable, more studies in this area are needed. Cyclobenzaprine is a central-acting muscle relaxant that is closely related to antidepressants. It is used in a topical concentration of 1–2% in patients with musculoskeletal and neuropathic pain. Currently there is no favorable data for its use as a topical agent.

Antidepressants

The two most commonly used topical tricyclic antidepressants are amitriptyline and doxepin. The actions of tricyclic antidepressants in the periphery include actions on sodium channels with local anesthetic properties, antihistaminergic, anticholinergic, and adrenergic contributing to putative mechanisms that may contribute to a peripheral mode of action when administered topically. These agents have been used for the treatment of a variety of painful neuropathic conditions, including PHN, DPN, and CRPS. The literature generally shows that higher concentrations of amitriptyline 5–10% were more likely to be successful in reducing pain than that of lower concentrations. In one study, 10% amitriptyline was associated with systemic side effects such as slower cognition and difficulty concentrating suggesting systemic absorption may be an integral component to analgesia. In a randomized peripheral neuropathic pain study, 3.3% topical doxepin was as efficacious as a combination of 3.3% doxepin and 0.075% capsaicin and superior to placebo. Doxepin 5%, available as a topical cream, is indicated for the treatment of pruritus. Amitriptyline, in various combinations with ketamine, capsaicin, and lidocaine, has shown some effectiveness in reducing peripheral neuropathic pain, proctodynia, and pain associated with radiation-induced dermatitis.

Table 27.2 summarizes the topical analgesics that have been approved for specific indications by the FDA.

Table 27.2 FDA-approved topical analgesics

Drug	Indication	Dosage	Brand name
Diclofenac sodium 1% gel	Osteoarthritis of joints amenable to topical treatment ("not evaluated for spine, hip, or shoulder")	2 (upper extremities) or 4 g (lower extremities) up to four times daily, total dose should not exceed 32 g per day	Voltaren Gel®
Diclofenac 1.3% patch	Topical treatment of acute pain due to minor strains, sprains, and contusions	One patch twice daily (180 mg diclofenac epolamine)	Flector®
Diclofenac sodium topical solution *1.5%*	Signs and symptoms of osteoarthritis of the knee(s)	16.05 mg/ml dropper, 40 drops to each knee four times daily	Pennsaid® (generic available)
Diclofenac sodium topical solution 2%	Signs and symptoms of osteoarthritis of the knee(s)	20 mg of diclofenac per 1 g of solution per actuation 2 actuations (40 mg) either into the hand and then onto the knee or directly to the knee twice daily	Pennsaid®
Lidocaine 5% patch	Pain associated with post-herpetic neuralgia	Maximum of 3 patches; up to 12 hours within a 24-hour period	Lidoderm® (generics available)
Capsaicin 8% patch	Management of neuropathic pain associated with post-herpetic neuralgia	Up to four patches for 60 minutes and repeat every 3 months or as warranted by the return of pain (not more frequently than every 3 months)	Qutenza®

Compounded Topical Analgesics

The use of compounded topical analgesics consisting of two or more agents has become increasingly popular. This is likely secondary to provider preference for using multimodal approaches to treat pain as well as the increased ease of obtaining these medications from compounding pharmacies. They are usually made in a gel or cream form which consists of a base that allows for maximal penetration through the lipophilic stratum corneum and the hydrophilic epidermis. These medications have been used to treat somatic, neuropathic, and even central pain syndromes. Although most data on the use of compounded agents is from case reports and retrospective studies, there has been some evidence of benefit for neuropathic facial pain, vulvodynia and chemotherapy-induced peripheral neuropathy. While these studies mostly focused on the combination of two or three drugs, there are providers who prescribe a combination of many more therapeutic agents. One popular formulation consists of ketamine 10%, diclofenac 1%, baclofen 2%, bupivacaine 1%, clonidine 0.2%, cyclobenzaprine 2%, gabapentin 6%, and pentoxifylline 3%. It is important to consider that the purpose of using a "compounded" medication is to address symptoms or disorders that require patient-specific alterations of medications not available through routine delivery systems. In December 2006, the FDA issued a warning to the compounding pharmacy industry regarding the wide-scale distribution of topical anesthetic rather than being developed for individual patients – particularly high-potency local anesthetics applied to large surface areas for extended periods of time. Even though there are some favorable studies using combination therapy, further research in this area is needed.

Gabapentin

The analgesic mechanism of action of gabapentinoids is the result of antagonism at the α2δ-1 subunit of voltage-gated calcium ion channels of sensory neurons. Topical concentrations are typically around 5–6% and have been used in the treatment of neuropathic pain. In a retrospective study, topical gabapentin was shown to provide significant pain relief in vulvodynia. Additionally, it possesses minimal adverse effects compared with those of systemic gabapentin.

Pentoxifylline

Pentoxifylline is phosphodiesterase inhibitor with various therapeutic effects, such as decreasing inflammation and increasing blood flow. It has been shown to be beneficial in a number of dermatological conditions but is only FDA approved for the treatment of intermittent claudication. Topical concentrations of 3–6% have been used in the treatment of a variety of conditions including osteoarthritis and neuropathic pain. There is no clear evidence for its use in these conditions.

Cannabinoids

Cannabinoids have attracted immense attention as potential analgesics, whose effects act through at least two receptors: (1) the cannabinoid-1 (CB-1) receptor, predominantly expressed in the central nervous system, and (2) the cannabinoid-2 (CB-2) receptor, predominantly expressed on cells of the immune system. Inhibition of inflammatory hyperalgesia by activation of both peripheral CB1 and CB2 cannabinoid receptors in preclinical models suggests a potential role for topical peripheral cannabinoid administration. With the widespread use of cannabinoids in a variety of pain conditions with reports of mixed results from the various potential modes of administration, it is anticipated that future randomized, controlled trials will clarify the role of cannabinoids in the treatment of painful conditions.

Opioids

Peripheral opioid receptors are abundant and proliferate on nociceptors in areas of inflammation via cellular immune responses, allowing endogenous opioid peptide release to modulate nociception and inflammation. Thus, the peripheral opioid system is an attractive target for analgesic development. Efficacy of topical morphine in the management of chronic OA-related pain has been reported; however, the presence of morphine metabolites in the urine raises doubts regarding a true peripheral mode of action in the study. Topical morphine is effective in skin ulcer-related pain in conditions such as calciphylaxis and scleroderma. The peripheral mu opioid agonist, loperamide, which does not cross the blood-brain barrier, has been successfully utilized in oral pain in the transplant setting of graft-versus-host disease. The preclinical development of peripheral opioid receptor agonists, particularly agents with limited ability for central nervous system penetration, holds the potential to retain many of the benefits of opioid therapy while limiting the adverse events associated with systemic use.

Over-the-Counter Topical Analgesics

A wide variety of topical analgesics are available without a prescription, sold to consumers "over the counter" (OTC). Generally, OTC topical agents are used, according to FDA labeling requirements, for the "temporary relief of minor pain" due to a variety of acute pain conditions, particular "muscle and joint aches, strains, and sprains." Common OTC topical agents have a combination of agents that produce superficial vasodilation via rubefacients, including camphor, menthol, benzoin resin, methyl salicylate (component of wintergreen), rapidly evaporating solvents such as alcohol and acetone, and an aromatic effect that creates a sensation of warmth that is intensified during the application process (e.g., "heat rubs"). Typically, a pharmacologically active component is added to the mixture, such as salicylates, capsaicin, and lidocaine. Clinical trial evidence suggests that the efficacy of topical OTC agents is stronger for acute pain than chronic pain and that the therapeutic effect is likely due to counterirritation effects versus a primary pharmacological mode of action. Single-agent preparations of lidocaine and capsaicin are available, and odor-free products are becoming increasingly popular that accommodate routine use. A variety of delivery methods are available which include patches creams, gels, foams, sticks, sprays and roll-ons.

Pearls and Pitfalls

- Some of the advantages of using a topical analgesics over oral analgesics are as follows:
  A. Local application directly over painful areas
  B. Fast onset of action
  C. Higher concentration of analgesic in the pain area
  D. Low or no systemic drug levels
  E. Reduction of systemic side effects
  F. Reduction of drug-drug interactions
  G. Ease of implementing in multimodal therapies
  H. Ease of combining more analgesics in one vehicle to obtain synergies

I. Improvement of compliance
J. Decreased risk of dependency or abuse

- Some of the limitations are as follows:
  A. Topical agents must have appropriate molecular size (small molecules) and physiochemical properties (aqueous/lipid solubility) for dermal and tissue preparation.
  B. Skin permeability may vary in the presence of tissue enzymes that metabolize drugs.
  C. Disease state may alter dermal absorption.
  D. Local skin reactions may occur in response to the drug or vehicle.
  E. Systemic side effects may occur with topical analgesics when associated with excessive use or when used in combination with factors that may increase absorption (such as concurrent use of heat, application to damaged skin, or with an occlusive dressing)
- Although site reactions are common with some topical preparations, they are generally mild, transient, and well tolerated.
- In the United States, ketamine is considered a controlled substance; therefore caution should be taken when prescribing this treatment as it does have abuse potential.
- Compounded drugs are not reviewed by FDA for safety and efficacy and are not FDA approved for specific indications. This means they do not have the standard warnings that accompany traditional drug labels. Compounded drugs may have a higher risk of adverse events compared to FDA-approved drugs, especially when not utilized with medical supervision. In particular, topical local anesthetics and NSAIDs can expose patients to significant systemic toxicity, even potentially fatal outcomes, when not utilized appropriately.
- Newer guidelines released by the American College of Rheumatology (ACR) recommend the use of topical NSAIDs, rather than oral NSAIDs, for the treatment of patients with hand or knee OA, who are aged >/= 75 years and have not responded to first-line acetaminophen treatment.
- There is supportive evidence for the use of topical NSAIDSs in the treatment of acute soft tissue injuries and chronic joint pain. Evidence also supports the use of capsaicin in PHN and lidocaine in the treatment of PDN and PHN. Other topical analgesics show poor or limited evidence to support their use in acute and chronic pain conditions.

Recommended Reading

1. Anitescu M, Benzon HT, Argoff CE. Advances in topical analgesics. Curr Opin Anaesthesiol. 2013;26(5):555–61.
2. Argoff CE. Topical analgesics in the management of acute and chronic pain. Mayo Clin Proc. 2013;88(2):195–205.
3. Arnstein PM. The future of topical analgesics. Postgrad Med. 2013;125(4 Suppl 1):34–41.
4. Barton DL, Wos EJ, Qin R, et al. A double-blind, placebo controlled trial of a topical treatment for chemotherapy-induced peripheral neuropathy: NCCTG trial N06CA. Support Care Cancer. 2011;19(6):833–41.
5. Boardman LA, Cooper AS, Blais LR, et al. Topical gabapentin in the treatment of localized and generalized vulvodynia. Obstet Gynecol. 2008;112(3):579–85.
6. Campbell CM, Kipnes MS, Stouch BC, et al. Randomized control trial of topical clonidine for treatment of painful diabetic neuropathy. Pain. 2012;153:1815–23.
7. Casale R, Symeonidou Z, Bartolo M. Topical treatments for localized neuropathic pain. Curr Pain Headache Rep. 2017;21(3):15.
8. Cassanueva B, Rodero B, Quintial C, et al. Short-term efficacy of topical capsaicin therapy in severely affected fibromyalgia patients. Rheumatol Int. 2013;33(10):2665–70.
9. Cline AE, Turrentine JE. Compounded topical analgesics for chronic pain. Dermatitis. 2016;27(5):263–71.
10. Derry S, Sven-Rice A, Cole P, Tan T, Moore RA. Topical capsaicin (high concentration) for chronic neuropathic pain in adults. Cochrane Database Syst Rev. 2013;2:CD007393.
11. Derry S, Moore R, Gaskell H, McIntyre M, Wiffen PJ. Topical nonsteroidal anti-inflammatory drugs for acute musculoskeletal pain in adults.Cochrane Database Syst Rev. 2015;6:CD007402.
12. Elikottil J, Gupta P, Gupta K. The analgesic potential of cannabinoids. J Opioid Manag. 2009;5(6):341–57.
13. Finch PM, Drummond PD. Topical treatment in pain medicine: from ancient remedies to modern usage. Pain Manag. 2015;5(5):359.
14. Flores MP, de Castro APC R, JDS N. Topical analgesics. Rev Bras Anestesiol. 2012;62(2):244–52.
15. Gálvez R, Navez ML, Moyle G, et al. Capsaicin 8% patch repeat treatment in nondiabetic peripheral neuropathic pain: a 52-week, open-label, single-arm, safety study. Clin J Pain. 2017;33(10):921–31.
16. Ho KY, Huh BK, White WD, Yeh CC, Miller EJ. Topical amitriptyline versus lidocaine in the treatment of neuropathic pain. Clin J Pain. 2008;24(1):51–5.
17. Joussellin É. Flector Tissugel® in the treatment of painful ankle sprain [in French]. J Traumatol Sport. 2003;20:1S5–9.
18. Katz NP, Gammaitoni AR, Davis MW, Dworkin RH. Lidocaine patch 5% reduces pain intensity and interference with quality of life in patients with postherpetic neuralgia: an effectiveness trial. Pain Med. 2002;3(4):324–32.
19. Keppel Hesselink JM, Kopsky DJ, Stahl SM. Bottlenecks in the development of topical analgesics: molecular, formulation, dose-finding, and phase III design. J Pain Res. 2017;10:635–6411.
20. Kulkantrakorn K, Lorsuwansiri C. Sensory profile and its impact on quality of life in patients with painful diabetic polyneuropathy. J Neurosci Rural Pract. 2013;4(3):267–70.
21. Mahoney JM, Vardaxis V, Moore JL, et al. Topical ketamine cream in the treatment of painful diabetic neuropathy a randomized, placebo-controlled, double-blind initial study. J Am Podiatr Med Assoc. 2012;102:178–83.
22. Massey T, Derry S, Moore RA, McQuay HJ. Topical NSAIDs for acute pain in adults. Cochrane Database Syst Rev. 2010. https://doi.org/10.1002/14651858.CD007402.pub2.
23. Peppin JF, Albrecht PJ, Argoff C, Gustorff B, et al. Skin matters: a review of topical treatments for chronic pain. Part two: treatments and applications. Pain Ther. 2015;4(1):33–50.
24. Quan D, Wellish M, Gilden DH. Topical ketamine treatment of postherpetic neuralgia. Neurology. 2003;60(8):1391–2.
25. Sawynok J. Topical analgesics for neuropathic pain in the elderly: current and future prospects. Drugs Aging. 2014;31(12):853–62.
26. Sawynok J. Topical and peripheral ketamine as an analgesic. Anesth Analg. 2014;119(1):170–8.
27. Sawynok J. Topical analgesics for neuropathic pain: preclinical exploration, clinical validation, future development. Eur J Pain. 2014;18(4):465–81.

Opioids for Chronic Non-cancer Pain

28

Jason E. Pope and Timothy R. Deer

Introduction

Chronic pain affects 100 million patients in the United States, creating a significant healthcare burden and public health concern. Moreover, past opioid medication treatments that were commonplace are now outside the scope of practice and considered significant practice deviations. How did the chronic pain space contribute to opioid prescribing and the current opioid epidemic? It began with a letter to the editor.

Historical Perspective

In a letter to the editor, retrospectively inspecting X,000 charts over an ill-defined timeline for various hospital admissions, the author noted that the "challenges with opioid abuse potential was low, as only 4 people were identified." As discussed in numerous analyses since, this letter to the editor was misquoted and served as one of the catalysts to suggest opioid therapy could be used as chronic, ongoing treatment with little risk or harm.

Once accepted falsely as fact, opioid-based therapy became more assessable. Events that propagated the treatment included:

1. Overwhelmed primary care offices
2. Pain declared by the Clinton Administration as the 5th vital sign
3. Pharmaceutical companies beginning to formulate tamper-resistant medications and long-acting formulations
4. Hospital credentialing and status based on positive feedback, specifically asking about pain treatment
5. Slow payer adoption of evidence-based refractory pain treatment options
6. Poor data sharing regarding prescription filling and prescribing doctors

A study in JAMA indicated that despite the medical decision to justify increasing opioid-based medications for patients in an effort to promote health activity, and well-being, so too did their morbidity and mortality. In March of 2016, the Center for Disease Control (CDC) elected to place a guidance document to help providers reduce or eliminate opioid prescribing for non-cancer pain, with limits of 50 morphine equivalents per day for non-cancer-related pain. Compliance testing is recommended and is reviewed in detail in another chapter. Compliance testing includes urine drug testing with available ranges of specificity and sensitivity, at varying testing intervals based on risk stratification. Current guidance includes prescribing no more than every 30 days, with face-to-face encounters, evaluating for analgesia, activities of daily living, adverse side effects, and aberrant drug-seeking behavior.

Before initiating or maintaining opioid-based therapy for chronic pain, non-pharmacologic strategies need to be employed. These include physical therapy and its ancillary treatments (massage ultrasound, etc.) and pharmacologic strategies that are not opioid related (neuropathic pain medication, nonsteroidal anti-inflammatory drugs). Treatment goals are required and focused on function. Vigilance is also necessary, including pharmacy board reporting review and compliance testing.

The CDC published guidance for clinicians on prescribing as follows: start low, go slow, begin with short-acting medications, and prescribe no more than needed (quantity and dose) and no more than typically 50 MME (morphine milligram equivalents). If dosing exceeds 50 MME to 90 MME, careful individual risks versus benefits need to be weighed. Greater than 90 MME needs to be avoided or carefully justified (Table 28.1).

J. E. Pope (✉)
Evolve Restorative Center, Santa Rosa, CA, USA

T. R. Deer
The Spine and Nerve Center of the Virginias, Charleston, WV, USA

T. R. Deer et al. (eds.), *Deer's Treatment of Pain*, https://doi.org/10.1007/978-3-030-12281-2_28

Table 28.1 CDC recommendations

1	Opioid is not the first-line therapy
2	Establish goals for pain and function
3	Discuss risks and benefits
4	Use immediate-release opioids when starting
5	Use the lowest effective dose
6	Prescribe short durations for acute pain
7	Evaluate benefits and harms frequently
8	Use strategies that mitigate risk
9	Review prescription drug monitoring programs
10	Use urine testing
11	Avoid concurrent opioid and benzodiazepine prescribing
12	Offer treatment for opioid use disorder

Thankfully, the reliance on systemic opioids is becoming less and less with innovation in the non-pharmacologic pain care therapies, including radio-frequency ablation and neuromodulation with spinal cord stimulation, while long-term delivery of opioids may be best suited as intrathecal therapy. Interestingly, there is clear data to suggest that patients on lower doses of opioids, either naively or weaned to less than 100 MME, have better success with advanced therapies and experience more sustainable treatment. Further, spinal cord stimulation seems to mitigate opioid increases.

Conclusion

Systemic opioid therapy for patients is challenging, balancing risks and benefits of a therapy that biologically has a short tenure with the development of tolerance. If these therapies are used vigilantly, with careful risk and harm assessment, along with compliance, they can be available ancillary tool in the treatment of pain. More high-quality evidence is needed.

Further, it is clear that chronic pain treatment is better managed sustainably by employing neuromodulation techniques. These therapies have high levels of evidence and have been shown to mitigate opioid consumption.

Recommended Reading

1. Han B, Compton W, et al. Non-medical prescription opioid use and use disorders among adults aged 18 through 64 years in the United States, 2003-2013. JAMA. 2015;314(4):1468–78.
2. https://www.cdc.gov/drugoverdose/pdf/guidelines_at-a-glance-a.pdf.
3. https://www.cdc.gov/mmwr/volumes/65/rr/rr6501e1.htmNNT versus NNH.
4. Levy RM. Neuromodulation: the "not-so-hidden" cure for the opioid crisis. Neuromodulation. 2017;20:519–24.
5. Sharan AD, Riley J, Falowski S, Pope JE, et al. Association of opioid usage with spinal cord stimulation outcomes. Pain Med. 2017;0:1–9.

29 Opioids for Cancer Pain and Hospice Care

Thomas P. Pittelkow and Halena M. Gazelka

Introduction

Pain is one of the most distressing and feared symptoms people encounter during their lifetime. The concept of cancer-associated pain only compounds the total pain patients experience in the domains of physical, psychological, spiritual, and social pains that accompany a cancer diagnosis. In fact, pain as a presenting symptom of malignancy is not uncommon in the advanced cancer state and often is a primary reason for patients to seek medical care. The prevalence of cancer-associated pain is wide-ranging, but reports suggest that over one-half of patients with cancer will have symptoms of pain at the time of diagnosis, and as the cancer progresses to an advanced state, this number often grows. Pain affects all domains of life, including activities of daily living, quality of life, sleep, interpersonal relationships, and affect. The concern for untreated or undertreated cancer pain may even lead to increased healthcare utilization and hospital admission. As is outlined in the World Health Organization (WHO) ladder of intensity-focused cancer-associated pain treatment, the use of opioid analgesic therapies sets the foundation for the treatment of cancer pain (Fig. 29.1).

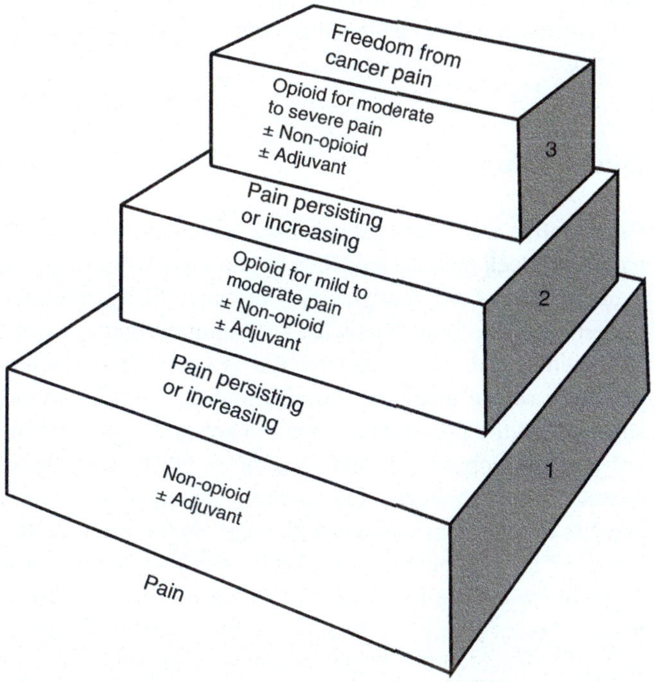

Fig. 29.1 As pain persists or increases, the next step should be assessed for implementation. (Adapted from WHO three-tiered ladder of cancer-associated pain relief. Reprinted from the World Health Organization. *WHO Cancer Pain Relief – a Guide to Opioid Availability*, 2nd ed. 1996. apps.who.int/medicinedocs/documents/s22085en/s22085en.pdf. Accessed 5 Oct 2018. With permission from the World Health Organization)

Background and Historical Perspective

History of Opioids in Cancer Pain

The application of opioid therapy for the treatment of pain in modern times has been around since the beginning of the ninetieth century, where the isolation of morphine from the opium plant by a German chemist created a new foundation of pain treatment. Given the profound analgesic effect of this medication, interest in its use for multiple medical conditions grew rapidly including both in the controlled setting of the operative room and in the community. Concerns over the psychophysiologic-dependent effects observed with the use of morphine and heroin led to legislative efforts in the early twentieth century to control its prescriptive use and the pharmaceutical interest in development of new medicines, like oxycodone, to find an analgesic with less physical dependence. It was not until the 1970s where legislative efforts created the Controlled Substance Act regulating medications in a tiered system of scheduled medicines based on therapeutic effect, perceived harmfulness, and potential for abuse and

T. P. Pittelkow (✉) · H. M. Gazelka
Division of Pain Medicine, Department of Anesthesiology and Perioperative Medicine, Mayo Clinic College of Medicine and Science, Rochester, MN, USA
e-mail: Pittelkow.thomas@mayo.edu; Gazelka.halena@mayo.edu

T. R. Deer et al. (eds.), *Deer's Treatment of Pain*, https://doi.org/10.1007/978-3-030-12281-2_29

addiction and the Drug Enforcement Agency to control the socially destructive problem of heroin addiction. Over the subsequent decades, the pendulum of opioid prescribing began to swing, from very conservative use in the 1980s to more liberal use in the 1990s and 2000s, particularly in the treatment of cancer-associated pain. The reported undertreatment of pain, particularly cancer pain, was a primary catalyst to advocate for the regular use of opioid therapy. Additionally, several studies that were published suggested the application of opioid therapy in the cancer population was different than non-cancer pain and that its potential for abuse and addiction was not as concerning as once thought. Proponents argued that the primary obligation to care for patients with cancer pain was to alleviate suffering and that all patients with cancer-associated had a human right to have access to opioid therapy.

Epidemiology

Pain is often a primary reason for a significant minority of patients to seek medical care thus prompting the discovery of a newly diagnosed malignancy. Although likely underreported, the symptoms of pain are so ubiquitous that it is truly unknown the number of patients that are prescribed opioids prior to a cancer diagnosis. Population-based studies would suggest that the prevalence of pain in newly diagnosed cancer patients approaches 50% and up to 80% of those in advanced cancer states. Interestingly, the type of cancer appears to matter, as patients with solid organ tumors of the head and neck, pancreas, bone, brain, and lung and hematologically based lymphoma tend to have the highest prevalence of pain. However, despite the known relationship of pain prevalence with the stage of cancer, a large majority of patients continue to report insufficient control of their pain, and in all cancer stages, there remain challenges with control of tumor burden and severe pain. This is particularly troubling given that patients who report high pain intensities often are at greater risk for pain-related interference with their daily activities and ability to enjoy life. The vast majority of reported pain in cancer patients is the result of tumor burden; however, the toxic effects of treatment and chronic health comorbidities also are confounding factors in the treatment of patients' reported pain.

Basic Principles of WHO Ladder of Cancer Pain

The World Health Organization (WHO) three-tier ladder approach to the treatment of cancer pain provides a hypothetical stepwise structure for clinicians to consider when implementing therapy options for patients with cancer pain, ranging from mild to severe pain. Typically, patients with cancer pain have already self-initiated Tier 1 strategies, as this embodies mild-to-moderate cancer-associated pain. This stage utilizes non-opioid analgesics, such as paracetamol or nonsteroidal anti-inflammatory (NSAIDs), which are coupled with an adjuvant if indicated for the pain symptoms. As the pain becomes more intense or poorly controlled, Tier 2 is categorized as moderate-to-severe cancer-associated pain. Most of these patients are believed to be relatively opioid naïve and have not achieved adequate analgesia with routine non-opioid and adjuvant therapies. In Tier 2 the WHO recommends trialing traditionally less potent opioid analgesics (e.g., codeine or hydrocodone) which typically are coupled with a non-opioid therapy and an adjuvant analgesic if indicated. The goal of pain-free living is the pinnacle of the ladder; however, this is often tempered by more realistic expectations to establish tolerable pain with little disruption of daily activities. Tier 3 encompasses patients with persistent severe cancer-associated pain who have failed to achieve adequate control on the lower tiers. Typically, the more potent conventional opioid therapies (e.g., morphine, hydromorphone, fentanyl, and methadone) are combined with a non-opioid and adjuvant medication. Historically speaking, the use of weak and strong opioid therapies was used in the WHO terminology, but this distinction was purely based on customary prescribing patterns and habitual practices rather than true fundamental pharmacologic differences among the pure mu-opioid agonists. Currently, cancer pain specialists advocate understanding the spectrum of opioid, non-opioid, and adjuvant medications available and ensuring that each patient has the right medication delivered at the right time.

Assessment and Application (Table 29.1)

As with any therapy in medicine, the use of opioid therapy in the treatment of cancer pain requires comprehensive assessment of the pain and allows the prescriber and patient to

Table 29.1 Application of opioid therapies for the management of cancer-associated pain

Primary management of cancer-associated pain
Focus on alleviation of patient suffering
Patient satisfaction with level of acceptable pain control
Detailed discussion regarding realistic expectations for pain control
Regular assessment and evaluation of pain control and therapeutic effects
Recognize holistic care of pain, including psychosocial, behavioral, spiritual, and emotional aspects of pain (i.e., total pain)
Alleviation of pain during the day and night, with movement and at rest
Regular conversation detailing the current pertinent medical information and current therapeutic efforts, including both expected and unexpected side effects

clarify the goals of pain treatment. The goal of any medical treatment is to individualize the therapy to balance the risk-benefit profile offering a favorable outcome and an improved quality of life within the broader scope of a patient's goals of care. This is particularly important in a patient with cancer, as often the pain can be treated with other therapies including chemotherapy, radiation therapy, surgery, or other disease-modifying agents. If routine attempts to correct a potentially remediable cause fail, then a trial or adjustment of opioid therapy should be considered, and often this is concurrent with the disease-directed treatment.

Cancer Survivorship

Increased surveillance and improved therapies, including targeted therapies, are contributing to significant improvement in cancer survivorship rates, with 5-year survival rates of greater than 60% for those diagnosed. This incredible improvement in survival all too often results in patients suffering from sequelae of their cancer or its treatment. Unfortunately, approximately 30% of survivors suffer from chronic pain, be it related to their cancer diagnosis and treatment or not. Often, it falls to primary care providers to resume responsibility for the long-term care of patients surviving cancer. They may feel ill equipped to manage the unique chronic pain issues of this population, who often suffer from medical comorbidities complicating treatment choices.

The transition from acute pain management during the treatment phase of cancer to the chronic pain management in survivorship can be challenging for patients and providers alike. Providers must be adept at evolving pain treatment plans from routine opioid prescribing to a more measured and thoughtful approach required for maintenance of chronic pain patients. Further, patients must adjust their expectations from the anticipation of immediate palliation of acute cancer-related pain and treatment-related pain to long-term management of what may be a chronic pain issue.

Unfortunately, all too often this deliberate transition is not addressed, and patients surviving malignancy have a high relative risk of remaining on opioids chronically. While long-term opioid therapy may be reasonable in many patients, there is evidence that lack of provider knowledge regarding other pharmacologic and non-pharmacologic therapies for chronic pain may play a significant role in persistent opioid therapy.

It is recommended that providers approach opioid therapy in cancer survivors with a structured approach much as they would in other patients suffering from other chronic pain. Screening for recurrent disease and/or second malignancy should be routine. Thereafter, pain management should proceed in a stepwise fashion, with appropriate diagnosis as a critical initial step. Referral to specialists, particularly pain specialists, may be significantly beneficial.

When opioids are considered for the treatment of post-malignancy pain, patients should be screened for risk of substance abuse and psychiatric comorbidities. A detailed discussion regarding the potential risks, benefits, and alternatives of therapy should be undertaken. Side effects and their treatment, especially constipation, should be reviewed. Opioid therapy should be initiated on a trial basis, with the goals of treatment, particularly in regard to functional status, delineated. Should chronic opioid therapy be undertaken, the management and monitoring should follow a structured approach as for any other patient on chronic opioid therapy. Discontinuation and weaning of therapy should be considered regularly, particularly if provider and patient goals are not being met or if there are concerns for misuse or diversion.

Surviving malignancy is a clear risk for prolonged opioid use, and while this may be appropriate for some patients and for some diagnoses related to cancer or its treatment, many patients may benefit from alternative strategies for chronic pain.

Uses and Indications

How Is Cancer Pain Different?

Cancer pain signaling pathways are based on the same neurophysiologic pathways that relay nociceptive information from the periphery to the thalamic interpretation center in acute and chronic pain. However, the fundamental cellular and molecular differences between cancer-associated pain and non-cancer pain are still being examined. The actual neural transmission, neuromodulation, and perceptual aspects of cancer pain are specific to cancer pain syndrome categories, including malignancy-related, cancer treatment-related, and non-cancer-related chronic health conditions (Table 29.2). In non-cancer pain diagnoses, typically there is an expected endpoint, i.e., recovery from postsurgical pain or management of chronic myofascial pain. The process of noxious stimuli that stems from cancer typically involves two types of pain, namely, that of nociceptive pain and neuropathic pain. Most often, the presence of mixed nociceptive and neuropathic pain is implicated; thus polyanalgesic efforts targeting multiple different receptors are the mainstay of treatment. Classically speaking, nociceptive pain responds well to opioid therapies, when compared to neuropathic pain where often non-opioid and adjuvant analgesics may be required to target a different subset of receptors to obtain adequate analgesia.

Malignancy-related cancer pain syndromes are responsible for the vast majority of symptoms observed in the cancer population. In particular, the presence of tumor invasion of

Table 29.2 Common causes of cancer pain: tumor burden, cancer treatment-related side effects, and chronic medical and psychiatric comorbidities

Cancer-related	Cancer treatment-related	Chronic comorbidities
Metastases Bone Soft tissue Visceral Leptomeninges Epidural invasion	Chemotherapy side effects Peripheral neuropathy Postherpetic neuralgia Avascular necrosis	Frailty, immobility, deconditioning
Nerve compression/ infiltration	Radiation therapy side effects Painful skin irritation Mucositis Tissue and nerve fibrosis/necrosis	Diabetic or hereditary neuropathy
Malignant bowel obstruction	Surgery side effects Postthoracotomy pain Postmastectomy pain Phantom limb pain	Psychosocial and psychiatric distress
Pathologic fracture		Arthritis – osteoarthritis or rheumatoid arthritis
Ischemia related to tumor		Headache disorders
Hemorrhage related to tumor		Chronic pain syndromes – fibromyalgia, CRPS

the bone, organ and soft tissue, muscle, and neurovascular structures yields increased noxious stimuli and thus increased pain perception. As the cancer changes over time, so will the pain, which again ultimately depends on the course of the disease itself. Commonly, but to a lesser extent, cancer pain is treatment-related, such as chemotherapy-induced peripheral neuropathy or postradiation pain syndromes, and often these challenging symptoms may last for years even after a cancer has been treated. Finally, chronic health conditions that are prevalent in the general population are also prevalent in the cancer population, so performing a thorough history and physical examination will yield a more definitive diagnosis to the etiologic basis and successful management. Regardless of the ultimate diagnosis, the primary goal is to help cancer patients live as long as they can by achieving adequate pain relief using simple and focused therapeutic treatment plans.

Treatment of Persistent and Incident Pain

Cancer pain has been shown in numerous settings to have a profound impact on patients' perceived quality of life, unfavorable psychosocial outcomes, and caregiver burden. Reports of pain are entirely consuming of cancer patients and their support systems, preventing the routine aspects of daily activities and simple cognitive tasks. Evidence would suggest that treatment of cancer pain with multimodal therapeutic strategies results in a clinically meaningful improvement in health-related quality of life. This type of outcome is best achieved when both constant persistent pain and incident-related breakthrough pain are well treated. Ideally, when treating patients with cancer pain, clinicians would rely on a longer-acting opioid therapy in either an oral, transdermal, or rectal form to allow the patient control of the moment-to-moment stable pain and would employ use of a shorter-acting opioid agent orally, parenterally, rectally, or subcutaneously to prevent acute flares of the transient acute exacerbation of pain with movement, transitions, repositioning, or even unprovoked spontaneous pain. For many cancer patients, the anticipation of breakthrough pain is all encompassing and impairs a sense of control due to the severe and paroxysmal nature of a flare. It is imperative that the clinician strive to help patients achieve an acceptable basal coverage of pain and titrate an optimal breakthrough dose, which is roughly 10–20% of the daily oral opioid dose.

Opioid Metabolism

Opioid therapy achieves analgesia through activation of opioid-specific receptors, specifically the mu-, delta-, and kappa-opioid receptors. Classically, the mu-opioid receptor is thought to be the primary receptor responsible for analgesia. There are several known subtypes of the mu-opioid receptor which likely explains the heterogenous variation in response to the various opioid therapies that are classically defined as mu-opioid agonists. The historical basis of treatment using opioid therapy for cancer pain traditionally has relied on pure mu-opioid agonists, but there are other agents that can be used including mu-opioid agonist-antagonists (i.e., buprenorphine and butorphanol) and multi-mechanism mu-opioid agonists (i.e., tramadol and tapentadol).

Traditionally, when offering an opioid-based analgesic therapy to cancer patients, clinicians would use a pure mu-opioid agonist that is short-acting, particularly in patients who are opioid naïve or have limited opioid exposure. The initial first step based on the WHO ladder of cancer pain treatment was often codeine given its perceived weak mu-opioid effect. Fortunately, after discovering that there are phenotypic variants in the population with vastly different metabolic processing speeds (i.e., slow, rapid, or ultrarapid metabolizer) due to the metabolic processing of the CYP2D6 isoenzyme of the hepatic cytochrome P450 system, this has led to a change in typical opioid prescribing habits. Clinicians have become more aware that many of the prescribed opioid therapies have active metabolites that may have unintended effects, so understanding and assessing the patient for medical comorbidities is essential. The goal of opioid therapy in cancer pain is to benefit from analgesic effects while minimizing the experience of adverse effects.

When considering opioid therapy, there is no medical literature on the superiority of one opioid over another in the treatment of cancer pain. The balance of analgesia with tolerable side effects is a discussion that is individualized to each patient. The clinician must understand the basics of opioid therapy including efficacy and safety and then apply it to each patient and assess how the individual's response in regard to analgesia, adverse effects, and tolerability. Given this information, the prototypic opioid for treatment of cancer pain is morphine. Morphine is offered as an immediate-release and long-acting sustained-release formulation. Morphine is hepatically metabolized via glucuronidation pathway (phase II metabolism) into two metabolites, morphine-6-glucuronide (M6G) and morphine-3-glucuronide (M3G). M6G is responsible for mu-opioid receptor analgesia, while M3G is neurotoxic and can elicit concerning effects such as myoclonus, agitation, and seizures. Morphine metabolites are renally excreted; thus close monitoring of patient's medical comorbidities and general health status is vital to ensuring acceptable outcomes with morphine opioid therapy. If renal function is changing or declining, consideration of an opioid with less reliance on the renal excretion or presence of active metabolites should be considered.

Hydromorphone, hydrocodone, oxymorphone, and oxycodone are all reasonable alternatives to morphine. These agents are all relatively more potent than morphine and also come in immediate-release and long-acting sustained-release formulations. Hydromorphone and oxymorphone are both metabolized via phase II glucuronidation by the UDP-glucuronosyltransferase 2B7 subtype, like morphine. Hydromorphone is converted into active metabolites hydromorphone-6-glucuronide (H6G) and hydromorphone-3-glucuronide (H3G). Similar to morphine, H6G is responsible for analgesia, and H3G is potently neurotoxic, and both are renally excreted. After its metabolism, oxymorphone does not produce an active metabolite that is believed to complicate treatment. Hydrocodone, like codeine, is somewhat unique in that it requires activation via phase I metabolism using the hepatic isoenzyme CYP2D6 to norhydrocodone and hydromorphone, which of course relies on phase II glucuronidation metabolism, and are renally excreted. The exact contribution of hydrocodone and its metabolites to the analgesic response remains uncertain, but certainly its use for moderate cancer pain is well documented. The parent drug oxycodone is responsible for the majority of its analgesic effects with negligible contributions from its metabolism via phase I reactions by the hepatic isoenzymes CYP3A4 to noroxycodone and by CYP2D6 to oxymorphone. Thus, when clinicians select an opioid for use in patients with renal impairment, they must understand and anticipate the changes in the parent opioid and metabolites and what effect both will yield when accumulated.

The use of fentanyl is favorable in patients with advanced renal disease as it is highly lipophilic and does not have any known active metabolites. Fentanyl is metabolized almost exclusively via phase I reactions via the hepatic isoenzyme CYP3A4 to its primary product of norfentanyl and is renally excreted. There is no evidence to suggest opioid toxicity with the use of fentanyl in advanced renal failure with uremia; however, caution is advised. In patients with limited enteral access, fentanyl is a unique opioid in advanced cancer states as it comes in parenteral, transdermal, and transmucosal formulations. It is advocated to use transdermal applications in an opioid-tolerant patient, given its lipid-soluble properties and potential to accumulate quickly depending on the body habitus. The transdermal route also has specific considerations, including the location of application on the body (requires subcutaneous adipose tissue for diffusion of medication), the rate of absorption can vary depending on skin temperature, and the high abuse potential given its rapid distribution and metabolism.

Opioid agonist-antagonist agents, such as buprenorphine, offer the clinician an opportunity to treat cancer pain in complex patients, who may struggle with prominent side effects of traditional opioid therapies and/or have a history of polysubstance abuse. Buprenorphine is primarily hepatically metabolized via phase I metabolism by the isoenzyme CYP3A4 resulting in an active metabolite norbuprenorphine. Buprenorphine and its metabolites are renally excreted. Both buprenorphine and its major metabolite norbuprenorphine have varying ranges of effect at the mu-, delta-, and kappa-opioid receptors, including partial agonist and antagonist effects. The unique properties of agonist-antagonist opioid therapies allow for a more favorable side effect profile, notably a ceiling effect for concerning side effects such as respiratory depression. Typically, the main limiting factor of opioid therapy is based on the side effect profile.

The multi-mechanism mu-opioid agonists, including tramadol and tapentadol, offer a dual mechanism of effect. The less potent activation of mu-opioid receptor compared to a pure opioid agonist offers an alternative to patients that are opioid naïve and opioid sensitive or tolerate limited exposure to pure opioid agonists. The other main mechanism of action inhibits reuptake of the monoamine neurotransmitters, including serotonin and norepinephrine, which have been shown to play a role in propagation and neuromodulation of chronic cancer pain states. Tramadol is hepatically metabolized via phase I isoenzymes CYP3A4 and CYP2D6 into the analgesic metabolite O-desmethyltramadol. Tapentadol, which is thought to have less selective serotonin reuptake inhibition compared to tramadol, is hepatically metabolized via phase I glucuronidation by UGT1A9 and UGT2B7 enzymes into a clinically inactive metabolite.

Opioid analgesics are the source of both significant benefit and adverse events. Clinicians must understand the basic metabolic aspects of each medication in order to balance the intended use with potential harm. Particularly in the cancer population, clinicians must regularly assess patients as health status and conditions are continually changing. We must continue to uncover new discoveries regarding the metabolism of opioid medications, including the various genetic polymorphisms of the cytochrome P450 system and the wide phenotypic expressions that exist, in order to provide cancer patients with the right medication, delivered at the right time, at the right dose to enhance the analgesic response and minimize the unintentional adverse events.

Evidence for Efficacy

Cancer Pain Management

The treatment of cancer pain requires comprehensive assessment and application of multimodal therapies. Many cancer patients have significant pain relief with disease-directed treatment. However, well over half of cancer patients report that their pain is not well controlled and often suboptimally managed. The undertreatment of cancer pain is likely a combination of multiple factors, including underestimation by clinicians, increasingly complex patient presentations, and concerns from both the clinician and patient regarding the use of opioid therapy. All cancer patients deserve a comprehensive and thorough assessment of their symptom burden to improve the ability to tailor therapy specific for the individual. When discussing implementation of opioid therapy, clinicians should discuss the rationale for opioid therapy, the benefits associated with opioid therapy, the typical risks and side effect profile of opioid therapy, and the role of opioid rotation and escalation. Ultimately, the goal of the clinician and healthcare team is to provide a comprehensive multimodal treatment plan to support the patient and their loved ones and provide a safe effective construct for improved cancer pain control.

Opioid Rotation

The use of opioid therapy when treating cancer pain is widely heralded as the standard of care. However, the heterogenous individual response to opioid receptor activation varies greatly. There is no standard for effective opioid dose. Although intuitively it may appear that serum levels should correlate with analgesia, this has not been shown in clinical studies. Thus, it is essential when using opioids in the treatment of cancer patients to understand that each individual fundamentally has their own individual minimally effective opioid dose required to achieve analgesia. A lack of response to one opioid therapy does not constitute a failure of all opioid therapies. Rather, a systematic approach must be taken to ensure that the patient is given an opportunity to try another opioid therapy.

Table 29.3 Basic "equianalgesic" table

	PO	IV/SQ	Relative potency
Morphine	30 mg	10 mg	1:3
Oxycodone	20 mg	N/A	–
Hydromorphone	7.5 mg	1.5 mg	1:5
Fentanyl	N/A	100 mcg	–
Oxymorphone	10 mg	1 mg	1:10

When deciding to rotate an opioid therapy due to poor efficacy, ensure that the patient appropriately used the medication as prescribed. Also, rule out any other cause that could be responsible for ill-effects mimicking opioid toxicity such as disease progression or metabolic derangements. After clinical assessment of the patient and their medical comorbidities, chose an opioid that is metabolized differently than the original opioid. Use an equianalgesic conversion table to calculate a total daily dose of the new opioid and reduce on an order of 30–50% for potential cross-tolerance (Table 29.3). Reassessment of pain characteristics should be detailed and focused and performed under close supervision. For cases that have been refractory to several opioid rotations or for very challenging cases, the application of methadone has been useful; however, methadone should be prescribed by an experienced clinician using appropriate dose equivalent calculations with appropriate monitoring and longitudinal care.

When prescribing opioid therapies, the practice of using a conservative percentage-based dose adjustment strategy of increases of 10–20% with each increase is utilized when pain is poorly controlled, as the dose-limiting factors when using opioids are the side effects. Unlike almost every other prescribed non-opioid and adjuvant medication for treatment of pain, there is no maximal daily dose. This unique property of the opioid therapies allows them to be prescribed to achieve analgesic effect without a ceiling dose. However, caution must be followed as the main limiting factor is the side effect profile.

Opioid Side Effects

The use of opioid therapy in the treatment of cancer pain can pose challenges due to dose-limiting side effects (e.g., sedation, constipation, nausea and vomiting, and myoclonus). Adverse side effect management is considered a core component of managing opioid therapy in cancer patients. Almost all opioid-naïve and opioid-sensitive cancer patients will experience some degree of slowed cognition in the early stages of therapy. This is typically a transient phenomenon, and efforts should focus on ensuring that there is not an underlying medical reason for the altered sensorium besides the opioid, such as disease progression. Occasionally, treatment of the sedation with modafinil or methylphenidate has been shown to help. The most ubiquitous side effect that the body will never become tolerant to is that of constipation. Appropriate bowel medications such as schedule stimulants and as needed laxatives are critical to preventing obstipation and bowel obstruction, and often escalation in the bowel regimen needs to follow an increased opioid dose. Opioid-induced nausea and vomiting is a complex series of multiple mechanisms occurring peripherally (impaired gut inertia) and centrally (activation of the chemoreceptor trigger zone and vestibular system). As with most side effects, this is typically transient, and opioid-induced nausea and vomiting is best treated with anti-dopaminergic agents. There is limited clinical data to suggest one opioid is less likely than another to reduce the risk of opioid-induced nausea and vomiting. Finally, one of the more distressing and concerning side effects is that of myoclonus. This clinical entity needs to be recognized and addressed with opioid reduction and rotation, hydration, and potentially benzodiazepine therapy if clinical signs of seizure are present. Opioid neurotoxicity is a spectrum of neuromuscular symptoms ranging from mild sedation to generalized seizure activity. Often, patients appear unwell, and the first thought is to increase opioid therapy. This only causes more neural activation and potentially provokes the phenomenon of opioid-induced hyperalgesia. Ultimately, treating the underlying cause by reducing and altering opioid therapy is crucial. In some cases, transitioning from an oral to intrathecal route is the best way to provide enhanced analgesia while limiting opioid-related side effects.

Of particular interest when using opioid therapy in the cancer population is the effect of immunosuppression. Opioids behave like cytokines modulating the pro-inflammatory milieu via alterations in the synthesis and receptor expression of the typical innate immune response systems through interaction with mu-opioid receptors in the peripheral and central nervous system. Studies have demonstrated a direct effect of opioid therapies binding to mu-opioid receptors on peripheral circulating immune cells such as lymphocytes, NK cells, and macrophages leading to an alteration of the typical immune response and reduced recruitment and activation of neutrophils to an area of infection. Opioids have indirect effects as well through activation of descending central nervous system pathways via the hypothalamic-pituitary-adrenal axis modulating glucocorticoids and sympathetic nervous system release of norepinephrine, which have been demonstrated to impair innate immune function. Interestingly, intrathecal opioids may not exert the same immunosuppressive effects as systemic opioid therapy given the lower dose typically needed to achieve analgesia.

Intrathecal Therapy

The treatment of refractory cancer pain or patients with significant opioid-related side effects with escalating doses of opioid therapy becomes unfruitful and potentially harmful. At some point along the care continuum, clinicians should consider application of an intrathecal drug delivery system (IDDS) to provide opioid therapy directly to the central source near the opioid receptors. The delivery of opioid medication to the neuraxis has been shown to provide substantial benefit to patients with cancer pain syndromes related to the bone, nerve, and viscera. The only FDA-approved opioid medication for use in IDDS is morphine. Unfortunately, there is no well-defined algorithm for clinicians to follow as to when to reach for IDDS in the cancer pain population. However, best practice guidelines have been published in recent years suggesting that an implant of an IDDS can improve cancer patients' symptom burden and quality of life, regardless of life expectancy. In summary, it is recommended to consider IDDS when conservative therapies have failed or patients are experiencing significant side effects from traditional opioid therapies. Comprehensive cancer pain care employing IDDS with routine medical management likely awards cancer patients with improved symptom control, reduced opioid-related side effects, and improved survival.

Opioid Pain Management and Hospice

Most cancer patients will experience pain during the course of their disease, and this is particularly common once palliative treatment has become the focus of care. One specialized form of palliative care, hospice care, is care at the end of life (when life expectancy is equivalent to 6 months or less). In the United States, the majority of hospice care is provided in private homes with family members serving as 24 hour caregivers. When asked what they fear most at the end of life, many patients respond that pain that is not controlled is their primary concern. Thus, it is vital that patients and families be educated on options for pain control and that hospice workers (consisting primarily of nurses) be vigilant in assessing for pain and experts at treating it. Each hospice has at least one physician medical director. It is that physician's responsibility to ensure that patients are eligible for hospice and that treatment plans are appropriate. Commonly this includes an aggressive plan for pain management, along with the management of other disease-related symptoms. Obviously, it is vitally important that pain be addressed with multimodal treatment including non-medication strategies and that sources of pain other than physical pain also be addressed, as psychological distress can exacerbate physical symptoms.

The mainstay of pain management on hospice has been opioids, for several reasons. First, pain at the end of life, especially due to advancing cancer, can be tremendously severe. Typically, the adjunctive meds recommended initially on the WHO ladder for pain control are not potent enough to manage this pain. Further, opioids can be rapidly titrated and delivered by multiple different routes in response to pain levels and the declining status of the patient. It has been estimated that greater than 70% of patients will require an alternate dose than orally to deliver pain medications at the end of life.

One of the merits of opioids is their flexibility in route of delivery and absorption. Commonly used administration routes for hospice patients include oral, transdermal, transmucosal, intravenous, subcutaneous, and rectal. Fentanyl, morphine, hydromorphone, and methadone can all be delivered in IV form at home through a CADD pump, either IV or subcutaneously, except in the case of methadone, which causes site irritation when administered subcutaneously. The primary advantages of subcutaneous opioid administration include rapid absorption and lack of need for intravenous access. Limiting factors include the need for opioid solution, necessity of a CADD pump for administration, and the inability to run high volumes (max of 5 mL/hour recommended to avoid "pooling" of medication). Further, the subcutaneous button must be changed, often on a weekly basis. Rectal administration can also provide a valuable alternative to other options, particularly when the oral route is lost, such as in patients with high-grade bowel obstruction. Advantages of rectal administration include ease of dosing (as the dose is consistent with the oral route), the ability to provide long-acting opioids (when placed intact into the rectum), the lack of need for IV access or CADD pump for administration, and good tolerance, although many patients and families may be hesitant to consider this route, at least initially. For many patients, the skillful ministrations of a physician adept at pain management will allow them to remain at home even as varied routes of administration and alternate opioids, if needed, are trialed.

Besides the typical oral, transdermal, transmucosal, IV, subcutaneous, and rectal routes of administration, some hospices are able to supply epidural administration of opioids in combination with local anesthetics. When available, this is most commonly performed at inpatient hospice facilities, rather than in patient homes, as many hospices simply do not have the resources to make this available on an outpatient basis. Epidural opioid administration can be extremely advantageous and allow for much smaller dosing of opioid than with other routes, especially when combined with local anesthetic. Obviously, the site of pain is an important consideration when considering epidural administration, as this is most useful for abdominal, pelvic, and lower extremity pain locations.

Besides pain, opioids are commonly used on hospice for the management of dyspnea. Approximately 50–70% of cancer patients experience dyspnea in the last weeks of life, and it is also common in multiple other disorders, such as restrictive pulmonary disease, congestive heart failure, COPD, etc. Dyspnea is a common symptom with complex mechanisms, depending on the disease state. While the administration of oxygen may relieve dyspnea and even be life prolonging in patients with hypoxemia, it has not been shown to prolong life or even to reliably relieve dyspnea in non-hypoxic patients. Further, oxygen therapy in these instances can be both burdensome and expensive. In these cases, the administration of opioids is the mainstay of treatment. In randomized controlled trials, morphine significantly outperformed placebo in the relief of dyspnea. Any opioid can be used to treat dyspnea, and most routes are equivalent. However, nebulized opioids have not been shown to be significantly effective and thus are best avoided. If patients are taking opioids for pain management, this will often assist with management of dyspnea, as well. For hospice patients, using a benzodiazepine in addition to the opioid may improve the benefit. Often, much lower doses of opioid are required to treat dyspnea in comparison to doses for pain management.

The mechanism by which opioids relieve dyspnea is not well understood. Studies have shown that naloxone can induce dyspnea, implicating endogenous opioid receptors, which are present throughout the peripheral and central nervous system. Likely the effects of opioids on dyspnea are multifactorial, just as the pathophysiology of dyspnea is felt to be, with effects on the work of breathing and on the medullary, carotid, and aortic chemoreceptors sensing hypercapnia and hypoxemia.

Main Points

1. The majority of patients with advanced cancer will experience pain.
2. Recognition of total pain (e.g., psychosocial, spiritual, emotional, and physical) is imperative to successful treatment.
3. Conventionally, the methodical application of multimodal analgesic therapy including opioid, non-opioid, and adjuvant therapies is based on the WHO analgesic ladder for treatment of cancer-associated pain.
4. The undertreatment of cancer pain is likely a combination of multiple factors, including underestimation by clinicians, increasingly complex patient presentations, and concerns from both the clinician and patient regarding the use of opioid therapy.

5. Full clinical assessment should include pain characterization, pain impact on quality of life domains, malignancy diagnosis and prognosis, and recognition of comorbid medical and psychiatric conditions.
6. Treatment of cancer pain patients requires understanding the etiology of the pain. Pain can originate from tumor burden, side effects of the disease-directed treatments, and non-cancer-related pain syndromes.
7. Initial opioid treatment of cancer-associated pain should begin with an immediate-release preparation of medication, and extended-release or transdermal preparations should be reserved for opioid-tolerant patients.
8. Clinicians and patients should work together to ensure a plan of care using opioid therapy is in place to grant excellent baseline pain control and anticipate breakthrough pain.
9. Surviving malignancy is a clear risk for prolonged opioid use, and while this may be appropriate for some patients and for some diagnoses related to cancer or its treatment, many patients may benefit from alternative strategies for chronic pain.
10. Options of opioid therapy to treat cancer-related pain include pure opioid agonists, opioid agonists-antagonists, and multi-mechanism opioid agonists.
11. Comprehensive multimodal cancer pain care often yields improved patient analgesia, outcomes, and quality of life.
12. Rotation of opioid therapies should occur when patients experience troublesome opioid-related adverse side effects, lack of analgesic response with appropriate titration, and notable changes in medical comorbidities that affect opioid processing.
13. Management of opioid-related side effects is an expected part of opioid therapy and should be discussed with patients.
14. Use of intrathecal drug delivery systems for treatment of cancer-related pain syndromes should be considered for patients with significant opioid-related side effect burden or refractory pain symptoms to conservative medical treatments.
15. The mainstay of pain management for patients enrolled in hospice has been opioids, as opioids can be rapidly titrated with excellent effect and delivered by multiple different routes to meet the needs of the dying patient.

Recommended Reading

1. Baldwin J, Cox J. Treating dyspnea: is oxygen therapy the best option for all patients? Med Clin North Am. 2016;100:1123–30.
2. Ben-Aharon I, Gafter-Gvili A, Paul M, Leibovici L, Stemmer SM. Interventions for alleviating cancer-related dyspnea: a systematic review. J Clin Oncol. 2008;26:2396–404.
3. Ben-Aharon I, Gafter-Gvili A, Leibovici L, Stemmer SM. Interventions for alleviating cancer-related dyspnea: a systematic review and meta-analysis. Acta Oncol. 2012;51:996–1008.
4. Bhaskar AK. Interventional management of cancer pain. Curr Opin Support Palliat Care. 2012;6:1–9.
5. Boland JW, Pockley AG. Influence of opioids on immune function in patients with cancer pain: from bench to bedside. Br J Pharmacol. 2018;175(14):2726-2736.
6. Brogan SE, Winter NB, Okifuji A. Prospective observational study of patient-controlled intrathecal analgesia: impact on cancer-associated symptoms, breakthrough pain control, and patient satisfaction. Reg Anesth Pain Med. 2015;40:369–75.
7. Bruel BM, Burton AW. Intrathecal therapy for cancer-related pain. Pain Med. 2016;17:2404–21.
8. Carlson CL. Effectiveness of the World Health Organization cancer pain relief guidelines: an integrative review. J Pain Res. 2016;9:515–34.
9. Cherny NI, Foley KM. Current approaches to the management of cancer pain: a review. Ann Acad Med Singap. 1994;23:139–59.
10. Cherny NI, Portenoy RK. The management of cancer pain. CA Cancer J Clin. 1994;44:263–303.
11. Chow R, Saunders K, Burke H, Belanger A, Chow E. Needs assessment of primary care physicians in the management of chronic pain in cancer survivors. Support Care Cancer. 2017;25:3505–14.
12. Deandrea S, Montanari M, Moja L, Apolone G. Prevalence of undertreatment in cancer pain. A review of published literature. Ann Oncol. 2008;19:1985–91.
13. Deer TR, Smith HS, Burton AW, et al. Comprehensive consensus based guidelines on intrathecal drug delivery systems in the treatment of pain caused by cancer pain. Pain Physician. 2011;14:E283–312.
14. Deer TR, Pope JE, Hayek SM, et al. The Polyanalgesic Consensus Conference (PACC): recommendations on intrathecal drug infusion systems best practices and guidelines. Neuromodulation. 2017;20:96–132.
15. Deer TR, Pope JE, Hayek SM, et al. The Polyanalgesic Consensus Conference (PACC): recommendations for intrathecal drug delivery: guidance for improving safety and mitigating risks. Neuromodulation. 2017;20:155–76.
16. Glare PA, Davies PS, Finlay E, et al. Pain in cancer survivors. J Clin Oncol. 2014;32:1739–47.
17. Greco MT, Roberto A, Corli O, et al. Quality of cancer pain management: an update of a systematic review of undertreatment of patients with cancer. J Clin Oncol. 2014;32:4149–54.
18. Hassenbusch SJ, Paice JA, Patt RB, Bedder MD, Bell GK. Clinical realities and economic considerations: economics of intrathecal therapy. J Pain Symptom Manag. 1997;14:S36–48.
19. Jacox A, Carr DB, Payne R. New clinical-practice guidelines for the management of pain in patients with cancer. N Engl J Med. 1994;330:651–5.
20. Kamal AH, Bull J, Kavalieratos D, Taylor DH Jr, Downey W, Abernethy AP. Palliative care needs of patients with cancer living in the community. J Oncol Pract. 2011;7:382–8.
21. Kay S, Husbands E, Antrobus JH, Munday D. Provision for advanced pain management techniques in adult palliative care: a national survey of anaesthetic pain specialists. Palliat Med. 2007;21:279–84.

22. Lemay K, Wilson KG, Buenger U, et al. Fear of pain in patients with advanced cancer or in patients with chronic noncancer pain. Clin J Pain. 2011;27:116–24.
23. Mercadante S, Porzio G, Aielli F, et al. Opioid switching from and to tapentadol extended release in cancer patients: conversion ratio with other opioids. Curr Med Res Opin. 2013a;29:661–6.
24. Mercadante S, Valle A, Porzio G, et al. Opioid switching in patients with advanced cancer followed at home. A retrospective analysis. J Pain Symptom Manag. 2013b;45:298–304.
25. Neal JM, Barrington MJ, Brull R, et al. The second ASRA practice advisory on neurologic complications associated with regional anesthesia and pain medicine: executive summary 2015. Reg Anesth Pain Med. 2015;40:401–30.
26. Pachman DR, Swetz KM, Mauck WD, et al. An exploratory pilot study of palliative medicine compared to anesthesia-pain consultation for pain in patients with cancer. J Support Oncol. 2011;9:113–9.
27. Paice JA. Cancer pain management: strategies for safe and effective opioid prescribing. J Natl Compr Cancer Netw. 2016;14:695–7.
28. Paice JA, Von Roenn JH. Under- or overtreatment of pain in the patient with cancer: how to achieve proper balance. J Clin Oncol. 2014;32:1721–6.
29. Paice JA, Portenoy R, Lacchetti C, et al. Management of chronic pain in survivors of adult cancers: American Society of Clinical Oncology Clinical Practice Guideline. J Clin Oncol. 2016;34:3325–45.
30. Pope JE, Deer TR, Bruel BM, Falowski S. Clinical uses of intrathecal therapy and its placement in the pain care algorithm. Pain Pract. 2016;16:1092.
31. Portenoy RK, Ahmed E. Principles of opioid use in cancer pain. J Clin Oncol. 2014;32:1662–70.
32. Ripamonti CI, Bandieri E, Roila F, ESMO Guidelines Working Group. Management of cancer pain: ESMO clinical practice guidelines. Ann Oncol. 2011;22(Suppl 6):vi69–77.
33. Sacerdote P. Opioids and the immune system. Palliat Med. 2006;20(Suppl 1):s9–15.
34. Shimm DS, Logue GL, Maltbie AA, Dugan S. Medical management of chronic cancer pain. JAMA. 1979;241:2408–12.
35. Singh H, Banipal RPS, Singh B. Assessment of adequacy of pain management and analgesic use in patients with advanced cancer using the brief pain inventory and pain management index calculation. J Glob Oncol. 2017;3:235–41.
36. Smith TJ, Staats PS, Deer T, et al. Randomized clinical trial of an implantable drug delivery system compared with comprehensive medical management for refractory cancer pain: impact on pain, drug-related toxicity, and survival. J Clin Oncol. 2002;20:4040–9.
37. Smith TJ, Coyne PJ, Staats PS, et al. An implantable drug delivery system (IDDS) for refractory cancer pain provides sustained pain control, less drug-related toxicity, and possibly better survival compared with comprehensive medical management (CMM). Ann Oncol. 2005;16:825–33.
38. Stearns L, Boortz-Marx R, Du Pen S, et al. Intrathecal drug delivery for the management of cancer pain: a multidisciplinary consensus of best clinical practices. J Support Oncol. 2005;3:399–408.
39. Sutradhar R, Lokku A, Barbera L. Cancer survivorship and opioid prescribing rates: a population-based matched cohort study among individuals with and without a history of cancer. Cancer. 2017;123:4286–93.
40. Temel JS, Greer JA, Muzikansky A, et al. Early palliative care for patients with metastatic non-small-cell lung cancer. N Engl J Med. 2010;363:733–42.
41. Vallejo R, de Leon-Casasola O, Benyamin R. Opioid therapy and immunosuppression: a review. Am J Ther. 2004;11:354–65.
42. Vissers KC, Besse K, Wagemans M, et al. 23. Pain in patients with cancer. Pain Pract. 2011;11:453–75.
43. Vuong S, Pulenzas N, DeAngelis C, et al. Inadequate pain management in cancer patients attending an outpatient palliative radiotherapy clinic. Support Care Cancer. 2016;24:887–92.
44. Wang J, Barke RA, Charboneau R, Roy S. Morphine impairs host innate immune response and increases susceptibility to *Streptococcus pneumoniae* lung infection. J Immunol. 2005;174:426–34.
45. Warner NS, Bendel MA, Warner MA, et al. Bleeding complications in patients undergoing intrathecal drug delivery system implantation. Pain Med. 2017;18:2422.
46. Wilson J, Stack C, Hester J. Recent advances in cancer pain management. F1000Prime Rep. 2014;6:10.

Pharmacogenetics and Pharmacogenomics of Pain Treatment

30

Piotr K. Janicki

Introduction

Pharmacogenetics and pharmacogenomics of analgesics constitutes a relatively new area of pharmacology of pain management and is focused on influence of the genetic variants on the drug response during both acute and chronic pain management. The words pharmacogenomics and pharmacogenetics are often used interchangeably; there is however a difference. PharmGKB, an internationally recognized scientific and clinical knowledge resource, has this definition on its website (*http://www.pharmgkb.org/page/faqs*): *In general, pharmacogenetics usually refers to how variation in one single gene influences the response to a single drug. Pharmacogenomics is a broader term, which studies how all of the genes (the genome) can influence responses to drugs. Based on this definition listed above, this chapter both analyzes the effect of variants in the single genes on the pain management and summarizes the effect of multiple variants in the genome on pain treatment.*

Background and Historical Perspective

The interindividual variability in the therapeutic response to analgesic drugs constitutes well-known factors impairing effective pain management. It is assumed that specific inherited genetic variants can predict a patient's response to drugs. For example, 12–60% of the variability in alfentanil response can be explained by genetics, as illustrated in an experimental pain study in twins showing that the strength of the correlation between genetics and thermal pain depended on the pain stimulus applied.

Pharmacogenetic information could possibly be used to tailor pain medication based on an individual's genetic background. Many potential genetic markers have been described, and the importance of genetic predisposition in analgesic efficacy and toxicity (in particular opioids) has been demonstrated in knockout mouse models and human twin studies. From the findings of transgenic mouse studies, over 400 genes have been implicated in pain transmission and response. Such predictors are especially of value for neonates and young children, in whom the assessment of efficacy or side effects is complicated by the inability of the patient to communicate this properly. The current problem is determining which of the many potential candidates to focus on for clinical implementation.

From the clinical and practical point of view, the effects of genetic polymorphism in different systems associated with opioid pharmacology (or any other drug category) can be classified into two general categories—pharmacokinetic (PK) and pharmacodynamic (PD) interactions. Pharmacokinetics is what the body does to the drug, whereas pharmacodynamics is what the drug does to the body. In order to diagnose the genetic factors, genetic laboratories usually provide the list of biomarkers which could be used to characterize polymorphic conditions of each patient. Pharmacogenomics could possibly be used to tailor pain medication based on an individual's genetic background. This chapter will analyze the influence of these most promising (or more clinically relevant) genetic factors on the analgesic response of pain drugs from different categories, with particular emphasis on pharmacogenomics interactions confirmed in multiple published clinical studies and offering most likely recommendations for future use of pharmacogenomics in individualized (personalized) pain management.

PK Genetic Biomarkers (or Genetics of Drug Metabolism)

Cytochrome P450 (CYP)

The majority of well-documented evidences and clinical trials for pain drugs are associated with polymorphic hepatic

P. K. Janicki (✉)
Department of Anesthesiology and Perioperative Medicine, Penn State College of Medicine, MS Hershey Medical Center, Hershey, PA, USA
e-mail: Pjanicki@pennstatehealth.psu.edu

T. R. Deer et al. (eds.), *Deer's Treatment of Pain*, https://doi.org/10.1007/978-3-030-12281-2_30

cytochrome P450 (CYP) activity (phase I metabolism) (Table 30.1). There have been 57 CYP functional genes identified in humans thus far. These genes are all highly polymorphic, and this contributes to the vast interindividual differences in drug metabolism. Each of these genes harbors hundreds of common and rare variants (minor allele frequencies in population more than 5% or less than 5%, respectively), coding and not coding. Copy-number variation (CNV) is common, so individuals may carry more or less than two copies of the same fully active gene. Thus, an enormous number of genetic permutations can potentially influence drug metabolism. Nongenetic factors, such as medications, also influence the activity of individual CYP enzymes. Given the degree of genetic variation and variability in enzyme activity over time, each person essentially has her/his own unique cytochrome profile.

Table 30.1 Cytochrome P450 metabolic pathways for most analgesic drugs on US market

Pain management		
Generic	Brand	Genes of interest
Alfentanil	Alfenta	CYP3A4/CYP3A5
Buprenorphine	Suboxone, Butrans	CYP3A4/CYP3A5
Carisoprodol[a]	Soma	CYP2C19
Celecoxib	Celebrex	CYP2C9
Codeine[a]	Various brands	CYP2D6
Cyclobenzaprine	Amrix, Flexeril	CYP3A4/CYP3A5, CYP1A2
Diclofenac	Voltaren, Pennsaid Zorvolex	CYP2C9
Dihydrocodeine[a]	Trezix, Synalgos-DC	CYP2D6
Dihydroergotamine	D.H.E. 45	CYP3A4/CYP3A5
Eletriptan	Relpax	CYP3A4/CYP3A5
Fentanyl	Actiq, Duragesic	CYP3A4/CYP3A5,
Flurbiprofen	Generic	CYP2C9
Frovatriptan	Frova	CYP1A2
Hydrocodone[a]	Hysingla, Norco, Lortab Vicodin	CYP2D6
Ibuprofen	Advil, Motrin	CYP2C9
Indomethacin	Indocin, Tivorbex	CYP3A4/CYP3A5
Ketamine	Ketalar	CYP3A4/CYP3A5
Lidocaine	Various brands	CYP1A2
Meloxicam	Mobic, Vivlodex	CYP2C9
Methadone (active portion)	Dolophine, Methadose	CYP2C19
Nabumetone	Relafen	CYP1A2
Naproxen	Aleve, Naprelan, Naprosyn	CYP2C9
Oxycodone[a]	Oxycontin, Percocet, Roxicet	CYP2D6
Piroxicam	Feldene	CYP2C9
Ropivacaine	Naropin	CYP1A2
Sufentanil	Sufenta	CYP3A4/CYP3A5
Tizanidine	Zanaflex	CYP1A2
Tolvaptan	Samsca	CYP3A4/CYP3A5
Tramadol[a]	Conzip Ultram	CYP2D6,
Zolmitriptan	Zomig	CYP1A2

[a]Indicates prodrug

Commercial tests typically focus on a few dozen common polymorphisms that influence the functional activity and expression of individual enzymes important for drug metabolism (e.g., CYP2D6, CYP2C19, CYP2C9, and CYP2B6), including wide range of drugs used in pain management (Fig. 30.1a and Table 30.1). Based on the genotyping results, an individual's metabolizer status is assigned as ultra-rapid (UM), extensive (normal) (EM), intermediate (IM), or slow (poor) (PM) (Table 30.2). Genotypes associated with being an extensive metabolizer are generally the most common fully functional alleles (so called wild-type alleles). Reported allele frequencies are based on studies of individuals from European and, to a lesser degree, Asian ancestry; African populations, which are highly diverse, are underrepresented in this research. An individual's profile of common CYP alleles is predictive, but not an absolute indicator of metabolizer status. Other undetected mutations in the same gene, including rare variants, can impact gene function. For example, in CYP2B6, low activity alleles operate in recessive fashion, so individuals with only one copy of the low activity CYP2B6*6 allele, which is quite common in some African populations, may also carry a different gene-disrupting variant that is not detected by standard testing. In this situation, the person is a compound heterozygote for low activity alleles and will be a slow metabolizer, contrary to the test results.

Out of over 50 CYP450 enzymes, only four account for over 90% of opioid metabolism: CYP3A4/5, CYP2C9, CYP2B6, and, most importantly, CYP2D6, for which most clinical data are available. CYP3A4/5 are the major hepatic enzymes for opioid metabolism accounting for 40–60% of all opioid metabolisms (Table 30.3). Unfortunately, there is not yet a widely available commercial test for CYP3A4/5, but the other two, CYP2C9 and CYP2D6, can be tested for common genetic defects which are technically referred to as "polymorphism" since the alleles on the gene may be altered or absent. Please note again that all commercial tests have been designed to detect only common polymorphisms—rare variants are not detected using commercial testing. The only way of detecting these variants is deep resequencing of the entire coding sequence (exons) of the target gene. Fortunately, unique characteristics and new knowledge regarding these three enzymes provide some simple screening questions that allow the opioid prescriber to have a high index of suspicion that a genetic opioid metabolic defects of the enzyme exist in a patient. CYP2D6, CYP2C9, and CYP2B6 genes have a poor, intermediate, and normal (extensive) metabolizer phenotype. CYP2D6 and CYP2C9 also have an UM phenotype. CYP3A4 has an IM and IM and NM phenotype, and CYP3A5 has a non-expresser, intermediate expresser, and expresser phenotype. For CYP3A5, the majority of patients are non-expressers, which is the equivalent of a poor metabolizer (Table 30.4).

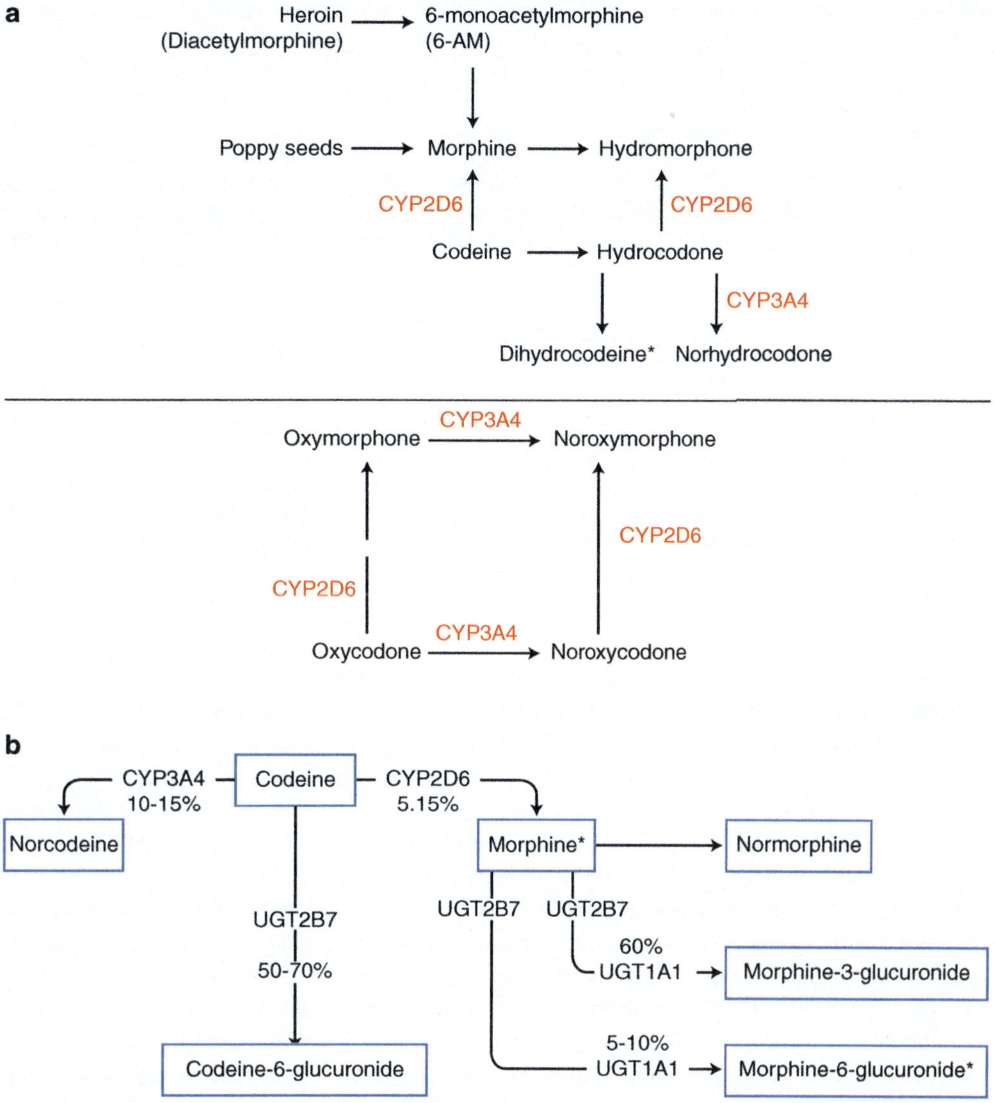

Fig. 30.1 Opiates and their main metabolic pathways. Upper panel (**a**): Shown in red are the major cytochrome P450 enzymes involved in phase I metabolism. Pattern of drug metabolites may reflect the genotype and associated metabolic phenotype of the patient. Actual proportions of individual metabolites might vary. Phase II reactions (e.g., glucuronide conjugation) are also prominent for some of opioid analgesics. Lower panel (**b**): Major metabolic pathways of cocaine by phase I and II reactions. The numbers indicate the percentage involvement of the give pathway of codeine metabolism. *indicate active metabolites of codeine

Table 30.2 Relationship between genotypes and phenotypes for CYP activity in opioid-metabolizing pathways

Enzyme variation	Opioid dosage	Laboratory terminology	Genomic correlation
Normal	Normal	Extensive (normal) metabolizers *EM or NM*	Wild-type homozygote or carrier of recessive variant
Overactive	Significantly increased	Rapid (or ultra-rapid) metabolizers *UM*	Carriers of more than two copies of alleles (copy number variants)
Underactive	Somewhat increased	Intermediate metabolizer *IM*	Two copies of decreased functional recessive allele or carrier of dominant dysfunctional allele
Inactive or absent	Decreased dose because of not metabolizing opioids, e.g., causing toxicity	Poor metabolizer *PM*	Two copies of recessive alleles or heterozygous carriers of dominant nonfunctional allele

Table 30.3 Drugs used in management of pain and their metabolic pathways in relation to polymorphic cytochrome P450 isoforms

CYP2D6	CYP2C9	CYP3A4/5	CYP2B6
Amitriptyline	Celecoxib	Codeine	Methadone
Codeine	Flurbiprofen	Diazepam	
Desipramine	Ibuprofen	Fentanyl	
Diazepam	Meloxicam	Hydrocodone	
Hydrocodone	Piroxicam	Oxycodone	
Imipramine		Methadone	
Methadone			
Nortriptyline			
Oxycodone			
Tramadol			
Venlafaxine			

The most frequently addressed candidate gene in the literature of pain is highly polymorphic CYP2D6. Over 100 different alleles have been discovered, of which approximately 25% lead to total loss of activity in vivo and 6% result

Table 30.4 Observed clinical consequences of interactions between opioid analgesics and polymorphic cytochrome P450

Opioid	CYP2D6 PM or inhibition	Patient is CYP2D6 UM*	CYP3A4 inhibition	CYP3A4 induction	CYP2B6 PM or inhibition
Codeine	Decreased analgesia (less morphine produced)	Increased analgesia (more morphine produced)	Mildly increased analgesia (more codeine and morphine)	Mildly decreased analgesia (less morphine and codeine	N/A
Hydrocodone	Possible decrease analgesia or increased toxicity (less hydromorphone metabolite)	Possible increased analgesia and toxicity (more hydromorphone present)	Increased analgesia and toxicity (more hydrocodone and hydromorphone)	Decreased analgesia (less hydrocodone and hydromorphone)	N/A
Oxycodone	Possible decrease analgesia or increased toxicity	Possible increased analgesia and toxicity	Increased analgesia and toxicity (more oxycodone and oxymorphone)	Decreased analgesia (less oxycodone and oxymorphone)	N/A
Methadone	Increase analgesia and toxicity risk	Decreased analgesia	Increased analgesia and toxicity risk	Decreased analgesia	Increased toxicity (QTc prolonged)
Tramadol	Decrease analgesia and increased risk of pro-serotoninergic side effects and seizures	Increased analgesia and toxicity	Slight increased analgesia and toxicity risk	Possible decrease analgesia	Slight increase analgesia and toxicity risk
Hydromorphone	N/A	N/A	N/A	N/A	N/A
Oxymorphone	N/A	N/A	N/A	N/A	N/A
Fentanyl	N/A	N/A	Decreased metabolism	N/A	N/A
Sufentanil	N/A	N/A	Decreased metabolism	N/A	N/A
Alfentanil	N/A	N/A	Decreased metabolism	N/A	N/A

**UM* = ultrametabolizer

in decreased activity. In the white population, 5–10% of individuals are a PM and 2–4% a UM. In the Asian population, CYP2D6 PMs are less common, but IMs are more common, with up to 20% of the Japanese population carrying the *10 decreased activity allele. In the African population, the frequently occurring *17 and *29 alleles also lead to an IM phenotype. These alleles are virtually absent in the white population. The most investigated and clinically relevant pharmacogenetic examples involving CYP2D6 polymorphism include prodrug activation pathways for codeine and tramadol. Codeine, hydrocodone, oxycodone, and tramadol are metabolized by CYP2D6 to active metabolites. The Clinical Pharmacogenetics Implementation Consortium guidelines provide *CYP2D6*-guided therapeutic recommendations to individualize treatment with tramadol and codeine. However, implementation guidelines for other opioids, which are more commonly used in real-world settings for pain management, are currently lacking. Hence, further studies are warranted to bridge this gap in our knowledge base and ultimately ascertain the role of pharmacogenetic markers as predictors of response to opioid analgesics.

Codeine is a prodrug, which is demethylated by the CYP2D6 enzyme to morphine, which has 200 times the affinity for the mu-opioid receptor (MOR) when compared to codeine (Fig. 30.1b for the entire metabolic pathway of codeine). The CYP2D6 enzyme is highly polymorphic, with over 100 alleles identified thus far. Some of these alleles can lead to inactivation, reduction in function, or duplication of the gene. These various genotypes have been described with their accompanying phenotypes. Two nonfunctioning alleles are associated with poor metabolism; one or two functioning alleles are associated with extensive metabolism, and duplicated alleles or an allele with a promoter function is associated with ultra-rapid metabolism (Fig. 30.2).

One early case report showed life-threatening opioid intoxication from codeine prescribed for cough in a patient with bilateral pneumonia, who was later found to have three functioning CYP2D6 alleles, consistent with ultra-rapid metabolism. Subsequent case reports described apnea in a child following oral codeine administration, later found to have CYP2D6 allele with a promoter function, and death in a child following codeine administration following adenotonsillectomy, who was found to have supratherapeutic levels of codeine and functional duplication of CYP2D6. A follow-up case report described several more fatal or life-threatening incidents in children taking codeine following adenotonsillectomy. One case report also revealed apnea leading to death in a nursing newborn of a mother taking codeine, who was found to have a genotype associated with ultra-rapid metabolism, and a case-control study demonstrated severe respiratory depression in breastfeeding newborns with mothers having an ultra-rapid metabolism genotype. Due to this mounting evidence, the Food and Drug Administration issued a black box warning for codeine in May 2013, listing it as contraindicated in pediatrics following adenoidectomy and/or tonsillectomy and adding a warning regarding breastfeeding mothers taking codeine. This has also led the Clinical Pharmacogenetics Implementation

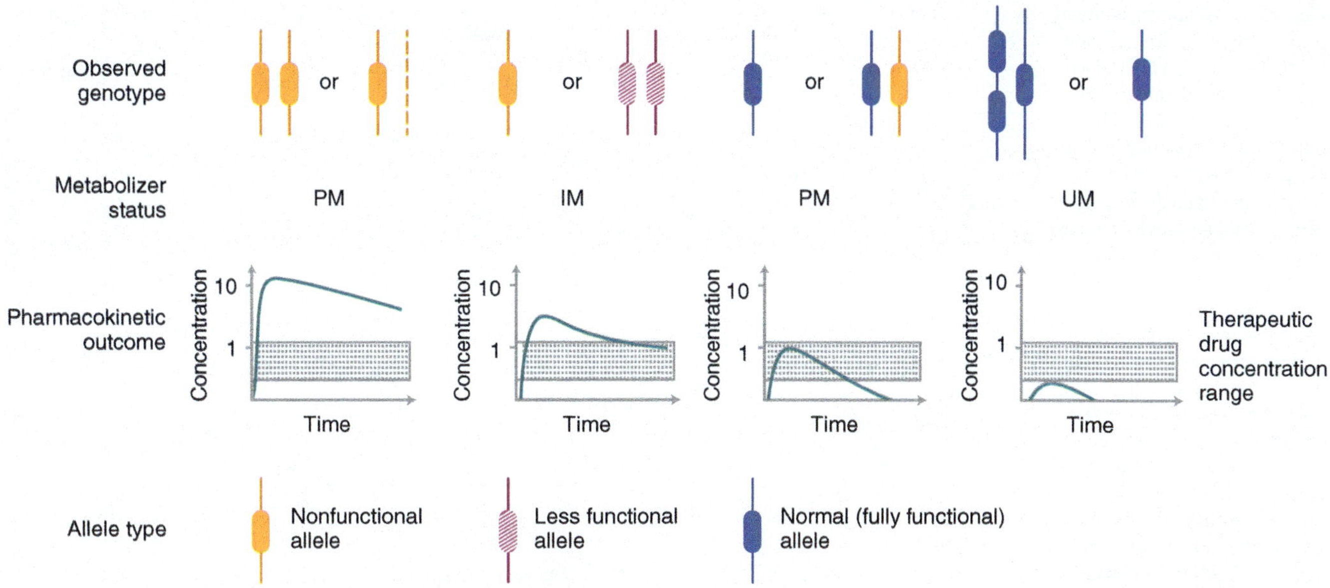

Fig. 30.2 Pharmacogenetic and pharmacokinetic correlation between number and type of alleles in the CYP2D6 gene and the associated metabolic status. (PM poor metabolizers, IM intermediate metabolizers, EM extensive metabolizers, UM ultrarapid metabolizers). Pharmacokinetic outcomes of the drugs metabolized by the CYP2D6 system are presented as their observed plasma concentrations (solid line) in relation to the expected plasma concentrations (dotted band)

Consortium to publish guidelines regarding the use of genotyping and the prescription of codeine and tramadol.

Like codeine, tramadol is also a prodrug metabolized by CYP2D6, which converts it to its active metabolite, O-desmethyltramadol, also referred to as M1, which has MOR activity. Experimental pain studies found that patients with genotypes associated with UM experienced reduced discomfort from experimental pain, accompanied by increased serum levels of the tramadol M1 metabolite, while patients with genotypes associated with poor metabolism had little clinical effect with minimally detectable tramadol metabolite (Fig. 30.3). In similar fashion to codeine, there are case reports that describe respiratory depression in patients taking tramadol that are later found to have an ultrarapid metabolizing genotype. The results of clinical trials vary, as patients with a PM genotype receiving tramadol following abdominal surgery required more additional/rescue opioids than patients with an EM genotype, whereas patients with a PM genotype receiving tramadol following knee arthroscopy attested to better analgesia than patients with an extensive metabolizing genotype. This suggests that during time of intense pain, the therapeutic effects of tramadol may rely more heavily on its opioid metabolite, but in time of less-severe pain, the non-opioid effects of tramadol itself may be more beneficial.

Other pathways such as CYP3A4/5 also may be involved in their metabolism but generally have smaller effect (Tables 30.3 and 30.4). These enzymes are especially relevant for inactivation of fentanyl, sufentanil, and alfentanil, where the inactive metabolites are formed via N-dealkylation. In contrast to CYP2D6, CYP3A4 is involved in the formation of the nonactive metabolites of codeine and tramadol, norcodeine, and *N*-desmethyltramadol, respectively. For oxycodone, 80% of this drug is converted by CYP3A4 to the inactive metabolite noroxycodone.

Opioids that avoid CYP450 metabolism include oxymorphone, hydromorphone, and morphine, making these good choices to avoid common metabolism-based drug interactions associated with cytochrome P450 polymorphism. Other drug classes highly dependent on the CYP2D6 pathway that are used adjunctively for pain include the tricyclic antidepressants (amitriptyline and nortriptyline) and duloxetine.

Recently, after extensively reviewing all published evidence in the pharmacogenomics of opioids in pain treatment, Matic et al. (2017) published the short list of 10 genes that are the most promising markers for clinical use in this context (Table 30.5).

Most nonsteroidal anti-inflammatory drugs (NSAIDs) are highly dependent on CYP2C9 for metabolism. Many NSAIDs are metabolized by the cytochrome CYP2C9. The gene coding for CYP2C9 is highly polymorphic, with over 50 variants identified. Two frequent allelic variants, CYP2C9*2 and CYP2C9*3, are found in poor metabolizers. The incidence of PM is highest in the Caucasian population.

CYP2C9 polymorphism may play a significant role in NSAIDs toxicity. Poor metabolizers have reduced CYP2C9 activity compared to wild type, resulting in reduced NSAID clearance, increased area under the plasma drug concentration–time curve, and possibly an increased risk of adverse

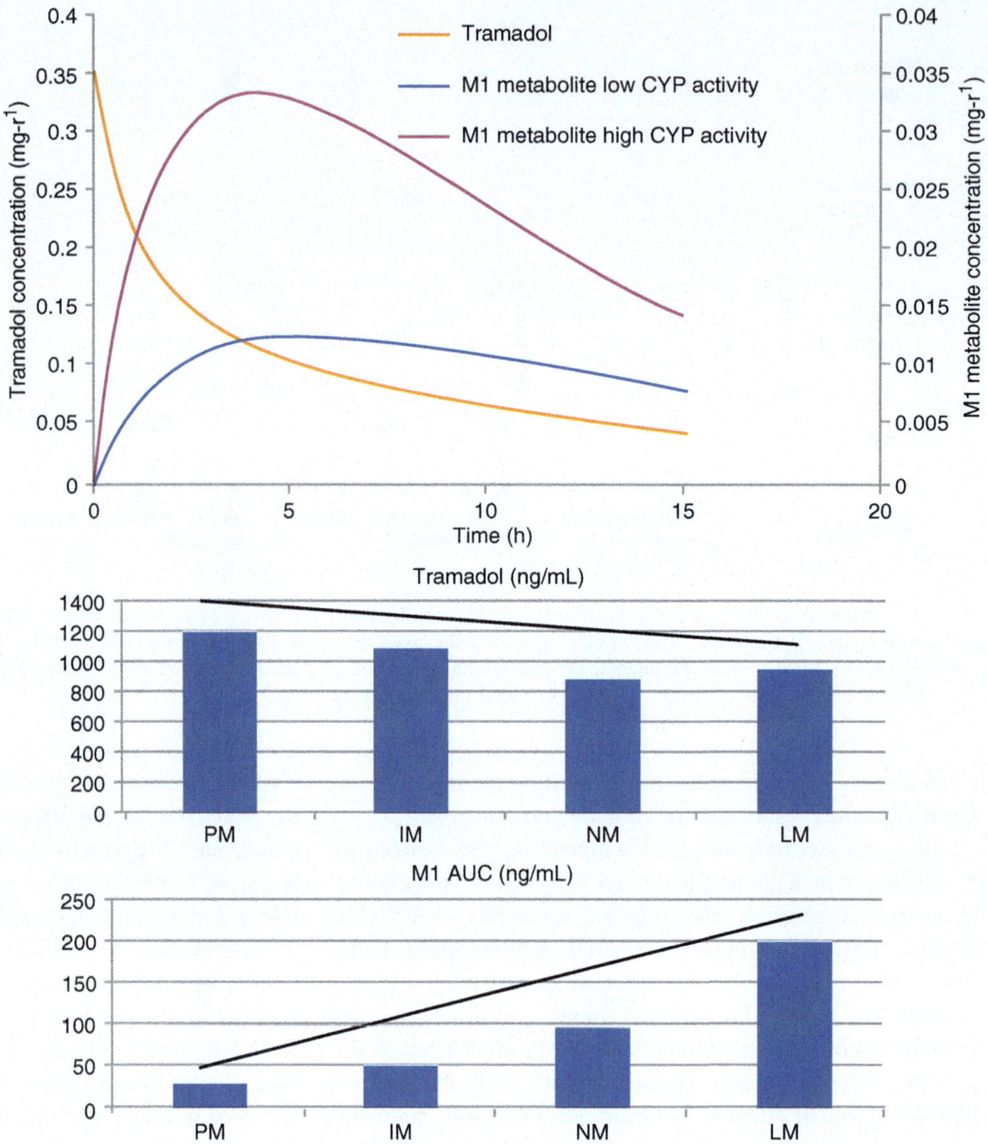

Fig. 30.3 Metabolic pathway of tramadol as a prodrug and its dependence on CYP2D6 genotype and phenotype in different types of CYP2D6-dependent metabolizers. (PM poor metabolizers, IM intermediate metabolizers, NM normal metabolizers, UM ultra rapid metabolizers). The upper panel presents simulated plasma concentrations of tramadol and its active M1 metabolite and its dependence on CYP2D6 metabolic activity. Lower panel presents area under the curve (AUC) for plasma concentrations of tramadol and active M1 metabolite in relation to the type of CYP2D6 metabolizers

Table 30.5 Short list of most likely candidate genes for clinical implementation of pharmacogenomics of opioids (full name of genes and their abbreviations)

Pharmacokinetic interactions
Cytochrome P450 family 2 subfamily D member 6 *(CYP2D6)*
Cytochrome P450 family 3 subfamily A member 4 *(CYP3A4)*
Cytochrome P450 family 3 subfamily A member 5 *(CYP3A5)*
UDP glucuronosyltransferase family 2 member B7 *(UGT2B7)*
ATP-binding cassette subfamily B member 1 *(ABCB1)*
ATP-binding cassette subfamily C member 1 *(ABCC3)*
Solute carrier family 22 member 1 *(SLC22A1)*
Pharmacodynamic interactions
Opioid receptor mu *(OPRM1)*
Catechol-O-methyltransferase *(COMT)*
Potassium voltage-gated channel subfamily *(KCNJ6)*

effects, although this is controversial. Case reports of patients treated with celecoxib showed that CYP2C9*3 homozygous patients had seven to ten times lower apparent clearance compared to patients with wild-type CYP2C9.24,25. A number of studies have also demonstrated a higher frequency of CYP2C9*2 and CYP2C9*3 in individuals who present with gastrointestinal bleeding following NSAID therapy. CYP2C8 polymorphisms may also influence variability in pharmacokinetics of NSAIDS, more specifically ibuprofen and diclofenac. Polymorphisms in this enzyme have been shown to change the clearing capacity leading to abnormally higher levels. CYP2C8 polymorphisms have also been implicated in gastrointestinal bleeds. One study examined the frequency of CYP2C8*3 allele in NSAID-induced gastrointestinal bleeds and found that it was significantly higher in NSAID users who experienced bleeds. This study also examined CYP2C9*2 and found that it also confers a higher risk of gastrointestinal bleed when taking NSAIDs.

Ketamine is an antagonist for N-methyl-D-aspartate receptors and is widely used as an analgesic, although it displays several other useful properties in anesthesia. There are several cytochrome enzymes that have been found to be involved in the N-demethylation of ketamine enantiomers. Some of these include CYP2B6, CYP2C9, and CYP3A4. Reviews on the variability between CYP2D6 and CYP2C19 poor and extensive metabolizers found no differences in side effects of ketamine, although these cytochromes have not been previously identified to be involved in the metabolism of ketamine. Further testing of CYP3A4 in a Swedish white population (comparing normal and slow metabolizers) showed no difference in the overall pharmacokinetics or in ketamine-related side effects.

Uridine Diphosphate Glucuronosyltransferase

Uridine diphosphate-glucuronosyltransferase (UGT) encompasses a group of phase II enzymes that are widely distributed throughout the human body and are involved in glucuronidation conjugation reactions. Morphine is primarily metabolized by UGT2B7 in the liver into two metabolites: morphine-3-glucuronide (M3G) and morphine-6-glucuronide (M6G). M3G is the major metabolite (90%) but does not confer an analgesic effect and may cause stimulatory effects such as allodynia, myoclonus, and seizure. The minor metabolite M6G (10%) is a potent analgesic but has poor permeability through the blood-brain barrier. When administered intravenously, it has a slower onset but longer duration of action compared to morphine and has lower rates of adverse effects.

A number of UGT polymorphisms have been investigated. One small trial involving neonates investigated the UGT2B7 900G.A SNP. The 900A allele is thought to confer greater UGT activity over the wild-type 900G allele. The investigators found that 900A carriers had relatively lower plasma morphine levels and higher M3G-morphine metabolic ratios, compared to wild type. These results suggest that patients with wild-type 900G/G have lower morphine glucuronidation rates and possibly respond better to morphine with lower adverse effects. Another trial, involving Japanese cancer patients and investigating the 802C.T SNP, found that patients with T allele had a lower frequency of nausea.

P-Glycoprotein Transporter ABCB1

The P-glycoprotein transporter ABCB1 is an ATP-dependent efflux transporter present in a variety of human tissues, including the gastrointestinal tract, kidney, liver, and brain. It is involved in the transport of a broad range of drug substrates and influences their plasma levels. It is coded by the highly polymorphic *ABCB1* gene, which has 38 identified single nucleotide polymorphisms (SNPs). One P-glycoprotein substrate is the prototypical opioid analgesic morphine. P-glycoproteins in brain capillary endothelial cells act as outward transporters for morphine across the blood-brain barrier, thereby influencing cerebrospinal fluid (CSF) morphine concentrations. The C3435T (rs1045642) allelic variant of ABCB1 reduces P-glycoprotein transporter function, resulting in increased CSF morphine concentrations. This variant has been associated with significant differences in interindividual pain relief achieved by morphine in cancer patients. Another study found that individuals with C3435T and G2677T/A variant alleles reported an increased antinociceptive effect from oxycodone. The respiratory depressive effects of morphine are also thought to be mediated by central nervous system MORs. The C3435T variant has been associated with increased respiratory depressive effects of fentanyl in Korean and Turkish adult patients. A recent study involving American pediatric patients showed a significant association between ABCB1 (rs9282564) polymorphism and postoperative respiratory depression, but not with the C3435T variant. A contradictory result was noted in a separate study, which showed patients with variant alleles had a lower frequency of adverse drug reactions, such as nausea and itching. Patients with combined wild-type genotype of 3435CC and 2677GG had significantly more adverse reactions. A possible explanation is the studied adverse reactions are affected by plasma opioid concentrations rather than CSF concentrations which appear to be associated with respiratory depression.

ABCC3

The *ABCC3* gene encodes the ATP-binding cassette subfamily C member 3 transporter, also known as Multidrug Resistance Protein 3. A study in mice genetically lacking *ABCC3* revealed that this transporter is involved in the efflux of M3G and M6G from the liver to the bloodstream. In a study of adult white individuals, 51 genetic variations were discovered, but only the promoter SNP_211C_T (rs4793665) was associated with significantly decreased *ABCC3* mRNA expression and alterations in the binding of transcription factors. A study in children undergoing adenotonsillectomy indicated that the_211C_T polymorphism was associated with lower M3G and M6G plasma concentrations. All patients with undetectable M6G concentrations were carriers of the T allele. More studies are needed to confirm this effect on the metabolism of morphine. Additionally, the *ABCC3* gene requires further screening for relevant genetic variants in other, non-Caucasian populations.

SLC22A6

Another drug transporter known to transport analgesics, particularly NSAIDs, is SLC22A6, human organic anion transporter 1. However, the clinical relevance for chronic pain treatment of its variation has not been clarified yet.

SLCO1B1

SLCO1B1, also known as OATP2, was shown to transport opioid peptides across blood-brain barrier; therefore, it is possible that genetic variability may have influence on the pain perception. This has not been clinically assessed yet, but immunofluorescence microscopy and uptake measurements were used to study localization and transport properties.

Dopamine transporter (DAT, SLC6A3) and glutamate transporter protein excitatory amino acid transporter 2 (SLC1A2, EAAT2) polymorphisms have also been reported to affect pain perception. Allele DAT∗10 was significantly underrepresented in patients with chronic daily headache associated with drug abuse when compared with the migraine-without-aura group, and A allele carriers of −181 A/C in EAAT2 polymorphism used significantly more analgesics than non-A carriers in migraine patients with chronic daily headache.

SLC22A1

The Organic Cation Transporter 1 (OCT1), encoded by the SLC22A1 gene, is primarily present on the sinusoidal membrane of hepatocytes. It is responsible for the uptake of positively charged compounds at physiological pH, such as morphine and the active metabolite of tramadol, O-desmethyltramadol. The role of SLC22A1 loss-of-function polymorphisms on tramadol PK and PD was emphasized by the finding of increased O-desmethyltramadol plasma concentrations and prolonged contraction of the eye pupils in healthy volunteers. Another study in adult postoperative patients on patient-controlled analgesia found that those with two inactive SLC22A1 alleles had higher O-desmethyltramadol area under the concentration curve (AUC) and lower tramadol consumption during the first 24 hours after surgery. In line with these observations, O-desmethyltramadol/tramadol metabolic ratios in newborn infants carrying the SLC22A1 low activity genotype were higher than those in infants carrying two SLC22A1 wild-type alleles. Organic cation OCT1 is expressed from the first postnatal day and increases quickly in the following months, which fits with the found genotype-phenotype correlation. In healthy volunteers with the previously mentioned deficient SLC22A1 alleles, an increase of 56% in morphine AUC after codeine administration was found. The association of these deficient SLC22A1 alleles with morphine was confirmed in a pediatric cohort with 220 children aged 6–15 years. The children with two loss-of-function alleles treated with intravenous morphine for postoperative pain had significantly lower clearance compared with patients with wild-type alleles. It has been proposed that these genetic variants could explain why children with a white background experienced more adverse events than African American children, in whom the variant alleles are less frequent. SLC22A1 deficient alleles may be especially relevant for patients carrying the CYP2D6 UM status: both genetic variants lead to an increase in morphine and O-desmethyltramadol plasma concentrations and subsequently increase toxicity risk.

The indication for genetic testing is the same for all PK biomarkers—the results of therapeutic drug monitoring are not within normal limits, and the drug is known to be metabolized by the enzyme being genotyped (tested). Other contributing factors—such as drug interactions, the timing of analysis relative to dose administration, compliance, prescribing error, and malabsorption—should be ruled out prior to testing. In pain management, therapeutic drug monitoring may apply to blood levels, urinary drug screening, and oral fluid/saliva sampling.

PD Genetic Biomarkers (or Genetics of Pharmacodynamics)

Generally speaking, the understanding of previously described PK biomarkers is more advanced than that of PD biomarkers. This is because PK genes can be analyzed and then the changes in blood levels of a drug secondary to the genetic variation can be objectively measured, allowing for a very clear cause-and-effect relationship. There are however several lines of evidences which might suggest that genetic factors could be involved in PD drug response in pain management.

Human μ (Micro or mu)-Opioid Receptor (MOR)

The gene encoding for MOR is known as OPRM1. A number of single nucleotide polymorphisms (SNPs) have been described in OPRM1, and the best characterized of these is A118G. It has been suggested that the G allele for OPRM1 may provide some protection against pain. One study found that the minor allele (G) was more likely to be present in a control group of opioid-naïve patients compared to patients with chronic pain treated with opioids. Another trial found that fentanyl requirements after cosmetic orofacial surgery were significantly reduced in patients carrying the OPRM1 minor allele variant. In the obstetric population, women with an A118G SNP, regardless of whether they are homozygous or heterozygous, have been demonstrated to have higher pressure pain thresholds than women with the wild-type allele. Another trial in the obstetric population found that women with the G variant were more responsive to intrathecal fentanyl. Other studies indicate that patients carrying the GG allele required higher opioid doses to achieve adequate pain relief. One trial examined MOR genotypes in cancer patients who had been treated with a stable dose of morphine over a period of at least 3 days. The investigators found that OPRM1 AA patients required an average morphine dose of 112 mg over 24 hours, while the AG group required an average dose of 132 mg, and the GG group required an average of 216 mg over the same time period. Although these data appear to contradict earlier studies, a possible explanation is that fentanyl has a higher binding affinity (threefold) compared to morphine and beta-endorphins for MOR. An increase in the binding affinity of beta-endorphins for the receptor may provide greater competition for morphine, thus resulting in higher doses required to displace beta-endorphin from MOR. At the very least, it suggests that people with A118G variant have different responses to opioids compared to those with the wild-type allele (Table 30.6).

Cyclooxygenase 1 and 2

Prostaglandin-endoperoxide synthase 1 and 2 (PTGS1 and PTGS2) are separate genes which encode cyclooxygenase 1 (COX)-1 and COX-2. Genetic variation in either of these enzymes can cause altered PD responses to NSAIDs. Certain SNPs are associated with altered expression of the PTGS2 transcript. In particular, a G → C polymorphism in the promoter region of the gene is associated with lower PTGS2 expression in individuals compared to those who inherit the homozygous major allele (G/G). Subjects with homozygous major allele reported lower pain intensities with rofecoxib treatment for 48 hours following surgery, compared to G/C or C/C subjects. This was not seen in those treated with ibuprofen. However, subjects with G/C or C/C genotypes reported decreased pain intensity with ibuprofen treatment at 48 hours following surgery, compared to G/G patients. This was not seen in subjects treated with rofecoxib. This is presumably because G/G patients have increased PTGS2 and increased COX-2 expression and therefore have an improved response to a COX-2 selective agent. On the other hand, patients who are heterozygous or homozygous for the minor allele (G/C or C/C genotype) may have reduced COX-2 expression and therefore experience greater benefit from a nonselective NSAID such as ibuprofen.

Table 30.6 OPRM1 gene 118A>G single nucleotide polymorphism in mu-opioid receptor and response

Parameter	Wild type, AA genotype (high sensitivity)	Heterozygote (G allele carrier, intermediate sensitivity)	Homozygous G alleles carrier (low receptor sensitivity)
Opioid dose and response	Normal	Normal to slightly increase opioid dose needed for pain relief	Increased opioid dose needed for pain relief, slight protection from opioid-induced nausea, and vomiting
Naltrexone response for alcohol dependence	Poorer response to naltrexone in alcoholics, increased risk of relapse	Typical rate in success of naltrexone to treat alcohol addition	Increase success to naltrexone treatment in alcoholics, including lower relapse rates
Opioid/ heroin addiction risk	Typical risk of opioid addiction in Asians	Increased risk factor of opioid addiction in Asians	Increased risk factor of opioid addiction in Asians

κ (Kappa)-Opioid Receptor and δ (Delta)-Opioid Receptor

The genes OPRK1 and OPRD1 encode the κ-opioid and δ-opioid receptor, respectively. Variations in OPRK1 and OPRD1 expression have been associated with dependence and addiction to various substances, including alcohol, opioids, heroin, and cocaine. Other allelic variation substitution have been associated with increased postoperative and chronic pain.

Catechol-O-methyl Transferase (COMT)

The catechol-O-methyl transferase (COMT) enzyme is responsible for the breakdown of biologically active catecholamines, such as dopamine, noradrenaline, and adrenaline. These are involved in numerous physiological processes, including the modulation of pain. Several polymorphisms have been identified within the COMT gene. The most widely studied variant is 158 Met, where a G to A nucleotide substitution at codon 158 results in an amino acid change from valine to methionine. Trials have demonstrated patients with Met/Met genotype have lower morphine requirements than those with a Val/Val expression. In children post adenotonsillectomy, it was demonstrated that the presence of any number of COMT SNPs, including 158 Met, was associated with a threefold greater likelihood of analgesic intervention compared to children who were homozygotes for major alleles. In addition, children with SNPs were also more likely to have increased pain postoperatively (Table 30.7).

KCNJ6

The G protein-activated inwardly rectifying potassium 2 (GIRK2) channel, encoded by the KCNJ6 gene, is one of the

Table 30.7 Opioid response and catechol-O-methyltransferase (COMT) activity related to the genetic polymorphism

COMT high activity (Val/Val)	COMT intermediate (Val/Met) and low activity (Met/Met)
Increased breakdown of neurotransmitters	Decreased breakdown of neurotransmitters
Higher pain threshold	Lower pain threshold
Decreased opioid receptor density	Increased opioid density
Increased opioid requirements	Decreased opioid requirements

downstream signaling effectors of the MOR. The effect of _1250G_A (rs6517442) and 1032A_G (rs2070995) on postoperative analgesia was assessed in adult patients undergoing gastrectomy and colectomy for gastric and colorectal cancer. Homozygous1032A allele patients and patients carrying the haplotype _1250G/1032A more often required rescue analgesia. Lower KCNJ6 mRNA expression levels were found in 1032AA individuals, while the _1250G_A SNP did not alter this expression. Another study on 1032A_G in chronic pain patients showed a trend in the same direction. In contrast to the adult postoperative study with the combined_ 1250G/1032A haplotype. Preterm infants with the _ 1250AA genotype who received either morphine or remifentanil needed more time to reach a pain-free state after endotracheal intubation. In an explorative analysis in adult white patients undergoing total knee arthroplasty, both_ 1250G_ A and 1032A were not associated with opioid dose. Of the 69 SNPs identified and analyzed in this study, significant hits were found with 8 other polymorphisms (rs1543754, rs858035, rs9981629, rs928723, rs2835925, rs2211843, rs1787337, rs2835930). These SNPs were combined in a genetic risk score and validated in a cohort with healthy individuals and patients with low back pain. Several SNPs in the KCNJ6 gene have been reported to be related to opioid response, but negative findings have been published as well. Therefore, the functional consequences of the mentioned variants and their relative effects on either mRNA or protein expression need to be further studied.

5-*HTT*

Genetic polymorphism of serotonin transporter (5-HTT) has been associated with alteration of pain pathways. For example, study in the healthy volunteers found that subjects with the triallelic 5-HTTLPR genotype coding for low 5-HTT expression gained better analgesic effect of remifentanil compared to those homozygous for the 5-HTTLPR LA allele. Low 5-HTT-expressing group compared to the high 5-HTT-expressing group exhibited significantly increased pressure pain and heat-pain thresholds. Association between inferred low 5-HTT expression and elevated thresholds to thermal pain was found in the healthy individuals. Similarly, homozygotes for variable-number tandem-repeat polymorphism suffered less from temporomandibular joint pain and dysfunction.

Melanocortin-1 Receptor Gene

Genetic studies in mice and humans revealed the modulatory effect of MC1R (melanocortin-1 receptor) gene variants on kappa-opioid receptor-mediated analgesia (e.g., after administration of pentazocine). It is unclear whether this gene affects basal pain sensitivity or the efficacy of analgesics acting at the more clinically relevant MOR. It was also demonstrated that MC1R gene mediates kappa-opioid analgesia in females only. This finding suggested that individuals with variants of the human MC1R gene, associated in our species with red hair and fair skin, might also display altered kappa-opioid analgesia. In this respect it was reported that women with two variant MC1R alleles displayed significantly greater analgesia from the kappa-opioid, pentazocine, than all other groups.

Main Points

1. There is currently insufficient evidence to justify routine pharmacogenetic testing for pain management, with exception of CYP2D6 genotyping for patients administered with codeine or tramadol and experiencing either lack of efficacy or adverse effects of therapy.
2. Variant spectrum of human CYP genes is extensive, and only a fraction of these variants has been characterized to date. Moreover, the multitude of very rare novel sequence variants indicates that the commonly used genotyping platforms are not satisfactory for determining the true genotype, which is critical information for personalized treatment with drugs influenced by CYP polymorphisms.
3. The future success of pharmacogenomic testing will depend upon more extensive sequencing strategies and the characterization of rare mutations with definite biological impact on treatment response, adverse effects, and pain pathology.

Recommended Reading

1. Agarwal D, Udoji MA, Trescot A. Genetic testing for opioid pain management: a primer. Pain Ther. 2017;6(1):93–105.
2. Bell GC, Donovan KA, McLeod HL. Clinical implications of opioid pharmacogenomics in patients with cancer. Cancer Control. 2015;22(4):426–32.
3. Fujikura K, Ingelman-Sundberg M, Lauschke VM. Genetic variation in the human cytochrome P450 supergene family. Pharmacogenet Genomics. 2015;25(12):584–94.
4. Kapur BM, Lala PK, Shaw JL. Pharmacogenetics of chronic pain management. Clin Biochem. 2014;47(13–14):1169–87.
5. Matic M, Jongen JL, Elens L, de Wildt SN, Tibboel D, Sillevis Smitt PA, van Schaik RH. Advanced cancer pain: the search for genetic factors correlated with interindividual variability in opioid requirement. Pharmacogenomics. 2017;18(12):1133–42.
6. Matic M, de Wildt SN, Tibboel D, van Schaik RHN. Analgesia and opioids: a pharmacogenetics shortlist for implementation in clinical practice. Clin Chem. 2017;63(7):1204–13.
7. Oosten AW, Matic M, van Schaik RH, Look MP, Jongen JL, Mathijssen RH, van der Rijt CC. Opioid treatment failure in cancer patients: the role of clinical and genetic factors. Pharmacogenomics. 2016;17(13):1391–403.

8. Owusu Obeng A, Hamadeh I, Smith M. Review of opioid pharmacogenetics and considerations for pain management. Pharmacotherapy. 2017. https://doi.org/10.1002/phar.1986. [Epub ahead of print].
9. Saba R, Kaye AD, Urman RD. Pharmacogenomics in pain management. Anesthesiol Clin. 2017;35(2):295–304.
10. Stamer U, Musshoff F, Kobilay M, Madea B, Hoeft A, Stuber F. Concentrations of tramadol and O-desmethyltramadol enantiomers in different CYP2D6 genotypes. Clin Pharmacol Ther. 2007;82(1):41–7.
11. Ting S, Schug S. The pharmacogenomics of pain management: prospects for personalized medicine. J Pain Res. 2016;9:49–56.
12. Webster LR, Belfer I. Pharmacogenetics and personalized medicine in pain management. Clin Lab Med. 2016;36(3):493–506.
13. Zanger UM, Klein K, Thomas M, Rieger JK, Tremmel R, Kandel BA, Klein M, Magdy T. Genetics, epigenetics, and regulation of drug-metabolizing cytochrome p450 enzymes. Clin Pharmacol Ther. 2014;95(3):258–61.

Part V

Interventional Treatment of Pain

Radiation Safety

31

Chong H. Kim, Torin Walters, and Vikram B. Patel

Introduction

Almost half of the radiation exposure experienced by the general population in the USA is from ionizing radiation from medical imaging. Ionizing radiation can be from X-rays or gamma rays, and as pain medicine has increasingly become more interventional, primarily with the aid of fluoroscopy, the need for basic understanding of radiation safety has become critical in optimal patient care.

Background and Historical Perspective

The use of fluoroscopy is a staple of interventional pain management, for accuracy and safety. Although the fluoroscopically guided procedures by pain physicians traditionally utilize relatively lower amounts of radiation compared to other specialties, newer procedures in neuromodulation and minimally invasive spine treatments may require greater exposures to radiation. More than ever before, radiation safety practices are necessary to ensure an optimal patient care environment.

The basic principles of fluoroscopy safety include justification and dose optimization. Both refer to maximizing patient benefit while minimizing risk to both patient and staff using the ALARA (as low as reasonably achievable) principle. The aim is to minimize the risk of radiation exposure or other hazard while keeping in mind that some exposure is inevitable, and therefore be acceptable. This philosophy is based on the assumption that any amount of radiation increases the potential risk of negative biological effects. X-rays were discovered in 1895 by Wilhelm Conrad Roentgen (1845–1923), who was a Professor at Wurzburg University in Germany. Roentgen's research included work with cathode-ray tubes where he observed a fluorescent glow of crystals. The tubes consisted of a glass envelope (bulb) with positive and negative electrodes. The air in the tube was evacuated, and when a high voltage was applied, the tube produced a fluorescent glow. Roentgen shielded the tube with heavy black paper and discovered a green colored fluorescent light by a material located a few feet away from the tube. He concluded that this new unknown or X-ray was capable of passing through the heavy paper covering and exciting the phosphorescent materials in the room. Roentgen also found that the new ray could pass through some substances and cast shadows of solid objects, such as tissue of humans, but not bones and metal objects. Roentgen's discovery at that time drew interest, by both scientists and laymen.

The discovery and use of X-rays in the late 1800 led to widespread experimentation and use that resulted in numerous reports of negative effects, such as hair loss and burns. Although some physicians reported the risks and side effects of radiation, many refuted the claims. The widespread and unrestrained use of X-rays led to serious injuries. Often injuries were not appropriately attributed to X-ray exposure, in part because of the slow onset of symptoms and due to the lack of knowledge. Some early experimenters did tie X-ray exposure and skin burns together. The first warning of possible adverse effects of X-rays came from Thomas Edison, William J. Morton, and Nikola Tesla who each reported eye irritations from experimentation with X-rays and fluorescent substances. By the end of the nineteenth century, the understanding of X-rays and radioactivity led to the science of radiation protection, also known as health physics.

Radiation exposure of tissue is quantified by the amount of absorbed dose or the amount of radiation that is deposited into the human tissue. Radiation exposure refers to the

C. H. Kim (✉)
MetroHealth/Case Western Reserve University, Department of PM&R, Cleveland, OH, USA
e-mail: ckim3@metrohealth.org

T. Walters
Department of Diagnostic Radiology, Joan C. Edwards School of Medicine, Marshall University, Senior Partner Radiology Inc, Huntington, WV, USA

V. B. Patel
Phoenix Interventional Center for Advanced Learning, Algonquin, IL, USA

T. R. Deer et al. (eds.), *Deer's Treatment of Pain*, https://doi.org/10.1007/978-3-030-12281-2_31

concentration of ionizing radiation in a specific volume of air, measured in roentgens (R). Absorption occurs when the human body is exposed to ionizing radiation, resulting in an interaction and energy transfer. The absorbed dose is described in gray (Gy) units (International System) or the older radian (rad) units (United States). One gray (1 J/kg) is equivalent to 100 rad. Rem (rad equivalent man) is a unit of exposure, while Gy is a unit of energy. One rem is equivalent to 0.01 sievert (Sv). Absorbed dose, measured in Gy or rads, is how much radiation is absorbed by a specific tissue. Effective dose, measured in Sv or rem, takes into account the particular sensitivity of the tissue or organ that absorbs the radiation and reflects the equivalent whole-body dose that would result in the equivalent risk from a nonuniform source of irradiation, such as fluoroscopy.

Risks of Radiation

The goal of radiation safety in the use of fluoroscopy is to minimize the absorbed dose to the skin and reduce radiation scatter from the patient to the physician and the staff. The skin typically absorb radiation from a direct beam at a rate of 2–5 rad/min but may be higher depending on the mode and intensity in which the radiation source is operated. The threshold for radiation injury, in relatively acute hypersensitivity conditions, to the skin is 3 Gy for temporary epilation, 6 Gy for erythema, and 15–20 Gy for desquamation, dermal necrosis, and ulceration. They can also be seen in additive exposure, over 6–12 months. The annual occupational limits of exposure are 5000 mrem to the body, 15,000 mrem to the lens, and 50,000 mrem to the extremities. There is no regulatory limits to the amount of radiation a patient may receive from medical procedure.

Risks of ionizing radiation involves the detachment of electrons from subatomic particles by electromagnetic waves at the atomic or molecular level. The risk levels are generally low in diagnostic and interventional procedures. Nevertheless, the ionizing radiation may cause DNA damage that increases the risk for future cancers. Radiation-induced cancers may develop decades after exposure and include myeloma, leukemia, lung cancer, thyroid cancer, breast cancer, bone cancer, and skin cancer. A case-cohort study showed left-sided tumor location in 86% of interventional cardiologists with brain cancer, while the general population has equal frequency. This finding is suggested to be significant as most cardiologists stand with their left side closest to the radiation source. In addition to cancers, radiation-induced cataracts along with detectable opacities are well documented. Relative risk of cataracts is 2.6–3.2 times higher for interventional specialists. There may be a genetic component of cataract development, which further elucidates some of the mechanisms behind DNA damage and response and repair pathways. Detectable opacities and cataracts have been observed in <1 Sv. Unfortunately, no clear threshold dose has been observed, although the latency period is inversely related to the exposure dose.

The cellular damage by ionizing radiation is proposed to be due to the production of free radicals, which can interfere with chemical bonds between molecules that regulate key cellular processes. Direct ionizing radiation can lead to DNA mutation, while indirect interaction can cause free radical damage to essential cell enzymes. The rate of cellular proliferation and cellular differentiation determines the susceptibility of the tissues to radiation injury. The systems with high cell turnover, such as blood-forming organs, are most sensitive, while nervous tissues with little or no cell turnover are the least sensitive (Table 31.1).

Current limits for occupational radiation exposure have been established at levels that will prevent acute radiation effects (erythema, epilation) and limit the risks of late effects, such as cancer or genetic damage, to very low, "acceptable" levels of comparable to non-radiation-related occupational risks. These limits can be found in Title 10, Part 20 of the Code of Federal Regulations. These limits are based on external, internal, and external-plus-internal exposures (Table 31.2). The shallow-dose equivalent is the external dose to the skin of the whole body or extremities from an external source of ionizing radiation. This value is the dose equivalent at a tissue depth of 0.007 cm averaged over and area of 10 cm^2. The lens dose equivalent is the dose equivalent to the lens of the eye from an external source of ionizing radiation. This value is the dose equivalent at a tissue depth

Table 31.1 Sensitivity of human organs and tissues

Radiation sensitivity	Organ or tissue
Very high	Embryonic tissue, lymphoid organs, bone marrow, blood, testes and ovaries, small intestine
High	Skin, lens and cornea of the eye, gastrointestinal organs (oral cavity, esophagus, stomach, rectum), bladder, uterus
Medium	Growing cartilage, growing bones, blood vessels
Low	Mature cartilage or bone, pituitary gland, lungs, thyroid, pancreas, kidneys, adrenal glands
Very low	Brain, spinal cord, muscles

Table 31.2 Annual occupational dose limits for adult workers

Limit	rem[a]	Sievert (sv)
Shallow dose equivalent, whole body	50	0.5
Shallow dose equivalent, max. extremity	50	0.5
Eye dose equivalent to the lens of the eye	15	0.15
Total organ dose equivalent	50	0.5
Total effective dose equivalent	5	0.05

[a]rem = the common unit of dose equivalent. Sievert is the S.I. dose equivalent unit
(100 rem = 1 sievert)

of 0.3 cm. The deep-dose equivalent is the whole-body dose from an external source of ionizing radiation. This value is the dose equivalent at a tissue depth of 1 cm. The total effective dose equivalent is the dose equivalent to the whole body.

The risk of developing cancer from medical imaging radiation exposure is generally small and depends on:

- Radiation dose – The lifetime risk of cancer increases, the larger the dose and the more X-ray exams a patient undergoes.
- Patient's age – The lifetime risk of cancer is larger for a patient who receives X-rays at a younger age than for one who receives them at an older age.
- Patient's sex – Women are at a somewhat higher lifetime risk than men for developing radiation-associated cancer after receiving the same exposures at the same ages.
- Body region – Some organs are more radiosensitive than others.

The deleterious effect ionizing radiation has on human tissue can be divided into two types: non-stochastic or stochastic effects. Stochastic effects are events that occur by chance and which may occur without a threshold level of dose, whose probability is proportional to the dose and whose severity is independent of the dose. In the context of radiation protection, the main stochastic effect is cancer and genetic effects. Stochastic effects occur by chance. Stochastic effects often show up years after exposure. As the dose to an individual increases, the probability that cancer or a genetic effect will occur also increases. However, at no time, even for high doses, it is certain that cancer or genetic damage will result. Similarly, for stochastic effects, there is no threshold dose below which it is relatively certain that an adverse effect cannot occur. In addition, stochastic effects can occur in individuals that have not been exposed to radiation above background levels. Simply put, the likelihood of cancer or genetic damage from a specific exposure cannot be determined. While it cannot be determined conclusively, it is often possible to estimate the probability that radiation exposure will cause a stochastic effect. It is estimated that the probability of having a cancer in the USA rises from 20% for non-radiation exposed workers to 21% for persons who work regularly without protective measures in radiation-exposed environment. The risk of developing solid cancers follows a linear pattern with increasing dose, although the age at which exposure takes place is highly relevant. A decline in radiosensitivity does take place with age, making young children more susceptible to radiation-induced malignancies. Although the malignancy risk for the population as a whole is 5%/Sv, this rises to 15%/Sv in a young girl and falls to 1%/Sv in a 70-year-old.

The probability for genetic defects is even less likely to increase for workers exposed to radiation. Studies conducted on Japanese atomic bomb survivors who were exposed to large doses of radiation found no more genetic defects than what would normally occur. However, data from the Radiation Effects Research Foundation on individuals exposed to radiation from the atomic bombs in Hiroshima and Nagasaki have shown an increased relative risk of developing malignancy (leukemia, oral cavity, esophagus, stomach, colon, lung, breast, ovary, urinary bladder, thyroid, liver, non-melanoma skin, and nervous system) as a result of radiation exposure. As such, multiple bodies, including the US Department of Health and Human Services, have classified ionizing radiation as a human carcinogen. Radiation-induced hereditary effects have not been observed in human populations, yet they have been demonstrated in animals. If the germ cells that are present in the ovaries and testes and are responsible for reproduction were modified by radiation, hereditary effects could occur in the progeny of the individual. Exposure of the embryo or fetus to ionizing radiation could increase the risk of leukemia in infants and, during certain periods in early pregnancy, may lead to mental retardation and congenital malformations if the amount of radiation is sufficiently high. The United Nations Scientific Committee on the Effects of Atomic Radiation (UNSCEAR) proposes a hereditary defect risk of between 0.3% and 0.8% per Sv.

Unlike stochastic effects, non-stochastic effects or deterministic effects are characterized by a threshold dose below which they do not occur. In other words, non-stochastic effects have a clear relationship between the exposure and the effect. In addition, the magnitude of the effect is directly proportional to the size of the dose. Non-stochastic effects typically result from very large doses of radiation received in a short amount of time, while the radiation-induced skin effects may make several weeks to manifest at lower doses. These effects will often be evident within hours or days. Examples of non-stochastic effects include erythema (skin reddening), skin and tissue burns, cataract formation, sterility, radiation sickness, and death. Each of these effects differs from the others in that both its threshold dose and the time over which the dose was received cause the effect (i.e., acute vs. chronic exposure).

Cases of non-stochastic effects due to radiation burns occurring to the hands or fingers have been reported. These cases occurred when a radiographer touched or came in close contact with a high intensity radiation emitter. Intensity on the surface of an 85 curie Ir-192 source capsule is approximately 1768 R/s. Contact with the source for 2 seconds would expose the hand of an individual to 3536 rems, and this does not consider any additional whole-body dosage received when approaching the source. Again, risk estimates of radiation-induced cancer from medical imaging are mainly based on extrapolation of existing data from Japanese survivors from the 1945 atomic bombings.

Safety

The primary tool for estimating radiation dose is the personal dosimeter and is reported as equivalent dose or as effective dose. The radiation dose cannot be directly measured and is estimated based on the data from the personal dosimeter.

Three guiding principles of radiation protection are justification, optimization, and limitations. Justification is defined as no practice involving exposures to radiation should be adopted unless it produces sufficient benefit to the exposed individual or to society to offset the detriment it causes. Justification requires evaluation and weighing of the needs for the use and exposure of radiation, along with risks and benefits. Discussion about the possible risks of ionizing radiation should be part of the consent process prior to any radiological procedure, such as fluoroscopy. The principle of optimization of radiation protection is defined as the source-related process to keep the magnitude of individual doses, the number of people exposed, and the likelihood of potential exposure as low as reasonably achievable below the appropriate dose constraints, with economic and social factors being taken into account. This process of optimization below constraint should be applied whatever the exposure situation, i.e., planned, emergency, and existing. Finally, limitations is defined as effective dose to individuals shall not exceed the dose limits recommended and also applies radiation safety for the operator and staff and to limit the scatter and total exposure.

The two basic types of radiation safety controls, engineered and administrative, are used to provide a safe working environment. Engineered controls include shielding, interlocks, alarms, warning signals, and material containment. Administrative controls include postings, procedures, dosimetry, and training.

Engineered controls such as shielding and door interlocks can be used to contain the radiation in a cabinet or a radiation vault, though these are not commonly used in interventional setting such as in a fluoroscopic procedure room. Fixed shielding materials are commonly high density concrete and/or lead. Door interlocks are used to immediately cut the power to X-ray generating equipment if a door is accidentally opened when X-rays are being produced. Warning lights are used to alert workers and the public that radiation is being used. Sensors and warning alarms are often used to signal that a predetermined amount of radiation is present. Safety controls should never be tampered with or bypassed.

Administrative controls supplement the engineered controls. These controls include postings, procedures, dosimetry, and training. It is commonly required that all areas containing X-ray-producing equipment or radioactive materials have signs posted bearing the radiation symbol and a notice explaining the dangers of radiation. Normal operating procedures and emergency procedures must also be prepared and followed. In the USA, federal law requires that any individual who is likely to receive more than 10% of any annual occupational dose limit be monitored for radiation exposure. Individual states may have different requirements. This monitoring is accomplished with the use of dosimeters, which are discussed in the radiation safety equipment section of this material. Proper training with accompanying documentation is also a very important administrative control.

Radiation protection can be divided into three areas, time, distance, and shielding. Decreasing the time for which the radiation beam is on, or the exposure time, decreases radiation exposure. This can also be influenced by reducing the fluoroscopy dose rate.

$$\text{Dose} = \text{Dose Rate} \times \text{Time}$$

The distance between the radiograph source and radiation exposure is inverse square in nature. The further the distance, the less the radiation exposure. For example, doubling the distance from the radiation source reduces the radiation exposure to one-fourth of the original dose.

$$\text{Inverse square law}: I_1 / I_2 = D_2^2 / D_1^2$$

I_1 = Intensity 1 at D_1
I_2 = Intensity 2 at D_2
D_1 = Distance 1 from source
D_2 = Distance 2 from source

Additionally, the radiation intensity is highest at the X-ray beam skin entrance surface. As a result, positioning the beam image intensifier as close to the patient as possible minimizes the radiation exposure. Also, if possible, the operator should be positioned on the side opposite of the tube when possible. Furthermore, scatter from the patient and radiation from the cover of the X-ray beam collimating device must also be considered and minimized.

Finally, shielding includes architectural, equipment mounted, and personal protective devices. The depth of penetration for a given photon energy is dependent upon the material density (atomic structure). The more subatomic particles in a material (higher Z number), the greater the likelihood that interactions will occur and the radiation will lose its energy. Therefore, the more dense a material is, the smaller the depth of radiation penetration will be. Materials such as depleted uranium, tungsten, and lead have high Z numbers and are therefore very effective in shielding radiation. Concrete is not as effective in shielding radiation, but it is a very common building material, and so it is commonly used in the construction of X-ray equipment installations.

The half-value layer (HVL) is useful for determining what thickness of a given material is necessary to reduce the exposure rate from a source to some level. At some point in the material, there is a level at which the radiation intensity becomes one-half that at the surface of the material. This depth is known as the half-value layer for that material. Each material has its own specific HVL thickness. Not only is the HVL material dependent, but it is also radiation energy dependent. This means that for a given material, if the radiation energy changes, the point at which the intensity decreases to half its original value will also change. As the energy of the radiation increases, the HVL value also increases.

Architectural shielding is built into the basic structure, into the walls of the room. Equipment-mounted shielding includes table-suspended drapes, ceiling-mounted shields, and lateral table-mounted shields. Lead skirt around the patient table significantly reduced scatter radiation, particularly to the groin, knee, and feet. Also, rolling and fixed transparent lead shields can be used for extra, portable protection. Additionally, disposable, lightweight, sterile radioprotective drapes, and pad forms can be placed on the patients once the field has been prepared outside of the beam path to reduce the radiation exposure to the operator.

Personal protective devices include lead aprons, thyroid shields, eyewear, and gloves. Traditionally, personal protective aprons protect the torso, from the chest to the thighs. Although aprons with sleeves or additional sleeve attachments are available, most do not protect the arms for legs below the knees. Also, some aprons do not protect the backs. When wearing the open aprons, the operator must ensure they are facing the direction of the radiation source. Traditionally, the aprons were made from 100% lead; however, composite and non-lead aprons and protective garments are now available. Radiation-attenuating materials, such as bismuth oxide and barium sulfate and rare-earth metals, are commonly used as non-lead options. Composites containing lead, tin, tungsten, and barium are also alternatives. Composite and non-lead shielding, though costlier, are lighter in weight. Composite aprons are 10–15% lighter than all lead aprons. No lead aprons are the lightest, 15–40% lighter. Most lead aprons weigh around 10 pounds. Lead aprons and thyroid shields should always be worn during radiation use. Personal protective lead aprons can be one- or two-piece options. Two-piece aprons are composed of separate vest and skirt. Aprons typically range from 0.25 to 0.5 mm lead equivalency. The lead equivalency of 0.25 mm allow approximately 10% of the radiation to pass through, while 0.5 mm has a transmission ratio of about 2%. Ergonomics are critical in the use of personal lead aprons, as risk of back injury have been reported. The lead aprons and garments should be placed on hangers, should not be folded and routinely inspected, visually and fluoroscopically to minimize and detect damages.

Eye wear is another essential component of personal radiation protection. Use of leaded glasses alone reduced the lens dose rate by a factor of 5–10. Lead glasses that shield against exposures from the side can lower doses by 2.5–4.5 times. All eye protection should have wraparound protection or side protection to limit scatter radiation as well as re-scatter from the operators head. Eye wear with the equivalent of 0.75 mm of lead attenuates 95% of the incident radiation against 120 keV X-rays (typically the highest energies encountered in most X-ray procedures). For lower energies, such as scattered X-rays, the attenuation effect is even greater. Additionally, ceiling-suspended shields and disposable radiation-absorbing pads can reduce eye dose by factors of 2–7. Some reports have raised concern that protection from lead glasses may be incomplete. Face shields and radio-absorbent surgical caps can also be considered.

Radiation protection for the hands include gloves and lotions. Lead and lead-free sterile gloves, sleeves, and heavy-duty mittens are available. The gloves have been shown to attenuate 25–38% of incident radiation against 120 keV direct beam X-rays. The gloves range from 0.2 to 0.4 mm in thickness. However, if the operator's hands are in the primary radiation beam, leaded gloves may not help reduce exposure. Recording systems in fluoroscopy require automatic exposure control for optimum image quality. Automatic brightness control (ABC) maintains intensifier exposure rates on the basis of subject thickness by adjusting various technique factors. As a result, the ABC will increase the radiation intensity when any shielding is placed in the primary beam. In this situation, radioprotective bismuth oxide containing lotion can be considered. However, as always, the most effective radiation protection is to avoid the primary beam.

Finally, last area for radiation protection is appropriate use of fluoroscopy. Most procedures are performed using a C-arm. The X-ray tube is usually below the patient, while the image intensifier is located above the patient. To minimize radiation exposure, the image intensifier should be positioned as close to the patient as possible. If possible, the case should be reviewed and prepared in advance to limit surprises and unnecessary use of fluoroscopy. The last image hold setting should be use. Low-dose settings will minimize the radiation exposure rate. The image should be kept within the patient's body limits. Collimation will improve image contrast by reducing scatter. Spot fluoroscopy, which enables a square or rectangular collimation of a region of interest within the general field, has been shown to have advantages over traditional collimation. Intermittent, "tap" fluoroscopy should be used whenever possible. Limited use of magnification, boost, or digital subtraction will aid in minimizing radiation exposure. Additionally, pulsed mode has been shown to reduce radiation exposure up to 75%, 83% when used with low-dose modes.

Summary of recommendations for personal radiation safety in the use of fluoroscopy are listed below.

Personal Radiation Safety

- Maximize equipment and room shielding to minimize radiation exposure.
- Always use personal radiation shielding.
- Position yourself to minimize radiation exposure.
- Avoid primary beam exposure.
- Minimize fluoroscopy time.
- Use low-dose-rate settings, including low frame rate.
- Use collimation.
- Limit magnification, use wide display mode if available.
- Review and prepare for the case in advance.
- Complete and stay current on radiation training and education.
- Wear dosimeters and monitor the dose.

Recommended Reading

1. Meisinger QC, Stahl CM, Andre MP, Kinney TB, Isabel G. Radiation protection for the fluoroscopy operator and staff. Am J Roentgenol. 2016;207(4):745–54.
2. Rathmell J. Atlas of image-guided interventions in regional anesthesia and pain medicine. Chapter 3. Radiation safety. Philadelphia: Lippincott Williams and Wilkins; 2006.

32 Radiofrequency Ablation

Chase A. Kissling, David Provenzano, Steven P. Cohen, and Eric T. Lee

Introduction and Most Common Uses of RFA

Radiofrequency ablation (RFA) has been used to treat chronic pain since the 1970s and is a frequently and increasingly employed interventional technique used for the treatment of axial spine and musculoskeletal pain conditions. This chapter will focus on the most common uses of RFA for chronic pain, including treating pain originating from the axial spine (including lumbar and cervical facet syndrome and sacroiliac joint dysfunction) and knee joint pain.

Facet joint, sacroiliac joint dysfunction, and osteoarthritis of the knee are common causes of pain that affect many individuals. Facet joint (zygapophysial)-mediated pain has been identified as a source of chronic axial spine pain. The prevalence of facetogenic pain in the cervical spine ranges from 45% to 55%. The lumbar facet joints are the primary etiology of axial low back pain in 15–45% of cases, depending on the age of the studied population. The prevalence of low back pain secondary to sacroiliac joint dysfunction ranges from 10% to 25%. Chronic knee osteoarthritis (OA) is one of the most common diseases of advanced age, and pharmacologic therapy is of limited value. It is projected that more than 59 million persons in the United States (18% of the population) will have osteoarthritis by 2020.

The number and types of published works varies between interventions. In this chapter, we will be presenting evidence primarily from randomized controlled trials (RCTs) prospective studies and systematic reviews when possible.

C. A. Kissling
Walter Reed National Military Medical Center, Bethesda, MD, USA

D. Provenzano (✉)
Pain Diagnostics and Interventional Care, Sewickley, PA, USA

S. P. Cohen
Department of Anesthesiology and Critical Care Medicine, Johns Hopkins School of Medicine, Baltimore, MD, USA

Department of Physical Medicine and Rehabilitation, Johns Hopkins School of Medicine, Baltimore, MD, USA

Department of Anesthesiology, Uniformed Services University of the Health Sciences, Bethesda, MD, USA

Department of Physical Medicine and Rehabilitation, Uniformed Services University of the Health Sciences, Bethesda, MD, USA
e-mail: scohen40@jhmi.edu

E. T. Lee
Musculoskeletal Care and Regenerative Medicine, St Charles Spine Institute, Thousand Oaks, CA, USA
e-mail: Eric.lee@summitpainalliance.com

Cervical Facet RFA

Anatomy

In the axial spine, the medial branches of the dorsal rami curve around the lateral aspect of the neck of the superior articular process. These articular branches pass above and below each respective zygapophysial joint (Figs. 32.1, 32.2, and 32.3). The third occipital nerve, which is the large superficial medial branch of the C3 dorsal ramus, is an exception. It crosses the lateral and dorsal aspect of the C2–C3 facet joint before passing upward to become cutaneous over the suboccipital area. Unlike the lower cervical facet joints, the third occipital nerve forms the sole innervation to the C2–C3 joint. The third occipital nerve has a diameter of 1.1–1.9 mm which makes it consistently larger than the lower cervical medial branches, all of which have a mean diameter of less than 1 mm.

Efficacy (Table 32.1)

A systematic review of fluoroscopically guided cervical medial branch thermal radiofrequency neurotomy by Engel et al. in 2016 yielded eight primary publications and found the majority of patients were pain-free at 6 months. The number needed to treat for complete pain relief at 6 months was 2 based on high quality studies according to the GRADE system. Twelve papers reported minor and temporary unwanted effects with no serious complications. The evidence of risk is of low quality according to the GRADE sys-

T. R. Deer et al. (eds.), *Deer's Treatment of Pain*, https://doi.org/10.1007/978-3-030-12281-2_32

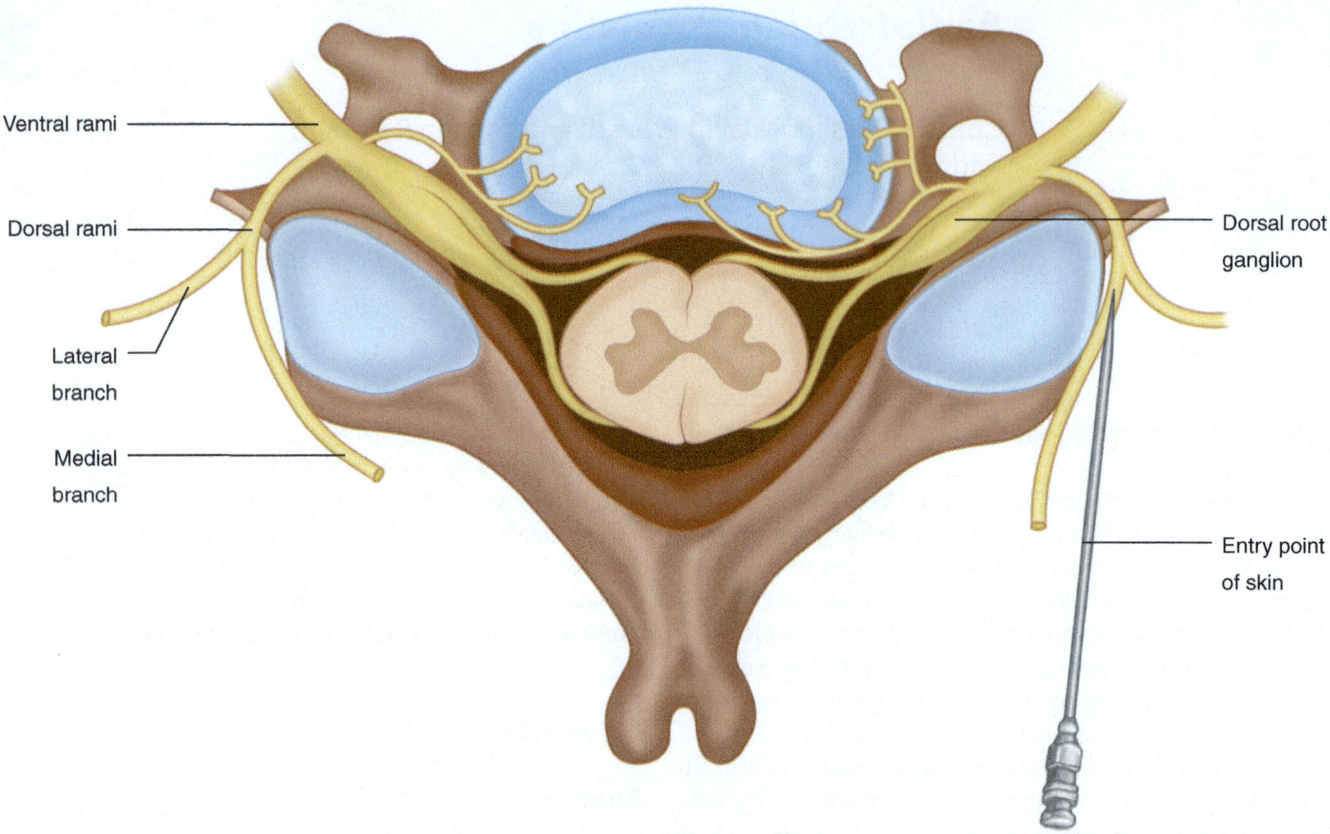

Fig. 32.1 Schematic drawing demonstrating the targets of radiofrequency neurotomy of cervical medial branch

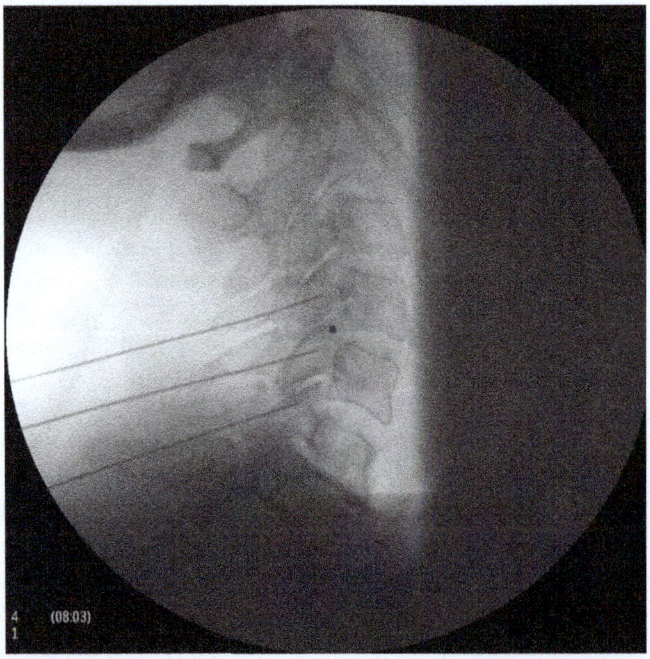

Fig. 32.2 Lateral radiographic demonstrating radiofrequency cannulae placed to lesion the C4, C5, and C6 medial branches for the C4–C5 and C5–C6 facet joints

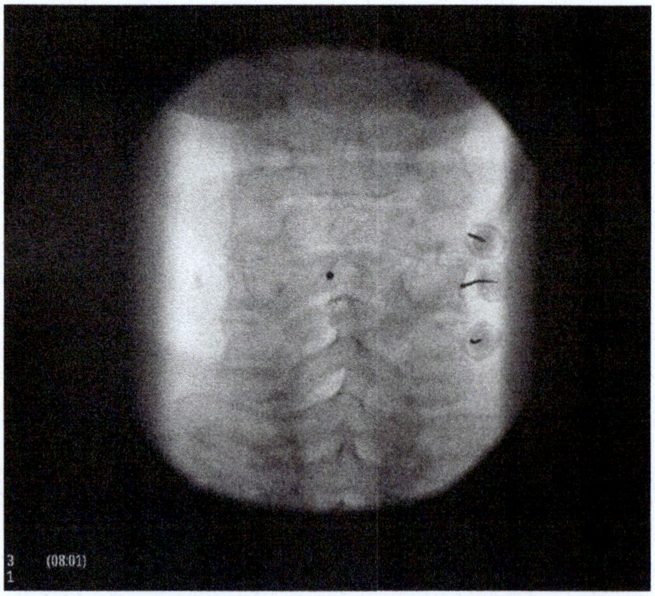

Fig. 32.3 Anterior-posterior radiograph demonstrating radiofrequency cannula placement for the C4, C5, and C6 medial branches for the C4–C5 and C5–C6 facet joints

Table 32.1 Prospective and randomized controlled trials for cervical radiofrequency for axial spine pain

Study author/characteristics	Radiofrequency technique	# of patients	Primary outcomes	Comments
Lord et al. 1998 RCT, double-blind, sham-controlled	Monopolar thermal RFA	24 pts. who failed conservative management confirmed with double-blind, placebo-controlled LA nerve blocks	RF denervation was found to be superior to sham, and a median time of 263 days elapsed before pain returned to at least 50% of the preoperative level in the RF group	Landmark evaluation Small sample size
Sapir et al. 2001 Prospective	Monopolar thermal RFA	46 pts. with cervical whiplash who failed conservative mgmt. and who achieved 80% reduction in pain with controlled comparative LA blocks divided into groups based on potential for monetary gain via litigation	66% of litigation group and 71% of non-litigation group reported relief with time to recurrence of 50% of baseline pain being 8 ± 2 months. There was a similar rate of recurrence in both groups	Small study size
Speldewinde 2011 Prospective	Monopolar thermal RFA	130 pts. selected with at least 2 fluoroscopically-guided diagnostic LA blocks who obtained at least 80% pain relief	76% overall success Average 88% pain relief for at least 12 months	Positive study
Macvicar et al. 2012 Prospective	Thermal RFA with parallel placement	104 pts. with neck pain selected who had complete relief following controlled comparative diagnostic LA blocks	74% and 61% of pts. achieved >80% relief for >6 mos in 2 practices. Relief lasted 17–20 months for first RFA, 15 months for repeat treatments	Positive study Rigorous inclusion criteria

LA Local anesthetic

tem. Another systematic review of cervical RFA literature by Falco et al. in 2012 (updated from 2009) evaluated four randomized controlled trials and six observational studies using USPSTF grading criteria. Based on one randomized, sham-controlled, double-blind trial and five observational studies, the authors concluded that indicated evidence to support cervical radiofrequency neurotomy was fair.

Lumbar Facet RFA

Anatomy

The lumbar facet joints are synovial joints formed by the superior and inferior articular processes of each respective vertebral body. In the lumbar spine, the superior articular facet is anterior and lateral to the inferior articular facet. The facets contribute 40% to torsional load resistance in the lumbar spine. The facet joints assist in resisting forward translation, rotation, compressive loads, and shearing forces generated in the lumbar spine. The target nerves (i.e., medial branches) and anatomic landmarks are subtly different in the lumbar spine compared to the cervical spine. The medial branch of each lumbar dorsal ramus runs caudally across the neck of the superior articular process, and the articular branches approach each joint from below and from above. At L5, it is the dorsal ramus itself that is amenable to ablation. The L1–L4 medial branches are held in position and covered by the mamillo-accessory ligament. The mamillo-accessory ligament is not a true ligament because it connects two points on the same bone: the accessory process located on the transverse process and the mammillary process located on the superior articular process. The medial branch is covered by the mamillo-accessory ligament distal to the middle of the neck of the superior articular process. Unlike the L1 through L4 medial branches, the L5 dorsal ramus exists in the groove formed by the sacral ala and the superior articular process of S1 and is not held in position by the mamillo-accessory ligament. Compared to the cervical spine, the orientation of the facet joints and nerves in the low back complicate the positioning of straight needles parallel to the nerves. The medial branches targeted are small—often less than 2 mm in diameter. Therefore, incorrect needle technique will result in the inability to lesion the targeted nerve. Figures 32.4 and 32.5

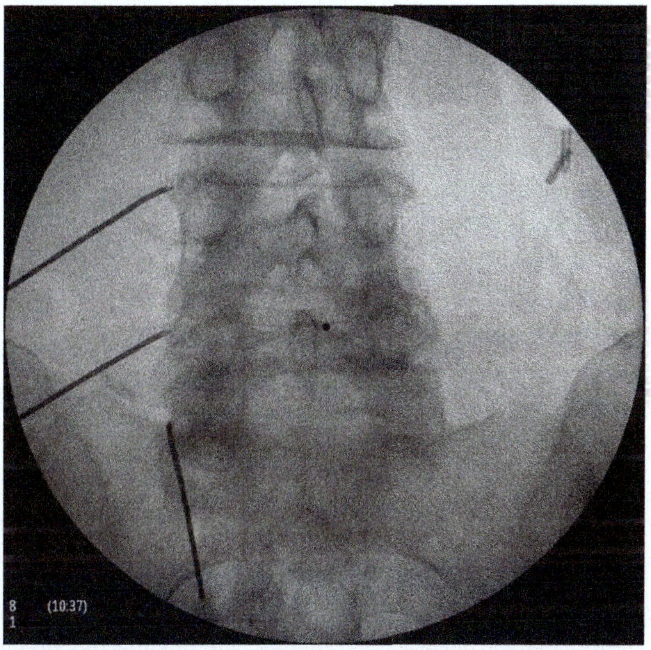

Fig. 32.4 Anterior-posterior radiograph demonstrating radiofrequency cannulae placement for the L3 and L4 medial branches and L5 dorsal ramus targeting the L4–L5 and L5–S1 facet joints

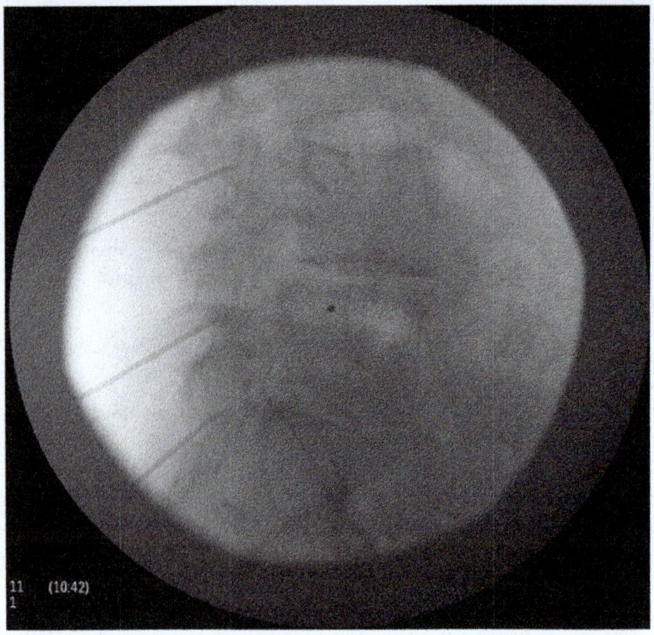

Fig. 32.5 Lateral radiograph demonstrating radiofrequency cannulae placement for the L3 and L4 medial branches and L5 dorsal ramus targeting the L4–L5 and L5–S1 facet joints

demonstrate placement of radiofrequency cannulae for the lumbar spine.

Efficacy (Table 32.2)

A meta-analysis of seven RCTs by Lee et al. in 2017 found a significant improvement in pain scores at 1 year in RFA treatment groups compared to sham. A Cochrane review of RFA for chronic low back pain in 2015 evaluated 23 studies. Twelve studies examined suspected facet joint pain, five studies likely disc pain, two studies SI joint pain, two studies radicular CLBP, one study suspected radiating low back pain, and one study CLBP with or without suspected radiation. The review authors found no high-quality evidence suggesting that RF denervation provides pain relief or functional improvement for patients with CLBP with high-quality evidence lacking. A 2014 review by Poetscher et al. looking at nine studies found low-to-moderate evidence favoring RFA for pain control with no sufficient evidence for cost-effectiveness and complications. In a systematic review of six RCT by Leggett et al. in 2014 examining lumbar facet RFA, five of six studies found statistically significant positive benefit to lumbar RFA. An updated systematic review by Falco et al. in 2012 that considered 11 RCTs and 14 observational studies found good to fair evidence for lumbar facet RFA. In another review by Bogduk et al. in 2009, three out of six studies on lumbar medial branch RFA for facet pain were considered significantly flawed. Among the three studies that were not considered flawed and showed definitive positive outcomes, two were observational, and one was a randomized controlled trial (RCT). The therapeutic efficacy of lumbar medial branch RF has been evaluated in both observational trials and RCTs. In the six RCTs, three contained technical flaws in both patient selection and surgical technique, which yields less reliable findings. Since then, one large randomized study has been published which found no efficacy for lumbar facet RFA; yet, this study was again flawed with regard to technical aspects (e.g., electrode placement and orientation), statistical analysis (i.e., interpretation of minimal clinically important differences), and non-stringent selection criteria (e.g., only one diagnostic block).

As alluded to above, an important factor influencing efficacy is placement of electrodes, which should ideally be placed parallel to the target nerve. Because of inherent challenges in maximizing lesion size, utilizing large electrodes and pre-injecting electrolytic fluids (i.e., fluid modulation) should be considered when performing monopolar RF ablation. Time of ablation also matters. Extending the duration of RF lesioning beyond 90 seconds has been shown by Provenzano et al. to maximize lesion size while limiting size variability.

Repeat RFA

The efficacy of repeat RFA should be briefly addressed. At least three retrospective and one prospective study have been done to assess repeat RFA, all showing a success rate of greater than or equal to 85% for repeated RFA treatments. The duration of pain relief of each treatment varied between 10 and 12 months with no statistical difference in pain relief duration for subsequent treatments.

Sacroiliac Joint RFA

Anatomy

The sacroiliac joint (SIJ) is a large joint that contains both ligamentous and intra-articular components. It is primarily innervated by the lateral branches of posterior primary rami sensory nerves, which derive from the L5 to S4 levels. A recent cadaveric study provided further insight into the innervation of the SI joint. Roberts et al. demonstrated that the SIJ innervation was from S1–S2 in all cases and S3 in 88% of cases, with L5 and S4 providing sensory input in less than 10% of cases. Based on the anatomy, optimal RF interventional techniques were proposed. These nerves cross between the transverse sacral tubercles (TST) one through three, with the greatest concentration between the second and third TST. Unlike in the cervical/lumbar spine,

Table 32.2 Prospective and randomized controlled trials for lumbar radiofrequency for axial spine pain

Study author/ characteristics	Thermal mono/bipolar or cooled RFA	# of patients	Primary outcomes	Comments
Juch et al. 2017 RCT, non-blinded	Thermal	681 pts. with chronic LBP, a positive diagnostic block for lumbar (251 pts) and SI joint pain (228 pts) unresponsive to conservative care	599 (88%) completed the 3 months follow-up; 521 (77%) completed the 12 month follow-up. The mean difference in pain intensity between RFA and control groups at 3 months was −0.18 (95%CI, −0.76 to 0.40) in the facet joint trial and − 0.99 (95%CI, −1.73 to −0.25) in the facet/SI joint combination trial	Negative study Significant methodological and statistical flaws including poor procedure technique
Van Tilburg et al. 2016 RCT, double-blind multicenter, sham-controlled	Thermal	60 with suggestive lumbar facet pain and positive diagnostic block. Sham group crossover at 3 months if no improvement	There was a statistically significant effect on the level of pain on DOS and at 1 month. However, there was no statistically significant difference with the passage of time between the groups (Group × Period). In the crossover group, 11/19 patients had a decrease in NRS of ≥2 at 1 month crossover ($p = 0.65$). There was no statistically significant difference in satisfaction with the passage of time between the groups (Group × Period). The independent factors 'Group' and 'Period' also showed no statistically significant difference. There was no statistically significant Group × Period effect for recovery	Positive but cannot reject null hypothesis
Nath et al. 2008 RCT, placebo-controlled	Thermal	40 pts. with back pain >2 years with no response to conservative treatment and positive diagnostic blocks	Significant improvement in back/leg pain and back/hip movement in the active treatment group at 6 months posttreatment, improved quality-of-life scores, and reduced use of analgesics. No significant complications were reported	Positive study Appropriate study design
Tekin et al. 2007 RCT, double-blind, sham-controlled	Thermal or pulsed RFA	60 pts (20 pulsed RF, 20 thermal RFA and 20 LA without RF) with chronic LBP unresponsive to conservative treatment, and a single positive diagnostic facet block (>50% pain reduction)	Patient satisfaction was excellent in 20%, good in 50%, moderate in 25%, and bad in 5% of patients in control group. In thermal RF group satisfaction was excellent in 65%, good in 30%, and moderate in 5% of patients. In the PRF group, satisfaction was excellent in 35%, good in 50% and moderate in 15% of patients. Patient satisfaction was lowest in control group ($P = 0.03$) and highest in CRF group ($P = 0.004$)	Positive study
Van Wijk et al. 2005 RCT, double-blind, sham-controlled	Thermal RFA	81pts with LBP >6 months with >50% reduction in pain with diagnostic block	The combined outcome measure showed no differences between RFA ($n = 40$; success 27.5%) and sham ($n = 41$; success 29.3%) ($P = 0.86$). The VAS pain score in both groups improved ($P = 0.001$). Global perceived effect improved after radiofrequency facet joint denervation compared to sham ($P = 0.05$). The other secondary outcome parameters showed no significant differences	-Technical and procedural flaws including perpendicular needle placement
Leclaire et al. 2001 Prospective double-blind RCT	Thermal RFA	70 pts. with LBP >3 months with good response to fluoroscopically guided diagnostic block	4 weeks, the Roland-Morris score had improved by a mean of 8.4% in the neurotomy group and 2.2% in the placebo group, showing a treatment effect of 6.2% ($P = 0.05$). At 4 weeks, no significant treatment effect was reflected in the Oswestry disability score (0.6% change) or the visual analog scale pain score (4.2% change). At 12 weeks, neither functional disability, as assessed by the Roland-Morris scale (2.6% change) and Oswestry Disability Index (1.9% change), nor the pain level, as assessed by the visual analog scale (−7.6% change), showed any treatment effect	Significant technical and procedural flaws including required pain relief > 24 hours with lidocaine diagnostic block
Van Kleef et al. 1999 Double-blind RCT	Thermal RFA	31 patients with CLBP>1 year with positive diagnostic block, 15 received RFA L3–L5, 16 received sham	8 weeks after treatment, 10 improved patients in the radiofrequency group ($n = 15$) and 6 in the sham group ($n = 16$). The unadjusted odds ratio was 3.3 ($P = 0.05$, not significant), and the adjusted odds ratio was 4.8 ($P < 0.05$, significant). The differences in effect on the visual analog scale scores, global perceived effect, and the Oswestry Disability Index scale were statistically significant. At 3, 6, and 12 months after treatment, there were significantly more improved patients in the radiofrequency group compared with the sham group	Positive study
Gallagher et al. 1994 RCT	Thermal	60 pts. with LBP > 3 months received diagnostic block. Those patients with positive or equivocal response were then randomized to RFA or sham. Pts with no relief excluded	Patients who showed improvement with diagnostic block had improved pain scores following RFA at 1 and 6 months. Pts with an equivocal block showed no improvement in pain scores	Significant technical and procedural flaws. Reinforces that a positive diagnostic block is important for positive outcome from RFA

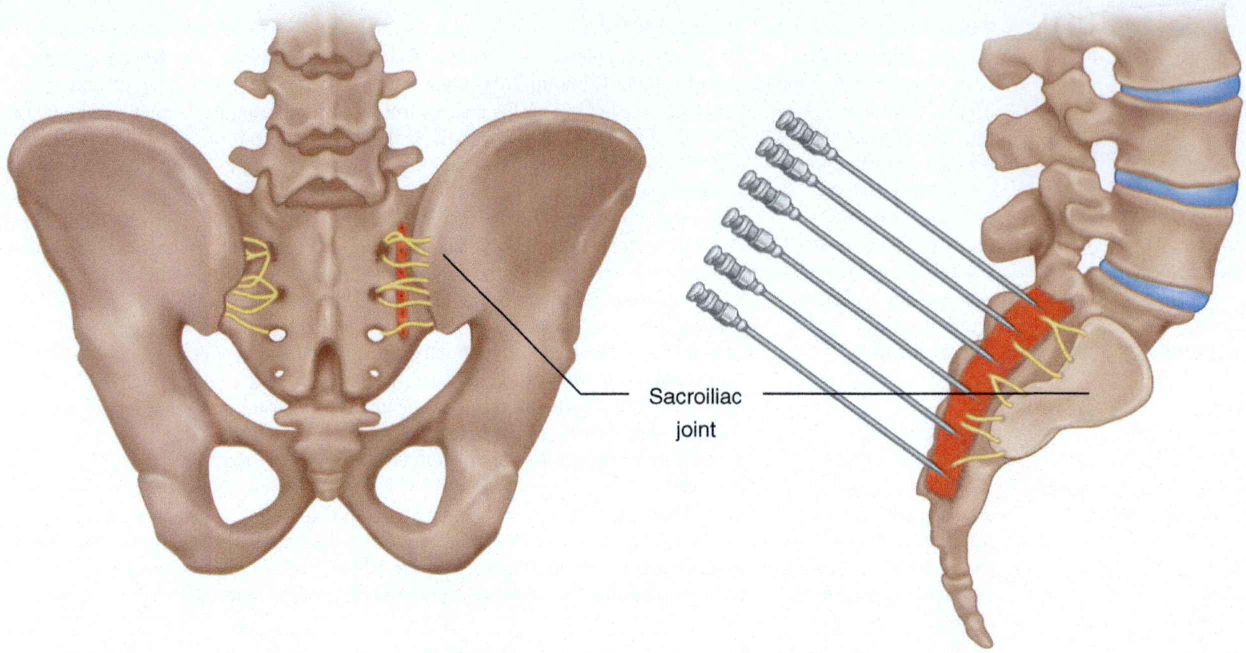

Fig. 32.6 Proper placement of cannulas for sacroiliac RFA

there is tremendous variation in nerve location from person to person, side to side, and level to level. The nerves may run along the bone or up to 8 mm superficial from the sacrum. Based on a cadaveric study of lateral branch sizes by Roberts et al. in 2014, the S2 branch is the largest at 0.86 mm ± 0.41 followed by S1 at 0.64 ± 0.16 mm, L5 at 0.51 mm, S3 at 0.38 ± 0.06 mm, and S4 (in one specimen) at 0.36 mm. In an experimental study by Dreyfuss et al., the authors found that lateral branch blocks more reliably block nociceptive stimuli from the posterior ligaments than the joint capsule, suggesting that extra-articular pathology may be more amenable to RFA.

Several RF techniques, which target the posterior innervation of the joint, have been developed to treat SI joint pain in addition to standard monopolar RFA. These include bipolar intra-articular RF, bipolar lateral branch RF, cooled RF ablation of the lateral branches, and sensory stimulation-guided SI joint RF. Ferrante et al. utilized an intra-articular bipolar leapfrog technique. Only 36.4% of individuals who underwent this procedure obtained at least a 50% decrease in visual analog scale (VAS) pain score for at least 6 months. In an attempt to improve results, a sensory stimulation-guided approach that targeted the L5 dorsal ramus sensory branch and the SI joint lateral branches was developed. Data from the retrospective review by Yin et al. indicated that 64% of individuals obtained a successful outcome, defined as greater than 60% consistent subjective relief and greater than 50% consistent decrease in pain score for a minimum of 6 months. Bipolar RF strip lesions have also been used to target the lateral branches. Burnham and Yasui treated the L5 dorsal ramus, in addition to three bipolar strip lesions at S1–S3 in nine patients. The procedure was associated with reductions in back/leg pain frequency and severity, analgesic usage, and high satisfaction scores for up to 12 months post-procedure. Figure 32.6 depicts proper placement of RFA probes for SIJ RFA.

Efficacy (Table 32.3)

A systematic review of sacral RFA by King et al. in 2015, looking at 15 studies (2 RCT, 4 prospective, 9 retrospective), found moderate evidence of effectiveness, which was limited in extent and duration. Another systematic review of two SIJ studies by Leggett et al. in 2014 evaluating cooled RFA found a statistically significant reduction in pain for the intervention group when compared with the control group. Three months post procedure, Cohen et al. found a 3.7-point reduction in pain within the intervention group, while the control group experienced only a 0.5-point reduction in pain. Three months post procedure, Patel et al. found a 2.4-point pain reduction in the intervention group and a 0.8-point pain reduction in the control group.

Table 32.3 Prospective and randomized controlled trials for sacroiliac radiofrequency for axial spine pain

Study author/ characteristics	Thermal monopolar/ bipolar or cooled RFA	# of patients	Primary outcomes	Comments
Juch et al. 2017 MINT trial RCT, non-blinded	Bipolar, cooled, and multielectrode	681 pts. with chronic LBP, a positive diagnostic block of the lumbar facet joints (251 pts), SI joint (228 pts) or a combination of facet joints, sacroiliac joints, and intervertebral disks (combination trial, 202 participants) unresponsive to conservative care	599 (88%) completed the 3 months follow-up; 521 (77%) completed the 12 months follow-up. The mean difference in pain intensity between RFA and control groups at 3 months was −0.71 (95%CI, −1.35 to −0.06) in the sacroiliac joint trial and − 0.99 (95%CI, −1.73 to −0.25) in the combination trial	Negative study Significant methodological flaws and technical flaws Lack of controlled diagnostic blocks Multiple RFA techniques examined Lack of L5 dorsal ramus treatment in the SI joint study
Van Tilburg et al. 2016 Multicenter RCT with crossover at 3 mos	Monopolar and bipolar	60 with suspected sacroiliac joint pain based on history and physical exam	No statistical difference in outcome between sham and RFA, with a similar percentage showing improvement in primary RFA (43.3%) vs crossover RFA (42.1%)	No difference in outcomes Two RF techniques examined
Cohen et al. 2008 RCT, placebo-controlled	Cooled	28 pts with positive diagnostic SI joint randomized to receive L4–L5 primary dorsal rami and S1–S3 lateral branch RFA vs sham	1, 3, and 6 months after the procedure, 11 (79%), 9 (64%), and 8 (57%) radiofrequency-treated patients experienced pain relief of 50% or greater and significant functional improvement	Positive study
Patel et al. 2012 RCT, placebo-controlled	Cooled	51 patients randomized in a 2:1 ratio to undergo lateral branch and sham RFA, respectively from L5–S3 RFA following two positive diagnostic blocks	3-month f/u, 47% of the treatment group and 12% in the sham group achieved treatment success. At 6 and 9 months, 38% and 59% in the treatment group achieved treatment success, respectively	In addition to SI joint screening blocks, all patients also experienced ≥75% pain relief following two prognostic L5 dorsal ramus and S1-3 lateral branch blocks
Burnham and Yasui 2007 Uncontrolled, prospective cohort	Bipolar RF strip lesions	Nine subjects with SIJ pain confirmed with diagnostic block treated with a series of RF strip lesions performed adjacent to the lateral dorsal foraminal aperture plus conventional monopolar lesioning at the L5 dorsal ramus.	8/9 satisfied, with significant reductions in back pain severity/ frequency; decreased analgesic intake and satisfaction with pain level	Positive study

It is worth stating that the available literature regarding SIJ RFA is extremely diverse in terms of patient selection, structures targeted, and RF technologies employed with very few high-quality RCT.

Knee RFA

Anatomy

The knee joint is innervated by the articular branches of the femoral, common peroneal, saphenous, tibial, and obturator nerves. The articular branches of these nerves, known as the genicular nerves, surround the knee and provide innervation to the joint. Genicular nerves' relevant branches include the superior lateral (SL), superior middle (i.e., contributes to subpatellar plexus), superior medial (SM), inferior lateral (IL), and inferior medial (IM). The most common targets for RFA include the SL, SM, and IM genicular nerves, which pass in periosteal areas connecting the shaft of the femur to bilateral epicondyles and the shaft of the tibia to the medial epicondyle in the subpatellar region. In individuals with a significant subpatellar component of pain, targeting the nerve branch from the vastus intermedius (i.e., superior middle branch) may be a useful therapeutic target. Due to its proximity to the common peroneal nerve, the IL branch has not been established as a safe therapeutic target. Hu et al. evaluated the anatomy of sensory patellar target nerves using transcutaneous electrical nerve stimulation (TENS) and correlated it with cadaveric dissection to determine optimal anatomic targets for blocks and RFA for superior and inferior knee pain. This study supports the target areas of the confluence of femur and medial and lateral epicondyles for superior and anterior knee pain and the confluence of the tibia and the medial epicondyle for inferior knee pain. It further suggested that in cases where there was insuffi-

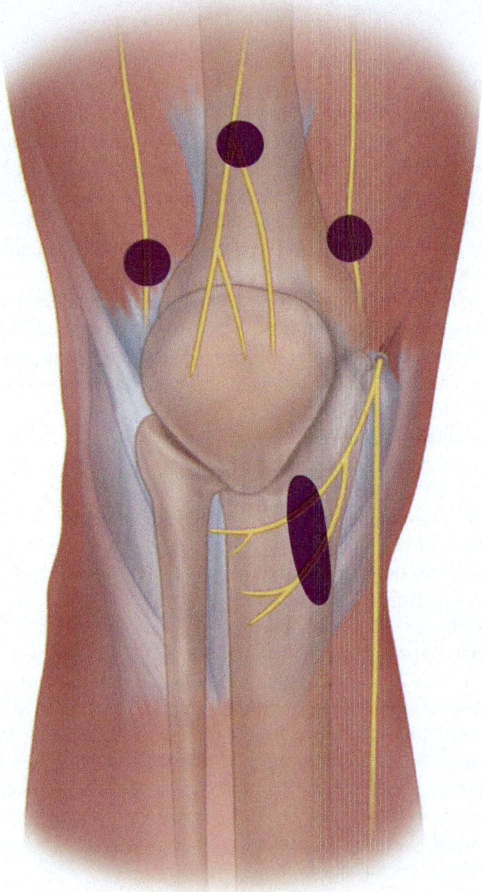

Fig. 32.7 Possible locations for cannula placement for geniculate RFA. Please note there is significant variability of geniculate nerve anatomy. These locations represent common targets based on prior studies

cient reduction in superior knee pain, treatment should be extended medially past the medial edge of the patella. The inferior border is the tibial tubercle. Franco et al. [13] suggested that the variability in nerve course means there is a greater chance of nerves being captured using a two-lesion approach; however, no clinical correlation of improved outcomes has been validated. In terms of the ideal depth of RF cannula, lateral fluoroscopic guidance should show the active tip in the middle one-third of the tibial and femoral shaft. Figure 32.7 depicts the ideal placement of probes for genicular RFA.

Efficacy (Table 32.4)

There are very few RCT to date, but a review of 17 publications by Gupta et al. in 2017 investigating thermal, cooled, and pulsed RFA found a low level of evidence supporting the superiority of any specific RFA procedure modality. The majority of the studies reported positive patient outcomes, but the inconsistent procedural methodology, inconsistent patient assessment measures, and small study sizes limited the applicability of any specific study to clinical practice. Another review by Bhatia et al. in 2016 that evaluated six publications utilizing conventioal thermal and cooled RFA showed an overall benefit of knee RFA compared to placebo based on low-quality evidence, with follow-up periods ranging from 3 to 12 months.

Safety/Complications

Although RF treatment can be associated with both minor and major complications, there is limited data documenting the occurrence of these complications. Following RF, the most common side effect of the treatment is a temporary exacerbation of pain secondary to an inflammatory response either of the heated nerves (i.e., neuritis) or the surrounding tissue, lasting from several days to 2 weeks.

Lord et al. audited 83 cervical medial branch RF procedures and recorded procedural side effects and complications. Following cervical medial branch RF, increased temporary postoperative pain occurred in 97% of cases, lasting a median duration of 10 days. Three-day post-RFA administration of diclofenac sodium has been shown to improve analgesia and patient satisfaction scores after conventional monopolar lumbar facet RF denervation. In addition, the injection of corticosteroids through the RF cannulae at the conclusion of the procedure has been shown to reduce post-procedure lumbar paraspinal tenderness. Corticosteroid is often injected with local anesthetic to prevent neuritis and has been shown along with pentoxifylline to decrease post-procedure pain compared to saline. However, there is some research suggesting that steroids injected before ablation may result in a decrease in lesion size.

Some patients may also experience transient dysesthesias of the skin over the operative area. These transient dysesthesias occur more frequently with cervical medial branch and sacroiliac joint lateral branch RF.

One of the most feared complications is damage to surrounding nontargeted spinal nerves. Methods to prevent this complication include precise anatomic placement of the RF cannula through fluoroscopic guidance in multiple views, motor testing, and a detailed understanding of lesion dimensions. This is especially relevant when methods are used to enhance lesion size, including cooled probe RF and fluid pre-injection. Retrograde lesioning has been shown to occur with fluid pre-injection prior to RF treatment.

In addition, the risk of toxicity to nontargeted tissues, including central and peripheral nervous system structures,

Table 32.4 Prospective and randomized controlled trials for geniculate radiofrequency for axial spine pain

Study author/ characteristics	Thermal mono/ bipolar or cooled RFA	# patients	Primary outcome results	Comments
Pineda et al. 2017 Prospective, observational, non-controlled	Thermal	25 pts who received US-guided RFA of SM, SL, and IM genicular nerves	The proportion of participants with improvement of 50% or greater in pretreatment VAS scores at 1, 6, and 12 months following intervention were 22/25 (88%), 16/25 (64%), and 8/25 (32%), respectively	Positive study No diagnostic blocks used
Shen et al. 2016 RCT	Thermal	54 patients with unilateral or bilateral knee pain >3 mos in duation with poor response to conservative treatment. 27 treated with RFA, 27 with conventional treatment with plasma and hyaluronidate	3-month follow-up found significantly increased scores for vitality, bodily pain, general health perceptions, physical functioning, and social role functioning by SF-36 and in pain, range of motion, stability, walking, and stair climbing by AKSS (all $P < 0.05$) in the RFA group. Controls received higher scores by AKSS in pain at the termination of treatments and in pain, range of motion, and walking at the termination of 3-month follow-up (all $P < 0.05$)	Overall positive No diagnostic block used
Choi et al. 2011 RCT, double-blind	Thermal	38 patients with severe knee OA >3 months with positive genicular diagnostic block unresponsive to conservative treatment randomized to genicular RFA vs sham	VAS pain scores lower in RFA group at 4 ($p < 0.001$) and 12 ($p < 0.001$) weeks compared with the control group. Oxford knee scores showed similar findings as VAS scores ($p < 0.001$). In the RF group, 10/17 (59%), 11/17 (65%), and 10/17 (59%) achieved at least 50% knee pain relief at 1, 4, and 12 weeks, respectively	Positive study
Ikeuchi et al. 2011 Prospective, non-randomized open label	Thermal	35 patients with chronic refractory OA knee pain assigned to RFA (18 pts) vs nerve block (17 pts)	Radiofrequency treatment significantly decreased knee pain as measured by VAS for 12 weeks compared with the control group. More patients in the RF group responded to the treatment than in the control group. The differences were statistically significant at 4 weeks, 8 weeks, and 12 weeks in pain VAS	Positive study

should also be considered prior to injecting specific fluids (e.g., high NaCl concentrations). Injected volumes of 0.5 mL for medial branch blocks have been shown to spread to adjacent nontargeted tissues including the neuroforamen. The RF active tips should be positioned safely away from the neuroforamen to avoid thermal lesioning of the spinal nerves.

Other complications that may occur specifically following cervical medial branch and third occipital nerve (TON) RF include ataxia and spatial disorientation. Ataxia and spatial disorientation are more common with cervical medial branch RF of the upper cervical levels, especially the TON, and are usually mild and self-limiting.

Other, more general/minor issues associated with RFA that merit mention include significantly prolonged fluoroscopy times and therefore radiation exposure in overweight patients and multifidus atrophy following lumbar RFA. There are challenges associated with placement of RFA electrodes in a patient with prior spinal hardware, and based on a cadaveric study by Gazelka et al., pedicle screws (both titanium and stainless steel) could serve as a possible source of thermal injury during RFA.

Technical Aspects for Improving RF Outcomes

All RFA (monopolar, bipolar, and cooled) utilize low-energy, high-frequency alternating current (300–500 Hz) to cause thermal destruction of tissue around the uninsulated electrode tip. The alternating current causes frictional heating of the tissue for conventional RF, and the time of lesioning, tip size, and set temperature all influence the final lesion size.

With monopolar RF, lesions are in the shape of a prolate spheroid, with coagulation occurring primarily in the radial direction perpendicular to the long axis of the electrode. Minimal lesioning occurs distal to the tip. Therefore, for monopolar RF, the cannula should ideally be placed with the shaft of the cannula parallel to the target nerve. When performing monopolar thermal RF, it is important to understand the maximum tolerable margin of error for specific cannulas and radiofrequency settings that will still allow for a lesion to incorporate the full diameter of the targeted nerve. The current interventional pain medicine monopolar lesion size is small, and the radius of the lesion is approximately one to two times the width of the electrode.

In bipolar RFA, a passive electrode replaces the grounding pad. Bipolar RF is employed when a larger lesion is required, and it has been used for such conditions such as sacroiliac joint dysfunction. When performing bipolar RF, it is important to understand specific configuration parameters that will influence lesion development. One parameter that is of crucial importance is the set interelectrode distance (IED). The goal is to choose an IED that will allow for ablation of the desired area while limiting destruction to nontargeted structures. In addition, the IED should be set to limit hourglass lesioning, which may result in missing the targeted structure. The maximum IED will depend on multiple configuration parameters including the size of the active tip, lesioning time, and the composition of any pre-injected fluid.

Recently, cooled probe radiofrequency ablation (RFA) has been used for the treatment of lumbar facet syndrome, sacroiliac joint dysfunction, and knee osteoarthritis. Compared to traditional thermal RFA, cooled RFA results in significant lesion development distal to the tip of the radiofrequency cannula. Lesioning distal to the tip is advantageous in certain anatomical areas, such as the sacroiliac joint, where perpendicular placement of the RF cannula is often required and there is significant variability in the number and location of nerves at each level. In cooled RFA, an internally cooled electrode is utilized which allows for continuous internal cooling of the tip with a perfusate. The internal perfusate serves as a heat sink and removes heat closest to the electrode, transferring it distally. Therefore, heating of the tissue nearest to the electrode is reduced, and greater current dispersion occurs, resulting in larger lesions.

In the quest for larger coagulation zones, methods to modulate the local tissue environment surrounding the RF cannula to allow for greater energy deposition have been investigated. The nerves innervating the facet joints have a diameter of less than 2 mm and are associated with anatomical variability. Therefore, the development of controlled and defined larger lesions may facilitate lesioning structures that are small and have variable courses, with the goal of reducing technical failures. The chemical composition of the pre-injected fluid has been shown to alter lesion size and development in both monopolar and bipolar RFA setups. Increasing the sodium chloride (NaCl) concentration of the pre-injected fluid has been shown to significantly increase power output and lesion size.

Future Study Design

The efficacy of RFA in literature is inconsistent. Few double-blind placebo RCTs have been performed, with most of the literature consisting of retrospective studies or case series. Differences in conditions studies, treatment parameters, selection criteria, and anatomical variations limit the interpretation of results.

The success rate of RFA depends on appropriate patient selection. Inappropriate selection criteria have contributed to poor outcomes. Prior studies addressing the efficacy of RFA either failed to appropriately screen patients or used single medial branch blocks or intra-articular injections of lidocaine or corticosteroid to screen patients, which may have actually self-selected placebo responders. Additionally, zygapophyseal joint pain accounts for a lower proportion of low back pain compared to neck/mid back pain, thus corrupting RF efficacy data if the cause of low back pain is misdiagnosed. Evidence on imaging of degenerative changes, in addition to positive historical and physical exam signs (e.g., pain not worsened by sitting, paraspinal tenderness), represents a good first step, followed by the use of controlled medial branch blocks to confirm diagnosis.

Genicular nerve RFA is relatively new, but it is quickly expanding as a treatment for refractory knee pain. As such, there are few studies to date. Further large-scale studies with longer follow-up periods are needed and forthcoming, not only in order to demonstrate the efficacy of RF genicular neurotomy but also to track any long-term adverse effects. Additionally, variations in the genicular nerves are still not well established, and such knowledge can influence future treatment and study design.

Conclusion

Radiofrequency ablation is an effective therapeutic treatment for spinal pain originating from cervical and lumbar facet, sacroiliac, and knee joints, although additional work on improving patient selection, extending the duration of relief, and limiting technical failures is needed. Methods to enlarge lesion size in a controlled manner to increase the likelihood of capturing the targeted nerve(s) in the coagulation zone should be studied in greater depth. It should be noted that although deductive reasoning suggests that an increase in lesion size should decrease the chance of missing a nerve, a direct association between increased lesion size and increased effectiveness has not been established. There remains a great need for prospective RCT examining the effectiveness of RFA in carefully selected patients using optimal technique that includes precise anatomical placement and the use of various maneuvers to maximize lesion size.

Pearls and Pitfalls

Pearls

- Research in RFA is variable with few well-designed studies, but overall evidence points to RFA as a safe and at least moderately effective solution for conservative resistant axial spine and knee OA pain.

- Appropriate patient selection is critical for determining which patients would best benefit from RFA. Diagnostics block should be performed and produce significant relief prior to RF treatment.
- Proper positioning of active tip parallel to target nerve is necessary to the maximize chance for successfully ablating the medial branches for the cervical and lumbar spine.
- The pre-injection of specific fluids, longer ablation times, and active cooling of RF tip can increase lesion size and assist in reducing technical failures.

Pitfalls

- Well-designed RCT with appropriate technique and patient selection are needed.
- Variable anatomic location of the target nerve can make proper positioning of the electrode challenging. Methods to enhance technical success include using equipment, pre-injection, and lesion settings to enhance lesion size while limiting damage to nontargeted structures.
- Improper placement of active tip can lead to the inadvertent ablation of motor nerves.

Recommended Reading

1. Bhatia A, et al. Radiofrequency procedures to relieve chronic knee pain an evidence-based narrative review. Reg Anesth Pain Med. 2016;41:501–10.
2. Bogduk N. International spine intervention society practice guideline for spinal diagnostic and treatment procedures. 2nd ed. San Francisco: International Spine Intervention Society; 2013.
3. Bogduk N, Macintosh J, Marsland A. Technical limitations to the efficacy of radiofrequency neurotomy for spinal pain. Neurosurgery. 1987;20(4):529–35.
4. Bogduk N, Dreyfuss P, Govind J. A narrative review of lumbar medial branch neurotomy for the treatment of back pain. Pain Med. 2009;10(6):1035–45.
5. Burnham RS, Yasui Y. An alternate method of radiofrequency neurotomy of the sacroiliac joint: a pilot study of the effect on pain, function, and satisfaction. Reg Anesth Pain Med. 2007;32(1):12–9.
6. Choi WJ. Radiofrequency treatment relieves chronic knee osteoarthritis pain: a double-blind randomized controlled trial. Pain. 2011;152:481–7.
7. Cohen SP, Hurley RW, Buckenmaier CC, Kurihara C, Morlando B, Dragovich A. Randomized placebo-controlled study evaluating lateral branch radiofrequency denervation for sacroiliac joint pain. Anesthesiology. 2008;109(2):279–88.
8. Cosman ER Jr, Gonzalez CD. Bipolar radiofrequency lesion geometry: implications for palisade treatment of sacroiliac joint pain. Pain Pract. 2011;11(1):3–22.
9. Cosman ER Jr, et al. Factors that affect radiofrequency heat lesion size. Pain Med. 2014;15:2020–36.
10. Engel A, et al. The effectiveness and risks of fluoroscopically-guided cervical medial branch thermal radiofrequency neurotomy: a systematic review with comprehensive analysis of the published data. Pain Med. 2016;17:658–69.
11. Falco FJ, et al. Systematic review of the therapeutic effectiveness of cervical facet joint interventions: an update. Pain Physician. 2012;15(6):E839–68.
12. Ferrante FM, King LF, Roche EA, Kim PS, Aranda M, Delaney LR, Mardini IA, Mannes AJ. Radiofrequency sacroiliac joint denervation for sacroiliac syndrome. Reg Anesth Pain Med. 2001;26(2):137–42.
13. Franco CD, et al. Innervation of the anterior capsule of the human knee: implications for radiofrequency ablation. Reg Anesth Pain Med. 2015;40(4):363–8.
14. Gallagher J, Petriccione dVP, Wedley J, Hamman W, Ryan P, Chikanza I, Kirkman B, Price R, Watson M, Grahame R, Wood S. Radiofrequency facet joint denervation in the treatment of low back pain: a prospective-controlled double-blind study to assess its efficacy. Pain Clin. 1994;7:193.
15. Gupta A, et al. Comparative effectiveness review of cooled versus pulsed radiofrequency ablation for the treatment of knee osteoarthritis: a systematic review. Pain Physician. 2017;20(3):155–71.
16. Haemmerich D. Biophysics of radiofrequency ablation. Crit Rev Biomed Eng. 2010;38(1):53–63.
17. Iannaccone F, et al. A review of long-term pain relief after genicular nerve radiofrequency ablation in chronic knee osteoarthritis. Pain Physician. 2017;20(3):E437–44.
18. Ikeuchi M, Ushida T, Izumi M, Tani T. Percutaneous radiofrequency treatment for refractory anteromedial pain of osteoarthritic knees. Pain Med. 2011;12:546–51.
19. Juch JN, et al. Effect of radiofrequency denervation on pain intensity among patients with chronic low back pain-the mint randomized clinical trials. JAMA. 2017;318(1):68–81.
20. Kornick C, Kramarich SS, Lamer TJ, Sitzman TB. Complications of lumbar facet radiofrequency denervation. Spine. 2004;29(12):1352–4.
21. Lau P, Mercer S, Govind J, Bogduk N. The surgical anatomy of lumbar medial branch neurotomy (facet denervation). Pain Med. 2004;5(3):289–98.
22. Leclaire R, Fortin L, Lambert R, Bergeron YM, Rossignol M. Radiofrequency facet joint denervation in the treatment of low back pain: a placebo-controlled clinical trial to assess efficacy. Spine. 2001;26(13):1411–6; discussion 1417.
23. Lee C-H, et al. The efficacy of conventional radiofrequency denervation in patients with chronic low back pain originating from the facet joints: a meta-analysis of randomized controlled trials. Spine J. 2017;17(11):1770–80.
24. Lord SM, Bogduk N. Radiofrequency procedures in chronic pain. Best Pract Res Clin Anaesthesiol. 2002;16(4):597–617.
25. Lord SM, Barnsley L, Wallis BJ, McDonald GJ, Bogduk N. Percutaneous radio-frequency neurotomy for chronic cervical zygapophyseal-joint pain. N Engl J Med. 1996;335(23):1721–6.
26. Lord SM, et al. Percutaneous radiofrequency neurotomy of the cervical medial branches: a validated treatment for cervical zygapophysial joint pain. Neurosurg Q. 1998a;8(4):288–308.
27. Lord SM, McDonald GJ, Bogduk N. Percutaneous radiofrequency neurotomy of the cervical medial branches: a validated treatment for cervical zygapophysial joint pain. Neurosurg Q. 1998b;8(4):288–304.
28. Macvicar J, et al. Cervical medial branch radiofrequency neurotomy in New Zealand. Pain Med. 2012;13:647–54.
29. Nath S, Nath CA, Pettersson K. Percutaneous lumbar zygapophysial (facet) joint neurotomy using radiofrequency current, in the management of chronic low back pain: a randomized double-blind trial. Spine. 2008;33(12):1291–7; discussion 1298.
30. Organ LW. Electrophysiologic principles of radiofrequency lesion making. Appl Neurophysiol. 1976;39(2):69–76.
31. Patel N, Gross A, Brown L, Gekht G. A randomized, placebo-controlled study to assess the efficacy of lateral branch neurotomy for chronic sacroiliac joint pain. Pain Med. 2012;13(3):383–98.
32. Pineda SM, et al. Analgesic effect and functional improvement caused by radiofrequency treatment of genicular nerves in patients

with advanced osteoarthritis of the knee until 1 year following treatment. Reg Anesth Pain Med. 2017;42(1):62–8.
33. Pino CA, Hoeft MA, Hofsess C, Rathmell JP. Morphologic analysis of bipolar radiofrequency lesions: implications for treatment of the sacroiliac joint. Reg Anesth Pain Med. 2005;30(4):335–8.
34. Poetscher AW, et al. Radiofrequency denervation for facet joint low back pain. A systematic review. Spine. 2014;39:E842–9.
35. Provenzano DA, Lassila HC, Somers D. The effect of fluid injection on lesion size during radiofrequency treatment. Reg Anesth Pain Med. 2010;35(4):338–42.
36. Provenzano DA, Lutton EM, Somers DL. The effects of fluid injection on lesion size during bipolar radiofrequency treatment. Reg Anesth Pain Med. 2012;37(3):267–76.
37. Provenzano DA, Liebert MA, Somers DL. Increasing the NaCl concentration of the preinjected solution enhances monopolar radiofrequency lesion size. Reg Anesth Pain Med. 2013;38(2):112–23.
38. Provenzano D, et al. The interaction between the composition of preinjected fluids and duration of radiofrequency on lesion size. Reg Anesth Pain Med. 2015;40(2):112–24.
39. Rambaransingh B, Stanford G, Burnham R. The effect of repeated zygapophysial joint radiofrequency neurotomy on pain, disability, and improvement duration. Pain Med. 2010;11:1343–7.
40. Roberts S, et al. Cadaveric study of sacroiliac joint innervation: implications for diagnostic blocks and radiofrequency ablation. Reg Anesth Pain Med. 2004;39(6):456–64.
41. Sapir DA, Gorup JM. Radiofrequency medial branch neurotomy in litigant and nonlitigant patients with cervical whiplash: a prospective study. Spine. 2001;26:E268–73.
42. Shen, et al. Radiofrequency thermocoagulation in relieving refractory pain of knee osteoarthritis. Am J Ther. 2017;24(6):e693–700.
43. Speldewinde GC. Outcomes of percutaneous zygapophysial and sacroiliac joint neurotomy in a community setting. Spine. 2011;12(2):209–18.
44. Tekin I, Mirzai H, Ok G, Erbuyun K, Vatansever D. A comparison of conventional and pulsed radiofrequency denervation in the treatment of chronic facet joint pain. Clin J Pain. 2007;23(6):524–9.
45. Van Eerd M, et al. Cervical facet pain. Pain Pract. 2010;10(2):113–23.
46. Van Kleef M, Barendse GA, Kessels A, Voets HM, Weber WE, De Lange S. Randomized trial of radiofrequency lumbar facet denervation for chronic low back pain. Spine. 1999;24(18):1937–42.
47. Van Tilburg CWJ, et al. Randomized sham-controlled double-blind multicenter clinical trial to ascertain the effect of percutaneous radiofrequency treatment for sacroiliac joint pain: three-month results. Clin J Pain. 2016a;32(11):921–6.
48. Van Tilburg CWJ, et al. Randomised sham-controlled double-blind multicentre clinical trial to ascertain the effect of percutaneous radiofrequency treatment for lumbar facet joint pain. Bone Joint J. 2016b;98-B:1526–33.
49. Van Wijk R, Geurts JWM, Wynne HJ, et al. Radiofrequency denervation of lumbar facet joints in the treatment of chronic low back pain: a randomized, double-blind, sham lesion-controlled trial. Clin J Pain. 2005;21:335–44.
50. Yin W, Willard F, Carreiro J, Dreyfuss P. Sensory stimulation-guided sacroiliac joint radiofrequency neurotomy: technique based on neuroanatomy of the dorsal sacral plexus. Spine. 2003;28(20):2419–25.

Basic Science of Radio Frequency

33

Tiffany Lin, Simon Willis, Dost Khan, and Maunak V. Rana

Background and Historical Perspective

Radiofrequency (RF) therapy had been used in the management of chronic painful conditions since the first documented treatment of trigeminal neuralgia with thermocoagulation of the gasserian ganglion by Kirschner in 1931. Kirschner applied a direct current of 350 mA to the gasserian ganglion utilizing a diathermy apparatus and a needle with an uninsulated tip under x-ray guidance yielding unpredictably sized lesions. The earliest RF lesion generators and electrodes were designed and constructed by B.J. Cosman, S. Aranow, and O.A. Wyss in the 1950s utilizing continuous-wave RF power sources within the frequency range of 0.1–1 MHz. These devices were developed with the purpose of producing RF thermal lesions, and amazingly today's commercial RF generators continue to utilize the same frequency range. Later, in 1965, Rosomoff et al. implemented higher-frequency currents in percutaneous radiofrequency cervical cordotomy procedures for intractable pain from various pathologies, producing more predictable lesion size. Over the years as RF technology has advanced, its clinical implications have grown not only within the realm of pain management but in other specialties as well.

T. Lin · M. V. Rana (✉)
Department of Anesthesiology and Critical Care, The University of Chicago, Chicago, IL, USA
e-mail: tlin@dacc.uchicago.edu; mrana@dacc.uchicago.edu

S. Willis
Department of Anesthesiology, University of Virginia School of Medicine, Charlottesville, VA, USA
e-mail: simon.m.willis@medstar.net

D. Khan
Department of Anesthesiology, Northwestern University Feinberg School of Medicine, Chicago, IL, USA
e-mail: dost.khan@northwestern.edu; dkhan@nm.org

Physics of Radio Frequency

RF relies on Ohm's law to generate the desired lesion or effect by manipulating current, voltage, impedance, and basic concepts of electromagnetism. Current is the transfer of energy from an electrical source and is measured in Hertz (Hz). Voltage is the force that drives the current and is measured in Volts. Impedance is the resistance to the flow of the current and is measured in Ohms (Ω). These concepts are represented by the following equation: $V = I \times R$, where V is the voltage, I is the current, and R is the impedance. The current in RF is administered as an alternating current within the kilocycle Hz range, as a lower frequency would result in noticeable pain during clinical use.

The setup of the RF circuit consists of a generator, a dispersive pad to return energy to the generator, an insulated introducer needle to prevent dispersal of energy outside of the targeted area, and an electrode with a thermocouple to provide a precise area of therapy with a temperature-regulated lesion. Furthermore, RF setups rely on a system of continuous impedance monitoring to ensure continuity of the electrical current. When the electrode is at the target site, current passes between the pad and the electrode. As current flows through body tissue, which acts as a resistor, ions within the tissue electrolytes are agitated, causing oscillation of molecules and production of friction and heat. Current spreads sideways from the electrode tip, where heat is produced in the tissue. Therefore, the tissue heats up the tip rather than the tip heating the tissue.

The biological changes that occur in tissue exposed to radiofrequency energy are thought to be secondary to the thermal effects, the high intensity electric fields, or a combination of the two. The electric field vector created around an RF electrode within a conductive, dielectric medium, such as human tissue, is governed by the classic Maxwell's Equations on electromagnetism. At the frequencies utilized in RF technology, electrical and magnetic fields are generated, with the magnetic field's effect being thus far clinically negligible. The current density that is responsible for clinical effect is a

T. R. Deer et al. (eds.), *Deer's Treatment of Pain*, https://doi.org/10.1007/978-3-030-12281-2_33

function of tissue electrical conductivity. Structures that readily conduct electrical energy such as nervous tissue and water will have higher current density than those structures with a lower conductivity, such as bone. Also, the coagulated tissue that is produced during continuous RF may serve to affect impedance as the resultant tissue may decrease the flow of energy into tissues.

The resulting temperature is governed by heat production and elimination. Heat production resulting from current flow is related to impedance (resistance to the alternating current) which varies widely from tissue to tissue. Heat elimination can be affected by tissue conductivity and vascularization of the tissue bed as blood flow carries heat away, known as the heat sink effect. Both in vitro and ex vivo models have shown that the presence of vessel simulation leads to smaller volume of tissue ablation. RF lesioning occurs in two phases. The first phase requires a large generator output to build up heat to desired tip temperature. During the second phase, the generator output gradually lowers until a steady level is reached, compensating for heat washout. Temperatures utilized for conventional RF generally range between 80 °C and 90 °C. However, irreversible neuronal disruption can occur above 44 °C, with cell structure destruction found to occur with 20 seconds or more of exposure at 45–50 °C, commonly referred to as the "lethal temperature range." Tissue exposure to temperature greater than 60 °C causes coagulation as well as protein and collagen denaturation, leading to cell necrosis. Higher temperatures may lead to side effects including hematoma, smoke, and gas formation, along with adherence of tissues to the probe. A temperature gradient exists from the central to the peripheral zone of a lesion. Some RF techniques specifically aim to expose the target structure to lower temperature zones to prevent deafferentation sequelae. Decreased temperature is also thought to have selective effect on small unmyelinated nerve fibers.

By applying radiofrequency to tissue, while controlling for temperature and lesion time, a lesion is produced. The lesion size and tissue injury can be related to the current density, which is current divided by the electrode surface area. For a given constant current, as the electrode surface area decreases in size, a greater current density, tissue heating, and resultant lesioning will occur. The size of the lesion is affected by many factors, which will be elaborated on in a later section.

Types of Radio Frequency

As RF technology has continued to advance, various forms of RF have developed with numerous applications and improving efficacy (see Table 33.1). Continuous RF is the conventional or standard form of RF therapy. It utilizes a current of 100–500 kHz applied in a continuous fashion to the target tissue. The continuous current produces a thermal lesion that interrupts nociceptive signal conduction and blocks pain signal transmission. Continuous RF, similar to other forms of RF, is nonselective and causes destruction in both sensory and motor nerve fibers. Three different types of continuous RF exist: monopolar, bipolar, and cooled. Pulsed radiofrequency will be discussed later in this chapter.

Table 33.1 Advantages and disadvantages based on RF modality

Type of RF	Advantages	Disadvantages
Conventional thermal (monopolar/ bipolar)	Less expensive equipment Longer history of clinical utility	Requires parallel placement to target nerve for optimal lesioning
Cooled RF	Larger lesion size generated Parallel or perpendicular approach to nerve may be performed Potentially increased duration of analgesia due to greater tissue coagulation	Increased potential for lesioning adjacent tissue Increased equipment costs
Pulse RF	Less risk of neuro-destruction Reduced risk of deafferentation pain Can potentially be used on peripheral nerves (i.e., intercostal, greater occipital)	Shorter duration of effect Requires repeat procedures more frequently Potential for minimal analgesic benefit

Monopolar RF represents the conventional RF therapy where the current flows between the probe electrode and the dispersive pad. With this technique the current generates heat at the active tip of the electrode and not distal to it. As the lesion is confined to an area at the tip of the electrode, the needle must be placed in a parallel fashion to the direction of the nerve and not perpendicular to it (see Figs. 33.1, 33.2, and 33.3).

In bipolar RF, current flows between two electrode probes without requirement of the dispersive pad. The electrodes are placed across the desired target, usually spaced up to 10–15 mm, resulting in a connecting brick-shaped lesion that spans these adjacent points (see Fig. 33.4). While monopolar RF is able to generate higher maximum ablation temperatures in less time, the volume of tissue ablated by bipolar RF is much larger while causing less vessel damage, possibly due to lower ablative temperature reached. In fact, a bipolar lesion is similar to three closely spaced monopolar lesions produced using the same generator setting and cannula size. Thus, bipolar RF helps to reduce number of lesions and cannula diameter, minimizing patient discomfort. Bipolar RF is also more forgiving toward inevitable operational imperfections as inter-lesion heating is robust to various departures from ideal parallel tip alignment. However, the active tip

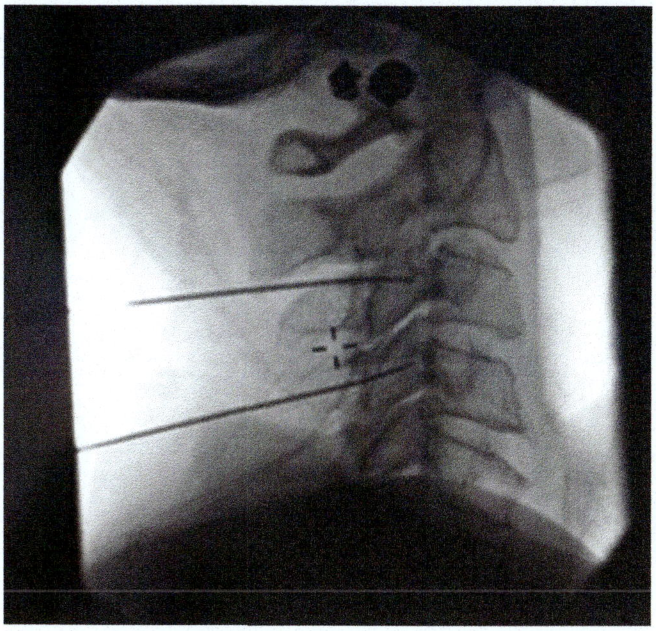

Fig. 33.1 Conventional RFA needle placement in parallel to cervical medial branches, during conduct of cervical medial branch RFA

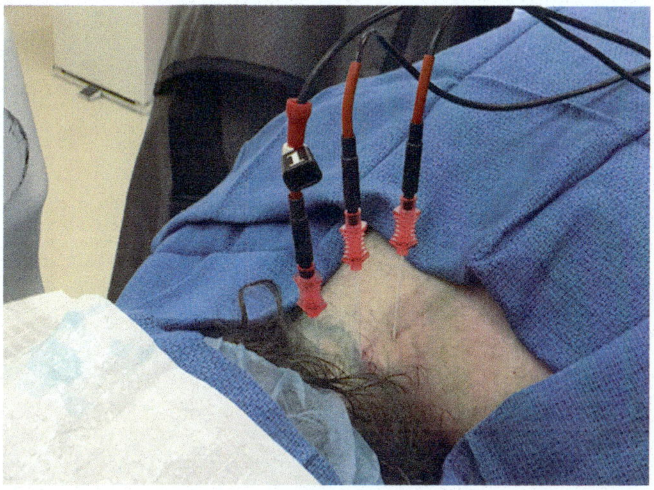

Fig. 33.2 Image of conventional RFA of cervical medial branches with the patient in prone position

length must be equal; otherwise alterations and less efficacious lesion geometry would result.

Cooled RF is a newer technology that was created with the intent of producing decreased heat at the electrode tip. The electrode is cooled via an internal perfusion system with water, while the RF heat develops around the electrode tip (see Fig. 33.5). Such cooling effect results in decreased impedance around the electrode tip with a theoretical delivery of higher energy, allowing for larger volume of tissue to be heated while avoiding excessive heating of tissue close to the electrode. Temperature at the electrode tip is maintained low, and RF heating takes place beyond the electrode tip and propagates spherically (see Figs. 33.6 and 33.7). Ex vivo studies have demonstrated the ability of cooled RF to achieve suitable temperatures to induce thermal transition of collagen and thermal neurolysis while showing no histologic evidence of damage to neural tissue in safety zones surrounding the targeted area. Cooled RF also generates larger lesions than bipolar RF.

Pulsed radio frequency (PRF) differs from conventional RF in that PRF is suggested to not lead to neural destruction. While heating of tissue does occur with PRF, the clinical effect does not rely on the generation of a heat lesion. Instead, PRF is thought to cause an alteration in the signal transduction of pain fibers. The distinction between PRF and conventional RF lies in the generator setting and the temperature achieved at the active tip. In PRF, pulses of 50 kHz current are delivered for 20 milliseconds at a frequency of 2 Hz (or every 0.5 seconds). The pauses between generated pulses allow for heat to dissipate through adjacent vascular structures, via conduction and convection, producing a lesion less than 42 °C that is insufficient to produce neural coagulation and irreversible tissue damage. Thus the average tissue temperature rise for the same RF voltage and probe electrodes is less in PRF than in conventional RF as the RF duration in PRF constitutes only a small fraction of the time between each pulse. Therefore, larger RF voltages can be used in PRF than in conventional RF without increasing the average tissue temperature around the electrode. In vitro studies have shown that PRF, when compared to conventional RF, leads to less tissue disruption and has a limited or temporary effect on impulse propagation in the nerve tissue. The greatest current density produced in PRF is distal to the active tip, allowing electrodes to be placed perpendicularly to the target nerve, shortening procedure time. PRF is believed to pose a lower risk of developing deafferentation pain than conventional RF. However, its duration of relief is generally much shorter and requires the procedure to be performed more often to obtain similar pain reduction levels as in conventional RF.

The exact mechanism of PRF is yet to be fully elucidated. PRF is believed to cause both short- and long-term changes in several neural markers. C-fos is a proto-oncogene that is expressed rapidly in response to an excitatory stimulus. It has been used as a marker for sensory neuron activation and may play a role in nociceptive transmission. Immunohistochemistry studies demonstrate an increased expression of C-fos in lamina I and II of the spinal cord in animals exposed to PRF vs conventional RF at the same temperature. Such elevated expression is present 7 days after stimulation, suggesting a sustained activation of a pain-inhibiting process. However, c-fos expression is sometimes non-specific in neuronal tissues. ATF3 (activating transcription factor 3) is a marker of neuronal cellular stress, specific to small diameter neurons such as Aδ and C fibers. Application of PRF to dorsal root

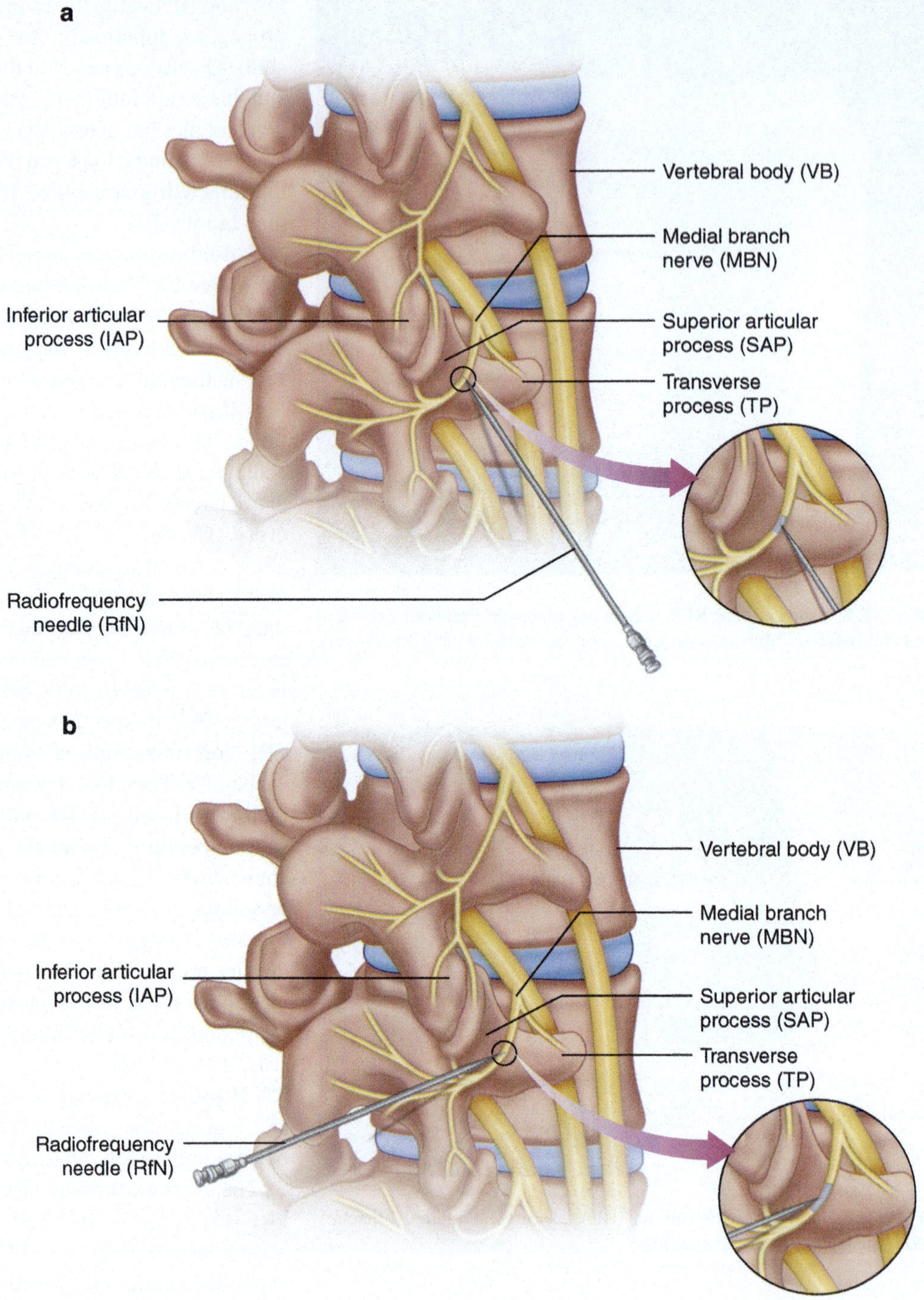

Fig. 33.3 Image (**a**) Needle placement perpendicular to medial branch nerve; Image (**b**) Needle placement parallel to medial branch nerve. With conventional RFA, needle placement parallel to the nerve yields larger surface of ablated tissue

ganglia has been shown to cause both short- and long-term upregulation of ATF3 in small caliber neurons, implicating PRF's role in targeting nociceptive neurons. Limited animal behavioral studies have also shown pain-relieving effect of PRF on mechanical hypersensitivity and thermal allodynia. Increased met-enkephalin level in the spinal cord 24 hours after PRF exposure implies a possible role for endogenous opioids. In addition, PRF effects have been found to be attenuated by $\alpha 2$ antagonists and SSRIs, suggesting PRF analgesic effect may involve descending noradrenergic and serotonergic inhibitory pathways. Lastly, a recent study by Yeh et al. demonstrates that PRF provides neuromodulation with a long-term anti-allodynic effect (up to 28 days) by inhibiting spared nerve injury-induced IGF2 and ERK1/2 activation that is responsible for inflammatory response and mechanical allodynia.

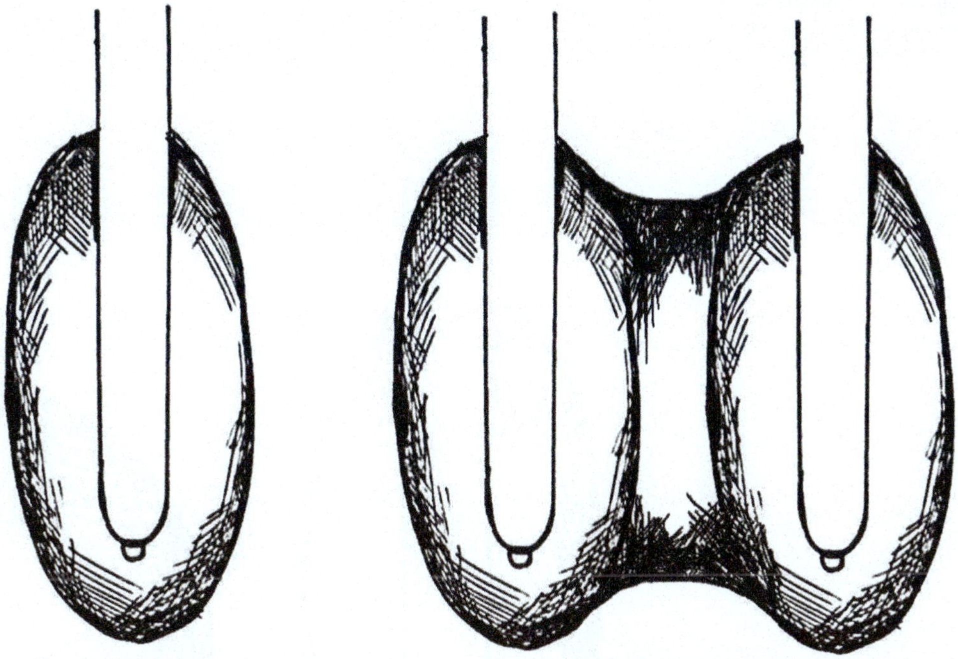

Fig. 33.4 Comparison of conventional monopolar vs bipolar lesion geometry

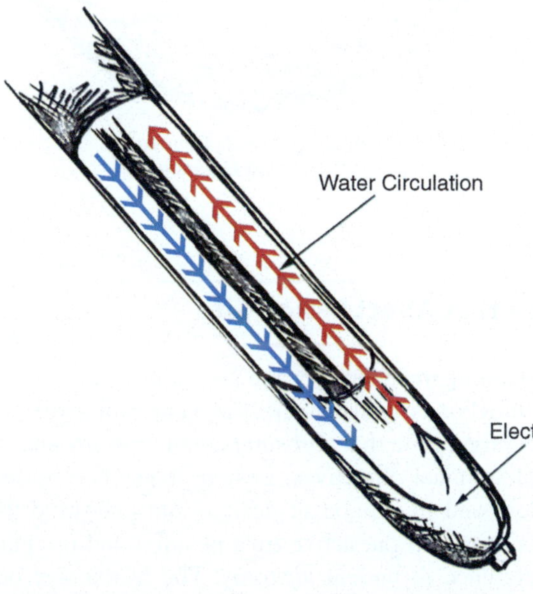

Fig. 33.5 Inner dynamics of a cooled radiofrequency needle, demonstrating flow of water reducing tissue impedance and therefore permitting for larger region of ablated tissue

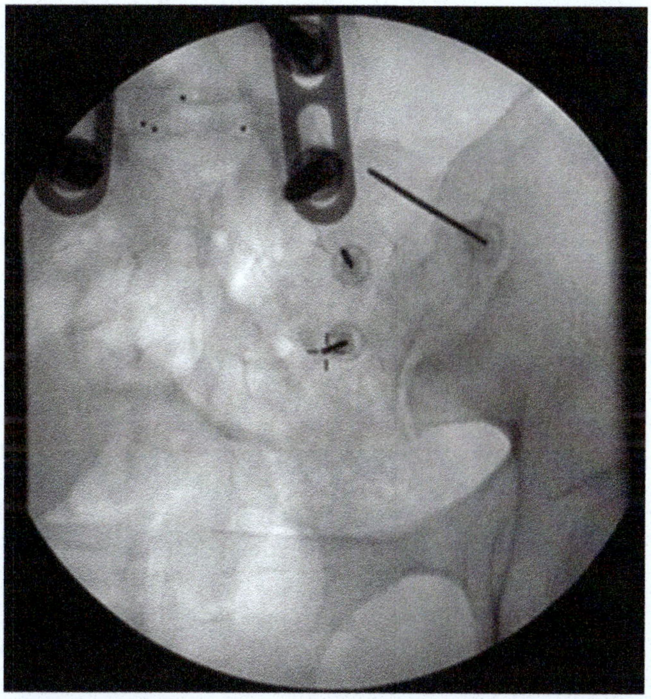

Fig. 33.6 Image of sacroiliac joint (SI joint) RFA with the cooled radiofrequency needles in place lateral to the sacral foramina

Histological Effects of RF

Many animal studies have been performed to evaluate the histological effects of conventional RF and PRF. 42 °C conventional RF lesions in rats result in endoneurial edema in the subperineurial and perivascular areas of the nerve. Light microscopy demonstrates transverse myelin fiber damage along with axoplasma separation, leading to impaired nerve transmission. Electron microscopy also confirms alternation of myelin configuration. Additionally, lamellar separation,

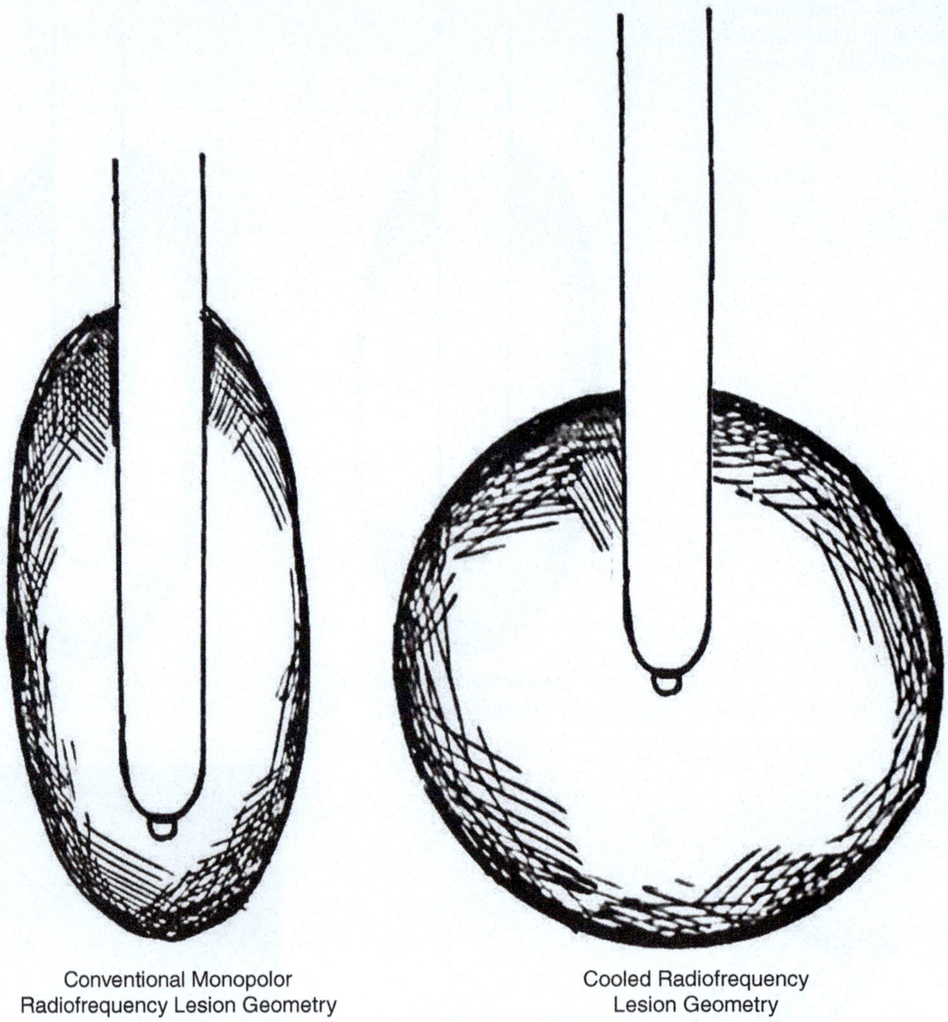

Fig. 33.7 Comparison of conventional monopolar vs cooled RF lesion geometry

protrusion of myelin, and accumulation of neurofilaments were found, pointing to neurodegeneration. However, these changes were transient in nature without progression to overt axonal injury. 80 °C conventional RF lesions caused coagulative necrosis and show significant endoneural edema with progression to Wallerian degeneration. Electron microscopy shows evidence of neurodegeneration, including epineurial thickening, lamellar separation, intra-axonal vacuolization, increased intracellular endoplasmic reticulum, and Schwann cell damage.

PRF only demonstrates relatively minor histological changes, such as the development of large vacuoles throughout the cytoplasm. The changes are restricted to the relatively smaller sized C and Aδ fibers as well, presumably because larger neurons are protected by their myelin sheath. Microscopic examination of PRF lesions has shown morphologic changes of mitochondria with abnormal mitochondrial membranes along with disruption and disorganization of microfilaments and microtubules.

Factors that Affect Lesion Size

Understanding the geometry and size of heat lesions generated with RF is critical for selecting generator settings and probe configuration that will suit patient anatomy and yield favorable clinical objectives. Lesion geometry determines the extent and likelihood of desired and undesired tissue changes based on the active tip's position and orientation with reference to patient anatomy. The lesion size determines the degree and likelihood of interventional success, complications, number of required lesions, methodological difficulty, procedure time, radiation exposure, tissue damage, and intra- or post-procedural pain. The advantage of a large lesion includes a decreased likelihood of missing a target nerve with an increased extent of nerves capture by each lesion. Achieving a large lesion also avoids incomplete neurolysis, improves degree and duration of pain relief, and decreases procedure time, X-ray exposure, and number of lesions required. The disadvantage of a large lesion includes increased likelihood and severity of damage to nontarget nerves, skin burns in thin patients, and post-procedural paresthesia. Side effects are related to the volume of the affected tissue, both target and surrounding structures. Because the target nerve cannot be visualized during the RF procedure with the use of fluoroscopy, successfully ablating it while limiting damage to nontarget structures depends on accurate placement of the electrode and working knowledge of the expected size and variability of the RF-induced lesion.

The size of an RF lesion can be affected by manipulating cannula tip sizes and generator settings. According to Cosman et al., large monopolar RF lesions can be generated by maximizing tip size (16 g/6 mm, 18 g/10 mm, or 16 g/10 mm), heating temperature (80–90 °C), and lesion time (2–3 minutes) within practical limits.

Lesion size can also be further enhanced by fluid injection via the cannulae prior to radiofrequency ablation. Increasing NaCl concentration in the preinjection fluid decreases impedance surrounding RF cannula, increasing power output. Provenzano et al. found that preinjection fluids with >3% NaCl increase lesion growth in all dimensions, most significantly in the horizontal plane with limited growth extension distal to the tip. While most of the lesion growth occurs by 90 seconds regardless of the presence of preinjection fluid, fluid pre-injection with >3% NaCl allows for continued lesion expansion throughout the 180-second cycle, resulting in larger lesions. Lidocaine, which is a standard pre-injectate to prevent procedural pain, when added to NaCl pre-injection fluid, does not significantly alter mean increases in lesion dimensions or modifications in electrical parameters. In bipolar RF, fluid preinjection also increases the inter-electrode distance that can be used to produce an optimal lesion.

Summary

The mechanism of analgesia and treatment after radiofrequency ablation is well-known and founded. As technology has developed from initial monopolar lesions, bipolar and cooled RF have resulted leading to use in various clinical indications. Additionally, the use of pulsed radio frequency, while not commonly used currently in the United States, has received world-wide support for the use in conditions where denervation pain would be a deleterious result. The theory behind RF highlights the conglomeration of electricity and magnetism for clinical care. The monopolar, bipolar, and cooled RF are via a conventional energy approach, with the cooled RF allowing for dissipation of energy to yield a larger lesion size for targeted tissue.

Pulsed RF, while yet to have a fully, elucidated mechanism has shown promise in certain clinical conditions. For more widespread use, the basic, mechanistic science behind PRF needs to be consistently assessed and presented, so that this technology may join the currently utilized approaches for interventional pain procedures.

Recommended Reading

1. Boxem KV, Huntoon M, Zundert JV, Patijn J, van Kleef M, Joosten EA. Pulsed radiofrequency: a review of the basic science as applied to the pathophysiology of radicular pain. Reg Anesth Pain Med. 2014;39:149–59.
2. Cosman ER, Dolensky JR, Hoffman RA. Factors that affect radio-frequency heat lesion size. Pain Med. 2014;15:2020–36.
3. Provenzano DA, Watson TW, Somers DL. The interaction between the composition of preinjected fluids and duration of radiofrequency on lesion size. Reg Anesth Pain Med. 2015;40:112–24.
4. Rae W, Kapur S, Mutagi H. Radiofrequency therapies in chronic pain. BJA Educ. 2011;11(2):35–8.
5. Sluijter M, Racz G. Technical aspects of radiofrequency. Pain Pract. 2002;2(3):195–200.

Cryotherapy

34

Maged Guirguis, Ian Hakkinen, Yamah Amiri, Jose Posas III, and Chong H. Kim

Introduction

Cryotherapy is an old therapy but a relatively new technique used to help manage pain in patients with neuralgic pain conditions. Ice and/or Cold forms of analgesia have long been used, and written records go back to the time of Hippocrates for their use. Current models of cryoablation to induce cryoneurolysis rely upon a cryoprobe that produces an ice ball to destroy axons leading to Wallerian degeneration. This nerve damage has led to pain relief across many different diseases. Outcomes have been reported as curative or provided relief from pain for up to months at a time.

Anatomy of the peripheral nerve consists of bundles of axons termed fascicles that are surrounded by different connective tissue layers. The outer layer is called the *epineurium* which surrounds the nerve and helps hold nerve fascicles together. Nerve fascicles are surrounded by the *perineurium* which holds the individual axons within them. Within the fascicles there is a layer which covers individual axons called the *endoneurium*. Blood supply to the nerve comes from the vasa vasorum and is located within the endoneurium and perineurium forming the blood-nerve barrier. Peripheral nerves can be classified as sensory, motor, or mixed.

Given the broad range of injuries that can occur to peripheral nerves in 1943, Sir Herbert Seddon came up with a classification scheme for nerve damage. The scale is eponymously named the Seddon scale which is composed of three types of nerve injury:

- Type 1: Neuropraxia is the most mild of nerve damage that results from nerve compression usually after blunt trauma. The axons remain intact but there is a loss of nerve conduction and some demyelination. Patients usually recover within hours to days, but in some cases, it can take weeks. EMG studies are usually negative.
- Type 2: Axonotmesis occurs when there is complete disruption of the axon and myelin sheath with preservation of the perineurium, epineurium, and endoneurium. Recovery is possible through Wallerian degeneration. EMG studies will show decreased conduction and muscle fasciculations.
- Type 3: Neurotmesis is the most severe and occurs when there is complete transection of the nerve. There is disruption of all three nerve sheath layers. Recovery is unlikely without the help of surgery. EMG studies will show no conduction through the nerve.

Cryoablation results in a nerve injury that falls into the classification as axonotmesis. The ice ball disruption of the nerve results in axon destruction followed by Wallerian degeneration that will occur within 3 weeks post insult. Wallerian degeneration consists of deterioration of the distal axon to the insult and proximal deterioration to the last node of Ranvier. Schwann cells and macrophages remove cellular debris and allow for the proximal axon to form a growth cone and regrow through the intact nerve sheath. Growth rates will vary but usually is considered to be at a rate of between 1 and 3 mm per day. Due to the type of nerve injury, cryoablation may not provide permanent relief in patients, but this can be overcome with changes and optimization of the temperatures that are used.

The exact mechanism for how cryoablation causes nerve insult is not exactly known. Cryoablation has been used to treat several cancers where tissues closest to the probe tip swell and disrupt the cell membranes. The extracellular space then forms a hyperosmotic state which causes peripheral cells to shift their fluid out of the cell. This process is followed by fluid shifts backward into the cells when the cooling process begins leading to disruption of their mem-

M. Guirguis (✉) · I. Hakkinen · Y. Amiri · J. Posas III
Pain Management, Ochsner Health System, New Orleans, LA, USA
e-mail: mguirguis@ochsner.org; jose.posas@ochsner.org

C. H. Kim
MetroHealth/Case Western Reserve University, Department of PM&R, Cleveland, OH, USA
e-mail: chkim@centerforpainrelief.com

T. R. Deer et al. (eds.), *Deer's Treatment of Pain*, https://doi.org/10.1007/978-3-030-12281-2_34

branes. For nerves it is thought that there is damage to the vasa vasorum leading to ischemic necrosis. Temperature range can help to determine what type of lesion and response will occur. At −20 °C there is little to no insult made to the nerve, while at temperatures below −140 °C, there can be permanent nerve destruction and scar formation. The optimal temperature for nerve ablation ranges between −60 °C and −100 °C. The cold temperatures also reduce the inflammatory response and destruction of the nerve. Unlike radiofrequency ablation where heat is used to induce nerve lesions, there is a lower risk of neuroma formation.

Background and Historical Perspective

The use of ice or cold for analgesia goes back to the time of Hippocrates and follows a basic principle that when cold is applied to a painful region analgesia is produced. The idea of pain relief with cryotherapy dates back to the twentieth century with the beginning of modern use of cryoprobes coming around in the 1960s. Dr. Irving Cooper a neurosurgeon used a cryoprobe to treat Parkinson's disease by targeted ablation in the thalamus. Further development of cryoprobes came from a South African ophthalmologist Dr. Selig Amoils who invented the first handheld cryoprobe. Cryoprobes now most commonly use nitrous oxide, liquid nitrogen, or argon to form an ice ball in targeted nerves leading to their destruction. One of the first major studies looked at postsurgical thoracotomy pain and the use of cryotherapy. The cryoablation of the nerves showed superior analgesic effect compared to nerve blocks using bupivacaine.

Procedure

Cryoprobes rely on gasses such as nitrous oxide with a micropore needle-based delivery system. When delivered the gas is rapidly ejected forming a high pressure system through the needle's micropore where it can expand and form an ice ball. The probe then warms up melting the ice ball and can be safely removed from the patient. Depending upon the probe, they can have a built-in nerve stimulator to identify the nerve and allow for focusing on the targeted nerve. Most probes are covered in Teflon proximally to the tip in order to help with localizing and focusing the temperature to the ice ball at the tip.

Temperature Optimization

Research on rabbit sciatic nerve helped to elucidate the correct temperature that will allow for axonotmesis to occur. The researchers looked at several temperatures, −20 °C, −60 °C, −100 °C, −140 °C, and −180 °C, which were used with the cryoprobe. At −20 °C there was no change in nerve function. As temperatures were lowered to −60 °C, nerve conduction was lost with eventual recovery. At −100 °C the nerve lost conduction and underwent Wallerian degeneration with eventual recovery. Further, at −140 °C and −180 °C, there was necrosis of the nerve and formation of scar tissue forming a more permanent nerve destruction. This study helped to give a recommended range for cryoneurolysis of between −60 °C and −100 °C to allow for recovery over time while still providing nerve disruption and analgesia.

Benefits and Future Use

Since the early uses of cryotherapy, the positive benefits have continued to show promise with other disease and analgesic uses. Cancers have been treated with insertion of a cryoprobe and frozen from the inside. Targeting of other nerves continues to be expanded upon including the occipital, trigeminal, and pudendal nerves. Being able to localize the nerves and understanding their anatomical landmarks have further enhanced the use of cryotherapy.

When paired with ultrasound, a small cryoprobe can be placed precisely to allow for accurate cryoneurolysis and prevent damage to surrounding tissues. Ultrasound guidance makes procedures easy to be done in the clinic setting without any needed radiographic imaging. Utilizing ultrasound has immense benefits for targeting and providing optimal production results. Ultrasound guidance is covered more in the occipital neuralgia section of this chapter. Analgesia for chronic pain will continue to evolve, and cryoablation has a great potential to be a new and leading treatment modality. Cryoablation has been shown here to be effective at reducing pain related to a myriad of diseases. Cryotherapy leaves patients pain free or without pain for months at a time all with minimal side effects from the procedure.

Uses and Indications

With the current opioid epidemic, it is more crucial than ever to utilize alternative pain management methods like cryoanalgesia. Since Dr. Cooper created the first modern cryoanalgesia probe in 1961, cryoanalgesia has further grown to treat a broad range of different medical conditions that often are debilitating for patients. Alternatives to cryoanalgesia include surgical resection, alcohol and phenol neurolysis, anticonvulsants, and radiofrequency ablation. Before treatment with cryoablation, it is often necessary to have a diagnostic nerve block with a reported 50% reduction in pain in the patient. This pre-procedure test will help to identify if the nerve is truly the etiological cause of the pain and avoid unnecessary procedures.

Table 34.1 Uses and efficacy of cryotherapy in select neuralgia and neurologic disease

Neuropathic condition	Paper	Efficacy as reported by patient
Intercostal neuralgia	Green et al. (2002) Lu et al. (2013)	Chronic pain secondary to thoracic surgery was shown to have a 50% reduction in patient's pain Nondivided intercostal muscle flap and intercostal nerve cryoanalgesia were compared for post-esophagectomy/post-thoracotomy pain, and it was found that up to 6 months, similar pain relief from both modalities was reported by patients
Occipital neuralgia	Kim et al. (2015)	Patients with greater than 75% pain relief from local anesthetic before cryoanalgesia showed increased duration (8.1 months) and greater pain relief than individuals with 50–74% response to local (4.1 months)
Trigeminal neuralgia	Dar et al. (2013) Pradel et al. (2002)	Instant pain relief for palliative pain management of secondary trigeminal neuralgia due to cancer that lasted from 2 weeks to 4 months in the three-patient study Significant pain relief for at least 6 months post cryoablation
Temporomandibular joint pain	Sidebottom et al. (2011)	17 patients with significant TMJ pain that failed medical and arthroscopic management found an average of 7-month pain relief that decreased VAS scores from 6.8 to 2 posttreatment
Hip adductor spasticity and obturator neuralgia	Kim et al. (1998)	2 case reports of patients with hip adductor spasticity resulting in pain and inability to ambulate finding pain relief and ability to walk post cryoablation
Intractable peroneal pain	Evans et al. (1981)	31 out of 40 patients reported improved pain relief for 30 days; and 11 of those patients had complete relief of symptoms
Phantom limb pain	Moesker et al. (2014)	3 out of 5 patients with phantom limb pain had 90–100% resolution of pain
Genitofemoral neuralgia	Fanelli et al. (2003)	10 patients with postherniorrhaphy neuropathic pain received cryoablation of ilioinguinal (4), genitofemoral (1), or combined (5) therapy. Results found an average 77.5% reduction in pain, 80% decrease in analgesic use, and 90% increase in daily function

With improved technique and more research, cryoanalgesia can provide an excellent alternative to current pain therapies. Currently cryotherapy is used secondary to many noninvasive treatments and an effort that effectively saves a patient from untreated pain and allow them to return to a normal life (Table 34.1).

Intercostal Neuralgia

Intercostal neuralgia relating to surgical incision and rib retraction can be debilitating for patients and lead to complications postoperatively. Research by Karmakar et al. in 2004 described post-thoracotomy pain to be likely a result from a combination of trauma to the intercostal nerves and myofascial pain. The group found that up to 50% of patients will develop post-thoracotomy pain syndrome and a further 30% will continue to experience pain 5 years post-op. Patients will mostly describe post-thoracotomy pain as mild, while others experience debilitation with changes to normal daily function.

In treating intercostal neuralgia, another group, Green et al. in 2002 examined 43 patients aged 26–84 who received cryoneurolysis for their chronic pain secondary to thoracotomy pain and postherpetic neuralgia. The group found that 3 months post cryoneurolysis, 50% of their subjects continued to have pain relief.

Cryoneurolysis had a positive patient analgesic report, but a more recent study from Ju et al. in 2008 compared the effectiveness of cryoanalgesia for postoperative thoracic pain to the current gold standard of thoracic epidural analgesia. The group used a randomized controlled study that segregated patients into epidural and cryoanalgesia groups. Results found no difference among the two groups in first 3 days post-op followed by an increased incidence of pruritus in the epidural group. In addition, they found high chronic pain incidences of 50 to 60% in both groups at 1 month, 3 months, 6 months, and 12 months post-op. Of note was that the group did find higher incidences of allodynia-like pain, pain intensity, and debilitation of daily activities in the cryoneurolysis group.

Another study by Lu et al. in 2013 compared cryoanalgesia to nondivided intercostal muscle flaps for treating postoperative thoracotomy pain in patients undergoing esophagectomies. In their randomized controlled study, 80 patients received a flap, and the other 80 received cryoanalgesia. Their findings showed that up to 6 months, both groups had no statistical difference in pain scores or the use of oral pain medication. While the flap group showed improved pain treatment at 6, 9, and 12 months, this could show that cryoanalgesia is an option in early pain management up to 6 months postoperatively.

Treating intercostal neuralgia continues to prove that further investigations are required in identifying factors for patients who show good response to cryotherapy. Although Ju et al. has shown debilitation and increased pain intensity, some patients did benefit from cryoanalgesia, which provides an alternative to individuals who are unable to receive a thoracic epidural. Furthermore, cryoanalgesia has been utilized by another group Kim et al. (2016) for Nuss procedures in the treatment of pectus excavatum. The group used thoracoscopic transthoracic cryoneurolysis to target five intercostal nerves and resulted in 1 month of adequate analgesia. The authors recommend further utilization of this method for Nuss procedure showing the growth of cryoanalgesia.

Occipital Neuralgia

Occipital neuralgia is characterized by the International Headache Society as a unilateral or bilateral paroxysmal, shooting or stabbing pain in the distribution of the greater, lesser, or third occipital nerves. It is commonly associated with tenderness over the involved nerves with patients also reporting feelings of diminished sensation or dysesthesia. Etiology is most commonly idiopathic; however, structural causes including but not limited to trauma, compression of the nerve or nerve roots, and upper cervical cord lesions have been implicated in some cases. It has been complex to treat and no standard of care has been established. Current treatments range from conservative treatment to medical management with severe cases requiring minimally invasive surgery. Conservative treatment includes avoidance of triggers, rest, hot or cold compresses, and relaxation, while medical management ranges from usage of NSAIDs, antiepileptics, TCAs, triptans, and calcium channel blockers. Patient refractory to conservative and medical management often seeks other methods of relief from minimally invasive, such as Botox injections, occipital nerve blocks, and radiofrequency ablation, to invasive surgeries that includes neurectomies or nerve stimulation implants.

Cryoneurolysis has been shown to achieve reliable and long-lasting pain relief in patients with other neuralgias. A positive diagnostic block is mandatory for success using this technique. It is well known that local anesthetic agents inhibit neural activity by interfering with voltage-gated sodium channels resulting in prevention of depolarization. This mechanism of action hinders pain transmission by nociceptive C fibers. An observational study by Kocer in 2016 reported patients who underwent a greater occipital nerve block with lidocaine and saline mixture had a decreased number of attacks with low severity. While these effects were temporary, there was still a significant difference between baseline and 6th month results with MIDAS scores of 31.87 ± 3.98 and 6.75 ± 2.76. In a retrospective study of peripheral nerve blocks ($n = 64$) utilizing bupivacaine as a local anesthetic, a 60% efficacy rate specifically for patients with occipital neuralgia ($n = 5$) was reported with an endpoint assessment time ranging from 1 to 48 months.

A retrospective study by Kim et al. in 2015 looked at 38 patients divided into 2 groups based on their response to local anesthetic injection. They found individuals who received cryoablation reported a greater than 75% pain reduction which was a statistically significant relief. In addition, they found an increased duration of relief with cryoablation for up to 8.1 months compared to 4.1 months in the group with 50–74% relief response from injectable nerve blocks. In addition, the group found greater relief in women than men; however, the study distribution included 10 men to 28 women. This study supports the reasoning that cryoablation can be utilized for occipital neuralgia. While standards have not been set, even when a patient received a minimal 50% relief, they still found 4 months of pain relief. In the complexity of treating occipital neuralgia, cryoablation provides another treatment option for patients.

Given the superficial nature and consistency of nerve location in relation to bony landmarks, ultrasound can be used to further localize and better target the nerve to cryotherapy. Ultrasound can identify muscles, ligaments, vessels, joints, and bony surfaces and most importantly can have direct visualization of thin nerves when using high-resolution transducers. Using this technique versus landmarks allows for targeting of the occipital nerve more proximally where it has not yet divided. This allows for a greater efficacy not only in diagnostic blocks but also during the cryoneurolysis procedure, ensuring the precise target has been reached. Utilization of Doppler sonography reduces risk of intravascular injection of local anesthetics or injury of vessels during the procedure. Visualization with ultrasound also allows the provider to observe the size of the occipital nerve before and after treatment to observe any changes in nerve size, edema surrounding the nerve (suggested by hypoechoic densities), or other signs of inflammation.

Trigeminal Neuralgia

Trigeminal neuralgia is characterized as an intense stabbing pain that lasts from seconds to minutes most commonly found in the border of the V2 and V3 distribution. It can be triggered by simple movements of the jaw as in eating and make everyday tasks excruciatingly painful. Etiology varies by patients and has been reported to be by entrapment of the nerve root, tumor invasion, cysts, and arteriovenous malformations. Treatment currently includes the use of antiseizure medications, botulinum toxin injections, and surgical decompression for refractory pain; cryoablation can provide an alternative. A group, Dar et al. in 2012 found the use of CT-guided cryoablation for rapid palliative pain relief for patients suffering from trigeminal neuralgia secondary to cancer. They used a selection criteria described by Callstrom and Charboneau that required (1) moderate to severe pain, (2) localized pain to no more than two sites, and painful metastatic lesions accessible to percutaneous ablative devices. Research results found that the three patients of their study had immediate relief lasting between 1 and 4 months based on patient for their trigeminal neuralgia.

Previous studies from another research group, Pradel et al. in 2002 reported 19 patients undergoing cryoablation who had failed carbamazepine treatment or experienced significant side effects. They found complete pain relief within 5 days of treatment and pain returned for 13 of the 19 subjects after 6–12 months of being without pain. The cryotherapy results show that when medical management has failed, cryotherapy can provide effective management for up to 6 months. The group's results reported that six patients remained pain-free, while the remainder had either repeated cryoablation or returned to lower doses of carbamazepine. Cryoanalgesia can provide significant improvement in patient's daily life with reduced pain, reduced drug dosages, and an effective alternative therapy.

Temporomandibular Joint Pain

Temporomandibular joint pain occurs from muscles of the temporomandibular joint leading to an aching, burning, throbbing, or stiff pain. Treatment includes rest and nonsteroidal anti-inflammatory medication. Treatment can progress to surgical arthrocentesis or open surgery in severe cases. Surgical treatment is mainly indicated when functional disability is also present with the pain. Sidebottom et al. in 2011 performed a retrospective study to investigate the use of cryoablation on 17 patients whose pain did not improve with medical or surgical arthroscopic management. The patients did not qualify for open surgical treatment, and thus cryoablation was attempted. The patients were included if they found adequate relief from nerve block using local anesthetic. Their findings include improved pain relief with a decreased visual analogue scale of 6.8 before treatment to 2 posttreatment. Pain relief was found to last for 7 months on average, and three patients had complete resolution of pain. When patients have exhausted all other treatment modalities, cryoablation shows promise providing adequate pain relief for at least 7 months.

Hip Adductor Spasticity and Obturator Neuralgia

Injuries to the central nervous system can result in chronic muscle spasticity and include stroke, multiple sclerosis, and trauma. Patients can develop chronic pain as a result of the injury and spasticity of their muscles. Treatment approaches include physical therapy, central-acting oral medications, surgical intrathecal pump implantation, injections, or surgery. In 1998 Kim et al. published a case report series that showed the benefits of cryotherapy. One patient suffering from lower limb muscle spasticity found benefit from implanted baclofen pump; however, their hip adductors continued to debilitate their ability to walk. Cryoneurolysis was performed on the obturator nerve and resulted in decreased spasticity with pain relief that lasted for 5 months.

Another patient in this cases series suffered from metastatic breast carcinoma that lead to blastic lesions along their posterior pelvic brim resulting in right medial thigh pain that left them wheelchair bound due to pain on exertion. The patient's analgesia therapy included fentanyl patches and oxycodone as needed with acetaminophen. Cryoanalgesia targeted to their obturator nerves to relieve their hip adductors and resulted in immediate relief and the ability to ambulate for 6 months with a cane. These cases provide evidence that spasticity can significantly interrupt a patient's daily life and cryoneurolysis can be a useful adjuvant therapy for patients who have refractive hip adductor pain or spasticity.

Genitofemoral Neuralgia

Genitofemoral neuralgia results in paresthesias and neuropathic pain distributed along the lower abdomen and medial aspect of the thigh. The painful distribution can include scrotal pain in males and labia majora pain in females. Campos et al. in 2009 used ultrasound-guided cryoablation of the femoral component of the nerve that provided a 47-year-old male immediate relief from his 3 months of left scrotal pain. His pain went from a 4/10 on the visual analogue scale to an acceptable 2/10 at 3-month follow-up. Furthermore, one study by Fanelli et al. in 2003, looked at ten patients with postherniorrhaphy neuropathic pain who had failed to find relief from noninvasive treatment but were able to find relief from cryoablation. Of these individuals, one underwent genitofemoral ablation, five underwent combined ilioinguinal/genitofemoral ablation, and the remaining four underwent ilioinguinal ablation. They found an average of 77% reduction in pain, 80% decrease in analgesic intake, and 90% increase in physical activity in this study group. Of the ten patients, seven found complete relief from cryoablation.

Intractable Perineal Pain

Sacral nerve roots are common sources of perineal pain that can result from many etiologies such as tumor invasion, trauma, osteoarthritis, bone spurs, or even somatized pain resulting from depression. Treatment progressing from conservative to invasive surgeries can now evolve with the addition of cryoablation. A study by Evans et al. in 1981 looked at 40 patients who were divided into 3 groups based on their source of pain: cancer, coccydynia, or perineal neuralgia. The patients had failed other therapies and underwent cryoablation for pain relief. The patients were followed up for 3 months after treatment, and 23 patients required only a single treatment for pain relief, while the rest required additional cryoablations as a result of inadequate pain relief or a return of pain. Seventy-eight percent of their patients found relief with 11 of those patients describing complete pain relief. The mean duration of relief was found to be 39 days and 16 days for the group that reported complete relief. In some patients, the range of relief lasted up to 180 days. Six patients did not receive adequate relief and underwent a second treatment where three found better pain control. When other pain management strategies fail, cryoablation is an alternative that could be utilized for sacral nerve-related pain.

Phantom Limb Pain

Phantom limb pain is a burning, sharp, pins and needle-type pain a patient may experience following limb amputation. The complexity of treating the pain is a result of the intricate feedback between the peripheral and central nervous systems. Sensory neurons are reported to be hyperexcitable as a result of inflammatory mediators released from local tissue. While the changes occur, standardized treatment has not been found yet. Cryoneurolysis might provide promise in this debilitating condition. A study by Moesker et al. in 2014 involved five patients with phantom limb pain that had their pain localized to the most distal nerve tract that corresponds to their nerve pain. With strong response from local anesthetic, they received cryoablation at the same location. The researchers followed the patients for a minimum of 6 months and two patients up to 5 years. In three of their patients, there was a 90–100% decrease in reported pain. Phantom limb pain has a multifactorial cause of pain that is poorly understood, which includes a psychological component. With the utilization of cryoanalgesia, increased support can be provided to patients suffering from phantom limb pain.

Future Uses

Lateral Femoral Cutaneous Nerve

Pain in the anterolateral thigh is often associated with the disease of meralgia paresthetica. It is caused by compression or entrapment of the lateral femoral cutaneous nerve (LFCN). Meralgia paresthetica presents with pain, numbness, and dysesthesia across the anterolateral thigh. Risk factors for developing the disease include obesity, diabetes, pregnancy, and surgery. Treatment for meralgia paresthetica ranges from conservative to invasive use of nerve ablation. Nerve ablation with radiofrequency ablation has shown promise for relieving persistent and treatment-resistant pain. Due to the success of radiofrequency ablation with meralgia paresthetica, it is likely that cryoablation of the LFCN will result in similar results. Currently cryoablation has been used with patient-specific success. More studies need to be done, and it is a promising treatment alternative for meralgia paresthetica.

Cryotherapy for Total Knee Arthroplasty Pain

Osteoarthritic knee pain is a chronic problem for many adults and results in nearly 30% of all doctor visits. The treatment options range from lifestyle changes and pharmacological treatment to surgical replacement of the knee. In both non-surgical and surgical management, the use of the cryotherapy has indications for treatment. The sensory nerves that can be targeted include the medial and intermediate femoral cutaneous branches of the femoral nerve along with the saphenous nerve and infrapatellar and sartorial branches. Using anatomical landmarks and the superficial nature of these nerves, a well-targeted cryoprobe can be used to reduce knee pain either without surgery or before and after surgical intervention. Given the nature of the narcotic epidemic, having cryotherapy as an alternative can help to prevent patients from requiring narcotic pain medicine.

Cryotherapy as an Adjunct for Tapering Opioids

Cryotherapy use is also being explored as an adjunct therapy during tapering of opioids in comprehensive opioid addiction treatment (COAT). Opioid therapy is associated with development of physical dependence and addiction. Even with acute low doses of opioids, patients are at an increased risk of developing opioid use disorder (OUD). Analgesic tolerance is linked to opioid-induced hyperalgesia, a paradoxical response where patients may become more sensitive to certain stimuli. Patients may experience pain to non-painful stimuli (allodynia), suggesting involvement of the sensory nerves. Cryoneurolysis has the potential to play a role in relieving pain such as allodynia, eliminating the need to increase opioid dosages in patients. Furthermore, by treating the source of the pain via cryotherapy, it is plausible that tapering of opioids in COAT would have a higher success rate.

Pearls and Pitfalls

- The use of cryotherapy is best done with a well-trained and knowledgeable physician of local anatomy and device use.
- The optimal temperature for targeting nerves is between −60 °C and −100 °C. This can be adjusted depending

upon the nerve and pain reduction required which can be upward of −180 °C to cause complete nerve destruction.

- Before cryotherapy a test diagnostic block is done using local anesthetic that requires a 50% reduction in pain before the use of cryotherapy is performed. This is done to rule out other causes of pain and increase the likelihood that the cryotherapy will target the right nerve.
- The procedure is often performed twice for two 2-minute periods of freezing to induce adequate nerve insult. It is important to let the ice ball that forms to thaw before removal of the probe to reduce the risk of complications.
- As with all procedures, there are risks that can result in complications such as pain, bleeding, infection, or damage to surrounding structures. When used near pleural tissue, there is the risk of pneumothorax. In addition permanent nerve damage can occur that may lead to neuritis, dysesthesia, or numbness of the overlying skin.
- Future directions for cryoablation include the addition of new diseases such as meralgia paresthetica, the further use of ultrasound guidance, and the use of handheld liquid nitrogen-based portable devices that can be used in clinic.
- Cryoablation has shown promise in other areas beyond pain and includes the treatment of cancer. Lung pleural tumors show great promise for treatment with cryoablation. Stage 1 renal cell carcinoma also has shown promise for treatment with cryoablation. Metastatic bone disease has also been treated in a palliative manner.

Recommended Reading

1. Cheng J. Cryoanalgesia for refractory neuralgia. J Perioper Sci. 2015;2(2):1–8.
2. Dar SA, Love Z, Prologo JD, Hsu DP. CT-guided cryoablation for palliation of secondary trigeminal neuralgia from head and neck malignancy. J Neurointerv Surg. 2013;5(3):258–63. https://doi.org/10.1136/neurintsurg-2012-010265.
3. Evans PJ, Lloyd JW, Jack TM. Cryoanalgesia for intractable perineal pain. J R Soc Med. 1981;74(11):804–9.
4. Fanelli RD, DiSiena MR, Lui FY, Gersin KS. Cryoanalgesic ablation for the treatment of chronic postherniorrhaphy neuropathic pain. Surg Endosc. 2003;17(2):196–200.
5. Green CR, Michael de Rosayro A, Tait AR. The role of cryoanalgesia for chronic thoracic pain: results of a long-term follow up. J Natl Med Assoc. 2002;94(8):716–20.
6. Kim PS, Ferrante FM. Cryoanalgesia: a novel treatment for hip adductor spasticity and obturator neuralgia. Anesthesiology. 1998;89(2):534–6.
7. Kim DH, Hwang JJ, Lee MK, et al. Analysis of the Nuss procedure for pectus excavatum in different age groups. Ann Thorac Surg. 2005;80(3):1073–7. PubMed PMID: 16122489.
8. Kim CH, Hu W, Gao J, Dragan K, Whealton T, Julian C. Cryoablation for the treatment of occipital neuralgia. Pain Physician. 2015;18(3):E363–8.
9. Lu Q, Han Y, Cao W, Lei J, Wan Y, Zhao F, Huang L, Li X. Comparison of non-divided intercostal muscle flap and intercostal nerve cryoanalgesia treatments for post-oesophagectomy neuropathic pain control. Eur J Cardiothorac Surg. 2013;43(3):e64–70.
10. Moesker AA, Karl HW, Trescot AM. Treatment of phantom limb pain by cryoneurolysis of the amputated nerve. Pain Pract. 2014;14(1):52–6.
11. Pradel W, Hlawitschka M, Eckelt U, Herzog R, Koch K. Cryosurgical treatment of trigeminal neuralgia. Br J Oral Maxillofac Surg. 2002;40(3):244–7.
12. Sidebottom AJ, Carey EC, Madahar AK. Cryoanalgesia in the management of intractable pain in the temporomandibular joint: a five-year retrospective review. Br J Oral Maxillofac Surg. 2011;49(8):653–6.
13. Trescot AM. Cryoanalgesia in interventional pain management. Pain Physician. 2003;6(3):345–60.

35 Chemodenervation: Neurolytic Blockade and Potent Neurotoxins for the Treatment of Cancer Pain

Puneet Sayal, Michael S. Leong, and David Copenhaver

Introduction

Intractable cancer pain continues to be a significant issue for oncological care. Although spread of disease may be controlled, symptom management for nausea, vomiting, lack of appetite, and pain control can be elusive. Opioids and nonopioid oral analgesics, alike, can help to a certain extent. Interventional treatments, such as chemodenervation, neurolytic blockade at targeted ganglia, or even intrathecal (IT) neurolysis, may need to be utilized once conventional systemic therapies have been tried and failed.

Neurolytic blockade at targeted ganglia with phenol or alcohol can significantly reduce pain and anxiety and depression about pain. The most commonly used blocks target pain in the abdomen or pelvis. These procedures have a low incidence of complications but are limited to the innervation of that specific ganglia and cannot always account for variations in innervation.

IT neurolytic blockade to the sympathetic chain and spinal cord can significantly reduce refractory pain from cancer and oral analgesic requirements. However, intrathecal neurolytic blockade is nonselective for sensory and motor neurons and can leave patients with transient (4.3%) or permanent paralysis (0.8%). Intrathecal neurolytic blockade has traditionally been performed using alcohol and phenol, and a hypobaric solution of alcohol will demonstrate rostral spread in the CSF, and a hyperbaric solution of phenol will spread caudally. Both alcohol and phenol, even with their potential distribution to the anterior motor nerve roots, leading to paresis, urinary retention, and paralysis, however, can produce an estimated 3–6 months of significant relief of cancer pain.

Modern alternatives from natural agents such as *Euphorbia* and soapwort, which are synthesized to resiniferatoxin (RTX) and saporin, respectively, offer durable IT analgesia for cancer pain, but avoid prolonged motor dysfunction. RTX, a TRPV1 agonist, and saporin, a ribosomal inactivating protein, may produce long-lasting pain relief for greater than 6 months after IT administration. The latter portion of this chapter will explore the history, data, and future studies of these novel natural compounds for cancer pain relief (Table 35.1).

Neurolytic Blockade

Neurolytic blockade is commonly employed in patients with a significant cancer pain burden, typically that is located in the abdomen or pelvis. Alcohol and phenol are the chemical agents used, and both act by denaturing protein and causing Wallerian degeneration. Alcohol and phenol can be used to denervate any peripheral nerve or nerve plexus and carry the significant risk of motor dysfunction. We will describe three procedures that target abdominal and pelvic cancer pain.

Celiac Plexus Neurolysis

The celiac plexus lies anterior to the abdominal aorta; is formed by the celiac, superior mesenteric, and aorticorenal ganglia; and innervates the liver, pancreas, gall bladder, stomach, spleen, kidneys, adrenal glands, and part of the intestine (from the gastroesophageal junction to the splenic flexure of the colon). The transcrural technique for the celiac plexus block involves using fluoroscopy to advance a 22 G spinal needle in an oblique trajectory to the ipsilateral

P. Sayal
International Spine, Pain & Performance Center, Washington, DC, USA
e-mail: Drsayal@isppcenter.com

M. S. Leong (✉)
Stanford Pain Management Center, Redwood City, CA, USA
e-mail: msleong@stanford.edu

D. Copenhaver
UC Davis Cancer Pain Management and Supportive Care, University of California, Davis Division of Pain Medicine, Davis, CA, USA
e-mail: dcopenhaver@ucdavis.edu

T. R. Deer et al. (eds.), *Deer's Treatment of Pain*, https://doi.org/10.1007/978-3-030-12281-2_35

Table 35.1 Comparing different neurolytic agents

Agent	Mechanism of action	Onset	Duration	Side effects
Alcohol	Denature proteins, Wallerian degeneration	Immediate to hours	Variable, 3–12 months	Motor dysfunction, neuritis
Phenol	Denature proteins, Wallerian degeneration	Immediate to hours, typically delayed relative to alcohol	Variable, 3–12 months – typically shorter than alcohol	Motor dysfunction, dysesthesias, local inflammatory response
RTX	TRPV1 receptor agonist	Peaks at 4 hours in animal models	24 hours in animal models	Inability to detect thermal pain and immune dysfunction in animal models
SAP	NK1 receptor antagonist	Slow onset, over weeks in animal models	Unclear duration	Unclear when used for neurolysis Fever, myalgias, hepatotoxicity, thrombocytopenia, and vascular leak syndrome when used in cancer treatment

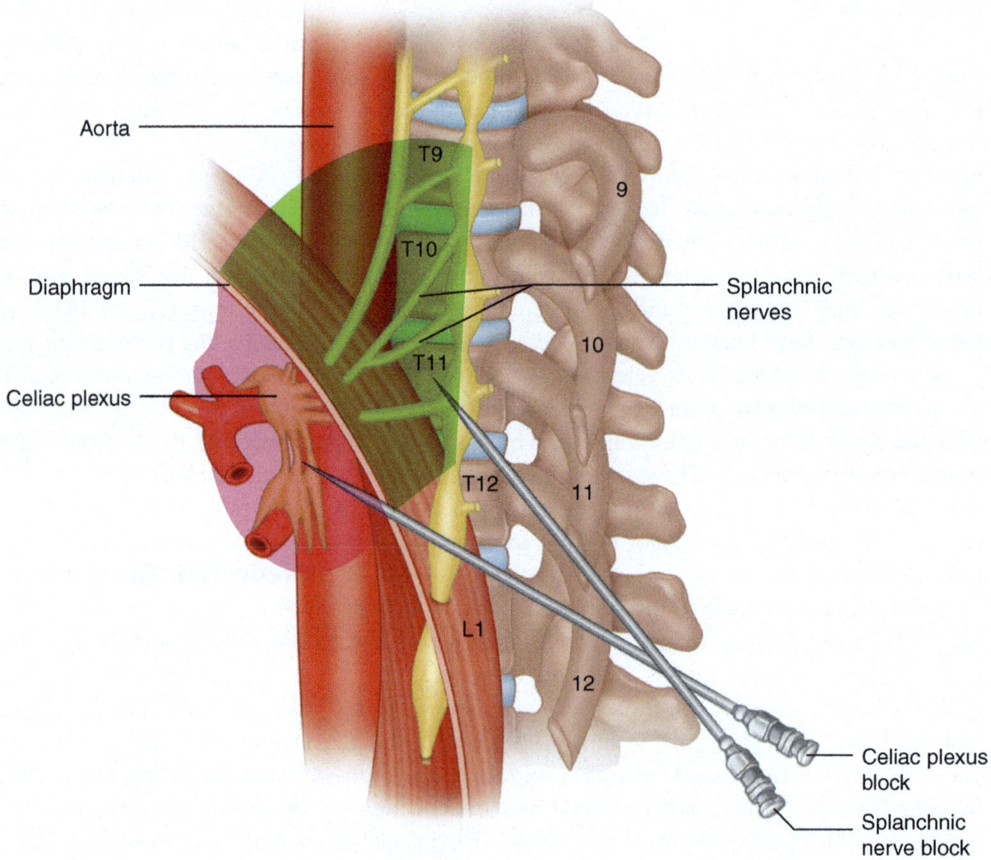

Fig. 35.1 Splanchnic and celiac plexus neurolysis

anterolateral prevertebral space anterior to the T12 or L1 vertebral bodies (Fig. 35.1). The needle is then advanced using either contrast dye or aspiration to identify when one has entered and exited anterior to the aorta. Contrast dye is then used to ensure adequate bilateral spread (a second needle may be placed on the contralateral side if bilateral spread is inadequate). A test dose of local anesthetic is injected to ensure there is no intravascular or intrathecal spread. This is then followed by the neurolytic agent.

Celiac plexus neurolysis carries the risk of hypotension, increased defecation, backache, neuritis, retroperitoneal bleeding, urinary retention, and serious neurologic compromise, including paraplegia. The reported complication rate is 1–2%.

Splanchnic Nerve Neurolysis

The splanchnic nerves carry visceral afferent information from the celiac plexus and therefore innervate the same organs. The splanchnic nerves lie in the retrocrural space. This procedure shares the initial approach with the celiac

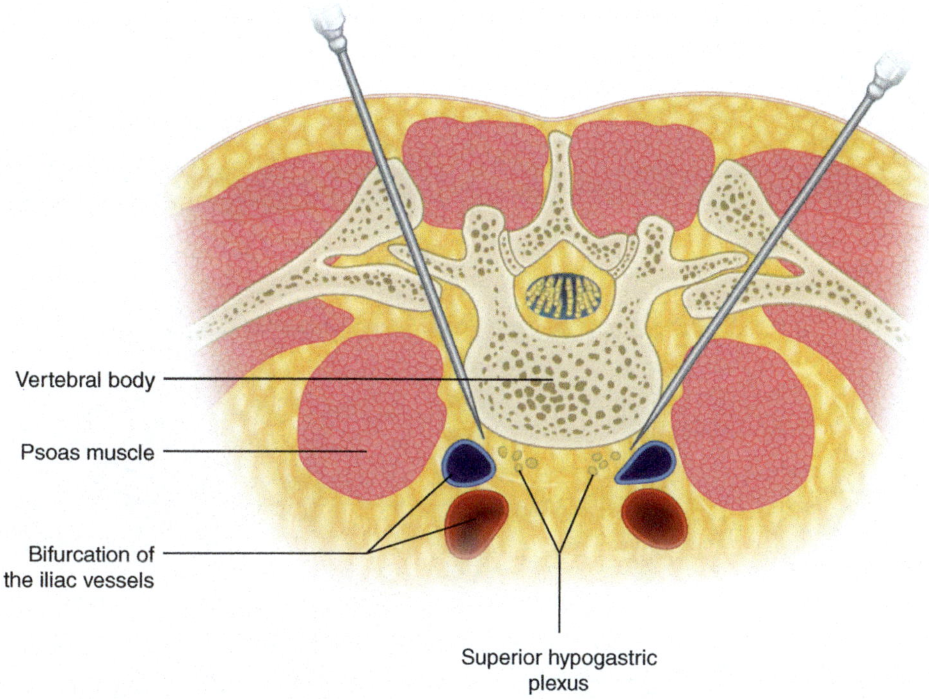

Fig. 35.2 Superior hypogastric plexus neurolysis

plexus neurolysis, a fluoroscopically guided oblique approach to the ipsilateral prevertebral space of T12 or L1. It is commonly performed with needles placed bilaterally (see Fig. 35.1). Contrast dye is then used to ensure bilateral spread in the prevertebral space and is followed by a test dose of local anesthetic to ensure no intravascular or intrathecal spread. This is then followed by the neurolytic agent.

Splanchnic nerve neurolysis carries the same risks as celiac plexus neurolysis. The reported complication rate is 1–2%.

Superior Hypogastric Neurolysis

The superior hypogastric plexus lies in the retroperitoneum, in the prevertebral space at the lower lumbar and superior sacral segments, and innervates the lower abdomen and pelvis. The most commonly described approach is a fluoroscopically guided posterolateral, transdiscal approach at the L5-S1 vertebral interspace. Prophylactic antibiotics are given. Using an oblique approach, lateral to the S1 superior articulating process (on either side) to avoid the intrathecal sac, the needle is advanced into and through the intervertebral disc and out the anterior aspect of the disc (Fig. 35.2). Correct positioning and bilateral spread is confirmed with contrast dye and fluoroscopy. A test dose of local anesthetic is given to ensure no intravascular or intrathecal spread. This is then followed by the neurolytic agent.

The risks of superior hypogastric neurolysis are the same as celiac plexus and splanchnic nerve neurolysis, except that it carries significantly lower risk of hypotension and increased defecation.

Ganglion Impar Neurolysis

The ganglion impar lies in the retroperitoneal space, immediately anterior to the sacrum at approximately the level of the sacrococcygeal junction, and innervates the perineum, distal rectum, anus, distal urethra, vulva, and distal third of the vagina. The most common approach is at the sacrococcygeal ligament. The needle is advanced using fluoroscopic guidance through the ligament until it is passes through to the anterior aspect (Fig. 35.3). Correct position is confirmed using contrast dye in the shape of a "reverse comma" to ensure no intravascular spread or bowel injury. This is then followed by the neurolytic agent.

Ganglion impar neurolysis carries the risks of infection, bleeding, neuritis, nerve injury, and damage to nearby organs (such as the rectum).

Resiniferatoxin (RTX)

History

RTX comes from the genus of plants called *Euphorbia*. RTX (*Euphorbia resinifera*) is a cactus-like plant that comes from Morocco and was synthesized by the Wender group at

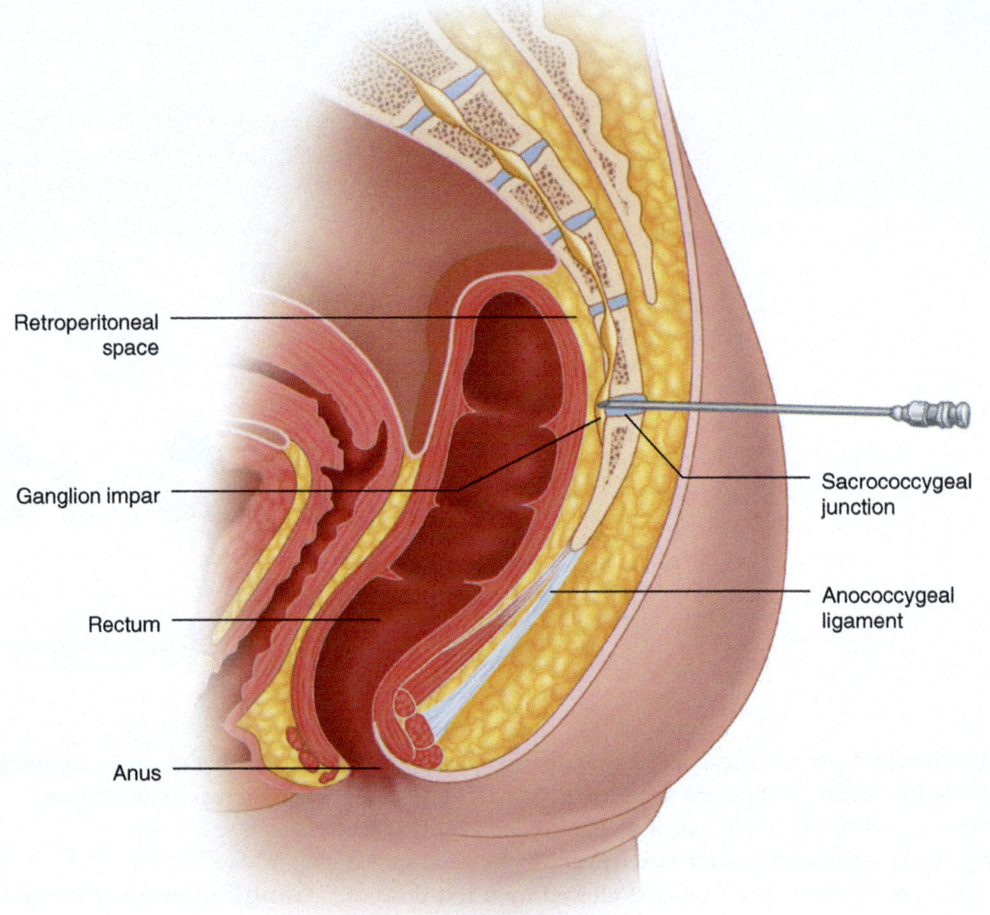

Fig. 35.3 Ganglion impar neurolysis

Stanford University in 1997. RTX is one of the most potent TRPV1 receptor agonists and potentially one of the best agents to treat inflammatory and intractable chronic pain.

Mechanism of Action

TRPV1 receptors are nonselective cation channels that are sensitized from noxious stimuli, leading to inflammatory conditions and pain. In chronic pain states, vanilloid (TRPV1) receptors are upregulated on neurons, have reduced stimulation thresholds, and cause an increased perception of pain. TRPV1 agonists activate and depolarize TRPV1 receptors, initially causing a burning sensation, and then ultimately are desensitized and become analgesic, particularly to neuropathic pain. Capsaicin, a less potent TRPV1 agonist than RTX, has been approved for the treatment of postherpetic neuralgia (Qutenza® (capsaicin) 8% patch) (Qutenza capsaicin, 8% patch, Acorda Therapeutics, NY). RTX, the most potent TRPV1 receptor agonist, is 1000–10,000 times more potent than capsaicin or 16 billion on the Scoville scale.

RTX can reduce chronic pain without affecting normal pain perception, sensation, or motor function.

Preclinical Data

From preclinical animal models, RTX has been shown to have robust effects on TRPV1 cells. RTX had instantaneous effects and induced a large influx of calcium and plasma membrane effect to DRG cells after treatment that was sustained.

Continued work demonstrated that either periganglionic DRG injections or IT injections would eliminate TRPV1-positive cells.

A single IT dose of RTX (1.2 mcg/kg) significantly attenuated thermal responses with a sharp decrease in VAS and duration through 14 weeks. Additionally, oral analgesics (opioids and NSAIDs) were substantially decreased.

Resiniferatoxin and Cancer Pain

In humans, RTX has been tested for treating cancer pain by IT injection. The US National Institutes of Health (NIH) opened a phase 1 study of IT RTX for treating severe refractory pain associated with advanced cancer, which was an open-label, single-site, dose escalation, safety study for

Table 35.2 NRS pain intensity (PI) scores after IT RTX administration

Patient	Pre-RTX NRS	Post RTX NRS (last recorded)	% improvement
1	7.3	6.1	15.5
2	8.3	3.8	54.0
3	8.4	6.0	28.8
4	8.0	5.4	32.1
5	9.0	8.7	9.6
6	8.6	7.9	8.3

patients with severe pain due to cancer, rated at an average numeric rating scale (NRS) of >6/10, over a 7-day window. The targeted pain area was mid-chest (T5 dermatome) or below, and RTX injections were performed via a spinal catheter from a standard epidural kit placed in the lumbar region (Table 35.2).

During this phase 1 trial, patients with intractable pain, associated with various cancer diagnoses, were enrolled. Intrathecal treatment with RTX produced significant and long-lasting pain relief, reduction of opioids, and profound increase in mobility. Overall, RTX in this study population has been well tolerated with no unexpected side effects.

Future Directions for Resiniferatoxin

A follow-up study is being developed by Scintilla Pharmaceuticals (Los Altos, California, USA) for treatment of patients with severe cancer pain using RTX with epidural administration in early 2017. Future studies could focus on neuropathic pain syndromes, such as refractory trigeminal neuralgia, postherpetic neuralgia, phantom limb pain, and complex regional pain syndrome.

Saporin

Pathophysiology

Substance P is a member of the tachykinin family and is involved in driving synaptic plasticity in the spinal cord. The neurochemical plexus has characteristic firing patterns and amplitudes that drive the development of synaptic change, and this may participate in the development of central sensitization.

Studies with knockout mice have shed further light on the role of substance P and the NK1 receptor, where a lack of the NK1 receptor allowed for reduction in noxious chemical signaling, including absent responses to capsaicin. Mice were also found to demonstrate general blunting in response to danger, reduced aggression, and less anxiety upon maternal separation. NK1 receptors receive a variety of input from excitatory neurotransmitters, most notably glutamate. A quest for a more targeted ligand, specific to the sensory pain concern, pointed to substance P.

Substance P has demonstrated a role in nociception at the spinal level. The inflammatory cascade has been noted to promote the upregulation of the NK1 receptor, specifically at the superficial levels of the dorsal horn (DH) of the spinal cord within nociceptive neurons.

Blocking NK1 receptors will reduce afferent input at the level of C-fibers, the DH, and reduce the potential for wind up. The understanding of neuropeptide receptor physiology, as it relates to the NK1 receptor and substance P, has led to novel drug development, including saporin, a ribosome-inactivating protein (RIP), due to its N-glycosidase activity. Saporin is extracted from the seeds of *Saponaria officinalis* (common name: soapwort).

Safety and Efficacy of Saporin

High frequency, afferent, noxious input drives release of substance P and activation of NK1 receptors at the DH. Intrathecal substance P-saporin (SP-SAP) is a targeted neurotoxin that produces selective destruction of superficial NK1 receptors in the spinal DH. SP-SAP appears to allow for a very selective destructive process, in contrast to other neurolytic agents.

Many toxicity studies in both rat and canine models have shown selective destruction occurring along the dorsal portion of the spinal cord and not the ventral surface. Additionally, when dogs were given larger doses of SP-SAP at 150 μg via an IT catheter, loss of motor neurons expressing the NK1 receptor was noted. This resulted in progressive lower limb paresis. SP-SAP certainly demonstrates efficacy in the development of a highly specific destructive lesion; however further studies will need to be assessed in order to assure appropriate dose and safety across species.

SP-SAP and Cancer Pain

In a landmark study in 2013, SP-SAP was used for analgesia for dogs suffering from cancer-related bone pain. Dogs that received SP-SAP had improved activity and pain scores when compared to controls. Although SP-SAP is a targeted neurolytic destructive agent, no deafferentation-related pain was noted. However, it was important to note that there were motor effects and ataxia in some of the dogs. The targeted neurolytic destruction of specific afferent pain pathways offers a novel opportunity for cancer pain and supportive care medicine.

The Future SP-SAP

Arthur Frankel and colleagues presented the first, human phase I trial utilizing *SP-SAP*. They concluded that *SP-SAP* appears to be safe for human use at doses less than 4 mcg.

Currently the agent is administered with a single-shot IT injection at the L5-S1 interspace, modeling the canine study from Brown and colleagues at the University of Pennsylvania. The consideration for more rostral delivery of the agent with an IT catheter may allow for a greater distribution of the agent and enhanced treatment effect. The study will continue with escalating doses to better discern the balance between analgesic benefit and toxicity.

Conclusion

As patients receive more sophisticated care for their cancer, patients are living longer with more advanced tumor burden. Living longer with multiple comorbid conditions and progressive cancer can allow for significant pain concerns. Furthermore, many patients suffer from intractable pain in the setting of cancer and end of life. This chapter summarized commonly used techniques for neurolytic blockade and discussed the promise of augmenting the supportive care armamentarium to include targeted neurochemical destructive agents, such as RTX and SP-SAP.

Recommended Reading

1. Ahluwalia A, et al. Impaired IL-1-1-induced neutrophil accumulation in tachykinin NK1 receptor knockout mice. Br J Pharmacol. 1998;124:1013–5. Print.
2. Ahmed DG, Mohamad MF, Mohamed SA. Superior hypogastric plexus combined with ganglion impar neurolytic block for pelvic and/or perineal cancer pain relief. Pain Physician. 2015;18:E49–56. Print.
3. Allen JW, et al. Safety evaluation of IT substance P-saporin, a targeted neurotoxin, in dogs. Toxicol Sci. 2006;91(1):286–98. Print.
4. Bley KR. TRPV1 agonist approaches for pain management. In: Gomtsyan A, Faltynek CR, editors. Vanilloid receptor TRPV1 in drug discovery: medicinal chemistry, biology, and therapeutic potential for chronic pain and pathological disorders. New York: John Wiley & Sons; 2010. p. 325–47. Print.
5. Brown DC, Agnello K. IT substance P-saporin in the dog: efficacy in bone cancer pain. Anesthesiology. 2013;119(5):1178–85. Print.
6. Brown DC, et al. Physiologic and antinociceptive effects of IT resiniferatoxin in a canine bone cancer model. Anesthesiology. 2005;103(5):1052–9. Print.
7. Candid K. IT neurolytic blockade for the relief of cancer pain. Best Pract Res Clin Anaesthesiol. 2003;17:407–42. Print.
8. Cao YQ, et al. Primary afferent tachykinins are required to experience moderate to intense pain. Nature. 1998;392:390–4. Print.
9. de Leon-Casasola OA, Kent E, Lema MJ. Neurolytic superior hypogastric plexus block for chronic pelvic pain associated with cancer. Pain. 1993;54(2):145–51. Print.
10. Frankel AE, et al. Preliminary results from a phase I study of substance P-saporin in advanced cancer patients with intractable pain. Cancer Res. 2016;76(14):CT030. Print.
11. Gerbershagen HU. Neurolysis. Subarachnoid neurolytic blockade. Acta Anaesthesiol Belg. 1981;32:45. Print.
12. Heiss J, et al. A phase 1 study of the IT administration of resiniferatoxin for treating severe refractory pain associated with advanced cancer. J Pain. 2014;15(4):S67. Print.
13. Iadarola M, Mannes A. The vanilloid agonist resiniferatoxin for interventional-based pain control. Curr Top Med Chem. 2011;11(17):2171–9. Print.
14. Karai L, et al. Deletion of vanilloid receptor1-expressing primary afferent neurons for pain control. J Clin Invest. 2004;113(9):1344–52. Print.
15. Koyyalagunta D, et al. The effectiveness of alcohol versus phenol based splanchnic nerve neurolysis for the treatment of intra-abdominal cancer pain. Pain Physician. 2016;19:281–92. Print.
16. Laird JMA, et al. Visceral hyperalgesia and acute responses to chemical but not mechanical visceral stimuli are abolished in NK1 receptor knockout mice. Neuroscience. 1998;24:881. Print.
17. Loev MA, et al. Cryoablation: a novel approach to neurolysis of the ganglion impar. Anesthesiology. 1998;88(5):1391–3. Print.
18. Mansikka H, et al. Neurokinin-1 receptors are involved in behavioral responses to high intensity heat stimuli and capsaicin-induced hyperalgesia in mice. Anesthesiology. 1999;90:1643–9. Print.
19. Olah Z, et al. Ligand-induced dynamic membrane changes and cell deletion conferred by vanilloid receptor 1. J Biol Chem. 2001;276(14):11021–30. Print.
20. Parker D, Grillner S. Activity-dependent metaplasticity of inhibitory and excitatory synaptic transmission in the lamprey spinal cord locomotor network. J Neurosci. 1999;19:1647–56. Print.
21. Parker D, Zhang W, Grillner S. Substance P modulates NMDA responses and causes long-term protein synthesisdependent modulation of the lamprey locomotor network. J Neurosci. 1998;18:4800–13. Print.
22. Qutenza® (capsaicin) 8% patch. Prescribing information; 2009. Print.
23. Watanabe A, Yamakage M. IT neurolytic block in a patient with refractory cancer pain. J Anesth. 2011;25(4):603–5. Print.
24. Weintraub A. Prickly painkiller. Sci Am. 2013. Print.
25. Wender PA, et al. The first synthesis of a daphnane diterpene: the enantiocontrolled total synthesis of (+)-resiniferatoxin. J Am Chem Soc. 1997;119(52):12976–7. Print.
26. Wiese AJ, et al. IT substance P-saporin in the dog: distribution, safety, and spinal neurokinin-1 receptor ablation. Anesthesiology. 2013;119(5):1163–77. Print.

Blockade of the Nerves of the Head and Face

36

Narayan R. Kissoon

Introduction

Peripheral nerve blocks have been used in the management of headache disorders and facial pain for several decades, and the observed effects are believed to be as a result of direct suppression of nociceptive input as well as modulation of the central pain pathways. These injections can be beneficial in primary headache disorders, secondary headache disorders, and cranial neuralgias when patients have failed conservative medical management, contraindications are present in the use of systemic medications, and/or unable to tolerate systemic medications. The choice of peripheral nerve injections depends on the headache syndrome, location of pain, presence of autonomic features, and response to prior injections. Peripheral nerve injections can be performed at bedside in the outpatient clinic, and proper technique is important to maintain safety and efficacy. Depending on the peripheral nerve block type, the use of ultrasound guidance can increase the safety and accuracy of the injection as well as potentially identify causative lesions such as proximal entrapment of the occipital nerve in occipital neuralgia. Growing evidence with randomized controlled trials has added support in the use of peripheral nerve blocks in the management of headache disorders, and appropriate use of peripheral nerve injections can improve clinical outcomes in craniofacial pain.

Background and Historical Perspective

Occipital neuralgia was the first cranial neuralgia to be routinely treated with peripheral nerve blocks. The first description was in 1969 by Arnold where a series of patients that presented with occipital pain had responded to occipital nerve blocks. Occipital nerve blocks continue to be the most commonly used peripheral nerve blocks used in the treatment of headache disorders. However, as evidence has grown supporting the use of occipital nerve blocks, injections targeting other cranial distributions (e.g., supraorbital nerve blocks, auriculotemporal nerve blocks, lesser occipital nerve blocks, and sphenopalatine ganglion blocks) have been incorporated into the management of headache disorders. Over time the use of peripheral nerve blocks has increased, and for decades peripheral nerve blocks have been used in the treatment of headaches and facial pain.

In headache disorders, the mechanism of action for peripheral nerve blocks has been believed to be related to suppression of nociceptive input and alteration of activity in second-order neurons of the trigeminocervical complex in the brainstem. This has been evident by longer than expected benefit based on the pharmacokinetics of local anesthetics and pain relief in distributions outside of the treated nerves. Intracranial structures in the anterior and middle fossa have innervation by the ophthalmic branch of the trigeminal nerve, and the posterior fossa has innervation by the upper cervical nerve roots. Primary afferent neurons from the greater occipital nerve synapse with second-order neurons in the C2 spinal segment, which also has trigeminal nerve afferent terminations that extend into the same C2 spinal segment. Relevant to the mechanism of action with occipital nerve blocks, input from the greater occipital nerve can alter activity in the primary afferents of the trigeminal nerve due to a convergence of input at the trigeminocervical complex. This convergence of sensory input from intracranial structures and cutaneous fibers innervating the entire scalp has been believed to be the mechanism to which suppression of input with anesthetic blocks alters the central pain pathways to provide long-term headache relief. Aside from modulation of the central pain pathways, peripheral nerve blocks have been suspected to act via direct suppression of activity in primary afferent fibers for cranial neuralgias.

N. R. Kissoon (✉)
Division of Headache, Department of Neurology, Mayo Clinic, Rochester, MN, USA

Division of Pain, Department of Anesthesiology, Mayo Clinic, Rochester, MN, USA
e-mail: kissoon.narayan@mayo.edu

T. R. Deer et al. (eds.), *Deer's Treatment of Pain*, https://doi.org/10.1007/978-3-030-12281-2_36

Uses and Indications

Primary Headache Disorders

Trigeminal Autonomic Cephalalgias: Cluster Headache and Beyond

Trigeminal autonomic cephalalgias are some of the most debilitating headache disorders to the extent that a subset of these headaches has been colloquially termed "suicide headaches." These are unilateral headaches in the frontal, temporal, or orbital region that are accompanied by autonomic features and/or agitation. The duration and frequency of attacks are used to differentiate the trigeminal autonomic cephalalgias. The most common of these headache disorders are cluster headaches. In the transitional period while trying to get cluster headaches in remission, the use of oral steroids or peripheral nerve blocks are potential treatment options to reduce the frequency of headache attacks during up-titration of the preventative therapy. Specifically, peripheral nerve injections can be useful as the bridging therapy in trigeminal autonomic cephalalgias when there is a contraindication to use of systemic steroids or the patient has already failed bridging treatment with oral steroids.

The choice of peripheral nerve injections depends on the distribution of headache, presence of autonomic features, and response to prior injections. Occipital nerve blocks are an initial option for patients naïve to peripheral nerve injections as some of the strongest evidence in the literature for nerve blocks in headache are studies evaluating the use of occipital nerve blocks in cluster headache (Table 36.1). In patients with chronic intractable cluster headache, the addition of either supraorbital nerve blocks or auriculotemporal nerve blocks could be used depending on the distribution of the headache. Alternatively, if autonomic phenomena (e.g., tearing, ptosis, redness, or congestion) are present, then sphenopalatine ganglion blocks either in place of occipital nerve blocks or in conjunction with occipital nerve blocks are potential options. Some evidence exists for the use of peripheral nerve blocks in other trigeminal autonomic cephalalgias (Table 36.1). From the literature, patients with hemicrania continua tend to respond better to supraorbital nerve blocks. Paroxysmal hemicrania has been shown to respond to sphenopalatine ganglion blocks, and short-lasting, unilateral, neuralgiform headache attacks with conjunctival injection and tearing (SUNCT) syndrome has responded to occipital nerve blocks.

Migraine

Migraine is the most common headache disorder seen in pain or headache clinics and is a syndrome characterized by a severe throbbing or pulsatile headache typically accompanied by nausea, photophobia, and phonophobia. In the acute setting, both episodic and chronic (>15 days a month of headache) migraine can present in status migrainosus after failing management with acute medical therapies, and peripheral injections can be helpful to prevent patients from going to the emergency department, prevent admission to the hospital, or shorten the hospital stay. Prolonged auras can be debilitating, and in patients with known history of migraine with aura whom are presenting with a typical aura, occipital nerve blocks have been shown to abort both prolonged and motor auras.

In chronic migraine, botulinum toxin injections have been shown to be very effective as preventative treatment, but patients often experience a "wearing off" phenomenon with an increase in frequency of headache several weeks before the next round of botulinum toxin injections. Alternating in between rounds of botulinum toxin injections with peripheral nerve blocks can be an option to minimize worsening of headache prior to the next round of botulinum toxin injections. If patients with chronic intractable migraine have failed medications and botulinum toxin injections, or have a contraindication, then a potential treatment option could be periodic nerve blocks as a preventative strategy but would limit the use of steroid in the injectate to no more than once every 3 months. Most headache medications are US Food and Drug Administration category C or worse, which makes migraine in pregnancy challenging to treat. Lidocaine is category B (unlike bupivacaine and most steroids), and so nerve blocks with lidocaine can be used safely in pregnancy. Older patients with migraine (or other headache disorders) often do not tolerate preventative medications or have a contraindication to these medications, and so peripheral nerve injections are a potential option for treatment.

With long-term use of periodic nerve blocks, would consider using a non-particulate steroid such as dexamethasone or alternate with local anesthetic-only injections. Evidence in the treatment of migraine has shown that local anesthetic-only injections have been just as effective as injections with steroid. Growing evidence has emerged for the use of peripheral nerve injections in migraine with randomized controlled trials supporting the use of both occipital nerve blocks and sphenopalatine ganglion blocks as an adjunctive treatment (Table 36.1). Similar to trigeminal autonomic cephalalgias, the distribution of headache, presence of autonomic features, and response to prior injections can help determine the choice of injection. Either occipital nerve blocks or sphenopalatine ganglion blocks are reasonable first options as blocks in treatment of refractory migraine.

Other Primary Headache Disorders

There is a limited role for the use of peripheral nerve injections in other primary headache disorders. In the literature, a single study investigated the treatment of frontal distribution tension headaches with occipital nerve blocks and did not demonstrate an improvement in the headaches (Table 36.1).

Table 36.1 Evidence for efficacy in primary headache disorders

Author, year, and (N)	Evidence	Peripheral nerve injections	Results
Cluster headache			
Ambrosini et al. 2005, (*N* = 23)	Randomized controlled	GON (LA/steroid) vs saline	GON > placebo with response >4 weeks in most
Leroux et al. 2011, (*N* = 43)	Randomized controlled	3 GON (steroid)	GON > placebo at 15 days
Costa et al. 2000, (*N* = 15)	Randomized controlled	SPG – 10% lidocaine vs 10% cocaine	10% lidocaine = 10% cocaine with cessation of HA after ~30 minutes in NTG-induced HA
Gaul et al. 2016, (*N* = 101)	Prospective	GON (LA/steroid)	GON > baseline at 1 week. Episodic cluster HA had better response than chronic cluster HA
Peres et al. 2002, (*N* = 14)	Open label	GON (LA/steroid)	GON > baseline at 1 week
Bigo et al. 1989, (*N* = 16)	Retrospective	GON (steroid)	Complete or partial response in 9 patients
Govindappagari et al. 2014, (*N* = 13)	Retrospective	GON, SON, STN, ATN	In pregnancy, INJ > baseline at 24 hours with pain relief up to 158 days
Afridi et al. 2011, (*N* = 22)	Case series	GON (LA/steroid)	GON > baseline for median of 21 days
Busch et al. 2007, (*N* = 15)	Case series	GON (LA only)	GON prolonged blink reflex 20 minutes after INJ
Felisati et al. 2000, (*N* = 20)	Case series	SPG (LA/steroid)	55% of patients responded with complete cessation of attacks for up to 24 months
Kittrelle et al. 2006, (*N* = 5)	Case series	SPG (LA)	80% of patients responded with 75% or greater pain relief within 3 minutes of block
Hemicrania continua			
Antonaci et al. 1997, (*N* = 7)	Prospective	GON, LON, SON	SON > GON and LON. Long-term effects past anesthetic effect not evaluated
Guerrero et al. 2012, (*N* = 9)	Retrospective	GON, SON	In indomethacin-intolerant patients, GON + SON > baseline ranging from 2–10 months
Androulakis et al. 2016, (*N* = 1)	Case report	Serial SPG (LA)	Resolution of continuous HA within 6 weeks
Paroxysmal hemicrania			
Antonaci et al. 1997, (*N* = 6)	Prospective	GON, LON, SON	No change acutely, but long-term effect not assessed
Morelli et al. 2010, (*N* = 1)	Case report	Serial SPG (LA/steroid)	In indomethacin-intolerant patient, SPG > baseline with benefit sustained at 4 months
SUNCT			
Pareja et al. 1995, (*N* = 9)	Retrospective	GON, SON ION, LNB	No difference from baseline, but limited information and not everyone received blocks
Choi et al. 2012, (*N* = 1)	Case report	3 weekly GON (LA/steroid)	Resolution of HA after 3rd GON
Porta-Etessam et al. 2010, (*N* = 1)	Case report	GON (LA/steroid)	Resolution of HA after 2 weeks
Migraine			
Ashkenazi et al. 2008, (*N* = 37)	Randomized controlled	GON + cervical TPI, LA/steroid vs LA	No difference between groups at 4 weeks, but high dropout rate (65% completed study)
Palamar et al. 2014, (*N* = 32)	Randomized controlled	GON with US at level of occiput, LA vs saline INJ	GON > placebo at 4 weeks
Dilli et al. 2015, (*N* = 69)	Randomized controlled	GON(LA/steroid) vs saline INJ	No difference between groups. Episodic and chronic migraine included in study
Inan et al. 2015, (*N* = 84)	Randomized controlled	4 weekly GON, then 2 monthly GON vs saline INJ	GON > placebo at 4 weeks
Gul et al. 2016, (*N* = 44)	Randomized controlled	4 weekly GON vs placebo	GON > placebo at 3 months
Cuadrado et al. 2016, (*N* = 36)	Randomized controlled	GON (LA) vs saline INJ	GON > placebo at 1 week
Cady et al. 2015, (*N* = 41)	Randomized controlled	Twice weekly SPG for 6 weeks, LA vs saline	SPG > placebo at 24 hours and > baseline at 6 months
Ashkenazi and Young 2005, (*N* = 19)	Prospective	GON ± cervical TPI (LA/steroid)	GON > baseline 20 minutes after INJ
Dimitriou et al. 2002, (*N* = 70)	Prospective	SON, STN (LA)	82% of patients had cessation of acute migraine attack within 15 minutes after INJ
Anthony 1992, (*N* = 50)	Retrospective	GON (LA/steroid)	HA free for mean duration of 32 days

(continued)

Table 36.1 (continued)

Author, year, and (N)	Evidence	Peripheral nerve injections	Results
Gawel and Rothbart 1992, (*N* = 184)	Retrospective	Single or multiple GON (LA/steroid)	GON > baseline up to 6 months after INJ
Caputi and Firetto 1997, (*N* = 27)	Retrospective	GON,SON (LA)	GON + SON > baseline at 6 months
Afridi et al. 2011, (*N* = 57)	Case series	GON (LA/steroid)	GON > baseline for median of 30 days
Kim et al. 2016, (*N* = 13)	Case series	GON (LA/steroid), then 10% lidocaine INJ	GON > baseline for mean of 148 days
Tobin and Flitman 2011, (*N* = 1)	Case report	GON (steroid)	GON > baseline for up to 3 weeks
Migraine aura			
Cuadrado et al. 2016, (*N* = 22)	Case series	GON (LA only)	Cessation in 50% of prolonged auras (>2 hours) + good response when aura <1 week
Rozen 2007, (*N* = 2)	Case report	GON (LA/steroid)	Cessation of motor auras within 5 minutes with baseline aura typically lasting up to 5–7 days
Tension headache			
Leinisch-Dahlke et al. 2005, (*N* = 15)	Open label	GON (LA/steroid)	In patients with frontal distribution HA, GON = baseline
Orgasmic headache			
Selekler et al. 2009, (*N* = 1)	Case report	GON (LA/steroid)	Resolution of HA after 10 weeks
Hypnic headache			
Rehmann et al. 2016, (*N* = 1)	Case report	Multiple GON (LA/steroid)	GON > baseline at 6 months

Abbreviations: *HA* headache, *NTG* nitroglycerin, *LA* local anesthetic, *GON* greater occipital nerve block(s), *LON* lesser occipital nerve block(s), *SON* supraorbital nerve block(s), *SPG* sphenopalatine ganglion nerve block(s), *ATN* auriculotemporal nerve block(s), *STN* supratrochlear nerve block(s), *LN* lacrimal nerve block(s), great auricular nerve block(s), *ITN* infratrochlear nerve block(s), *INJ* injection(s), *TPI* trigger point injection(s)

Some case reports have shown benefit in less common disorders such as hypnic headache and primary headache associated with sexual activity. The role of peripheral nerve injections is unclear in these other headache disorders but could be considered if the headaches are refractory to medication management or the patient has been suspected of having a comorbid secondary headache syndrome.

Secondary Headache Disorders

Cervicogenic Headache

Cervicogenic headache is a result of referred pain from cervical structures innervated by the upper three cervical spinal nerves. Typically, these headaches are in an occipital distribution with posterior to anterior radiation of pain provoked by head movements or digital palpation of cervical musculature and/or accompanied by reduced range of motion in the neck. Imaging findings of a disorder of the cervical spine and response to treatment directed at a cervical structure or its nerve supply are supportive of the diagnosis. Cervicogenic headaches are often unilateral, side-locked, and non-throbbing in character but can be bilateral and have migrainous features or present with comorbid migraine. Evidence primarily supports the use of occipital nerve blocks in cervicogenic headache (Table 36.2), and the use of peripheral nerve injections can prevent or postpone the need for more invasive procedures such as cervical spine injections, neuroablative procedures, or joint arthrodesis.

These patients are typically older (age > 50), and occipital nerve blocks are a potential treatment option for patients where systemic medications are not a treatment option. Some patients with cervicogenic headache present with a history of traumatic injury (e.g., whiplash injury) and have accompanying post-concussive symptoms. There is evidence supporting the use of occipital nerve blocks in the treatment of post-concussive headache. Disruption of the cervical structures can occur after craniotomy (e.g., suboccipital or microvascular decompression). Post-craniotomy headaches can be refractory to medication management, and peripheral nerve injections can be another option in these often medically intractable headaches. However, caution needs to be observed to prevent intradural injection as a result of a skull defect.

Medication Overuse Headache

Medication overuse often confounds a headache presentation and can make other headache disorders difficult to treat. These rebound headaches can develop with regular overuse of acute headache medications for durations greater than 3 months. This can occur when triptans, opioids, butalbital, and combination analgesics are used more than 9 days a month or when acetaminophen and NSAIDs are used more than 14 days a month. Treatment options include counseling regarding cessation of overuse, bridging with short course of systemic steroids or naproxen (long-acting NSAID), or peripheral nerve injections. Patients often have difficulties with cessation of medication overuse on their own or are unable to bridge with systemic medications, whereby leaving

Table 36.2 Evidence for efficacy in secondary headache disorders

Author, year, and (N)	Evidence	Peripheral nerve injections	Results
Cervicogenic HA			
Inan et al. 2001, (*N* = 28)	Randomized controlled	2 GON vs C2/3 nerve block without image guidance	GON > baseline at 2 months with no difference between groups after 1 week
Naja et al. 2006, (*N* = 50)	Randomized controlled	Nerve stimulation-guided GON + LON, ± FN (LA vs saline)	GON + LON > placebo at 2 weeks. GON and LON in all patients. Not all received FN
Pingree et al. 2017, (N = 14)	Prospective	US-guided GON at level of C2	GON > baseline at 4 weeks. Both cervicogenic HA and occipital neuralgia included in study
Naja et al. 2006, (*N* = 47)	Prospective	Multiple nerve stimulation-guided GON + LON, ± FN	GON > baseline at 6 months. GON and LON in all patients. Not all received FN
Vincent et al. 1998, (*N* = 41)	Prospective	GON (LA)	GON > baseline at 1 week even with small volume of LA (1–2 mL)
Bovim and Sand 1992, (*N* = 24)	Prospective	GON or SON (LA)	GON > baseline at 30 minutes. Pain relief in cervicogenic HA > migraine and tension HA. Pain relief in GON > SON
Anthony 2000, (*N* = 180)	Retrospective	GON + LON (steroid)	GON > baseline for mean of 23.5 days. Unclear if LA was used
Yi et al. 2005, (*N* = 4)	Case series	GON (LA only)	Patients with comorbid migraine, GON > baseline ranging from 10 days to 2 months
MOH			
Karadas et al. 2017, (*N* = 105)	Randomized controlled	Cessation of MOH vs 1 GON vs 3 GON (LA only)	GON > cessation of MOH at 4 months. GON + stopping MOH improved long-term outcomes
Tobin and Flitman 2009, (*N* = 108)	Retrospective	Multiple GON (LA/steroid)	GON > baseline at mean of 5.5 weeks. Failure rate was higher with MOH than without MOH
CSF leak			
Naja et al. 2009, (*N* = 50)	Randomized controlled	Multiple GON (LA only) vs medical management	In PDPH, GON > medical management at 8 days
Matute et al. 2008, (*N* = 2)	Case report	GON	In PDPH, HA resolved after GON in 1 patient + other discharged within 48 hours of GON
Niraj et al. 2017, (*N* = 1)	Case report	GON (LA/steroid)	In spontaneous intracranial hypotension, GON > baseline in a 3-month period
Kent and Mehaffey 2016, (*N* = 3)	Case series	SPG (LA)	In PDPH, SPG > baseline for 48 hours preventing need for blood patch
Post-concussive HA			
Hecht 2004, (*N* = 10)	Retrospective	GON (LA/steroid)	GON had good response for >24 hours

Abbreviations: *HA* headache, *MOH* medication overuse headache, *PDPH* postdural puncture headache, *LA* local anesthetic, *GON* greater occipital nerve block(s), *LON* lesser occipital nerve block(s), *SON* supraorbital nerve block(s), *SPG* sphenopalatine ganglion nerve block(s), *FN* facial nerve block(s)

peripheral nerve injections (either occipital nerve blocks and/or nerve blocks in the distribution of headache) as a viable option to allow for cessation of medication overuse. At the time of presentation, these patients are frequently not being treated with a preventative medication, and peripheral nerve injections can be a bridge to allow time for the preventative medication to become effective over the course of several weeks. Given the difficult to treat nature of medication overuse headache, the presence of medication overuse can conversely limit the efficacy of peripheral nerve injections in treatment of other comorbid headache disorders.

CSF Leaks

Orthostatic headaches raise concern for the possibility of CSF leaks. The most common type is related to dural puncture after percutaneous procedures such as lumbar puncture, inadvertently after interventional procedures (most commonly epidural injections), or neuro-axial surgeries. Alternatively, patients can present insidiously with headache related to spontaneous intracranial hypotension. The headaches often have migrainous features, and patients can have a history of traumatic injury. Imaging can show pachymeningeal enhancement, flattening of the pons, brain sag, extradural fluid collections, and/or meningeal diverticula related to focal dural thinning and dehiscence. In some cases, the patients can present with aphasia, dementia, cranial nerve deficits, and/or even with a paradoxical headache due to an acquired Chiari I malformation. Most cases of post-dural puncture headaches resolve with conservative management (e.g., fluid hydration and caffeine), but refractory severe headaches require intervention and are most commonly treated with an epidural blood patch. Depending on the timing of the headache (e.g., weekends or holidays), resources of the medical center, and patient preference, an epidural blood patch may not be an option or readily available for treatment of the CSF leak. In these instances, occipital nerve blocks and sphenopalatine ganglion blocks have been shown to be a potential alternative treatment (Table 36.2).

Other Secondary Headache Disorders

Typically with secondary headache disorders, the underlying cause should be treated as peripheral nerve injections will have limited efficacy. However, if the secondary cause has been adequately treated (e.g., infection, mass lesions, or other cause), then the presence of a comorbid primary headache disorder or medication overuse should be considered. When conservative medical managements fails, peripheral nerve blocks of the head can be a viable treatment option as outlined above.

Cranial Neuralgias, Neuropathy, and Face Pain

Occipital Neuralgia

Occipital neuralgia is characterized by paroxysmal pain in the occipital distribution that is shooting, stabbing, or sharp in quality and with tenderness at the emergence or distribution of the nerves as outlined by the diagnostic criteria of the International Classification of Headache Disorders. Pain relief with local anesthetic block is part of the diagnostic criteria. While by strict International Classification of Headache Disorders criteria these would be considered alternative diagnoses, there are case reports in the literature of secondary causes of occipital neuralgia related to compression, vascular malformations, atlantoaxial joint arthrosis syndrome, neurosyphilis, or demyelinating lesions in multiple sclerosis. Initially, entrapment at the level of the trapezius was the proposed mechanism, but anatomical studies have demonstrated more proximal regions of potential entrapment within the suboccipital muscles either as the nerve courses in fascial planes or within the belly of the muscles. In most cases of occipital neuralgia, a cause is not found. Occipital nerve blocks have been effective in providing pain relief in occipital neuralgia in conjunction with medical management. Ultrasound performed at the time of the injection can be useful to identify potential areas of entrapment and can provide needle guidance to the regions more likely to be affected based on current anatomical studies.

Trigeminal Distribution Pain

Facial pain can be challenging to treat, and all cases require advanced imaging to exclude secondary causes. Of the facial pain syndromes, trigeminal neuralgia has several therapeutic options. Trigeminal neuralgia is characterized by sudden, recurrent, unilateral, and brief, electric shock-like episodes of pain in distributions of one or more branches of the trigeminal nerve (more often V2 or V3 distribution). The patients are typically over the age of 50, and vascular compression is the most common cause of trigeminal neuralgia. For patients that do not respond to anticonvulsant therapy, microvascular decompressions can be curative even if a compressive vascular loop is not found on MRI and compressive vascular lesions have been found only at time of surgery. Alternatively, medically intractable trigeminal neuralgia may respond to injections or neuroablative procedures directed at the gasserian ganglion for those that are not surgical candidates. However, these injections are invasive (potentially painful) and if the pain is in isolated branches of the trigeminal nerve, then peripheral injections (e.g., supraorbital, infraorbital, and mental nerve blocks) in the distribution of pain may be options that could be performed at bedside. The finding of anesthesia (often with history of dental procedures) would be suggestive of trigeminal neuropathy and would be indicative of a more difficult to treat pain syndrome but can still respond to peripheral nerve injections. Evidence exists supporting the use of peripheral nerve injections for distal branches of the trigeminal nerve with supraorbital neuralgia, infratrochlear neuralgia, lacrimal neuralgia, auriculotemporal neuralgia, and lacrimal neuralgia (Table 36.3). Occipital nerve blocks have shown some benefit in trigeminal distribution pain likely due to the convergence of input at the trigeminocervical complex, but the subset of patients with persistent idiopathic facial pain are less likely to respond to injections (Table 36.3).

Evidence for Efficacy

In the past several years, the evidence for the use of peripheral nerve blocks has grown substantially with the most robust data supporting the use of occipital nerve blocks. There are randomized controlled trials supporting the use of occipital nerve blocks for the treatment of cluster headache, migraine, cervicogenic headache, medication overuse headache, and post-dural puncture headaches (Tables 36.1, 36.2, and 36.3). Given that occipital nerve blocks are part of the diagnostic criteria for occipital neuralgia, evidence is limited regarding efficacy due to the challenges in designing a randomized trial. In addition to occipital nerve blocks, sphenopalatine ganglion blocks have randomized trials demonstrating efficacy in both cluster headache and chronic migraine (Table 36.1). The remaining peripheral nerve injections have prospective and retrospective studies supporting the use (Tables 36.1, 36.2, and 36.3), but based on the purported mechanism of action for nerve blocks in craniofacial pain, the occipital nerve block data could be translated to support the use of other peripheral nerve injections depending on the distribution of pain.

Table 36.3 Evidence for efficacy in cranial neuralgias/neuropathy

Author, year, and (N)	Evidence	Peripheral nerve injections	Results
Occipital neuralgia			
Pingree et al. 2017, ($N = 14$)	Prospective	US-guided GON at level of C2	GON > baseline at 4 weeks. Both cervicogenic HA and occipital neuralgia included in study
Anthony 1992, ($N = 50$)	Retrospective	GON (LA/steroid)	HA free for mean duration of 31 days
Sahai-Srivastava and Subhani 2010, ($N = 89$)	Retrospective	GON (LA/steroid)	Side effects with 5% lidocaine >1% lidocaine and no long-term efficacy data presented
Zipfel et al. 2016, ($N = 7$)	Retrospective	US-guided GON at intermediate site	GON > baseline for majority at 3 months. Grouped with other types of craniofacial pain
Aubry et al. 2016, ($N = 45$)	Retrospective	CT-guided GON (LA/steroid) at one or two sites	GON > baseline for mean of 7.7 months + GON at first bend of nerve more effective
Kastler et al. 2015, ($N = 37$)	Retrospective	CT-guided GON (LA/steroid) at first bend of nerve	GON > baseline for mean of 9.16 months
Vanderhoek et al. 2015, ($N = 2$)	Case reports	Multiple GON (LA/steroid) with US at level of occiput	Pain relief for 4 weeks up to 3 months
Trigeminal distribution pain			
Mulero et al. 2012, ($N = 8$)	Prospective	SON (LA)	Complete pain relief lasting from 2 to 6 months
Villar-Quiles et al. 2017, ($N = 7$)	Prospective	ITN (LA)	Complete pain relief for 2 weeks up to 16 months
Jurgens et al. 2012, ($N = 25$)	Retrospective	GON (LA/steroid)	GON > baseline for mean of 27 days. Pain relief in trigeminal neuralgia/neuropathy > idiopathic persistent facial pain
Sjaastad et al. 1999, ($N = 5$)	Case series	SON	SON > baseline for up to 3 weeks
Speciali and Goncalves 2005, ($N = 6$)	Case series	ATN	Pain relief with blocks, but duration of effect not outlined
Weatherall 2008, ($N = 1$)	Case report	GON (LA/steroid)	GON > baseline at 8 weeks
Cuadrado et al. 2017, ($N = 3$)	Case series	LN (LA)	LN > baseline for >2 months

Abbreviations: *HA* headache, *LA* local anesthetic, *GON* greater occipital nerve block(s), *LON* lesser occipital nerve block(s), *SON* supraorbital nerve block(s), *SPG* sphenopalatine ganglion nerve block(s), *ATN* auriculotemporal nerve block(s), *LN* lacrimal nerve block(s), *ITN* infratrochlear nerve block(s)

Pearls and Pitfalls

Occipital Nerve Block

Landmark-Based Technique

Pearls

- *Positioning*: Sitting position with head and neck flexed onto a pillow on the table.
- *Anatomical landmarks*: The emergence of the greater occipital nerve is typically located 1/3 of the distance lateral from the external occipital protuberance to the mastoid process along the nuchal ridge. The lesser occipital nerve can typically be found 2/3 of the way lateral from the occipital protuberance to the mastoid process along the nuchal ridge. Area of maximal tenderness can help denote location of occipital nerve, and injection at site of maximal tenderness can improve efficacy (Fig. 36.1).
- *Needle*: 1 ½ inch 22 G needle. Larger needle may cause more initial discomfort, but a larger bore than 25 G needle can increase the speed of injection. Alternatively, a 2 inch 25 G needle can be used, which can be helpful if the proceduralist intends for a field block with coverage of the lesser occipital nerve distribution.
- *Injectate*: With an initial injection, use of a particulate steroid such as triamcinolone or methylprednisolone, often at a dose of 10–20 mg, could be considered. However, the use of a non-particulate steroid such as dexamethasone (at an equivalent dose) is safer and can minimize the risk of skin atrophy or inadvertent intravascular injection. With serial injections a non-particulate steroid or local anesthetic-only injection should be considered. Typically, the steroid is diluted with a 1:1 mixture of local anesthetic consisting of 1% lidocaine (short acting) and 0.5% bupivacaine (long acting). A higher volume (up to 6 mL) of injectate can be used in hopes of lateral spread to treat the lesser occipital nerves and can also account for variable anatomy.

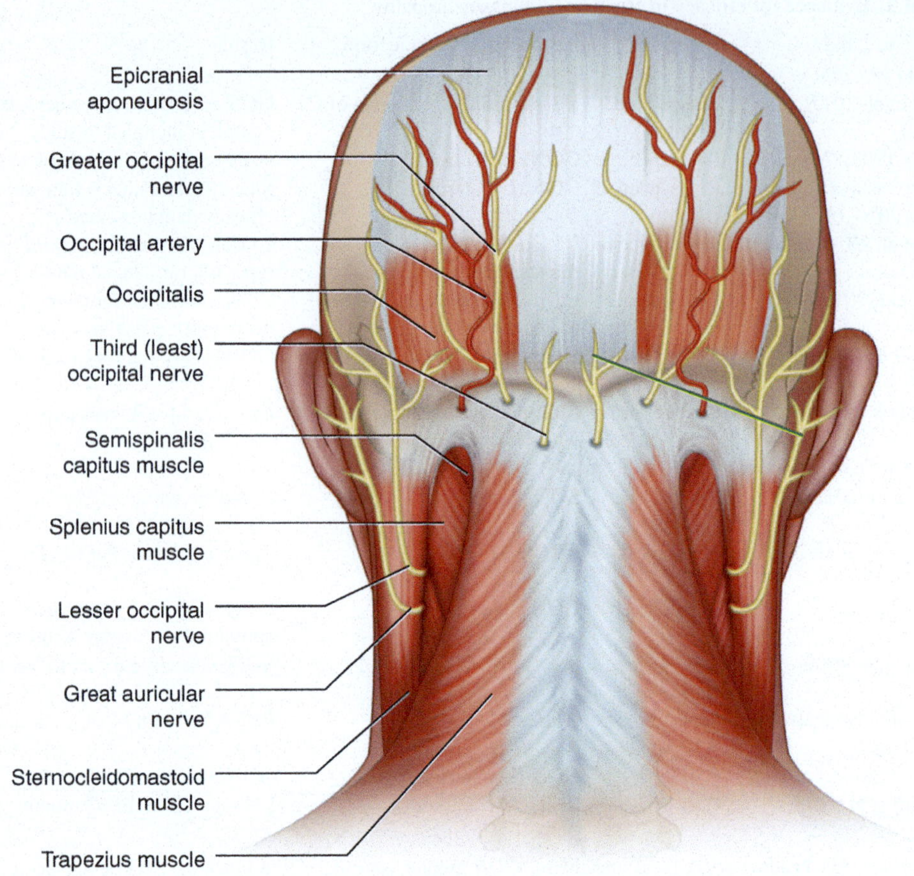

Fig. 36.1 The emergence of the greater occipital nerve can be found 1/3 the distance lateral from the external occipital protuberance to the mastoid process along the line shown

- *Technique*: After the suspected area of emergence for the occipital nerve is palpated, marked, and prepped with a disinfectant (typically chlorhexidine), a needle is introduced with a cephalad approach toward the occiput until it touches the periosteum. The needle is withdrawn a few millimeters, and after negative aspiration, the injectate is spread in a fanlike distribution along the nuchal ridge (3–4 mL). If desired in order to get a more extensive field block, the needle could then be directed with a shallow approach in the subcutaneous plane parallel to the nuchal ridge and directed toward the mastoid process where the remaining injectate (1–2 mL) is injected along the linear plane as the needle is withdrawn between the mastoid process and occipital protuberance (Fig. 36.1).

Pitfalls

- Landmark-based occipital nerve blocks should be avoided in patients with prior history of suboccipital decompression, presence of skull defect, ventricular shunt placement, deep brain stimulation, or occipital nerve stimulation. In select cases, occipital nerve blocks could be considered, but preferably with ultrasound guidance.
- To prevent skin atrophy or hair loss, the use of non-particulate steroid or local anesthetic-only blocks should be considered with serial nerve blocks. If steroids are used, then avoid injections any more frequent than once every 3 months.
- Indication can help dictate whether or not to consider ultrasound guidance. In general with primary headache disorders (e.g., migraine and cluster headache), landmark-guided injections can be sufficient as the mechanism is via suppression of nociceptive input. Similarly in secondary headache disorders like medication overuse headache and CSF leaks where the likely mechanism of action is suppression of nociceptive input, landmark-based injections may be worth trying initially. In secondary headache disorders like cervicogenic headache and occipital neuralgia, ultrasound guidance may be the preferable method and can help assess for proximal compression/entrapment of the greater occipital nerve.

Ultrasound-Guided Greater Occipital Nerve Block at the Level of C2

Pearls

- *Positioning*: Prone with head and neck flexed.
- *Anatomical landmarks*: The C2 level is identified as the linear ultrasound transducer is moved caudally from the

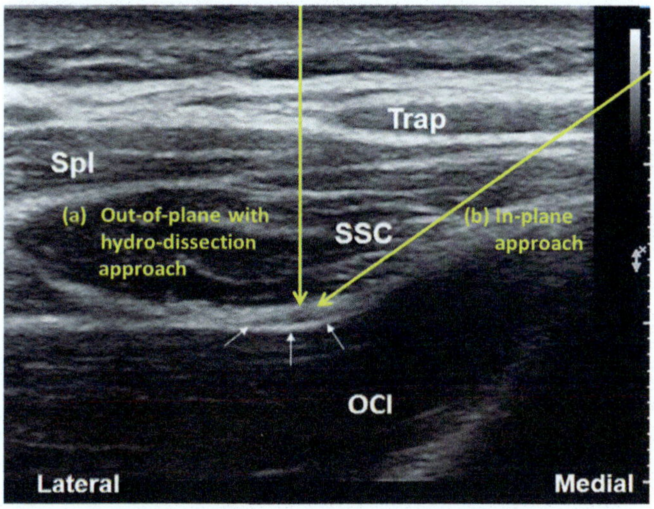

Fig. 36.2 Short axis view of the greater occipital nerve (white arrows) as it courses cephalad in between the obliquus capitis inferior (OCI) and semispinalis capitis (SSC) muscles. With the injection, an (**a**) out-of-plane approach with hydro-dissection or (**b**) in-plane approach with a medial to lateral trajectory can be used with the needle. Trap, trapezius muscle; Spl, splenius muscle. (Reproduced from Narouze [9])

external occipital protuberance until the first bifid spinous process is visualized. Once this C2 spinous process is identified, then the ultrasound transducer is moved laterally with the lateral edge of the transducer aimed at the transverse process of C1 to visualize the obliquus capitis inferior muscle. After emerging from the suboccipital triangle, the greater occipital nerve can be visualized as it courses cephalad between the obliquus capitis inferior and semispinalis capitis muscles (Fig. 36.2).

- *Needle*: 22 or 25 G needle. The length of the needle depends on the circumference of the patient's neck and may need a longer needle up to 2 inches in length for patients with a significant amount of adipose tissue.
- *Injectate*: The use of a non-particulate steroid such as dexamethasone (typically 4–5 mg) is safer and can minimize the risk of inadvertent intravascular injection. Similar to the landmark-based injections, the steroid is typically diluted with a 1:1 mixture of 1% lidocaine and 0.5% bupivacaine. With the more proximal location of injection using ultrasound guidance, a smaller volume of 3–4 mL is typically used when compared to landmark-based injections due to the closer proximity to the spinal cord and concerns for neuro-axial spread.
- *Technique*: After being prepped with sterile solution and identification of the greater occipital nerve between the obliquus capitis inferior and semispinalis capitis muscles with a linear transducer, Doppler ultrasound is used to identify any vascular structures that could be in the way of the needle trajectory. A needle is then introduced and advanced with a medial to lateral approach or in an out-of-plane approach with hydro-dissection until the tip or area of hydro-dissection is visualized in the fascial plane between the obliquus capitis inferior and semispinalis capitis muscles. The injectate is infiltrated around the greater occipital nerve along the fascial plane between the two muscles under direct visualization.

Pitfalls

- Careful assessment of needle tip position is needed to prevent inadvertent neuro-axial spread of injectate.
- Ultrasound guidance can increase safety of occipital nerve blocks in patients with history of craniotomy, but risk is still increased, and caution is important.

Supraorbital/Supratrochlear Nerve Block

Pearls

- *Positioning*: Supine.
- *Anatomical landmarks*: The location of the supraorbital nerve as it emerges from the supraorbital foramen can be identified by palpating the superior border of the orbit for the supraorbital notch, which typically is located along the mid-pupillary line (Fig. 36.3).
- *Needle*: ½–¾ inch, 27 or 30 G needle.
- *Injectate*: The use of a non-particulate steroid such as dexamethasone (typically 2–3 mg) can minimize the risk of skin atrophy or hair loss. When used with occipital nerve blocks for primary headache disorders, could consider anesthetic-only injections with long-acting local anesthetic (often 0.5% bupivacaine) for a total volume of 0.5–0.75 mL.
- *Technique*: After being prepped with a disinfectant (often an alcohol swab), the needle is introduced at the superior margin of the orbit, just slightly above the brow line, and advanced several millimeters into the subcutaneous tissue. After negative aspiration, the injectate is injected into the supraorbital region for a total volume of up to 0.5 mL. The needle can then be withdrawn, but not enough to exit the skin and redirected medially with an angle to obtain a supratrochlear nerve block where an additional 0.25 mL could be injected.

Pitfalls

- Be sure to apply pressure following removal of the needle to prevent periorbital hematoma formation.
- Take caution to prevent from entering the orbit, and use the index finger of the free hand without the syringe (careful to avoid inadvertent needle stick) to palpate the superior margin of the orbit while having the needle directed cephalad.
- Use of steroids in trigeminal distribution nerve blocks can put the patient at risk for skin atrophy.

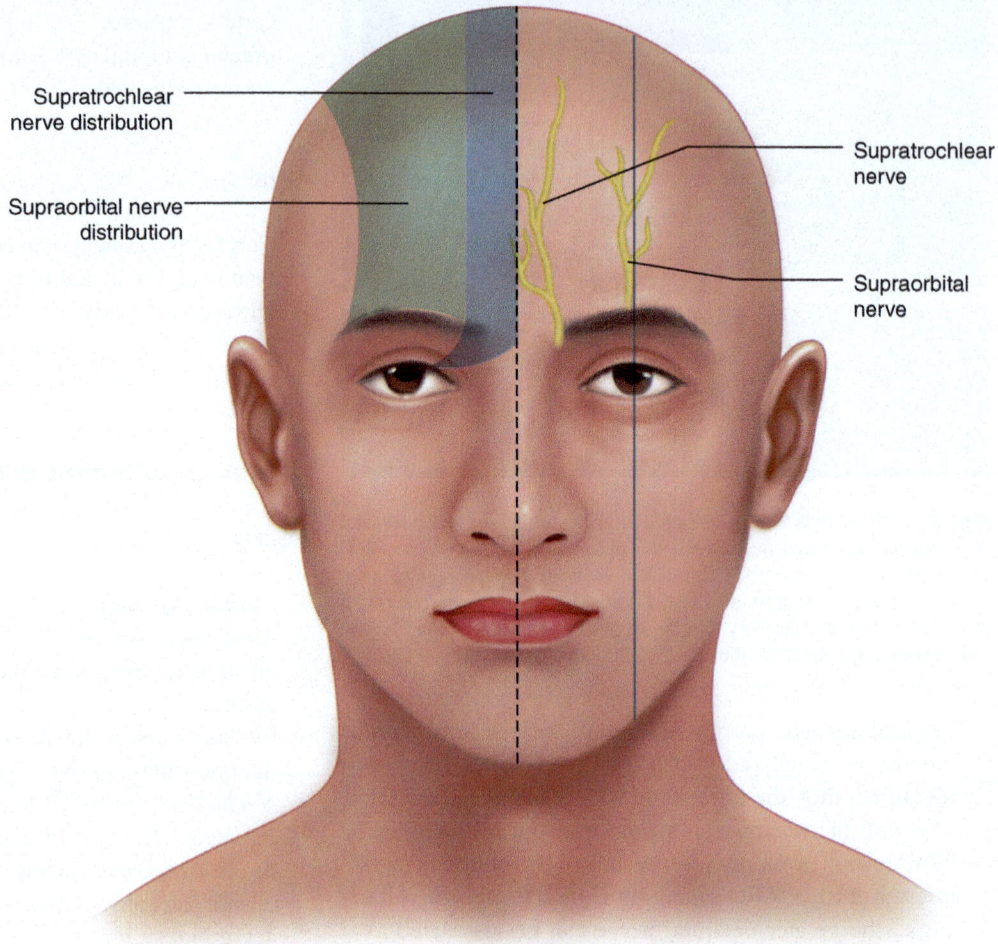

Fig. 36.3 The supraorbital nerve emerges from the supraorbital notch along the mid-pupillary line, and the supratrochlear nerve emerges inferior and medially to the supraorbital notch along the edge of the orbit

Sphenopalatine Ganglion Nerve Block (Transnasal Approach)

Pearls

- *Positioning*: Supine with the neck extended in a sniff position.
- *Anatomical landmarks*: The sphenopalatine ganglion is located in the pterygopalatine fossa, which is a couple millimeters deep to the lateral nasal mucosa at the level of the middle turbinate (Fig. 36.4). Topical application of local anesthetic to the posterior wall of the nasopharynx can diffuse through the nasal mucosa to allow for a noninvasive method to block the sphenopalatine ganglion.
- *Needle*: None. Commercially available sphenopalatine ganglion block catheters or a long applicator with cotton swab tip can be used.
- *Injectate*: Local anesthetic only and often 4% topical lidocaine is used.
- *Technique*: Initially, a small amount (0.25–0.5 mL) of topical lidocaine can be injected in the nares to anesthetize the path of the catheter or cotton tip applicator. When using the catheter, a lubricating jelly can be used to coat the tip of the catheter to reduce discomfort during insertion. The catheter is connected to a 3 mL syringe filled with injectate. During insertion the inner catheter is retracted and inserted along the superior border of the middle turbinate (often with a directional indicator on the catheter facing cephalad). The catheter is advanced until met with light resistance when it comes into contact with the posterior pharynx. The catheter is retracted 5 mm and the inner catheter is advanced fully. The catheter is rotated medially (so catheter tip is located laterally) to ensure coverage of the mucosa of the lateral wall where the sphenopalatine ganglion is adjacent and then 1–2 mL of local anesthetic is injected. Alternatively, a cotton tip applicator can be used where the cotton tip is soaked with 4% lidocaine and advanced in the same trajectory as the catheter method. Once the cotton tip reaches the posterior pharynx, the applicator is left in place for 20–30 minutes. During this time, the 4% topical lidocaine can be applied to the end of the applicator and dripped down the applicator into the nasopharynx.

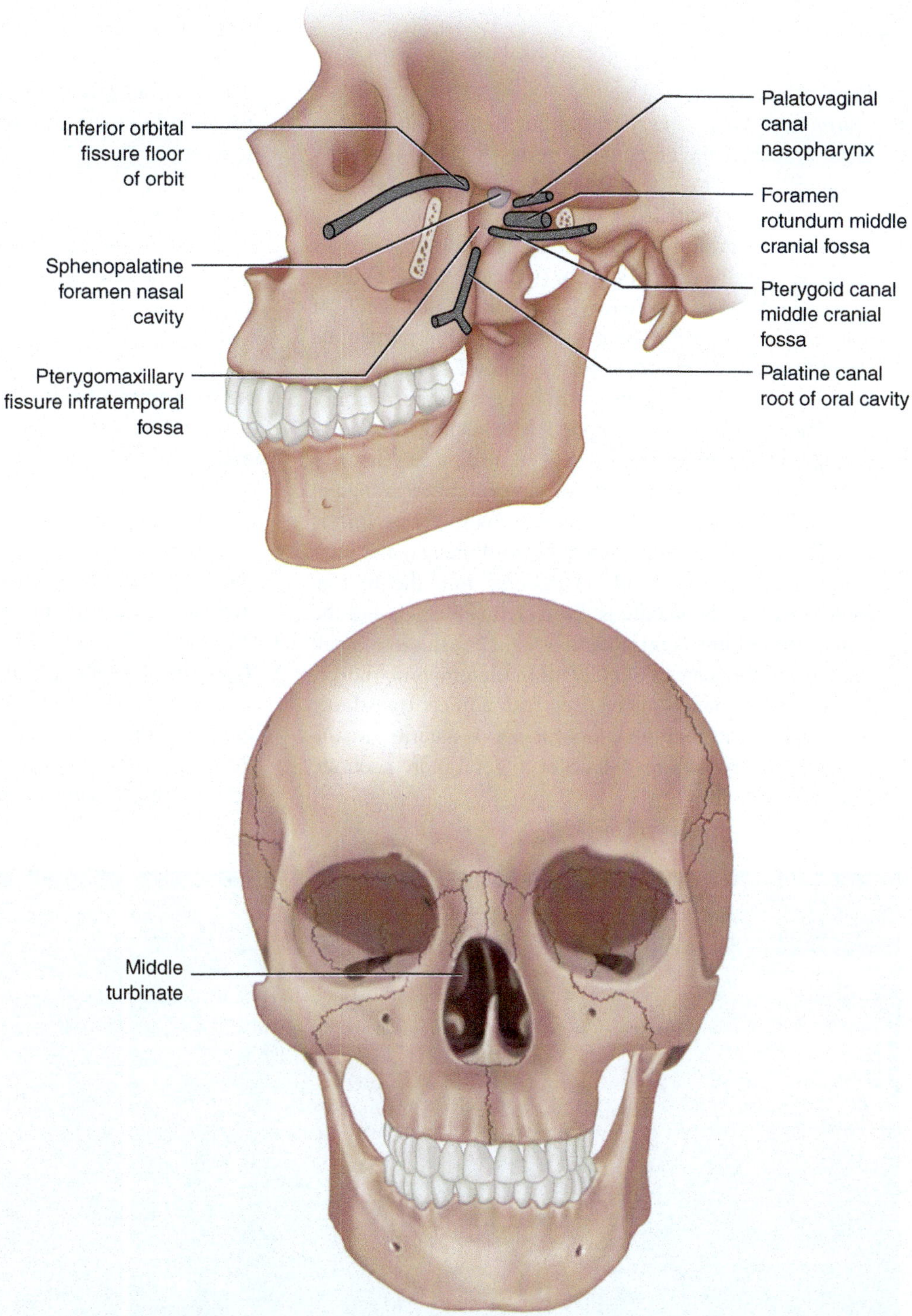

Fig. 36.4 The sphenopalatine ganglion lies within the pterygopalatine fossa, which is a couple millimeters deep to the lateral nasal mucosa at the level of the middle turbinate

Pitfalls

- The injection can cause difficulties with swallowing due to anesthesia of the posterior pharynx and so would advise patient to avoid eating for several hours (duration of local anesthetic) after the sphenopalatine ganglion block.
- The transnasal sphenopalatine ganglion blocks should be avoided in patients with a history of sinus surgery, septal deformities, nasopharyngeal surgery, or pituitary surgery (transsphenoidal approach) due to altered anatomy.

Auriculotemporal Nerve Block

Pearls

- *Positioning*: Supine.
- *Anatomical landmarks*: The auriculotemporal nerve is a distal branch of the mandibular nerve (V3) that lies anterior to the temporal artery at the level of the tragus.
- *Needle*: ¾–1 ½ inch, 25 or 27 G needle.
- *Injectate*: To minimize the risk of skin atrophy or hair loss, the use of anesthetic only (typically 0.5% bupivacaine) would be preferred for a total volume of 1–2 mL. If a steroid is considered, then would use a non-particulate steroid such as dexamethasone (typically 2–3 mg).
- *Technique*: At the level of the tragus, the temporal artery is palpated. After being prepped with disinfectant solution, the needle is introduced several millimeters anterior to the temporal artery just above the zygomatic arch, and the needle is advanced until the underlying periosteum is met. The needle is withdrawn a few millimeters, and after negative aspiration, 1 mL is injected into the region. Following this the needle is redirected cephalad, and the remaining volume is injected in a fanlike fashion to block the distal branches of the auriculotemporal nerve. Ultrasound guidance can be used with a linear transducer to visualize the auriculotemporal nerve anterior to the pulsating temporal artery in order to get a more accurate injection (Fig. 36.5).

Pitfalls

- With close proximity to the temporal artery, aspiration for blood is important to help prevent intravascular injection. The use of ultrasound guidance can be helpful to visualize the blood vessels and minimize the risk of intravascular injection.
- At times it can be difficult to get coverage of the area of pain with a proximal block, and redirection of needle cephalad or the addition of a trigger point injection/field block to area of pain in the temporal region can be of benefit.

Mental Nerve Block

Pearls

- *Positioning*: Supine.
- *Anatomical landmarks*: The mental nerve emerges from the mental foramen, which is along the mid-pupillary line and can be identified by palpation.
- *Needle*: ¾–1 ½ inch, 25 or 27 G inch needle.
- *Injectate*: Anesthetic only (typically 0.5% bupivacaine) or with non-particulate steroid such as dexamethasone (typically 2–3 mg) for a total volume of 2–3 mL.
- *Technique*: The mental foramen is identified by palpation and prepped with disinfectant solution. A needle is

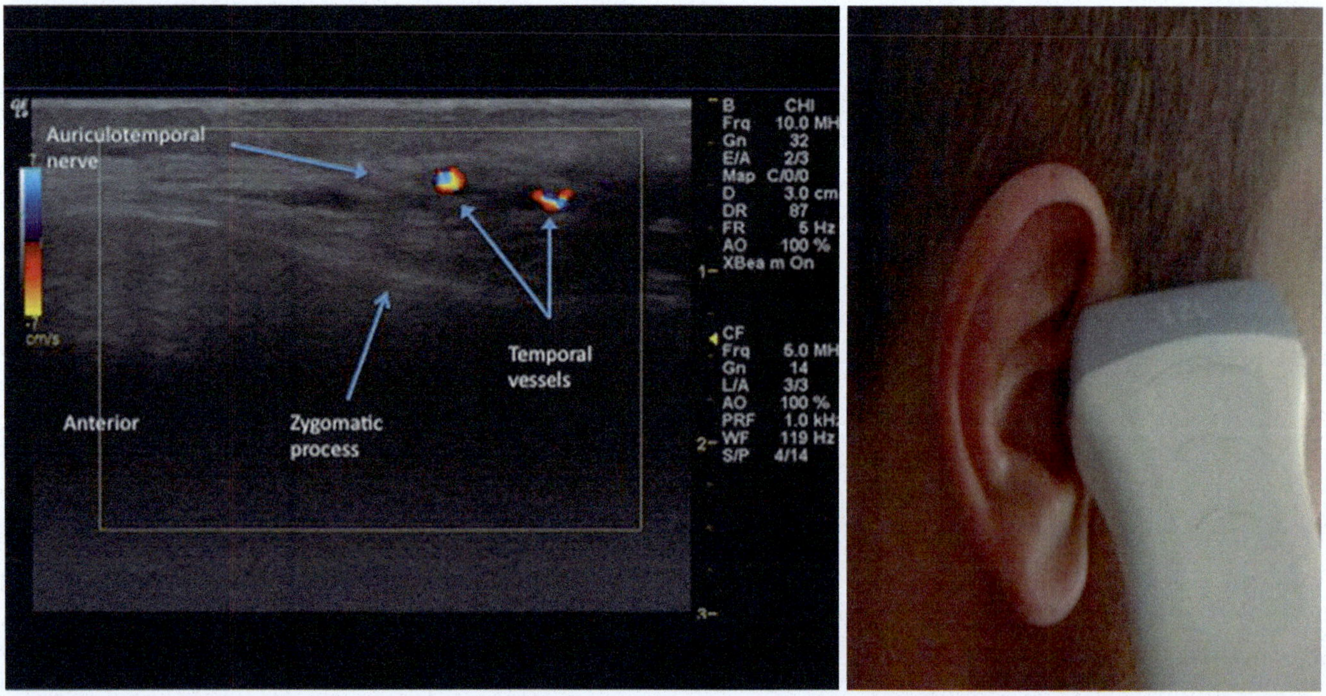

Fig. 36.5 The auriculotemporal nerve lies anterior to the temporal artery and can be identified with a short axis view of the temporal artery at the level of tragus. (Reproduced from Narouze [9])

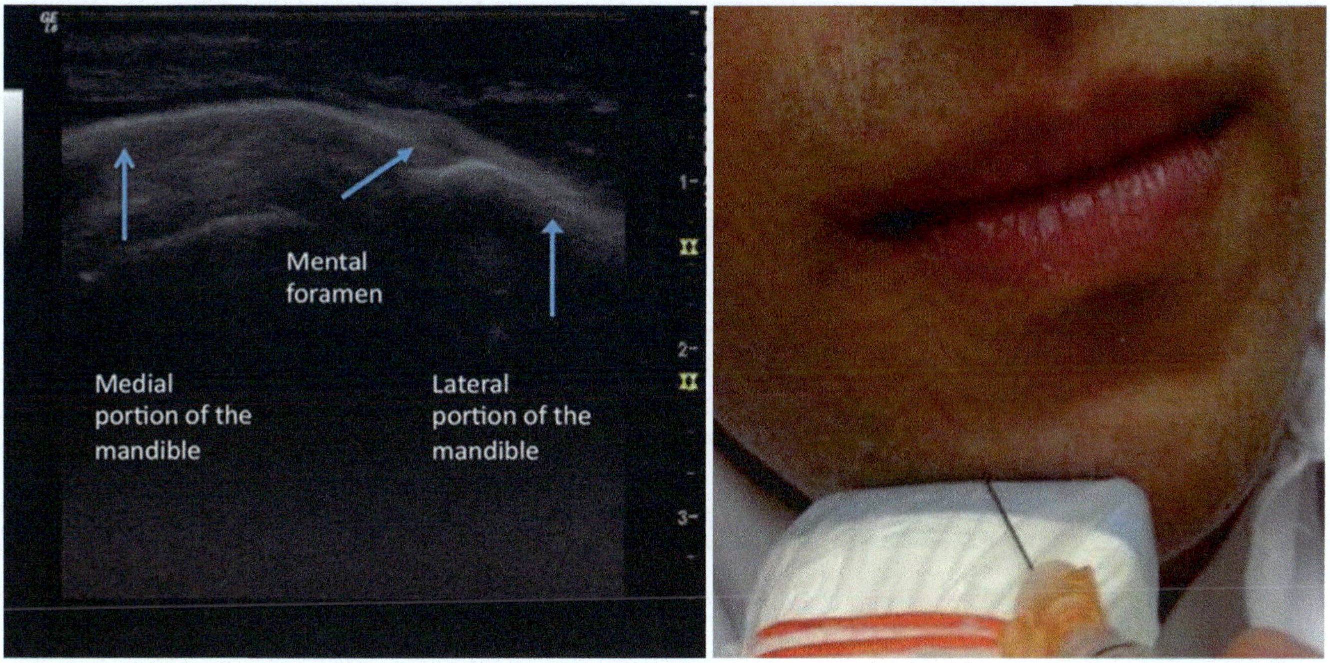

Fig. 36.6 The mental nerve can be found along the mid-pupillary line, and ultrasound can be used to identify the mental foramen in order to avoid intraforaminal injection. (Reproduced from Narouze [9])

introduced and advanced slightly medial to avoid entering the mental foramen. After touching periosteum and negative aspiration, the needle is withdrawn several millimeters, and the injectate is spread in a fanlike fashion near the mental foramen. Ultrasound guidance with a linear transducer can be helpful to prevent intraforaminal injection (Fig. 36.6).

Pitfalls

- Intraforaminal injection into the mental foramen can cause nerve compression or impingement.
- Use of steroid could potentially cause skin atrophy or hair loss.

Infraorbital Nerve Block

Pearls

- *Positioning*: Supine.
- *Anatomical landmarks*: The infraorbital nerve emerges from the infraorbital foramen, which is along the mid-pupillary line and can be identified by palpation along the inferior margin of the orbit.
- *Needle*: 0.75–1.5 inch, 25 or 27 G needle.
- *Injectate*: Anesthetic only (typically 0.5% bupivacaine) or with a non-particulate steroid such as dexamethasone (typically 2–3 mg) for a total volume of 2–3 mL.
- *Technique*: The infraorbital foramen is identified by palpation and prepped with disinfectant solution. A needle is introduced and advanced slightly medial to avoid entering the infraorbital foramen. Ultrasound guidance with a linear or "hockey stick" transducer in a transverse orientation resting along the zygomatic bone and maxilla can be helpful for identification of the nerve and prevent the need to touch periosteum (Fig. 36.7). With the use of ultrasound, the needle can be advanced in an out-of-plane approach or with an in-plane, lateral to medial, approach, and the injectate can be infiltrated around the nerve taking precaution to avoid intraforaminal injection (Fig. 36.7). Alternatively, without ultrasound, the needle could be advanced until gentle contact is made with the periosteum. The needle is then withdrawn a few millimeters, and after negative aspiration, the injectate is spread in a fanlike fashion around the nerve.

Pitfalls

- Extra care should be taken to avoid injection into the orbit (or structures within the orbit such as the globe). The orbital plate of the inferior orbit is comprised of delicate bony structures. Proper precautions (e.g., shallow depth of needle and angulation of needle trajectory) can prevent any orbital trauma or inadvertent injection of orbital structures.
- The use of steroids can cause skin atrophy particularly with repeated injections.

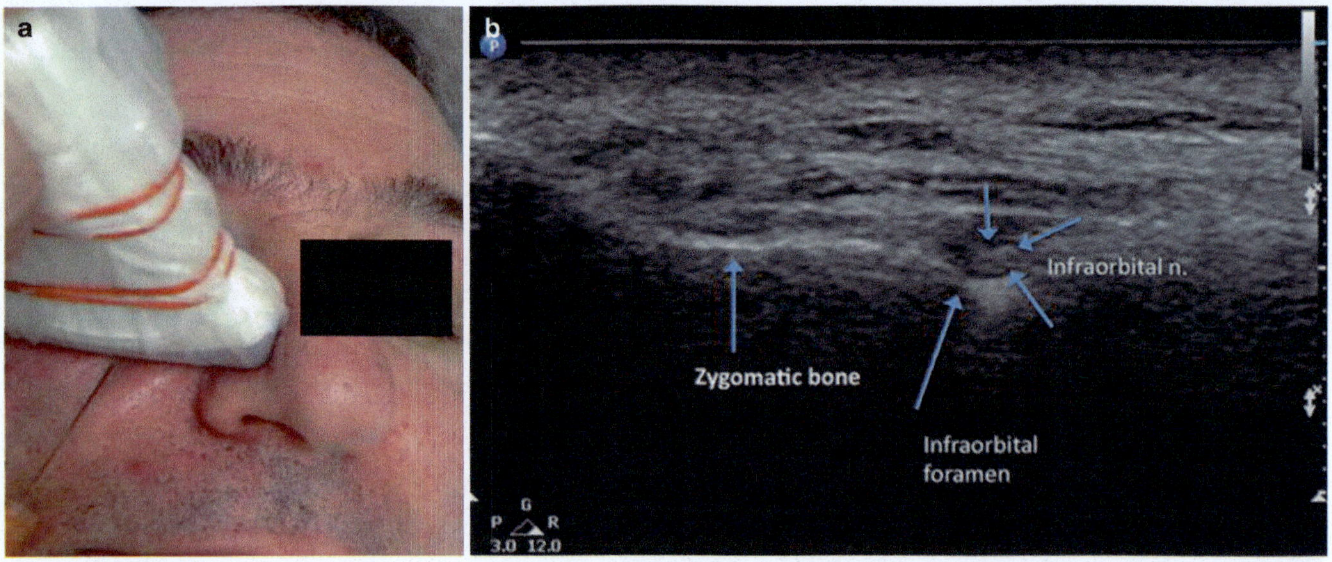

Fig. 36.7 The ultrasound transducer can be placed in a (**a**) transverse orientation and rested along the zygomatic bone and maxilla in order to visualize the (**b**) infraorbital nerve. (Reproduced from Narouze [9])

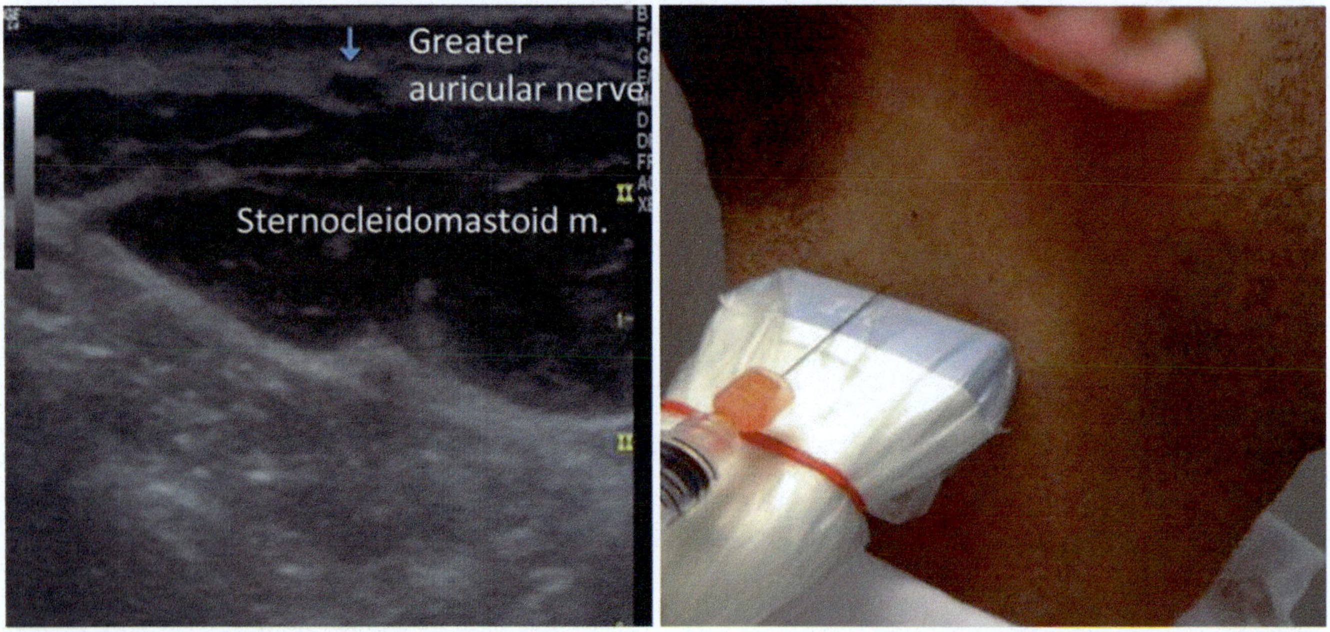

Fig. 36.8 With ultrasound, the great auricular nerve can be identified as it superficially courses over the sternocleidomastoid muscle to achieve a more proximal nerve block. (Reproduced from Narouze [9])

Great Auricular Nerve Block

Pearls

- *Positioning*: Sitting position with the head and neck flexed onto a pillow on the table or prone.
- *Anatomical landmarks*: Mastoid process behind the ear.
- *Needle*: 1 ½ inch, 22 or 25 G needle
- *Injectate*: Same injectate as occipital nerve block (see above), but with a total volume of 3–4 mL.
- *Technique*: The mastoid process is palpated, and after being prepped with disinfectant solution (typically chlorhexidine), the needle is inserted until encountered by periosteum. The needle is withdrawn a few millimeters, and after negative aspiration, the injectate is spread in a fanlike fashion while directing the needle medially toward the lobe of the ear. Ultrasound guidance (with transducer in a transverse orientation) can be used to properly identify the nerve and follow the great auricular nerve as it traverses superficial to the sternocleidomastoid to obtain a more proximal block (Fig. 36.8).

Pitfalls

- Extra caution should be taken with patients that have a history of mastoidectomy to avoid inadvertent needle insertion through bony defects. Ultrasound guidance is preferred with the surgical history to aid in more accurate needle positioning.
- In some instances, a great auricular nerve block can be obtained with a larger volume occipital nerve block (field block using 6 mL volume) due to lateral spread of injectate, and so if pain is in multiple nerve distributions (e.g., greater, lesser, and greater auricular nerve distributions), then a single injection can be effective without the need for multiple skin insertion sites.

Recommended Reading

1. Ambrosini A, Vandenheede M, Rossi P, Aloj F, Sauli E, Pierelli F, et al. Suboccipital injection with a mixture of rapid- and long-acting steroids in cluster headache: a double-blind placebo-controlled study. Pain. 2005;118(1–2):92–6.
2. Ashkenazi A, Blumenfeld A, Napchan U, Narouze S, Grosberg B, Nett R, et al. Peripheral nerve blocks and trigger point injections in headache management - a systematic review and suggestions for future research. Headache. 2010;50(6):943–52.
3. Blumenfeld A, Ashkenazi A, Napchan U, Bender SD, Klein BC, Berliner R, et al. Expert consensus recommendations for the performance of peripheral nerve blocks for headaches--a narrative review. Headache. 2013;53(3):437–46.
4. Cady R, Saper J, Dexter K, Manley HR. A double-blind, placebo-controlled study of repetitive transnasal sphenopalatine ganglion blockade with tx360((R)) as acute treatment for chronic migraine. Headache. 2015;55(1):101–16.
5. Leroux E, Valade D, Taifas I, Vicaut E, Chagnon M, Roos C, et al. Suboccipital steroid injections for transitional treatment of patients with more than two cluster headache attacks per day: a randomised, double-blind, placebo-controlled trial. Lancet Neurol. 2011;10(10):891–7.
6. Mulero P, Guerrero AL, Pedraza M, Herrero-Velazquez S, de la Cruz C, Ruiz M, et al. Non-traumatic supraorbital neuralgia: a clinical study of 13 cases. Cephalalgia. 2012;32(15):1150–3.
7. Naja ZM, El-Rajab M, Al-Tannir MA, Ziade FM, Tawfik OM. Occipital nerve blockade for cervicogenic headache: a double-blind randomized controlled clinical trial. Pain Pract. 2006;6(2):89–95.
8. Naja Z, Al-Tannir M, El-Rajab M, Ziade F, Baraka A. Nerve stimulator-guided occipital nerve blockade for postdural puncture headache. Pain Pract. 2009;9(1):51–8.
9. Narouze SN. Interventional management of head and face pain: nerve blocks and beyond. New York: Springer; 2014. xvi,. p. 154.
10. Narouze S. Occipital neuralgia diagnosis and treatment: the role of ultrasound. Headache. 2016;56(4):801–7.
11. Palamar D, Uluduz D, Saip S, Erden G, Unalan H, Akarirmak U. Ultrasound-guided greater occipital nerve block: an efficient technique in chronic refractory migraine without aura? Pain Physician. 2015;18(2):153–62.
12. Pingree MJ, Sole JS, O' Brien TG, Eldrige JS, Moeschler SM. Clinical efficacy of an ultrasound-guided greater occipital nerve block at the level of C2. Reg Anesth Pain Med. 2017;42(1):99–104.

37 Ganglion Blocks of the Head and Face

Reda Tolba and Tyler Nix

Sphenopalatine Ganglion

Background

The sphenopalatine ganglion (SPG), also known as Meckel's ganglion and pterygopalatine ganglion, is of importance to pain clinicians because of its role in headache disorders and facial neuralgias. One of four parasympathetic ganglia located in the head, the SPG houses the greatest number of neurons outside the brain that, in part, have a role in the trigemino-autonomic reflex. Axons from the ganglion innervate and control blood flow to the nasal mucosa and lacrimal glands, with symptoms such as congestion and rhinorrhea occurring during times of parasympathetic hyperactivity.

Its superficial location in the back of the nasopharynx allows for a relatively simple intervention, which was first performed by Greenfield Sluder in 1908 for the treatment of unilateral facial pain associated with mucosal congestion and lacrimation that he described as sphenopalatine neuralgia. Sluder took a transnasal approach that first involved the application of a 20% cocaine solution that was placed on the posterior portion of the middle turbinate for several minutes along with the use of nitrous oxide. Sluder would then transverse the nostril with a 4.5 inch needle and inject a "2% silver nitrate solution, 0.4% gaseous formaldehyde solution, 0.5% phenol solution with a 1% iodine wash," which he would repeat several times in some cases. Over time this technique would be used for the treatment of several conditions with varying degrees of success, including vascular spasms, low back pain, ear ache, and temporomandibular joint dysfunction.

Today the SPG block is seen as an effective tool to help manage patients who suffer from conditions that fall within the category known as trigeminal autonomic cephalgias (TACs), a term coined in 2004 by the International Headaches Society that encompasses a group of primary headaches that are unilateral, follow the distribution of the trigeminal nerve, and are associated with symptoms associated with parasympathetic activation. Cluster headaches (CH), also known as histamine headache and cranial autonomic syndrome, are included within this classification, and it has been shown that it can be managed in both acute and chronic situations through SPG blockade. This was first demonstrated by Devoghel et al. and was soon followed by Barre in 1982. Barre found success in managing nitroglycerin-induced CH acutely by intranasal application of cocaine. In 1985 a small study performed by Kittrelle showed equal benefit with 4% lidocaine when compared to 10% cocaine solution for aborting acute CH. The anesthetic effect, as opposed to the sympathomimetic effect specifically linked to cocaine and not lidocaine, was shown to be key; although the exact mechanism for how lidocaine or cocaine worked was not known, it was theorized that by blocking the SPG, there was a reduced incidence of intracranial vasodilation through parasympathetic activation.

Studies showing the effectiveness of SPG blockade for treating other headache disorders and facial neuralgias have been increasing over the past decade, mostly with mixed results. Several controlled, randomized trials have looked into the effectiveness of intranasal lidocaine for treating migraines with typical features that include aura, phonophobia, and photophobia. Subjects given intranasal 4% lidocaine were shown to have brief remission of symptoms, but this was generally not sustained for over an hour. Similar results were seen when using this technique for other headache disorders including postdural puncture headache and tension-type headaches too. Trigeminal neuralgia, postherpetic facial neuralgias, and other forms of atypical facial pain are also indications for SPG blockade, although more research is needed to justify its use.

R. Tolba
Wake Forest Baptist Medical Center, Winston Salem, NC, USA

T. Nix (✉)
Anesthesiology Department, Ochsner Health System, New Orleans, LA, USA
e-mail: Tyler.nix@ochsner.org

T. R. Deer et al. (eds.), *Deer's Treatment of Pain*, https://doi.org/10.1007/978-3-030-12281-2_37

Anatomy

The SPG is located within the pterygopalatine fossa (PPF) and is approximately 1.5 mm posterior to the maxillary sinus, which allows for easy access with respect to topicalization and/or injection. Its boundaries are further defined by the pterygoid canal posteriorly, the sphenopalatine foramen medially, and a lateral wall formed by the pterygomaxillary fissure. Sensory, parasympathetic and sympathetic projections converge within this area providing input to the SPG.

The SPG is suspended within the PPF from two ganglionic projections of the maxillary branch (V2) of the trigeminal nerve (V). These two are sensory branches that do not synapse within the SPG but rather pass directly to the lesser and greater palatine nerves that supply sensation to the uvula, tonsils, soft and bony palate, as well as the mucosa of the buccal cavity.

Preganglionic parasympathetic fibers derive from the superior salivatory nucleus in the pons and travel within the nervus intermedius of the facial nerve (VII). These fibers ultimately pass through the Vidian nerve to the SPG where they synapse with postganglionic fibers, which use the trigeminal nerve as a pathway to promote the secretomotor function of the lacrimal glands as well as the glands of the nasal cavity and upper pharynx.

The sympathetic fibers that pass through, but do not synapse within the SPG, counteract the parasympathetic innervation derived from the facial nerve. These fibers originate from the superior cervical ganglion and join the greater petrosal nerve after passing through the superior cervical ganglion. The sympathetic postganglionic fibers then transverse through the PPF and send projections to the nasal and pharyngeal mucosa as well as the lacrimal glands.

Pathophysiology

The strongest studies showing the clinical value of SPG blockade have been graded 1C for the treatment of cluster headaches and migraine headaches and atypical facial pain and head pain. Observational studies are not being too far behind in rating. It's hypothesized that the SPG plays an important and unique role in expression of cranial autonomic symptoms that are often seen in TACs, such as cluster headaches. Stimulation of the superior salivatory nucleus by trigeminal afferents leads to activation of postganglionic parasympathetic neurons within the SPG, which causes cerebral vasodilation and increased cerebral blood flow through the release of vasoactive intestinal peptides and nitric oxide in dural blood vessels. As a result it's thought that this leads to plasma protein extravasation, which causes neurogenic inflammation and activation of trigeminal nociceptors that we sense as facial pain. By blocking the SPG, it's possible that this activation may come to a halt and could lead to the cessation of headache symptoms.

Techniques for Sphenopalatine Ganglion Block

Several techniques exist to accomplish a SPG block that range in invasiveness, imaging requirements, and potential risks. Local anesthetics frequently used are 4% cocaine, 2–4% lidocaine, or 0.5% bupivacaine. Current American Society of Anesthesiologists (ASA) guidelines are to be followed if procedural sedation is to be used to make the patient more comfortable during the block. These monitors include noninvasive blood pressure monitoring, pulse oximetry, and EKG; end-tidal CO_2 monitoring may be necessary as well depending on patient's comorbidities and the amount of sedation given.

Absolute contraindications that exist, regardless of technique, include local infection at or around site of injection (skin or paranasal sinus) as well as coagulopathy. If procedural sedation is to be used then NPO status must be verified in order to minimize an aspiration event. Relative contraindications include anatomic abnormalities and ability for patient to cooperate during the procedure, specifically staying still, in order to avoid misplacement of the needle.

Prior to obtaining consent, it's also important to make sure the patient understands the potential complications that may arise with a SPG block. Infection and bleeding at site of needle insertion are potential complications that arise with any invasive procedure. If too much pressure is placed on the lateral nasal wall, then a patient may experience epistaxis for a brief period of time, especially if the procedure is performed in the winter months given indoor heating may dry the nasal mucosa. Complications unique to this procedure revolve around the anatomic relationship of the SPG to the maxillary artery. Local anesthetic injection into the maxillary artery can lead to severe consequences that include hemodynamic instability, bradycardia, and mental status changes. The physician performing the block and their colleagues assisting with the procedure must be able to recognize signs and symptoms of local anesthetic systemic toxicity (LAST) as well as how to manage the condition if it occurs, although this should be a rare event given standard technique of aspiration prior to injection along with the volume of anesthetic injected for this procedure.

Intranasal Approach

Considered the simplest and most tolerable, the intranasal approach, also known as the anterior approach, consist of taking a cotton-tipped applicator coated in topical anesthetic and placing it posterior to the middle nasal turbinate. The zygomatic arch is used as a reference point to help guide the applicator along the middle turbinate as these two structures are parallel. A nasal speculum can be used to distend the nare in order to allow for larger applicator to be used for the procedure. Once placed in the correct position, the local anesthetic should be absorbed through the mucosa, which is adjacent to the SPG. Applicator is generally left within the nasal passage for up to 30 minutes to allow for maximal absorption.

Patency of each nare should be assessed prior to performing an intranasal approach to ensure that the cotton-tipped applicator will be able to be placed within the nasal passage without any undue trauma. Gentle pressure to the applicator while twisting it is considered the most effective technique to help lead to proper placement. Sedation may be required along with the use of lidocaine jelly to help numb the nasal passage.

Transoral Approach

Also known as the greater palatine foramen approach, this technique has been utilized by dentists for years to help assist in tooth extractions that occur in the anterior maxillary region. By extending the patient's neck and having them open their mouth as wide as possible, the physician is able to feel along the medial gum line of the third molar to help appreciate a dimple on the hard palate that represents the location of the greater palatine foramen. A curved dental needle is inserted at this area and passed through the foramen in order to reach the SPG, which is approximately 2.5 cm superior and slightly posterior to the foramen. Aspiration must be performed prior to injection to ensure that you do not aspirate heme or cerebrospinal fluid.

This technique is considered more difficult compared to the intranasal approach, and results can vary given the uncertainty of needle placement. Facial paresthesia may be induced as the maxillary nerve is directly cephalad to the SPG. Intraorbital hematoma is also more common with this approach given a needle is transversing a highly vascular area that contains terminal branches of the maxillary artery. Furthermore, patient discomfort is expected as the foramen contains a nerve trunk within a space that has little compliance.

Lateral Infratemporal Approach (Infrazygomatic Approach) (Figs. 37.1 and 37.2)

Commonly referred to as the infrazygomatic approach, this technique requires the utilization of C-arm fluoroscopy to help place a cannula in the superior portion of the pterygopalatine fossa. This allows for direct administration of local anesthetic to the SPG as opposed to diffusion of local anesthetic across mucous membranes as seen with the intranasal approach and also helps confirm proper placement of medicine that isn't seen with the transoral approach. A *percutaneous fluoroscopically guided infrazygomatic approach* to the sphenopalatine ganglion for both diagnostic blocks and radiofrequency ablation is used by interventional pain physicians. A lateral fluoroscopic view of the face is obtained with the c-arm by superimposing the two rami atop each other. A skin wheal is created inferior to the zygomatic arch and anterior to the mandible. Then a 22 or 25 gauge 3.5 inch spinal needle is then inserted coaxially with lateral fluoroscopic guidance. The needle is then advanced superiorly and medially toward the pterygopalatine fossa utilizing lateral and AP fluoroscopic guidance. The needle tip will terminate just lateral to the ipsilateral nasal wall (confirm with AP view). Following final needle positioning, 0.2 mL of contrast material is injected under live fluoroscopic imaging to rule out intravascular spread. Aspiration is then performed, and if negative for heme and CSF, then injection of local anesthetic (0.5–1 mL of lidocaine 1%) is given. Most common complication is paresthesia from contact with the maxillary nerve.

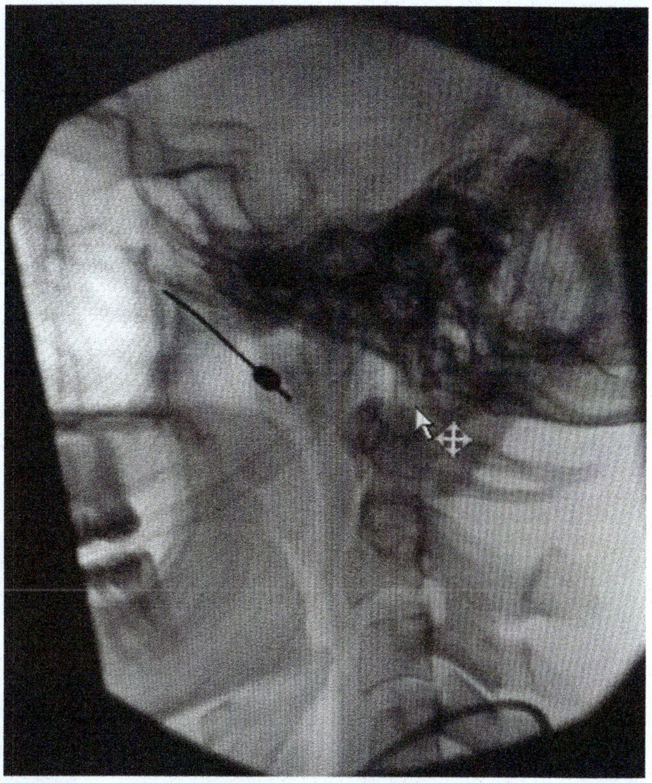

Fig. 37.1 Fluoroscopic lateral view image showing the needle in the pterygopalatine fossa as the target for sphenopalatine ganglion block

Future Treatment Options

Sphenopalatine ganglion blockade with local anesthetics using any of the described techniques above can now be

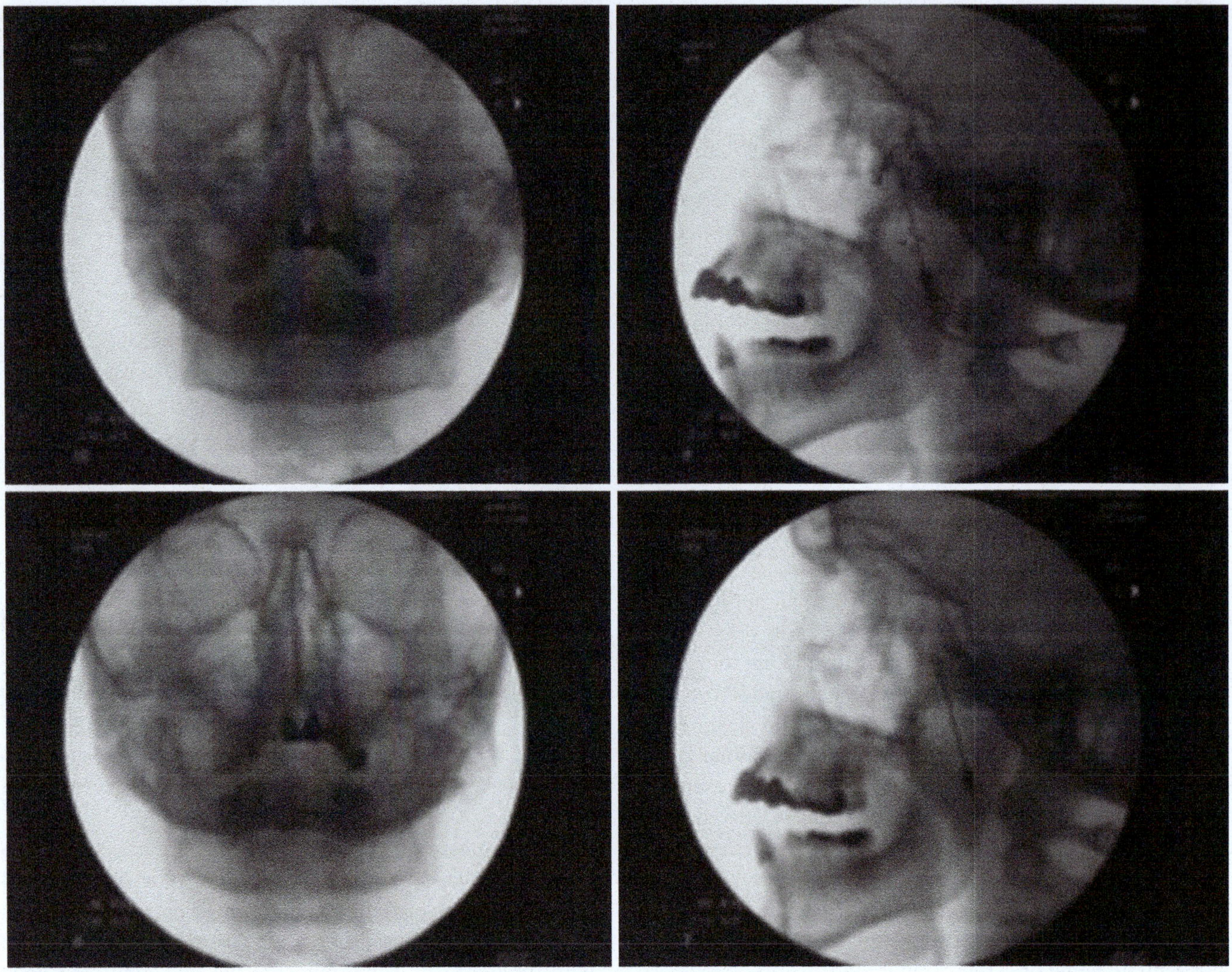

Fig. 37.2 Percutaneous fluoroscopic views: Needle courses medially toward the ipsilateral nasal wall. (Reproduced from Bolash R., Tolba R. (2017) Sphenopalatine ganglion. In: Pope J., Deer T. (eds) *Treatment of chronic pain conditions*. Springer, New York, NY)

seen as a trial for patients to help assess whether this helps treat their TAC or facial neuralgia. If so, further treatment options are available and continue to be developed to help deliver longer-lasting results as opposed to the temporary relief seen with local anesthetics. Radiofrequency ablation is becoming a more popular option as is chemical ablation with destructive substances such as alcohol and phenol. The continued advancement in managing headache and facial pain disorders is important because of the cost burden it places on our healthcare system. Headache disorders are estimated to have a direct cost burden of around $11 billion along with an indirect cost burden of $13 billion annually through short-term disability and worker's compensation. Finding an easy and effective means at treating this through sphenopalatine ganglion blockade is therefore very important in reducing healthcare expenditure within the United States.

Gasserian Ganglion

Background

The gasserian ganglion, also known as the trigeminal ganglion or the semilunar ganglion, is a cluster of nerve cell bodies located within Meckel's cave in the middle cranial fossa that gives rise to the three branches of the trigeminal nerve – opthalmic (V1), maxillary (V2), and mandibular (V3). The branches have efferent motor fibers that are used to innervate muscles involved in facial expression and muscles of mastication, as well as afferent sensory fibers that transmit sensation from the face, teeth, oral mucosa, and anterior two thirds of the tongue. Its role in our perception of facial pain has led to interventional treatments being created over the years to help deal with a variety of disorders that include trigeminal neuralgia, TMJ joint syndrome, and postherpetic neuralgia to name a few. The historical background behind gasserian ganglion blockade isn't as old compared to SPG blockade, but that hasn't prevented physicians from seeking a variety of therapies targeted at this area to treat both typical and atypical facial pain.

Gasserian ganglion blockade is most commonly performed for the treatment of trigeminal neuralgia, also known as tic douloureux, which presents as a sharp pain in the mandibular nerve distribution. Pharmacological treatment is first line, but it has been reported that up to 25% of patients do not respond to such treatment. Nader et al. have demonstrated that injection of local anesthetic and steroids to the area of the gasserian ganglion is an effective form of managing trigeminal neuralgia as well as other forms of atypical facial pain that cannot be attributed to a different disorder. Treatment of ophthalmic postherpetic neuralgia can be accomplished as well with a gasserian ganglion blockade, which is otherwise difficult to manage with medications that include anticonvulsants and antidepressants.

Anatomy and Techniques for Blockade

The three branches of the trigeminal nerve that arise from the gasserian ganglion exit through three distinct foramina – superior orbital fissure (V1), foramen rotundum (V2), and foramen ovale (V3) (Fig. 37.3). The foramen ovale is of particular interest for gasserian ganglion blockade, which is done under sedation and thus requires the physician to follow ASA guidelines just like for a SPG block. Unlike the SPG block, it is not advised to perform this without the use of imaging guidance. Studies have shown that this can be effectively performed with the use of fluoroscopy, ultrasound, or computed tomography.

Ultrasound-guided gasserian ganglion block is becoming a popular technique as noted by the literature, but it is still more common to have this procedure performed under fluoroscopic x-ray guidance. The key anatomical landmark to obtain under x-ray is the foramen ovale, which can be seen by obliquing away from the nose at 20–30° followed by a 30–35° tilt in the caudio-cranial direction (Fig. 37.4). This "tunnel vision" technique should present the foramen ovale just medial to the mandible and superior to the petrous ridge. A 10 cm, 22 gauge B-bevel needle can then be directed toward the foramen ovale in a controlled fashion, and once the needle passes through the base of the skull, contrast should be injected to confirm location, which should help highlight Meckel's cave. Aspiration must then be performed and be negative for both heme and CSF prior to injection of local anesthetic and/or non-particulate steroid. Proper placement will often elicit a mandibular nerve paresthesia. Patients should be monitored for a short duration after the procedure to ensure that none of the local anesthetic reached the CSF, which could create a high spinal and lead to hemodynamic and respiratory compromise. If a patient receives relief with this procedure, then further treatment options may be provided to help produce longer-lasting results, such as chemical neurolysis, radiofrequency ablation, and even neuromodulation.

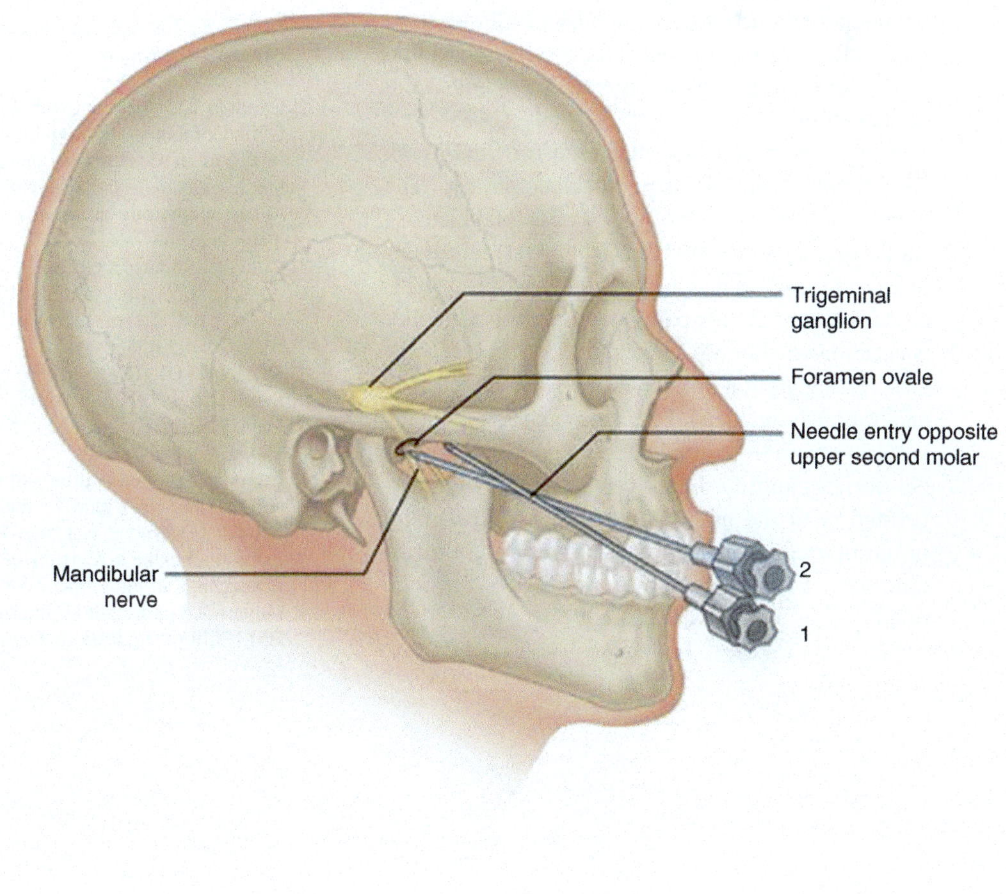

Fig. 37.3 Anatomy of trigeminal nerve and technique of the block from entry site: AP and lateral views relative to mouth and pupil. (Reproduced from Jusino E., Guirguis M. (2017) Trigeminal nerve block. In: Pope J., Deer T. (eds) *Treatment of chronic pain conditions*. Springer, New York, NY)

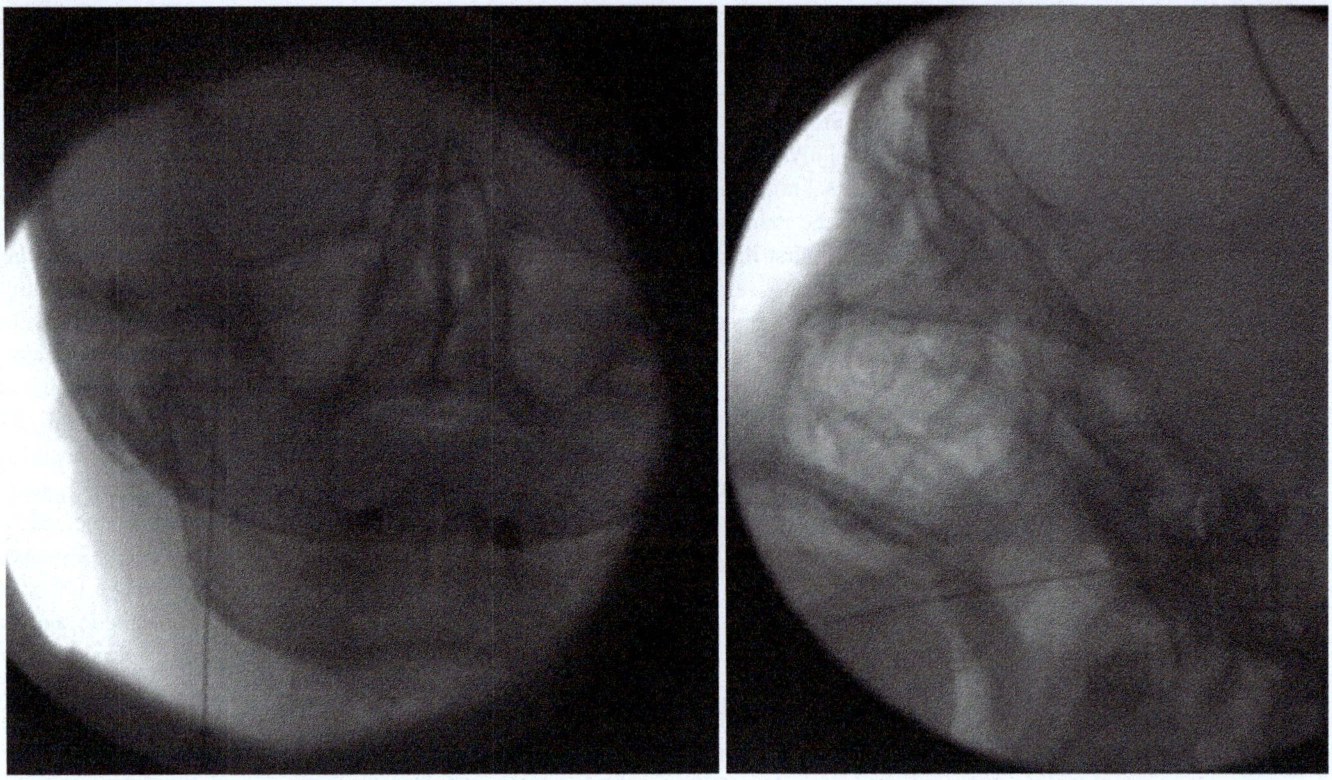

Fig. 37.4 Radiographic image: trigeminal nerve block. (Reproduced from Jusino E., Guirguis M. (2017) Trigeminal nerve block. In: Pope J., Deer T. (eds) *Treatment of chronic pain conditions*. Springer, New York, NY)

Clinical Pearls

- Sphenopalatine (SPG) ganglion block can be used as an effective tool to help manage patients who suffer from different headache disorders and facial pain conditions.
- The two common approaches used for SPG block are intranasal and infrazygomatic approach. The latter is performed under fluoroscopic guidance.
- Radiofrequency ablation and chemical neurolysis of the SPG with phenol or alcohol can be considered for longer-lasting pain relief if temporary relief was achieved after SPG block.
- Gasserian ganglion block can be used as diagnostic and therapeutic method to help manage patients suffering from trigeminal neuralgia.
- Gasserian ganglion block can be effectively performed with the use of fluoroscopy, ultrasound, or computed tomography. The key anatomical landmark to obtain under x-ray is the foramen ovale.

Recommended Reading

1. Bolash R, Tolba R. Sphenopalatine ganglion. In: Pope J, Deer T, editors. Treatment of chronic pain conditions. New York: Springer; 2017.
2. Candido KD, Germanovich A, Ghaly RF, Gorelick GH, Knezevic NN. Computed tomography scan-guided Gasserian ganglion injection of dexamethasone and lidocaine for the treatment of recalcitrant pain associated with herpes simplex type 1 infection of the ophthalmic division of the trigeminal nerve. Anesth Analg. 2011;112:224–7.
3. Cohen S, Ramos D, Grubb W, Mellender S, Mohiuddin A, Chiricolo A. Sphenopalatine ganglion block: a safer alternative to epidural blood patch for postdural puncture headache. Reg Anesth Pain Med. 2014;39:563.
4. D'Alessio DJ. Trigeminal neuralgia: a practical approach to treatment. Drugs. 1982;24(3):248.
5. Day M. Sphenopalatine ganglion analgesia. Curr Rev Pain. 1999;3(5):342–7.
6. Edvinsson L. Innervation and effects of dilatory neuropeptides on cerebral vessels. Blood Vessels. 1991;28:35–45.
7. Felisati G, Arnone F, Lozza P, et al. Sphenopalatine endoscopic ganglion block: a revision of a traditional technique for cluster headache. Laryngoscope. 2006;116:1447–50.
8. Guyatt G, Gutterman D, Baumann MH, Addrizzo-Harris D, Hylek EM, Phillips B, Raskob G, Lewis SZ, Schunemann H. Grading

strength of recommendations and quality of evidence in clinical guidelines: report from an American college of chest physicians task force. Chest. 2006;129(1):174–81.
9. Hawkins K, Wang S, Rupnow MF. Indirect cost burden of migraine in the United States. J Occup Environ Med. 2007;49:368–74.
10. Huang J, Zhongge N, Finch P. Gasserian ganglion and retrobulbar nerve block in the treatment of ophthalmic postherpetic neuralgia: a case report. Pain Pract. 2017;17(7):961–7. https://doi.org/10.1111/papr.12547. Epub 2017 Feb 25.
11. Jusino E, Guirguis M. Trigeminal nerve block. In: Pope J, Deer T, editors. Treatment of chronic pain conditions. New York: Springer; 2017.
12. Khonsary SA, Ma Q, Villablanca P, Emerson J, Malkasian D. Clinical functional anatomy of the pterygopalatine ganglion, cephalgia and related dysautonomias: a review. Surg Neurol Int. 2013;4:S422–8.
13. Kittrelle JP, Grouse DS, Seybold ME. Cluster headache. Local anesthetic abortive agents. Arch Neurol. 1985;42:496–8.
14. Maizels M, Scott B, Cohen W, Chen W. Intranasal lidocaine for treatment of migraine: a randomized, double-blind, controlled trial. JAMA. 1996;276:319–21.
15. Maksymowicz W. Treatment of trigeminal neuralgia by glycerol gangliolysis of the trigeminal ganglion. Neurol Neurochir Pol. 1987;21:45–8.
16. Mohammadkarimi N, Jafari M, Mellat A, Kazemi E, Shirali A. Evaluation of efficacy of intra-nasal lidocaine for headache relief in patients refer to emergency department. J Res Med Sci. 2014;19:331–5.
17. Moiseiwitsch J, Irvine T, Hill C. Clinical significance of the length of the pterygopalatine fissure in dental anesthesia. Oral Surg Oral Med Oral Pathol Oral Radiol Endod. 2001;92:325–8.
18. Nader A, Kendall MC, De Oliveria GS, Chen JQ, Vanderby B, Rosenow JM, Bendok BR. Ultrasound-guided trigeminal nerve block via the pterygopalatine fossa: an effective treatment for trigeminal neuralgia and atypical facial pain. Pain Physician. 2013;16(5):537–45.
19. Nappi G, Moskowitz MA. Cluster headache and trigeminal autonomic cephalgias: general aspects. Handbook of clinical neurology. 2011;97(3rd series):387–8.
20. Narouze SN. Role of sphenopalatine ganglion neuroablation in the management of cluster headache. Curr Pain Headache Rep. 2010;14(2):160–3.
21. Narouze S, Kapural L, Casanova J, Mekhail N. Sphenopalatine ganglion radiofrequency ablation for the management of chronic cluster headache. Headache. 2009;49(4):571–7.
22. Robbins MS, Robertson CE, Kaplan E, Ailani J, Charleston L, Kuruvilla D, Blumenfeld A, Berliner R, Rosen NL, Duarte R, Vidwan J, Halker RB, Gill N, Ashkenazi A. The sphenopalatine ganglion: anatomy, pathophysiology, and therapeutic targeting in headache. Headache J Head Face Pain. 2016;56:240–58.
23. Ruskin AP. Sphenopalatine (nasal) ganglion: remote effects including "psychosomatic" symptoms, rage reaction, pain, and spasm. Arch Phys Med Rehabil. 1979;60:353–9.
24. Rusu MC, Pop F. The anatomy of the sympathetic pathway through the pterygopalatine fossa in humans. Ann Anat. 2010;192:17–22.
25. Shah R, Racz G. Long-term relief of posttraumatic headache by sphenopalatine ganglion pulsed radiofrequency lesioning: a case report. Arch Phys Med Rehabil. 2004;85:1013–6.
26. Sluder G. The anatomical and clinical relations of the sphenopalatine ganglion to the nose. N Y State J Med. 1909;90:293–8.
27. Sluder G. Nasal neurology, headaches and eye disorders. St. Louis: CV Mosby; 1927.
28. Stechison MT, Brogan M. Transfacial transpterygomaxillary access to foramen rotundum, sphenopalatine ganglion, and the maxillary nerve in the management of atypical facial pain. Skull Base Surg. 1994;4:15–20.
29. Talman WT, Corr J, Dragon DN, Wang D. Parasympathetic stimulation elicits cerebral vasodilation in rat. Auton Neurosci. 2007;133(2):153–7.
30. Tator CH, Rowed DW. Fluoroscopy of foramen ovale as an aid to thermocoagulation of the Gasserian ganglion; technical note. J Neurosurg. 1976;44:254–7.
31. Tsui BC. Ultrasound imaging to localize foramina for superficial trigeminal nerve block. Can J Anaesth. 2009;56:704–6.
32. Uddman R, Hara H, Edvinsson L. Neuronal pathways to the rat middle meningeal artery revealed by retrograde tracing and immunocytochemistry. J Auton Nerv Syst. 1989;26:69–75.
33. van Kleef M, Slujter M, van Zundert J. Radiofrequency treatment. In: Benzon H, Rathmell JP, Wu CL, Turk DC, Argoff CE, editors. Raj's practical management of pain. 4th ed. Philadelphia: Elsevier; 2008. p. 1063–78.
34. Waldman SD. Sphenopalatine ganglion block – 80 years later. Reg Anesth. 1993;18(5):274–6.
35. Yang I, Oraee S. A novel approach to transnasal sphenopalatine ganglion injection. Pain Physician. 2006;9:131–4.
36. Yarnitsky D, Goor-Aryeh I, Bajwa ZH, Ransil BI, Cutrer FM, Sottile A, Burstein R. Possible parasympathetic contributions to peripheral and central sensitization during migraine. Headache. 2003;43(7):704–14.

Destructive Procedures of the Head and Face

38

Xiang Qian and Anuj Aggarwal

Introduction

Destructive procedures of the head and neck can provide diagnostic and therapeutic options for patients suffering from orofacial pain. Orofacial pain affects more than 35 million adults in the United States alone, with important impacts on healthcare, productivity, and quality of life. Orofacial pain, unlike many other pain syndromes, has different features when compared to pain syndromes arising from spinal pathology, with its own unique anatomical pathways such as the trigeminal system.

Trigeminal neuralgia (TN), a severe neuropathic condition and one of the most common subtypes of orofacial pain, involves the trigeminal afferents. It helps represent the different pathophysiological considerations of orofacial neuropathic conditions compared to other neuropathies, such as the higher proportion of myelinated to unmyelinated fibers compared to other spinal nerves. This has implications for the presence of myelinated thermoreceptive afferents found in the face and mouth which are otherwise not found in nonprimates and may be secondary to the higher density of sensory receptors on the face found in humans and other primates. In addition, the trigeminal system has a unique central relay system that can lead to unique presentations; for example, transection of the inferior alveolar nerve (V3 branch innervating the low teeth) can induce hypersensitivity outside the classical distribution of the nerve in an area such as the upper lip (V2 territory). Further compounding this are findings in animal studies suggesting the lower threshold for sensitization and inflammation of the orofacial tissues. Expanding further out from the trigeminal system, the orofacial region is disproportionately represented in the somatosensory cortex, posing unique challenges for treatment. This is further compounded by the complex anatomy involved in orofacial pain with a plethora of sites that can be the source of pain including the teeth, temporomandibular joint, mucosa, sinuses, salivary glands, and referred pain from other sites including the eyes and ears (Fig. 38.1).

In addition to this, the orofacial region has unique significance in daily function necessary for eating, speaking, and drinking and thus can significantly negatively impact an individual's quality of life. Trigeminal neuralgia offers a window in which to understand the wide variety of orofacial pain syndromes due to its extensive innervation of the orofacial region, of which more than 20 distinct ones have been characterized. Despite significant investigation, the etiology of TN is not fully understood; however, dysfunction of the myelin sheath has been the focus of much investigation. Trigeminal neuralgia is often divided into classical TN when clinical examination, imaging studies, and laboratory studies are generally unremarkable and secondary TN when it is due to an identifiable disease process. Secondary causes of TN, which in studies have accounted for approximately 10% of TN cases, include multiple sclerosis which can have bilateral presentation, posterior fossa tumors including meningiomas, and tumors in the trigeminal nerve itself. Like other orofacial pain conditions, TN patients unfortunately often suffer for months to years prior to appropriate diagnosis.

In general, orofacial pain is mostly neuropathic in presentation and comes with four different features: (1) pain associated with nerve damage, (2) pain from an organic source such as a tumor, (3) pain secondary to vascular etiologies and associated with migraine-like headaches, and (4) burning, unremitting pain with no identifiable etiology or inciting event. These presentations are most amenable to destructive procedures as possible treatment options. In contrast, other orofacial pain syndromes, such as atypical facial pain (AFP: "persistent facial pain that does not have the characteristics of the cranial neuralgias and is not attributed to another disorder," according to ICHD-2, International Classification of Headache Disorders, Second Edition), are

X. Qian (✉)
Department of Anesthesiology, Perioperative and Pain Medicine, Stanford University, Stanford University Pain Management Center, Redwood City, CA, USA
e-mail: xqian@stanford.edu

A. Aggarwal
Department of Anesthesiology, Perioperative and Pain Medicine, Stanford University, Redwood City, CA, USA
e-mail: akaggarw@stanford.edu

T. R. Deer et al. (eds.), *Deer's Treatment of Pain*, https://doi.org/10.1007/978-3-030-12281-2_38

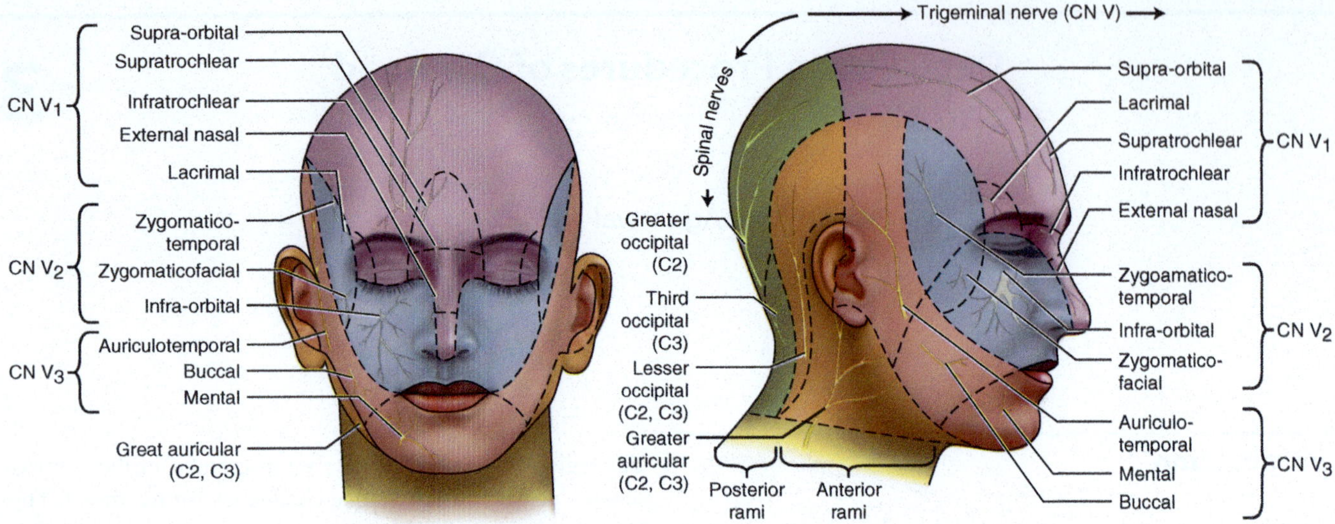

Fig. 38.1 Innervation of the head and face

often a combination of various pathophysiological mechanisms including both biological and psychological factors, and as such interventional management can be a part of their management but needs to be offered with caution.

Though the following discussion of interventional strategies in this chapter will be focused on the aforementioned conditions, it should be mentioned that a comprehensive discussion and evaluation of orofacial pain includes consideration of tooth-related orofacial pain, temporomandibular disorders, painful oral mucosal lesions, psychosomatic diseases, sinonasal disorders, salivary gland diseases, and cardiac toothache. A complete discussion of these conditions and their various treatments is out of the scope of this chapter; however, they should be part of any comprehensive evaluation.

Upon diagnosis of an orofacial pain syndrome, a series of therapeutic options become available. Often, the first line of treatment is medical management. As many newer pharmacological agents have become available, possibilities exist for either monotherapy or polypharmacy. Interventions are available for patients who are intolerant of medication therapy or whose pain is extreme and unremitting in spite of medication therapy. Secondary causes must be explored in all patients because, if such causes are discovered, surgical interventions may supersede medical options. Each medication or intervention is associated with side effects and potential risks. These pitfalls must be weighed based on each individual's medical conditions, lifestyle, age, personal preference, and past therapies. The patient must be well-informed about both medical and interventional options as soon as the diagnosis is made. Percutaneous interventional procedures such as radiofrequency ablation (RFA), glycerol rhizotomy (GR), and percutaneous balloon (PBC) of the trigeminal ganglion and its branches are some of the most commonly used interventional procedures as they avoid exposure to general anesthesia, provide successful short-term results, and are available to people with significant comorbidities. These procedures may be performed using conventional fluoroscopic, ultrasound, or CT-guided imaging, including combined flat panel CT and fluoroscopy. Surgical options include stereotactic radiosurgery such as Gamma Knife and microvascular decompression (MVD), of which MVD remains a cornerstone of treatment for trigeminal neuralgia. The V2 and V3 branches of the trigeminal nerve are most commonly affected and are thus the most frequent targets for intervention. Expanding further, radiofrequency ablation and cryotherapy of distal peripheral nerves of the trigeminal ganglion can be targeted for more focused treatment. Ultrasound treatment has greatly expanded the safety and ability to perform these procedures.

In this chapter, we will start with the trigeminal nerve to serve as a reference, from which to explore the history, use, and indications of destructive procedures for a variety of painful conditions in the head and face, and proceed distally to its branches and peripheral locations.

Trigeminal Nerve

Background and History

The first attempted percutaneous treatment of TN occurred in 1911, when Harris injected the trigeminal ganglion with alcohol. Two years after Harris described his approach, Rethi treated patients with electrocoagulation of the trigeminal nerve and ganglion. The procedure was associated with a high complication rate including unintended nerve damage, bleeding, and damage to surrounding structures secondary to limitations in electrode design and temperature control. In 1914, Hartel described a method for accessing the foramen ovale, which is the basis for percutaneous procedures still in use today.

In 1974, Sweet and Wepsic described radiofrequency treatment of the trigeminal roots. Their method used short-acting anesthetics to allow for more precise lesion creation using more precise electrical stimulation and temperature monitoring. Over the next few decades, Nugent further refined the radiofrequency technique by using a fine cordotomy-type electrode. Tew and Taha introduced curved thermistor-tipped electrodes, which achieved high rates of pain relief with fewer complications.

Glycerol rhizotomy dates to the late nineteenth century, when physicians injected various agents such as chloroform and osmic acid next to nerve trunks. Although reports indicated that this method was effective in producing pain relief, the effect was transient and often accompanied by significant weakness, sensory loss, and dysesthesias. Glycerol rhizotomy therapy was refined in 1981 by Hakanson when his team was exploring the use of stereotactic radiotherapy for TN treatment. Hakanson used glycerol as a vehicle to suspend tantalum dust and then injected this into the trigeminal cistern. Hakanson later found that injection of glycerol alone caused pain relief. The exact mechanism of action of glycerol is incompletely understood. Studies have suggested its hypertonicity causes a rapid rate of change in intracellular osmolarity, resulting in axonal demyelination and fragmentation.

Percutaneous balloon compression was discovered in the 1950s when Taarnhoj described his surgical methodology for decompressing the dorsal trigeminal root. Later, Shelden and Pudenz reported their surgical method for decompression of the second and third nerve divisions. In working to decompress the trigeminal ganglion, they found that the effectiveness of their technique derived from the resultant injury to the posterior trigeminal root posterior to the ganglion. It was not until 1983, when Mullan and Lichtor described compression of the trigeminal ganglion with a percutaneously inserted Fogarty balloon catheter, that PBC became a viable treatment option. Studies in rabbits revealed that compression seems to preferentially affect the medium and large myelinated pain fibers, sparing small fibers, allowing for recovery of motor and sensory function, and preservation of the corneal reflex.

Many elements of percutaneous intervention have remained true to the techniques described by their pioneers. All three percutaneous procedures (RF, GR, and PBC) rely on Hartel's landmarks to gain access to the foramen ovale. Much effort has been devoted to improving visualization and navigation to the foramen ovale. Although fluoroscopy has been the imaging modality of choice, newer studies have demonstrated the potential usefulness of computed tomography (CT), flat panel CT, ultrasonography, and neuronavigation systems, especially for patients with anatomic variants. Recent advances in ultrasonography have allowed these techniques to be done without x-ray guidance, though it remains the gold standard.

Though percutaneous techniques have become more common, MVD surgery remains a cornerstone of treatment of trigeminal neuralgia with excellent results. MVD is a non-destructive procedure with low risk of facial sensory loss and subsequent dysesthesias or anesthesia dolorosa that is believed to be addressing the underlying primary pathology: vascular compression. Horsley first proposed an open surgical procedure involving sectioning the roots of the trigeminal nerve in 1891. Dandy in the 1920s and 1930s did so in the posterior cranial fossa and advanced the theory of compression of the nerve by vascular structures. This work unfortunately was not advanced until the 1960s and 1970s, when Gardner and Janetta elaborated on further anatomic abnormalities. Work on MVD continued to expand with development of safer operative and anesthetic techniques and the expanded use of microsurgical techniques, and as such, MVD has now become a widely accepted treatment for TN. Since the 2000s, with the advancement in imaging techniques and delivery of targeted radiation, Gamma Knife radiosurgery (GKRS) has become an option for minimally invasive destruction of the trigeminal nerve and a treatment option for TN.

Percutaneous Interventions for Trigeminal Neuralgia

Traditionally, fluoroscopic guidance has been utilized to address the trigeminal ganglion. A submental view is achieved, and with careful Ipsilateral oblique of the C-arm, the foramen ovale is identified via the classic trans-foramen ovale Hartel technique. The needle is then advanced into the foramen ovale and further advanced to the Meckel's cave where the trigeminal ganglion lies. From here, which ever technique desired is utilized.

For RFA, once the needle is in place, the patient can be awakened, and sensory and motor responses tested. Detailed mapping then occurs to guide lesion placement and minimize sensory and motor side effects (as shown in Fig. 38.2). Radiofrequency lesions are typically made at a maximum 55–60 °C to 80–90 °C for 30–120 seconds. For PBC, the operator percutaneously inserts a balloon catheter through the foramen ovale into Meckel's cave and inflates it for 1–10 minutes. For GR, small amount of glycerol (~0.2–0.4 ml) is injected into Meckel's cave with the patients in a seated position, and they remain in the same

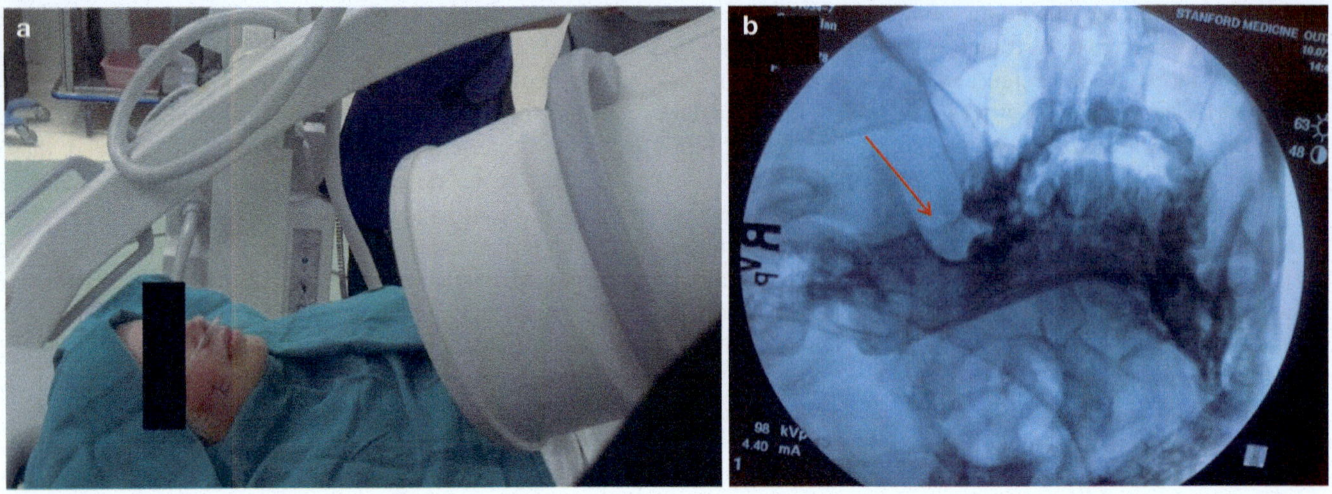

Fig. 38.2 (**a**) Submental view: needle insertion site (noted by red start) at about 2 cm lateral to the side of the corner of the mouth. (**b**) Foramen ovale (noted by red arrow) visualized under fluoroscopy

position for 1–2 hours. Among these techniques, RFA provides the most targeted ablation to individual sub-branches of trigeminal nerve.

Pain relief with RFA is generally high with most studies reporting greater than 95% or complete pain resolution. Rates of pain control and the duration of pain relief consistently correlate with the degree of sensory loss. A prospective study of 154 patients found that a high degree of sensory loss predicted a low rate of pain recurrence but the highest rate of dysesthesia. In contrast, patients with mild sensory loss had the highest pain recurrence rates and the lowest rates of dysesthesia. In a series of 1600 patients, rates of anesthesia dolorosa ranged from 0% to 12%. Another study demonstrated rates of corneal anesthesia from 1% to 20.3%. Rates of masseter weakness with RFA ranged from 3% to 29%. Few studies have examined predictors of outcomes after RFA treatment, though a recent study found that outcomes were significantly better for patients with isolated V3 vs V2 pain.

Less common in practice, clinical investigations of GR demonstrate that approximately 90% of patients have complete or immediate pain relief following glycerol injection, and 77% have good or excellent pain control after a 10-year follow-up. Facial sensory loss may occur following glycerol rhizotomy: 32% to 48% are mild, 13% are moderate, and 6% are dense.

Pain relief following PBC is usually immediate but can be delayed by a week after the procedure. Numbness in the V2 and V3 distribution occurs in approximately 80% of patients but is typically mild and often improves with time. Pain relief is immediate in 92% to 100% of patients, and recurrence rates are reported as 19% to 32% over 5 to 20 years.

All percutaneous procedures come with a risk of infection, bleeding, cerebrospinal fluid leak, and anesthesia dolorosa. Percutaneous interventions are not appropriate for patients who cannot tolerate an awake procedure or, in the case of RFA, are unable to cooperate with the necessary localization stimulation. There is a greater risk of the trigeminal depressor response and hypotension and bradycardia when PBC is used. Thus, PBC is contraindicated in patients with cardiovascular disease. RFA provides more precise lesioning than GR or PBC. Most patients following PBC have some degree of pterygoid weakness, which is also mild and resolves after weeks to months; however, in rare cases the unilateral symptomatic jaw weakness is permanent, and thus this procedure is contraindicated for patients with preexisting contralateral jaw weakness.

Percutaneous interventions offer pain relief for TN that is immediate with varying durability and a generally favorable side effect profile. However, treatment selection remains an inexact science in the absence of high-quality outcomes data. The majority of studies are retrospective and highly variable in their patient populations, treatment technique, and reported outcomes. Studies include varying numbers of patients with atypical pain, MS, and bilateral TN. Most series also include varying percentages of patients who have had multiple ablative treatments.

Although the general technique for each procedure is similar, each technique has operator-dependent technical variations that limit comparisons:

1. RF: Type of electrode, delivery of energy, and location of lesioning.
2. GR: The method for cisternography varies as does the volume of glycerin injected.
3. PBC: The level of pressure and duration compression.

A lack of standardization in pain relief outcomes and definition of complications also limits comparisons of techniques. An additional complicating factor is whether patients

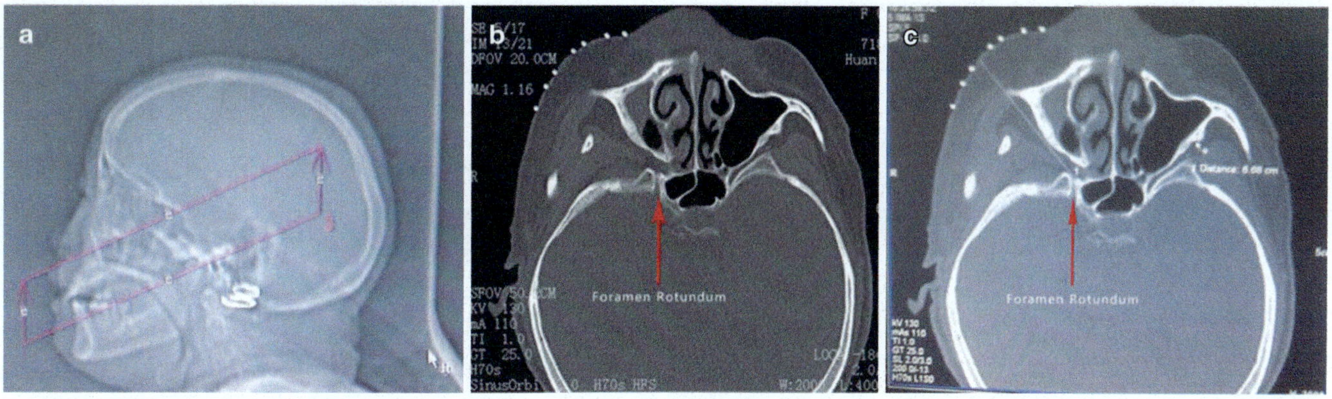

Fig. 38.3 Foramen ovale approach with CT guidance. (**a**) CT scan is utilized to help localize foramen rotundum in patients. Characteristics of the scanogram include semi-coronal position, orientation parallel to the plane connecting external acoustic pore and ipsilateral maxillary third molar bone. (**b**) The CT scan that captured simultaneously the foramen rotundum and its external and internal openings was used to design needle puncture route. Note that the white dots on the left top maxillary surface are transactional view of the positioning grid. (**c**) Computer-simulated needle puncture route was generated, which includes needle entry angle, path, and distance from the needle entry point to the external opening of foramen rotundum

require medications postoperatively to achieve complete pain control. Finally, there is high variability in the duration of follow-up. Although Kaplan-Meier analyses are able to partially control for such variability, the variability in outcomes reporting for TN makes defining the exact time of pain recurrence difficult. These factors hamper the use of single-modality studies in comparisons of outcomes across treatment modalities.

Recent Advances in Percutaneous Treatment of Trigeminal Neuralgia

Although fluoroscopy remains the predominant method of image guidance for percutaneous procedures, skull base anatomy is complex, which often makes fluoroscopic guidance difficult. This becomes even more challenging when an individual trigeminal sub-branch (e.g., V1 or V2) nerve block is desired. Manipulation of the needle within Meckel's cave can be very painful to the awake patient and technically difficult, often necessitating general anesthesia and prolonged fluoroscopy time. For example, for V2 trigeminal neuralgia patient, failure to position the needle properly can lead to treatment failure or serious complications such as nonspecific lesion to V3 or V1 branch, intracranial hemorrhage, and infection. An alternative approach has since been developed to target V2 through foramen rotundum under CT guidance where V2 nerve branch exits the cranium, and subsequently crosses the pterygopalatine fossa, and enters the orbit through the inferior orbital fissure. Approaching through the foramen rotundum, rather than the foramen ovale, has the potential to simplify targeted treatment of the maxillary branch of the trigeminal nerve in TN patients, decrease the median time for needle placement, and minimize intraoperative patient discomfort.

In this CT-guided approach, the patient is positioned supine, and the head is taped gently to prevent accidental head movement. A positioning grid is placed over the cheek on the painful side. Oblique coronal scanning is conducted with the scanning frame parallel to the plane connecting external acoustic pore to ipsilateral maxillary third molar bone. The resulting CT image frame simultaneously captures the foramen rotundum (FR) and its external and internal openings. The intrinsic ruler of the CT scanner is used to measure the distance from the needle entry point to the external opening of FR or FO as well as to determine the needle entry angle. The skin and subcutaneous tissues are anesthetized, and a 10 cm 22 gauge radiofrequency needle is inserted and advanced along the predetermined path based on the angle and depth previously measured. Intermittent CT guidance is used until reaching the external opening of the FR or FO. With this approach, when compared with the classic approach through the FO, it appears to be able to not only provide similar pain relief up to at 1-year follow-up visit but also with fewer adverse effects, except for facial hematoma and facial numbness, which are no worse than the classic approach. CT guidance also lowers procedure duration time and is better tolerated by the patients (Figs. 38.3 and 38.4).

Microvascular Decompression and Gamma Knife Radiosurgery for Trigeminal Neuralgia

Among patients who develop TN younger than 65 years, surgery is considered the definitive treatment for TN, specifically MVD, given its favorable outcomes. Studies have indicated that upward of 50% of patients stop responding to drug therapy and a similar proportion eventually undergo surgical intervention. Studies show that patients with paroxysmal and more sharply delineated distribution of their pain

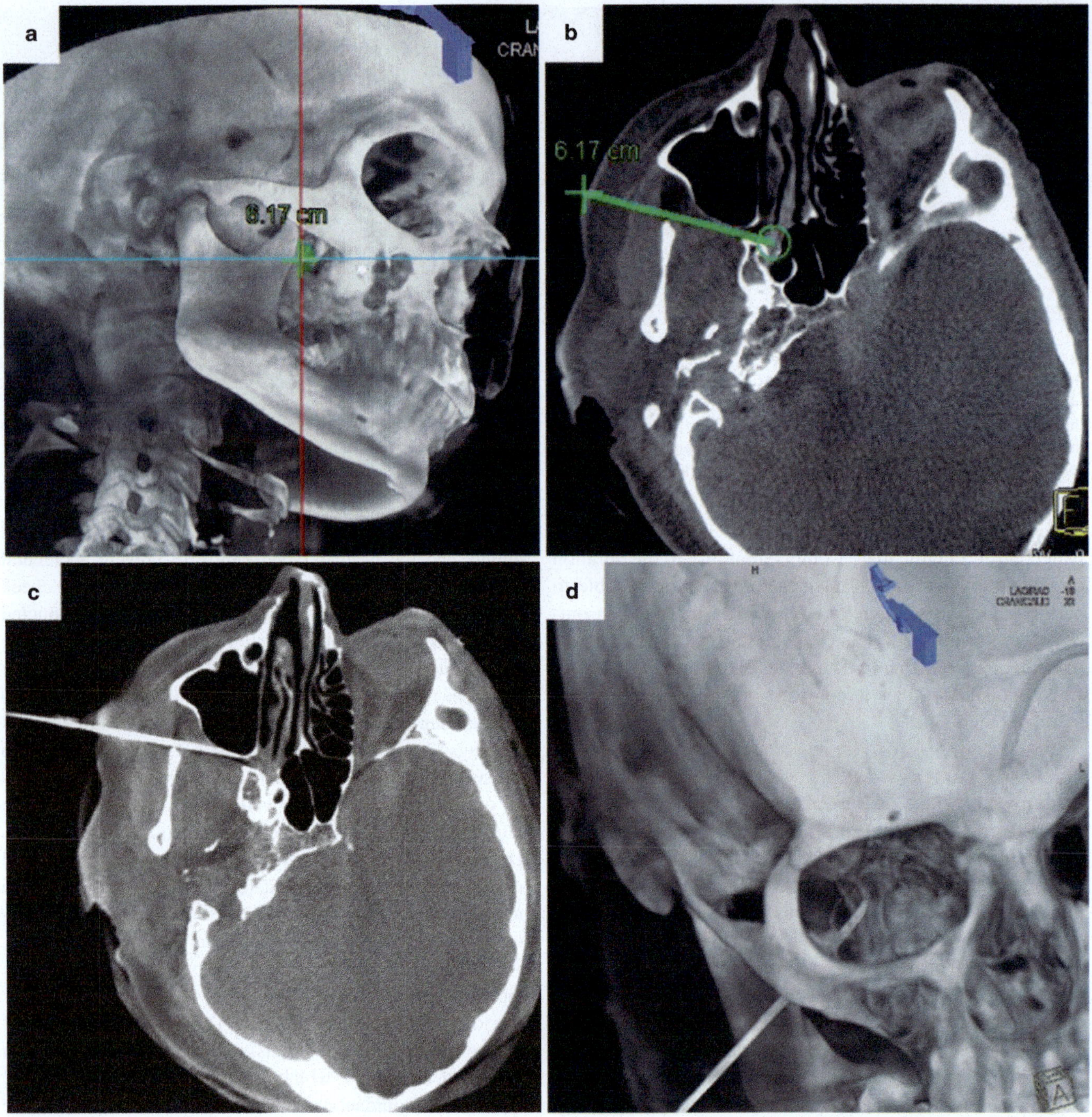

Fig. 38.4 Percutaneous infrazygomatic needle access of foramen rotundum in patients with V2 TN under regular flat panel C-arm CT guidance. The C-arm CT is then used to select a needle path to the foramen rotundum (FR) using needle guidance software, and a lesion depth is calculated (**a, b**). The needle is then positioned in a bulls-eye approach targeting the selected depth, with a postpositioning CT performed to confirm the needle location prior to treatment as depicted on this multiplanar reformatted CT image (**c**). A 3D reconstructed image displays the needle in position within the foramen rotundum (FR) (**d**)

as opposed to diffuse pain tend to respond more favorably to surgical intervention. When to consider surgical intervention remains an open question, though studies indicate that earlier intervention may offer better outcomes, it is generally considered appropriate to trial at least two different medications prior to consideration of more interventional techniques and practice guidelines which have been jointly published by the American Academy of Neurology and the European Federation of Neurological Societies.

Today, two major surgical approaches (aside from percutaneous procedures discussed already) exist: MVD and Gamma Knife radiosurgery (GKRS). Historically, open rhizotomy or tractotomy have been utilized as surgical treatments, but these techniques have been largely abandoned.

Recent advances in imaging and posterior fossa exploration techniques have led to frequent discovery of a vascular vessel impinging on the trigeminal nerve root in which cases simple decompression of the artery from the nerve root has produced long-lasting relief. Neurovascular compression can often be shown on imaging, and advances combining MRI and MRA scans into a three-dimensional image volume along with intraoperative findings have a sensitivity of nearly 95%. Microvascular decompression surgery is performed under general anesthesia and requires a 3 cm craniotomy behind the ear with retraction of the dura to expose the trigeminal nerve and the compressing vascular elements as the nerve enters the pons. Most commonly, Teflon felt is used to separate the nerve from the offending vessel. In cases where no evidence of neurovascular compression is found, neurolysis can be performed by the surgeon which involves separating the fibers of the nerve as it enters the pons. Complications of MVD include risks associated with general anesthesia making it an unfavorable option for older patients or those with significant cardiac or pulmonary comorbidities, and mortality rates are reported at less than 0.5%. Possible morbidity, ranging from 1% to 5%, includes dizziness, facial palsy, cerebrospinal fluid leak, meningitis, stroke, hemorrhage, anesthesia dolorosa, and issues with hearing. Microvascular decompression surgery, which remains one of the most widespread treatment for TN, has an excellent track record of success with proper patient selection. Various studies have shown a success rate of 87–98% with immediate relief, with sustained success in approximately 80% of patients at 2 years. Studies with further follow-up have shown success in 55–68% of patients after 8–10 years.

Gamma Knife radiosurgery, one of the newest techniques to treat TN, involves the use of high-energy photons concentrated into targeted rays to deliver a focused radiation dose to the trigeminal nerve root resulting in destruction of the nerve. Efficacy has been reported to be similar to percutaneous procedures, with 60% of patients reporting immediate relief and 75% of patients reporting at least 50% relief after 18 months. At 2–3 years, 25% of patients have reported recurrence, increasing to 50% at 4 years. Unlike MVD or percutaneous procedures, a significant number of patients reported delayed relief onset over the course of 3–12 weeks. All studies report an excellent safety profile, with the most common comorbidity anesthesia dolorosa at similar rates to percutaneous procedures.

Peripheral and Distal Targets of Facial Innervation

Trigeminal Nerve Branches

1. Maxillary Nerve (V2)

Trigeminal neuralgia can be treated and targeted more distally at the maxillary and mandibular branches. Blockade of the branches of the trigeminal nerve has classically been done with image guidance (either fluoroscopic or CT guidance) utilizing the pterygoid plate (to target V2) and accessing the trigeminal ganglion via the foramen ovale (to target V3).

Targeting the maxillary branch can be done with landmark-based techniques with an extraoral and intraoral approach. For the extraoral approach, the coronoid notch is identified with the needle placed perpendicular to the skin at the notch close to the middle of the zygoma and then advanced until the lateral pterygoid plate is encountered at approximately 4–5 cm after which the needle is redirected anterior and superiorly. The needle should then continue to be advanced within the pterygopalatine fossa until paresthesia of the maxillary branch is elicited. To better assist the extraoral approach, fluoroscopic guidance is often used to identify the midpoint of the zygomatic arch, the mandibular condyle, the coronoid process, and the mandibular notch areas and advance the needle as described as seen in Fig. 38.5.

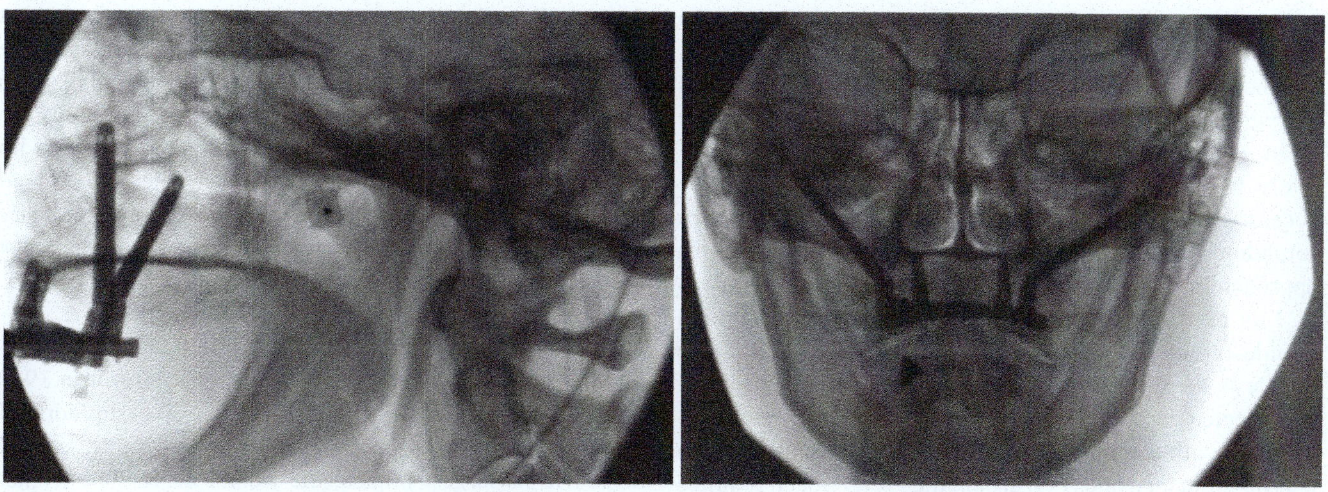

Fig. 38.5 Extraoral fluoroscopic approach for maxillary block

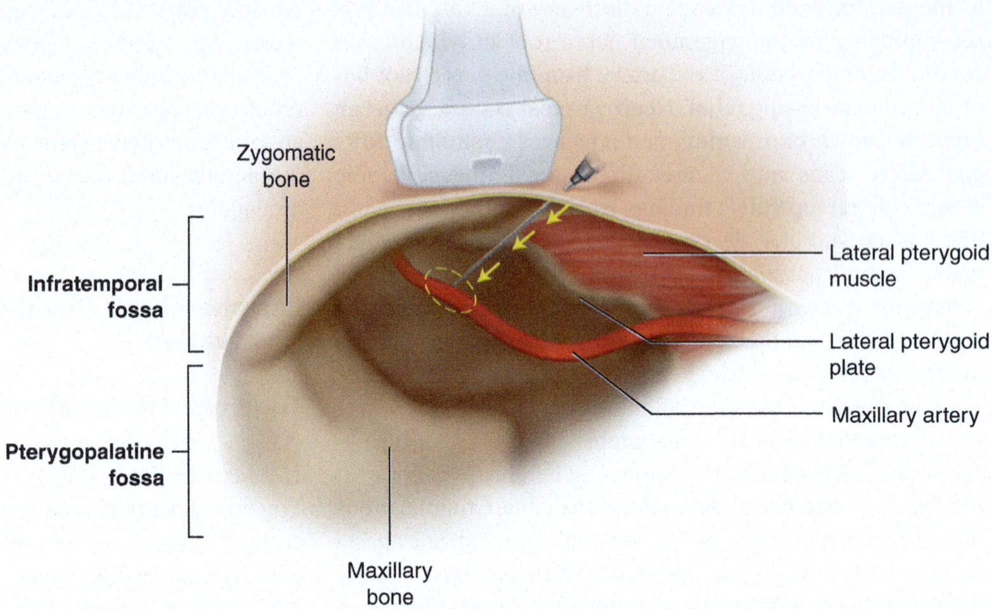

Fig. 38.6 Ultrasound-guided approach for maxillary block. Using a linear probe, the zygomatic bone, lateral pterygoid muscle, lateral pterygoid plate, maxillary bone, and maxillary artery are visualized just below the zygomatic bone and superior to the mandibular notch anterior the mandibular condyle. The needle can be visualized in real time as it is inserted in plane medial to lateral toward the pterygopalatine fossa, advancing toward the maxillary artery just deep to the lateral pterygoid muscle and plate

For the intraoral approach, the cheek at the angle of the mouth is retracted by the hand until the upper molar is seen; the needle should then be placed at the mucosa over the teeth and advanced tangentially to the maxillary tuberosity with contact with the bone at 3–4 cm. Aside from this oblique intraoral approach, there is also the pterygomaxillary and posterior palatinal intraoral approach.

Recently, Nader et al. described a novel ultrasound guidance technique, which allows real-time visualization and imaging of vascular structures, lateral pterygoid plate, and maxillary artery, to access the pterygopalatine fossa, opening opportunities to access the maxillary V2 nerve, sphenopalatine ganglion, and petrosal nerves. In lateral decubitus position, a linear probe is placed below the zygomatic bone and superior to the mandibular notch anterior to the mandibular condyle, allowing visualization of the zygomatic bone, lateral pterygoid muscle, lateral pterygoid plate, maxillary bone, and maxillary artery. A needle can then be visualized in plane medial to lateral toward the pterygopalatine fossa, advancing toward the maxillary artery just deep to the lateral pterygoid muscle and plate as shown in Fig. 38.6.

In addition to the aforementioned techniques to selectively target the V2 branch, the V2 branch can also be accessed via an infrazygomatic approach via the foramen rotundum (FR) as described in the previous section. This approach is performed using a flat panel CT, where the dyn-aCT is used to select a needle path to the FR using an iGuide program and resulting in a calculated depth. The needle is then positioned in a trajectory directly targeting the selected depth. CT scanning is then used to confirm the needle location prior to treatment. When compared to the classic foramen ovale (FO) group, the FR approach requires shorter procedure time, has good clinical outcome with less complication, and presents an alternative when an isolated V2 branch block is desired.

2. Mandibular Nerve (V3)

The mandibular branch innervates both the muscles of mastication and sensation of the lower third of the face. The landmark-guided extraoral approach is the same for the mandibular V3 nerve as for the maxillary V2 nerve. Once the needle encounters the lateral pterygoid plate, the needle is moved posteriorly off the lateral pterygoid plate until paresthesia is obtained. This approach can be augmented with fluoroscopic guidance to identify the coronoid notch and pterygoid plate. An intraoral approach involves retracting the cheek with the index finger to visualize the second upper molar tooth. A needle is then advanced above the mucosa of the second upper molar toward the infratemporal plate toward the midpoint of the zygomatic arch to contact the infratemporal plate at approximately 4–5 cm. Ultrasound guidance, similar to the maxillary nerve approach, allows for real-time visualization by placing the probe below the zygoma and just above the mandibular notch anterior to the mandibular condyle with identification of the zygomatic approach, lateral pterygoid muscle, lateral pterygoid plate, mandible, and maxillary artery, and the injection can then be performed in plane just deep to the lateral pterygoid muscle.

3. Supraorbital and Supratrochlear Nerve (V1 Branch)

Supraorbital neuralgia was first described by Beyer in 1949 as a rare cause of extracranial headache. The supraorbital nerve arises from the ophthalmic branch of the trigeminal nerve via its largest branch, the frontal nerve. The frontal nerve runs along the roof of the orbit and divides into a lateral branch, the supraorbital nerve, and, a smaller, medial branch, the supratrochlear nerve. The supraorbital nerve provides sensation to the lateral forehead, upper eyelid, and anterior scalp, while the supratrochlear nerve innervates the medial forehead, nasal bridge, and medial third of the upper eyelid. Often, supraorbital neuralgia presents as unilateral forehead pain with tenderness over the supraorbital notch, and its etiology is often multifactorial. Known causes can include trauma to the forehead, tight fitting eyewear and helmets, or sinus infections with secondary edema. To target the supraorbital nerve, a linear probe can be placed on the supraorbital ridge in transverse position to visualize the supraorbital notch to allow access via out of plane, making this nerve a target for both radiofrequency lesioning and cryoablation. An out of plane approach has been shown to have a 94% success rate, and repeated studies have shown superiority of ultrasound-guided techniques to landmark-based techniques. When injecting, care should be taken to apply pressure on the upper eyelid to prevent dissection of solution into the loose tissues of the upper eyelid.

4. Infraorbital Nerve Block (V2 Branch)
Infraorbital nerve blocks are useful for the management of infraorbital neuralgia, a pain condition often due to herpes zoster in the V2 distribution, facial bone fractures, and facial malignancies. The infraorbital nerve derives from the maxillary nerve; it enters of orbit via the inferior orbital fissure coursing along the floor of the orbital to exit via the infraorbital foramen to innervate the lower eyelid, lateral nare, and upper lip. The infraorbital nerve gives off the superior alveolar nerve to innervate the upper incisor, canine, and gingiva. In seated or supine position, a linear ultrasound probe can be placed on the zygomatic bone in transverse position to identify the infraorbital notch; the nerve can then be blocked in an out of plane technique, taking care not to insert the needle into the notch itself. For patients with a positive response, cryoablation and radiofrequency treatment can be successfully utilized for longer-term benefit.

5. Zygomaticotemporal Nerve (V2 Branch)
The zygomaticotemporal nerve, a branch of the maxillary division of the trigeminal nerve, originates in the pterygopalatine fossa and enters the orbit through the inferior orbital fissure and travels along the lateral wall where the nerve divides to the zygomaticotemporal and zygomaticofacial nerves. The zygomaticotemporal division travels along the inferolateral portion of the orbit, going through a bony canal in the zygomatic bone and then entering the temporal fossa to ascend between the bone and temporalis muscle. It should be noted that anatomical studies have found that this nerve communicates with both the facial and auriculotemporal nerves. Previous research as shown the resection of the corrugator supercilii muscle and destruction of the zygomaticotemporal nerve has been shown to improve migraine headaches. The nerve should be targeted at its emergence from the deep temporal fascia located approximately 1.5 cm posterolateral and 0.5 cm cephalad to the lateral orbital commissure. Approximately 2 cm posterolateral from this point the needle should be inserted, using the index figure to mark the point of emergence. Cryoablation and radiofrequency ablation can be utilized for longer-term relief.

6. Auriculotemporal Nerve Block (V3 Branch)
Auriculotemporal nerve blocks can be used to treat atypical facial pain, herpes zoster pain involving the external auditory meatus, or temporomandibular joint pain. Though rarely diagnosed, it may represent a common cause of trigeminal headaches as a review study looking at manual palpation to elicit headaches mapped 42.6% of such trigger regions in the auriculotemporal distribution. In addition to trigeminal headaches, auriculotemporal syndrome, also known as Frey syndrome, was first described in 1923 as unilateral hyperhidrosis and flushing of the ear and cheek with stimulation of the parotid gland while eating or drinking. Frey syndrome has been found to involve the auriculotemporal as well as greater auricular nerve. The auriculotemporal nerve derives from the mandibular nerve, traveling through the parotid gland and then between the temporomandibular joint and external auditory meatus to innervate the pinna, external auditory meatus, and the temporomandibular joint with continuation with the temporal artery to innervate the temporal and lateral scalp. First described in 2007 by Shankar and Brethauer, the auriculotemporal nerve can be targeted with ultrasound guidance by placing a linear probe just above the origin of the zygomatic process to visualize the temporal artery, with the nerve just anterior to the artery. For patients with a positive response, cryoablation or radiofrequency ablation can be successfully utilized for longer-term benefit.

7. Mental Nerve (V3 Branch)
The mental nerve can be targeted for mental nerve neuralgia, facial bone fractures, malignancies, or atypical facial pain. Bell first described mental nerve neuralgia in 1830 with numbness below the chin in a case report secondary to bony metastasis in the left mandible from breast cancer. Similar case reports were published by Calverley and Mohnac who coined the term numb chin syndrome in 1963 in five patients from metastatic cancer. The mental nerve is a branch of the mandibular nerve arising from the mental foramen in the mandible at level of the second premolar to innervate the medial aspect of the chin. The nerve can be visualized with ultrasound guidance by utilizing a linear probe along the lower border of the mandible in transverse position.

The nerve can be accessed out of plane with visualization of the mental foramen. Radiofrequency lesioning or cryoablation offer therapeutic options for the mental nerve.

8. Inferior Alveolar Nerve (V3 Branch)
Intraoral malignancies and post-traumatic neuralgias secondary to dental procedures can result in inferior alveolar neuralgia. The inferior alveolar nerve originates from the mandibular nerve at the entry to the mandibular canal and provides sensation to the molars, premolars, and gingiva. It has two branches, the incisor branch innervating the canines and incisors and the mental branch which arises from the foramen to innervate the lower lip and gingiva. To target the inferior alveolar nerve, the anterior margin of mandible just above the last molar serves as the landmark. The needle is advanced at the inner surface of the mandible in the submucosa. This can be a target for cryoablation and radiofrequency neuromodulation.

Facial Nerve Targets Not Branches of the Trigeminal Nerve

1. Greater and Lesser Occipital Nerve
Greater and lesser occipital nerve blocks are useful both for the diagnosis and treatment of occipital neuralgia, which was first described in 1821 by Beuto et al. The greater occipital nerve anatomically derives from the dorsal primary rami of the second and third cervical nerves, piercing the fascia below the superior nuchal ridge and traveling with the occipital artery to supply sensation to the medial portion of the posterior scalp on the ipsilateral side to the vertex. In contrast, the lesser occipital nerve anatomically derives from the ventral rami of the second and third cervical nerves, traveling along the posterior border of the sternocleidomastoid muscle to innervate the lateral portion of the posterior scalp to the pinna of the ear.

Blockade of these nerves can be performed in either sitting or prone position, aided with flexion of the cervical spine. By palpation the occipital artery can be located at the superior nuchal ridge with the greater occipital nerve found just medial to the artery. The lesser occipital nerve can then be blocked by directing laterally and just inferiorly. These procedures can also be performed under fluoroscopic guidance. More recently, studies have demonstrated that ultrasound guidance improves efficacy and reduces the risk of inadvertent vascular injection. Ultrasound-guided block at the level of C2 as the nerve travels just superficial to the obliquus capitis inferior and just below the semispinalis capitis muscles demonstrated higher success of injections in cadaveric studies compared to traditional techniques. To perform this, the ultrasound probe should be placed midline over the occiput to identify C1 and C2. When C2 is identified with its bifid spinous process, the transducer should be moved laterally to visualize the suboccipital muscles and then have the lateral end of the transducer tilted cephalad to have the transducer in line with the inferior oblique muscle in long axis. This obtains a short axis view of the semispinalis capitis muscles, allowing differentiation between it and the obliquus capitis muscles, with the greater occipital nerve found in the fascial plane in between.

For patients who respond to diagnostic blocks with local anesthetic and steroid, pulsed radiofrequency neuromodulation, continued radiofrequency ablation, or cryoablation can be implemented to extend therapeutic benefit. Ultrasound has been shown to improve success of greater occipital nerve blocks; in one study, blind injections had a success of 30.8% compared to 76.9% with ultrasound-guided blocks. CT-guided techniques have been described as well, with needle placement for C2 between the posterior arches of C1 and C2 and for C3 at the lateral aspect of the C2-C3 foramen just anterior the base of the C3 superior facet. Li and colleagues have also described surgical micro decompression with a success rate of 89.5%. Surgical excision has also been described by Ducic and colleagues with a success rate of 41%.

2. Greater Auricular Nerve
The greater auricular nerve derives from the primary ventral ramus of the second and third cervical nerves by penetrating the fascia just inferior and lateral to the lesser occipital nerve; it becomes more superficial upon curving around the sternocleidomastoid muscle to innervate the ear, external auditory canal, angle of the jaw, and skin over the parotid glands with the posterior auricular nerve as the terminal branch. To access the nerve, with slight cervical flexion, a linear probe should be placed in transverse oblique orientation over the sternocleidomastoid muscle to allow visualization of the greater auricular nerve superior and lateral to the sternocleidomastoid muscle. The superficiality of the nerve makes it an excellent target for radiofrequency lesioning and cryoablation. It should be noted that surgical sectioning of the sensory auricular branch has been utilized for otalgia; however, as with any such treatment of a peripheral nerve, neuroma formation is a concern.

3. Glossopharyngeal Nerve
The glossopharyngeal nerve can cause pain in the ear, base of tongue, tonsillar fossa, and beneath the angle of the jaw. One of the first descriptions comes from 1910 by Weisenburg who identified the case as "an unusual tic douloureux" in a patient with pain in the throat and ear. Over the years, two

predominant types have been described, an oropharyngeal type caused by swallowing or talking and a tympanic type caused by sound or touch over the outer auditory canal. In addition to this, vagoglossopharyngeal neuralgia has been described with associated features of asystole and syncope.

The glossopharyngeal nerve, a mixed sensory, motor, and autonomic nerve, arises from the medulla oblongata, traveling laterally to exit through the jugular foramen to pass through the internal jugular vein and the internal carotid and then to course medially behind the styloid process (see Fig. 38.7). Due to the close correlation with the vagus nerve, a small minority of patients will have significant vagal symptoms with glossopharyngeal pain. Vascular impingement has been implicated in glossopharyngeal neuralgia which is treated by microvascular decompression of the posterior cerebral artery. In other patients, an elongated styloid process can lead to pain as well (Eagle's syndrome) and is another potential surgical target.

Surgical treatment can be employed for patients with an elongated styloid or microvascular decompression of the glossopharyngeal nerve. Aside from surgical intervention, nerve blocks and neurolysis can be utilized to treat pain arising from the glossopharyngeal nerve. There are two approaches, intraoral and extraoral. The intraoral approach is based on anatomic landmarks, with the glossopharyngeal nerve found inferior to the tonsillar pillar via the palatoglossal fold. The extraoral approach allows for various interventions, including radiofrequency neuromodulation and neurolysis, utilizing the styloid process as the primary landmark. Under fluoroscopic guidance, the glossopharyngeal nerve is classically accessed percutaneously through the jugular foramen (JF).

Telischak et al. reported a lateral cervical approach to access the SP using CT guidance rather than the classical JF approach (cranial nerves including glossopharyngeal nerve, vagus nerve, and accessory nerve pass through together at the level of JF). The classical JF approach can be complicated by injuries to the nearby vagus nerve, spinal accessory nerve, and the internal carotid artery. In the lateral cervical approach, the initial needle skin entry point is approximately 1 cm below the ipsilateral earlobe, with the final needle position at or overshooting the styloid process posteriorly by 1–5 mm, where cranial nerves glossopharyngeal nerve, vagus nerve, and accessory nerve have sufficiently separated from each other, with glossopharyngeal nerve being most adjacent to the distal part of SP. With this approach Telischak et al. have minimized unwanted complications such as damage to neurovascular tissue and dural folds (Fig. 38.8).

The first description of ultrasound-guided treatment comes from Bedder and Lindsay in 1989 to treat pain secondary from cancer of the throat and tongue. For ultrasound guidance, placing a linear probe just inferior to the earlobe in a transverse oblique position between the mastoid and the angle of the mandible visualizes the styloid process just medial to the mastoid process. The nerve is then accessed in an out of plane technique by first touching the styloid process and then redirecting posteriorly. For patients with a positive response, radiofrequency lesioning can be utilized for therapeutic innervation.

Fig. 38.7 Glossopharyngeal nerve anatomy

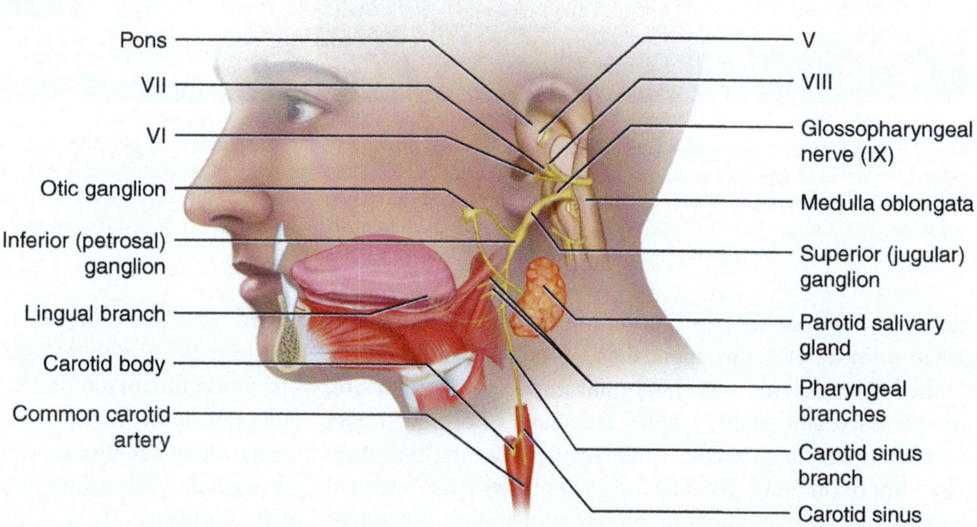

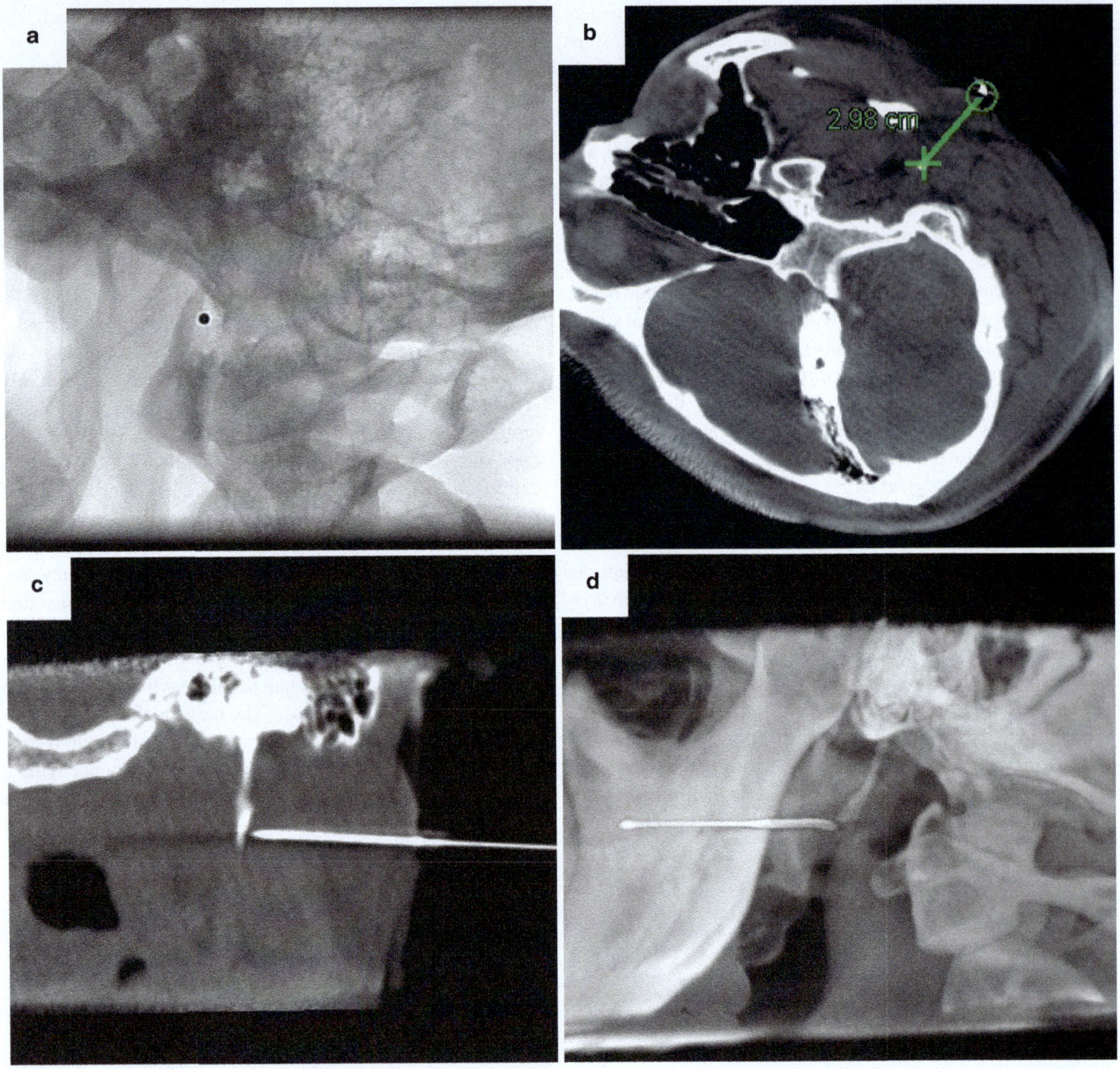

Fig. 38.8 CT-guided glossopharyngeal nerve block A BB marker is placed on the skin (**a**), and a flat panel C-arm CT is performed. The C-arm CT is then used to select a needle path using needle guidance software, and a lesion depth is calculated (**b**). The needle is then positioned in a bulls-eye approach targeting the selected depth, with a post-positioning CT performed to confirm the needle location prior to treatment as depicted on this multiplanar reformatted CT image abutting the styloid process (SP) (**c**). A 3D reconstructed image displays the needle in position adjacent to the styloid process (SP) (**d**)

Summary Orofacial pain is common but often under recognized disease, affecting more than 35 million adults in the United States alone, with important impacts on healthcare, productivity, and quality of life. Treatment of orofacial pain is multimodal, with medical management as first-line therapy. Approximately 30–50% of patients will fail medical therapy and are candidates for interventions, such as percutaneous ablation procedure (RFA, GR, PBC, etc.), Gamma Knife radiosurgery, MVD, and others. Fluoroscopy remains the predominant method of image guidance for percutaneous ablation procedures. However, skull base anatomy is complex, which often makes fluoroscopic guidance difficult and necessitates other imaging-guided techniques, such as CT and ultrasound. In this chapter, we have summarized the history, use, imaging technique, and indications of destructive procedures for a variety of painful conditions in the head and face, including trigeminal neuralgia, glossopharyngeal neuralgia, and others.

Recommended Reading

1. Anderson LC, Vakoula A, Veinote R. Inflammatory hypersensitivity in a rat model of trigeminal neuropathic pain. Arch Oral Biol. 2003;48(2):161–9.
2. Barker FG 2nd, Jannetta PJ, Bissonette DJ, Larkins MV, Jho HD. The long-term outcome of microvascular decompression for trigeminal neuralgia. N Engl J Med. 1996;334(17):1077–83.
3. Bennett, C. R., & Giovannitti, J. A., Jr. (1998). Neural blockade of oral and circumoral structures. Neural blockade in clinical anesthesia and management of pain, 3rd. Philadelphia: Lippincott Williams & Wilkins, 528.
4. Blumenfeld A, Nikolskaya G. Glossopharyngeal neuralgia. Curr Pain Headache Rep. 2013;17(7):343.
5. Bowsher D. Trigeminal neuralgia: an anatomically oriented review. Clin Anat. 1997;10(6):409–15.
6. Burchiel KJ, Slavin KV. On the natural history of trigeminal neuralgia. Neurosurgery. 2000;46(1):152–4; discussion 154–5.
7. Casey KF, Jannetta PJ. History of trigeminal neuralgia. In: Trigeminal neuralgia, vol. 3. Oxford: Oxford University Press; 2010.
8. Cheng JS, Lim DA, Chang EF, Barbaro NM. A review of percutaneous treatments for trigeminal neuralgia. Neurosurgery. 2014;10(Suppl 1):25–33; discussion 33.
9. Eboli P, Stone JL, Aydin S, Slavin KV. Historical characterization of trigeminal neuralgia. Neurosurgery. 2009;64(6):1183–6; discussion 1186–7.
10. Eller JL, Raslan AM, Burchiel KJ. Trigeminal neuralgia: definition and classification. Neurosurg Focus. 2005;18(5):E3.
11. Gusmão S, Oliveira M, Tazinaffo U, Honey CR. Percutaneous trigeminal nerve radiofrequency rhizotomy guided by computerized tomography fluoroscopy. Technical note. J Neurosurg. 2003;99(4):785–6.
12. Haines SJ, Jannetta PJ, Zorub DS. Microvascular relations of the trigeminal nerve. An anatomical study with clinical correlation. J Neurosurg. 1980;52(3):381–6.
13. Larsen A, Piepgras D, Chyatte D, Rizzolo D. Trigeminal neuralgia: diagnosis and medical and surgical management. JAAPA. 2011;24(7):20–5.
14. Lichtor T, Mullan JF. A 10-year follow-up review of percutaneous microcompression of the trigeminal ganglion. J Neurosurg. 1990;72(1):49–54.
15. Nader A, Kendall MC, De Oliveria GS, Chen JQ, Vanderby B, Rosenow JM, Bendok BR. Ultrasound-guided trigeminal nerve block via the pterygopalatine fossa: an effective treatment for trigeminal neuralgia and atypical facial pain. Pain Physician. 2013;16(5):E537–45.
16. Pollock BE. Surgical management of medically refractory trigeminal neuralgia. Curr Neurol Neurosci Rep. 2012;12(2):125–31.
17. Trescot AM. Peripheral nerve entrapments: clinical diagnosis and management. Cham: Springer International Publishing; 2016.
18. Vadivelu N, Vadivelu A, Kaye AD. Orofacial pain: a clinician's guide. Cham: Springer International Publishing; 2014.
19. Wang JY, Bender MT, Bettegowda C. Percutaneous procedures for the treatment of trigeminal neuralgia. Neurosurg Clin N Am. 2016;27(3):277–95.

39 Interlaminar Approach for Cervical Epidural Steroid Injection

Sanket Pathak and Andrew Ng

Introduction

Cervical epidural steroid injection (CESI) is a frequently performed intervention for neck pain. The prevalence of chronic neck pain is estimated to be between 30% and 50%. As with back pain, neck pain carries with it significant societal and economic impacts and is the fourth leading cause of disability according to a report on the state of U.S. health.

Background and Historical Perspective

The first reported use of epidural steroid was in 1952 when Robecchi and Capra used hydrocortisone to treat lumbar disc herniation. Shortly thereafter, in 1961, Jean Thierry-Mieg described the first cervical epidural steroid injection to treat cervicobrachial neuralgia. Today, interlaminar CESI is commonly performed to deliver steroids into the epidural space.

Therapeutic CESI's are performed either through an interlaminar or transforaminal approach. The main difference between the two approaches lies in the anatomic deposition of steroid solution, as interlaminar CESI delivers steroids close to the pathology site while transforaminal CESI delivers steroids at the specific spinal nerve root level. The interlaminar approach is more commonly performed due to lower risk for injection into a radiculomedullary which has been associated with anterior spinal artery syndrome, spinal cord infarction, and vertebral artery occlusion. However, interlaminar CESI has its own unique complications such as dural puncture and direct spinal cord injury.

S. Pathak
Department of Anesthesiology, Thomas Jefferson University Hospital, Philadelphia, PA, USA
e-mail: Sanket.Pathak@jefferson.edu

A. Ng (✉)
Department of Anesthesiology, Jefferson Pain Center, Thomas Jefferson University Hospital, Philadelphia, PA, USA
e-mail: Andrew.Ng@jefferson.edu

Uses and Indications

Cervical epidural steroid injections are used to treat cervical radicular pain secondary to cervical disc herniation, cervical spondylotic neuroforaminal stenosis, and cervical spinal stenosis. Other pathologies which may benefit from CESI include chronic pain secondary to cervical post-laminectomy syndrome, cervical discogenic pain, cervicogenic headaches, post-herpetic neuralgia, phantom limb pain, and complex regional pain syndrome (Table 39.1). The underlying mechanism for radicular pain was first thought to be secondary to mechanical nerve compression. Herniated cervical intervertebral discs produce inflammatory and pain mediators such as phospholipase A_2, metalloproteinases, nitric oxide, interleukin-6, and prostaglandin E_2 which can cause spinal nerve irritation and chemical radiculitis. One proposed mechanism of action for CESI is to attenuate the inflammatory response.

Relevant Anatomy

The cervical spinous processes are attached to the lamina at an angle of 15–20°, making the interlaminar approach to the midline perpendicular. The most prominent cervical spinous process is C7, and this serves as an important landmark for

Table 39.1 Indications for cervical interlaminar epidural steroid injections

Indications for interlaminar CESI:
Cervical radiculitis secondary to:
Cervical disc herniation
Cervical spondylotic neuroforaminal stenosis
Cervical spinal stenosis
Other pain syndromes
Cervicogenic headaches
Cervical discogenic pain
Cervical post-laminectomy syndrome
Post-herpetic neuralgia
Phantom limb pain
Complex regional pain syndrome

T. R. Deer et al. (eds.), *Deer's Treatment of Pain*, https://doi.org/10.1007/978-3-030-12281-2_39

reference. The needle first encounters skin, followed by subcutaneous tissue, supraspinous ligament, interspinous ligament, ligamentum flavum, and, finally, the epidural space. The epidural space is a potential space containing spinal nerve roots, internal vertebral venous plexus, connective tissues, segmental blood supply, epidural fat, and lymphatics. The epidural veins are positioned laterally at the level of each cervical vertebral body. Therefore, venous puncture is more likely to occur if the epidural needle is positioned laterally. In approximately 50% of the population, the ligamentum flavum is unfused in the midline, and the interspinous ligament is either absent or thin in the cervical spine. Therefore, the practitioner may experience subtle loss of resistance and the risk of an inadvertent dural puncture with the midline interlaminar approach. The epidural space in the cervical spine is narrower in comparison to the lumbar spine. Most practitioners will enter at the C6–C7 or C7–T1 interspace since it has the widest epidural space of approximately 3–4 mm. Rathmell et al. published a recent consensus guideline recommending that interlaminar CESIs be performed at C7–T1 interspace, but preferably not higher than the C6–C7 interspace. The upper cervical segmental levels have narrow epidural space, therefore increasing risk of needle penetration and injury to the dural sac and spinal cord.

Technique

Prior to any procedure, the practicing physician should review the patient's pertinent cross-sectional imaging, including magnetic resonance imaging (MRI) or computed tomography (CT). The optimal positioning for the procedure is prone with arms by the hips. A pillow is placed under the chest to facilitate cervical spine flexion, therefore opening the cervical interspaces. The fluoroscope is positioned above the cervical spine with a slight caudal angulation of 15–20° under anteroposterior (AP) view. The needle entry site overlying the cervical interspace is then anesthetized with 2–3 ml of 1% lidocaine. An 18 or 20 G 3 ½ in Touhy needle is then inserted. A longer needle length may be required in patients with increased body habitus. Care is taken to slowly advance the needle through the skin and underlying ligaments until it is finally seated in the interspinous ligament where most resistance is met. Repeated AP fluoroscopic images can be taken to ensure midline tracking of the needle. Lateral or contralateral oblique views can also be obtained to determine needle depth. A loss of resistance syringe filled with a few milliliters of preservative-free normal saline or air is then attached to the epidural needle. The needle hub is held between the left thumb and index finger, while the palm of the left hand is firmly placed on the patient to reduce uncontrolled needle movements if the patient unexpectedly moves. Both epidural needle and loss of resistance syringe are advanced 1–2 mm at a time. With the right index finger, pressure is placed on the plunger of the loss of resistance syringe until a loss of resistance is felt, signifying entry into the epidural space. At this point, 1 ml of nonionic contrast is injected into the needle through an extension tubing under live fluoroscopy to confirm epidural contrast spread and visualize any potential intravascular uptake (Fig. 39.1). Epidural contrast spread should also be verified with a lateral or contralateral oblique view of the cervical spine (Fig. 39.2). Digital subtraction can be also used to reduce risk of intravascular injection. After epidural needle position is confirmed, 2–4 ml of mixture containing steroids (6–12 mg of betamethasone sodium phosphate and acetate or 8–16 mg of dexamethasone) and preservative-free saline is injected depending on the spread of contrast. The needle is then removed.

Evidence for Efficacy

Compared to the transforaminal CESI, the interlaminar approach has been more thoroughly investigated through multiple randomized clinical trials (RCT's) and systematic reviews (Table 39.2). Overall, there appears to be good evidence supporting cervical interlaminar injections in the treatment of radicular pain secondary to disc herniation and fair evidence in the treatment of pain secondary to spinal stenosis. Manchikanti et al. reviewed five moderate to high quality RCT's assessing pain relief and functional status in patients with either disc herniation or spinal stenosis that received cervical interlaminar injections with or without fluoroscopic guidance. All of these studies demonstrated positive results with pain relief and functional status improvement. In particular, two of the high-quality trials performed under fluoroscopy demonstrated greater than 50% pain relief and improvement in functional status 1 year after receiving interlaminar cervical epidural steroid injections in both cervical disc herniation population and central spinal stenosis population.

In another systematic review, Manchikanti et al. examined long-term efficacy of interlaminar CESIs in the populations of cervical disc herniation, spinal stenosis, discogenic pain, and post-surgery syndrome. Out of the seven manuscripts included, four were considered high methodological quality with one high quality study in each of the aforementioned pathology groups. This demonstrated Level II evidence for the efficacy of these injections based on the American Society of Intervention Pain Physicians (ASIPP) grading of evidence.

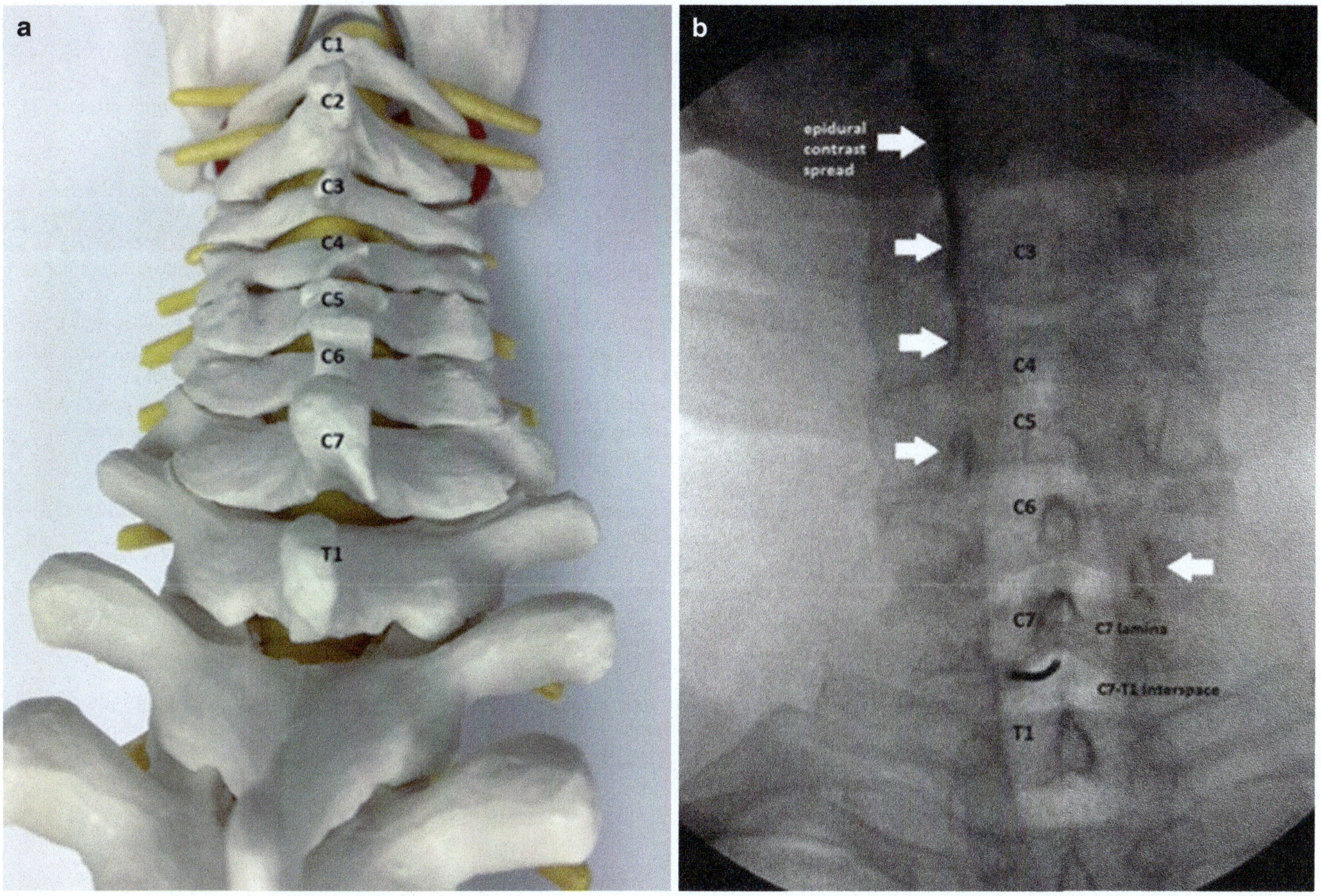

Fig. 39.1 (**a**) Cervical spine model in relation to anteroposterior fluoroscopic view. (**b**) 18 G Tuohy needle is positioned in the C7-T1 interspace. Epidural contrast spread is visualized along the lateral aspects of the epidural space indicated with arrows

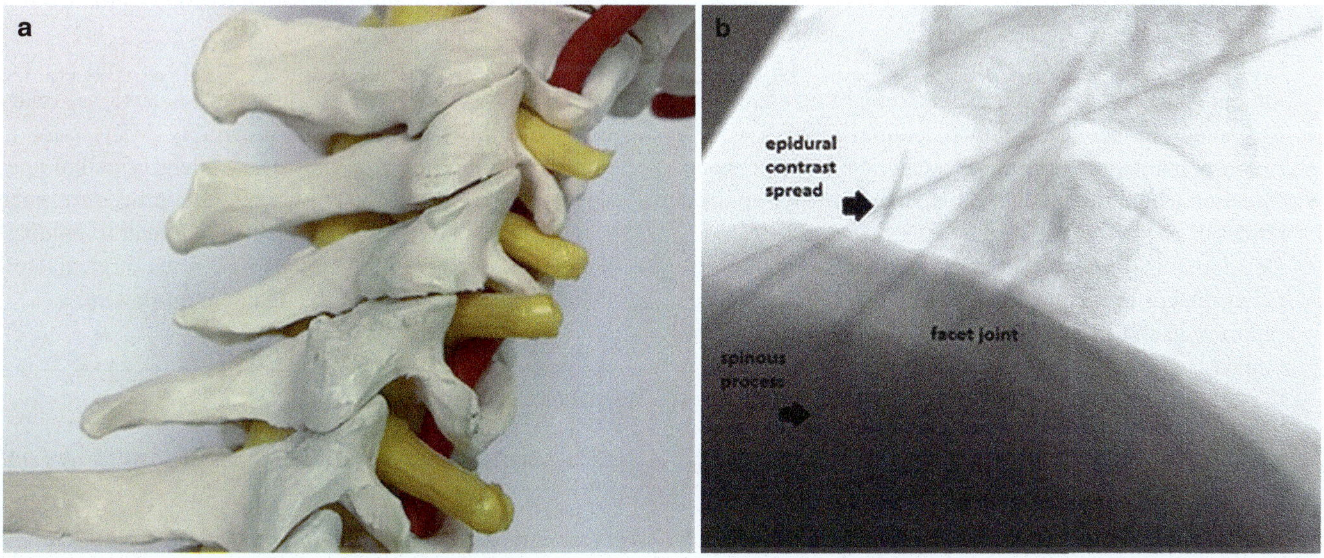

Fig. 39.2 (**a**) Cervical spine model in relation to lateral fluoroscopic view. (**b**) Epidural contrast spread is seen along the posterior aspects of the spinal canal indicated with arrows

Table 39.2 Summary of studies demonstrating interlaminar cervical epidural steroid injection efficacy

Author, study type	Condition	Study description	Outcome
Manchikanti et al. (RCT) 2012	Disc herniation or radiculitis	One hundred twenty patients undergoing multiple fluoroscopic guided interlaminar CESI over 2 years. Sixty patients received LA, and 60 patients received LA with steroid	>50% pain relief and functional status improvement in majority of both groups(77% and 80%, respectively) at 2 years
Manchikanti et al. (RCT) 2012	Central spinal stenosis	Sixty patients undergoing fluoroscopic guided interlaminar CESI. Thirty patients received LA, and 30 patients received LA with steroid	Significant pain relief (>50%) in 87% for both group. Functional status improvement in both groups, 77% and 87%, respectively
Castagnera et al. (RCT) 1994	Disc herniation or radiculitis	Twenty-four patients undergoing blind interlaminar CESI. Fourteen patients received LA with steroid, and 10 patients received LA, steroid, and morphine	Long-term pain relief in both groups (78.5% and 80%, respectively) with mean of 43 months' relief following single injection.
Stav et al. (RCT) 1993	Disc herniation or radiculitis	Forty-two patients undergoing blind interlaminar CESI. Twenty-five patients underwent epidural steroid injection with lidocaine, and 17 patients underwent steroid with lidocaine injection into neck muscles	Sixty-eight percent of epidural treated patients reported good and very good pain relief vs. 11.8% in neck muscles group
Pasqualucci et al. (RCT) 2007	Disc herniation or radiculitis	Forty patients comparing continuous (20) vs. single epidural injection (20)	Significant increase in pain control (>80%) and pain-free sleep in 17/20 patients in both groups
Manchikanti et al. (RCT) 2014	Cervical discogenic pain	One hundred twenty patients undergoing fluoroscopic guided interlaminar CESI. Sixty patients received LA, and 60 patients received LA with steroid	>50% pain relief and functional status improvement in majority of both groups (78% and 75%, respectively) at 2 years
Manchikanti et al. (RCT) 2012	Cervical post-surgery syndrome	Fifty-six patients undergoing multiple fluoroscopic guided interlaminar CESI. Twenty-eight patients received LA vs. 28 patients received LA with steroid	>50% pain relief and functional status improvement in 87% and 72% of patients, respectively, after 2 years

RCT randomized control trial, *CESI* cervical epidural steroid injection, *LA* local anesthetics

Pearls and Pitfalls

Although complications are rare in CESIs, the practitioner should still be mindful of the following:

- Dural puncture with subsequent development of headaches. Incidence of dural puncture is higher compared to lumbar spine due to the unique anatomy of cervical spine ligaments and the narrow dorsal epidural space.
- Epidural hematoma resulting in spinal cord compression
- Infection leading to arachnoiditis, meningitis, or epidural abscess
- Development of severe spinal cord and brain injuries. Quadriplegia related to direct needle trauma has been reported in the literature. Intravascular injection of particulate steroid can coalesce and occlude vasculature in the cervical spine

The following precautions should be considered to ensure patient safety when performing these procedures:

- Avoid deep sedation or general anesthesia to allow continuous patient feedback in the event of needle misplacement. If the patient develops paresthesia suggesting nerve root or cord puncture, the needle is immediately removed and the procedure is aborted.
- The use of non-particulate steroid (dexamethasone) or low-particulate steroid (betamethasone sodium phosphate and acetate) is recommended to minimize vascular occlusion.
- Verify if the patient has a history of bleeding disorder or if the patient is on anticoagulation therapy to reduce risk of epidural hematoma.
- The physician performing the procedure should personally review the patient's advanced cross-sectional imaging preferably (either CT or preferably MRI) prior to performing the injection in order to identify pathologies that preclude patients from obtaining the procedure, such as high-grade spinal stenosis, which can lead to epidural space effacement after injection or previous surgical laminectomy which disrupted the ligamentum flavum.

Recommended Reading

1. Collighan N, Gupta S. Epidural steroids. Br J Anaesth. 2010;10(1):1–5.
2. Huston CW. Cervical epidural steroid injections in the management of cervical radiculitis: interlaminar versus transforaminal, a review. Curr Rev Musculoskelet Med. 2009;2:30–42.
3. Manchikanti L, Falco FJ, Diwan S, Hirsch JA, Smith HS. Cervical radicular pain: the role of interlaminar and transforaminal epidural injections. Curr Pain Headache Rep. 2014;18(1):389.
4. Manchikanti L, Nampiaparampil DE, Candido KD, Bakshi S, Grider JS, Falco FJ, Sehgal N, Hirsch JA. Do cervical epidural injections

provide long term relief in neck and upper extremity pain? A systematic review. Pain Physician. 2015;18:39–60.
5. Mehta P, Syrop I, Singh JR, Kirschner J. Systematic review of the efficacy of particulate versus nonparticulate corticosteroids in epidural injections. PM R. 2017;9(5):502–12.
6. Rathmell JP, Benzon HT, Dreyfuss P, Huntoon M, Wallace M, Baker R, Riew KD, Rosenquist RW, Aprill C, Rost NS, Buvanendran A, Kreiner DS, Bogduk N, Fourney DR, Fraifeld E, Horn S, Stone J, Vorenkamp K, Lawler G, Summers J, Kloth D, O'Brien D Jr, Tutton S. Safeguards to prevent neurologic complications after epidural steroid injections: consensus opinions from a multidisciplinary working group and national organizations. Anesthesiology. 2015;122(5):974–84.
7. Woods BI, Hilibrand AS. Cervical radiculopathy: epidemiology, etiology, diagnosis, and treatment. J Spinal Disord Tech. 2015;28(5):E251–9.

Cervical Transforaminal Epidural Injections

40

Anish Sethi and Dajie Wang

Introduction

Cervical radicular pain is a common cause of neck and upper extremity pain, affecting approximately 83 per 100,000 people per year. For individuals affected by this, the most common cause of cervical radiculitis was cervical spondylosis in 68.4% of cases and cervical disk herniation in 21.9% of cases. Both pathologies can produce anatomic stenosis resulting in impingement or compression of nerve roots or the spinal cord. The etiology varies by patient age, with intervertebral disk herniation common in younger persons and spondylosis predominating in the older age group. Cervical spondylosis is present in 75% of patients older than 65 years of age.

Patients with cervical radiculopathy often present with neck pain with radicular upper extremity pain, weakness, and deep tendon reflex depression. The pain description ranges from a dull ache to a severe burning pain. As the radiculopathy progresses, the pain radiates to the upper or lower arm and into the hand, along the sensory distribution of the involved nerve root.

Initial treatment typically consists of conservative management options. Conservative treatment includes physical therapy, therapeutic exercises and stretches, and activity modification. Nonsteroidal anti-inflammatory medications and adjuvants such as muscle relaxants may be initiated. If there is minimal improvement with conservative treatment, cervical epidural steroid injections may be performed. Symptoms refractory to conservative therapy or symptoms consistent with cervical myelopathy necessitate consideration for surgical intervention. Current treatment strategies typically involve a gradual progression in the invasiveness of intervention, progressing from less to more invasive interventions only in refractory cases.

Cervical epidural steroids may be administered utilizing either the interlaminar or transforaminal approach. The transforaminal injection approach provides a direct route for medication delivery to the neuroforamen to target pathology. The interlaminar approach may fail to deliver adequate volumes of medication to areas of foraminal narrowing and pathology located distally in the anterolateral epidural space or neuroforamen. Medication may instead spread to areas of lower resistance to liquid flow, such as spreading through the dorsal epidural space with the interlaminar approach.

Background and Historical Perspective

In 1952, Robecchi and Capra reported the treatment of lumbar disk herniation with periradicular hydrocortisone. This is the first documented use of epidural steroids targeted at an inflamed nerve root. The use of cervical epidural steroids for cervical radiculopathy has been documented in articles dating back to 1961. It is unclear when the first cervical transforaminal epidural steroid injection (TFESI) was performed. The primary rationale for administering epidural corticosteroids is attributed to the anti-inflammatory affect. Cervical herniated disk specimens have demonstrated increased levels of hyperalgesic inflammatory markers, matrix metalloproteinase activity, nitric oxide, prostaglandin E2, and interleukin-6. In addition, phospholipase A2 also plays a role in nerve root inflammation and may even be neurotoxic. Epidural steroids have been shown to inhibit phospholipase A2 activity. Corticosteroids alter cell-mediated activity and cytokines, which has been implicated in the pathogenesis of radicular pain.

Corticosteroids have actions other than anti-inflammatory effects. Corticosteroids stabilize nerve membranes by inhibiting ectopic impulses and ion conductance and hyperpolarizing spinal neurons. Corticosteroids have been shown to inhibit C fiber transmission, which may explain relief of symptoms in non-inflammatory states.

Local anesthetic mixed with the corticosteroid may have additional benefits beyond the direct anesthetic affects. Lidocaine has been shown to have anti-inflammatory effect on nucleus pulposus-induced nerve injury. Lidocaine has been demonstrated to increase intra-radicular blood flow in

A. Sethi · D. Wang (✉)
Chronic Pain Medicine, Department of Anesthesiology, Thomas Jefferson University Hospital, Philadelphia, PA, USA
e-mail: dajie.wang@jefferson.edu

T. R. Deer et al. (eds.), *Deer's Treatment of Pain*, https://doi.org/10.1007/978-3-030-12281-2_40

an animal compressed nerve root model, which may improve intraneural metabolism and reduce inflammatory mediators.

Uses and Indications

Cervical transforaminal epidural steroid injections can be utilized to treat cervical radiculopathy, oftentimes after failure of conservative treatment including physical therapy, activity modification, and medications. Epidural injection in the cervical spine can be performed by either the interlaminar or transforaminal approach. Cervical transforaminal epidural steroid injections utilizes a small-volume injection that directly targets the compressed nerve root as it exits the neuroforamen, which is frequently the site of pathology.

The performance of cervical transforaminal epidural steroid injections can serve both a diagnostic and therapeutic purpose. While a combination of clinical examination, imaging, and electromyography may help identify the pathologic vertebral level, interventional pain specialists can perform diagnostic cervical TFESI's to confirm the precise causative symptomatic spinal level. The presence of pain relief by injecting local anesthetic and steroids at a level can assist in surgical planning. In addition, Costandi et al. demonstrated that a patient's response to cervical TFESI can be used to predict surgical outcomes.

Technique

Prior to starting the procedure, the physician should review any existing imaging in order to properly ascertain the anatomy of affected portions of the cervical spine. Prior to the procedure, intravenous access should be obtained, and the patient should be placed on standard monitors. The patient is positioned supine on the fluoroscopy table. A blanket is placed under the patient's head in order to keep the neck parallel to the table, and the patient is prepped and draped in a sterile manner.

Lateral fluoroscopic images should be obtained of the cervical spine (see Fig. 40.1). After the targeted neurofora-

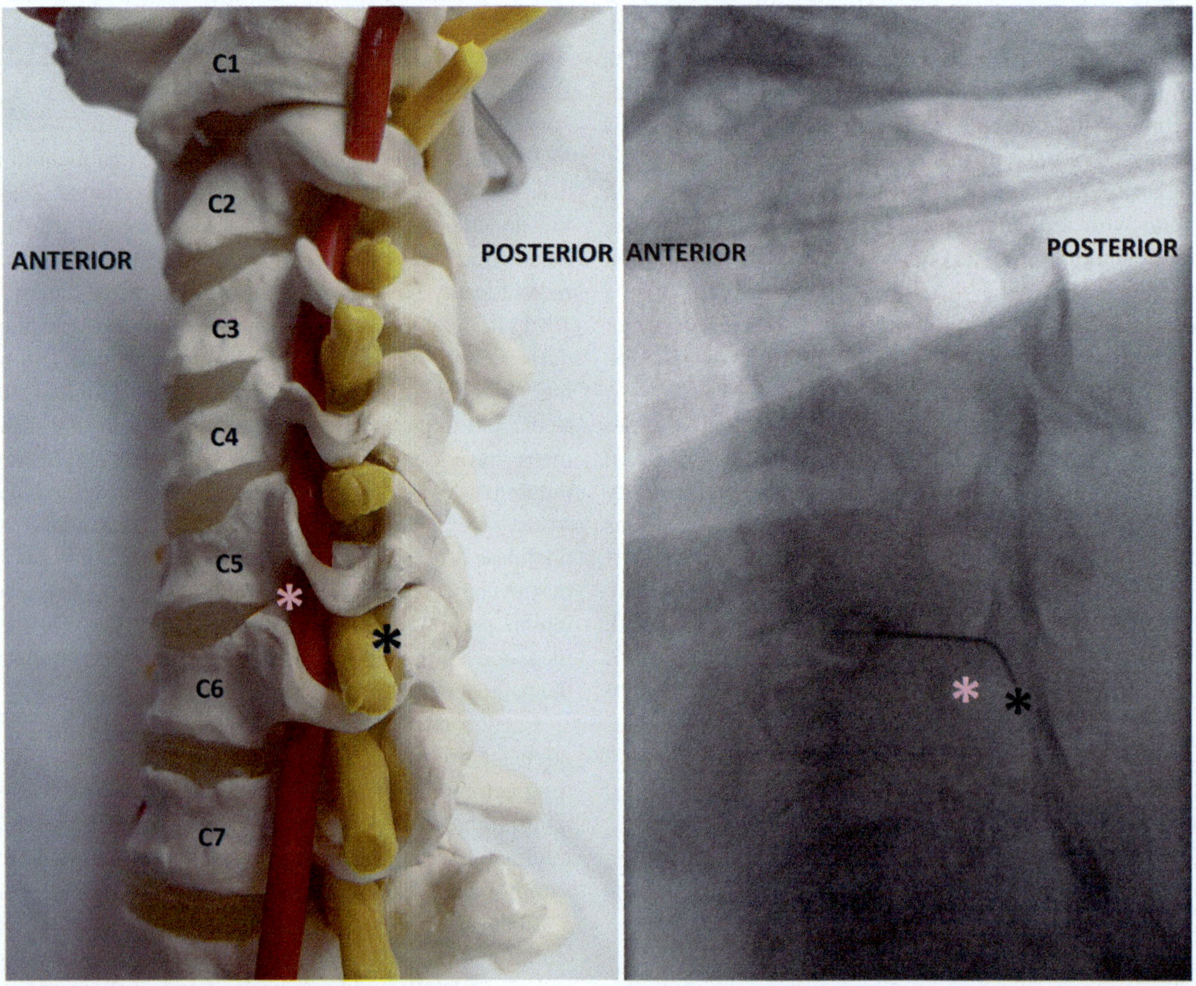

Fig. 40.1 *Left:* Spine model illustrating location of spinal nerve roots in relationship to neuroforamen. Note the vertebral artery running in the anterior portion of the neuroforamen. *Right:* Lateral fluoroscopic image obtained during left C5-C6 transforaminal epidural steroid injection targeting the C6 nerve root. The pink marker corresponds to needle entry point in the anterior foramen, and the black marker corresponds to the needle target in the posterior neuroforamen

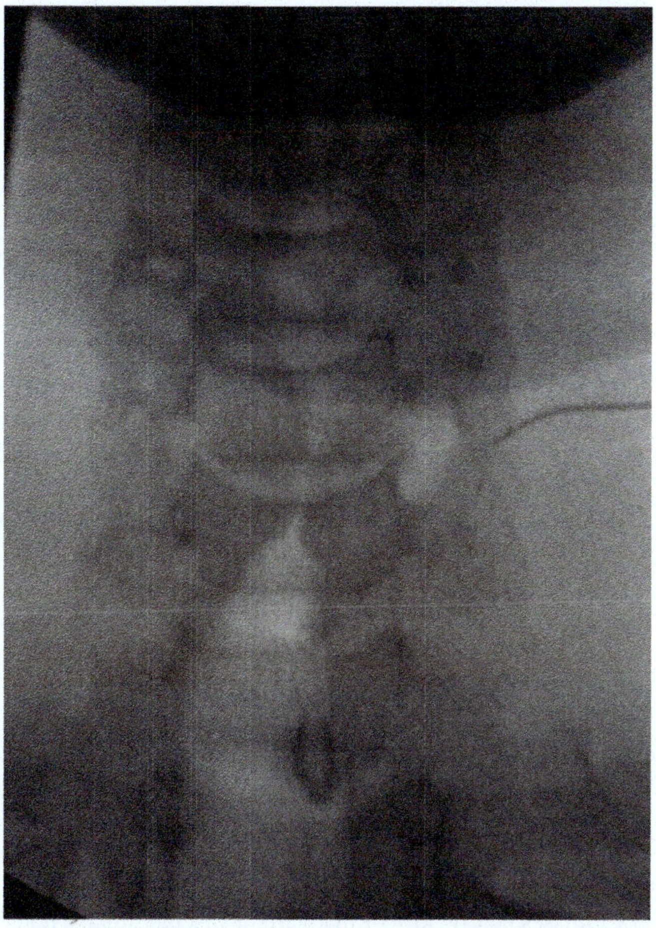

Fig. 40.2 AP fluoroscopic view of needle position during left C5-C6 transforaminal epidural injection. The needle tip should be lateral to the border of the uncovertebral joint

men is identified, the visualization of the neuroforamen is optimized by rotating the fluoroscope. The midpoint of the anterior neuroforamen is marked and used as the needle entry site. A skin wheal with local anesthetic at the needle entry site should be performed. The spinal needle should be advanced toward to posterior midpoint of the neuroforamen. After the needle is positioned in the posterior-lateral aspect of the neuroforamen, it is then further advanced into the neuroforamen under the AP fluoroscopic view. The needle tip should be placed slightly beyond the lateral border of uncovertebral joint (see Fig. 40.2). In lateral view, the needle tip should be in the mid-to-posterior portion of the affected neuroforamen. If the nerve is contacted, the needle should be slightly retracted off the nerve. Extension tubing should be attached to the needle hub; radiologic contrast should be injected under live fluoroscopy. While this occurs, it is important to check for spread of contrast over the nerve root (see Fig. 40.3). More importantly, inadvertent intravascular, intrathecal, or subdural spread should be monitored. If any of these occur, the needle should be retracted, and the procedure should be aborted. The needle may be slightly repositioned to obtain adequate nerve-root spread.

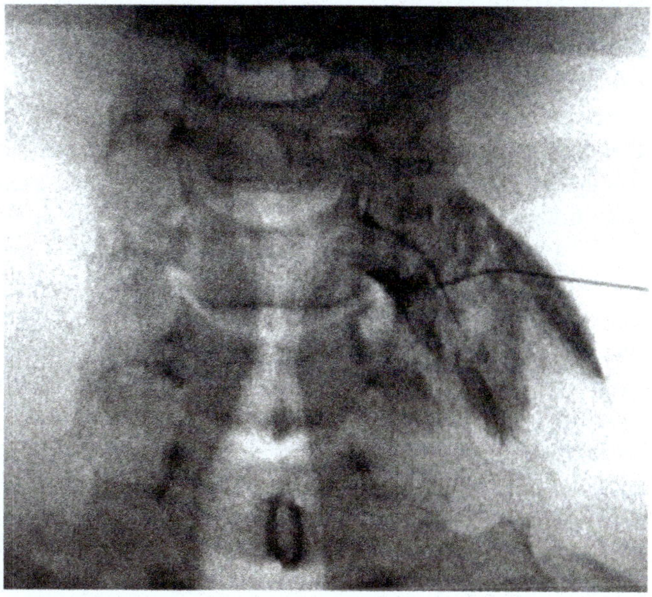

Fig. 40.3 AP fluoroscopic view taken during left C5-C6 transforaminal epidural injection, during injection of contrast, with spread of contrast along the left C6 nerve root. Note small amount of contrast spread in left paraspinal musculature as well

Ideally, contrast should outline the affected nerve root, with no evidence of vascular spread. Techniques to avoid intravascular injection, including intermittent aspiration, digital subtraction angiography, and administration of a test dose, will be covered later in this chapter. If there are no issues with needle placement, steroids may be injected slowly into the area. Frequent imaging and patient querying should be performed throughout the needle placement and injection process to minimize the risk of complications.

Evidence for Efficacy

The efficacy of transforaminal cervical epidural steroid injections for patients experiencing radicular symptoms has been demonstrated through multiple studies. However, most of these are non-randomized or retrospective studies. Additionally, there are studies that indicate that cervical ESIs may either delay or prevent patients from undergoing surgical intervention.

Compared to the interlaminar approach, the transforaminal approach has the advantage of being able to place medication adjacent to the nerve root implicated in causing pain. Stojanovic et al. demonstrated that medication spread in interlaminar ESI was unilateral in 51% of cases and ventral in only 28% of cases. Foraminal stenosis, disk herniations, and epidural fibrosis can potentially hinder the flow of medication from the interlaminar approach to reach the effected nerve root. Vallee et al. prospectively studied 32 subjects with radicular cervical pain unresponsive to medical therapy who underwent cervical TFESI and noted that greater than 50% pain relief occurred in 56% of patients at 6 months' follow-up.

Slipman et al. retrospectively studied 20 patients who underwent cervical TFESI for radicular pain due to cervical spondylotic foraminal stenosis. Follow-up was performed at a mean time of 21.2 months. This study showed that 60% of patients had good to excellent results from an average of 2.2 TFESIs. The subjects' pain scores decreased from 6.9 to 2.0.

Kolstad et al. studied 21 patients with unilateral cervical radiculopathy secondary to disk herniation or spondylosis confirmed by MRI or myelography. The subjects received two cervical TFESIs at a 2-week interval while awaiting operative treatment. After receiving the injection treatment, 5 of the 21 patients decided to cancel their surgery due to significant clinical improvement. In addition, they noted a statistically significant reduction in radicular pain score.

Anderberg et al. conducted a prospective, randomized study in which 40 patients with unilateral radicular pain and cervical spondylosis confirmed by MRI were enrolled. Patients were randomized for treatment with steroids/local anesthetic or saline/local anesthetic, and follow-up was performed at 3 weeks. Subjective improvement in sustained pain relief occurred for eight subjects in the steroid group and seven subjects in the saline group. There were no statistically significant differences in short-term pain control from the epidural steroids. This study suggested that beneficial effect can be achieved for radicular pain in selected patients, and perhaps local anesthetic alone may also provide sustained pain relief.

Several studies evaluated patients who are in the planning phase of surgical intervention. Lin et al. retrospectively studied 70 patients with radicular pain from disk herniation who underwent a trial cervical TFESI, prior to surgical intervention. Mean follow-up was at 13 months, and 65.33% of subjects had good to excellent relief according to Odom's criteria. Additionally, 63% of subjects had significant relief of their symptoms and did not wish to proceed with surgery. There were favorable results obtained in patients who were over age 50 and had symptom duration for less than 100 days. There were no complications reported from cervical TFESI in this study.

While cervical TFESI is typically performed with fluoroscopy, it may also be performed with CT guidance or ultrasound guidance. Desai et al. followed 50 patients for 3 months after CT-guided cervical selective nerve root block and reported a statistically significant reduction in pain and disability for at least 3 months. Cyteval et al. collected retrospective data on 30 patients who underwent CT-guided cervical TFESI and was able to demonstrate a statistically significant 51% improvement in pain scores 2 weeks postinjection and a significant improvement in 6-month pain scores.

Pearls and Pitfalls

The transforaminal approach was developed to deliver medication directly to the affected nerve root. In the hands of experienced interventionalists, the complication rate for cervical TFESI was reported as 0.32–1.6% in two studies which evaluated over 1000 injections. Possible complications with cervical TFESI include dural puncture, trauma to the spinal nerve, infection, side effects of radiation exposure, vasovagal reaction, and allergic and anaphylactic reaction to the medication. Few case reports exist on the more devastating complication of spinal cord vascular injury resulting in infarction and neurological deficit. In a few cases, catastrophic complications included quadriplegia and even death. While no registry exists regarding complications, these several case reports highlighted the potential catastrophic adverse outcomes.

There is a growing body of evidence to suggest that the major causative agent of neurologic infarct is due to the inadvertent injection of particulate corticosteroids into the vertebral artery or radiculomedullary artery, resulting in microembolic ischemia or infarction. As a result, multiple strategies are employed by interventional pain physicians to avoid this complication. Aspiration for blood is a simple technique that can be employed. However, while it was shown to have high specificity, it had low sensitivity. Utilizing intermittent fluoroscopy to identify vascular uptake of contrast misses nearly 50% of inadvertent vascular uptake noted during live fluoroscopy. As such, it would be beneficial to utilize live fluoroscopy to observe dynamic spread of contrast.

Digital subtraction angiography (DSA) was shown to increase the rate of intravascular detection from 18% to 33%, nearly doubling the detection rate. In DSA, blood vessels are better-visualized in a bony or dense soft tissue environment. DSA images are produced by "subtracting" a pre-contrast fluoroscopic image from later images that were obtained after the contrast is administered. This results in bony structures and spinal instrumentation becoming "subtracted," generating an unobscured image of blood vessels. This can assist in identifying any potential intravascular contrast uptake.

The use of an anesthetic test dose can be utilized to detect potentially dangerous intravascular injections. The test dose is performed by injecting a small amount of local anesthetic after confirming appropriate needle placement with the use of other modalities (e.g., contrast spread, DSA, etc.). A positive test dose would be evidenced by signs of intravascular local anesthetic injection, including perioral numbness, tinnitus, dizziness, motor deficits, parasthesias, or CNS changes. These side effects are typically short-lived. The purpose of the test dose is to prevent potentially harmful injections of intravascular particulate. Smuck et al. studied 678 cervical TFESIs and found a positive test dose in four cases (0.59%). While this is a small number of individuals, the test dose had most likely prevented potentially catastrophic complications.

Another risk that exists during cervical TFESI is inadvertent subdural or intrathecal injection, due to the close proximity to spinal cord anatomical structures. The subdural layer in the cervical region is larger compared to the subdural layer in the lumbar region, making the risk of accidental subdural injection higher in the cervical spine. With inadvertent subdural injection, only a small volume of local anesthetic solution is required to produce significant neurological and hemodynamic complications, including loss of consciousness, severe hypotension, bradycardia, and even cardiac arrest.

Proper needle placement is critical in avoiding potential complications from cervical TFESI. Conventionally, the ideal position within the foramen is mid-to-posterior foramen, in order to avoid potential vertebral artery injection. However, as demonstrated in a cadaveric study by Huntoon, 21 out of 95 intervertebral foramina dissected had an arterial vessel in the posterior aspect of the foramen. In addition, while the vertebral artery is typically located in the anterior foramen, radiographic studies indicate that vertebral artery anomalies are present in 7.6% of patients. Critical arteries located in the posterior aspect of the foramen may be vulnerable to injection or injury during cervical TFESI. The vertebral artery may be avoided by coaxial to the foramen over the posterior aspect of the foramen. As studied by Huntoon, the likelihood of encountering a radicular artery during cervical transforaminal injection appears to be greatest at the lower cervical-spinal levels (C5-T1). In addition, the caliber of the radicular artery as it enters the foramen at the level of the C8 spinal nerve is large enough to allow placement of a 22-gauge needle within the lumen. The inherent variability in vessel anatomy as well as the rich blood supply within the foramen necessitates extreme caution during needle placement. Needle placement should always be confirmed with fluoroscopy guidance.

Needle size itself has not shown to decrease the incident of intravascular injection during transforaminal epidural steroid injection. Smuck et al. demonstrated that there was no statistical difference in the rate of vascular injection between different gauges of needles. In addition, the same study suggested that compared to long-bevel needles, short-bevel needles do not reduce the risk of inadvertent vascular injection in transforaminal epidural injections.

Many practitioners subscribe to light conscious sedation during needle placement, especially during injection. This allows real-time feedback from the patient regarding pain, neurologic or mental status changes, or any focal deficits that may occur during injection. In addition, needle manipulation after contrast injection should be limited. Given the anatomy of the blood vessels, miniscule changes in needle position can cause the needle to migrate into a blood vessel lumen. Oftentimes, utilizing extension tubing can limit needle movement while performing syringe changes.

Much debate has existed regarding the type of steroid injected, primarily regarding particulate (e.g., triamcinolone, methylprednisolone) versus non-particulate (e.g., dexamethasone) steroids. Particulate steroid particles are larger than red blood cells, and there is concern for inadvertent arterial injection of particulate steroids leading to microembolic ischemia. Animal studies suggest that intravascular particulate steroid injection can cause serious neurologic deficits, while animals injected with non-particulate steroids experienced no neurologic compromise [H]. Tiso et al. presented a case of quadriparesis and brainstem herniation after inadvertent intra-arterial injection of particulate corticosteroid during cervical TFESI. Light microscopy data provided evidence that methylprednisolone and triamcinolone had a tendency to coalesce into large aggregates of greater than 100 μm. This data becomes especially relevant when one considers that arterioles are 10–15 μm and capillaries are 5–8 μm.

In order to compare the efficacy of particulate versus non-particulate steroids, Dreyfuss et al. compared outcomes from 30 subjects with cervical radiculopathy, half of the subjects received cervical TFESI with non-particulate dexamethasone, while the remaining half received cervical TFESI with particulate triamcinolone. While both groups exhibited statistically and clinically significant improvements, the difference between the groups was not significantly different. The authors concluded that given a lack of major difference between the two steroids, it would be prudent to utilize non-particulate agents in order to avoid potential vascular occlusion. A multidisciplinary team of specialty stakeholders was assembled by the US Food and Drug Administration in order to enhance of the safety of epidural steroid injections. The team published guidelines in 2015, which unanimously approved that only non-particulate steroids be used in therapeutic cervical transforaminal injections.

Recommended Reading

1. Anderberg L, Annertz M, Persson L, Brandt L, Säveland H. Transforaminal steroid injections for the treatment of cervical radiculopathy: a prospective and randomised study. Eur Spine J. 2007;16(3):321–8.
2. Benzon HT, Huntoon MA, Rathmell JP. Improving the safety of epidural steroid injec-tions. JAMA. 2015;313:1713–4.
3. Costandi SJ, Azer G, Eshraghi Y, et al. Cervical transforaminal epidural steroid injections: diagnostic and therapeutic value. Reg Anesth Pain Med. 2015;40(6):674–80.

4. Desai A, Saha S, Sharma N, Huckerby L, Houghton R. The short- and medium-term effectiveness of CT-guided selective cervical nerve root injection for pain and disability. Skelet Radiol. 2014;43(7):973–8.
5. Dreyfuss P, Baker R, Bogduk N. Comparative effectiveness of cervical transforaminal injections with particulate and nonparticulate corticosteroid preparations for cervical radicular pain. Pain Med. 2006;7(3):237–42.
6. Hoeft MA, Rathmell JP, Monsey RD, Fonda BJ. Cervical transforaminal injection and the radicular artery: variation in anatomical location within the cervical intervertebral foramina. Reg Anesth Pain Med. 2006;31(3):270–4.
7. Huntoon MA. Anatomy of the cervical intervertebral foramina: vulnerable arteries and ischemic neurologic injuries after transforaminal epidural injections. Pain. 2005;117:104–11.
8. Huston CW. Cervical epidural steroid injections in the management of cervical radiculitis: interlaminar versus transforaminal. A review. Curr Rev Musculoskelet Med. 2009;2(1):30–42.
9. Kolstad F, Leivseth G, Nygaard OP. Transforaminal steroid injections in the treatment of cervical radiculopathy. A prospective outcome study. Acta Neurochir. 2005;147(10):1065–70.
10. Lin EL, Lieu V, Halevi L, Shamie AN, Wang JC. Cervical epidural steroid injections for symptomatic disc herniations. J Spinal Disord Tech. 2006;19(3):183–6.
11. Ma DJ, Gilula LA, Riew KD. Complications of fluoroscopically guided extraforaminal cervical nerve blocks. An analysis of 1036 injections. J Bone Joint Surg Am. 2005;87(5):1025–30.
12. Mclean JP, Sigler JD, Plastaras CT, Garvan CW, Rittenberg JD. The rate of detection of intravascular injection in cervical transforaminal epidural steroid injections with and without digital subtraction angiography. PM R. 2009;1(7):636–42.
13. Okubadejo GO, Talcott MR, Schmidt RE, et al. Perils of intravascular methylprednisolone injection into the vertebral artery. An animal study. J Bone Joint Surg Am. 2008;90(9):1932–8.
14. Radhakrishnan K, Litchy WJ, O'Fallon WM, et al. Epidemiology of cervical radiculopathy. A population-based study from Rochester, Minnesota, 1976 through 1990. Brain. 1994;117(Pt 2):325–35.
15. Rathmell JP, Aprill C, Bogduk N. Cervical transforaminal injection of steroids. Anesthesiology. 2004;100(6):1595–600.
16. Rathmell JP, Benzon HT, Dreyfuss P, et al. Safeguards to prevent neurologic complications after epidural steroid injections: consensus opinions from a multidisciplinary working group and national organizations. Anesthesiology. 2015;122:974–84.
17. Rowlingson JC, Kirschenbaum LP. Epidural analgesic techniques in the management of cervical pain. Anesth Analg. 1986;65(9):938–42.
18. Rozin L, Rozin R, Koehler SA, et al. Death during transforaminal epidural steroid nerve root block (C7) due to perforation of the left vertebral artery. Am J Forensic Med Pathol. 2003;24(4):351–5.
19. Slipman CW, Lipetz JS, Jackson HB, Rogers DP, Vresilovic EJ. Therapeutic selective nerve root block in the nonsurgical treatment of atraumatic cervical spondylotic radicular pain: a retrospective analysis with independent clinical review. Arch Phys Med Rehabil. 2000;81(6):741–6.
20. Smuck M, Yu AJ, Tang CT, Zemper E. Influence of needle type on the incidence of intravascular injection during transforaminal epidural injections: a comparison of short-bevel and long-bevel needles. Spine J. 2010;10(5):367–71.
21. Smuck M, Maxwell MD, Kennedy D, Rittenberg JD, Lansberg MG, Plastaras CT. Utility of the anesthetic test dose to avoid catastrophic injury during cervical transforaminal epidural injections. Spine J. 2010;10(10):857–64.
22. Stojanovic MP, Vu TN, Caneris O, Slezak J, Cohen SP, Sang CN. The role of fluoroscopy in cervical epidural steroid injections: an analysis of contrast dispersal patterns. Spine. 2002;27(5):509–14.
23. Thierry-mieg J. Cervical epidural injections of corticoids in hyperalgiccervico-brachial neuralgias. 1st cervical epidurographical pictures. Rev Rhum Mal Osteoartic. 1961;28:451–3.

Diagnostic Cervical Nerve Root Blocks

41

Kiran K. Koneti and Ashish Gulve

Introduction

Cervical radiculopathy is a disabling condition frequently encountered in pain medicine practice. Average annual age-adjusted incidence is estimated to be about 0.1% of population. Female gender and white race were implicated as potential risk factors in a recent study of US military personnel. Cigarette smoking, axial load bearing and prior lumbar radiculopathy may also predispose patients to cervical radiculopathy. The classical clinical picture includes neck pain with radiation of pain to the arm and fingers corresponding to the dermatomes involved. Paraesthesias in arm and hand in conjunction with diminished muscle tendon reflexes, sensory disturbances and/or motor weakness with dermatomal/myotomal distribution are also common. In some patients radiating symptoms may not be present, and pain may be isolated to the shoulder. Pain may not always be the presenting complaint, as sensory or motor deficits may present without pain. The cervical radiculopathy can be due to degenerative conditions such as cervical disc prolapse alone (in about 20–25% of cases). Nevertheless the most common cause of root compression at the cervical level is narrowing of the foraminal space secondary to spondyloarthrosis. The most common level of root compression is usually C7, followed by C6. It is more commonly due to a combination of factors, which include disc herniation, osteoarthritis of uncovertebral and facet joints, decreased disc height and spondylolisthesis of cervical vertebrae – collectively known as cervical spondylosis. Less common causes include nerve root compression by tumour or due to cervical trauma.

The natural course of radiculopathy due to degenerative aetiologies is generally favourable, with a majority of patients reporting spontaneous resolution of symptoms over a period of time with physical therapy and/or oral medication. In a study involving a cohort of 51 patients with cervical radiculopathy managed nonoperatively, review at 10 years revealed that 42% were asymptomatic, 30% had mild symptoms and 28% had moderate symptoms. Similar natural resolution of symptoms was also reported in a large population-based study from Rochester, Minnesota.

A minority of patients, in whom natural resolution of symptoms is not seen, do end up having persistent disabling pain requiring some form of intervention. Surgical treatment, because of the well-known drawbacks, including perioperative complications, limitation of range of motion and/or adjacent segment degeneration, is generally reserved for unremitting and severe pain in patients in whom nonoperative treatments have failed. One effective modality of treatment for patients with unremitting pain is injection of steroid and local anaesthetic in the nerve root foramen into the periradicular space – 'cervical selective nerve root block' (CSNRB).

Besides ameliorating radiculopathy due to disc herniation and cervical spinal stenosis, CSNRB can improve symptoms temporarily prior to surgery or improve persistent pain after discectomy. Furthermore, the technique can be used for both diagnostic and therapeutic purposes.

Diagnostic Rationale

Spinal nerve segmental level of involvement may not be discernible owing to variability of pain referral patterns. Additionally, imaging studies or electrodiagnostic studies may not elucidate the segmental level of involvement. Diagnostic selective spinal nerve blocks (SSNB) are often called spinal nerve root blocks (SNRB); however, because anaesthetic is placed directly on the spinal nerve and not directly on the nerve root, correct anatomical nomenclature dictates that the procedure be called a selective spinal nerve block. A selective nerve root block is a spinal procedure in

K. K. Koneti
Department of Anaesthetics, Sunderland Royal Hospitals, Sunderland, UK

A. Gulve (✉)
Department of Pain Management, The James Cook University Hospital, Middlesbrough, UK
e-mail: ashishgulve@nhs.net

T. R. Deer et al. (eds.), *Deer's Treatment of Pain*, https://doi.org/10.1007/978-3-030-12281-2_41

which anaesthetic is placed on a specific nerve root of the spine to help identify the exact source of leg or arm pain. The injection is similar to a transforaminal epidural steroid injection, but in a selective nerve root block, there is no attempt to have the medication enter the epidural space. Rather, the aim is strictly to cover the offending nerve root.

SSNBs corroborate well with surgically confirmed pathology (87–100%) and prove favourable when compared with EMG, CT or myelography in predicting the level of lesion. Positive SSNBs provide important prognostic information about surgical outcome. Even when appropriately limited volumes of anaesthetic were not used, negative responses to blocks possessed predictive value. Lack of pain relief from a technically successful diagnostic nerve root block would accurately predict failure of a permanent surgical procedure.

Diagnostic Indications

Selective spinal nerve blocks (SSNBs) test the hypothesis that the spinal nerve transmits or is the pain source. To maintain diagnostic specificity, local anaesthetic is instilled along a spinal nerve and not onto adjacent structures or the epidural space. SSNB is a diagnostic test performed to identify a segmental level when negative or equivocal imaging studies are associated with clinical findings of nerve root irritation. Typically diagnostic cervical nerve root blocks are useful when the clinical picture is not clearly determining the exact culprit cervical nerve root level. Diagnostic blocks, despite their incompletely proven validity, are helpful in determining level of the surgery, guiding subsequent therapy and predicting if the patient would benefit from the surgery or not. These are particularly useful if radicular symptoms prove refractory to conservative interventions and surgery is being considered.

Therapeutic Injection Rationale

Therapeutic SNRBs do have some role especially if surgery is not considered or if patient is refusing surgery and still looking for pain control options. However, there is a need for combining steroid along with the local anaesthetic to extend the duration of pain relief. There is also role for action on the dorsal root ganglion in modulating the pain. Due to the multifactorial nature of the pain, the transforaminal epidural steroid injections (TFESIs) can be very helpful in the management of cervical radicular symptoms. Transforaminal epidural injections deposit medication along the affected nerve root and into the anterior epidural space at the site of inflammation. Cervical spinal stenosis (central or foraminal) and herniated nucleus pulposus can induce nerve root inflammation. Inflammation of the nerve root induces neurophysiologic and histologic changes that can result in radicular symptoms. Corticosteroid reduces morphologic and functional nerve root changes, and lidocaine decreases nerve root inflammation while increasing intraradicular blood flow. While there are no randomized controlled trials, efficacy studies for cervical transforaminal injections are ongoing. Recent studies have revealed that these injections can decrease pain and help patients avoid surgery. Evidence for cervical TFESI for axial neck pain is limited. Investigation has also demonstrated equal efficacy with particulate or non-particulate corticosteroid. This may be valuable when considering the risk associated with intravascular injection of particulate matter.

Therapeutic Indications

Cervical transforaminal epidural steroid injections can be performed for upper extremity radicular symptoms refractory to conservative interventions including medications and physical therapy. With severe limitation of function, one could perform the injection prior to the initiation of more conservative options to facilitate physiotherapy and rehabilitation therapies. There is no role for a series of cervical transforaminal epidural injections given without regard to the response of the initial or previous injection. A subsequent injection may be considered in a patient with partial or temporary pain relief from a previous injection. While there is limited evidence in the area of repeat injections, consensus indicates that, with rare exception, injections should be limited to three in a 6-month period or four in a year. These should ideally be spaced by at least 14 days to assess full response and minimize adrenal suppression.

Contraindications

Absolute

- Bacterial infection: systemic or localized at injection site
- Coagulopathy/bleeding diathesis: due to anticoagulants or haematological disease
- Anaphylaxis to local anaesthetic/injecting substance

Relative

- Allergy to injectants
- Steroid psychosis
- Pregnancy
- NSAIDS, aspirin or other antiplatelet agents (e.g. Ticlid, Plavix, Coumadin, Trental, Pletal, heparin, Lovenox, Innohep, Fragmin, Normiflo, Persantine, Aggrenox, *Ginkgo biloba*, Orgaran and Danaparoid)
- Hyperglycaemia, adrenal suppression, immunocompromised patient or congestive heart failure

Complications

Potential complications include but are not limited to:

- Infection (epidural abscess, discitis, meningitis, arachnoiditis, osteomyelitis, sepsis)
- Bleeding (epidural and subdural hematoma)
- Cardiovascular (dysrhythmias, congestive heart failure, hypotension, bradycardia, vasovagal reaction)
- Respiratory (over sedation, central nervous system trauma, excessive intrathecal or epidural local anaesthetic injection, pneumothorax, recurrent laryngeal nerve injury)
- Urologic (urinary retention, incontinence)
- Neurologic injury (direct neural trauma, compression from hematoma or abscess, radicular or vertebral artery trauma, embolization of particulate steroids or air, stroke, spinal cord injury, seizure)
- Dural puncture (spinal headache, uncal herniation, arachnoiditis, spinal block)
- Adverse local anaesthetic drug reaction (CNS and cardiovascular toxicity, restlessness, anxiety, incoherent speech, light-headedness, perioral paraesthesia, blurred vision, tremors, drowsiness, seizures, cardiac arrest, excessive intrathecal or epidural local anaesthetic injection resulting in spinal block or arm weakness)
- Adverse steroid reaction (facial flushing, injection site hypopigmentation, subcutaneous fat atrophy, increased appetite, fluid retention, gastritis, malaise, euphoria, insomnia, headache, immunosuppression, aseptic meningitis, arachnoiditis, congestive heart failure, increased intraocular pressures, adrenal insufficiency, steroid myopathy, rapid mood swings such as becoming aggressive, irritable and short-tempered, mania, hyperglycaemia, hypertension, epidural lipomatosis, menstrual irregularity)
- Allergic reaction (to non-ionic contrast agent allergy, local anaesthetic, corticosteroid, or latex causing urticaria, laryngeal oedema, bronchospasm, anaphylaxis)

Potential post-procedural complaints include but are not limited to:

- Vasovagal reaction (hypotension, bradycardia, nausea, pallor, diaphoresis, syncope)
- Pain (injection site, radicular, corticosteroid flare)
- Headache (corticosteroids, dural puncture)

Prerequisites for the Procedure

History and Physical Examination

A detailed history and physical examination are required to exclude non-radicular pain and to exclude any contraindications. Pain maps are used to establish the dermatomes involved and select the target nerves in the first instance. A history and physical examination including full neurological examination are required to record baseline data concerning the location and extent of pain, including a visual analogue score, and quality of life measures. This technique should be avoided if there is any evidence motor weakness.

Consent

Informed consent is essential. Similar to any invasive procedure, they carry the nominal risk of vasovagal syncope, infection, bleeding and allergic reaction. Patients can get temporary motor block on the injected side and also increased tingling and numbness due to sensory blockade. Some can experience numbness of the neck and face due to local anaesthetic infiltration of the skin resulting in blockade of superficial/deep cervical plexus branches. Risks of accidental nerve or spinal cord injury and very rare risk of paralysis need to be discussed. Accidental intravascular injection especially in vertebral or segmental arteries can lead to fits. Some patients can get transient hypotension. Steroids would generally be used in therapeutic rather than diagnostic injections. Steroid-related side effects listed in the complications need to be discussed with patient. Post-dural puncture headache, though rare, with a technically sound procedure, has been reported after nerve root blocks due to puncture of dural sleeves. After upper cervical blocks, the patient is likely to suffer a sense of ataxia transiently. These risks should be explained to the patient who should be advised of the precautions to be taken. The lower cervical root injections also pose risk of sympathetic block of the stellate ganglion and should be careful to warn the patient and watch for the same.

The patient should be advised that the procedure is a diagnostic one and should not be confused with a therapeutic procedure. They should be advised that they may or may not obtain relief and especially if the pain is not related to the nerve root being injected. Patients will need to monitor and record the duration and extent of any symptom relief. Immediate pain relief following the procedure needs to be assessed and documented prior to discharge of the patient. It is not unusual to have temporary increase in pain after the local anaesthetic effect has waned.

Location

Ideal to perform the procedure in a sterile environment (operating theatre/dedicated treatment suites) with adequate monitoring facilities. The minimal monitoring standards include monitoring with pulse oximetry, NIBP and ECG. Usually done as day-case procedures in many parts of the world. Full resuscitation facilities and staff trained in resuscitation should be available.

Sedation

Sedation by IV or oral route is not recommended for diagnostic procedures because it can alter the patient's interpretation of the pain relief and could compromise the diagnostic accuracy of the injection. Separating the pain relief duration which is usually short lasting from the procedure and sedation is difficult to determine and can lead to false-positive response.

Resuscitation Equipment

Although misadventure attributable to the agents injected is extremely unlikely, given the small doses injected for cervical nerve root blocks, it is safer to perform the procedure in a facility fully equipped with proper resuscitation facilities and personnel trained to do resuscitation. At the very least, the operator is equipped to deal with possible allergic reactions to local anaesthetic agents.

Materials

A. *Equipment and supplies*
   1. Fluoroscopy/CT guidance/ultrasound machine
   2. 22–25 gauge spinal or Chiba needle
   3. Medication and contrast syringes (various sizes with labels)
   4. Physiological monitoring
   5. Connection tubing (optional so that contrast can be injected during live fluoroscopic visualization or digital substraction angiography to confirm proper anatomical and extra-vascular needle placement)
   6. Skin marker (optional)

B. *Medications*
   1. Sedation should be avoided.
   2. Resuscitation drugs.

C. *Injectate agents*
   1. Non-ionic radiographic contrast medium (e.g. Iohexol, Niopam 300 or Omnipaque 240).
   2. Local anaesthetic or other agent (optional).
   3. Volumes range from 1 ml to 5 ml. Common agents includes lidocaine 1–2% or bupivacaine 0.125–0.50%. Low volumes of injection would improve diagnostic accuracy.
   4. Corticosteroids – Only non-particulate preservative free steroids should be used. Agents commonly used include but are not limited to dose equivalent of betamethasone sodium phosphate and betamethasone acetate (6–18 mg) and dexamethasone (Decadron Phosphate). For a diagnostic block, corticosteroids should be avoided.

Technique

A. *Preparation*

Physiologic monitoring and intravenous access is recommended. Skin is prepared with usual antiseptic preparation in a wider area around the needle entry point and covered by sterile drape (ideal to have transparent one) without suffocating the patient with the drape. The authors use chlorhexidine gluconate and isopropyl alcohol for preoperative skin prep.

B. *Target identification*

Thorough anatomical knowledge and better understanding of the pathology are essential. Interpretation of the image guidance is equally important. However, to achieve precision and avoiding complications, which at times can be potentially fatal with cervical nerve root injections, various techniques have evolved over decades. Fluoroscopy is still widely used even though there are limitations with this guidance and more recently it is enhanced with other techniques as described below.

Fluoroscopic Guidance

There are various techniques that have been described for fluoroscopic guided blocks in clinical practice. The preferred technique by the authors is oblique/prone/supine technique.

Patient is positioned lateral oblique, or patient prone with image intensifier oriented oblique. Target is posterior aspect of cervical intervertebral foramen of exiting spinal nerve. A cephalad to caudad tilt can maximize the intervertebral foramen opening. In contrast to the lumbar transforaminal approach, it is not necessary to target immediately under the pedicle, but instead any needle position along the posterior aspect of the intervertebral foramen (safe zone) is appropriate (Figs. 41.1, 41.2, 41.3, and 41.4).

The literature describes many positions on how these blocks are successfully performed using various radiological guidance with differing sizes of needles to improve outcomes and reduce complications. Table 41.1 summarizes some of the published studies in the recent past.

CT Guidance

Due to a lack of alternatives, CSNRB was conducted in the last decades mainly using fluoroscopy. However, fluoroscopy is limited in terms of visualizing the soft tissue structures of the neck. Various complications associated with the fluoroscopic-guided CSNRB including cerebellar infarct, spinal

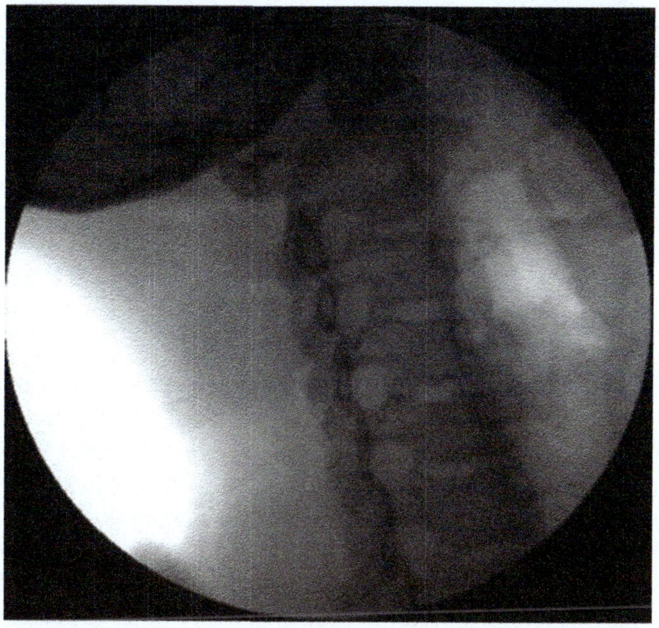

Fig. 41.1 Right-sided cervical neural foraminal view

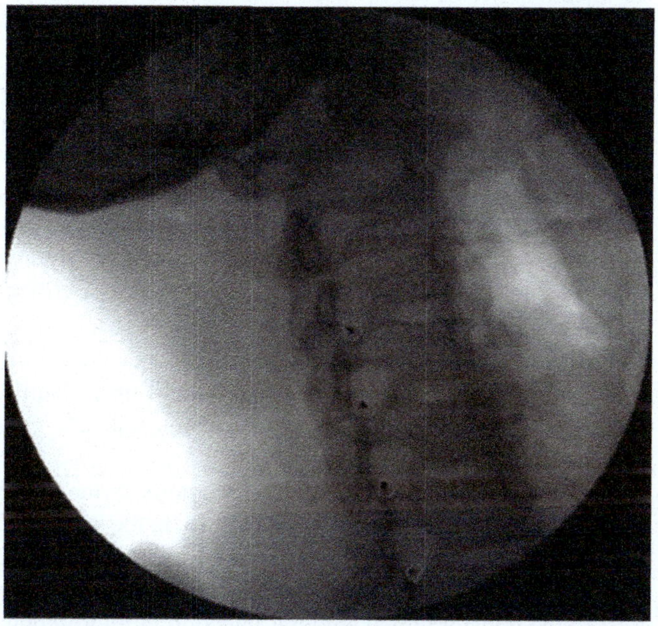

Fig. 41.2 Ideal needle positions for cervical nerve root blocks

cord infarct, quadriplegia and death have been reported and mainly attributed to particulate steroid or air embolism. However, complications associated with cervical injections, such as spinal cord or brainstem damage, seem to be rare with fluoroscopy. One study of a series of more than 1000 blocks showed a major adverse events rate of less than 1% and minor complication rate of 1.66%. Nevertheless, the difficulties of this procedure are exacerbated by the fact that fatal complications, especially vascular injuries like dissections, may not

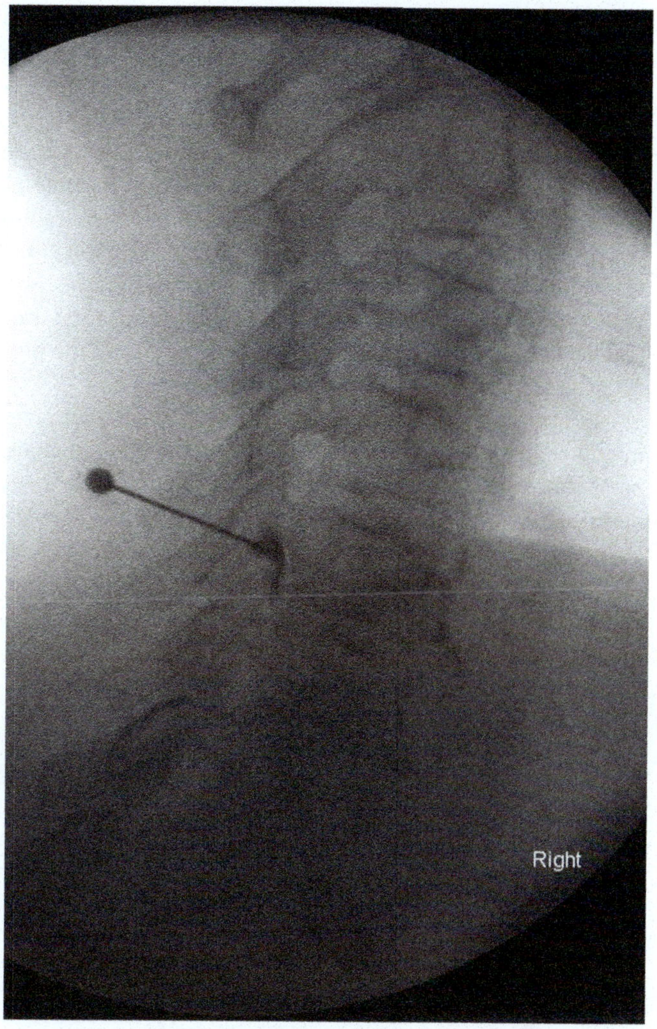

Fig. 41.3 Contrast spread oblique view

cause immediate clinical symptoms and are difficult to visualize with fluoroscopic. In contrast, Nakagawa et al. reported that ultrasound guidance might be useful for CSNRB by improving nerve and vascular localization.

Jee et al. have demonstrated that ultrasound-guided selective nerve root block and fluoroscopy-guided transforaminal block for the treatment of radicular pain in the lower cervical spine are equally effective in pain relief and functional improvement. They found ultrasound provided the benefit of real-time imaging without exposure to radiation. Nevertheless, ultrasound guidance enables only limited prepuncture planning and provides inherent technical limitations like the visualization of anatomical structures underneath the bony surface.

Pedicelli et al. describe the multi-slice CT-guided approach as the 'clinical gold standard' technique, as it provides highly detailed axial images, characterized by high spatial and contrast resolution, but without real-time procedure control. They also published that needle trajectory in hypertrophic bony overgrowth was superior using a 3D-rotational angiographic unit compared to fluoroscopy. A recent study performed by Kranz et al. evaluated CT fluoroscopy for cervical interlaminar epidural steroid injection. In 53 injections reviewed, there were no immediate symptomatic complications. A single case of thecal sac penetration was identified, which had occurred during an injection at the C5–C6 level. In conclusion, it seems the better the prepuncture planning, the tissue visualization of the target area and the needle control is, the safer and more reliable the procedure can be done.

All prior described techniques for preinterventional planning, needle control and visualization of the target area have been shown to have some benefits and some drawbacks as described above. Despite attractive features of CT-guided techniques compared to fluoroscopy, including direct visualization of soft tissue planes, vital organs, neural and vascular structures and the precise anatomic localization with millimetre accuracy, all techniques lack the possibility of multidimensional puncture guidance. From the reports described above, it seems, greater accuracy of needle visualization and better tissue resolution have to be traded with the inability to have excellent needle control or vice versa.

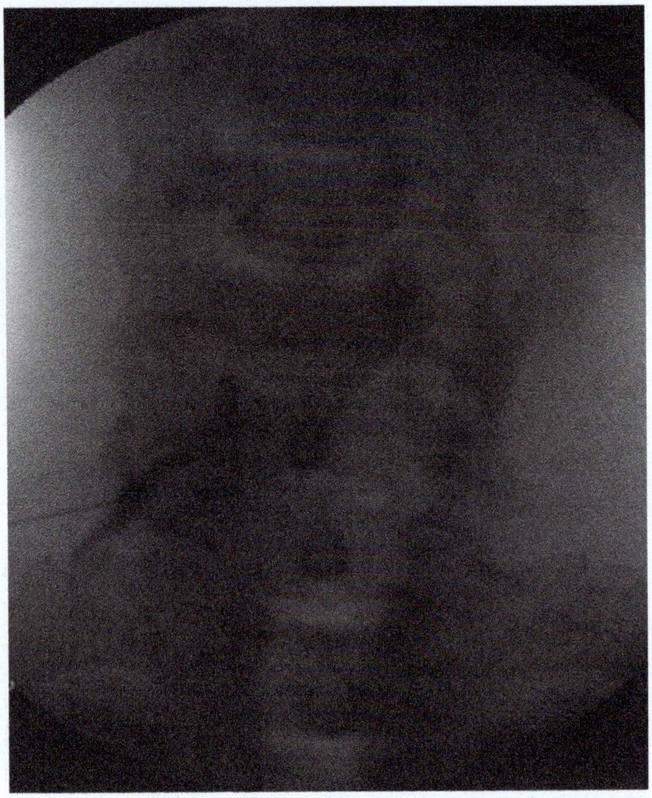

Fig. 41.4 A-P contrast spread

Ultrasound Guidance

Ultrasound use in chronic pain has been progressive in the last decade. Ultrasound guidance for cervical spine procedures is evolving rapidly as ultrasound provides direct visualization and imaging of various soft tissues without any radiation exposure. Hence, it is an appealing option to consider for CSNRBs, where there is a magnitude of critical soft tissue structures in a compact, very vascular area. Ultrasound imaging allows the real-time imaging of needle advancement and monitoring of injectate spread, hence increasing the accuracy of the block and minimizing the risk of intravascular injection. Moreover, the added benefit is its use in identifying the associated pathology or aberrant anatomy contributing the pain problem.

The few reported fatal complications of vertebral artery injury or brainstem and spinal cord infarction have been attributed to either vasospasm or unintentional arterial injection of particulate steroid with embolus formation which has been unavoidable with traditional techniques using fluoroscopy or CT guidance. A potential shortcoming in the fluoroscopic technique is that the needle may puncture a critical contributing vessel to the anterior spinal artery in the posterior aspect of intervertebral foramen. In this scenario, the ultrasound offers distinctive advantage in real-time identification of vessel puncture and spread of the injectate than after effect with fluoroscopy.

The target in ultrasound-guided technique is the nerve root or, more specifically, the ventral ramus, in the transverse process groove between the anterior and posterior tubercles. Hence, it is extraforaminal selective nerve root block in contrast to the transforaminal epidural injection in fluoroscopy-guided technique. Use of ultrasound for cervical nerve root injections requires expertise and should not be taken lightly. The needle is advanced in real time up to the extraforaminal

Table 41.1 Some of the CSNRBs from literature depicting patient position, radiological guidance, size of needle and outcomes with pain relief

Author	No of patients/injections	Position of patient	Approach	Guidance	Needle size/contrast	Pain relief
Morvan (1988)	51/71	Sitting	Anterolateral	X-ray	21G/No contrast	14% satisfactory
Bush (1996)	68/170	N/A	Lateral	X-ray in few	21G/22G	81% complete relief
Slipman (2000)	20/44	Supine	Lateral	X-ray	22G/Contrast	60% good to excellent
Vallee (2001)	32/41	Sitting	Anterolateral	X-ray	21G/No contrast	62% significant
Cyteval (2004)	30/30	Supine	Anterolateral	CT	22G/Contrast	60% good to excellent
Wagner (2005)	~200	Supine	Anterolateral	CT	25G/Contrast	N/A

area to avoid any vascularity within the foramen, and the injectate spread is monitored. The high-resolution ultrasound machine offers better visualization of the superficial structures of the neck to target the nerves. The advent of needles with better visualization under ultrasound has enabled to use thinner, blunt needles to avoid serious complications. It is very important to keep the tip of the needle in plane and under vision in the image throughout the advancement and visually check for negative aspiration for blood/CSF before injecting the injectate.

C. *Needle placement*

The needle punctures the skin over the target, and the shaft of the needle is directed along the axis of the x-ray beam towards the posterior aspect of the intervertebral foramen. Determine depth by rotating the image intensifier to AP, allowing for visualization of medial distance instead of using 'bone contact' to determine medial distance. Bone contact may be used in part for depth determination, but not in isolation, because, in isolation, it may increase the likelihood of thecal penetration. Approximately 0.25–0.5 ml contrast is injected during lateral or oblique, and AP fluoroscopic visualization is performed to confirm needle placement. Ideal to obtain digital subtraction angiography to detect any small vessel contrast uptake, which is sometimes difficult to detect in traditional fluoroscopy. If contrast is observed to flow proximal to the intervertebral foramen within the epidural space, then the adjacent infrasegmental spinal nerves may also be anaesthetized, potentially decreasing the procedure's diagnostic specificity.

'Two-Needle Technique'

Kumar et al. described this novel technique. The patient is placed in the lateral position on the operating table with the symptomatic side facing up. One or two pillows are placed under the head to prevent lateral flexion of the cervical spine. The neck is slightly extended and the patient is requested to depress both shoulders. This position helps to visualize the entire cervical spine in a majority of patients. The image intensifier is centred on the relevant level and tilted by 20–30° in order to obtain oblique projections of the cervical spine. This would show the neural foramen end-on. A metallic pointer is placed transversely on the patient's neck, so that it projects at the upper border of the nerve root foramen of the level to be injected and parallel to the disc space. A horizontal line is drawn on the skin at this level. A vertical line is drawn joining the posterior borders of the lateral masses of the adjacent vertebrae. Intersection of these lines gives the entry point for the needle, which overlies the bulk of the trapezius muscle and falls in the posterior triangle of the neck. For the 'two-needle technique', a 0.9 mm internal diameter/125 mm length needle as the 'outer needle' and 0.45 mm internal diameter/150 mm needle as the 'inner needle' are selected. The outer needle is well suited to negotiate the skin, deep fascia and muscle layers without bending. The 0.9 mm needle with stylet is introduced through the entry point on the skin and directed using image guidance through the bulk of the trapezius muscle, keeping it posterior to the neurovascular bundle of the neck. The needle is advanced under fluoroscopic guidance until the tip of the needle is just anterolateral to the posterior border of neural foramen, without actually entering it. An AP view is also obtained at this stage. The stylet is removed and the inner needle is inserted through the lumen of the outer needle. The inner needle is advanced with caution, to enter the nerve root canal under image guidance, observing the patient's response. In a majority of patients, radicular pain is reproduced at this point, which usually matches their clinical symptoms. Aspiration is attempted with a 5 ml syringe to ensure that the needle tip is not in any blood vessel. 0.2–0.5 ml of radio-opaque dye is injected through the inner needle to obtain an epidurogram, showing spread of the contrast medium along the nerve root (Figs. 41.5 and 41.6).

D. *Injection*

After confirmation of extravascular needle placement, with optimal contrast flow along the suspect cervical spinal nerve and into the epidural space, injectant is introduced. Typically, total volume of 0.5–2.0 ml of local anaesthetic and corticosteroid is injected. For purely diagnostic blocks, a smaller volume of anaesthetic (0.5–1.0 ml) should be used to increase diagnostic specificity. Care is made to avoid injecting against resistance as this may indicate the needle tip to be in a wrong place. Although most case reports of severe complications involved the use of particulate steroids.

Post-procedure Care

It is important to save the fluoroscopic images showing the final position of the needle in true A-P, oblique and lateral views before any injectate and after the injectate and document them. With the removal of the needle, the skin is cleaned to remove the antiseptic and any blood. A small adhesive dressing can be applied to the puncture sites. If the patient complains of any untoward side effects following the procedure, appropriate action must be taken. Vasovagal episodes may occur. These are managed with pulse and blood pressure monitoring, rest in the supine position and occasionally using atropine.

It is also important to watch for any untoward respiratory depression and loss of consciousness during and immedi-

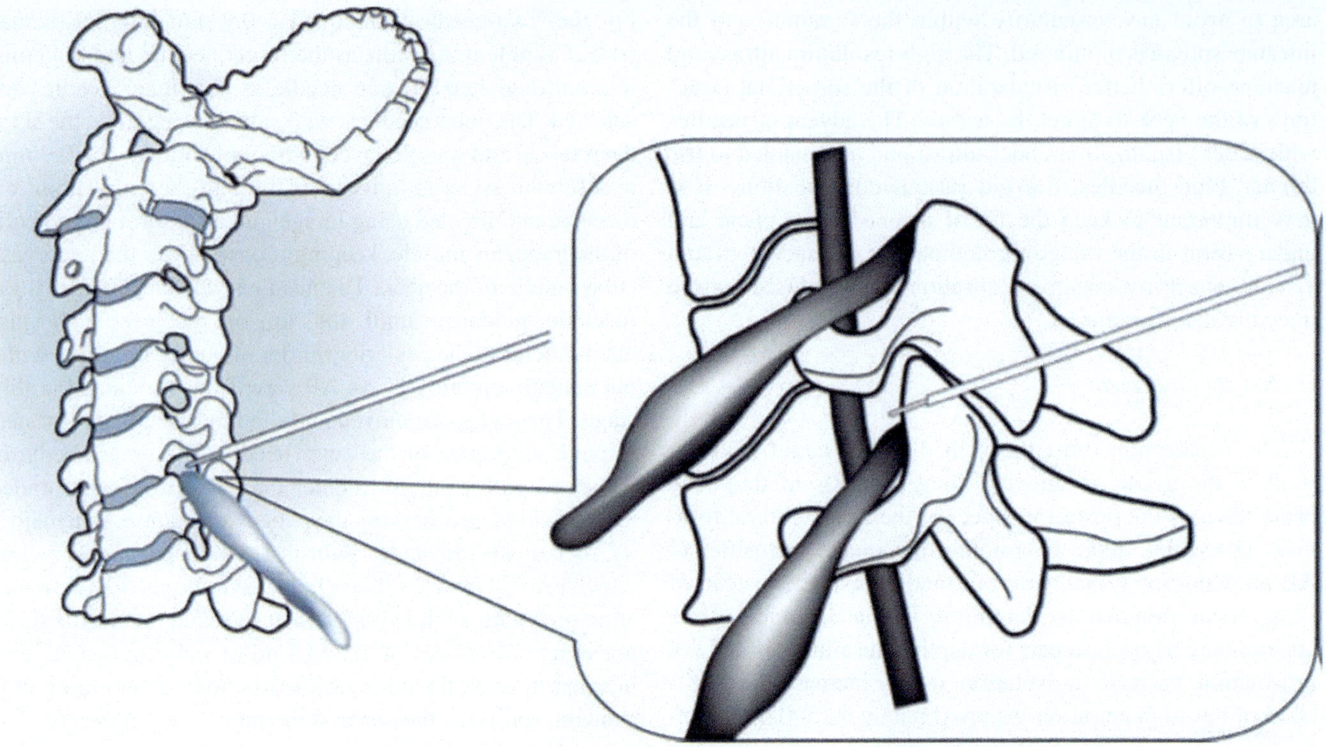

Fig. 41.5 Two-needle technique: schematic diagram showing relationship between the tip of needle, the nerve root and the vertebral artery at the nerve root foramen. The safe zone refers to the postero-superior quadrant of nerve root foramen as seen on oblique view. (Reprinted from Kumar, N. & Gowda, Cervical foraminal selective nerve root block: a 'two-needle technique' with results. V. *Eur Spine J* (2008) 17: 576. https://doi.org/10.1007/s00586-008-0600-6. © Springer-Verlag 2008)

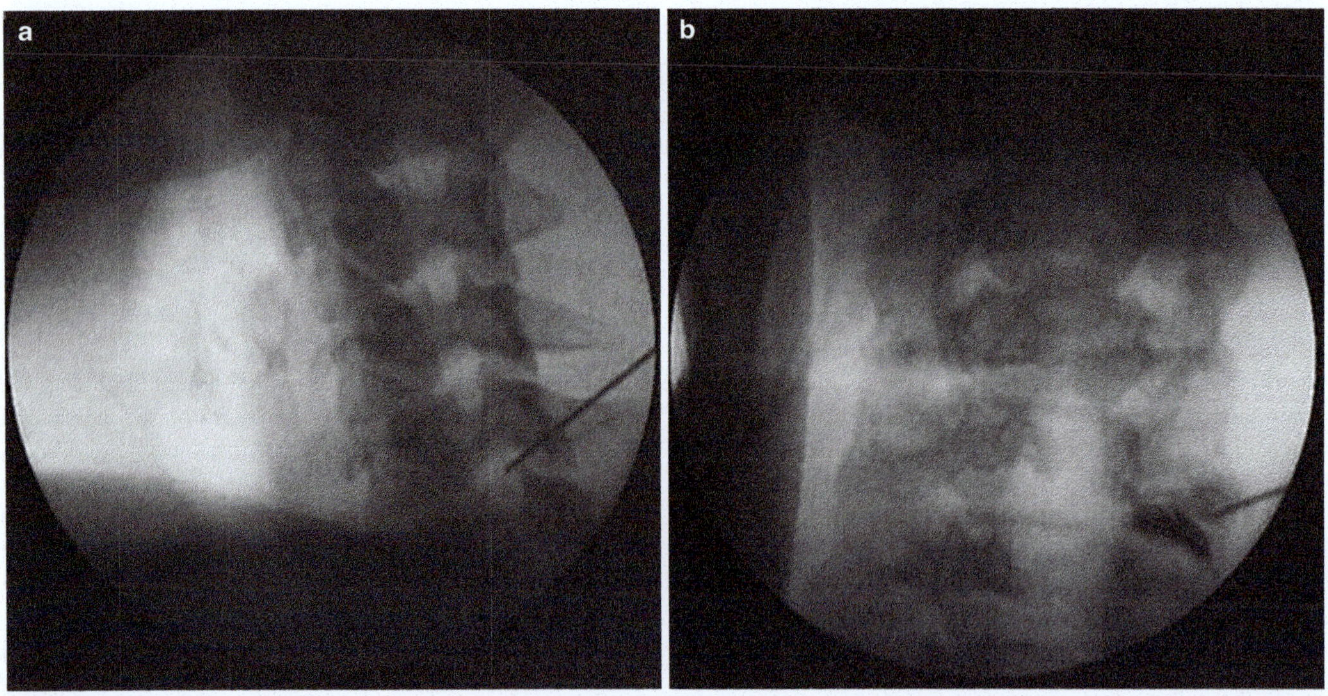

Fig. 41.6 (**a**) End-on view of the neural foramen seen on oblique X-ray. Tip of the needle is in the postero-superior quadrant of the foramen. (**b**) AP view of the same showing epidurogram. (Reprinted from Kumar, N. & Gowda, Cervical foraminal selective nerve root block: a 'two-needle technique' with results. V. *Eur Spine J* (2008) 17: 576. https://doi.org/10.1007/s00586-008-0600-6. © Springer-Verlag 2008)

ately after the procedure. Patients should be warned of the impending sensory loss and possible motor block and appropriate care for the duration of the symptoms, which can sometimes last up to 24 hours.

Documentation

The discharge documentation should include:

- Detailed account of the procedure along with drugs used and any immediate complications encountered.
- Details of immediate post-procedure pain relief (anatomical distribution and magnitude of pain relief).
- The follow-up or further appointment and necessary evaluation forms to be filled by patient need to be given.
- Contact details of the designated physician who performed the procedure and patient should there be any unusual symptom or pain following the procedure. Fever and tenderness greater than that, which might be ascribed to a needle track, may be signs of infection and need early intervention.
- To monitor the extent and duration of any relief that ensues. To this end a pain diary is helpful. However, critical are the time when the pain starts to return and the time that it returns to its former, accustomed intensity.
- If relief occurs, the patient should carefully attempt those movements and activities of daily living that customarily are restricted by pain, in order to determine if these movements and activities can be resumed while pain-free and record them.

Assessment

For diagnostic purposes, following completion of the injection, the patient is asked to rate their typical pain while attempting to provoke usual symptoms. Significant pain relief (75–100%) lasting equal to or greater than the expected duration of the anaesthetic suggests a positive response.

Conclusion

The cervical selective nerve root blocks are advanced spine procedures and not to be taken lightly. It is important to have a thorough understanding of the anatomy, anatomical changes with pathology, interpretation of imaging techniques and good working knowledge with fluoroscopic-guided nerve blocks in other areas of the spine.

Although no system is perfect in the current available options, a combination of these might overcome the disadvantages of each on its own. Hence, use of ultrasound for preplanning along with real-time contrast fluoroscopy with digital subtraction imaging might increase the precision along with use of blunt tip needle; non-particulate steroids for therapeutic blocks could reduce the serious or fatal complications.

Recommended Reading

1. Brouwers PJ, Kottink EJ, Simon MA, Prevo RL. A cervical anterior spinal artery syndrome after diagnostic blockade of the right C6-nerve root. Pain. 2001;91:397–9.
2. Bush K, Hillier S. Outcome of cervical radiculopathy treated with periradicular/epidural corticosteroid injections: a prospective study with independent clinical review. Eur Spine J. 1996;5:319–25.
3. Cyteval C, Thomas E, Decoux E, Sarrabere MP, Cottin A, Blotman F, Taourel P. Cervical radiculopathy: open study on percutaneous periradicular foraminal steroid infiltration performed under CT control in 30 patients. AJNR Am J Neuroradiol. 2004;25:441–4.
4. Derby R, Kine G, Saal JA, et al. Response to steroid and duration of radicular pain as predictors of surgical outcome. Spine. 1992;6:S176–83.
5. Dillin W, Booth R, Cuckler J, Balderston R, Simeone F, Rothman R. Cervical radiculopathy. A review. Spine. 1986;11:988–91.
6. Dooley JF, McBroom RJ, Taguchi T, et al. Nerve root infiltration in the diagnosis of radicular pain. Spine. 1988;13:79–83.
7. Dreyfuss P, Baker R, Bogduk N. Comparative effectiveness of cervical transforaminal injections with particulate and non-particulate corticosteroid preparations for radicular pain. Pain Med. 2006;7(3):237.
8. Eubanks JD. Cervical radiculopathy: non-operative management of neck pain and radicular symptoms. Am Fam Physician. 2010;81:33–40.
9. Haueisen DC, Smith BS, Myers SR, et al. The diagnostic accuracy of spinal nerve injection studies. Clin Orthop Relat Res. 1985;198:179–83.
10. Hogan QH, Abram SE. Neural blockade for diagnosis and prognosis. A review. Anesthesiology. 1997;86:216–41.
11. Jee H, Lee J, Kim J, Park K, Lee W, et al. Ultrasound-guided selective nerve root block versus fluoroscopy-guided transforaminal block for the treatment of radicular pain in the lower cervical spine: a randomized, blinded, controlled study. Skelet Radiol. 2013;42(1):69–78.
12. Karasek M, Bogduk N. Temporary neurologic deficit after cervical transforaminal injection of local anesthetic. Pain Med. 2004;5:202–5.
13. Kolstad F, Leivseth G, Nygaard O. Transforaminal steroid injections in the treatment of cervical radiculopathy. A prospective outcome study. Acta Neurochir. 2005;147:1065–70.
14. Kranz PG, Raduazo P, Gray L, Kilani RK, Hoang JK. CT fluoroscopy- guided cervical interlaminar steroid injections: safety, technique, and radiation dose parameters. Am J Neuroradiol. 2012;33:1221–4.
15. Krempem JF, Smith BS. Nerve root injection: a method for evaluating the etiology of sciatica. J Bone Joint Surg Am. 1974;56A:1435–44.
16. Kuijper B, Tans JTJ, Schimsheimer RJ, Van Der Kallen BFW, Beelen A, et al. Degenerative cervical radiculopathy: diagnosis and conservative treatment: a review. Eur J Neurol. 2009;16:15–20.
17. Kumar N, Gowda V. Cervical foraminal selective nerve root block a "two needle technique" with results. Eur Spine J. 2008;17:576–84. https://doi.org/10.1007/s00586-008-0600-6.
18. Lee MH, Cha YD, Song JH, An YM, Han JU, et al. Transient quadriplegia after fluoroscopic-guided selective cervical nerve root

block in a patient who received cervical interbody fusion – a case report. Korean J Anesthesiol. 2010;59(Suppl):S95–8.
19. Lees F, Turner JW. Natural history and prognosis of cervical spondylosis. Br Med J. 1963;2(5373):1607–10.
20. Lestini WF, Wiesel SW. The pathogenesis of cervical spondylosis. Clin Orthop Relat Res. 1989;239:69–93.
21. Lin EL, Lieu V, Halevi L, Shamie AN, Wang JC. Cervical epidural steroid injections for symptomatic disc herniations. J Spinal Disord Tech. 2006;19:183–6.
22. Ma DJ III, Gilula LA, Riew KD. Complications of fluoroscopically guided extraforaminal cervical nerve blocks an analysis of 1036 injections. J Bone Joint Surg Am. 2005;87:1025–30.
23. Macnab I. Negative disc exploration: an analysis of the causes of nerve root involvement in sixty-eight patients. J Bone Joint Surg Am. 1971;53A:5891–903.
24. McCarron RF, Wimpee MW, Hudkins PG, et al. The inflammatory effects of nucleus pulposus. A possible element in the pathogenesis of low back pain. Spine. 1987;12:760–4.
25. Morvan G, Monpoint D, Bard M, Levi-Valensin G. Direct intraforaminal injection of corticosteroids in the treatment of cervicobrachial pain. In: Interventional radiology in bone and joint. Vienna: Springer; 1988. p. 253–7.
26. Murphy RW. Nerve roots and spinal nerves in degenerative disk disease. Clin Orthop Relat Res. 1977;129:46–60.
27. Nachemson A. Newest knowledge of low back pain: a critical look. Clin Orthop Relat Res. 1992;279:8–20.
28. Nakagawa M, Shinbori H, Ohseto K. Ultrasound-guided and fluoroscopy assisted selective cervical nerve root blocks. Masui. 2009;58:1506–11.
29. North RB, Kidd DH, Zahurak M, et al. Specificity of diagnostic nerve blocks: a prospective, randomized study of sciatica due to lumbosacral spine disease. Pain. 1996;65:77–85.
30. Olmarker K, Rydevik B, Nordborg C. Autologous nucleus pulposus induces neurophysiologic and histologic changes in porcine cauda equina nerve roots. Spine. 1993;18:1425–32.
31. Olmarker K, Byord G, Cornfjord M, et al. Effects of methylprednisolone on nucleus pulposus- induced nerve root injury. Spine. 1994;19:1803–8.
32. Pedicelli A, Verdolotti T, Pompucci A, Desiderio F, D'Argento F, et al. Interventional spinal procedures guided and controlled by a 3D rotational angiographic unit. Skelet Radiol. 2011;40:1595–601.
33. Radhakrishnan K, Litchy WJ, O'Fallon WM, Kurland LT. Epidemiology of cervical radiculopathy. A population-based study from Rochester, Minnesota, 1976 through 1990. Brain. 1994;117(Pt 2):325–35.
34. Roth D, Mukai A, Thomas P, et al. Cervical radiculopathy. Dis Mon. 2009;55:737–56.
35. Saal JS, Saal JA, Yurth EF. Nonoperative management of herniated cervical intervertebral disc with radiculopathy. Spine. 1996;21:1877–83.
36. Scanlon GC, Moeller-Bertram T, Romanowsky SM, Wallace MS. Cervical transforaminal epidural steroid injections: more dangerous than we think? Spine. 2007;32:1249–56.
37. Schoenfeld AJ, George AA, Bader JO, et al. Incidence and epidemiology of cervical radiculopathy in the United States military: 2000 to 2009. J Spinal Disord Tech. 2012;25(1):17–22.
38. Schutz H, Lougheed WM, Wortzman G, et al. Intervertebral nerve-root in the investigation of chronic lumbar disc disease. Can J Surg. 1973;16:217–21.
39. Slipman CW, Lipetz JS, Jackson HB, Rogers DP, Vresilovic EJ. Therapeutic selective nerve root block in the nonsurgical treatment of atraumatic cervical spondylotic radicular pain: a retrospective analysis with independent clinical review. Arch Phys Med Rehabil. 2000;81:741–6.
40. Stanley D, McLaren MI, Euinton HA, et al. A prospective study of nerve root infiltration in the diagnosis of sciatica: a comparison with radiculography, computed tomography, and operative findings. Spine. 1990;6:540–3.
41. Tiso RL, Cutler T, Catania JA, Whalen K. Adverse central nervous system sequelae after selective transforaminal block: the role of corticosteroids. Spine J. 2004;4:468–74.
42. Vallee JN, Feydy A, Carlier RY, Mutschler C, Mompoint D, Vallee CA. Chronic cervical radiculopathy: lateral approach periradicular corticosteroid injection. Radiology. 2001;218:886–92.
43. van Akkerveeken PF. The diagnostic value of nerve root sheath infiltration. Acta Orthop Scand. 1993;64:61–3.
44. Wagner AL. CT fluoroscopic-guided cervical nerve root blocks. Am J Neuroradiol. 2005;26(1):43–4.
45. Wallace MA, Fukui MB, Williams RL, Ku A, Baghai P. Complications of cervical selective nerve root blocks performed with fluoroscopic guidance. AJR Am J Roentgenol. 2007;188:1218–21.
46. Windsor RE, Storm S, Sugar R, Nagula D. Cervical Transforaminal injection: review of the literature, complications, and a suggested technique. Pain Physician. 2003;6:457–65.
47. Wolff AP, Groen GJ, Crul BJ. Diagnostic lumbosacral segmental nerve blocks with local anesthetics: a prospective double-blind study on the variability and interpretation of segmental effects. Reg Anesth Pain Med. 2001;26:147–55.
48. Yabuki S, Kikuchi S. Nerve root infiltration and sympathetic block. Spine. 1995;20:901–6.
49. Yabuki S, Kawaguchi Y, Nordborg C, et al. Effects of lidocaine on nucleus pulposus-induced nerve root injury. Spine. 1998;23:2383–9.

Cervical Facet Joint Injection and Medial Branch Blocks

42

Ajax Yang, Jonathan Hagedorn, Sameer Jain, and Jay M. Shah

Introduction

Neck pain is a common cause of chronic pain and disability. It is the third most common chronic pain condition in the United States and fourth leading cause of disability worldwide. Neck pain is associated with several comorbidities, including back and joint pain, headache, and depression. The annual prevalence ranges between 15% and 50% with lifetime prevalence estimates as high as 67%. It occurs more frequently in women and prevalence peaks in middle age. Facet arthropathy accounts for 33–65% of total cases, more frequently at the mid- and low-cervical levels (C4–C7). While lumbar facet joint arthropathy has received much of the attention in the past, cervical facet joint pain is becoming increasingly identified and studied.

Despite the impressive achievement in modern-day high-resolution and three-dimensional imaging technology, imaging alone cannot meaningfully confirm or negate the presence or the absence of facet arthropathy as the cause of neck pain. The limitation of using imaging to identify the source of pain is especially problematic in multilevel spinal spondylosis, degenerative disc disease, or facet arthropathy where the pain generators are equivocal, or the presence of a spinal defect cannot explain the pain distribution and symptomatology.

A. Yang (✉)
Department of Rehabilitation Medicine, Icahn School of Medicine at Mount Sinai, New York, NY, USA

J. Hagedorn
Department of Pain Medicine, Mayo Clinic, Rochester, MN, USA

S. Jain
Department of Pain Medicine, Pain Treatment Centers of America, Little Rock, AR, USA

J. M. Shah
Department of Pain Medicine, Weill-Cornell Tri-Institutional Pain Program, New York, NY, USA

Background and Historical Perspective

First described in 1988, the most reliable way to diagnose a painful cervical facet joint is by injecting local anesthesia into the joint itself or the medial branch nerves that innervate the joint. Both methods have proven reliable; however, stronger research exists surrounding medial branch blocks for cervical facet pain. Regardless of technique, the main objective of either method is to provide pain relief of the affected joint and in doing so localize the joint as the source of the neck pain.

Innervation of the C4 through C7/T1 cervical facet joints involves the medial branches from the cervical dorsal rami. The C4 through C8 vertebral levels each receive dual facet joint innervation from the medial branch above and below the specific level. The medial branches of the C3 dorsal ramus are slightly different. The deep medial branch courses inferiorly to the C3–C4 facet joint in a fashion similar to other medial branches. However, the superficial medial branch of C3, also known as the third occipital nerve, takes a lateral course to the C2–C3 facet joint. Thus, pain from the C2–C3 facet joint can be blocked at the lateral aspect of the joint, and pain from the C3–C4 joint and lower can be blocked at the waist of the articular pillars above and below the joint.

Unfortunately, no particular signs or symptoms are significantly associated with cervical facet dysfunction. These patients will typically present with uni- or bilateral axial neck pain without radiation. If radiation is present, it rarely extends past the shoulder. The patient may describe limitations in neck extension and rotation. There is an absence of neurological symptoms. Pain may be reproducible with pressure over the facet joints.

Uses and Indications

Intra-articular cervical facet block (ICFB) and cervical medial branch block (CMBB) are considered when patients present with persistent (lasting longer than 3 months in duration), dis-

T. R. Deer et al. (eds.), *Deer's Treatment of Pain*, https://doi.org/10.1007/978-3-030-12281-2_42

abling neck pain, cervicogenic headache, or postlaminectomy pain syndrome recalcitrant to conservative management. These blocks are both diagnostic and therapeutic. The diagnostic value of the blocks lies in their selective, comparative, and reversible palliation directed at the suspected pain generator(s). The patients are instructed to observe relief from a specific symptom following blocks. The gold standard, a positive block, is considered with at least 80% pain relief lasting greater than 2 hours after lidocaine was injected followed by bupivacaine that provided 3 hours or longer of pain relief compared to lidocaine. This comparative two-step process using two distinct local anesthetics is crucial to reduce false positive block findings and enhance diagnostic accuracy. Although ICFB and CMBB are often intended as a confirmatory precursor to the more durable neurolysis techniques or even surgery, cervical diagnostic blocks, at times, can be therapeutic and long lasting in certain patient populations.

The decision to proceed with a diagnostic ICFB versus CMBB depends on many factors. The intra-articular approach may be preferred in the following situations:

1. When a facet synovial cyst is suspected to be a source of pain. The spinal synovial cyst can be drained followed by intra-articular injection.
2. When radiological evidence overwhelmingly supports one particular facet as the pain generator.

CMBB can be considered over intra-articular facet block in scenarios where:

1. The facet joint space is severely arthritic, obliterated, or fused.
2. The radiologic or clinical evidence to support the involvement of a particular facet joint is equivocal.
3. Rhizotomy or radiofrequency ablation is considered.
4. The patient has a high bleeding risk and concerns for hematoma formation exist. Although it has been reported, generally the chance of epidural hematoma development is meager; however, each facet joint space is contiguous with the epidural space. Therefore, epidural hematoma risk following intra-articular facet injection cannot be eliminated entirely.

Intra-articular Cervical Facet Block (ICFB)

Steps to perform the posterior method:

1. Place the patient in a prone, chin-tucked position with a pillow supporting the patient's chest and anterior shoulders. It is helpful to maintain depressed scapular position bilaterally by placing the patient's hands under the thighs in preparation for obtaining a lateral view.
2. Cleanse posterior neck up to the hairline and drape the surrounding area using strict sterile technique.
3. Under fluoroscopic guidance, obtain the anterior-posterior (AP) view before tilting the scope caudally to optimize superior and inferior articular process viewing and to remove parallax. Mark the skin entry point roughly two segments caudal to the lateral aspect of the target facet.
4. Anesthetize the skin and superficial tissue using 1% lidocaine.
5. Carefully advance the 22 or 25 gauge spinal needle in a cephalad and lateral direction toward the facet articulating interface. AP and lateral views are required to ensure that the needle trajectory (toward the articular pillar and the intra-articular space) is maintained.
6. Lateral view is used to ensure the needle tip stays within the posterior aspect of neural foramen.
7. Approximately 0.1–0.2 cc contrast can be injected to confirm intra-articular needle tip placement before introducing local anesthetic agent. This is elective and is based on the preference of the physician.

Steps to perform the lateral method:

1. The patient is positioned in the lateral decubitus position with the treatment side up and a pillow under the head.
2. Instruct the patient to maintain bilateral scapular depression to allow clear lateral fluoroscopic visualization.
3. The lateral neck is cleaned and draped sterilely.
4. Rotate the fluoroscope anteriorly and posteriorly to delineate the target facet joint as the image of the more proximal joint moves in the direction in which the fluoroscope is rotated. Square the target segment with parallax removed. Cephalad and caudal scope angulation may further enhance the image.
5. Once the optimal view is obtained, mark and anesthetize the skin and superficial tissue using 1% lidocaine.
6. Insert a 22 or 25 gauge spinal needle toward the target articular superior or inferior processes.
7. Small adjustments are made to manipulate the needle tip to "walk off" into the target joint space.
8. A small amount of contrast is used for intra-articular needle tip placement confirmation before injecting local anesthetic.

Cervical Medial Branch Blocks (CMBB)

Steps to perform the posterior method:

1. Place the patient in a prone, chin-tucked position with a pillow supporting the patient's chest and anterior shoulders. It is helpful to maintain depressed scapular position bilaterally by placing the patient's hands under the thighs in preparation for obtaining a lateral view.

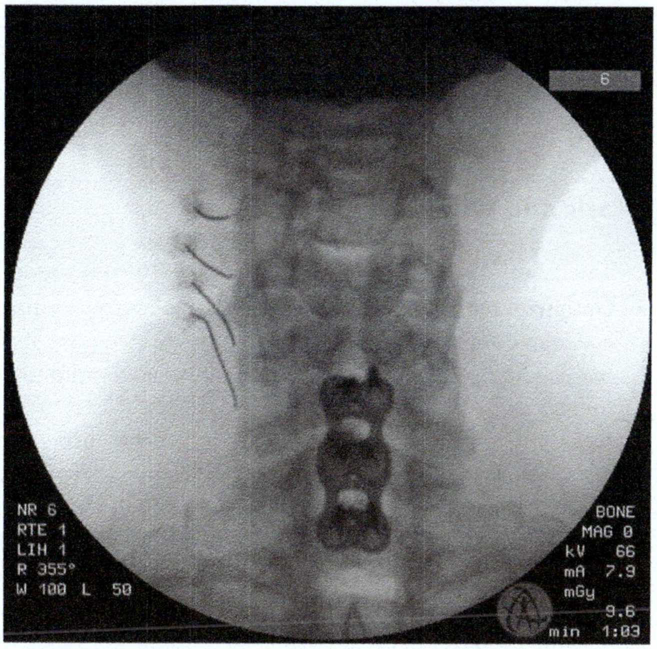

Fig. 42.1 Anterior-posterior view of cervical medial branch blocks

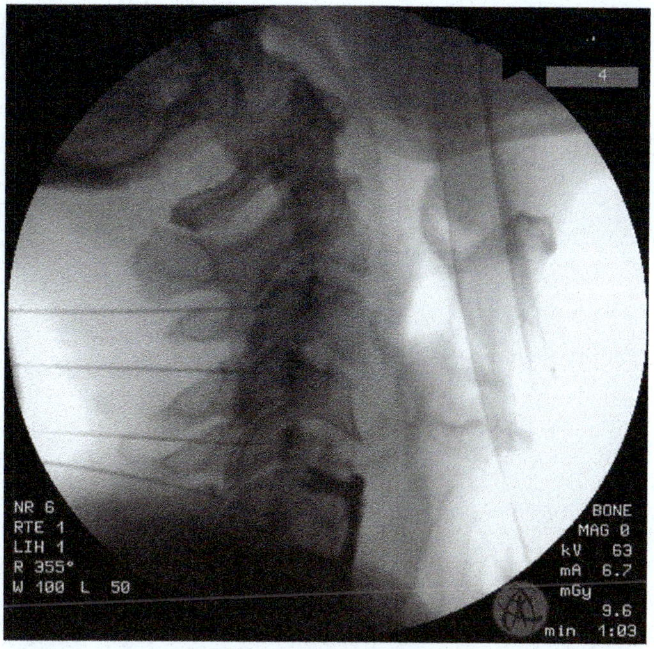

Fig. 42.2 Lateral view of the posterior approach to cervical medial branch blocks. The needle tips are placed in the center of the articular pillars

2. Cleanse the posterior neck up to the hairline, and drape the surrounding area using strict sterile technique.
3. Direct the beam in the AP direction to visualize the posterior aspects of the articular pillar waists, and identify the target joint. A small ipsilateral oblique of the fluoroscope may enhance the needle trajectory view.
4. Center the image.
5. Mark and anesthetize the skin and superficial tissue using 1% lidocaine.
6. A 22 or 25 gauge spinal needle is used to puncture the skin and advanced toward the most concave portion of the target vertebral segment (the waist), located midway between the superior and inferior articular pillars, where medial branches are found (Fig. 42.1).
7. A lateral view is used to confirm and visualize the depth of the needle tip (Fig. 42.2).
8. Oblique the fluoroscope to circumvent the shoulders, and reestablish the needle tip position when targeting segments below C6.
9. A small amount of contrast can be used for further needle tip confirmation before injecting low volume (0.3 cc) local anesthetics.

Steps to perform the lateral method:

1. The patient is positioned in the lateral decubitus position with the treatment side up and a pillow under the head. Alternatively, the patient may be supine.
2. Prepare and drape the injection site using strict sterile technique.
3. Project the fluoroscopic beam laterally to bring the articular pillars (trapezoid shaped) into view.
4. The ipsilateral and contralateral articular pillars can be clearly delineated by manipulating the fluoroscope as the image of the more proximal joint moves in the direction in which the scope is rotated. Square and center the target segment with parallax removed. Cephalad and caudal angulation may further enhance the image quality.
5. Mark and anesthetize the skin.
6. Enter the neck from the posterolateral direction, and insert a 22 or 25 gauge spinal needle toward the center of trapezoidal area (Fig. 42.3).
7. The patient's shoulders may obscure lateral views below C6. An oblique fluoroscope view can be used to circumvent the shoulders and reestablish the needle tip position.
8. Once the needle tip directly contacts the articular pillar, an AP view is used to solidify the positioning of the needle tip abutting laterally against the articular process.
9. Maintain the needle trajectory directly at the C7 articular process to prevent C8 nerve root and vertebral artery injury when approaching the C7 medial branch.
10. A small amount of contrast can be used for further needle tip confirmation before injecting low volume (0.3 cc) local anesthetics.

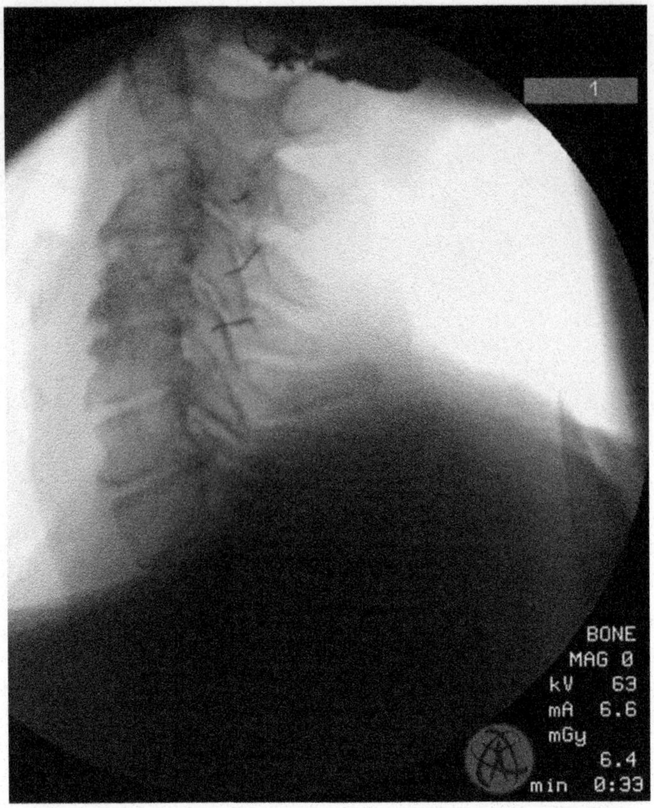

Fig. 42.3 Cervical medial branch blocks using the lateral approach

Evidence for Efficacy

(Table 42.1.)

Pearls and Pitfalls

- Optimize intermittent biplanar fluoroscopic visualization and move the needle in small increments to ensure that the needle tip location is known at all times to minimize injury risks.
- Excessive medially directed needle trajectory during the posterior approach to ICFB may result in epidural or dural puncture and spinal cord injury.
- Similarly, violating the anterior joint capsule may result in injury to the dorsal root ganglion, radicular/vertebral artery, or spinal cord.
- Use the posterior approach when targeting lower joints to minimize pneumothorax and neurovascular risks.
- The posterior approach to ICFB is generally safer to perform, but the lateral method is technically more forgiving.
- The posterior method to ICFB is recommended in patients with large shoulders.

Table 42.1 Cervical medial branch blocks and cervical intra-articular cervical facet injection evidence

Reference	Study design	Intervention	Size	Outcomes measures	Results
Manchikanti et al. (2006, 2008, 2010)	Randomized, double-blind, active-control	Fluoroscopic-guided cervical medial branch block	120 participants evenly divided into (1) local anesthetics with steroid (LA+S) and (2) local anesthetics (LA) only groups	Neck Pain Disability Index, numeric pain scores, medication use and baseline functional status at baseline, 3, 6, and 12 months. Injections were administered when pain increased and functional capacity decreased by 50%, respectively	Significant pain improvement at 12 and 24 months: 85% of local anesthetics only group and 92% (at 12 months)/93% (at 24 months) of steroid plus local anesthetics group. Functional status improvement: 63% of LA group and 68% of LA+S group had >50% in Neck Disability Index improvement at 12 months. The improvement sustained at 24 months: 70% of LA group and 75% of LA+S group
Manchikanti et al. (2004)	Prospective, observational	Fluoroscopic-guided medial branch block	100 participants underwent medial branch block with local anesthetics only or local anesthetics with steroid. Option to repeat injections	Pain scores, Oswestry Disability Index, functional and psychological status at 3, 6, and 12 months	Significant improvement observed in pain relief (92% at 3 months, 82% at 6 months, 56% at 12 months) and in functional and psychological status
Barnsley et al. (1994)	Randomized double-blind, active-control	Fluoroscopic-guided cervical facet joint injection	41 individuals following whiplash (median injury duration: 39 months) underwent intra-articular facet injection with local anesthetics or steroid	Pain scores	Median pain relief greater than 50% in steroid and local anesthetics groups were 3 and 3.5 days, respectively. No significant differences detected

Table 42.1 (continued)

Reference	Study design	Intervention	Size	Outcomes measures	Results
Park and Kim (2012)	Randomized, active-control	Fluoroscopic-guided cervical facet joint injection	400 patients with chronic neck myofascial pain and cervical facet referred pain pattern were divided into facet joint injection with conservative management (Group 1) and conservative management only (Group 2) groups	Cervical range of motion (ROM), pain score and headache symptoms	Group 1 had increased cervical ROM, increased mean pain reduction, and decreased tension-type headaches compared with Group 2. Younger individuals in Group 1 also had longer pain relief

- Limit cervical facet injectate volumes to less than 1 cc, and deliver the injection at a slow rate to prevent facet joint capsule rupture.
- Steroid is not required for CMBB.
- There are four options for injectate:
  - 1% lidocaine
  - 2% lidocaine
  - 0.25% bupivacaine
  - 0.5% bupivacaine
- To minimize the likelihood of a false positive, the authors advocate using a smaller volume (0.3 cc) and higher local anesthetic concentration (2% lidocaine or 0.5% bupivacaine) during CMBB.
- The use of low injectate volumes during CMBB is particularly important from a diagnostic standpoint for cervical medial branch radiofrequency ablation preparation.
- Double comparative blocks (lidocaine and bupivacaine) are the gold standard method to diagnose facetogenic pain. The patient must also respond concordantly for a positive block. However, a diagnostic block is considered positive when a patient reports a 50% pain improvement.
- Instruct the patient to use a written pain diary to track block efficacy.

Recommended Reading

1. Barnsley L, Lord SM, Wallis BJ, Bogduk N. The prevalence of chronic cervical zygapophyseal joint pain after whiplash. Spine (Phila Pa 1976). 1995;20:20–6.
2. Binder AI. Neck pain. BMJ Clin Evid. 2008;2008:1103.
3. Bogduk N, Marsland A. The cervical zygapophysial joints as a source of neck pain. Spine. 1988;13(6):610–7. PMID: 3175750.
4. Cohen SP. Epidemiology, diagnosis, and treatment of neck pain. Mayo Clin Proc. 2015;90(2):284–99. PMID: 25659245.
5. Fejer R, Kyvik KO, Hartvigsen J. The prevalence of neck pain in the world population: a systematic critical review of the literature. Eur Spine J Off Publ Eur Spine Soc Eur Spinal Deform Soc Eur Sect Cerv Spine Res Soc. 2006;15(6):834–48. PMCID: PMC3489448.
6. Fernández-de-las-Peñas C, Hernández-Barrera V, Alonso-Blanco C, Palacios-Ceña D, Carrasco-Garrido P, Jiménez-Sánchez S, Jiménez-García R. Prevalence of neck and low back pain in community-dwelling adults in Spain: a population-based national study. Spine. 2011;36(3):E213–9. PMID: 21079541.
7. Hechelhammer L, Pfirrmann CWA, Zanetti M, Hodler J, Boos N, Schmid MR. Imaging findings predicting the outcome of cervical facet joint blocks. Eur Radiol. 2007;17(4):959–64.
8. Hogg-Johnson S, van der Velde G, Carroll LJ, Holm LW, Cassidy JD, Guzman J, Côté P, Haldeman S, Ammendolia C, Carragee E, Hurwitz E, Nordin M, Peloso P, Bone and Joint Decade 2000-2010 Task Force on Neck Pain and Its Associated Disorders. The burden and determinants of neck pain in the general population: results of the Bone and Joint Decade 2000-2010 Task Force on Neck Pain and Its Associated Disorders. Spine. 2008;33(4 Suppl):S39–51. PMID: 18204398.
9. Jackson RP, Jacobs RR, Montesano PX. 1988 Volvo award in clinical sciences. Facet joint injection in low-back pain. A prospective statistical study. Spine. 1988;13(9):966–71.
10. Manchikanti L, Manchikanti KN, Damron KS, Pampati V. Effectiveness of cervical medial branch blocks in chronic neck pain: a prospective outcome study. Pain Physician. 2004;7(2):195–201.
11. Manchikanti L, Damron K, Cash K, Manchukonda R, Pampati V. Therapeutic cervical medial branch blocks in managing chronic neck pain: a preliminary report of a randomized, double- blind, controlled trial: clinical trial NCT 0033272. Pain Physician. 2006;9:333–46.
12. Manchikanti L, Singh V, Falco FJE, Cash KM, Fellows B. Cervical medial branch blocks for chronic cervical facet joint pain: a randomized, double-blind, controlled trial with one-year follow-up. Spine. 2008;33(17):1813–20.
13. Manchikanti L, Singh V, Falco FJ, Cash KA, Fellows B. Cervical medial branch blocks for chronic cervical facet joint pain: a randomized double-blind, controlled trial with one-year follow-up. Spine (Phila Pa 1976). 2008;33:1813–20.
14. Manchikanti L, Singh V, Falco FJE, Cash KA, Fellows B. Comparative outcomes of a 2-year follow-up of cervical medial branch blocks in management of chronic neck pain: a randomized, double-blind controlled trial. Pain Physician. 2010;13:437–50.
15. Manchukonda R, Manchikanti KN, Cash KA, Pampati V, Manchikanti L. Facet joint pain in chronic spinal pain: an evaluation of prevalence and false-positive rate of diagnostic blocks. J Spinal Disord Tech. 2007;20(7):539–45.
16. Park SC, Kim KH. Effect of adding cervical facet joint injections in a multimodal treatment program for long-standing cervical myofascial pain syndrome with referral pain patterns of cervical facet joint syndrome. J Anesth. 2012;26:738; Published online May 31, 2012.
17. Schwarzer AC, Aprill CN, Derby R, Fortin J, Kine G, Bogduk N. The false-positive rate of uncontrolled diagnostic blocks of the lumbar zygapophysial joints. Pain. 1994;58(2):195–200.
18. Stanley D, McLaren MI, Euinton HA, Getty CJ. A prospective study of nerve root infiltration in the diagnosis of sciatica. A comparison with radiculography, computed tomography, and operative findings. Spine. 1990;15(6):540–3.
19. Velickovic M, Ballhause TM. Delayed onset of a spinal epidural hematoma after facet joint injection. SAGE Open Med Case Rep. 2016;4:2050313X16675258.

Cervical Facet Radiofrequency Neurotomy

43

Jay M. Shah, Jonathan Hagedorn, Ajax Yang, and Sameer Jain

Introduction

Neck pain is the third most common chronic pain condition in the United States, which in conjunction with low back pain, leads to annual healthcare expenditures approaching $90 billion. It is also the fourth leading cause of disability worldwide. It's annual prevalence rate ranges between 15% and 50%, and lifetime prevalence rate is as common as 67%. Cervical facetogenic pain is estimated to be responsible for 36% to 60% of neck pain cases. It is more common in the lower cervical levels [1–10].

Background and Historical Perspective

The diagnosis of cervical facet-mediated pain typically relies on the use of local anesthetic blocks, either an intra-articular facet joint injection or a block of the nerves supplying the facet joint (i.e., the dorsal primary rami or medial branches). Because of the high rates of false-positive results following local anesthetic blocks, before proceeding with cervical facet radiofrequency ablation, many physicians will perform "double blocks" to more accurately identify the facet as a pain generator.

Once a diagnosis of facetogenic pain is established, the use of cervical medial branch radiofrequency neurotomy (CMBRFN) can be performed to provide long-term pain relief. This treatment modality uses an electric current to disrupt the nerves from the cervical facet joints, thereby interrupting the nociceptive signals from the joints. The duration of pain relief is determined by the denervation to the nerves, as to whether it was a partial or full thickness treatment. Pain relief from cervical radiofrequency ablation has been shown to last longer than 12 months in 58–74% of correctly diagnosed patients.

It wasn't until 1996 that robust data was published regarding the efficacy of cervical radiofrequency ablation. This RCT showed positive results with significantly more patients achieving pain relief from radiofrequency ablation than a similarly performed sham procedure. Additional studies have further established positive results demonstrating the efficacy of cervical medial branch radiofrequency ablation in providing pain relief for cervical facetogenic pain.

Potential complications from cervical radiofrequency ablation include needle placement into the vertebral artery, intervertebral foramen, and spinal canal. Deafferentation pain and post-ablation neuritis are also possible complications. Post-procedure pain at the ablation site is usually transient. When performing the procedure at the third occipital nerve, a set of distinct complications can occur, including ataxia, numbness, dysesthesias, dizziness, and hypersensitivity [11–18, 20].

Uses and Indications

Cervical medial branch radiofrequency neurotomy (CMBRFN), also known as cervical radiofrequency facet rhizotomy, facet ablation, or facet denervation, is a minimally invasive percutaneous procedure for the treatment of chronic degenerative neck pain and cervicogenic headache. CMBRFN is a nerve denervation procedure utilizing electric current alternating at the frequency of radio waves to coagulate the pain-generating nerves from the cervical zygapophysial or facet joints and thereby interrupting nociceptive transmission from these joints. The target nerves are the medial branches of one more of the cervical dorsal rami and/or the third occipital nerve. Relieving pain

J. M. Shah (✉)
Department of Pain Medicine, Weill-Cornell Tri-Institutional Pain Program, New York, NY, USA

J. Hagedorn
Department of Pain Medicine, Mayo Clinic, Rochester, MN, USA

A. Yang
Department of Rehabilitation Medicine, Icahn School of Medicine at Mount Sinai, New York, NY, USA

S. Jain
Department of Pain Medicine, Pain Treatment Centers of America, Little Rock, AR, USA

T. R. Deer et al. (eds.), *Deer's Treatment of Pain*, https://doi.org/10.1007/978-3-030-12281-2_43

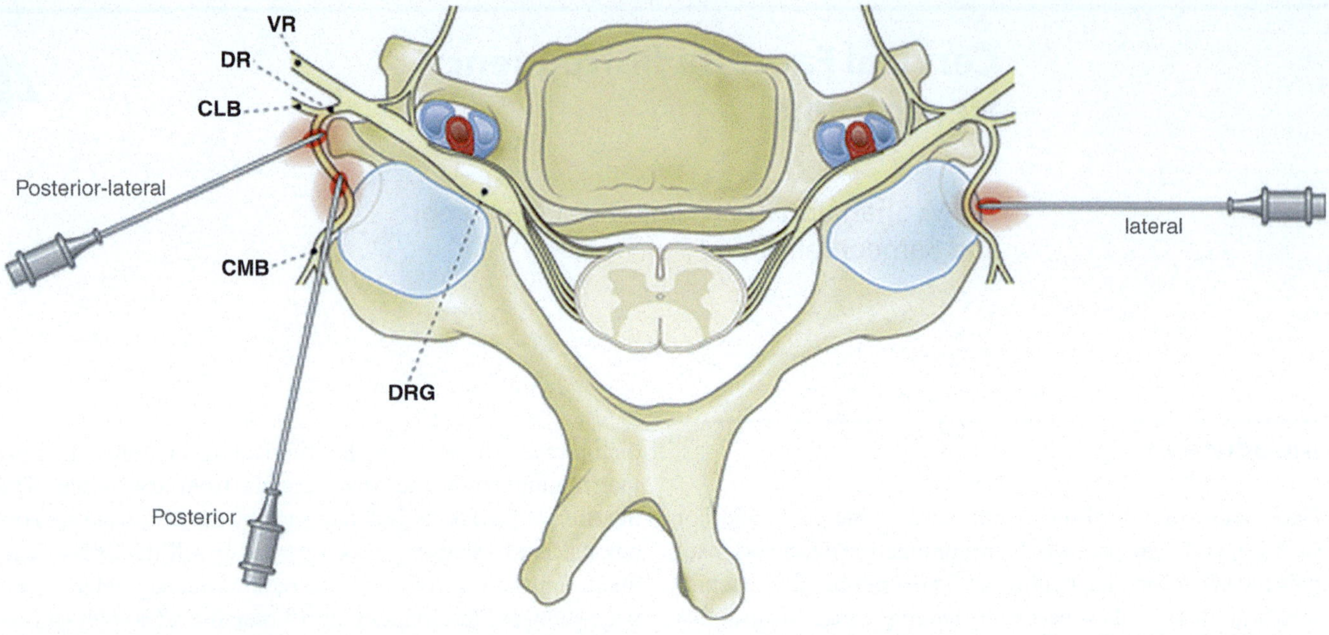

Fig. 43.1 The three currently used techniques for radiofrequency denervation of the cervical medial branch: the posterolateral, the posterior, and the lateral approach. VR ventral ramus of the cervical segmental spinal nerve, DR dorsal ramus of the cervical segmental spinal nerve, CLB cervical lateral branch from the dorsal ramus, CMB cervical medial branch from the dorsal ramus, DRG dorsal root ganglion. (Reproduced from Van Eerd M, Lataster A, Sommer M, Patijn J, et al. A modified posterolateral approach for radiofrequency denervation of the medial branch of the cervical segmental nerve in cervical facet joint pain based on anatomical considerations. *Pain Practice*. 2017; October; 5(8). With permission from JohnWiley and Sons)

in the cervical spine by performing CMBRFN is based on the finding that the recurrent sensory branch of the exiting nerve root has a consistent anatomic pathway that can be targeted to create radiofrequency lesions under fluoroscopic imaging.

A specialized needle electrode is placed immediately adjacent and parallel to the target nerve and is connected to a radiofrequency (RF) generator that delivers the alternating current to the body through a dispersion pad. The resulting electric field concentrates near the tip of the electrode and heats the surrounding tissue, thus coagulating the adjacent nerve. This process can be repeated to produce multiple RF lesions along each nerve target. These nerves are coagulated one at a time, with a maximum of three nerves denervated in any one application of the procedure (Fig. 43.1).

Common sources of pain that respond to CMBRFN include cervical disc degeneration, cervical and thoracic facet degeneration, soft tissue and facet injury from cervical whiplash, and cervical post-laminectomy pain. Although pain impulses ultimately pass through the recurrent sensory branches, they also pass through other structures including the sympathetic chain, meningeal nerve, and sino-vertebral nerve, creating a multi-segmental sensory plexus with rich innervation. Thus, targeting just a single branch of the recurrent sensory nerve alone may be insufficient to effectively denervate the multiple other afferent pathways, and this may account for the failures CMBRFN.

Diagnostic medical imaging modalities have been investigated as a means of diagnosing cervical facetogenic pain, but none have been validated. Radiographic appearances simply do not correlate with cervical pain. Studies have shown that plain X-ray, computerized tomography (CT), and magnetic resonance imaging findings are not useful for diagnosing painful cervical joints. No imaging modality provides valid diagnosis of a painful cervical joint.

Studies using comparative medial branch blocks (MBBs) and third occipital nerve blocks (TONBs) show cervical facetogenic pain accounts for 60% of chronic neck pain after whiplash. When headache is the dominant symptom after whiplash, pain referred from the C2–C3 facet joint (third occipital neuralgia) accounts for 53% of cases. Due to fact that cervical facets are a common cause of chronic neck pain and cervicogenic headache, CMBRFN is an intervention that is highly utilized for appropriated selected patients who respond with effective pain relief from comparative MBBs.

There have been various techniques and approaches of CMBRFN described in the literature. These techniques can be classified based on the position of the patient (prone, supine, lateral), on the position of the C-arm (lateral, antero-posterior, oblique), or on the trajectory of the RF probe toward the anatomical planes of the neck (posterolateral, lateral, posterior). There are three commonly utilized interventional approaches for CMBRFN that have been classified based on the needle trajectory toward the anatomical planes

Table 43.1 Considerations regarding interventional approaches for CMBRFN

Technique	X-ray direction	Patient position	Pros	Cons
Posterolateral	Oblique	Supine	Eye contact/communication with patient Shorter procedure time Small and single lesion at site with less anatomic variation of the CMB	Not tunnel view Angle of needle not exactly parallel to the CMB
Posterior	AP	Prone	Needle parallel to the CMB Multiple lesions with higher chance of targeting CMB Validated in a RCT [22]	Prone position: Less patient communication Multiple lesions may lead to muscle weakness Longer procedure time
Lateral	Lateral	Supine or lateral	Coaxial technique easier to perform	Point lesion with needle perpendicular to CMB More anatomic variation with this approach and less likely to target full thickness of CMB

as follows: the posterolateral technique, the posterior technique, and the lateral technique (Table 43.1, Fig. 43.2).

It has been consistently noted in the literature that the location of the CMB is at the anterior line of the facet column. The anterior line is defined as the line connecting the two superior articular processes. The CMB runs in the middle of the anterior line. From the anatomical studies, we can conclude that the CMB splits off early from the dorsal ramus just above the posterior tubercle midway between the anterior line between two adjoining facet joints (Fig. 43.2). From there, the CMB runs over the waist of the facet column with an interindividual variation of its course.

In properly selected cases, pain relief has been consistently reported in 70% of the cases with relief lasting between 6 months and 1 year. Should the pain return after a successful initial procedure, a repeat procedure has been shown to have a similar success rate.

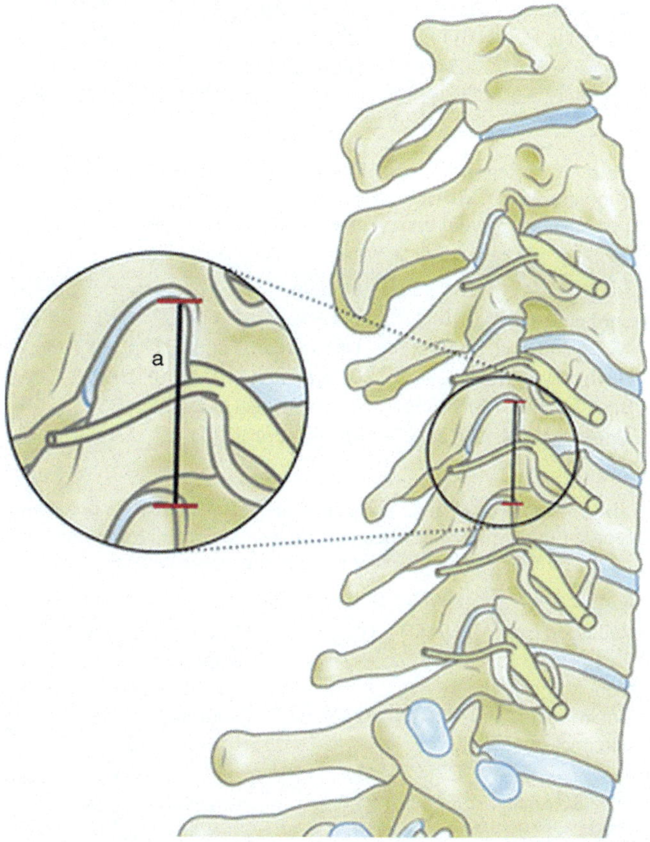

Fig. 43.2 Illustration of the anterior line (a) defined as the line connecting the most anterior tips of two consecutive superior articular processes. The medial branch nerves extend around the lateral margin of the midportion of the articular pillar at each respective level. The only exception is the C7 medial branch, which extends around the pillar slightly higher, just below the articular facets. The cervical medial branch passes through the half of this anterior line. (Reproduced from Van Eerd M, Lataster A, Sommer M, Patijn J, et al. A modified posterolateral approach for radiofrequency denervation of the medial branch of the cervical segmental nerve in cervical facet joint pain based on anatomical considerations. *Pain Practice*. 2017; October; 5(8). With permission from JohnWiley and Sons)

Evidence for Efficacy

The diagnosis of cervical facet-mediated pain is established by facet joint block or facet nerve blocks. The underlying principle for these tests is that local anesthetic block of the affected joint or its nerve supply (CMB) will lead to pain relief and pain-free movement of the affected joint. Single blocks, however, result in high false-positive rates varying from 27% to 63%. Double controlled local anesthetic blocks are recommended and have a specificity of 88% and sensitivity of 54% resulting in few false-positive diagnoses, but a high false-negative rate. The prevalence of facet joint pain based on double comparative blocks is estimated to range from 33% to 65% in patients with chronic neck pain. Clinical trials that employed dual controlled or placebo controlled MBB to select patients for RFN protocol with a 70% cutoff value for pain relief had reported successful outcomes in 60% to 74% of patients with chronic neck pain.

Current literature evaluating the correlation between CMBRFN and response to controlled CMB blocks suggests that overall, current diagnostic criteria for selecting patients for RFN based on MBB responses are less than optimal. Furthermore, a randomized multicenter-controlled trial evaluating the cost-effectiveness of RFN with 0, 1, or 2 diagnostic MBBs suggests that proceeding to radiofrequency denervation without a diagnostic block may be the most cost-effective treatment paradigm. Prospective multicenter clinical trials are needed to further optimize patient selection criteria prior to CMBRFN.

Tables 43.2, 43.3, and 43.4 highlight the current evidence base regarding the efficacy, success rates, and common complications regarding CMBRFN.

Table 43.2 Reported rates of success (defined as near complete resolution of pain) 6 months after CMBRFN of patients selected by analgesic responses to comparative medial branch blocks

Study	Design	Levels		Pain relief
Lord et al. (1995) [19]	Observational	C5–C7	7/10	70%
Lord et al. (1995) [19]	Explanatory	C3–C7	7/12	58%
McDonald et al. (1999) [24]	Observational	C3–C7	16/28	57%
Govind et al. (2003) [15]	Observational	C2–C3	32/49	65%
Barnsley et al. (2005) [1]	Observational	C2–C7	16/35	46%
MacVicar et al. (2012) [22]	Observational	C2–C7	71/104	68%

Table 43.3 Reported rates of success (defined as abolition of pain) 12 months after CMBRFN of patients selected by analgesic responses to comparative medial branch blocks [21]

Study	Design	Levels		Pain relief
Lord et al. (1995) [19]	Observational	C5–C7	4/10	40%
McDonald et al. (1999) [24]	Observational	C3–C7	10/28	36%
Govind et al. (2003) [15]	Observational	C2–C3	10/49	20%
Barnsley et al. (2005) [1]	Observational	C2–C7	9/35	26%
MacVicar et al. (2012) [22]	Observational	C2–C7	53/104	51%

Table 43.4 Risks and complications of CMBRFN procedures recorded in the literature, their prevalence (95% confidence intervals), and the references in which they were first documented [21]

Risks	Levels	Frequencies	Notes	References
Radiation risks	C2–C7	100%	Minimal	Lord (1998)
Post-procedure pain	C2–C7	98%	Temporary	Lord (1998)
Cutaneous numbness	C2–C3	97%	Enduring	Govind (2003)
	C2–C7	47%		Lord (1998)
Dizziness and ataxia	C2–C3	95%	Temporary	Govind (2003)
	C2–C7	23%		Lord (1998)
Dysesthesias	C2–C3	55%	Temporary	Govind (2003)
	C2–C7	30%		Lord (1998)
Pruritis	C2–C3	9%	Temporary	Govind (2003)
Post-procedural infection	C2–C7	3%	Temporary	Barnsley (2005) [1]
Vasovagal syncope	C2–C7	2%	Temporary	Lord (1998)
Neuritis	C2–C7	2%	Temporary	Lord (1998)
Dermoid cyst	C2–C7	1%	Enduring	Lord (1998)
Kobner's phenomenon	C2–C7	1%	Enduring	Lord (1998)

Pearls and Pitfalls

CMBBs as a Diagnostic Predictor for CMBRN Success

- CMBBs test to establish or exclude the presence of facetogenic pain, as well as enable appropriate patient selection for subsequent RFN with efficacious outcomes.
- Concordant response to controlled MBB, by definition, is long-lasting relief following bupivacaine but short-lasting relief following lidocaine.
- The commonly implemented diagnostic paradigm, while providing a strategy to treat spinal pain, may overlook the complexity of chronic spinal pain in that facet joint pain rarely occurs in isolation and follows or accompanies multiple other pain generators such as degenerative disc changes and secondary alterations in spinal biomechanics [24–27].
- Previous studies have found no difference in RF outcomes between cutoff values of 50% and 70%, suggesting a diagnostic cutoff percentage of pain relief of 70% higher to ensure successful RFN outcomes [25–27].

Technical Considerations for Safety and CMBRFN Optimization

- CMBRFN abolishes the pain for long periods by denaturing the chemical components of nociceptive A-delta and C nerve fibers and preventing conduction through them.
- It does not destroy the target nerves. They remain intact anatomically and over time they reinnervate and recover; then the pain returns, although it can be abolished again by repeat treatments.
- A major factor determining the quality and duration of effect is the length of the target nerve coagulated through its full thickness during RFN. The length of nerve coagulated is in turn influenced by variations in the neuroanatomy of the nerves, in particular, variation in their diameters and courses, and the sizes of lesions created in the procedure.
- RF lesions placed over the TON have less chance of coagulating the full thickness of the nerve for a satisfactory length than do lesions at other levels. Knowledge of the anatomic variability can lead to development of a modified treatment technique, allowing for the variations by placing larger RF lesions over a wider range of positions.
- The size of RF lesions is governed by the diameter (or gauge) of the RF electrode used to create them, the length of its active tip, the temperature it reaches, and the time the heat is applied by it.

- While serious complications of neural and vascular injuries must be recognized as risks of cervical RFN (Table 43.4), the adherence to the established and published procedural guidelines can help prevent these complications. The most important safety factor stipulated in those guidelines is that the procedure should not be done under general anesthesia [21–28]
- Patients undergoing CMBRFN must be awake and responsive so they can report the unusual sensations that will result from inaccurate electrode placement with appropriate sensory and motor testing prior to beginning RF ablation.
- The anatomy of the cervical articular pillars predicates how an electrode should be inserted. Because the concavity of the articular pillar slopes caudally and posteriorly, electrodes directed to nerves over the lateral aspect off the pillar should be inserted along a cephalad-anterior slope (Figs. 43.1 and 43.2).
- If a direct posteroanterior parasagittal approach is used, the lateral flange of the superior articular process of the target pillar and any osteophytes stemming from it may prevent the electrode from being placed correctly on targeted nerves located along the upper half of the pillar.
- To avoid neural damage on lateral branches, the needle tip should not pass the posterior tubercle on a lateral view or 2–3 mm behind the posterior margin of the intervertebral foramen on an oblique view.

Recommended Reading

1. Barnsley L. Percutaneous radiofrequency neurotomy for chronic neck pain: outcomes in a series of consecutive patients. Pain Med. 2005;6:282–6.
2. Barnsley L, Lord SM, Wallis BJ, Bogduk N. The prevalence of chronic cervical zygapophysial joint pain after whiplash. Spine. 1995;20(1):20–5; discussion 26. PMID: 7709275.
3. Binder AI. Neck pain. BMJ Clin Evid. 2008;2008. pii: 1103. PMCID: PMC2907992.
4. Bogduk N. International Spinal Injection Society guidelines for the performance of spinal injection procedures. Part 1: zygapophysial joint blocks. Clin J Pain. 1997;13(4):285–302. PMID: 9430809.
5. Bogduk N, Dreyfuss P, Baker R, Yin W, Landers M, Hammer M, Aprill C. Complications of spinal diagnostic and treatment procedures. Pain Med. 2008;9(suppl 1):S11–34.
6. Cohen SP. Epidemiology, diagnosis, and treatment of neck pain. Mayo Clin Proc. 2015;90(2):284–99. PMID: 25659245.
7. Cohen SP, Bajwa ZH, Kraemer JJ, Dragovich A, Williams KA, Stream J, Sireci A, McKnight G, Hurley RW. Factors predicting success and failure for cervical facet radiofrequency denervation: a multi-center analysis. Reg Anesth Pain Med. 2007;32(6):495–503. PMID: 18035295.
8. Cohen SP, Williams KA, Kurihara C, Nguyen C, Shields C, Kim P, Griffith SR, Larkin TM, Crooks M, Williams N, Morlando B, Strassels SA. Multicenter, randomized, comparative cost-effectiveness study comparing 0, 1, and 2 diagnostic medial branch (facet joint nerve) block treatment paradigms before lumbar facet radiofrequency denervation. Anesthesiology. 2010;113:395–405. PMID: 20613471.
9. Cohen SP, Strassels SA, Kurihara C, Griffith SR, Goff B, Guthmiller K, Hoang HT, Morlando B, Nguyen C. Establishing an optimal "cutoff" threshold for diagnostic lumbar facet blocks: a prospective correlational study. Clin J Pain. 2013;29:382–91. PMID:23023310.
10. Derby R, Melnik I, Lee JE, Lee SH. Correlation of lumbar medial branch neurotomy results with diagnostic medial branch block cutoff values to optimize therapeutic outcome. Pain Med. 2012;13:1533–46. PMID: 23126379.
11. Dieleman JL, Baral R, Birger M, Bui AL, Bulchis A, Chapin A, Hamavid H, Horst C, Johnson EK, Joseph J, Lavado R, Lomsadze L, Reynolds A, Squires E, Campbell M, DeCenso B, Dicker D, Flaxman AD, Gabert R, Highfill T, Naghavi M, Nightingale N, Templin T, Tobias MI, Vos T, Murray CJL. US spending on personal health care and public health, 1996–2013. JAMA. 2016;316(24):2627–46. PMCID: PMC5551483.
12. Engel A, Rappard G, King W, Kennedy DJ, Standards Division of the International Spine Intervention Society. The effectiveness and risks of fluoroscopically-guided cervical medial branch thermal radiofrequency neurotomy: a systematic review with comprehensive analysis of the published data. Pain Med. 2016;17(4):658–69. PMID: 26359589.
13. Fejer R, Kyvik KO, Hartvigsen J. The prevalence of neck pain in the world population: a systematic critical review of the literature. Eur Spine J. 2006;15(6):834–48. PMCID: PMC3489448.
14. Fernández-de-las-Peñas C, Hernández-Barrera V, Alonso-Blanco C, Palacios-Ceña D, Carrasco-Garrido P, Jiménez-Sánchez S, Jiménez-García R. Prevalence of neck and low back pain in community-dwelling adults in Spain: a population-based national study. Spine. 2011;36(3):E213–9. PMID: 21079541.
15. Govind J, King W, Bailey B, Bogduk N. Radiofrequency neurotomy for the treatment of third occipital headache. J Neurol Neurosurg Psychiatry. 2003;74(1):88–93. PMCID: PMC1738184.
16. Hogg-Johnson S, van der Velde G, Carroll LJ, Holm LW, Cassidy JD, Guzman J, Côté P, Haldeman S, Ammendolia C, Carragee E, Hurwitz E, Nordin M, Peloso P, Bone and Joint Decade 2000–2010 Task Force on Neck Pain and Its Associated Disorders. The burden and determinants of neck pain in the general population: results of the Bone and Joint Decade 2000–2010 Task Force on Neck Pain and Its Associated Disorders. Spine. 2008;33(4 Suppl):S39–51. PMID: 18204398.
17. Holz SC, Sehgal N. What is the correlation between facet joint radiofrequency outcome and response to comparative medial branch blocks? Pain Physician. 2016;19(3):163–72. PMID:26359589.
18. Kweon TD, Kim JY, Lee HY, Kim MH, Lee YW. Anatomical analysis of medial branches of dorsal rami of cervical nerves for radiofrequency thermocoagulation. Reg Anesth Pain Med. 2014;39(6):465–71. PMID: 25304480.
19. Lord SM, Barnsley L, Bogduk N. Percutaneous radiofrequency neurotomy in the treatment of cervical zygapophysial joint pain: a caution. Neurosurgery. 1995;36:732–9.
20. Lord SM, Barnsley L, Wallis BJ, Bogduk N. Chronic cervical zygapophysial joint pain after whiplash. A placebo-controlled prevalence study. Spine. 1996;21(15):1737–44; discussion 1744–1745. PMID: 8855458.
21. Lord SM, Barnsley L, Wallis BJ, McDonald GJ, Bogduk N. Percutaneous radio-frequency neurotomy for chronic cervical zygapophyseal-joint pain. N Engl J Med. 1996;335(23):1721–6.
22. MacVicar J, Borowczyk JM, MacVicar AM, Loughnan BM, Bogduk N. Cervical medial branch radiofrequency neurotomy in New Zealand. Pain Med Malden Mass. 2012;13(5):647–54. PMID: 22458772.

23. Manchikanti L, Manchikanti KN, Pampati V, Brandon DE, Giordano J. The prevalence of facet-joint-related chronic neck pain in postsurgical and nonpostsurgical patients: a comparative evaluation. Pain Pract. 2008;8(1):5–10. PMID: 18211589.
24. McDonald GJ, Lord SM, Bogduk N. Long-term follow-up of patients treated with cervical radiofrequency neurotomy for chronic neck pain. Neurosurgery. 1999;45(1):61–7; discussion 67–68. PMID: 10414567.
25. Palea O, Andar HM, Lugo R, Granville M, Jacobson RE. Direct posterior bipolar cervical facet radiofrequency rhizotomy: a simpler and safer approach to denervate the facet capsule. Cureus. 2018;10(3):e2322. PMID: 26359589.
26. Sapir DA, Gorup JM. Radiofrequency medial branch neurotomy in litigant and nonlitigant patients with cervical whiplash: a prospective study. Spine. 2001;26(12):E268–73. PMID: 11426167.
27. Speldewinde GC. Outcomes of percutaneous zygapophysial and sacroiliac joint neurotomy in a community setting. Pain Med Malden Mass. 2011;12(2):209–18. PMID: 21143762.
28. Van Eerd M, Lataster A, Sommer M, Patijn J, van Kleef M. A modified posterolateral approach for radiofrequency denervation of the medial branch of the cervical segmental nerve in cervical facet joint pain based on anatomical considerations. Pain Pract. 2017;17(5):596–603. PMID: 26359589.

Intercostal Nerve Block

44

Reda Tolba and Alexander Fontenot

Introduction

The intercostal nerves innervate the skin and musculature of the chest and abdominal wall supplying sensation to the major portions of the thorax and abdomen. Intercostal nerve blocks are fairly simple to perform and can provide excellent analgesia. They can supply relatively well-defined anatomical coverage, making them both excellent diagnostic tools and reliable therapeutic procedures. In addition, the intercostal nerve block has been shown to provide perioperative opioid sparing, improved pulmonary mechanics, and reduced central nervous system depression.

Background and Historical Perspective

The intercostal nerve block (INB) was first described by Heinrich Braun in 1907 in effort to treat acute and chronic pain of posterior and anterior portions of the superficial thorax and upper abdomen. However, it was not until the 1940s where clinicians discovered that INBs could favorably effect a reduction in pulmonary complications and in opioid requirements after upper abdominal surgery. Today, INBs are used in a variety of acute and chronic pain conditions affecting the torso and abdomen, as well as, less frequently, in breast and minor chest wall surgeries, and in combination with celiac plexus blockade and abdominal operations, in combination with light sedation or general anesthesia.

While many consider epidural anesthesia the best method of providing analgesia to the torso, it requires greater technical skills and has potential side effects including hypotension, urinary retention, and risk of nerve root or spinal cord injury. In addition, widespread use of anticoagulants often results in contraindication of epidural procedures. The interpleural block has also been suggested as a reliable method with the advantage of a localized sympathetic block; however, its disadvantage of shorter efficacy and, ultimately, higher plasma concentration of local anesthetic makes it a less desirable choice to ICBs in perioperative analgesia and anesthesia.

R. Tolba (✉)
Wake Forest Baptist Medical Center, Winston Salem, NC, USA

A. Fontenot
Anesthesiology Department, Ochsner Health system, New Orleans, LA, USA
e-mail: alexander.fontenot@ochsner.org

Uses and Indications

Indications

Intercostal nerve blocks have been shown to provide relief following post-traumatic and postoperative pain, as well as in chronic malignancy of the torso and nonmalignant pain involving the thoracic wall. Local anesthetic blocks of the intercostal nerves can also be used for diagnostic purposes when there is uncertainty surrounding the etiology of one's pain and a thoracic or visceral source is suspected.

Additional indications of INBs are listed below:

1. Postoperative pain management following thoracotomy, sternotomy, or upper abdominal wall surgery
2. Post-rib fracture pain
3. Cancer pain
4. Mastectomy and breast surgery pain
5. Chest wall pain following acute herpes zoster or postherpetic neuralgia
6. Prior to percutaneous thoracostomy or nephrostomy tube placement
7. Idiopathic intercostal neuralgia
8. Costochondritis
9. Abdominal wall pain

Studies have shown INBs' use for post-thoracotomy pain offers advantages in decreased need for parenteral or oral opioids perioperatively, as well as preserving effort-dependent pulmonary function (FEV_1 and peak expiratory

T. R. Deer et al. (eds.), *Deer's Treatment of Pain*, https://doi.org/10.1007/978-3-030-12281-2_44

flow rate) when compared to opioid analgesia. Blockade of two dermatomes above and two below the level of surgical incision is typically required.

The first three intercostal nerves also innervate sensation portions of the upper arm and axilla, while the lower intercostals from T6 to T12 innervate muscles of the upper abdomen and overlying skin (Fig. 44.1). Hence, INBs at the appropriate levels can control symptoms in the affected dermatome, further decreasing reliance on opioid analgesics which can be useful in cases where one needs to avoid respiratory depression or mental status changes.

If consideration for destruction of the intercostal nerve is being given, this technique can be used in a prognostic manner to indicate the degree of motor and sensory impairment that patient's may experience. Destruction of the intercostal nerve is occasionally indicated for palliation of cancer pain, including pain secondary to invasive tumors of the chest, ribs, or upper abdominal wall.

Finally, continuous INB local anesthetic infusion has also been demonstrated for perioperative analgesia to reduce the incidence of chronic post-thoracotomy neuralgia. Of note studies have not shown a significant difference between bupivacaine vs lidocaine infusions in providing superior pain relief.

Contraindications

While there are few absolute contraindications to an intercostal nerve block, there are a few specific scenarios in which extra attention may be warranted prior to block placement. These include the following:

1. Any patient in which pneumothorax would be particularly hazardous such as those with ongoing respiratory decompensation, those with single lung on the side of a planned procedure, patients on positive pressure ventilation, and postsurgical patients
2. Severe coagulation abnormalities
3. Local infections
4. Lack of expertise and resuscitation equipment
5. Lack of short-term plan to wean from the ventilator

Intercostal Nerve Anatomy

There are three layers of intercostal muscles, external, internal, and innermost intercostal muscles, which are all incomplete and thin layers of muscle and tendinous fibers. The neurovascular bundle lies in between the internal and innermost intercostal muscles in the costal groove. The neurovascular bundle enters the intercostal space between the parietal pleura and the internal intercostal membrane initially and then between the internal and innermost intercostal membrane. Although most of the textbooks describe the location of neurovascular bundle in the costal groove, one cadaver study showed that the neurovascular bundle was subcostal in only 17% of the cases and, in the remaining 73% of the cases, it was midway between the ribs.

The intercostal nerves (ICNs) originate from the anterior division of the 12 paired thoracic nerve roots which are associated closely with the thoracic ribs. Once the thoracic nerve roots emerge from the intervertebral foramen, they divide into the posterior cutaneous rami, the paired gray and white rami communicantes, and the ventral rami. The posterior cutaneous rami supply the facet joints as well as the skin and muscle of the paravertebral region. The paired gray and white rami communicantes pass anteriorly to contribute to the sympathetic chain. Finally, the ventral rami form the intercostal nerves.

As the ICN approaches the angle of the rib, it emerges inwardly between the parietal pleura and the internal intercostal membrane initially and then between the internal and innermost intercostal membrane. Shortly prior to reaching the midaxillary line, the lateral cutaneous branch is given off. This lateral cutaneous nerve splits into posterior and anterior divisions which innervate the skin of the chest wall from the scapular line to the midclavicular line. The intercostal nerve continues traveling anteriorly within the costal groove and, as it approaches the midline, pierces the overlying muscles and skin to terminate as the anterior cutaneous branches which innervate the anterior chest and abdominal wall. At times, the terminal branches of an intercostal nerve can cross the midline and provide sensory innervation to the contralateral chest and abdominal wall (Fig. 44.2).

Technique

Prior to any regional anesthetic procedure, preparation is important for the procedure to be safely performed. This requires attaining an adequate history and physical exam to assess the patient's airways, respiratory, and cardiac status. In addition, resuscitation should be nearby. Finally, intravenous access should be attained, and ECG, pulse oximetry, and blood pressure monitoring should be established before going forward.

Landmark Technique

This technique can be performed in the prone, as well as the lateral or sitting positions. The prone position is typically preferred, particularly if bilateral blocks are to be performed. After lying prone, the patient's arms are allowed to hang loosely off the sides of the table in an effort to permit the scapula to rotate laterally. The rib to be blocked is then identified by palpating

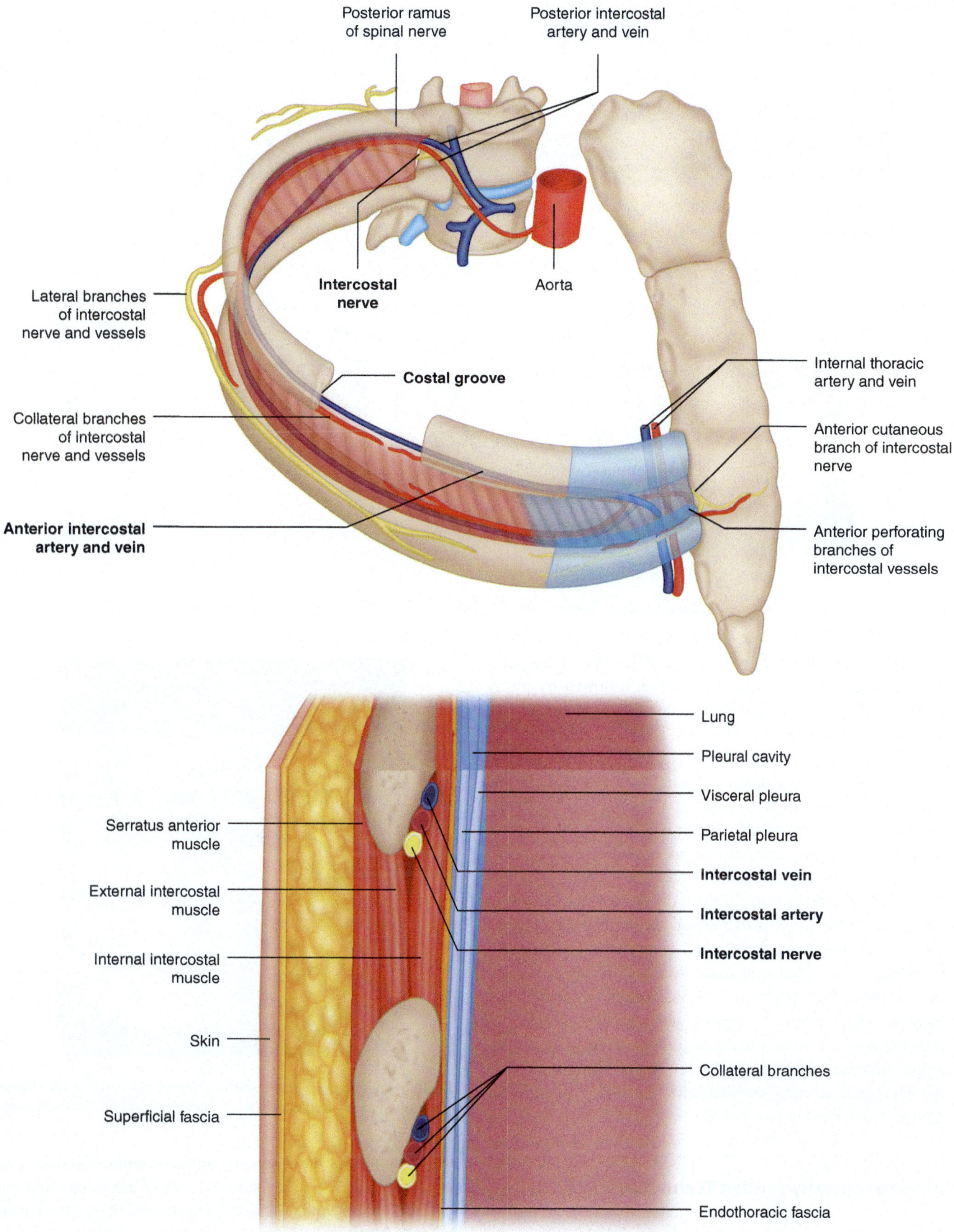

Fig. 44.1 Distribution of the thoracic dermatomes

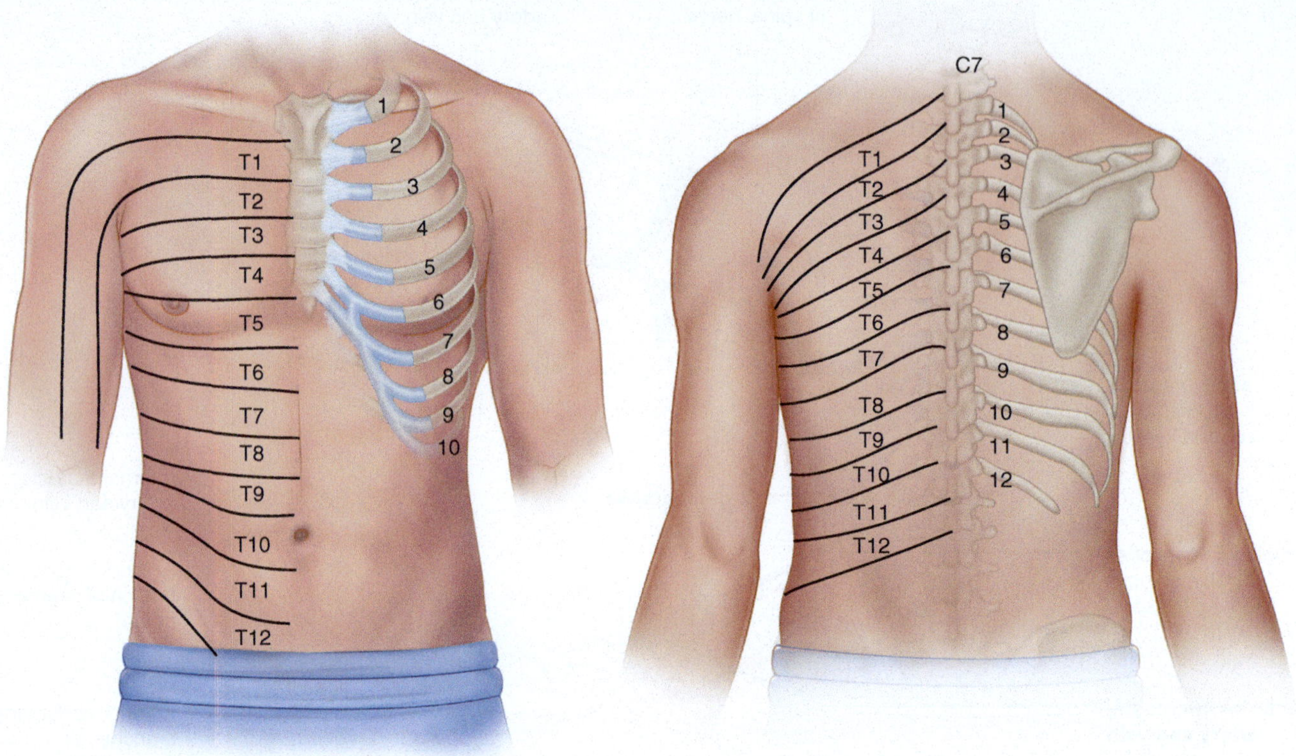

Fig. 44.2 Anatomy of the intercostal nerve block as it relates to the neurovascular bundle and surrounding structures

the nerves' path along the posterior axillary line. The skin is then prepared with an antiseptic solution followed by placement of the operator's middle and index finger on the rib near the site of needle insertion. After skin is anesthetized with 1 cc of lidocaine 1% a 22 gauge 3.5 inch spinal needle is inserted and advanced perpendicular to the skin between the middle and index fingers toward the middle of the rib until the needle impinges on the bone. Once the bone is contacted, the needle is withdrawn into the subcutaneous tissue where the skin and subcutaneous tissue are retracted with the palpating fingers. The needle is subsequently walked off the inferior margin of the rib where the needle is then advanced 2 mm deeper, placing the needle in proximity to the costal groove which contains the intercostal nerve. Following aspiration, 3–5 mL of local anesthetic such as 1.0% preservative-free lidocaine is injected. The local anesthetic can be combined with steroids if there is an inflammatory contributor to the ongoing pain. As there is overlapping intercostal innervation of the chest and abdominal wall, the intercostal nerves above and below the region of suspected pain will also need to be blocked.

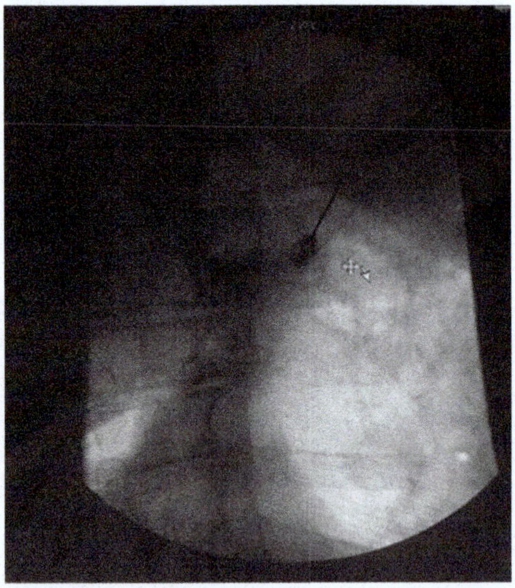

Fig. 44.3 Fluoroscopic image showing intercostal nerve block. Please note position of the needle underneath the rib and proper contrast spread

Fluoroscopically Guided Technique (Fig. 44.3)

For this technique, the patient is again placed in the prone position with the arms hanging off the side of the fluoroscopy table. The skin is first prepared with antiseptic solution. The rib to be blocked is then identified using fluoroscopy and the operators' index, and middle fingers are placed on the rib near the site of the needle insertion. A 22 gauge, 11/2 inch needle is attached to a 12 mL syringe and advanced perpendicular to the skin using fluoroscopic guidance directed toward the middle of the rib until the needle impinges on the bone. As with the landmark technique, once the bone is contacted, the needle is withdrawn into the subcutaneous tissue where the skin and subcutaneous tissue are retracted with the palpating fingers. The needle is subsequently walked off the inferior margin of the rib where the needle is then advanced 2 mm deeper, placing the needle in proximity to the costal groove which contains the intercostal nerve. Following negative aspiration for blood or air, 1–2 mL of contrast medium is injected for needle tip confirmation. Once appropriate needle tip placement is established, 3–5 mL of local anesthetic such as 1.0% preservative-free lidocaine with or without steroids is injected.

Ultrasound-Guided Technique (Fig. 44.4)

Narouze and Peng et al. have described the following technique: the patient is placed in the prone position where the appropriate rib is palpated. A 6–13 Hz linear transducer is placed in the short axis to the ribs so that two consecutive ribs are simultaneously observed. The ribs are identified as hyperechoic curvilinear line. Structures to be identified are external, internal, innermost intercostal muscles and the pleura. The pleura is identified as a prominent hyperechoic line with gliding action during respiration. The target intercostal nerve lies between the internal and innermost intercostal muscles; however the innermost intercostal muscle appears ill-defined layer of muscle, so needle target is the internal intercostal muscle. After localizing the skin with

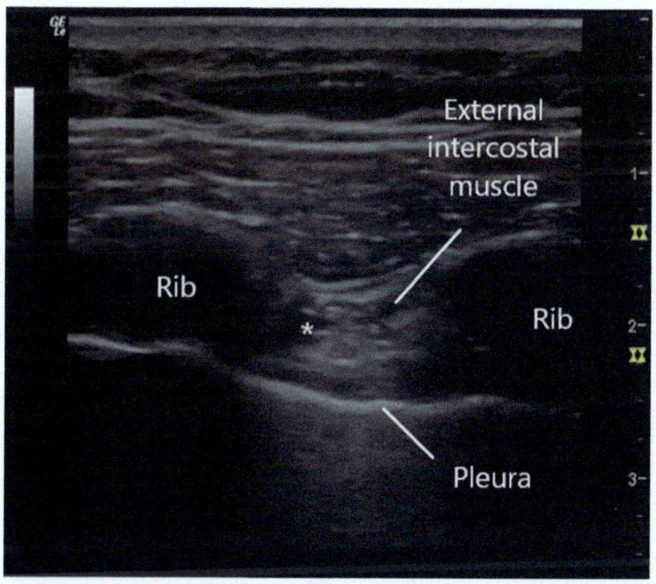

Fig. 44.4 Ultrasound image showing in asterixis the needle target for ultrasound-guided intercostal nerve block deep to the external intercostal muscle. Please note the depth of the pleura in relation to the rib and target area

1 cc of 1% lidocaine, a 22 gauge needle can be inserted either in-plane or out-of-plane just deep to the internal intercostal muscle or into the intercostal muscle. In-plane technique is preferred as it is easier to visualize the whole needle as it is advanced, which should be placed 2–3 mm proximal to the pleura. The needle entry site is the upper margin of the rib one level caudal to the targeted intercostal nerve. Advancing the needle should be slow and direct visualization. It is advised to inject small amount of solution upon reaching the external intercostal muscle to confirm needle tip position before further advancement. Precision is required and caution not to advance the needle too deep to avoid pleural puncture and pneumothorax. The needle is then slowly advanced a few millimeters further into the internal intercostal muscle, or in the plane between the internal and innermost intercostal muscle, if the latter can be visualized. The spread of local anesthetics is visualized in real time, as it is injected. If the injectate is seen pushing the external intercostal muscle upward, the needle position is still superficial. Usually 2–5 mm of local anesthetics is injected and is sufficient to block the intercostal nerve with minimal local anesthetic toxicity. When a pneumothorax is present, the pleura no longer glides with respiration (loss of gliding sign).

Complications

The intercostal nerve block is not without its own set of risks and complications. One of the most concerning potential issues is pneumothorax secondary to lack of operator experience and subsequent failure to control needle depth. The rate of occurrence, however, as detected by chest radiograph, is below 1%. Tension pneumothorax and the need for tube thoracostomy are exceedingly rare, although it should be noted that the risks of pneumothorax and lung injury are increased in patients who had prior chest surgery. Similarly, with lower thoracic intercostal nerve blocks, the peritoneum or retroperitoneum may be punctured causing such complications as liver subcapsular hematoma formation. Ultrasound guidance may assist in better needle tip control and potentially decreasing the occurrence of these complications.

Absorption of local anesthetic from the intercostal space can occur rapidly with peak arterial plasma concentrations developing in less than 5–10 minutes. Hence, local anesthetic toxicity can rarely occur as a result of bolus dosing secondary to rapid uptake from the vascularized intercostal space leading to sequelae including arrhythmias and seizures.

Other, less severe complications of intercostal nerve blocks include hypotension, secondary to central spread of the local anesthetic, as well as respiratory depression secondary to effective nerve block following administration of systemic opioids.

Of note, single-shot intercostal nerve blocks typically only provide adequate analgesia for approximately 6–8 hours; therefore, perineural catheter placement should be considered as an alternative when longer-lasting analgesia is required.

Clinical Pearls

- The intercostal nerve block can be utilized to manage acute and chronic pain of the thorax and upper abdomen.
- Intercostal nerve blocks are contraindicated when the threat of pneumothorax could be life-threatening as well as in patients with severe hemostatic deficiencies.
- In those with minor hemostatic abnormalities, intercostal nerve blocks may be a better-suited alternative to neuraxial blocks.
- Practitioners should develop a consistent method of hand and needle control for performing the intercostal nerve block.
- The benefit of ultrasound guidance in reducing the number of block-associated complications has not been studied in depth.
- Post-procedure evaluation and early detection of complications is essential.

Recommended Reading

1. Bhatia A, Peng PWH. Intercostal nerve block, Chapter 21. In: Narouze S, editor. Atlas of ultrasound-guided procedures in interventional pain management. Amherst: Springer; 2010. p. 285–90.
2. Fraifeld EM. Intercostal nerve blocks. In: Deer TR, Leong MS, Buvanendran A, editors. Comprehensive treatment of chronic pain by medical, interventional, and integrative approaches: the American Academy of Pain Medicine textbook on patient management. New York: Springer; 2013. p. 381–6.
3. Gulati A. Intercostal nerve block. In: Diwan S, Staats PS, editors. Atlas of pain medicine procedures. New York: McGraw-Hill; 2015. http://accessanesthesiology.mhmedical.com/content.aspx?bookid=1158&sectionid=64179235. Accessed 1 Aug 2017.
4. Hardy PAJ. Anatomical variation in the position of the proximal intercostals nerve. Br J Anaesth. 1988;61:338–9.
5. Harmon D, Barrett J. Intercostal block. In: Harmon D, Barrett J, Loughnane F, Finucane B, Shorten G, editors. Peripheral nerve blocks and peri-operative pain relief. Oxford: Saunders; 2011. p. 229–33.
6. Hill D. Peripheral nerve blocks: practical aspects. In: Breivik H, Campbell W, Eccleston C, editors. Clinical pain management: practical applications and procedures. London: Arnold; 2003. p. 216.
7. Ho AH, Karmakar MK. Intercostal nerve block. In: Hadzic A, editor. NYSORA textbook of regional anesthesia and acute pain management. New York: McGraw-Hill; 2007. http://accessanesthesiology.mhmedical.com/content.aspx?bookid=413&sectionid=39828196. Accessed 1 Aug 2017.
8. Peng P, Narouze S. Ultrasound -guided interventional procedures in pain medicine: a review of anatomy, sonoanatomy and procedures. Part 1: non-axial structures. Reg Anesth Pain Med. 2009;34:458–74.
9. Rohit R, Tureanu L, Molloy RE. Intercostal nerve block. In: Benzon HT, Raja SN, Liu SS, Fishman SM, Cohen SP, editors. Essentials of pain medicine. 3rd ed. St. Louis: Elsevier; 2017. p. 589–90.
10. Waldman SD. Intercostal nerve block. In: Waldman SD, editor. Atlas of pain management injection techniques. St. Louis: Elsevier; 2017. p. 370–5.

Thoracic Transforaminal Epidural Access

45

Alan Gonzalez Cota

Introduction

Thoracic transforaminal epidural steroid injections were developed as an equivalent to lumbar level techniques. They have been received with skepticism and are perceived as technically demanding with an increased risk of complications; thus, a group of patients with thoracic radiculopathy is left with limited options for pain relief. The medical literature is limited to reports and techniques of catastrophic neurological injury. The current chapter is limited to the technique of thoracic transforaminal epidural access. The diagnostic validity, therapeutic effect and safety of Thoracic transforaminal epidural steroid Injections (Thoracic TF-ESI) have not been studied well.

Background and Historical Perspective

The objective of thoracic transforaminal access is to place a needle in close proximity with a thoracic spinal nerve, exiting the paraspinal space to deliver an active agent. This procedure is technically demanding.

The delivery of corticosteroids into the thoracic epidural space has only been reported using the interlaminar approach, with low complication rates. In regard to efficacy, a prospective randomized study of interlaminar local anesthesia only versus local anesthesia plus corticosteroid found 71% improvement and 80% improvement in the numeric rating scale at 2-year follow-up. The limitations of this study are the lack of true controls (non-active agent) and reporting of group data only.

A. Gonzalez Cota (✉)
A.I.M. Interventional Spine Division, Rockville, MD, USA

Legacy Pain Management Rehabilitation, Bethesda, MD, USA

KureSmart Pain Management, Annapolis, MD, USA

Uses and Indications

Despite the lack of medical evidence (positive or negative) in peer-reviewed journals, blockade of thoracic spinal nerves may be a useful alternative in the treatment of intractable thoracic neuropathic pain and various other conditions, such as radicular pain from disk herniation, posthoracotomy or postlaminectomy pain, and postherpetic neuralgia.

Extensive experience in fluoroscopy-guided spinal procedures is recommended before attempting this technique. In addition, familiarity with life support equipment is a necessity, and it should be readily accessible.

Pearls and Pitfalls

Transforaminal Epidural Access Technique

- The physician should avoid this technique in patients unwilling to consent to the specific risks, such as possibility of neurological injury or paralysis, contrast medium anaphylaxis, uncooperativeness during the procedure, concurrent use of anticoagulants, pregnancy, severe anatomical changes from spondylosis or surgery, local or systemic infection, or allergy to local anesthetics used, contrast or to corticosteroids.
- The patient is placed in the prone position, with arms overhead. Ribs are accurately counted from cranial-to-caudal or caudal-to-cranial, and the level to be injected is marked.
- In the classic (or retroneural) technique (Fig. 45.1), first, a true AP view is obtained by "squaring off" the end plates at the level of interest. The target landmark is the inferior aspect of the transverse process at the junction with the lamina. The thoracic spinal nerve lies ventral to this landmark. Under AP view, a curved 22 g or 25 g needle is advanced to this target after local anesthesia of the overlying tissues is performed. After contact with the lamina at its junction with the transverse process using

T. R. Deer et al. (eds.), *Deer's Treatment of Pain*, https://doi.org/10.1007/978-3-030-12281-2_45

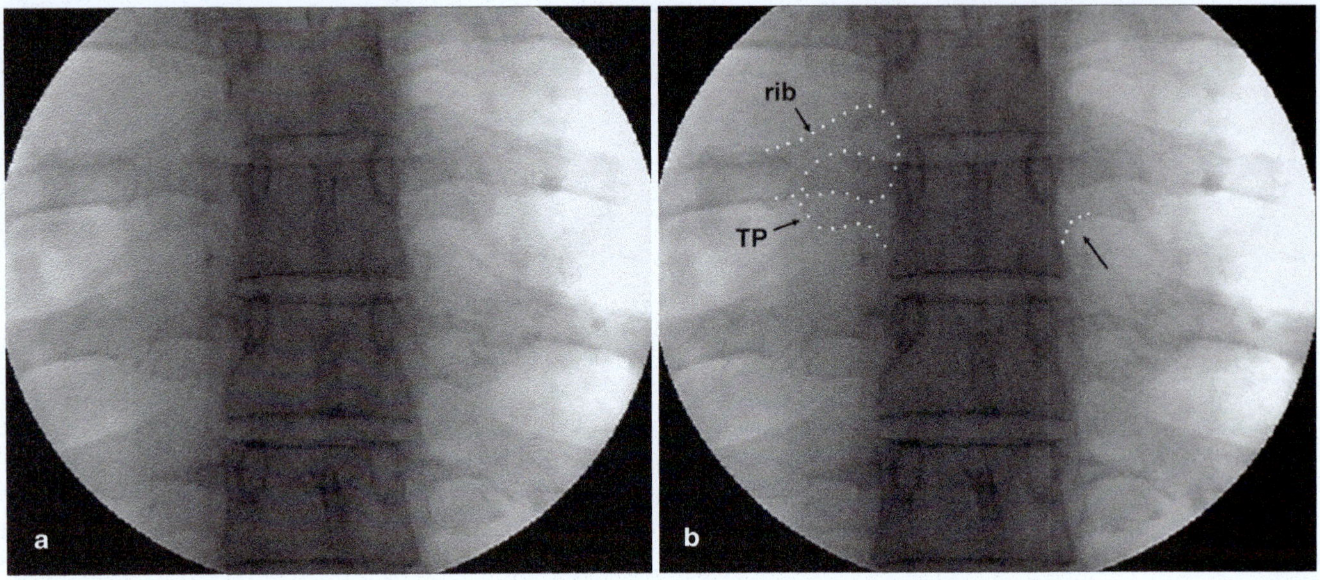

Fig. 45.1 (**a**) Retroneural Approach. (**b**). Locate the inferomedial margin of the (TP) as it merges with the lamina (L). Reproduced with permission from Bogduk N (ed). Practice Guidelines for Spinal Diagnostic and Treatment Procedures, 2nd edn. International Spine Intervention Society, San Francisco, 2013

intermittent fluoroscopy, the needle is rotated to the lateral edge of the lamina without advancing it into the foramen. The concavity of the needle should point medially without leaving the lamina. Then a precise lateral view (90°) should show the tip of the needle at the dorsal aspect of the neuroforamen. If this position is not detected, the needle should be withdrawn to touch the dorsal lamina under an AP view. If the needle is in fact on the dorsal neuroforamen, the needle is advanced with the curve pointing medially (away from the pleura). Then, under frequent intermittent fluoroscopy, the needle is advanced until the tip rests at the junction between the middle and posterior third of the foramen. The fluoroscope is repositioned to an AP view prior to contrast injection. The ideal location in this view is slightly medial to the lateral border of the lamina and lateral to the pedicle. Live contrast injection (Fig. 45.2) is advocated as minimum standard, and digital subtraction may be superior, although no studies are available to confirm this fluoroscopic modality.

- The most studied technique to date is with an oblique approach. A report of 198 cases by Rosas found only one case of uncomplicated pneumothorax, which resolved spontaneously.
- The oblique approach is based on an anatomical "box." The advantage of this technique is that it does not require readjustment from the lamina into the foramen. This target box is bounded by rib head laterally, pedicles and lamina medially, and pedicles superior and inferior (Fig. 45.3).
- To perform the oblique technique, first, the end plates of the desired level are aligned with the x-ray beam ("squared off"). An oblique view is obtained around 30° to the ipsilateral side when the head of the ribs has separated from the pedicles. The head of the rib can be identified where it forms the costovertebral joint. If the lamina medial to the head of the rib is not identified easily, it can be found by tracing medially to the mid-pedicular plane. An infraneural approach is then used after anesthetizing the underlying tissues. The target point is identified at the opposite side of the disk space, between the head of the rib and the lamina. At all times the needle needs to stay in line with the x-ray beam ("barrel view"). At least, it should remain between the lines formed by the proximal border of the head of the ribs medially and laterally to the pedicle line. A small bend can be useful if bony elements are encountered. Final advancement is done in the lateral view to avoid disk puncture (Fig. 45.4). If paresthesia is encountered, the needle should be withdrawn slightly. If paresthesia cannot be avoided with small repositioning, the procedure should be aborted.
- Once the target position is achieved in the classic or the oblique technique, contrast media is used to identify potential needle misplacement (Fig. 45.5). The needle is in the inferior aspect of the target box, this approach may contact, but should not enter the disk. Live contrast injection in the AP view first and then in the lateral view is advocated as a minimum safety standard. Digital subtraction may be superior, although no studies are available to confirm superiority of this fluoroscopic modality. If no vascular or extraforaminal uptake is noted initially, more contrast can be given to outline the silhouette of the target nerve and its dural sleeve.
- Then a test dose of lidocaine (2%) is recommended. If this procedure is undertaken for diagnostic purposes,

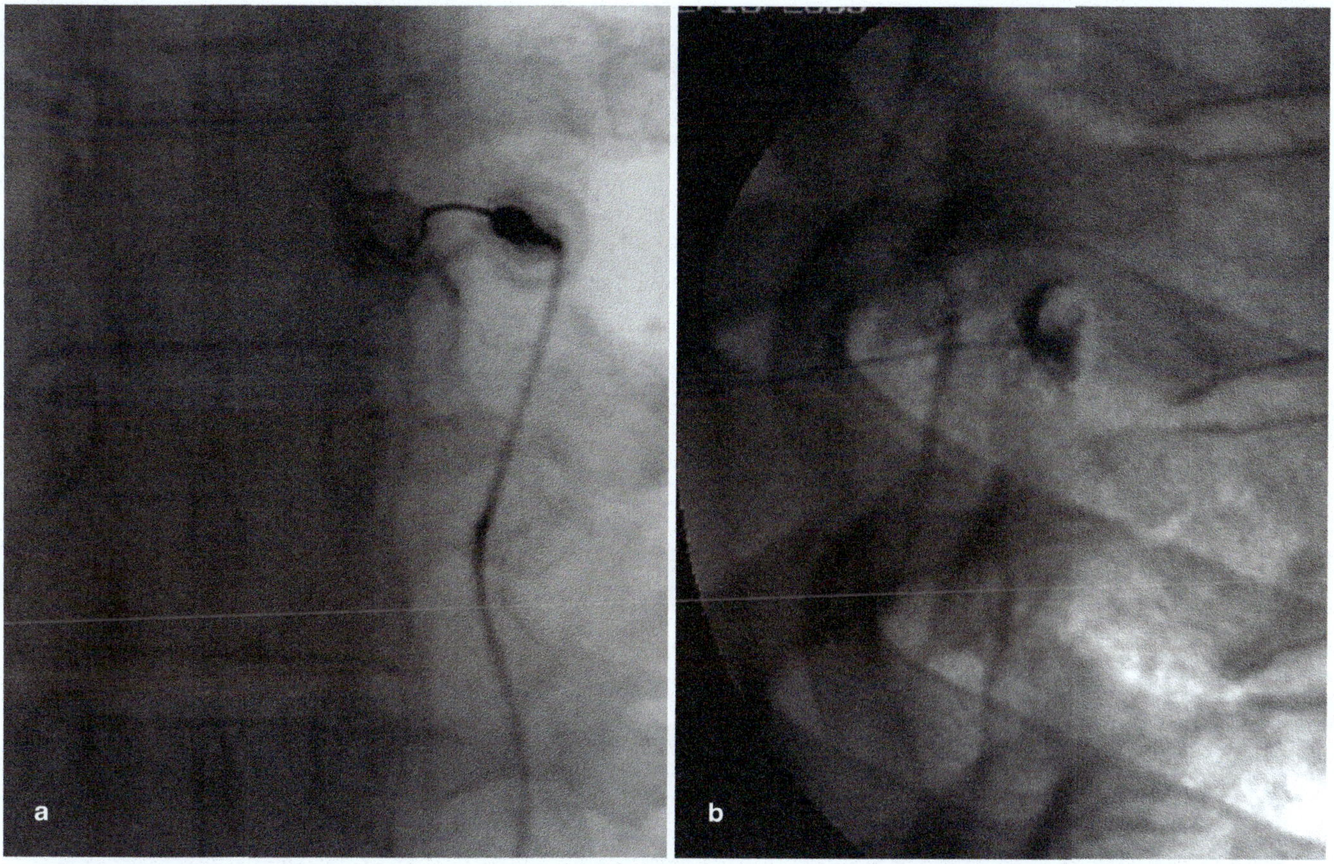

Fig. 45.2 **Retroneural Approach**. Anteroposterior view (**a**), Lateral View (**b**). Reproduced with permission from Bogduk N (ed). Practice Guidelines for Spinal Diagnostic and Treatment Procedures, 2nd edn. International Spine Intervention Society, San Francisco, 2013

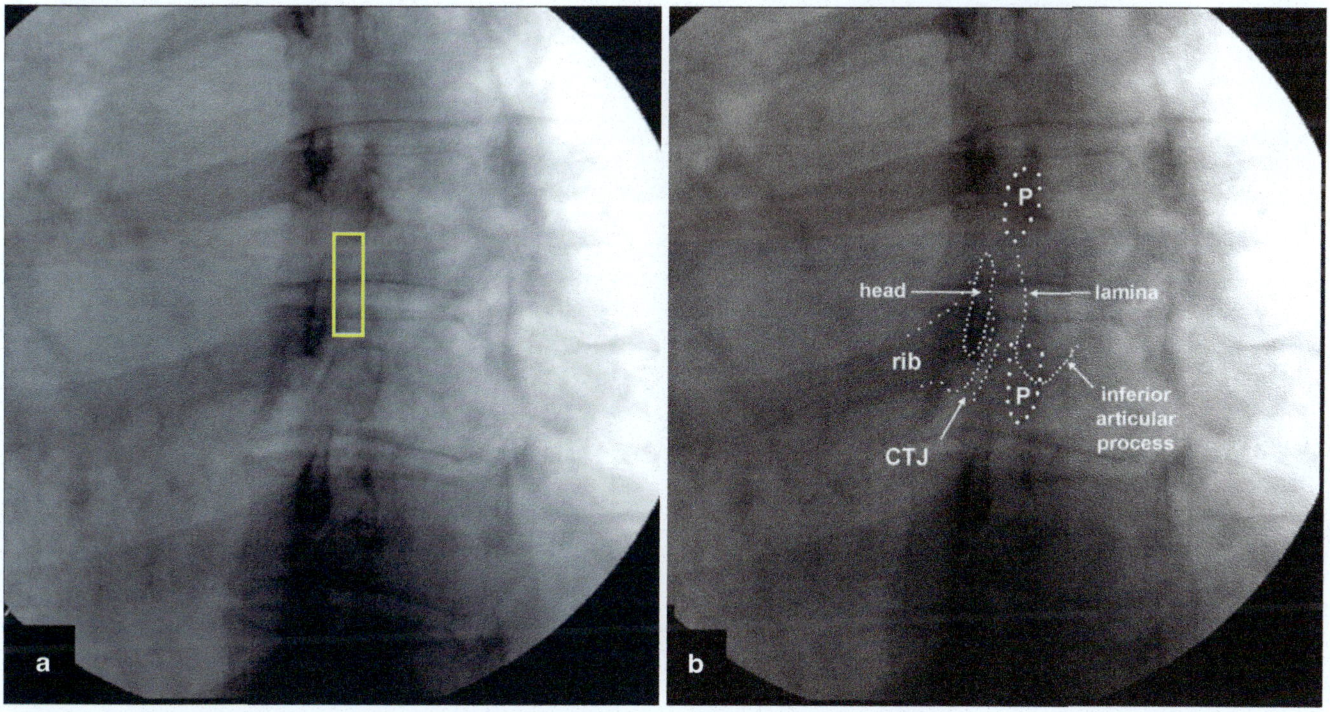

Fig. 45.3 **Oblique Approach**. "The Box" (**a**), fluoroscopic landmarks (**b**). Reproduced with permission from Bogduk N (ed). Practice Guidelines for Spinal Diagnostic and Treatment Procedures, 2nd edn. International Spine Intervention Society, San Francisco, 2013

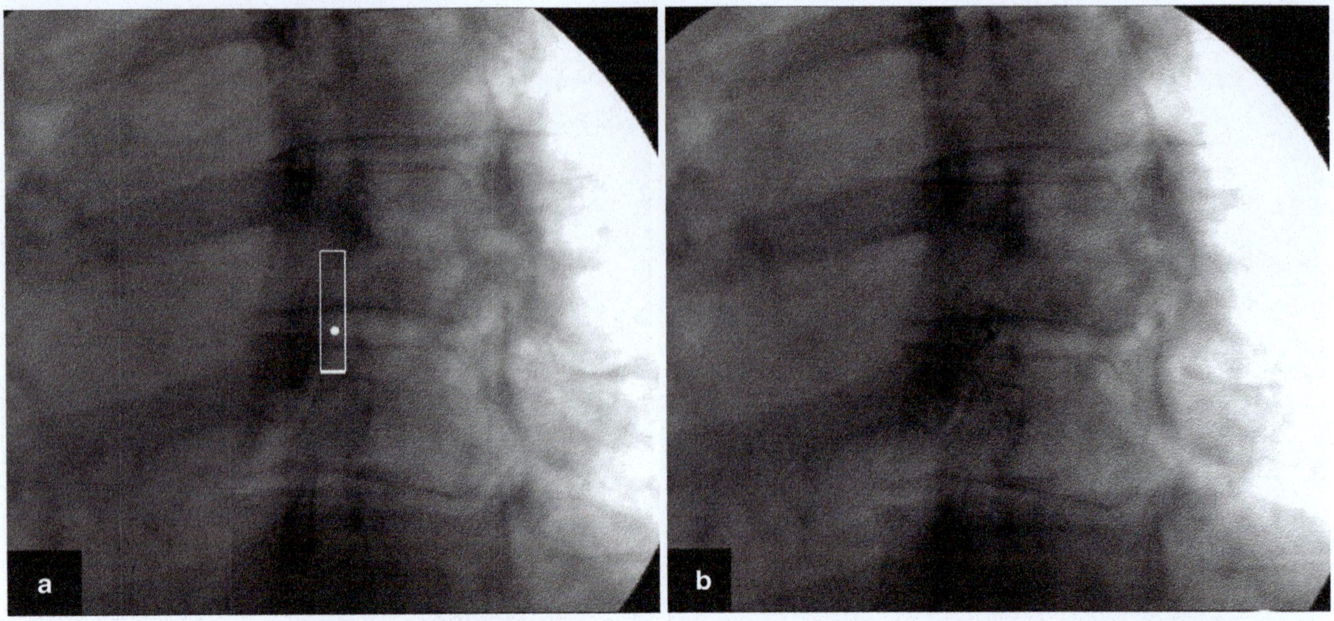

Fig. 45.4 **Infraneural oblique approach**. Needle target (**a**), Needle Placement (**b**). Reproduced with permission from Bogduk N (ed). Practice Guidelines for Spinal Diagnostic and Treatment Procedures, 2nd edn. International Spine Intervention Society, San Francisco, 2013

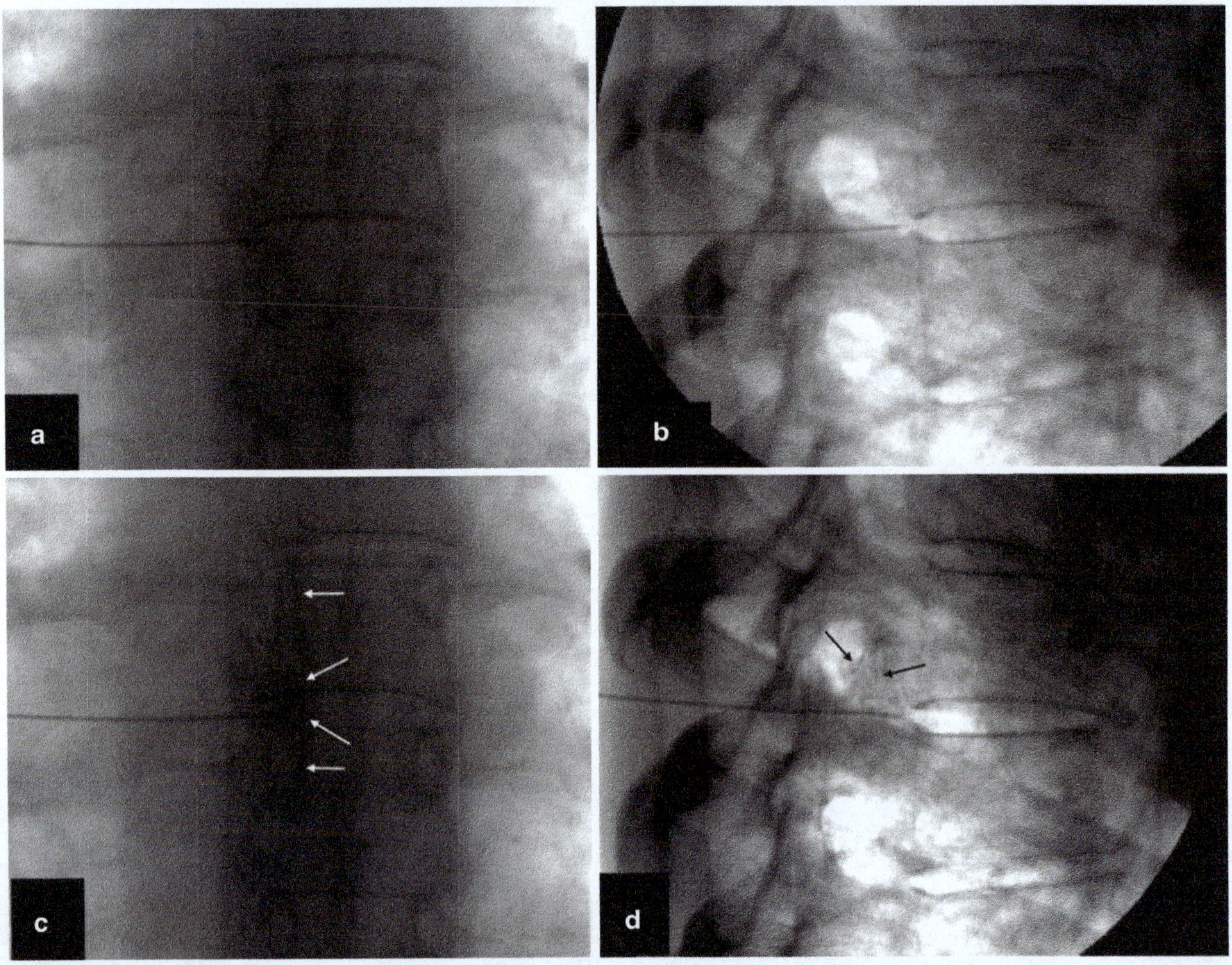

Fig. 45.5 Infraneural oblique approach. AP pre-contrast (**a**), Lateral pre-contrast (**b**), AP contrast injection (**c**), lateral contrast injection (**d**). Reproduced with permission from Bogduk N (ed). Practice Guidelines for Spinal Diagnostic and Treatment Procedures, 2nd edn. International Spine Intervention Society, San Francisco, 2013

corticosteroids should be avoided. If the pain physician decides to use a corticosteroid for a therapeutic purpose, particulate steroids should be avoided due to their association with small artery embolization (see Chap. 26, Injectable Corticosteroids).

Pitfalls

- The trajectory near the pleura and lungs is specific to the thoracic transforaminal needle technique.
- Vascular penetration should be recognized promptly to avoid potential embolization of the blood supply to the spinal cord or cauda equina, especially with the use of particulate steroids.
- If the patient coughs or moves unexpectedly during needle placement, the pain physician should recognize the early signs of pneumothorax.
- If contrast medium cannot be used because of a known anaphylactic reaction, this procedure should not be performed.
- Baseline data should be collected before the procedure, and the analgesic effects of the injection should be recorded ("pain diary").
- If there are any doubts about a pleural puncture, an AP and lateral chest x-ray can be obtained while monitoring the patient with continuous pulse oximetry.
- The patient should not travel by airplane for at least 3 days post-procedure, as the lower atmospheric pressure in the cabin can augment a subclinical pneumothorax.

Recommended Reading

1. Bogduk N, editor. Practice guidelines for spinal diagnostic and treatment procedures. 2nd ed; International Spine Intervention Society, San Francisco, 2013.
2. Glaser SE, Falco FJE. Paraplegia following a thoracolumbar transforaminal epidural steroid injection. Pain Physician. 2005;8:309–14.
3. Manchikanti L, Abdi S, Atluri S, et al. An update of comprehensive evidence-based guidelines for interventional techniques of chronic spinal pain: part II: guidance and recommendations. Pain Physician. 2013;16:S49–283.
4. Manchikanti L, Cash KA, McManus CD, et al. Thoracic interlaminar epidural injections in managing chronic thoracic pain: a randomized, double-blind, controlled trial with a 2-year follow-up. Pain Physician. 2014;17:E327–38.
5. Rosas HG, Gilula LA. Performing thoracic transforaminal injections: a new technique. Radiology. 2010;254:595–600.
6. Wang A, Pilgram TK, Gilula LA. Immediate complications and pain relief associated with 296 fluoroscopically guided thoracic foraminal nerve blocks. AJR Am J Roentgenol. 2011;197:1410–6.

Thoracic Interlaminar Epidural Steroid Injection

46

Christian Peccora

Introduction

Injections of local anesthetic with or without steroids into the epidural space have been shown to significantly decrease both acute and chronic pain along the dermatomes subserved by nerve roots traversing this area. There are numerous pathologies that can cause pain in or originating from the thoracic spine. Radicular pain can radiate along thoracic dermatomes and thus result in pain anywhere from the chest to the lower abdomen. Pain from other structures of the thoracic spine can cause axial pain or pain that radiates along the flanks and anteriorly. The anti-inflammatory effects of steroids and analgesia from local anesthetics infused via a thoracic epidural injection provide both diagnostic and therapeutic benefit for patients experiencing these kinds of pain. Though thoracic pain and thoracic stenosis resulting in radicular pain are less commonly encountered than similar painful pathologies in the cervical and lumbar spine, thoracic pain can be just as severe and can affect breathing and daily function. Therefore, having thorough familiarity with the anatomy, technique, and potential benefits and complications related to thoracic epidural steroid injections gives a pain physician an important tool to combat what can be severe pain of the thoracic spine, chest, and abdomen.

Background and Historical Perspective

Treatment of pain via injection of medication into the epidural space was described in the early twentieth century. A variety of medications have been researched and employed for epidural injections. The use of this procedure expanded to address both acute and chronic pain, and there has been a significant proliferation of the use of steroid and local anesthetic epidural injections for the treatment of chronic radicular pain in recent decades.

C. Peccora (✉)
Texas Pain Consultant Associates, Houston, TX, USA

The overall prevalence of thoracic back pain is notably less than cervical or lumbar pain in multiple analyses, but some studies suggest it could affect as much as 15% of the population. With regard to the chronic pain population specifically, there is some variation in the estimates of frequency of thoracic pain, but some studies suggest it could be as high as one-third of these patients. Regardless of the proportion affected, the disability associated with thoracic pain can be significant for the patient. Therefore, having the ability to successfully perform an interlaminar thoracic epidural steroid injection for the indications discussed below is a valuable skill for pain physicians to master.

Thoracic epidural steroid injections are not the only tool for managing thoracic pain. Indeed, a multimodal approach is more likely to provide long-term pain relief. The management of thoracic pain can include physical therapy, medication therapy, chiropractic techniques, acupuncture, and massage. In cases where thoracic epidural steroid injections fail to provide sufficient relief, facet joint injections, surgery, and other options can be considered.

Uses and Indications

There are multiple indications for thoracic epidural steroid injections, and some of these are different from the indications for epidural injections for pain control in the cervical or lumbar spine. Some of the indications for thoracic injections have not been studied rigorously, but they have logical underpinnings and analogous pathologies in the lumbar and cervical regions that have been studied in more detail. One of the more common indications is radicular pain of a thoracic nerve root. While disc herniations resulting in stenosis are less common in the thoracic spine, even a small or moderate herniation can result in pain or cause more notable stenosis when combined with spondylolisthesis, osteophytes, ligamentum flavum hypertrophy, scoliosis, facet arthropathy, facet joint cysts, and other anatomic changes. Herniation of the nucleus pulposus can generate an inflammatory

T. R. Deer et al. (eds.), *Deer's Treatment of Pain*, https://doi.org/10.1007/978-3-030-12281-2_46

response that results in both localized and radicular pain, and this pain may be addressed via deposition of steroids and local anesthetic in the epidural space. Spondylosis or other causes of neuroforaminal stenosis resulting or narrowing of the lateral canal or neural foraminae can cause radicular pain, and injectate can spread anterolaterally toward affected foraminae.

Acute herpes zoster and postherpetic neuralgia can cause severe, debilitating pain that sometimes fails to respond to neuropathic medications, antivirals, and topical lidocaine. A thoracic epidural steroid injection at the level of the affected dermatome can provide significant relief and serves as an alternative or complement to a costovertebral block. Postherpetic neuralgia affects thoracic dermatomes more frequently than other dermatomes. Indeed, there is some evidence that performing an epidural injection during an episode of acute herpes zoster can decrease the probability that postherpetic neuralgia will occur.

There are other indications for thoracic epidural steroid injections. Though rigorous randomized controlled trials have not been done and one study showed no significant improvement, this procedure is used to treat post-thoracotomy pain syndrome. Other neuropathic pain involving the chest, such as chronic postoperative pain after breast surgery, can be addressed with this procedure. As some neuropathic pain syndromes are difficult to diagnose based on history and clinical presentation, a thoracic epidural steroid injection can provide diagnostic value for both the patient and the physician.

Preoperative preparations for this procedure are not extensive. Pain level and location should be clearly documented prior to the procedure so that adequate assessment of efficacy is possible. After informed consent is obtained, appropriate monitors in accordance with American Society of Anesthesiology guidelines are placed if sedation is to be used. Even if sedation is not used, appropriate monitors of blood pressure, oxygenation, heart rate, and respiratory rate are recommended as inadvertent intrathecal or intravascular administration of local anesthetic can have significant cardiovascular, respiratory, and other effects, including hypotension, dyspnea, nausea, and agitation (see Pearls and Pitfalls below). Resuscitation equipment should be readily available to handle an emergent situation. The patient is placed comfortably in a prone position on the operating table compatible for fluoroscopy. A pillow may be placed under the mid to lower chest to accentuate the kyphosis of the region and optimize the interlaminar opening. The thoracic region near the expected injection site is generously prepped and draped in a sterile manner. Some practitioners place a sterile cover over their fluoroscope to decrease the risk of contamination of the field as multiple views are obtained and the physician's hands can come in close proximity to the unit during the performance of the procedure.

The technique used for epidural access at the thoracic level is similar to that employed in the lumbar and cervical levels in some ways but quite different in others. The skin overlying the target is anesthetized with 1–2 cc of 1% lidocaine being careful not to insert the needle too deeply before obtaining confirmatory fluoroscopic images as the epidural space and even the lungs can be quite superficial in thin patients. The epidural space is approached by advancing a needle through the skin, subcutaneous tissues, supraspinous ligament, interspinous ligament, and ligamentum flavum to access the epidural space between the laminae of the vertebral levels at or near the suspected pathology (Fig. 46.1). Eighteen- or 20-gauge Tuohy needles are commonly used. If a clear interlaminar space is visible, advancement directly into the spinous ligaments near the midline can occur (Fig. 46.2). Fluoroscopic images employing a caudad tilt are

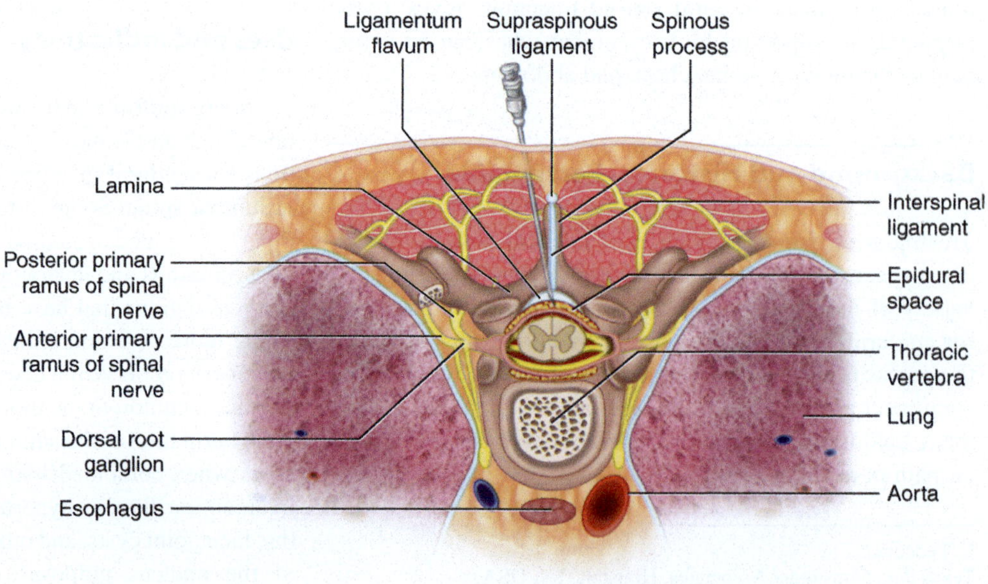

Fig. 46.1 Illustrated depiction of the needle advanced from the skin to the epidural space showing the different levels. A paramedian approach is employed

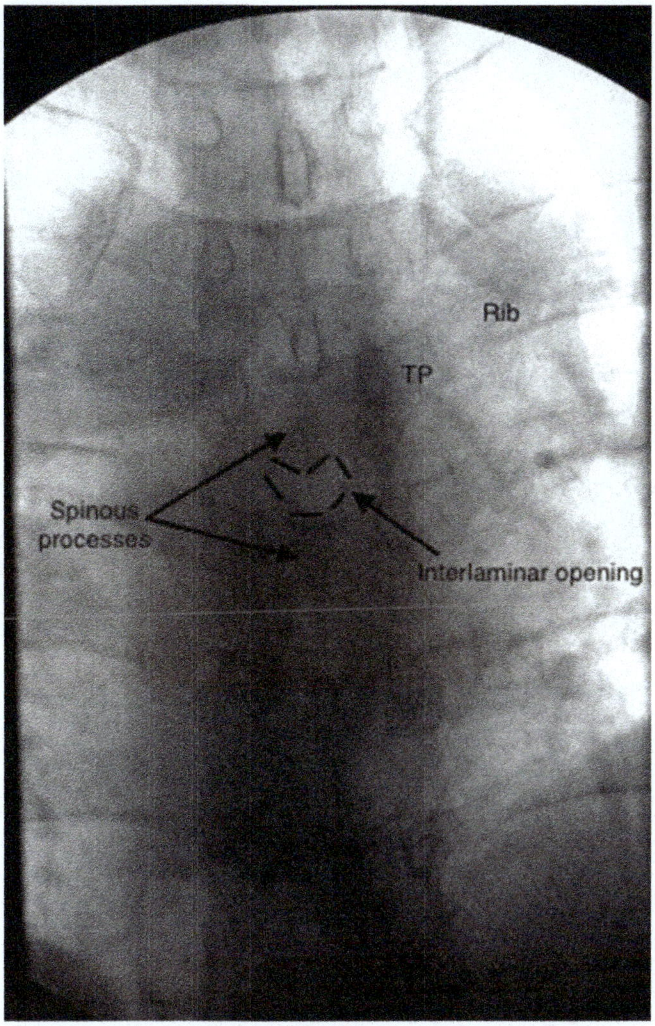

Fig. 46.2 AP view demonstrating pertinent anatomy, including interlaminar space. TP transverse process

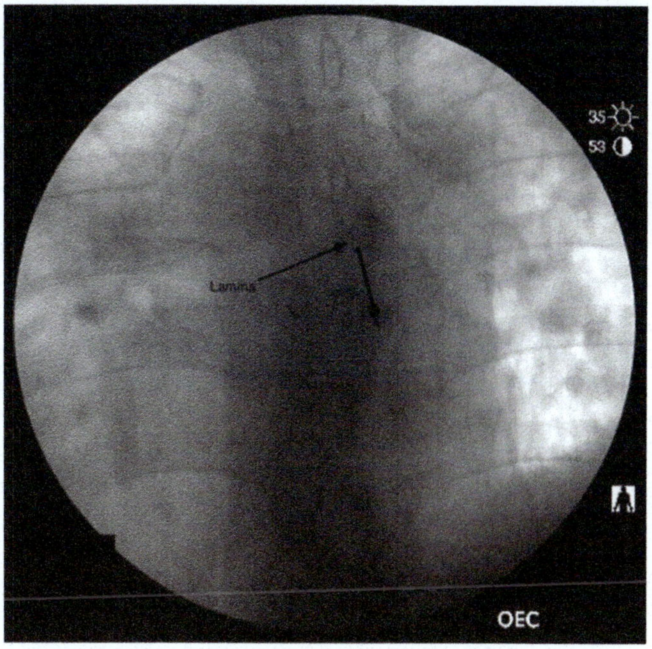

Fig. 46.3 AP view with needle. The lamina with which the needle can make contact and be "walked off" into the interlaminar epidural space is denoted

advised to maximally open the interlaminar space and allow visualization of a possible needle trajectory. This caudad tilt view will often reveal whether a paramedian or midline interlaminar approach is advisable. The angulation of spinous processes and other anatomic considerations may make a midline approach infeasible; this is discussed in further detail below. If anatomic considerations make interlaminar visualization suboptimal, the needle can be purposefully directed onto the lamina of the inferior vertebra at the level in question at a point lateral to the spinous process allowing one to avoid the spinous process and thus facilitate entry into the epidural space. This also allows the physician to assess the depth of insertion near where one would expect engagement with the ligamentum flavum to occur. The needle can then be walked off the lamina superiorly to engage the ligamentum flavum and advanced into the epidural space (Fig. 46.3). Of note, encountering the lamina with the needle can be painful, and a small amount of lidocaine can be deposited at the site to decrease pain as the needle is walked off the bone. Though the needle is commonly aimed toward the midline, it can be slightly deviated to the left or right to address unilateral symptomatology. When aiming for the bilateral spread of injectate, one must keep in mind that the ligamentum flavum sometimes is not fused at the midline in the thoracic spine, so an entry point slightly lateral to midline may provide improved safety during needle advancement use of the loss of resistance (LOR) technique. The epidural space in this region can be about 3–5 mm in width (though this naturally varies depending on the degree of stenosis), and the spinal cord is of course present at this level. Therefore, it is important the patient be sufficiently awake and cooperative to communicate any discomfort or paresthesia she or he may be feeling.

As mentioned above, anatomic considerations unique to the thoracic spine have important implications for performing a thoracic interlaminar epidural steroid injection. Though the spinous processes attach to the laminae in a fairly horizontal orientation in the cervical and lumbar spine, the spinous processes are steeply angled, in some cases to about 60°, particularly in the mid thoracic region near T5–T8. As such, a midline approach may be difficult. A paramedian approach ipsilateral to the painful side or aimed toward midline to address bilateral symptoms can be employed, as is commonly done when this technique is performed blindly for surgical analgesia. One must be aware of the fact that false loss of resistance may occur if the needle is superficial to the ligamentum flavum, particularly since a paramedian approach may cause the needle to avoid engagement in the supraspinous and interspinous ligaments.

Fluoroscopic guidance can be optimized to compensate for the increased difficulty of thoracic epidural steroid injections due to the presence of lung fields, ribs, and steeply angled spinous processes. It is important to familiarize oneself with the approximate locations of the ligamentum flavum, spinolaminar line, epidural space, and spinal cord on contralateral oblique and lateral fluoroscopic images (Figs. 46.4, 46.5, 46.6, and 46.7) so as to be able to advance the needle confidently to minimize false losses of resistance superficially while also ensuring the needle does not advance too deeply before the loss of resistance technique is employed. The use of a lateral view can help provide evidence that the needle is indeed in the epidural space as contrast spread has a characteristic appearance when the needle is properly placed. A lateral view can be complicated in the thoracic spine, however, because overlying structures, particularly the lung fields and ribs, obscure the views of spinal structures. Contralateral oblique (CLO) views can provide a clearer image of the region at which the needle approaches the epidural space. Contralateral oblique approaches have been studied in the cervical and lumbar spine wherein the fluoroscope beam is parallel to the lamina and thus establishes a clear spinolaminar line before which the needle will not enter the epidural space. If a needle is placed lateral to the midline, the needle may advance well beyond the beginning of where the epidural space appears to be on a lateral image because the ligamentum flavum follows the counters of the laminae in an anterolateral direction. Studies in the cervical and lumbar spine suggest that the optimal CLO angles are 50° and 45°, respectively, contralateral to the side where the needle will enter the epidural space. While this has not been studied in the thoracic spine, one can presume it is somewhere between these two numbers (Figs. 46.4 and 46.6). One can more confidently advance the needle to the spinolaminar line and thus avoid checking for loss of resistance too early, which minimizes the risk of false loss of resistance posterior to the epidural space (Figs. 46.8 and 46.9). Again, this

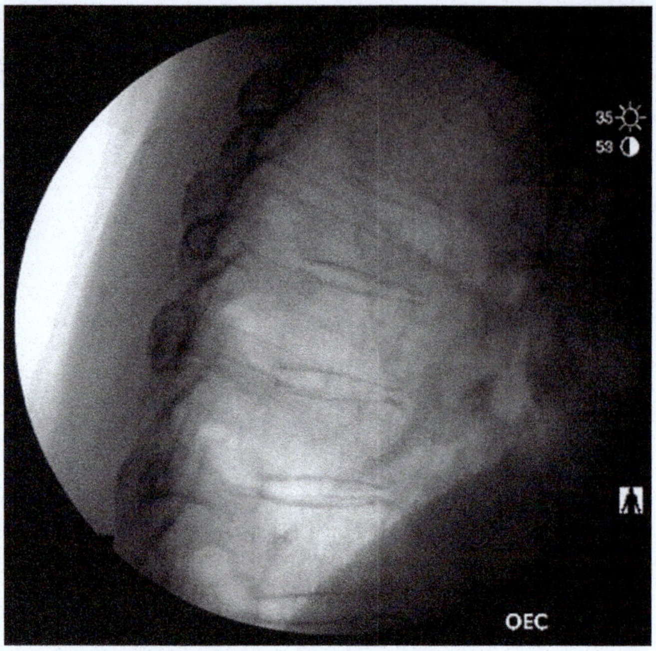

Fig. 46.5 Lateral view with fluoroscopy

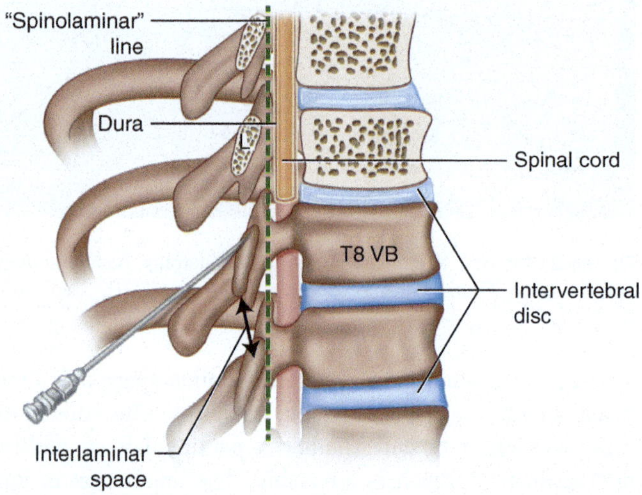

Fig. 46.6 Artistic adaption of contralateral oblique view. IVD intervertebral disc, SC spinal cord

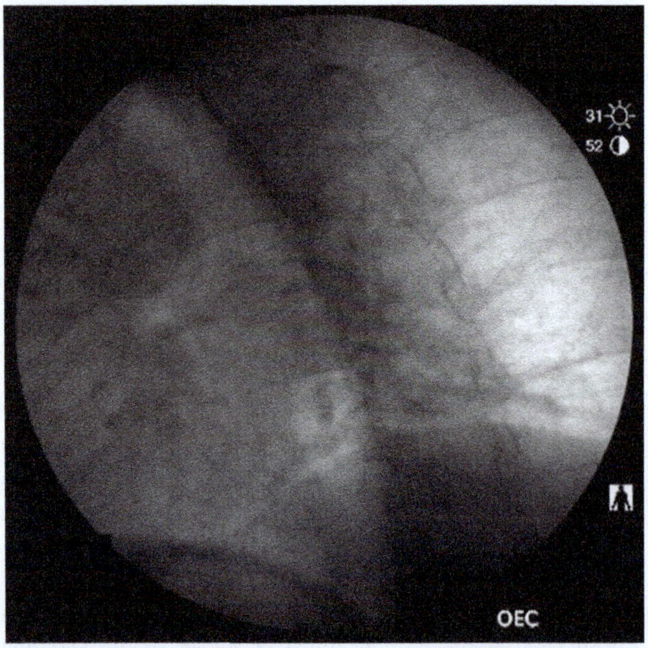

Fig. 46.4 Contralateral oblique view with fluoroscopy (roughly at 45–50°)

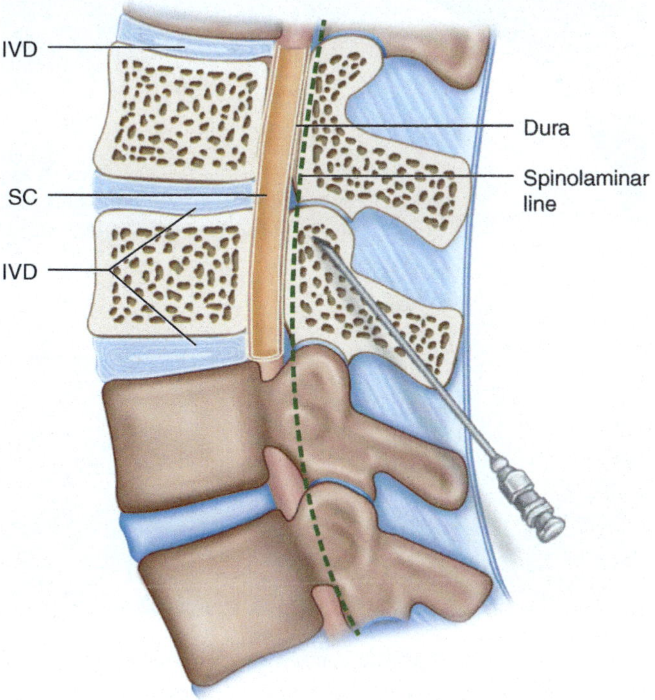

Fig. 46.7 Artistic adaptation of lateral view. SC spinal cord, IVD intervertebral disc

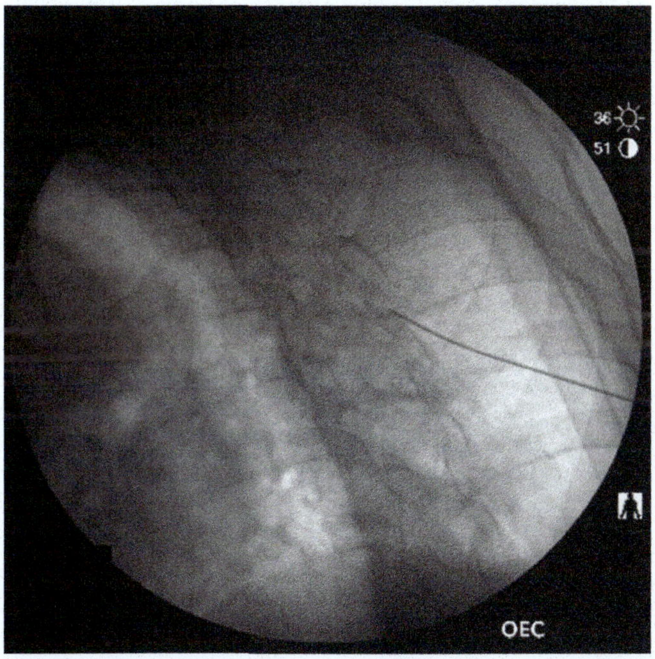

Fig. 46.8 Contralateral oblique view showing needle advancement toward spinolaminar line (roughly at 45–50°)

is particularly important when paramedian approaches avoid interspinous ligaments and thus the typical changes in resistance one has with a midline approach.

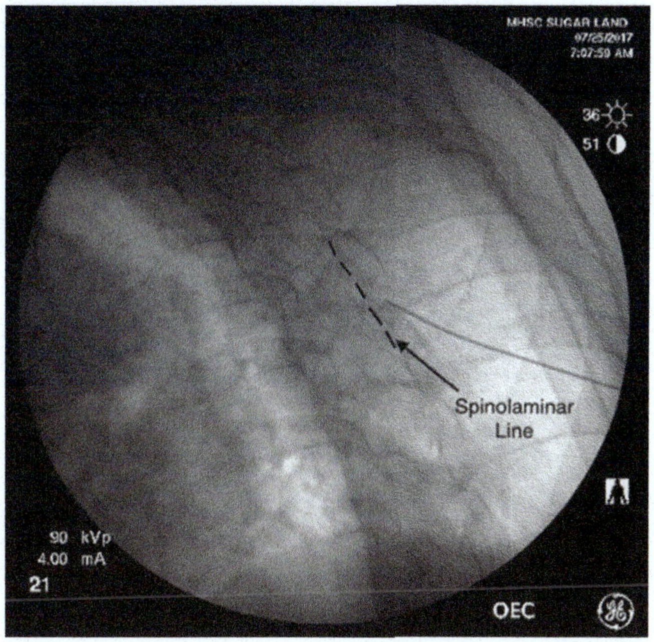

Fig. 46.9 Labeled contralateral oblique view showing needle advancement toward spinolaminar line (roughly at 45–50°)

The experienced practitioner can detect the resistance encountered as the needle engages the spinous ligaments and ligamentum flavum, and the approximate location of these structures can be deduced with fluoroscopic imaging. Once this engagement occurs, a glass or plastic syringe filled with air or a small amount of sterile normal saline is attached to the needle, and pressure is applied to the plunger to gauge resistance. The possibility of pneumocephalus via inadvertent injection of air into the intrathecal space causes many physicians to use at least a small amount of normal saline with LOR technique. Once the needle enters the epidural space, there is a notable decrease in resistance, which allows one to easily advance the plunger through the barrel of the syringe. At this point, a syringe with contrast is attached to the needle via tubing so as to minimize needle movement. Contrast is injected, and if contrast flow is appropriate, the physician can inject the desired medication into the epidural space.

Injection of 0.5–1 cc of contrast helps provide further evidence that the needle tip is in the epidural space and not posterior to it, intrathecally placed, or in a blood vessel. AP, contralateral oblique, and lateral views have characteristic contrast spread when the needle has been successfully situated in the posterior epidural space (Figs. 46.10, 46.11, and 46.12). Epidural adipose tissue and vasculature result in an asymmetric flow of contrast. Indeed, globules of adipose tissue can sometimes be detected in the fluoroscopic image after contrast injection (Fig. 46.10). If contrast spreads predominantly anteriorly toward the vertebral bodies on fluoroscopy, is not asymmetric, or appears to

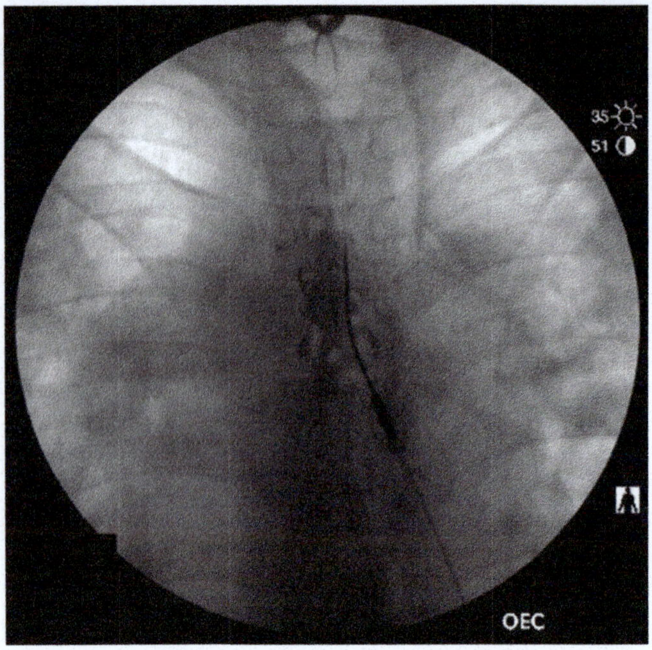

Fig. 46.10 AP view with contrast denoting the epidural space. Note the asymmetric spread and presence of adipose tissue "bubbles"

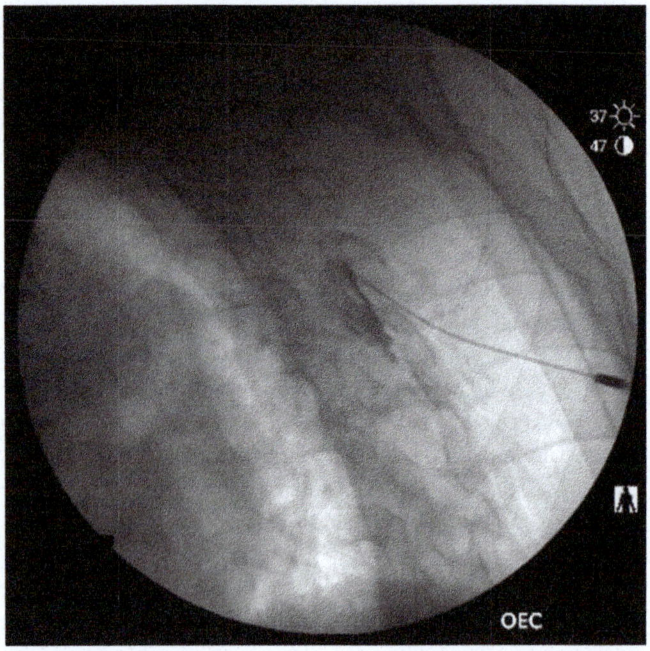

Fig. 46.11 Oblique view with contrast spread denoting the epidural space

provide myelographic outlines, there should be concern for intrathecal placement. Of note, if the needle is placed relatively far from midline, some contrast could be spreading into the lateral gutter and thus appear to be anterior on lateral fluoroscopic view while still remaining in the epidural space.

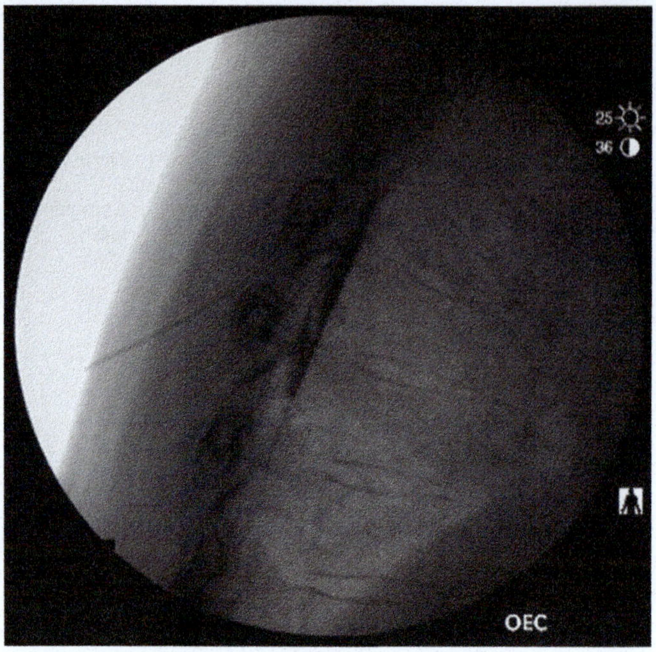

Fig. 46.12 Lateral view with contrast spread denoting the epidural space

Evidence for Efficacy

Multiple studies have shown efficacy of lumbar epidural steroid injections for treatment of radicular pain, particularly in the setting of acute radiculitis. These findings have been widely regarded as applicable to similar conditions in other parts of the spine, including the thoracic region. There is a paucity of evidence for the use of thoracic epidural steroid injections for the treatment of thoracic back pain, radiculopathy, and the other aforementioned indications for this procedure. A couple of the studies specific to the treatment of thoracic back pain via thoracic epidural steroid injections are summarized below and referenced at the end of this chapter if the reader desires further study.

A systematic review of studies looking at the efficacy of thoracic epidural steroid injections with and without steroids only found two studies that met inclusion criteria. One study was a randomized, active-control study and the other a prospective, blinded study. The evidence of efficacy from the randomized trial was fair with regard to treatment of thoracic pain from all causes. The study showed 80–85% of patients with discogenic, thoracic disc herniation, or radiculitis got 50% or greater pain relief even at 12 months. The prospective study evidence was considered limited or poor, but this study only analyzed efficacy of this procedure for post-thoracotomy pain syndrome.

A randomized, double-blind, controlled study with 2-year follow-up analyzed efficacy of thoracic epidural steroid injections in patients with function-limiting mid and upper back pain where thoracic facet arthropathy and intercostal neuritis had been excluded. A successful outcome was defined as a 50% improvement in numerical rating scale of pain and an analysis of changes in Oswestry Disability Index to account for improvements in function for at least 3 weeks. Patients who were successfully treated were then tracked for 2 years. On average, they received five to six thoracic epidural injections during the 2 years. The study compared thoracic epidural steroid injections with local anesthetic alone to the same with local anesthetic and steroid. Of the patients who received local anesthetic alone, 71% had a successful outcome. Patients treated with local anesthetic and steroid had a greater than 80% success rate. And of the patients who have a successful initial outcome as defined above, 80% and 86% had successful outcomes at 2 years of follow-up in each of the two treatment arms. The average pain scores at baseline were 7.7–7.9. After 24 months, they were 3.3–3.6. At all-time intervals measured in between, the patients also had pain scores averaging 3.2–3.5. Oswestry Disability Indices improved from 29.5 at baseline to 12.5–13.8. There was also a significant reduction in opioid usage at 2 years in the successfully treated patients. Though there were statistically significant differences in primary outcomes from baseline, multiple outcomes did not have a statistically significant difference between the local anesthetic and steroid and local anesthetic alone groups. Complications were rare. Of the 606 procedures performed in the study, there were only two subarachnoid punctures, no postoperative headaches, one person with postoperative pain at the site of the injection that was due to muscle spasm and resolved in a few hours, and one with pain in a lower extremity for a few months.

As this last study suggests, what medications should be included in the injectate needs to be studied further and has been a matter of much debate. Some studies have shown no difference in outcomes when epidurals are performed with steroids compared to when local anesthetic is used alone, while others suggest there may be a difference. This is further complicated by the fact that the mechanism of action of steroids in treating radicular pain or other causes of spinal pain such as disc herniations and facet arthropathy is unclear. Part of the mechanism of action may be via increasing anti-inflammatory proteins and decreasing the activity of pro-inflammatory proteins such as phospholipase A2, cyclooxygenase-1, and cyclooxygenase-2 and thus the production of inflammatory mediators. Even if one believes there is sufficient evidence for the use of steroids, which steroid to use is a matter of debate as well. There is concern regarding accidental intravascular injection of particulate steroid resulting in ischemic injury to the spinal cord and nerves subserved by the artery in question. Indeed, there is an increasingly strong consensus that non-particulate steroid should be used at levels above L2, particularly if using a transforaminal approach. This is especially the case for thoracic procedures where one commonly finds the artery of Adamkiewicz.

Pearls and Pitfalls

- Interlaminar thoracic epidural steroid injections, like epidural injections at other levels of the spine, are most commonly used to treat neuropathic pain, though of course in this case affecting the thoracic dermatomes.
- The anatomic considerations of the thoracic spine may make the utilization of certain fluoroscopic views potentially advantageous to safely administer the injectate and minimize the risk of injury to nerves. Lung fields, ribs, and the angulation of the spinous processes make performing an interlaminar epidural steroid injection and obtaining clear fluoroscopic views more complex in the thoracic than other levels of the spine.
- A paramedian approach is more commonly used for thoracic interlaminar injections than the same procedure at other levels of the spine because of the notable caudad angulation of the spinous processes in the thoracic spine.
- The contraindications and complications related to thoracic epidural steroid injections are the same as this procedure at other levels of the spine and are delineated below.

Contraindications to this procedure are local infection at the site of injection, uncorrected coagulopathy, patient refusal or lack of cooperation, increased intracerebral pressure, poorly controlled diabetes if steroids are to be employed, and allergy to the contrast or medications to be administered unless preoperative precautions and medications are provided. Relative contraindications include pregnancy, immunosuppression, and systemic infection.

Though complications are relatively rare, this procedure carries various risks. An adverse reaction to the medications, including hyperglycemia and hypertension due to steroids, numbness or weakness from local anesthetic administration, and allergic reaction to contrast or the medications administered, is possible. Systemic absorption of steroids and adrenocortical suppression or the development of Cushingoid features would be unusual except for when frequent epidural doses are administered. An epidural steroid injection allows for steroid to be deposited at the site where nerve irritation or other pathology is causing pain and thus one potentially avoids the systemic side effects of higher doses of steroids via an oral route. It is important to avoid intravascular placement of the needle as systemic effects of local anesthetic can lead to altered mental status, seizures, and cardiac arrhythmias. Intravascular injection of particulate steroid risks spinal cord infarction, though the risk is likely less with an interlaminar than a transforaminal approach and the use of non-particulate steroids such as dexamethasone. Intrathecal deposition of local anesthetic could result in a total spinal anesthetic depending on level of entry, volume and type of injectate, and the position of the patient. Infection can occur both in the skin and subcutaneous tissues and in the form of an epidural abscess; careful sterile protocol should be observed during this procedure. Bleeding and epidural hematomas have been reported that require immediate evaluation by a spine surgeon and possible evacuation. Risk mitigation of patients on blood thinners is discussed below. Spinal cord injury from direct needle trauma and injection of a medication or contrast into nerve tissue has been reported. The concomitant neurologic sequelae can be devastating, and the risk is increased with heavily sedated patients. It is recommended that patients be sufficiently awake to be able to answer questions during the procedure, including whether they are experiencing pain or paresthesias. A complication unique to thoracic epidural steroid injections that is not encountered in its lumbar and cervical counterparts is pneumothorax. This is a rare complication especially if the procedure is done under fluoroscopy since the needle would need to have diverged significantly from its intended track for this to occur. More minor things to watch for after the procedure include muscle and tissue soreness, particularly if bone was encountered repeatedly during the injection, and pain at the injection site. Ice and anti-inflammatory medications are usually sufficient to address this pain. Lastly, a post-dural puncture headache (PDPH) can occur if the dura is violated during the procedure.

Treatment of PDPH initially involves conservative measures such as increased caffeine and fluid intake, acetaminophen-/butalbital-/caffeine-containing medications, rest in the recumbent position, and possibly other pain medications such as NSAIDs. Though the vast majority of PDPH cases resolve on their own, an epidural blood patch can provide more immediate relief.

With more patients on an increasingly varied number of blood thinners in the last decade, various guidelines have been published regarding when to stop blood thinners for this procedure. The "Guidelines for Interventional Spine and Pain Procedures in Patients on Antiplatelet and Anticoagulant Medications" published by the American Society of Regional Anesthesia and Pain Medicine are often used when making these decisions. Indeed, a convenient application was developed for use on mobile devices that allows a physician to find how long an anticoagulant should be stopped and when it should be resumed based on the procedure, risk stratification, and medication. Thoracic interlaminar epidural steroid injections are considered an intermediate risk procedure, though certain conditions, including old age, concomitant use of other anticoagulants, renal dysfunction, liver disease including cirrhosis, and history of bleeding, can result in the procedure being regarded as high risk.

If severe stenosis exists at a particular level and/or no cerebrospinal fluid can be visualized surrounding the spinal cord, the injection should be performed at another nearby level and allow for spread of injectate to multiple nearby levels. This helps decrease the chance of further nerve compression and deficits or worsening pain that could be caused by increasing epidural pressure in a severely stenotic region.

Recommended Reading

1. Benyamin RM, Wang VC, Vallejo R, Singh V, Helm S II. A systematic evaluation of thoracic interlaminar epidural injections. Pain Physician. 2012;15(4):E497–514.
2. Deer TR, Leong MS, Buvanendran A, et al. Epidural (cervical, thoracic, lumbar caudal) block/injections. In: Treatment of chronic pain by interventional approaches, the American Academy of Pain Medicine textbook on patient management. New York: Springer; 2014.
3. Diwan S, Staats PS. Interlaminar epidural steroid injections: cervical, thoracic, lumbar, and caudal. In: Atlas of pain medicine procedures. New York: McGraw-Hill Companies, Inc.; 2015.
4. Furman MB. Atlas of image-guided spinal procedures. Philadelphia: Elsevier; 2018.
5. Manchikanti L, Cash KA, Mcmanus CD, Pampati V, Benyamin RM. Thoracic interlaminar epidural injections in managing chronic thoracic pain: a randomized, double-blind, controlled trial with a 2-year follow-up. Pain Physician. 2014;17(3):E327–38.
6. Rathmell JP. Interlaminar epidural injection. In: Atlas of image guided intervention in regional anesthesia and pain medicine. 2nd ed. Philadelphia: Wolters Kluwer/Lippincott Williams & Wilkins Health; 2012.

Thoracic Facet and Medial Branch Blocks

47

Rebecca A. Sanders

Introduction

While axial pain in the upper and mid back is less common compared to the cervical and lumbar regions, thoracic pain can be debilitating and has a prevalence of approximately 15% in the general population. Pain emanating from the thoracic facets accounts for 34–48% of these thoracic pain cases.

Thoracic zygapophyseal (facet or z-) joints are paired posterolateral articular structures at each vertebral level that allow axial range of motion and stability. Each joint is richly innervated and reinforced by a collagenous, fibrous capsule that provides resistance to prevent extremes of axial motion, particularly flexion. Similar to other synovial joints, thoracic facet joints are prone to inflammation, trauma, injury, and degeneration. Such pathology often leads to pain and restricted thoracic movement. Thoracic facetogenic pain may be modulated by multiple mechanisms, including capsular stretch and release of pro-inflammatory mediators. Inflammatory fluid causing capsular enlargement or chronic degeneration with osteophyte formation can cause regional nerve impingement.

Thoracic facet intra-articular injection and thoracic medial branch blocks are diagnostic and potentially therapeutic tools providers may choose in patients with mid and upper back pain. Intra-articular facet joint injections require image guidance for accurate needle placement within the facet capsule, after which an injectate is deposited. A local anesthetic is injected for diagnostic information, which is obtained based on the patient's pain response following administration. Corticosteroid is often added for therapeutic, anti-inflammatory properties.

Each thoracic facet joint inputs sensory information via the medial branch of the dorsal rami of the spinal nerve at and above the level of interest. Precise blockade of these medial branches can assist in the diagnosis of facetogenic thoracic pain and is often predictive of pain response to medial branch radiofrequency ablation. Medial branch blocks can also be employed for therapeutic purposes; in which case, local anesthetic with or without adjuvant medication is deposited along the medial branch nerve.

Background and Historical Perspectives

In 1987, Peter Wilson published a case series of 17 patients with thoracic pain of unknown etiology in which 13 patients experienced immediate and 9 experienced prolonged pain improvement following fluoroscopically guided intra-articular thoracic facet blocks at the level of maximal pain. In this report, he was the first to publically hypothesize thoracic facets as a potential pain generator, similar to that already accepted in the lumbar and cervical spine.

Subsequent investigation has focused on thoracic facet referral patterns, anatomical course and distribution of thoracic medial branches, prevalence of thoracic facet joint syndrome in patients with upper and mid back pain, and clinical efficacy of therapeutic medial branch blocks.

Chua et al. first described the anatomic foundation of thoracic facetogenic pain. Published in 1995, this manuscript described the anatomical course of thoracic medial branches based on 84 medial branches dissected on 4 cadavers. Figure 47.1 summarizes the anatomical distribution of the medial branch nerves at all thoracic levels. This publication was the first to refute the assumption that thoracic medial branch nerves followed a similar course observed in the lumbar spine (described by Bogduk in 1979). Prior to this report, thoracic medial branch blocks were performed at the junction of the transverse process and superior articular process.

Chua et al. established that thoracic medial branch nerve location was consistent among cadaveric specimen but varied among thoracic levels. For T1–T4 and T9–T10, the medial branch crossed the superolateral corners of each

R. A. Sanders (✉)
Department of Pain Management, Kansas Spine and Specialty Hospital, Wichita, KS, USA

T. R. Deer et al. (eds.), *Deer's Treatment of Pain*, https://doi.org/10.1007/978-3-030-12281-2_47

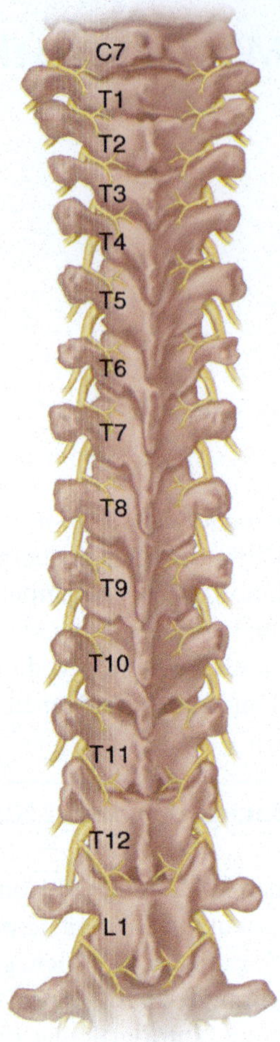

Fig. 47.1 Anatomical course of thoracic medial branch nerves in four cadaveric models dissected and described by Chua et al.

transverse process and then coursed inferiorly and medially along the transverse process. For T5–T8, the medial branch assumed a similar path; however, it most often did not contact the transverse process and instead was superiorly displaced and could be seen suspended in the intertransverse space. The T11 medial branch passed along the lateral surface at the base of the superior articular process. The T12 medial branch followed a similar course of that of the lumbar medial branches. In summary, the superolateral aspect of the transverse emerged as purposed anatomical target for thoracic medial branch blocks above the T11 medial branch. For T11 and T12 medial branch blocks, the target remained similar to that of lumbar medial branch blocks.

The prevalence of thoracic spine pain due to thoracic facet pathology has been determined to be 34–48% based on three clinical studies by Manchikanti et al. In a 2002 study, 46 patients with chronic thoracic pain (duration greater than 6 months) underwent diagnostic medial branch blocks to the most painful thoracic levels with lidocaine administration. Thirty-six patients experienced greater than 80% pain relief and underwent a confirmatory block with bupivacaine, of which 22 sustained pain improvement. Therefore, the prevalence of thoracic facetogenic pain was calculated to 48% in this population with a false positive rate of 58%. This study did not comment on the vertebral levels tested or the positive rates at individual thoracic levels.

In a 2004 prospective study evaluating prevalence of facetogenic neck and mid back pain, 72 patients with chronic thoracic pain were included in the mid back cohort. Following a similar pattern of controlled, staged diagnostic medial branch blocks with lidocaine and bupivacaine, prevalence was calculated as 42% for the thoracic cohort. Additionally, 64% of the mid back cohort had bilateral thoracic facet involvement.

Lastly, a prospective evaluation of 500 patients with chronic cervical, thoracic, or lumbar facetogenic pain underwent medial branch blockade with lidocaine and went on to have a subsequent blockade with bupivacaine if he or she experienced greater than 80% pain relief. For the thoracic subgroup, 34% experienced at least 80% pain improvement following both diagnostic blocks.

A series of publications investigating pain referral patterns following image-guided injections to targeted thoracic facet joints in order to produce joint distention have established thoracic facet joint referral patterns. These investigations support thoracic facet joints as a potential cause of scapular and posterior chest wall pain; however, there is substantial overlap of referral patterns among thoracic facet joints.

In 1994, Dreyfuss et al. published T3–T4 through T10–T11 referral patterns based on pain location noted in nine normal volunteers following thoracic facet joint distention with contrast material. For each thoracic facet distended, most intense pain typically radiated laterally and to one segment inferior to the joint injected. In these nine volunteers, pain never extended beyond the posterior axillary line, 2.5 vertebral segments inferiorly or 0.5 segments superiorly. Figure 47.2 provides a visual representation of pain patterns derived by Dreyfuss et al. when pressurizing T3–T4 through T10–T11 facet joints.

In 1997, Fukui et al. mapped referral patterns for C7–T1, T1–T2, T2–T3, and T11–T12 in patients with suspected facetogenic pain undergoing injections to these joints. Pain pattern was recorded following distention of joint with contrast medium. Again, significant overlap was noted, specifically in the upper thoracic region. Following T11–T12 facet distention, pain was noted in the corresponding paravertebral region and occasionally radiated to the iliac crest. Pain in the suprascapular region was noted with distention of C7–T1 and T1–T2, and midscapular radiation occurred with all three upper thoracic facet injections. Figure 47.2 summarizes the pain patterns established by Fukui et al.

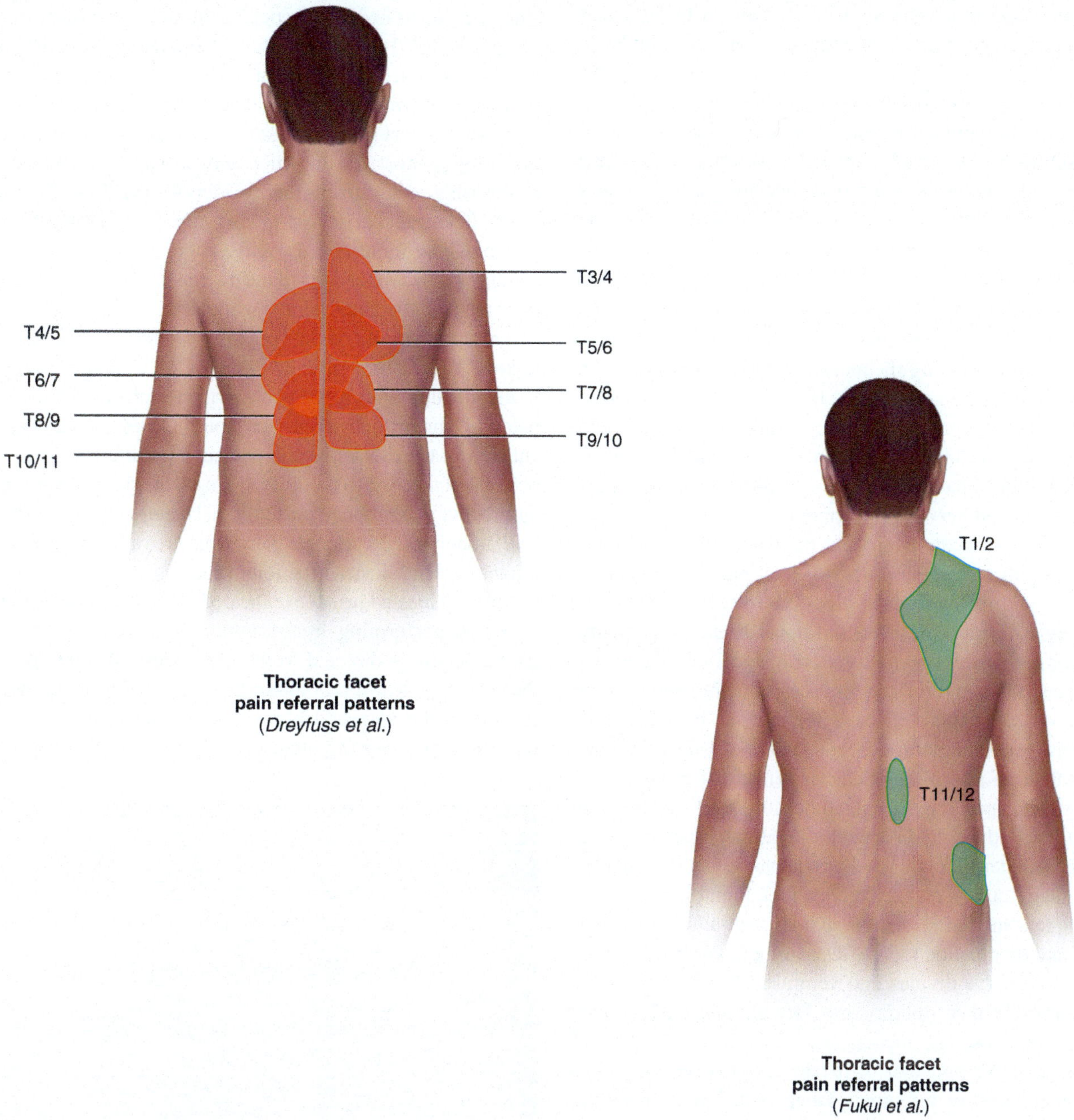

Fig. 47.2 Thoracic facet referral patterns in normal volunteers as determined by Dreyfuss et al. and Fukui et al.

Uses and Indications

Intra-articular thoracic facet injections and thoracic medial branch blocks are clinically used for diagnosis and/or treatment of upper to mid back pain, posterior chest wall pain, and scapular pain, particularly in those cases of limited response to conservative treatment measures. Pain improvement following one or multiple thoracic medial branch blocks is often a prerequisite to neurolysis.

Clinical diagnosis of thoracic facet pathology is often elusive because historical elements, physical exam, radiographic, and biomarker tools lack sensitivity and specificity. Thoracic facet pathology is considered in patients with concordant paravertebral tenderness in typical pain location without neurological features. Because thoracic facets are richly innervated with free nerve endings and encapsulated and unencapsulated nerve fibers, they are prone to generating pain but are also primed for diagnostic assessment following controlled blockade with local anesthetic at individual levels.

Thoracic facet joints are susceptible to deterioration from repetitive strain and use. This in part explains why thoracic facetogenic arthropathy and pain increase with advancing age. As part of the "three joint complex"—which includes the paired posterior facet joint and intervertebral disk that jointly function to allow regulated axial range of motion—thoracic facet joints are particularly vulnerable to escalated "wear and tear" following intervertebral disk degeneration. In a similar fashion, thoracic facet joints may become pain generators following a thoracic vertebral fracture. Thoracic facet interventions should be considered in patients with acute fractures appropriately treated with vertebral augmentation procedures and those with pain in the subacute and chronic phases.

Thoracic facet joints may be affected by inflammatory arthropathies, including rheumatoid arthritis, reactive arthritis, and ankylosing spondylitis. In cases of joint distention from fluid accumulation, capsular expansion, and osteophyte or synovial cyst formation, pain may spread beyond the expected referral pattern because of central canal or foraminal intrusion and nerve impingement.

Because historical, exam, and radiographic findings have limited ability to identify facetogenic pain, intra-articular injections and medial branch blocks are accepted means for obtaining a diagnosis for mid and upper back pain. In either procedural approach, administration of local anesthetic with or without adjuvant medications—most commonly a corticosteroid—is a potential treatment for thoracic facet-generated pain. Intra-articular thoracic facet injection of 1–2 mL of injectate containing a local anesthetic is sensitive for the diagnosis; however, specificity is limited because joint rupture is not uncommon and results in spread to adjacent structures which may be pain generators, including the paraspinal musculature, ligamentum flavum, and epidural and foraminal spaces.

Thoracic medial branch blockade is an alternative diagnostic and therapeutic tool. After exiting the neural foramen, each spinal nerve divides into ventral and dorsal roots. The dorsal root further divides into lateral, intermediate, and medial branches. The medial branch from the corresponding spinal nerve and that of the level above provides sensory innervation of a thoracic facet joint. Local anesthesia of these two medial branches provides sensory blockade for the individual facet joint. False positive rate of diagnostic medial branch blocks for thoracic facet pain is as high as 53% and attributed to placebo response, spread of local anesthetic to adjacent painful structures, and/or use of procedural sedation. Intravascular injectate administration and patient challenges in distinguishing between post-procedural and chronic pain lead to false negative responses.

Procedural Technique

Intra-articular facet joint injections and medial branch blocks are typically performed with fluoroscopic guidance. Ultrasound may be used an adjuvant modality. One cadaver study demonstrated intra-articular thoracic facet injections in 16 of 20 (80%) ultrasound-guided injections to facet joints T1–T2 through T10–T11. An associated technical description for preforming these injections with the modality was provided. A curvilinear transducer was used to first identify the inferior-most rib and then moved superior and medial to the rib's axial attachment to identify the T11–T12 facet joints. The transducer was moved superiorly along the sagittal plane to identify successive thoracic facet joints. The needle was advanced in-plane to the transducer as it was directed into the facet joint capsule.

Facets joints are most vertically oriented in the thoracic region. The inferior articular process of a thoracic vertebra in conjunction with the superior articular process of the level below forms an individual facet joint. Given the vertical orientation in the thoracic spine, the superior articular process is positioned anterior to the joint space, while the inferior articular process is positioned posteriorly. Therefore, anteroposterior (AP) imaging superimposes these structures and does not reveal a joint opening. Instead the joint space must be estimated and is typically located just above the pedicle of the lower vertebra.

When performing intra-articular injections, a 22 or 25 gauge needle is directed to the approximated joint space in the AP view while maintaining visualization of the needle tip within the vertebral bone shadow and advancing in an inferior to superior orientation, as demonstrated in Fig. 47.3.

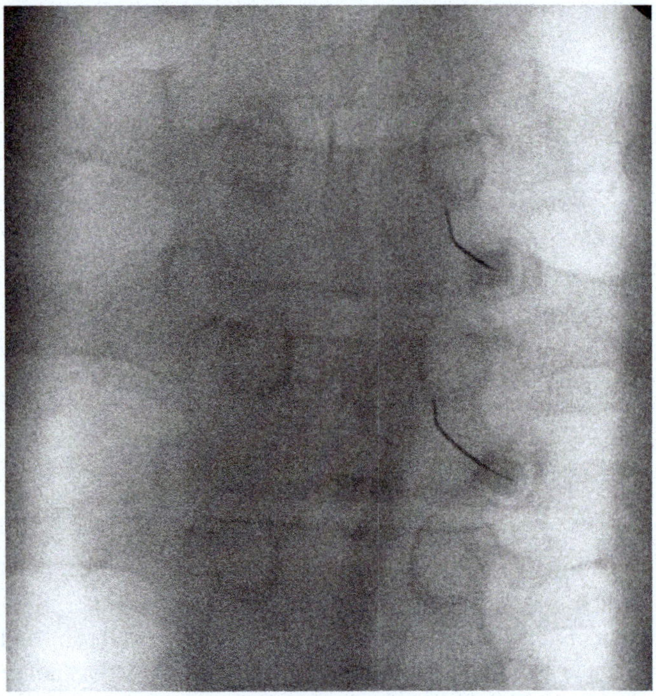

Fig. 47.3 Anteroposterior (AP) fluoroscopic image of right T4–T5 and T5–T6 facet injections. A 25 gauge needle has been advanced from an inferior to superior direction with needle tip approaching the location of joint space, which is typically located just above the pedicle of lower vertebral level

Next, a contralateral oblique image is obtained to visualize the joint opening. The needle should be located inferior to the joint space and advanced into the capsule. Contrast medium is injected with live fluoroscopy in either the contralateral oblique or AP view to assess final needle location. Intra-articular contrast spread is demonstrated in the contralateral oblique and AP views in Figs. 47.4 and 47.5, respectively. Once an arthrogram is noted, injectate is administered.

At lower thoracic facet levels, facet joint orientation transitions to the sagittal alignment characteristic of the lumbar region. This transition point classically occurs between T11–T12 and T12–L1. At this level, procedural approach mimics that of a lumbar facet joint injection. In the thoracic region, paired posterior joints have slightly varied orientation. In general, the right-side facet joint is posited more vertically and frontally.

Thoracic medial branch blocks are performed with fluoroscopic guidance and ideally without procedural sedation if diagnostic information is to be obtained. For each desired facet joint, the medial branch from the corresponding spinal nerve and the spinal nerve from the level above must be blocked. (For example, to provide sensory blockade to the T3–T4 facet, medial branches from the T2 and T3 spinal nerves must be blocked. These nerves are located along the superolateral corners of the T3 and T4 transverse process, respectively.)

The medial branch arises from the dorsal root shortly after it exits the intervertebral foramen and descends along the lateral aspect of the intertransverse space. The medial branch of T1 to T3 and T9 and T10 characteristically descend across the dorsal surface of the inferior transverse process, while the medial branches of T4 through T8 remain suspended in the intertransverse space. Figure 47.6 outlines pertinent anatomical bony landmarks and approximates location of the medial branch nerve when viewing the thoracic spine with AP imaging.

After the appropriate levels are identified, a 22 or 25 gauge needle is advanced to the target as suggested by Chua et al. and summarized in Fig. 47.1. For T1 through T10 medial branches, the needle tip is positioned at the superolateral corner of the inferior transverse process. While no bony landmark approximates the location of the T4 through T8 medial branches, the superolateral corner is a suitable target

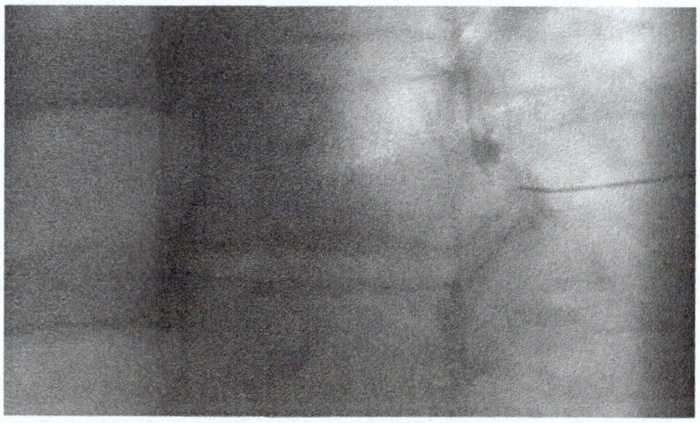

Fig. 47.4 Contralateral oblique image of right T4–T5 facet joint injections following contrast administration. Joint space is visualized in contralateral oblique view with needle penetration of the posterior and inferior aspect of the joint capsule

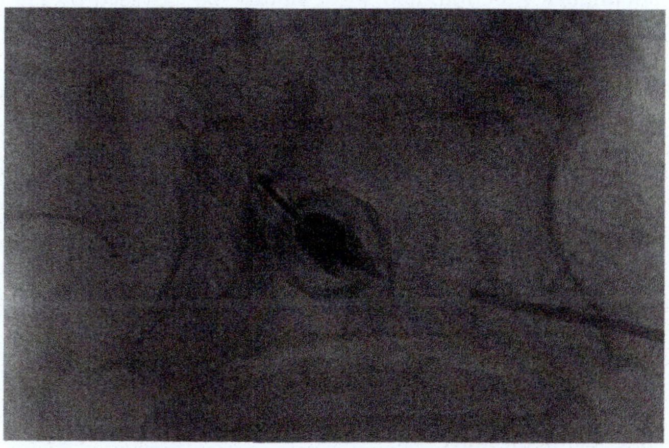

Fig. 47.5 AP image of contrast medium within a thoracic facet joint

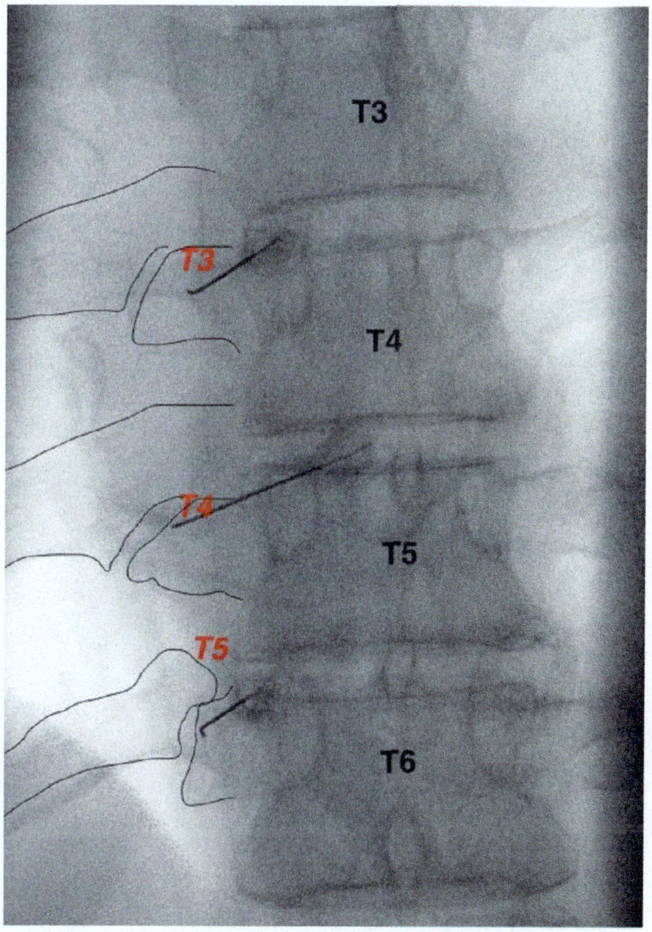

Fig. 47.6 AP fluoroscopic image of thoracic spine. Vertebral levels enumerated and approximated location of corresponding medial branch nerve indicated by red label

for needle placement to avoid pneumothorax with the goal of achieving injectate spread superiorly along the expected nerve location. The junction of the base of the superior articular process and the transverse process is the target for T11 and T12 medial branches. After needles are placed to the target location, 0.2 mL contrast medium is administered to confirm injectate spread will encompass the expected nerve location and avoid intravascular uptake. Figure 47.7 demonstrates final needle position for medial branch blocks for left T4–T5 and T5–T6 facet joints.

Because of the high false positive rate following medial branch blockade, repeated procedures with concordant pain response improve diagnostic accuracy in determining thoracic facet origin pain. Typically, the first blockade involves lidocaine administration, and those patients with at least 70% pain relief for the expected anesthetic duration of lidocaine proceed to a second blockade with bupivacaine. Facetogenic pain is diagnosed in those patients who then experience at least 70% pain improvement with pain relief lasting longer with bupivacaine administration compared to that experienced with lidocaine.

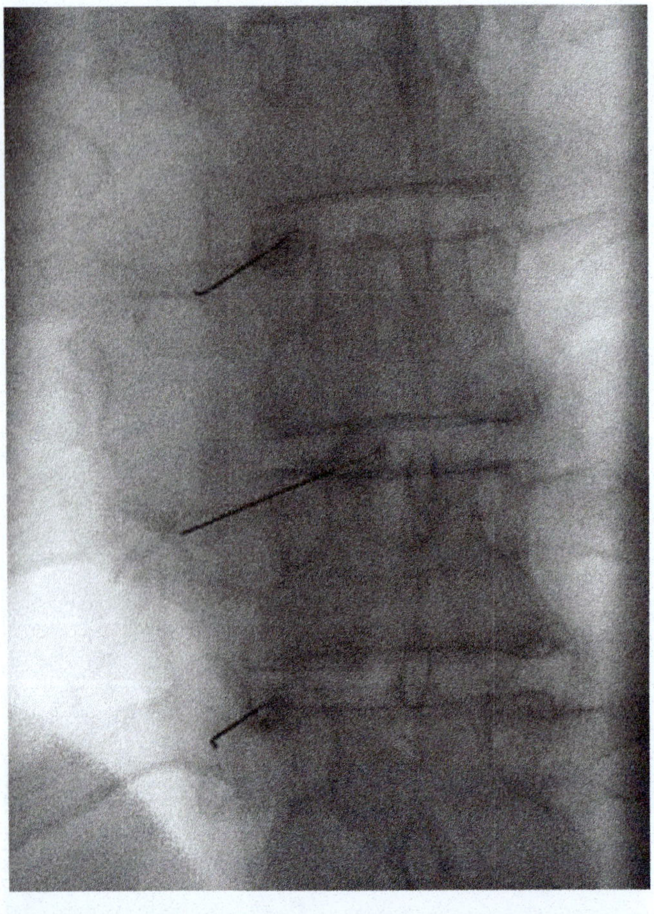

Fig. 47.7 AP fluoroscopic image of medial branch blocks for left T4–T5 and T5–T6 facet joints (medial branch nerve of T3, T4, and T5). A 25 gauge needle is positioned at superolateral corner of each transverse process

Thoracic facet and medial branch blocks are considered "intermediate-risk" procedures when following guidelines outlined by Norouze et al. in Interventional Spine and Pain Procedures in Patients on Antiplatelet and Anticoagulant Medications.

Evidence of Efficacy

Thoracic intra-articular facet joint injection response rate has not been clinically studied following Wilson's initial report of 9 of 17 patients with chronic thoracic spine pain experiencing greater than 1-month pain relief following joint injection with local anesthetic and steroid. Efficacy in the thoracic region has been extrapolated from studies concluding clinical success following intra-articular cervical and lumbar facet injections. Corticosteroids are well-established modulators of pain transmission via C fibers in addition to their immune-suppressive function. This is the basis for intra-articular corticosteroid administration, particularly in clinical scenarios of joint degeneration, trauma, injury, or other inflammatory processes.

In contrast, prospective trials have assessed thoracic medial branch block efficacy. These studies are outlined in Table 47.1. A recent systemic review of effectiveness of facet joint interventions for chronic spinal pain determined there is level II evidence for thoracic facet medial branch blocks for long-term pain and functional improvement.

In a prospective observational study, 55 consecutive patients with chronic, refractory thoracic facet pain determined by controlled diagnostic blocks received thoracic medial branch blocks with bupivacaine alone or with Sarapin and steroid additives. Patient pain scores, Oswestry Disability Index, Pain Patient Profile, and employment status were obtained at baseline and followed at 3, 6, 12, 24, and 34 months following initial intervention. On average, each patient received three to four procedures per year, which were based on return of pain symptoms. Approximately 70% had a minimum of 50% pain relief at 1, 2, and 3 years. The cohort exhibited statistically significant improvement in psychological, function, and work status—as assessed by Pain Patient Profile, Oswestry Disability Index, and employment status—at 1, 2, and 3 years compared to baseline.

In a series of publications, Manchikanti et al. described patient outcomes following a double-blinded, randomized prospective trial of 100 patients with chronic thoracic pain unresponsive to conservative treatments and diagnosed as thoracic facet pain based on a series of medial branch blocks, first with lidocaine and repeated with bupivacaine, with at least 80% pain improvement following each procedure and relief lasting longer following bupivacaine administration. The 100 included patients were randomized to receive thoracic medial branch blocks with bupivacaine or bupivacaine and betamethasone.

Table 47.1 Efficacy table. Therapeutic thoracic medial branch blocks

Author and year	Study type	Number and description of participants	Intervention	Outcomes measured	Results	Notes
Manchikanti, 2006	Prospective observational	55 consecutive patients; diagnosed with chronic, refractory thoracic facet pain[a]	Medial branch block (MBB) with bupivacaine or bupivacaine with Sarapin and Depo-Medrol	Pain score (NRS) Oswestry Disability Index (ODI) Patient Pain Profile (PPP) Work status	Patients with >50% pain relief: 3 and 6 months: 71% 12 months: 76% 24 months: 71% 36 months: 69%	Individual thoracic levels not specified On average, patients received 3–4 MBB procedures per year; as determined by return of pain or decline of functional status
				All obtained at baseline and 3, 6, 12, 24, and 36 months	Statistically significant functional improvement (ODI reduction >40%): at 12, 24, and 36 months	
					Statistically significant psychological improvement (PPP): at 12, 24, and 36 months	
Manchikanti, 2008	Prospective, randomized, double-blinded	48 consecutive patients, diagnosed with chronic, refractory thoracic facet pain[a]	Group A (*n* = 24) MBB with 0.25% bupivacaine	NRS ODI Opioid dose Work status	Patients with >50% pain relief at 12 months: Group A—79% Group B—79%	No placebo group for control Average number of MBB procedures in 1 year: Group A—3.4 Group B—3.2
			Group B (*n* = 24) MBB with 0.25% bupivacaine + 0.15 mg betamethasone	All obtained at baseline and 3, 6, and 12 months	Statistically significant functional improvement (ODI reduction >40%): Group A—88% Group B—88% No significant opioid dose decrease in either group In both groups, employment status did not statistically improve but clinical noted	Number of joints involved: 2–29% 3–40% 4–17% 5–21% Bilateral—69%
Manchikanti, 2010	Prospective, randomized, double-blinded	100 consecutive patients, diagnosed with chronic, refractory thoracic facet pain[a]	Group A (*n* = 50) MBB with 0.25% bupivacaine	NRS ODI Opioid dose Work status	Patients with ≥50% pain relief and ODI reduction ≥50% at 12 months: Group A—76% Group B—82%	No placebo control group Average length of pain improvement following MBB procedure: Group A—15.8 weeks Group B—13.6 weeks
	1-year follow-up		Group B (*n* = 50) MBB with 0.25% bupivacaine + 0.15 mg betamethasone	All obtained at baseline and 3, 6, and 12 months	Opioid dose and unemployment decreased in both groups but did not reach statistical significance	

(continued)

Table 47.1 (continued)

Author and year	Study type	Number and description of participants	Intervention	Outcomes measured	Results	Notes
Manchikanti, 2012	Prospective, randomized, double-blinded	100 consecutive patients, diagnosed with chronic, refractory thoracic facet pain[a]	Group A ($n = 50$) MBB with 0.25% bupivacaine	NRS ODI Opioid dose Work status	Patients with ≥50% pain relief and ODI reduction ≥50% at 24 months: Group A—80% Group B—84%	No placebo control group 78% of patients in Group A and 80% patients in Group B reached 2-year follow-up
	2-year follow-up		Group B ($n = 50$) MBB with 0.25% bupivacaine + 0.15 mg betamethasone	All obtained at baseline and 3, 6, 12, and 24 months	Opioid dose and unemployment decreased in both groups, but did not reach statistical significance	Average number of MBB procedures over the 2-year period: Group A—5.6 Group B—6.2

[a]Diagnosis based on staged diagnostic medial branch blocks to most painful thoracic level(s); patients with at least 80% pain relief following lidocaine administration proceeded to second block with bupivacaine administration. Those patients with at least 80% pain relief and pain relief last longer following bupivacaine administration compared to lidocaine were given thoracic facet pain diagnosis

Outcome measures included Numeric Rating Scale (NRS), Oswestry Disability Index, opioid dose, and work status; all were measured at baseline and 3, 6, 12, 18, and 24 months following initial intervention. Over the 2-year study period, patients averaged a total of six procedures. Both groups showed significant improvement in pain and function, and there was no statistical difference between the two treatment groups. At 2-year follow-up, greater than 50% pain improvement was reported by 80% of patients randomized to receive bupivacaine only blocks and 84% of patients who received bupivacaine and steroid. Both groups exhibited statistically significant functional improvement compared to baseline, as measured by Oswestry Disability Index. Again, no significant difference was noted between treatment groups. Opioid dose decreased but not in a statistically significant fashion. While there was no significant change in work status, all eligible patients were employed at 1-year and 2-year follow-up intervals. This publication series concluded that intermittent therapeutic medial branch blockade with or without steroid is an effective treatment for thoracic facet origin pain.

Thoracic facet-based procedures are a consideration for patients with persistent pain following thoracic compression fractures. One small case series of two patients with thoracic compression fractures exhibited significant and long-lasting pain improvement—based on verbal analog pain score—following fluoroscopically guided thoracic facet injections at the corresponding vertebral level.

Complications stemming from fluoroscopically guided thoracic facet joint nerve (medial branch) injections were evaluated as a subgroup in a prospective study evaluating 7500 episodes with 43,000 nerve blocks of the cervical, thoracic, and lumbar spine. The thoracic cohort consisted of 950 encounters and a total of 5821 levels. Minor, local bleeding occurred in 75% of encounters, which was statistically more common compared to cervical and lumbar procedures. Intravascular penetration was noted in 6% of causes, statistically less common compared to the cervical spine. Transient, local nerve root irritation occurred in one patient (0.03%), and there were no encounters resulting in nerve damage, spinal cord irritation, epidural hematoma, infection, vasovagal reaction, or facial flushing. This prospective study concluded that major complications were extremely rare, while minor complications—particularly localized bleeding—were common.

In a 3-year prospective study evaluating the rate of intravascular penetration during medial branch procedures, 1290 thoracic medial branch blocks were performed, and 0.7% involved intravascular penetration. Intravascular penetration in the thoracic region was statistically less common compared to the cervical and lumbar spine.

Pearls and Pitfalls

- Prevalence of thoracic facet-mediated pain in patients with thoracic pain is 34–48%.
- Thoracic facet interventions (intra-articular or medial branch blocks) are useful diagnostic tools because history, exam, and imaging findings lack specificity and sensitivity for diagnosing facet origin pain.
- Significant inflammation or joint hypertrophy may result in radicular symptoms due to foraminal or central canal narrowing.
- Consider multilevel procedures due to significant overlap in referral patterns of each thoracic facet joint.
- Consider thoracic facet-based procedures for patients with persistent pain in the setting of thoracic vertebral fracture and adequate treatment with vertebral augmentation therapy and in patient with subacute and chronic vertebral fractures.

- Thoracic facet joints are vertically oriented. Transition to sagittal orientation found in lumbar region typically occurs between T11–T12 and T12–L1.
- When performing a thoracic facet joint injection, first obtain AP imaging and advance needle in an inferior to superior direction to the estimated joint space, which is just above the ipsilateral pedicle of lower level. Then, obtain a contralateral oblique view to visualize joint opening, and advance the needle into the joint capsule.
- When performing upper and mid thoracic medial branch blocks, ideal target is the superolateral corner of the transverse process.
- For the T11 and T12 medial branch nerves, the target is analogous to that for lumbar medial branches at the junction of the root of the superior articular process and the root of the transverse process.
- To avoid false positive responses in diagnostic thoracic medial branch blocks, use a low volume of local anesthetic (0.5 mL) to avoid spread to adjacent structures, which may be pain generators.
- When advancing a needle in the thoracic spine, always maintain the needle tip within the bone shadow to reduce risk of pneumothorax. In the case of intra-articular facet injections, the needle tip should remain within the vertebral body shadow. In medial branch blocks, the needle tip should remain within the bony shadow of the respective thoracic transverse process.
- In high-risk patients with bilateral thoracic facetogenic pain, consider staged, unilateral procedures due to risk of pneumothorax.
- For patients on antiplatelet and anticoagulation therapy, thoracic facet and medial branch block procedures are considered "intermediate risk."

Recommended Reading

1. Atluri S, Singh V, Datta S, et al. Diagnostic accuracy of thoracic facet joint nerve blocks: an update of the assessment of evidence. Pain Physician. 2012;15:483–96.
2. Bogduk N, editor. Thoracic medial branch blocks. In: International spine intervention society practice guidelines for spinal diagnostic and treatment procedures. 2nd ed. San Francisco; 2013. p. 293–8.
3. Bogduk N, editor. Thoracic zygapophysial intra-articular access. In: International spine intervention society practice guidelines for spinal diagnostic and treatment procedures. 2nd ed. San Francisco; 2013. p. 283–91.
4. Chua WH, Bogduk N. The surgical anatomy of thoracic facet denervation. Acta Neurochir. 1995;136:140–4.
5. Dreyfuss P, Tibiletti C, Dreyer SJ. Thoracic zygapophyseal joint pain patterns. A study in normal volunteers. Spine. 1994;19:807–11.
6. Fukui S, Ohseto K, Shiotani M. Patterns of pain induced by distending the thoracic zygapophyseal joints. Reg Anesth. 1997;22:332–6.
7. Manchikanti L, Manchikanti K, Manchukonda R, et al. Evaluation of therapeutic thoracic medial branch block effectiveness in chronic thoracic pain: a prospective outcomes study with minimum of 1-year follow up. Pain Physician. 2006;9:97–105.
8. Manchikanti L, Singh V, Falco J, et al. Effectiveness of thoracic medial branch blocks in managing chronic pain: a preliminary report of a randomized, double-blind controlled trial. Pain Physician. 2008;11:491–504.
9. Manchikanti L, Singh V, Falco J, et al. Comparative effectiveness of a one-year follow-up of thoracic medial branch blocks in management of chronic thoracic pain: a randomized double-blind active controlled trial. Pain Physician. 2010;13:535–48.
10. Manchikanti L, Singh V, Falco FJ, et al. The role of thoracic medial branch blocks in managing chronic mid and upper back pain: a randomized, double-blind, active-control trial with a 2-year followup. Anesthesiol Res Pract. 2012;2012:1.
11. Manchikanti L, Kaye AD, Boswell MV, et al. A systemic review and best evidence synthesis of the effectiveness of therapeutic facet joint interventions in managing chronic spinal pain. Pain Physician. 2015;18:535–82.

Radiofrequency Ablation in the Thoracic Spine

48

Eric T. Lee and Chane Price

Introduction

Radiofrequency ablation (RFA) has long been an established treatment for chronic axial spine pain, more specifically facet zygapophysial syndrome. One of the most commonly targeted areas are the lumbar spine due to its increased weight-bearing which often leads to facet degeneration and pain. The cervical spine that also is a frequent source of pain with its increased mobility is also an area often treated by RFA. Thoracic facet-mediated pain, though not as common due to the reduced mobility and weight-bearing as compared to the cervical and lumbar spine, respectively, affects a considerable number of people as well. Targeting of the thoracic medial branch for treatment can be effective in reducing mid back pain.

Background and Historical Information

The first known use of radiofrequency ablation (RFA) was in 1931 when Kirschner treated trigeminal neuralgia with thermocoagulation of the gasserian ganglion. In the late 1950s, the first commercial radiofrequency (RF) machines became available. More recently, over the past 17 years, the use of RFA therapy has become more common for the treatment of cervical, thoracic, and lumbar zygapophyseal joint pain. In a systematic review, the evidence for pain relief with radiofrequency neurotomy of medial branch nerves is moderate to strong for the axial spine. In the thoracic spine, there are level II evidence for thoracic facet joint nerve blocks and evidence supporting radiofrequency neurotomy for long-term improvement.

E. T. Lee (✉)
Musculoskeletal Care and Regenerative Medicine, St Charles Spine Institute, Thousand Oaks, CA, USA

C. Price
Interventional Pain Physician, University of Miami, Coral Gables, FL, USA

In 1987 thoracic facet joints were identified as a source of chronic mid back and upper back pain. The pain patterns from these joints were studied more closely and described in the mid-1990s. The prevalence of thoracic pain has been estimated around 15% of the general population in contrast to 56% reporting low back pain and 44% reporting neck pain. Thoracic facet joints have been implicated as the source of chronic pain in the mid back or upper back in 34–42% of patients when using the modified criteria of the International Association for the Study of Pain (IASP). This number ranges from 34% to 48% of the patients based on the responses to controlled diagnostic medial branch blocks. Thoracic zygapophyseal joint pain can be treated in various ways including, but not limited to, medial branch nerve blocks, intra-articular facet injections, and medial branch nerve neurotomy or radiofrequency ablation (RFA).

There is evidence to support therapeutic facet joint interventions primarily in the form of medial branch blocks, whereas it is not as established for intra-articular injections. Though currently there is limited evidence for radiofrequency neurotomy at thoracic level, due to lack of randomized clinical trials, however, there is literature supporting its use which should not be underutilized in clinical practice. The purpose of this chapter is to better understand the role of radiofrequency neurotomy of the medial branch nerves for therapeutic treatment of axial thoracic back pain often related to facet joint disease.

Uses and Indications

Use: To Treat Thoracic Back Pain

Appropriate indications for radiofrequency ablation include facet-mediated thoracic back pain. Although this pain is most often axial in nature, there may be referred pain patterns that form a variety of pain-inducing conditions that can benefit from medial branch therapy. The goal of radiofrequency

T. R. Deer et al. (eds.), *Deer's Treatment of Pain*, https://doi.org/10.1007/978-3-030-12281-2_48

ablation is to disrupt the pain sending capabilities of nerves and proper targeting of medical branches and the conditions that transmit pain via them can allow for effective treatment.

Indications

- Spondylosis
- Spondylolisthesis
- Facet arthropathy (arthritis)
- Mid back pain
- Post back surgery pain
- Thoracic axial pain
- Thoracic facet syndrome

Thoracic facet-mediated pain responds equally to radiofrequency treatments as well. The first step is ensuring an accurate diagnostic medial branch block.

Preoperative contraindications as with all invasive procedures conditions are considered contraindications

Preoperative workup. In addition to appropriate medical clearance, proper medical workup such as physical exam, imaging, and diagnostic testing should be carried out to ensure proper patient selection and safety.

Anatomical Considerations

It is worth noting the anatomic features specific to the medial branch in the thoracic spine. Facet-mediated pain is transmitted via the medial branch of the dorsal rami, as with other areas of the axial spine. The medial branch anatomy in the thoracic spine from T1 through T12 may vary in location, and it is important to keep in mind when performing the procedure. The medial branches generally are located near the confluence of the transverse process and superior articulating process (SAP) on the vertebral body. There are significant variations, however, in terms of likelihood of location depending on which segment of the thoracic spine is being targeted.

For T1–T4 the medial branches lie toward the superior lateral aspect of the transverse process.

For T5–T8 the medial branches are more inconsistent in their location and can be found from the proximal 1/3 and slightly superior to the transverse process.

For T9–T10 the medial branches lie toward the superior lateral aspect of the transverse process.

For T11–T12 the medial branches are located close to the confluence of the SAP and transverse process (Figs. 48.1, 48.2, and 48.3).

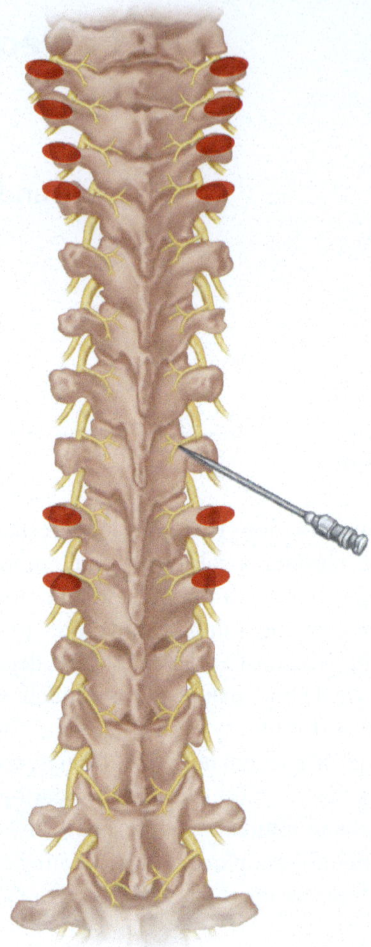

Fig. 48.1 T1–T4, T9–T10 (*red*-colored area most likely target location for medial branch)

Technical Considerations

Given the fact of the varied course of the medial branch in the thoracic spine, it is worth describing the operative technique to maximize efficacy of RFA treatment.

It is important to reiterate that the cannula should be placed to give the maximum chance for radiofrequency lesion to cross and fully cover the path of the medial branch.

After initial fluoroscopic guidance in anterior/posterior orientation, to identify the junction of the superior articulating process and the transverse process, a 20 or 22G 100 mm, with 5 mm or 10 mm, active tip RF cannula is advanced toward the aforementioned target.

Once periosteum was contacted, at the superior medial border of the transverse process, the cannula should be rotated and walked off following the superior border of the

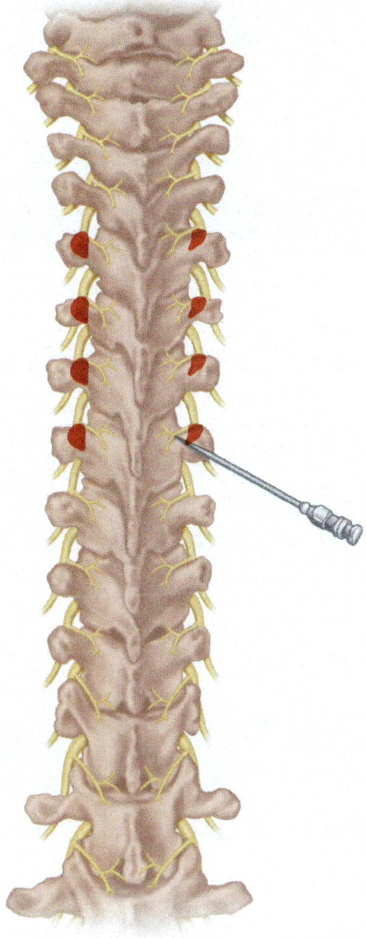

Fig. 48.2 T5–T8 (*red*-colored area most likely target location for medial branch)

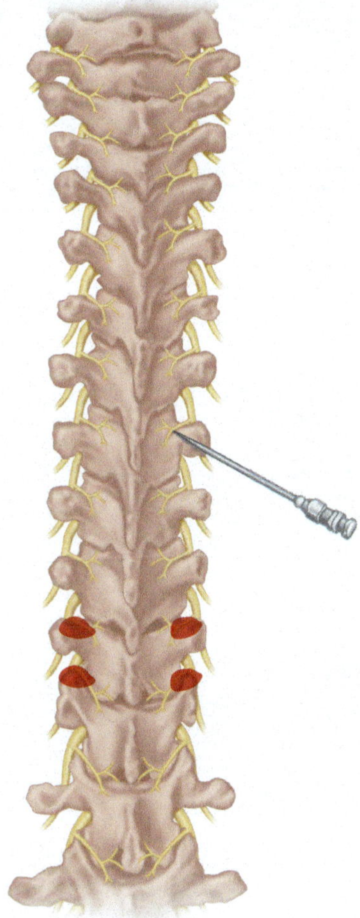

Fig. 48.3 T11–T12 (*red*-colored area most likely target location for medial branch)

transverse process and advanced about 2–3 mm until the needle lay in the proper position. Angle of advancement varies depending on which level of the vertebra is being targeted.

For T1–T4 and T9–T10, the RF cannula should be angled to ensure the active tip of the electrode covers the superior lateral edge of the transverse process.

For T5–T8 the RF cannula should be angled toward proximal 1/3 of the transverse process and directed slightly cephalad.

For T11–T12 the RF cannula should be angled toward the confluence of the SAP and transverse process.

A lateral fluoroscopic image should be obtained to confirm depth and needle placement.

As with all radiofrequency procedures, proper needle placement is essential. Placing the cannulas to maximize therapeutic lesioning of the targeted medial branch is imperative. Given the fact in most RF cannulas project the majority of their lesion lateral to the active tip, a more parallel to the target nerve placement of the electrode increases lesion officiation. Studies also support lesioning times 90 s or greater increase size.

Post procedure steroid injection may decrease chance neuritis and irritation (Figs. 48.4, 48.5, and 48.6).

Evidence for Efficacy (Table 48.1)

There are a limited number of studies on the efficacy of classic RF in thoracic facet-mediated pain. Stolker et al. evaluated 40 patients with thoracic pain symptoms who underwent 51 percutaneous RF facet denervation. Twenty-four underwent the procedure on the left side, 21 on the right

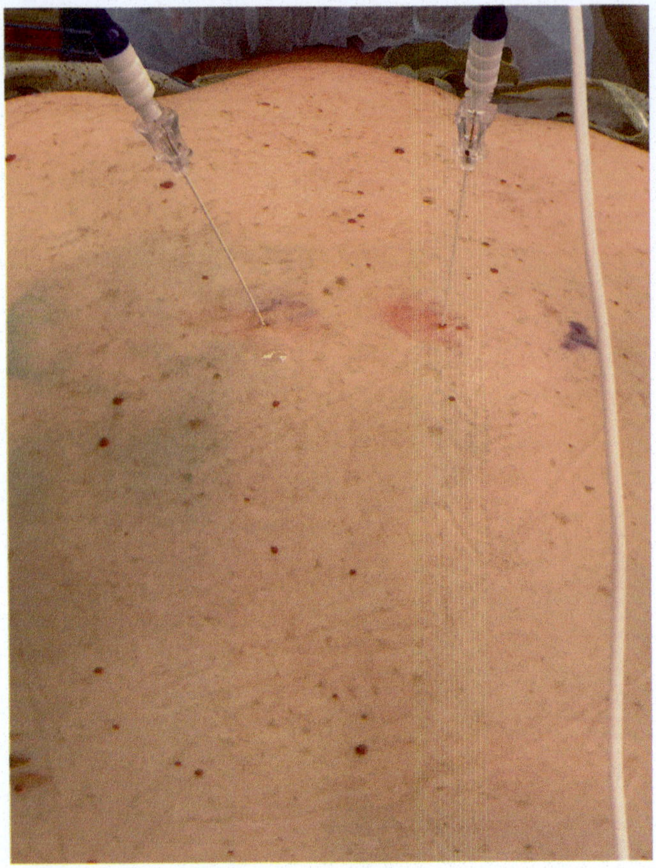

Fig. 48.4 Picture of *skin entry* with *wire*

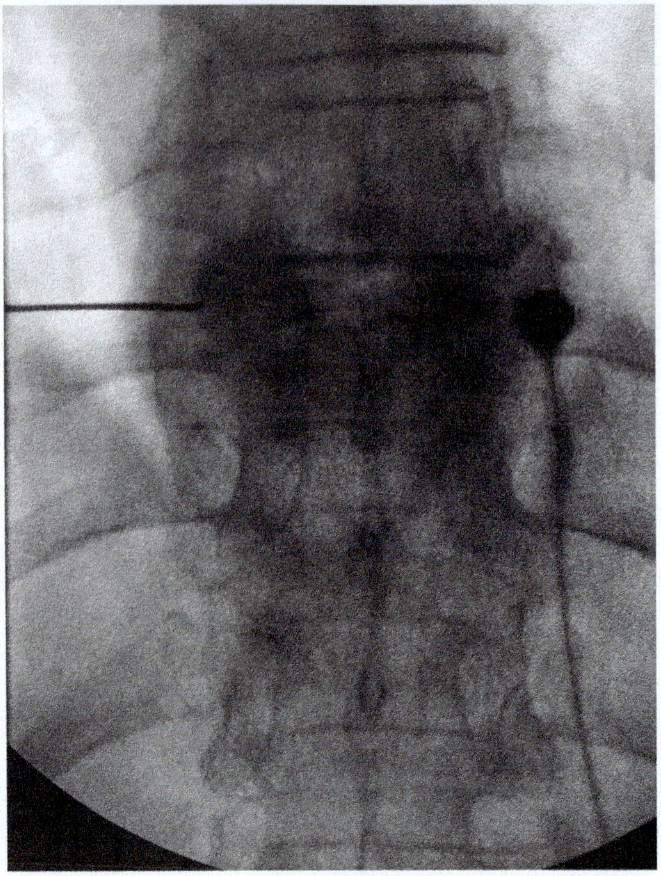

Fig. 48.5 Fluoroscopic bilateral T9 RFA

side, and 6 bilaterally. They showed that 82% of the patients had 50–75% reduction in pain symptoms 2 months after the intervention. The long-term relief was also considerable. In another study, Tzaan and Tasker noted a success rate of 40% in 15 patients who received one RF treatment of the ramus medialis (medial branch) of the thoracic rami dorsales.

Pearls and Pitfalls

Pearls

- Initial imaging should be done in AP plane to accurately count the vertebral level starting from either T1 or T12.
- Use of multiple angles under fluoroscopy of the transverse process with the superior articular process of the vertebrae improves safety and efficacy of the procedure.
- Altered entry angles from more lateral, or caudal approach, of the RF cannula may help align the active tip lesion with the medial branch target.
- Prior to lesioning, sensory testing, while monitoring impedance and response, helps ensure no unwanted lesioning and correct anatomical position in the mid back.
- Prior to lesioning, motor testing monitoring, impedance, and response to confirm needle placement and helps ensure no unwanted motor involvement.

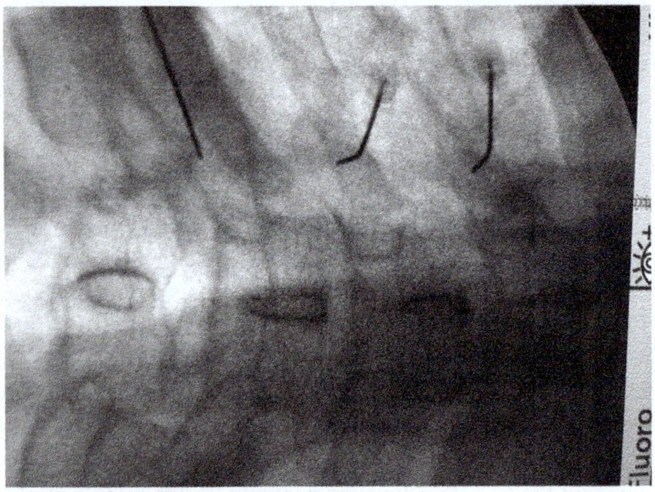

Fig. 48.6 T2–T4 cannula placement

- Be aware that patients on blood thinning medications have increased risk for neuraxial hematomas and other bleeding complications.
- An increase in the amount of energy, time, and temperature may also increase the lesion size.
- Given the fact that the thoracic spine confluence of the superior articulating process is slightly shorter than those in the lumbar spine, and transverse proves are in either a

Table 48.1 Evidence for efficacy

Study	Study design	Type of therapy	Total # of patients/study conducted	Primary outcome
Manchikanti et al. 2010	Randomized, double-blinded, controlled trial	Local anesthesia with or without steroid for z-joint pain in the thoracic region	100	90% of patients reported significant pain improvement at 12 months
Atluri et al. 2008	Systematic review	Diagnostic and therapeutic therapy for thoracic FJ pain	RCT: 1 original study with MBNB and 2 systematic reviews included Observational: 2 systematic reviews, 1 MBNB, 2 RF neurotomies	MBNBs' level of evidence is level I or level II-1 and recommendation is 1A or 1B. Positive evidence for medial branch nerve blocks, no positive evidence for intra-articular thoracic facet injections or medial branch neurotomy
Stolker et al. 1993	Observational	Thoracic medial branch neurotomy	40	2-month follow-up: 47.5% were pain free, 35% had greater than 50% pain relief, 17.5% had no pain relief 18–54-month follow-up: 44% were pain free, 39% greater than 50% pain relief, 17% no relief
Tzaan et al. 2000	Observational	Facet joint denervation with generalized anesthesia vs local anesthesia	90	No significant difference between the two groups, first procedure provided 41% of patients 50% or greater pain relief, repeat procedure did not change the outcome

lateral or cephalad-lateral orientation, the medial branches are often more superficial than those found in the lumbar spine. In order to more closely place the active tip of the cannula close to these nerves, there may be a need to make a more shallow caudal to cephalad angle of approach.

Pitfalls

- Large-volume diagnostic medial branch blocks give inaccurate prediction of RF lesioning.
- Anatomical variation of medial branch location dependent on which level is being targeted. Careful attention should be paid to maximize efficacy of the therapy.
- Complications: there is an increased risk of pneumothorax for all thoracic procedures noted. Use proper guidance under fluoroscopy and avoid advancing too deep to minimize this risk.
- The medial branch target in the thoracic spine may be more superficial than targets in the lumbar spine due to curvature of spine and decreased superficial soft tissues, which may increase the risk of cutaneous burns.

Recommended Reading

1. Atluri S, et al. Systematic review of diagnostic utility and therapeutic effectiveness of thoracic facet joint interventions. Pain Physician. 2008;11(5):611–29.
2. Boswell MV, et al. A systematic review of therapeutic facet joint interventions in chronic spinal pain. Pain Physician. 2007;10(1): 229–53.
3. Chua WH, Bogduk N. The surgical anatomy of thoracic facet denervation. Acta Neurochir [Wien]. 1995;136:140–4.
4. Dreyfuss P, Tibiletti C, Dreyer SJ. Thoracic zygapophyseal joint pain patterns. A study in normal volunteers. Spine (Phila Pa 1976). 1994;19(7):807–11.
5. Fukui S, Ohseto K, Shiotani M. Patterns of pain induced by distending the thoracic zygapophyseal joints. Reg Anesth. 1997;22(4):332–6.
6. Manchikanti L, et al. Comparative effectiveness of a one-year follow-up of thoracic medial branch blocks in management of chronic thoracic pain: a randomized, double-blind active controlled trial. Pain Physician. 2010;13(6):535–48.
7. Manchikanti KN, et al. An update of evaluation of therapeutic thoracic facet joint interventions. Pain Physician. 2012;15(4): E463–81.
8. Manchikanti L, et al. Assessment of the escalating growth of facet joint interventions in the medicare population in the United States from 2000 to 2011. Pain Physician. 2013;16(4):E365–78.
9. Manchikanti L, et al. A systematic review and best evidence synthesis of the effectiveness of therapeutic facet joint interventions in managing chronic spinal pain. Pain Physician. 2015;18(4):E535–82.
10. Provenzano DA, Lassila HC, Somers D. The effect of fluid injection on lesion size during radiofrequency treatment. Reg Anesth Pain Med. 2010;35(4):338–42.
11. Provenzano DA, Liebert MA, Somers DL. Increasing the NaCl concentration of the preinjected solution enhances monopolar radiofrequency lesion size. Reg Anesth Pain Med. 2013;38(2):112–23.
12. Speldewinde G. Outcomes of percutaneous zygapophysial and sacroiliac joint neurotomy in a community setting. Pain Med. 2011;12(2):209–18.
13. Stolker RJ, Vervest AC, Groen GJ. Percutaneous facet denervation in chronic thoracic spinal pain. Acta Neurochir. 1993;122(1–2):82–90.
14. Tzaan WC, Tasker RR. Percutaneous radiofrequency facet rhizotomy–experience with 118 procedures and reappraisal of its value. Can J Neurol Sci. 2000;27(2):125–30.
15. Walega D, et al. Third-degree burn from cooled radiofrequency ablation of medial branch nerves for treatment of thoracic facet syndrome. Pain Pract. 2014;14(6):e154–8. https://doi.org/10.1111/papr.12222. Epub 2014 May 2.

Lumbar Interlaminar Epidural Injection

49

Ioannis M. Skaribas, Jennifer L. Erian, Dustin Reynolds, and Elena E. Skaribas

Introduction

Lumbar interlaminar epidural steroid injections (LESIs) represent the most commonly performed procedure in chronic pain medicine. This procedure involves accessing the epidural space percutaneously with a needle via a posterior approach. As indicated by the nomenclature, the needle insertion and advancement are between (inter) the posterior bony plates of the vertebral body (lamina).

In chronic pain medicine, the lumbar interlaminar epidural injection is to inject corticosteroids into the epidural space for anti-inflammatory purposes. Although the procedure can be performed blindly utilizing anatomical landmarks and the loss of resistance technique, the medical standard of care is the real-time utilization of fluoroscopic imaging to promote accuracy and minimize risk.

Historical Perspectives

The discovery of the epidural neuraxial technique has changed the face of modern medicine not only with its use in the field of obstetrics but also in acute and chronic pain. Although commonly and mistakenly credited to August Bier, the father of spinal anesthesia, the first lumbar epidural injection was initially described by American neurologist James Leonard Corning. After having described the anesthetic properties of cocaine in 1884, Corning injected it for the very first time (1885) into the lumbar epidural space of a human volunteer using an approach between the spinous processes. In 1921, Spanish surgeon Fidel Pagés described a lumbar paramedian approach to the epidural space, an approach that was later popularized in 1933 by Italian surgeon, Achille Mario Dogliotti. Dogliotti expanded the previous work by Forestier and Sicard and in 1933 introduced the "Dogliotti's principle," effectively describing the "loss of resistance technique" that we recognize and practice to this day. The invention of the Tuohy needle by Ralph L. Huber (1940) and its further popularization by Edward Boyce Tuohy (1945) further advanced the applications of this interlaminar approach to the epidural space in both anesthesia and pain medicine. Fluoroscopy was not used for the procedure until the 1980s when it was recognized that despite the level of expertise and checkpoints, there was still a high rate of incorrect placement.

Anatomical Considerations

The epidural space is a potential expandable, nonuniform space extending from the foramen magnum cephalad to the sacral hiatus caudad. Although a cylindrical continuum, it is divided for practical procedural purposes in posterior, anterior, and lateral compartments. It contains septa, the internal vertebral venous plexus of Batson, adipose and areolar tissue, lymphatics, and arteries as well as the spinal nerve roots. It surrounds the spinal meninges and is bounded anteriorly by the posterior longitudinal ligament, laterally by the pedicles and the intervertebral foramina and posteriorly by the ligamentum flavum and the anterior surface of the lamina (Fig. 49.1). The ligamentum flavum is composed of left and right ligament flava fused in the middle and is thicker in the lumbar region compared to cervical and thoracic. The distance from the skin to the lumbar ligamentum flavum where the loss of resistance is elicited varies between 3 and 8 cm. The epidural space is cylindrical and narrower anteriorly and wider posteriorly. At its widest, it is 5–6 mm posteriorly at L2 level. Because of the triangular anatomy of the spinal canal that makes it

I. M. Skaribas (✉) · J. L. Erian · D. Reynolds
Expert Pain P.A., Department of Anesthesiology, McGovern Medical School, The University of Texas Health Science Center at Houston, Houston, TX, USA
e-mail: skaribasmd@expertpaincare.com; Jennifer.L.Franke@uth.tmc.edu; dustin.l.reynolds@uth.tmc.edu

E. E. Skaribas
Southern Methodist University, Dallas, TX, USA
e-mail: eskaribas@smu.edu

T. R. Deer et al. (eds.), *Deer's Treatment of Pain*, https://doi.org/10.1007/978-3-030-12281-2_49

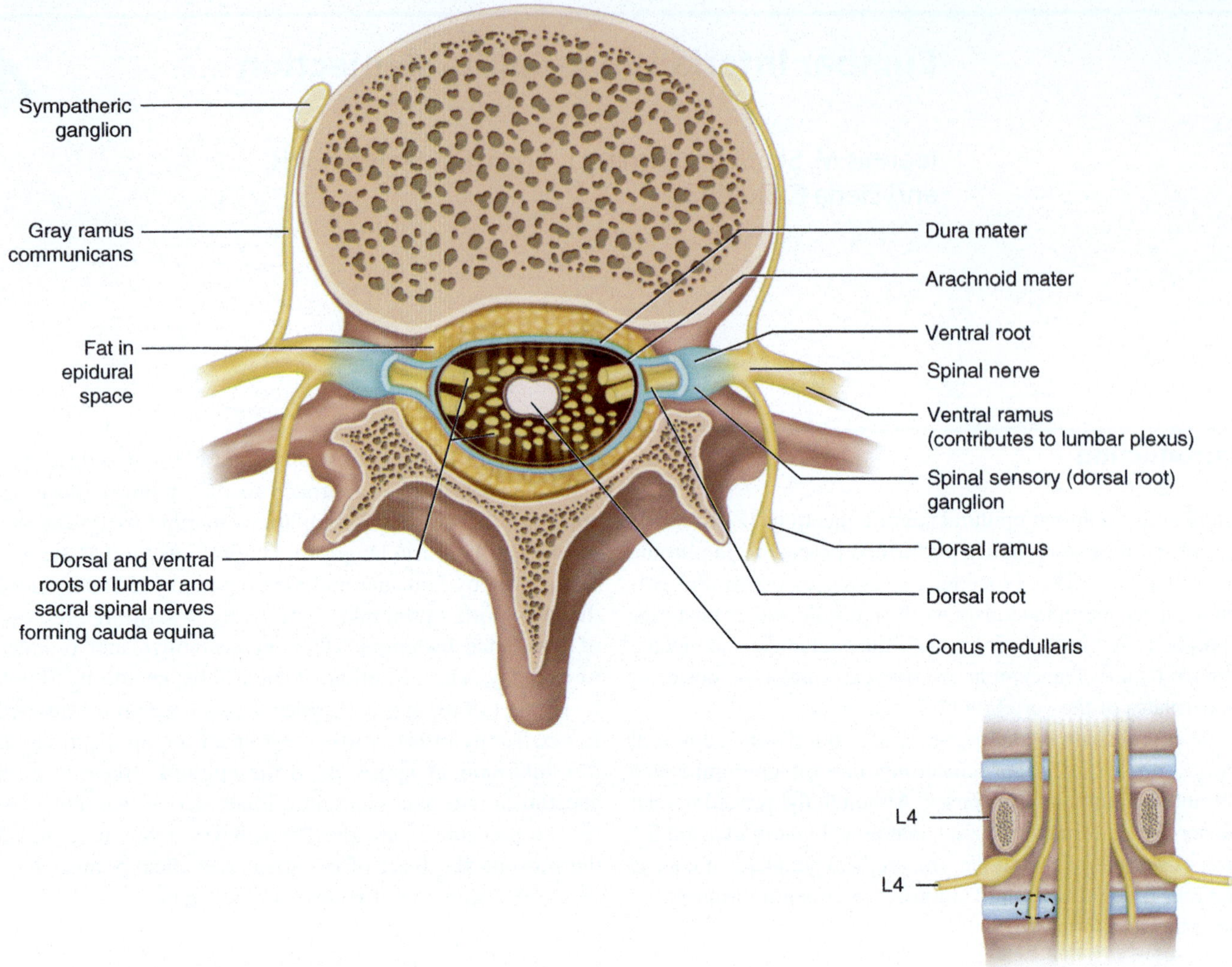

Fig. 49.1 Cross-sectional view of the lumbar spine and anatomical contents

narrower laterally, the midline is the safest point of entry into the lumbar epidural space with a needle. When identifying macroscopic anatomical landmarks, a horizontal line connecting the superior margins of the iliac crests correlates to the L4–L5 interspace. The spinal cord terminates at the L1–L2 level. From the conus terminalis arises the cauda equina, which occupies the lumbar cistern and consists of the second through fifth lumbar nerves, the first through fifth sacral nerves, and the coccygeal nerve. A lumbar interlaminar epidural steroid injection can be performed in a paramedian or midline fashion and involves a posterior insertion of an epidural needle between the laminae of two adjacent vertebrae and into the lumbar epidural space (Fig. 49.2).

Indications

1. Lumbar radiculopathy (sciatica) (unilateral, bilateral, or multilevel due to disc herniation or multifactorial lumbar spine degeneration)
2. Spinal stenosis (symptomatic mild/moderate spinal stenosis or severe spinal stenosis not meeting surgical criteria)
3. Chronic low back pain that has failed to or has responded poorly to previous conservative treatment
4. Neurogenic claudication
5. Lumbar failed back surgery syndrome(FBSS)
6. Discogenic low back pain
7. Postherpetic neuralgia

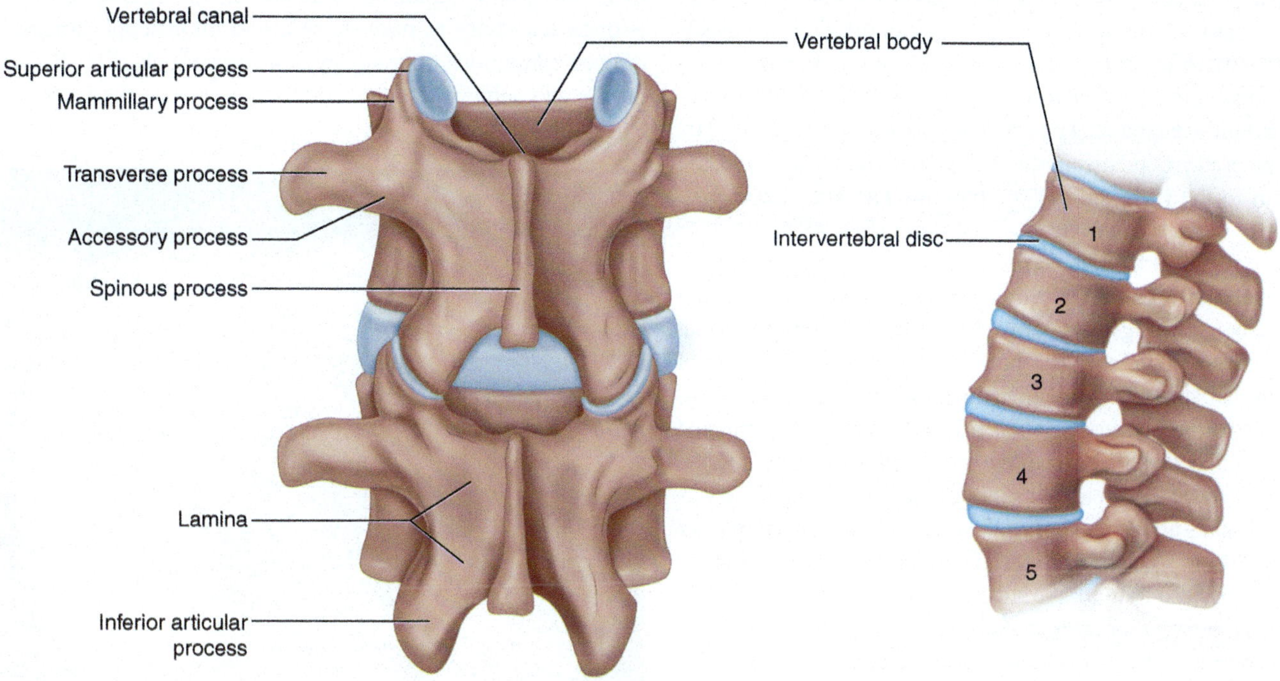

Fig. 49.2 Posterior view of the lumbar spine at L3–L4 level

Contraindications

1. Infection (local or systemic)
2. Anticoagulation
3. Systemic coagulopathy
4. Immunosuppression
5. Patient refusal or uncooperative patient
6. Pregnancy

Description of the Procedure

An interlaminar lumbar epidural steroid injection is an elective procedure and should be performed in an outpatient setting. Full availability of cardiopulmonary resuscitating equipment and medications is mandatory. The patient should always have intravenous access secured. Standard American Society of Anesthesiologists (ASA) monitoring should be applied. American Society of Regional Anesthesia (ASRA) guidelines for interventional spine procedures in patients on antiplatelet or anticoagulant medications should be observed. Although the administration of an anesthetic is optional since these cases can be performed with just local anesthesia, the clear majority in the United States is performed under monitored anesthesia care (MAC) with administration of a combination of an intravenous sedative (midazolam) and an intravenous opioid (fentanyl). Both medications should be used in small amounts (2–4 mg midazolam and/or 50–100 mcg of fentanyl). This combination provides for adequate sedation and patient comfort while at the same time maintains spontaneous respiratory status without loss of consciousness. Any anesthetic that induces loss of consciousness (propofol) should be avoided since a nonresponsive, noncommunicative patient cannot provide feedback and warnings of impending injury. This is particularly significant for any ESIs above the conus terminalis where potential injury to the spinal cord can be devastating. The pain management physician performing the procedure should never be the one administering the anesthetic. Informed consent after explanation of risks and benefits is always obtained, and the area is marked in the preoperative area.

The patient is placed in a prone position resting his head comfortably. One or more pillows or commercially available wedges are placed under the patient's lower abdomen to decrease the lumbar lordosis and optimize accessibility to the epidural space. The arms are positioned in arm rests. The operator is positioned to the left of the patient and the C-arm to the right side of the patient. The anesthesia provider is located at the head of the table (Fig. 49.3).

The patient's back is prepped and draped in a sterile manner. Preferably, DuraPrep is utilized since ChloraPrep has specific label warnings. A C-arm is introduced initially without any oblique angulation to obtain posterior-anterior views of the lumbar spine. Caudad or cephalad tilt is occasionally necessary to align the vertebral plates of the interspaces of interest and optimize visualization of the interlaminar opening into the epidural space. By identifying the spinous processes of the vertebral bodies above and below the intervertebral space that we are targeting, we can identify the interlaminar spaces of interest and proceed to mark the superimposed skin with a marker, utilizing a serat or similar surgical instrument. Next, the marked skin and the subcutaneous tissue are infiltrated with a short-acting local anesthetic, usually 5–10 cc of 1% lidocaine. A coaxial fluoroscopic technique is utilized. A Tuohy needle (20 or 18 gauge) is used, and it is advanced percutaneously until it is imbedded into the interspinous ligament. If there is intention to preferentially spread the injectate into the right or left epidural space, then the Tuohy needle is directed in an interlaminar paramedian approach (Fig. 49.4). A loss of resistance (LOR) 10 cc syringe containing 2–3 cc of preservative free saline is attached to the Tuohy needle, and the needle is advanced utilizing the LOR technique as well as fluoroscopic posterior-anterior and lateral views until there is advancement through the ligamentum flavum and LOR is obtained. It is often necessary to perform repeated fluoroscopic imaging or even continuous fluoroscopy to accurately place the Tuohy needle and achieve the desired trajectory. Once the LOR has

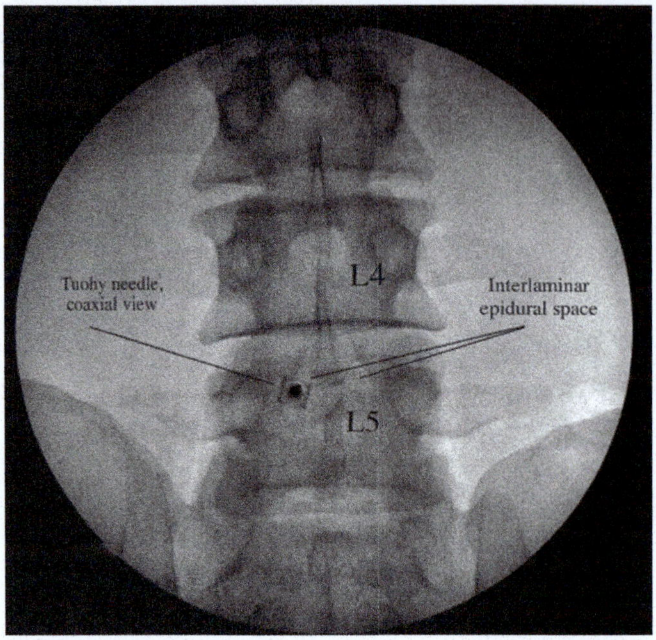

Fig. 49.4 Posterior-anterior view of the lumbar spine during a left paramedian L4–L5 epidural steroid injection. The interlaminar epidural space is easily fluoroscopically identified between the right and left laminae and the spinous process, representing the target area that the Tuohy needle needs to access. This is a left paramedian approach aiming to preferentially spread the injectate to the left paramedian epidural space upon injection. The Tuohy needle is placed in a perfect coaxial trajectory as demonstrated by the fluoroscopic image

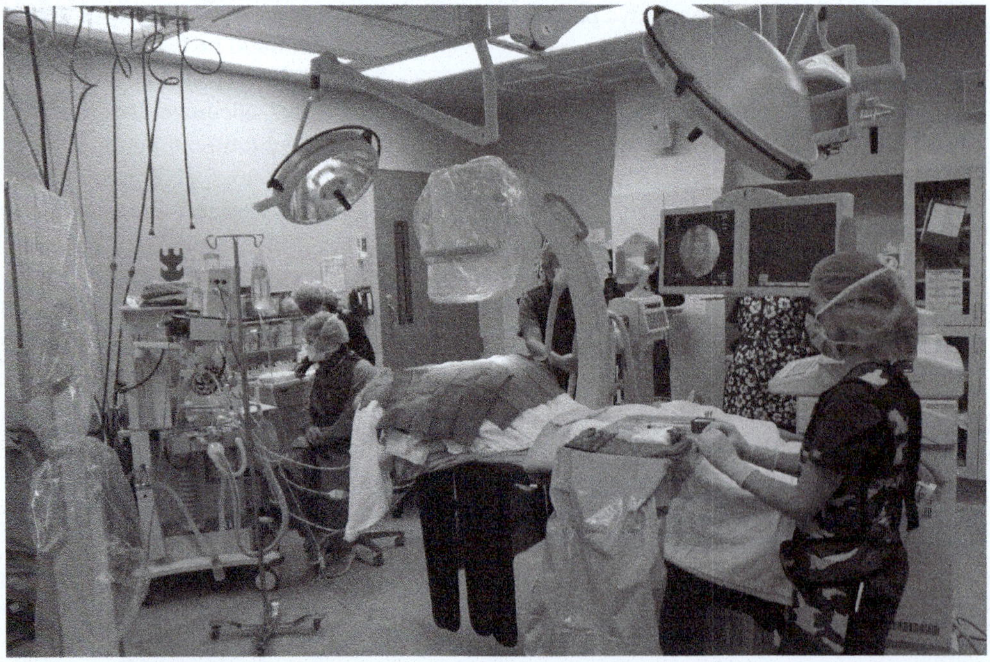

Fig. 49.3 Operating suite layout and patient placement for a lumbar epidural steroid injection. Patient is placed prone on the operating table with the fluoroscopy C-arm over the lumbar spine in a P-A orientation. The fluoroscopic C-arm and viewing tower are located at the right side of the patient. The anesthesia team and equipment are located at the head of the table

been obtained, 1–2 cc of an iodinated nonionic radiographic contrast most commonly Omnipaque (iohexol 180 or 240 mg/ml) is injected to obtain an epidurogram and confirm spread into the targeted areas of the epidural space and the avoidance of intravascular spread. The interlaminar approach allows for multidimensional epidural spread of the injectate in the path of least resistance (Figs. 49.5 and 49.6). This radiographic contrast injection should be performed under continuous real-time fluoroscopy to confirm absence of intravascular uptake. If intravascular absorption is obtained, then the needle needs to be removed and reinserted in a different location either in the same interspace or one interspace above or below. Following the contrast injection and after epidural spread has been verified with anterior-posterior and lateral views (Fig. 49.7), the corticosteroid mixture is injected. The type of mixture of the injectate that individual practitioners utilize varies significantly. A common practice is to utilize a mixture of a local anesthetic such as 0.25% bupivacaine or 0.25% ropivacaine mixed with 1–2 cc of 40 mg/cc Depo-Medrol (methylprednisolone) to a total volume of 4–5 cc. Other commonly used corticosteroids are Kenalog (triamcinolone), dexamethasone, and betamethasone. The steroid dosing per injection should be limited to 15 mg of dexamethasone, 40–80 mg of triamcinolone, 40–80 mg of methylprednisolone, and 12 mg of betamethasone.

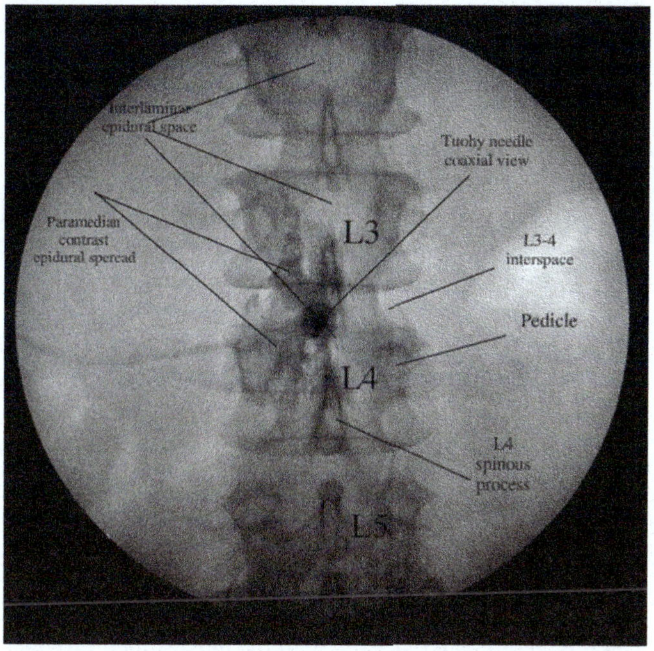

Fig. 49.6 Posterior-anterior view of a lumbar interlaminar left paramedian epidural injection at L3–L4 with coaxial needle placement. Spread of the dye to the left epidural space superimposes the vertebral bodies above and below the needle. The classic fluoroscopic epidural pseudo-honeycomb pattern is noted because of dye spread between the different components of the epidural space

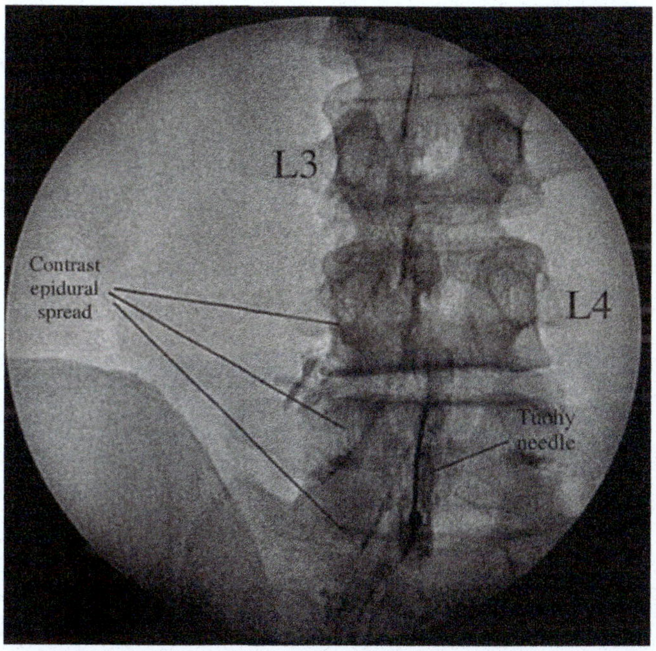

Fig. 49.5 Lumbar interlaminar epidural steroid injection with left paramedian spread of contrast dye. Midline placement of the Tuohy needle is noted with entry at the L4–L5 interlaminar epidural space. The spread of contrast to the left lumbar epiradicular space and multiple nerve roots follows the "path of least resistance" principle

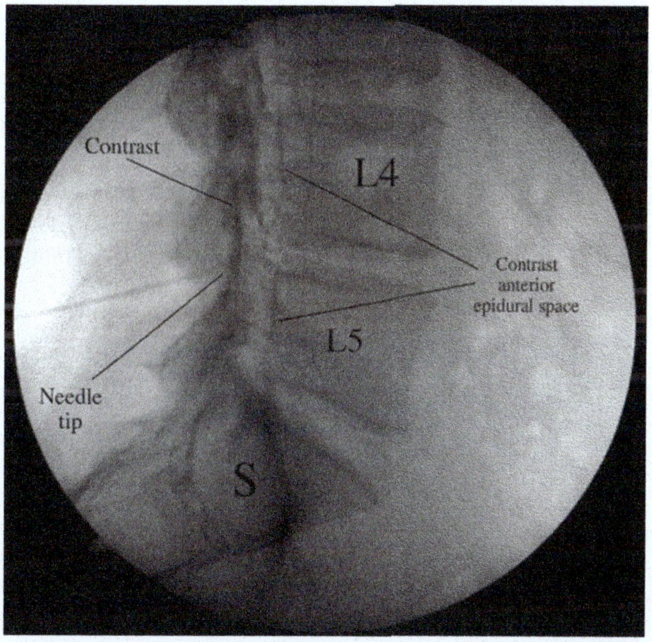

Fig. 49.7 Lateral fluoroscopic view of an L4–L5 interlaminar epidural injection. The tip of the Tuohy needle can be identified entering the L4–L5 epidural space. There is spread of the dye in both the posterior and anterior lumbar epidural space forming the so-called railroad sign typical of a successful lumbar epidural

Complications

Risks of lumbar interlaminar epidural injections are rare and can range from transient discomfort to death. This laundry list of complications includes spinal cord injury, dural puncture, post-dural puncture headache, intrathecal injection, intravascular injection, stroke, epidural hematoma, epidural abscess, chemical or bacterial meningitis, arachnoiditis, increased pain, paraplegia, disability, vasovagal syncope, discitis, soft tissue infection, osteomyelitis, retinal hemorrhage, transient blindness, and even death. Below we will explore some of these complications by groups according to subcategories including complications due to technique, underlying coagulopathy or use of anticoagulants, infectious processes, and reactions to medications.

Dural Puncture

Dural puncture is a risk even with the most skilled provider. Inadvertent dural puncture may be immediately evident if there is CSF backflow out of the Tuohy needle or the classic "swirl pattern" seen in the loss of resistance syringe during aspiration. This may subsequently cause a post-dural puncture headache due to loss of cerebrospinal fluid. Despite negative aspiration, subarachnoid and subdural injection cannot be ruled out. Epidurals performed under fluoroscopy will reveal a rapid uptake of the injected contrast dye if it is in the intrathecal space. Intrathecal injection can occur if the provider fails to recognize incorrect placement of the epidural needle. Local anesthetics injected intrathecally can result in a high spinal requiring hemodynamic and ventilatory support. Additionally, if the needle is placed between the dura and arachnoid in the subdural space, there can be a delayed total spinal, and this has been reported up to 20 minutes' postinjection (Fig. 49.8).

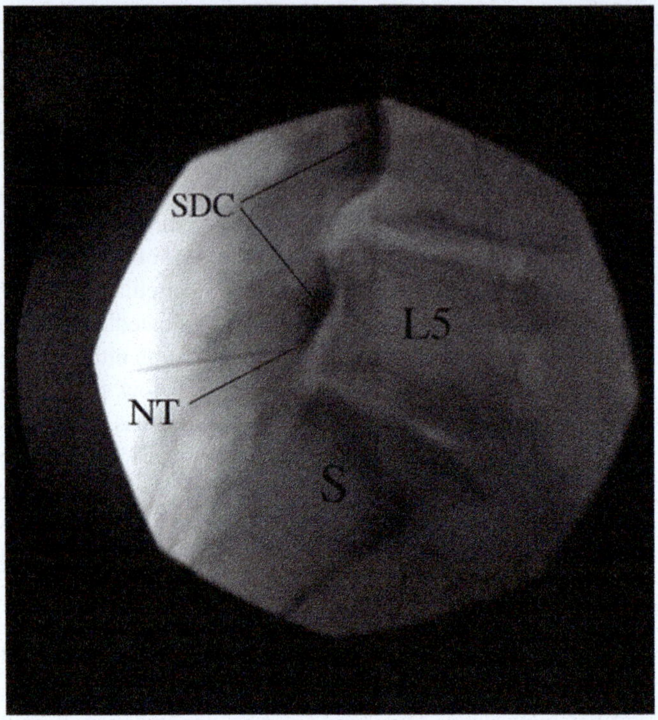

Fig. 49.8 Lateral fluoroscopic view of a lumbar interlaminar subdural injection. The subdural spread of the contrast follows a long posterior linear spread with a segmental loculated pattern of dye accumulation above and below the intervertebral spaces. The dye extends toward, but does not reach, the anterior epidural space

Intravascular Injection

Even with negative aspiration, intravascular placement cannot be ruled out. Contrast dye can be injected, and if intravascular, there will be rapid vascular uptake and disappearance of the dye highlighting the course of the vasculature. This will be less rapid when injected into the venous system compared to an arterial injection. Intravascular injection of local anesthetics can cause local anesthetic toxicity and even cardiovascular collapse requiring advanced cardiac life support. Not only can intravascular injections occur with inadvertent contact with an artery but can also cause shearing of the vessel and or spasm. Damage to vasculature particularly arterial damage can result in permanent neurologic damage due to interruption of the blood supply to the spinal cord. In most individuals, the artery of Adamkiewicz is found at the level of T8 to L3 and supplies the anterior spinal cord. Damage to this artery can cause permanent motor deficit or anterior spinal artery syndrome.

Neurological Injury

Direct damage to both the spinal cord and spinal nerves can be secondary to needle trauma. It is possible that a true loss of resistance may not be appreciated due to gaps in the ligamentum flavum and/or a soft ligament, and the epidural needle may be advanced too far. It is critical to stop the procedure if the patient complains of severe pain either during needle placement or when depositing the injectate. Therefore, it is imperative that the patient undergoing this procedure should always maintain a level of consciousness and can communicate and answer questions always. Inadvertent contact with the spinal cord or nerve roots can cause transient paresthesia and pain or even permanent nerve damage. The patient may not always complain of pain or other symptoms of injury.

Intradiscal Injury

Needle trauma to the intervertebral disc is a very rare complication and can produce various discogenic-related symptoms.

Anticoagulation and Neuraxial Complications

Complications can be secondary to anticoagulation despite adherence to guidelines provided regarding discontinuation of anticoagulation prior to neuraxial procedures. It is imperative to follow these guidelines; however, this must be in coordination with the primary prescriber. The risks and benefits must be weighed on an individual basis to determine if discontinuing anticoagulation is safe to perform the epidural steroid injection. The American Society of Regional Anesthesia (ASRA) has set forth anticoagulation guidelines for use in neuraxial procedures. Despite adhering to these recommendations, one must be cognoscente of potential complications and management as they are not fail-safe.

An epidural hematoma can develop due to bleeding from either the venous plexus or arteries in the epidural spaces that have been inadvertently damaged during needle placement. When the bleeding is severe enough to cause a hematoma and subsequent spinal cord or nerve root compression, signs of symptoms may be present. These include pain, paresthesias, weakness, or bowel and bladder dysfunction. Spinal cord compression is a surgical emergency no matter the underlying mechanism.

Complications Due to Medications

Steroids alone have their own complications and side effects. They can cause diabetes or hyperglycemia, hypertension, psychological manifestations, adrenocortical suppression, Cushing's syndrome, increased risk of infection, avascular necrosis of joints, pruritus, and nausea. When particulate steroids are used for epidural injection and they are accidentally injected intravascular, this can lead to emboli or infarction. If steroids are unintentionally injected into the intrathecal space, there is risk of developing adhesive arachnoiditis.

Side effects of local anesthetic include seizures, heart block, arrhythmias, and cardiovascular collapse. Local anesthetic injected directly into the spinal cord can cause spinal cord damage. In the event of intrathecal injection of local anesthetic as mentioned above, this can result in a high spinal.

Infection

Infection in the epidural space can result in an epidural abscess or meningitis. Aseptic technique during the procedure is critical. Compounded medications can lead to serious infections. Risk of infection is highest in immune-compromised individuals but can occur in any patient. Skin flora can be tracked to the epidural space during needle placement if the skin is not properly cleaned and/or if sterility is lost at any time during the procedure. If a patient complains of headache and light sensitivity, one must be vigilant of other causes which can be life-threatening including early signs of meningitis. It must not always be disregarded as simply a post-dural puncture headache. Just like with other infections caused by skin flora, the commonest culprits include *Staphylococcus aureus* and *Staphylococcus epidermidis* and *Streptococcus*.

Pearls and Pitfalls

1. When performing paramedian interlaminar injections, stay close to midline.
2. Utilize lateral fluoroscopic views to confirm needle placement and epidural spread.
3. When utilizing monitored anesthesia care, limit sedation to the minimum necessary and always keep the patient responsive.
4. Encourage communication with the patient and all staff involved.
5. Consider changes and corrective steps including terminating the procedure if the patient complains of pain during injection of the contrast dye or medication.
6. Limit steroid dosing per session to 15 mg dexamethasone, $\leq$80 mg triamcinolone, $\leq$ 80 mg methylprednisolone, or 12 mg betamethasone, or equivalent corticosteroid.
7. Consider particulate free steroids such as dexamethasone as first-line steroid for ESIs performed at a L3 level or above.
8. No "series of 3." Evaluate the patient after each lumbar epidural steroid injection.

Recommended Reading

1. Benzon H, Rathmell JP, Wu CL, Turk DC, Argoff CE. Raj's practical management of pain. 4th ed. Philadelphia: Mosby; 2013
2. Deer TR. Treatment of chronic pain by interventional approaches: the American Academy of Pain Medicine textbook on patient management. New York: Springer, American Academy of Pain Medicine; 2013.
3. Gorelick PB, Zych D. James Leonard Corning and the early history of spinal puncture (abstract). Neurology. 1987;37(4):672–4.

4. Narouze S, Benzon HT, Provenzano DA, Buvanendran A, De Andres J, Deer TR, Rauck R, Huntoon MA. Interventional spine and pain procedures in patients on antiplatelet and anticoagulant medications: guidelines from the American Society of Regional Anesthesia and Pain Medicine, the European Society of Regional Anaesthesia and Pain Therapy, the American Academy of Pain Medicine, the International Neuromodulation Society, the North American Neuromodulation Society, and the World Institute of Pain. Reg Anesth Pain Med. 2015;40(3):182–212.
5. Ranson M, Pope J, Deer T. Reducing risks and complications of interventional pain procedures. Chapter 13, complications of Epidural Injections. Philadelphia: Saunders; 2012.
6. Rathmell JP, Benzon HT, Dreyfuss P, Huntoon M, Wallace M, Baker R, Riew KD, Rosenquist RW, Aprill C, Rost NS, Buvanendran A, Kreiner DS, Bogduk N, Fourney DR, Fraifeld E, Horn S, Stone J, Vorenkamp K, Lawler G, Summers J, Kloth D, O'Brien D, Tutton S. Safeguards to prevent neurologic complications after epidural steroid injections. Anesthesiology. 2015;122(5):974–84.
7. Cousins MJ, Bridenbaugh PO. Neural blockade in clinical anesthesia and management of pain. 3d ed. chapter 7. Philadelphia: Lippincott Williams & Wilkins; 1998.

Lumbar Transforaminal Epidural Corticosteroid Injections

50

Nicholas J. Bremer and Mark N. Malinowski

Introduction

The accepted indication for L-TFESIs is for pain associated with mediated membrane irritability from inflammation. Inflammation may be from mechanical compression of the nerve roots or local mediators associated with soft tissue damage (e.g., annular disk tear). Mechanical compression of the nerve roots results from either foraminal or central canal stenosis or both. Foraminal stenosis occurs as a result of facet hypertrophy, disk disease, or, less frequently, cysts associated with the facet or nerve sheath. Central canal stenosis can occur as well by disk disease but may also result from ligamentum flavum overgrowth. While older populations typically have multifactorial etiologies for radiculitis, younger patients classically present with an isolated disk herniation. Similarly, older populations present with slow progression of symptoms, while younger patients may present with a history of a well-defined event.

Complications associated with the injection of the epidural space are wide ranging and can result in severe neurologic impairment and death. Much of the debate surrounding technique and medication is driven by reports of complications. The most severe complications include compressive lesions such as epidural hematoma and epidural abscess, spinal cord infarctions and paralysis, aseptic meningitis, stroke, and death. While this procedure is widely used, the skilled practitioner who is well trained may not be exempt from disastrous outcomes. Diligence is paramount when identifying appropriate candidates during the pre-procedure evaluation period.

Compressive lesions result in substantial post-procedural complications. These include infections and hematoma formation. Sterile technique is essential, and the use of proper hand care and sterile gloves, sterile field preparation and barriers, and proper masking is considered the gold standard. Special circumstances such as the immunocompromised patient, the poorly controlled diabetic, and those patients with active infections warrant reconsideration for injection appropriateness. Similarly, proper preparation of the injectate under USP and FDA guidelines with the use of single-dose vials is critical as there have been reports of severe infection and death due to contaminated products. Furthermore, patients who have an active coagulopathy must be addressed prior to injection. The American Society of Regional Anesthesia and Pain Medicine has provided appropriate guidelines for the periprocedural management of antiplatelet and anticoagulation medications. Holding or discontinuation of these medications should be done in conjunction with the appropriate specialist whereby the risk of stopping the medication does not outweigh the benefit of the planned procedure. Patients with underlying qualitative or quantitative platelet disorders or other organic coagulopathies should be optimized before the procedure is indicated. A full list of contraindications is listed in Table 50.1.

The use of particulate and non-particulate steroid has been a source of debate. Of particular concern is the use of particulate medications in the presence of vascular structures. There have been reports of paralysis and spinal cord infarction due to the inadvertent arterial injection of particulate steroid. Technical modifications of the procedure have been implemented to pro-

Table 50.1 Absolute and relative contraindications to lumbar transforaminal epidural corticosteroid injections

Absolute contraindications	Relative contraindications
Lack of informed consent	Concurrent anticoagulation usage
Pregnancy (due to radiation)	Immunosuppression
Systemic infection	Minor allergy to injectate
Localized infection over injection site	Anatomic aberrations preventing access
Severe allergy to injectate	Coexisting disease-preventing injection
Maximal steroid dose reached	
Patient cannot cooperate	

N. J. Bremer (✉)
Center for Pain Relief, Spine and Nerve Centers of the Virginias, Charleston, WV, USA
e-mail: Nicholas.Bremer@CenterforPainRelief.com

M. N. Malinowski
Adena Spine Center, Chillicothe, OH, USA

T. R. Deer et al. (eds.), *Deer's Treatment of Pain*, https://doi.org/10.1007/978-3-030-12281-2_50

mote safety, including preferential use of blunt-tipped needles, injection of radiocontrast administration, continuous fluoroscopy, and digital subtraction angiography (DSA). The concept of the "safe triangle" supraneural approach to the TFESI has been suggested to be safer than other approaches. Additionally, some would argue the interlaminar epidural or caudal epidural approach is a safer alternative to the transforaminal approach. However, no one modification has been proven superior to another, and the physician must weigh all circumstances prior to performing the injection.

Periprocedural sedation is also another area of controversy. Patient satisfaction, patient expectations, and safety come to a crossroad and create an unpleasant quandary for the physician. Of particular concern is the potential for undetected complications in the sedated patient. Trypanophobia and other anxieties may warrant periprocedural anxiolysis. However, it is the author's opinion and preference that an awake and communicating patient provides the best opportunity to monitor for complications. Furthermore, patients who are awake are less likely to develop disinhibition to their surroundings, a situation that is particularly concerning in the prone position during the procedure. Disinhibited patients in the prone position may react to uncomfortable stimulation and may lead to dural or spinal cord puncture.

Background and Historical Perspective

The administration of corticosteroid into the epidural space is a procedure that has long been used in the practice of pain management with reported use dating to the 1950s. Since then, epidural steroid injections (ESIs) have been performed in millions of people worldwide for the treatment of radiating pain from the spine. Historically, prior to the use of fluoroscopy, caudal injections through the sacral hiatus and interlaminar injections were the techniques of choice. Landmark approaches unaided by fluoroscopy have given way to move directed fluoroscopic-guided interventional techniques. The use of ESIs has more than doubled over the last decade, including with the transforaminal approach.

Controversy involving proper nomenclature for this injection exists. Despite consistent recommendation from the Spine Intervention Society, authors and physicians alike continue to incorrectly refer to transforaminal epidural injections as selective nerve root blocks, nerve root sleeve blocks, and others. This recommendation is based on the actual anatomic description of the injections.

It is useful to consider the transforaminal approach in relation to the other two approaches to the epidural space. The transforaminal approach is preferred by many interventionalists for several reasons. While epidural adhesions or fibrosis may hinder medications reaching the desired target in the caudal and interlaminar approaches, the transforaminal approach delivers high concentrations of medication directly at the presumed pain generator, maximizing potential patient benefit but also diagnostic value. In patients with prior lumbar surgery, where interlaminar access through the prior incision site would be technically challenging due to disrupted tissue planes, the transforaminal approach can be utilized. In addition, volume of injectate with the transforaminal approach is less than the caudal or interlaminar approaches, which also increases diagnostic value when compared to those approaches. Finally, caudal and interlaminar approaches have higher incidence of intravascular or extradural placement.

Uses and Indications

The role of transforaminal epidural steroid injections can be classified as either diagnostic or therapeutic. In modern medical practice, indications for decompressive surgery are principally in the realm of objective neurologic deficit, such as motor weakness, change in reflexes, and, of course, cauda equina syndrome.

Radiculitis—that is, nerve root inflammation alone—is thought to be the underlying pathophysiology of radicular pain. Nerve roots are often inflamed from, for example, the inflammatory cytokines released in an acute disk herniation. True radiculopathy—that is, neurologic signs (numbness, abnormal reflexes, motor weakness) emanating from a nerve root—is often compressive in nature. The difference is subtle but important, as the radiculitis rarely is a surgical indication, while radiculopathy may certainly involve a surgical option. However, surgeons who plan on decompressive surgery for radicular pain, alone, may find transforaminal epidural steroid injections helpful in eliciting the specific level to be addressed, with the associated predictive value in surgical planning.

The therapeutic benefit of transforaminal epidural steroid injections is less controversial in modern practice. An aspect of TFESIs that is particularly useful is in patients for whom anterior spread of medications would be helpful. Such a situation exists in the setting of discogenic pain any manner of disk posterior movement from the annulus, from protrusion, herniation, extrusion to full sequestration. TFESIs have been shown to have more reliably deliver injectate to the anterior epidural space (see Table 50.2 for a complete list of indications).

Evidence for Efficacy

The use of L-TFESIs has been shown to be an effective means to treat nerve root compression. Although arguably one of the commonest performed procedures in pain management, there is little level 1 evidence to support this procedure. While there is substantial debate regarding pro-

Table 50.2 Indications for lumbar transforaminal epidural corticosteroid injections

Diagnosis of radiculitis or radiculopathy to aid in surgical planning
Treatment of discogenic pain (by blocking sinuvertebral nerve)
Treatment of disk bulging, protrusion, herniation, extrusion, or sequestration
Treatment of compression of spinal nerve roots
Treatment of radiculitis (nerve root inflammation causing pain)
Treatment of nerve root infection (e.g., herpes zoster)
Treatment of lumbar spinal stenosis

cedure approach and nature of the injectate, a number of level 2 studies and other reviews exist that support the use of L-TFESI as a viable, nonsurgical option.

In 2009, Buenaventura published a systemic review of the available literature with respect to low back and radicular pain. He found that based on the US Preventive Services Task Force, the evidence was at level II-1 for short-term relief and level II-2 for long-term relief, meaning evidence obtained from well-designed controlled trials without randomization or well-designed cohort or case-control analytic studies, preferably from more than one center or research group. Other grading scales have since been described by the USPSTF.

In 2012, Manchikanti and colleagues published a review of the available literature. Of the 70 studies that were identified, 27 studies met inclusion criteria for methodological quality assessment with 15 randomized trials (with 2 duplicate publications) and 10 non-randomized studies. For both disk herniation and spinal stenosis, the evidence quality was either good or fair. Good meaning the evidence includes consistent results from well-designed, well-conducted studies in representative populations that directly assess effects on health outcomes; fair meaning the evidence is sufficient to determine effects on health outcomes, but the strength of the evidence is limited by the number, quality, or consistency of the individual studies, generalizability to routine practice, or indirect nature of the evidence on health outcomes.

Later, in 2015, Manchikanti and colleagues provided a critical review of published data and previous reviews of the effectiveness of epidural injection with and without corticosteroid for the treatment of lumbar spinal stenosis. This group addressed several studies to include a high-publicized study from 2014 reporting that ESI was inferior to either conservative care or surgical decompression. The author concluded that injection of the epidural space with or without corticosteroid provided significant improvement in pain and function for the treatment of lumbar spinal stenosis. Lastly, the degree of response to lumbar transforaminal epidural steroid injection has been shown to be more impactful and longer lasting with mild to moderate foraminal stenosis as compared to severe foraminal stenosis.

Pearls and Pitfalls

The paresthesia approach or eliciting radicular pain to localize proper needle position may seem simultaneously both intuitive and counterintuitive. There is little doubt of the needle position if the patient reports a radicular pain upon needle insertion; however there is no evidence to support improved accuracy or outcomes using this technique. Notwithstanding that lack of evidence, some physicians continue to use this practice in spite of availability of advanced imaging. With modern fluoroscopic techniques, there may be little need to use direct trauma to insinuate proper needle placement.

Patient selection is another opportunity to ensure positive outcomes. Certainly, attempting transforaminal access in a patient with severe neuroforaminal stenosis would prove frustrating for the physician and painful or even dangerous for the patient. In the presence of severe stenosis, the physician may choose an alternative approach to performing the procedure. Similarly, other structural deformities complicating the approach, to include severe foraminal stenosis, may respond to patient positioning, i.e., lumbar flexion using an abdominal roll or pillow.

Vascular spread of the injectate is a serious concern, especially if the needle is malpositioned in an artery. Some physicians are taught that aspiration prior to injection is a reliable method to detect intravascular spread. On the contrary, this is not a reliable choice as aspiration may create enough of a negative force such to draw the vascular wall against the needle tip, thereby suggesting an extravascular position. Similarly, continuous fluoroscopy (e.g., "live" fluoroscopy) with the use of contrast may provide a beneficial alternative; the advent of DSA is an excellent choice to detect unwarranted needle position. However, even DSA cannot reliably distinguish between venous and arterial uptake.

Procedure

Several approaches for lumbar transforaminal access have been described. For all approaches, written informed consent is obtained, and the patient's lower extremity strength is assessed for post-procedure comparison. The patient is then positioned prone on the fluoroscopy table. Use of a fluoroscope is not only best practice but currently a standard of care, with landmark techniques giving way to this more precise technology. Other patient positions can be utilized, such as the lateral position, but makes fluoroscope movement more difficult, particularly with tilting cephalocaudal directions. The skin overlying the lumbar spine is sterilized, and a sterile field is created. It would be prudent to choose a needle as narrow as physician comfort will allow and of a non-cutting tip variety, such as a "Chiba" needle, to minimize any potential nerve injury upon actual nerve contact.

Chlorohexidine preparation is recommended given its superior antimicrobial activity, as well as sterile gloves and syringes for injection of radiocontrast agent and injectable pharmacotherapy. Emergency carts with resuscitative medications and equipment ought to be readily available, along with a physician or other provider present capable of recognizing and treating complications.

The original and oldest utilized method is the subpedicular "safe triangle" technique. It is the most widely reported in the literature, and still most commonly utilized technique, so much so that it can be considered the standard approach. It will be the technique discussed in detail here. Other techniques have been reported that place the needle tip in various other positions and are termed supraneural, retroneral, and infraneural.

The first step in the subpedicular technique involves squaring off the one or two vertebral end plates cephalad to the targeted neural foramen in the anteroposterior roentogram projection. Imagining the pedicle itself is considered to be a clockface, the target point would immediately caudad to the "6 of clock" position on the pedicle, such that the needle tip position would be cephalad to the nerve itself but hugged underneath the pedicle.

This radiographic position ensures a high probability of success of placing the needle within the "safe triangle." The fluoroscope is then set oblique on the ipsilateral side, to bring the ventral aspect of the superior articular process midway between the anterior and posterior aspects of the vertebral body superior end plate, the "Scotty dog formation" (see Fig. 50.1).

The "safe triangle" is termed as such to refer to the fact that the targeted nerve is unlikely to lie within its bounds. As described by Boduk, the safe triangle is "formed by a transverse line tangential to the lower margin of the pedicle, a sagittal line tangential to the lateral margin of the pedicle, and a hypotenuse passing obliquely inferiorly and laterally from the inferior medial corner of the pedicle, tangential to the curvature of the pedicle at that corner" (see Fig. 50.2).

However, the artery of Adamkiewicz (arteria radicularis magna, ARM) also enters the spinal canal through the neuroforamen, usually in close proximity to the dorsal foot ganglion. This artery can enter the spinal canal anywhere between T7 and L4 but typically entered from T9 to L1 on the left (80% of the time). Within the neural foramen, the ARM is positioned in the cephalad or middle portion, ventral and superolateral to the dorsal root ganglion. Because of this variability, some physicians prefer to advance the needle inferior and lateral to the pedicle.

With this in mind, the injection mechanics start with a skin wheel, made with lidocaine 1% or 2%, with or without epinephrine. The needle is then passed in coaxial fashion to the target point within the safe triangle. Depth of the needle is best assessed in the lateral projection and the needle tip not extending more ventral than approximately the "6 o'clock" position on the pedicle in the lateral projection (see Fig. 50.3).

At this point, the fluoroscopy is positioned in the anteroposterior projection. After negative aspiration for blood or CSF, 0.25–0.5 cc of radiocontrast agent is injected slowly

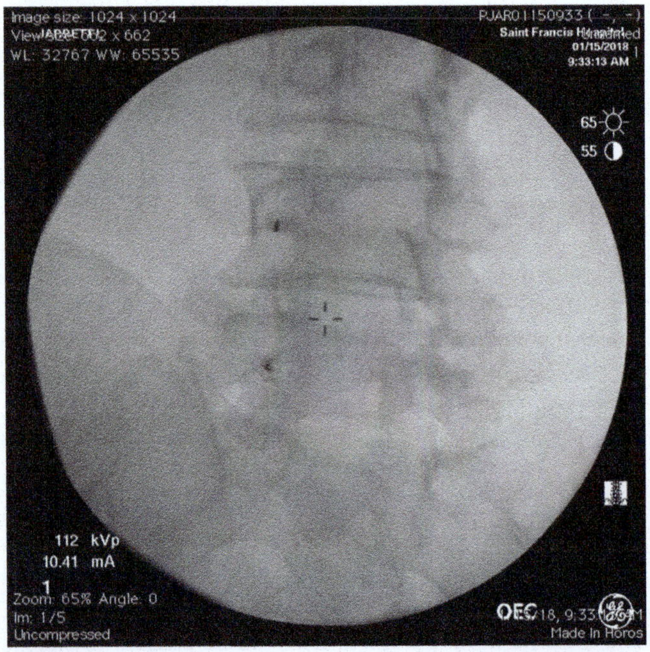

Fig. 50.1 The "Scotty Dog" with needles viewed in the coaxial beam targeting the left L4 and L5 nerve roots in the oblique fluoroscopic projection

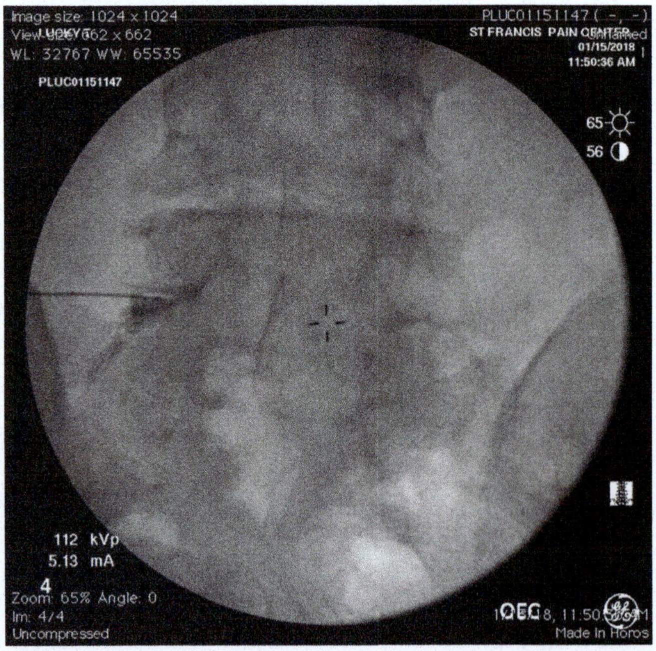

Fig. 50.2 Final position of the needle within the "safe triangle" in the anteroposterior projection

under live anteroposterior fluoroscopy with uptake being observed. Any vascular uptake would require repositioning of the needle. Spread of the radiocontrast agent along the path of the nerve foot and into the epidural space confirms proper positioning (see Fig. 50.4).

While some authors suggest eliciting paresthesia as proof of proper needle position, it certainly is not necessary and could potentially cause unnecessary injury. The injectate is then administered slowly in 0.5 cc aliquots while alerting the patient to articulate any discomfort in the back or legs. If any discomfort is noted, the needle is simply withdrawn slightly and injecting again after negative aspiration.

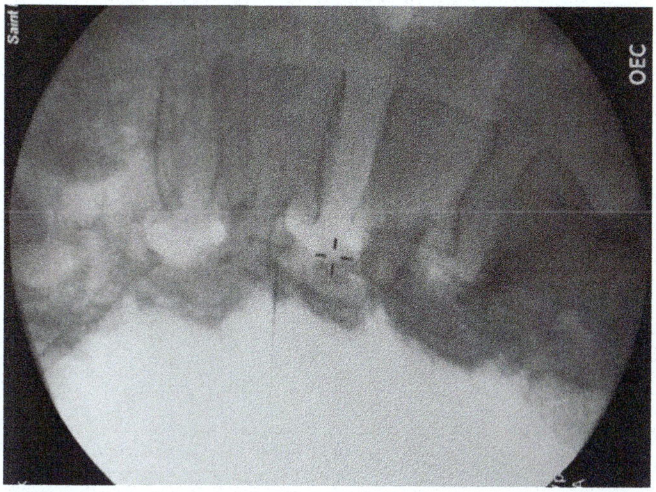

Fig. 50.3 Proper position of the needle tip at "6 o'clock" relative to the pedicle in the lateral projection

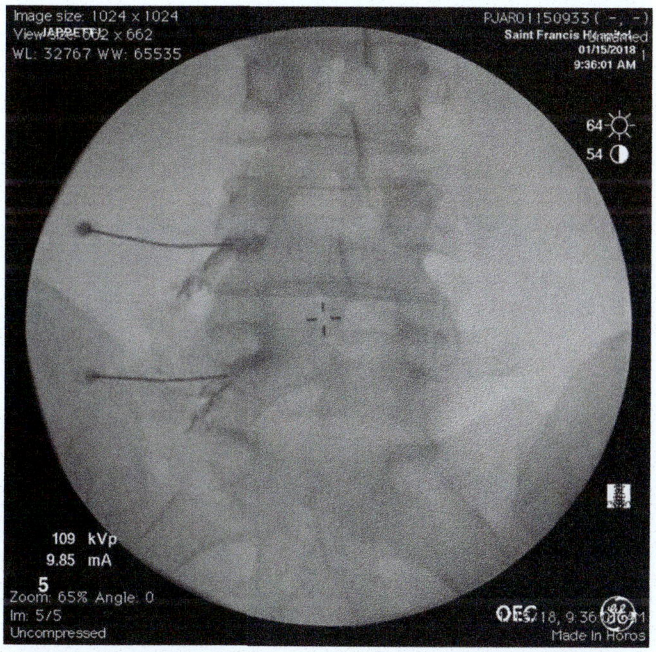

Fig. 50.4 Classic radiocontrast spread along the nerve root into the epidural space in the anteroposterior projection

Another approach is the infraneural approach. This is typically done with a blunt-tipped needle. As described previously, the patient requires the same pre-procedure evaluation. The patient is then placed in a prone position with a pad or pillow underneath the abdomen to create a slight flexion. After the sterile field is created, the lumbar spine is imaged in anterior to posterior view. The lumbar disk level of interest is identified, and a cephalad angle is used to square the superior end plate of the inferior vertebral level. An oblique tilt is achieved to approximately 25–30 degrees to bring the superior articulating process (SAP) of the inferior level into view. The skin overlying this area is anesthetized with local anesthetic solution. Typically, a 14-gauge introducer angiocatheter is advanced to approximate the SAP. The sharp needle is then removed leaving the catheter in place. Typically, a 20–22-gauge blunt nerve block needle is then advanced through the catheter whereby the tip is advanced around the SAP. Lateral view is then used to guide the blunt-tipped needle to the ventral epidural space and in position inferior to the nerve of interest. Nonionic contrast media is then administered in small amounts either using continuous fluoroscopy or DSA. The injectate is then delivered, and then the needle and catheter are removed from the patient together.

In spite of the lack of high-level evidence, there is preponderance of level 2 data in support of the use of L-TFESI for the diagnosis and treatment of radiculitis. There is substantial controversy surrounding the choice of GCC and approach to foraminal entrance, and no one technique or medication has been shown to be superior to another. Successful management of the patient with lumbar radiculitis lies in patient's choice and pre-procedural preparation, knowledge of anatomy, and vigilance on the part of the physician to recognize indications and prevent adverse outcomes through extensive knowledge of potential known complications.

Recommended Reading

1. Acarolglu E, Nordin M, Randhawa K, Chou R, Cote P, Mmopelwa T, Haldeman S. The Global spine care initiative: a summary of the guidelines on invasive interventions for the management of persistent and disabling spinal pain in low - and middle-income communities. Eur Spine J. 2018; epublished https://doi.org/10.1007/s00586-017-5392-0.
2. Bogduk. Practice guidelines for spinal and diagnostic and treatment procedures 2nd Edition. San Francisco: International Spine Intervention Society; 2013. p. 459–557.
3. Buenaventura RM, Datta S, Abdi S, Smith HS. Systematic review of therapeutic lumbar transforaminal epidural steroid injections. Pain Physician. 2009;12(1):233–51.
4. Chang M, Lee D. Outcome of transforaminal epidural steroid injection according to the severity of lumbar foraminal spinal stenosis. Pain Physician. 2018;21:67–72.

5. Feeley I, Healy E, Noel J, Kiely P, Murphy T. Particulate and non-particulate steroids in spinal epidurals: a systematic review and meta-analysis. Eur J Spine. 2017;26:336–44.
6. Fenton D, Czervionke L. Image-guided spine intervention. Philadephia: Saunders; 2013. p. 73–126.
7. Leung S, Chau W, Law S, Fung K. Clinical value of transforaminal epidural steroid injection in lumbar radiculopathy. Hong Kong Med J. 2015;21(5):394–400.
8. Liu J, Zhou H, Lu L, Li X, Jia J, Shi Z, Yao X, Wu Q, Feng S. Effectiveness of transforaminal versus caudal routes for epidural steroid injections in managing lumbosacral radicular pain. A systematic review and meta-analysis. Medicine. 2016;95(18):1–11.
9. Lutz GE, Vad VB, Wisneski RJ. Fluoroscopictransforaminal epidural steroids: an outcome study. Arch Phys Med Rehabil. 1998;79:1362–6.
10. Makkar J, Singh P, Jain D, Goudra B. Particulate versus non-particulate steroids for transforaminal epidural steroid injections: a systematic review and meta-analysis of the current literature. Pain Physician. 2016;19:327–40.
11. Manchikanti L, Hirsch J. Neurological complications associated with epidural steroid injections. Curr Pain Headache Rep. 2015;19:1–10.
12. Manchikanti L, Buenaventura RM, Manchikanti KN, Ruan X, Gupta S, Smith HS, Christo PJ, Ward SP. Effectiveness of therapeutic lumbar transforaminal epidural steroid injections in managing lumbar spinal pain. Pain Physician. 2012;15(3):E199–245.
13. Manchikanti L, Kaye A, Manchikanti K, Boswell M, Pampati V, Hirsch J. Efficacy of epirdural steroid injections in the treatment of lumbar central spinal canal stenosis: a systematic review. Anesth Pain Med. 2015;5(1):1–15.
14. Mehta M, Salmon N. Extradural block: confirmation of the injection site by x-ray monitoring. Anaesthesia. 1985;40:1009–12.
15. White AH, Derby R, Wynne G. Epidural injections for diagnosis and treatment of low back pain. Spine. 1980;5:78–86.

Lumbar Facet and Medial Branch Block

51

Sameer Jain, Jonathan Hagedorn, Jay M. Shah, and Ajax Yang

Introduction

Chronic low back pain (LBP) is among the most prevalent causes of medical disability in the world. About two-thirds of the population suffers from LBP at some point in their life. In the year 2016, LBP was the leading cause of years lived with disability (YLD) in the United States. In the year 2013, low back and neck pain conditions accounted for the third-highest healthcare expenditure with estimated spending of $87.6 billion. This number is expected to rise as the US population ages and hence poses an immense economic burden. Therefore, the importance of appropriately treating LBP cannot be understated. The causes of LBP are complicated and often multifactorial, making their diagnosis and management a challenge for physicians.

The zygapophysial (facet) joint is a common source of LBP. Interventions for facet joint pain are the second most commonly performed pain procedures after epidural steroid injections and represented approximately 37% of all pain interventions in 2006. The facet joints are a pair of true synovial joints formed from the superior articular process of one vertebra and the inferior articular process of the vertebra above. The position of the joint relative to sagittal and coronal planes determines its function. The higher joints in lumbar region are oriented in a sagittal plane and provide resistance to axial rotation. The lower facet joints being more coronally oriented offer protection from flexion and shearing forces. The degeneration of these joints over time is a common source of facet pain.

The medial branch is the terminal division of the posterior ramus, which provides sensory innervation to the facet joint. Each facet joint is innervated by the medial branch chronic low back pain (LBP): of the same level and at the level above (e.g., L3 to L4 facet joint is innervated by L2 and L3 medial branches). The medial branch is usually chronic low back pain (LBP): located at the junction of the transverse process below and the superior articular process.

Background and Historical Perspective

Prevalence of facetogenic LBP ranges considerably based on age. In individuals aged 31–40 years, the prevalence is estimated between 15 and 20%, but in the 51–60-year-old group, it is nearly 45%. The diagnosis of lumbar facet pain can be difficult due to its vague presentation and clinical course. Patients will usually complain of chronic LBP with or without radiation into the groin or thighs. The pain is often described as off-center and is worsened with extension, lateral bending, rotation, or walking uphill. Pain is typically worse in the mornings and associated with stiffness. Even with imaging, a thorough history, and clinical examination, a diagnostic block may be the only consistent method to determine the diagnosis of lumbar facet joint syndrome.

Goldthwait first described lumbar facet joints as a source of back pain in 1911. In 1933, Ghormley coined the term "facet syndrome" describing it as a LBP with or without radiation, worsened by twisting or rotatory strain to the lumbosacral spine. Eight years later, in 1941, it was reported that facet joints may be a primary source of back pain, separate from nerve compression. But, it wasn't until 1963 that researchers injected hypertonic saline into facet joints and reproduced LBP. This provided the basis for early researchers to use fluoroscopic guidance to inject facet joints with steroids and local anesthetics for pain control.

S. Jain (✉)
Department of Pain Medicine, Pain Treatment Centers of America, Little Rock, AR, USA

J. Hagedorn
Department of Pain Medicine, Mayo Clinic, Rochester, MN, USA
e-mail: hagedorn.jonathan@mayo.edu

J. M. Shah
Department of Pain Medicine, Weill-Cornell Tri-Institutional Pain Program, New York, NY, USA

A. Yang
Department of Rehabilitation Medicine, Icahn School of Medicine at Mount Sinai, New York, NY, USA

T. R. Deer et al. (eds.), *Deer's Treatment of Pain*, https://doi.org/10.1007/978-3-030-12281-2_51

Uses and Indications

Facet syndrome is a difficult diagnosis to make because of the multifactorial nature of LBP. Multiple conditions including nerve entrapment syndrome, discogenic pain, spinal stenosis, and osseous abnormalities can cause axial LBP and mimic facetogenic pain. Imaging studies may be suggestive of facet syndrome, but they are not conclusive. In patients with facet joint syndrome, distension of the facet joint with saline or contrast will reproduce the pain, while injection of local anesthetic into the facet joint will relieve it. Provocation of pain is not reliable and may cause unnecessary discomfort to the patient. Relief of pain with injection of local anesthetic is the gold standard for diagnosis of facet joint syndrome. Blockade of the medial branch nerves supplying the corresponding facet joint can also be used to diagnose facet joint syndrome.

Intra-articular (IA) facet joint injections were traditionally used as a therapeutic modality for treatment of facet joint pain. However, recent studies have demonstrated that IA facet joint injections are therapeutically inferior to radiofrequency ablation (RFA) of the medial branch nerves for the treatment of facet syndrome and should mainly be used for diagnostic purposes.

Indications for facet and medial branch blocks may be as follows:

- The primary indication for lumbar facet and medial branch blocks is to confirm the diagnosis of facet syndrome. Patient with lumbar facet syndrome will characteristically have axial LBP, which is typically worse in the morning, may radiate across the low back, and may or may not be accompanied with focal tenderness over the facet joint. A greater than 50–80% improvement in pain with these blocks can be considered diagnostic for facet syndrome.
- Most elderly patients with LBP have multilevel facet disease on imaging and diffuse back pain when examined clinically. Facet and medial branch blocks are indicated to diagnose the exact source of the patient's pain for presurgical evaluation.
- Alternatively, the patient may have normal radiographic findings. Facet and medial branch blocks can be used in this instance to uncover the etiology of the LBP.
- Temporary pain relief with facet and medial branch blocks may provide a prognostic value to predict a positive outcome with RFA.

Technique

Lumbar Intra-articular Facet Injection

Prior to starting the procedure, the physician should review any existing imaging in order to properly ascertain the anatomy of the affected portions of the lumbar spine. The patient is positioned prone on the fluoroscopy table with the head turned to one side. After the affected facet joint is visualized with the C-arm, it is angled obliquely 25–30 ° from the sagittal plane allowing direct visualization of the facet joint.

The skin and subcutaneous tissues overlying the targeted facet joint are anesthetized using 1–2 ml of 1% lidocaine. A 22-gauge, 3.5 inch spinal needle is used to carry out the block. The needle is placed through the skin, advancing it toward the joint space keeping it coaxial with the axis of the X-ray path. The needle is advanced until it is seated within the joint space. The position of the needle within the joint space can be confirmed by injecting 0.1–0.2 ml of contrast (Fig. 51.1). Once the needle tip is confirmed to be intra-articular, 0.5 ml of local anesthetic is injected into the joint space (in diagnostic blocks). If a therapeutic block is performed, then a combination of steroid and local anesthetic may be used.

Lumbar Medial Branch Block

Medial branch nerves supplying the facet joint are located in the groove between the transverse process and the superior articular process. The patient is positioned prone on the fluoroscopy table with the head turned to one side. After the affected facet joint is visualized with the C-arm, it is angled obliquely 25–30 ° from the sagittal plane allowing direct visualization of the facet joint as well as the junction between the transverse process and the superior articular process.

The skin and subcutaneous tissues overlying the targeted facet joint are anesthetized using 1–2 ml of 1% lidocaine. A 25-gauge, 3.5 inch spinal needle is used to carry out the block. The needle is placed through the skin, advancing it toward the junction of the transverse process and superior articular process keeping it coaxial with the axis of the X-ray path. The needle is advanced until it reaches the target (Fig. 51.2). Once the needle tip is at the target, 0.5 ml of local anesthetic is injected and the needle is removed.

The patient is instructed to assess the pain relief obtained after the diagnostic block over the next few hours. A block is considered to be diagnostic for facetogenic pain if the patient achieves over 50–80% pain relief.

Evidence for Efficacy

There have been a number of randomized, non-randomized, and observational studies published over the course of time evaluating the efficacy of intra-articular (IA) lumbar facet joint injections and lumbar medial branch blocks both as a therapeutic and diagnostic modality for the treatment of facetogenic LBP. Most studies recognized the use of these blocks for diagnostic purposes; however, the opinion about their use as a therapeutic option for facetogenic LBP was

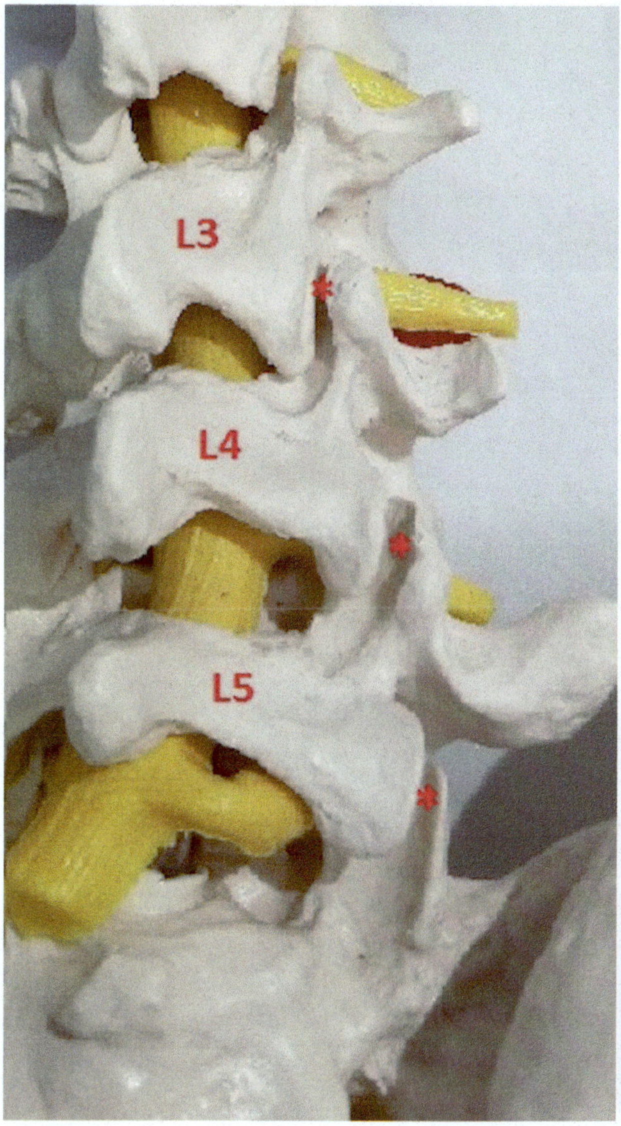

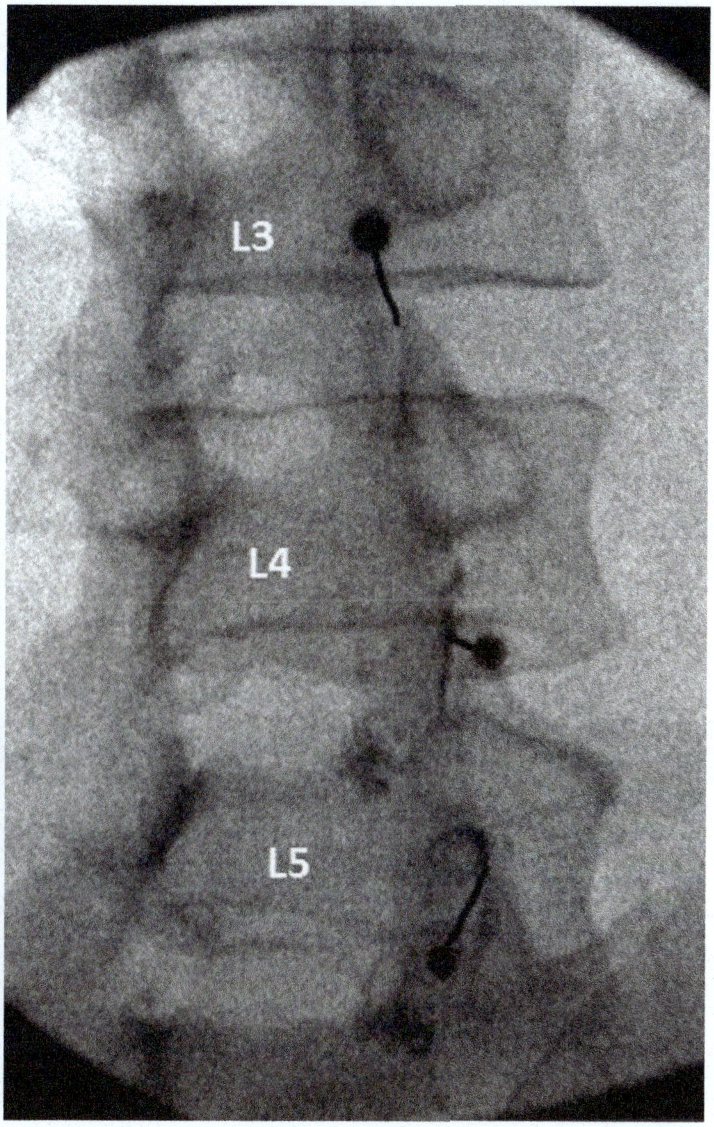

Fig. 51.1 *Left*: Spine model illustrating the needle target marked with an asterisk (*). *Right*: Oblique fluoroscopic image obtained during right L3–L4, L4–L5, and L5–S1 intra-articular facet joint injection. Final needle tip position prior to contrast injection can be visualized at the L3–L4 facet joint. The L4–L5 facet joint depicts the image obtained after the intra-articular injection of contrast

mixed. A review of randomized clinical trials regarding the efficacy of lumbar intra-articular and medial branch blocks can be found in Table 51.1.

Marks et al. published the results of a randomized trial comparing the efficacy of IA facet joint injections and medial branch blocks. Eighty-six patients with chronic refractory LBP were randomly assigned to receive either IA facet injection or medial branch block, using local anesthetic and steroid. There was no significant difference in the immediate response. The duration of response after facet joint injection was found to be marginally longer than after medial branch block ($p < 0.05$, 1 month after infiltration), but for both groups, the response was usually short-lived; by 3 months only two patients continued to report complete pain relief. Authors of the study concluded that facet joint injections and medial branch blocks may be of equal value as diagnostic tests, but neither is a satisfactory treatment for chronic LBP.

Carette et al. conducted a randomized, placebo-controlled trial to evaluate the therapeutic efficacy of injecting methylprednisolone acetate into the facet joints in chronic LBP patients. Patients with chronic LBP who reported immediate relief of their pain after injections of local anesthetic into the facet joints were randomly assigned to receive under fluoroscopic guidance injections of either methylprednisolone acetate (20 mg; $n = 49$) or isotonic saline ($n = 48$) in the same facet joints. After 1 month, none of the outcome measures evaluating pain, functional status, and back flexion differed clinically or statistically between the two study groups. No statistical difference was found again at the 3-month evaluation. Eleven patients (22%) in the methylprednisolone group

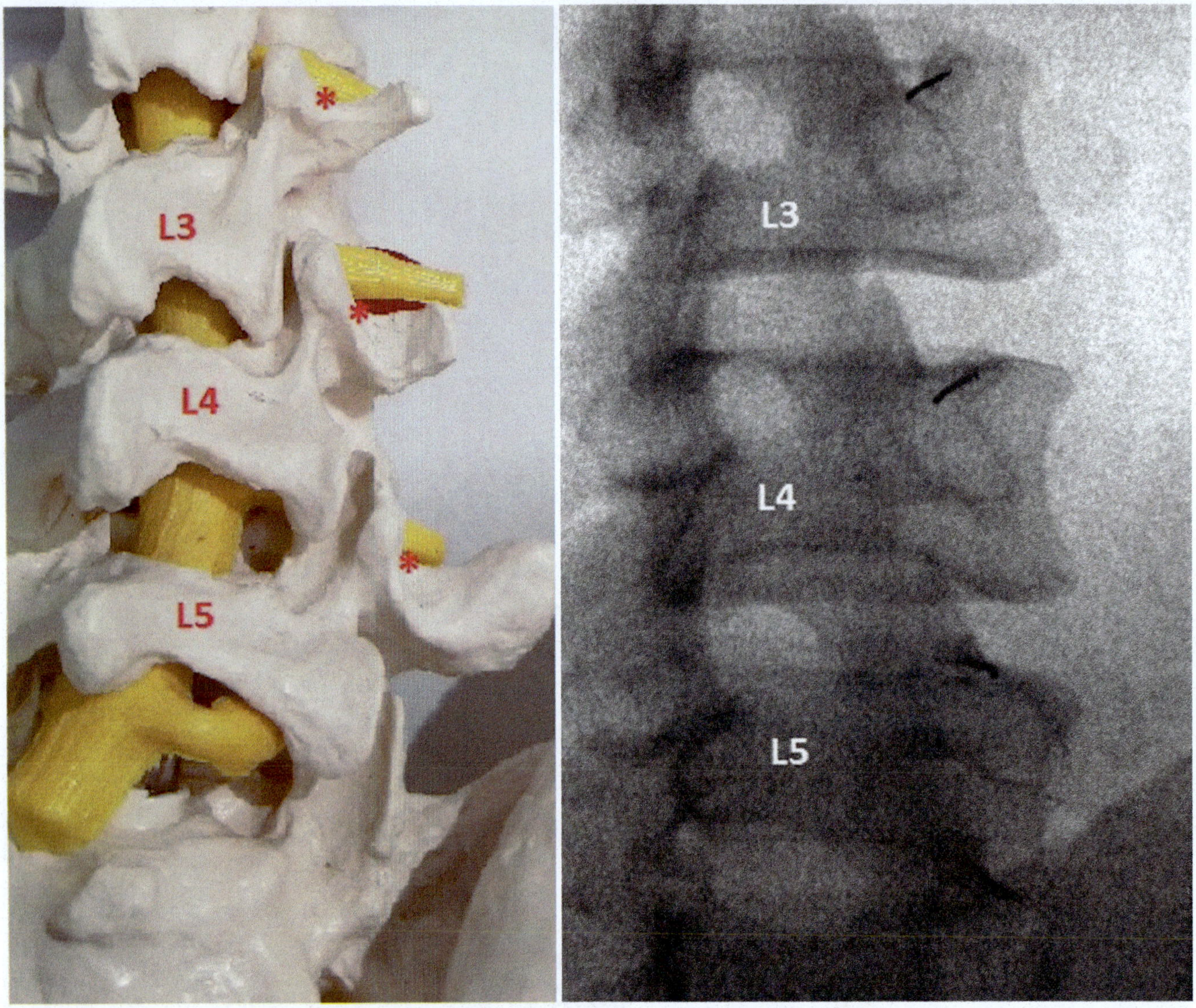

Fig. 51.2 *Left*: Spine model illustrating the needle target marked with an asterisk (*). *Right*: Oblique fluoroscopic image obtained during right L3–L4, L4–L5, and L5–S1 medial branch block. Final needle tip position lies at the junction of the superior articular process and the transverse process

and five patients (10%) in the placebo group had sustained improvement at 6-month evaluation ($p = 0.19$). Carette et al. concluded that injection of methylprednisolone into the facet joints has little therapeutic value in chronic LBP patients.

Fuchs et al. conducted a randomized, controlled, blind-observer clinical study of 60 patients to investigate the efficacy and safety of IA lumbar facet sodium hyaluronate (SH) injection compared with IA lumbar facet glucocorticosteroids (triamcinolone acetonide, TA) in the treatment of chronic non-radicular lumbar pain. The patients were randomly assigned to two groups to receive 10 mg SH or 10 mg TA IA per facet joint. After baseline evaluation, patients in each group received one IA injection each week for the first 3 weeks in a different lumbar facet joint. Patients reported lasting pain relief, better function, and improved quality of life with both treatments, at 3- and 6-month evaluation. Authors of the study concluded that IA lumbar facet SH and steroid injections are effective in the treatment of non-radicular chronic LBP.

Manchikanti et al. published the results of a double-blind, randomized, and controlled trial to evaluate the therapeutic efficacy of lumbar medial branch blocks (with or without steroids) in patients with a confirmed diagnosis of lumbar facet joint pain. The study included 120 patients randomized in 1:1 ratio to receive medial branch block with local anesthetic only (group I) or with local anesthetic and steroid (group II). Both groups were also divided into two categories, each with the addition of sarapin. The inclusion criterion was based upon a positive response to diagnostic controlled, comparative local anesthetic lumbar facet joint block. The patients

Table 51.1 Outcomes of randomized trials evaluating efficacy of lumbar IA facet blocks and MBBB

Study	Study design	Number of patients (N) and selection criteria	Control	Interventions	Follow-up period	Outcome measures	Results	Conclusion
Marks et al. (1991)	Randomized trial	$N = 86$; chronic LBP >6 months refractory to conservative management	–	IA facet injection ($n = 42$) vs MBBB ($n = 44$)	1 and 3 months	Pain relief	Both procedures provided good pain relief at 1 month f/u; only 2 patients had continued relief at 3 months	IA facet injection and MBBB are good diagnostic tools, however no therapeutic efficacy
Carette et al. (1991)	Randomized, double-blind, controlled trial	$N = 97$; patients with chronic LBP reporting immediate pain relief after injection of LA into the facet joint	IA facet injection of isotonic saline	IA facet injection of sodium chloride or methylprednisolone	1, 3, and 6 months	VAS, MPQ, MSIP	11 (22%) patients in methylprednisolone group and 5 (10%) in saline group had sustained improvement at 6 months; $p = 0.19$	IA facet steroid injections have no therapeutic value
Fuchs et al. (2005)	Randomized, double-blind, active-control trial	$N = 60$; patients with chronic LBP were included	Active-control study with no control group	IA facet injection of HA vs glucocorticosteroid injection	3 and 6 months	VAS, RMQ, ODI, short form-36	Patients reported lasting pain relief, better function, and improved quality of life with both treatments	IA facet HA and glucocorticosteroid injections have good therapeutic efficacy
Manchikanti et al. (2010)	Randomized, double-blind, active-control trial	$N = 120$; patients with chronic facetogenic LBP with positive response to diagnostic MBBB	MBBB with LA only	MBBB with LA alone ($n = 60$) or LA and steroids ($n = 60$). Both groups were also divided into two categories each with the addition of sarapin	3, 6,12, 18, and 24 months	NRS, ODI, employment status, opioid intake	Significant pain relief was shown in 85% in LA group and 90% in LA with steroids group at the end of the 2-year study period in both groups, with an average of 5–6 total treatments	Effectiveness demonstrated with MBBB with LA with or without steroids
Ribeiro et al. (2013)	Randomized, double-blind, active control	$N = 60$; patients with a diagnosis of facet joint syndrome	Triamcinolone acetonide Intramuscular injection of six lumbar paravertebral points	IA injection of six lumbar facet joints with triamcinolone hexacetonide	1, 4,12, and 24 weeks	Pain VAS, pain VAS during extension of the spine, Likert scale, IPS, RMQ, 36-Item Short-Form Health Survey	Pain VAS and VAS with spine extension improved in both groups over time ($p < 0.001$) with no difference between the groups, RMQ showed superiority of IA facet injection over systemic steroids at week 12 ($p = 0.01$), and Likert scale showed superiority of IA facet joint injections over systemic steroids at week 1 ($p = 0.03$)	Both treatments are effective in the treatment of facet joint pain with slight superiority of IA facet injections over systemic steroids

(continued)

Table 51.1 (continued)

Study	Study design	Number of patients (N) and selection criteria	Control	Interventions	Follow-up period	Outcome measures	Results	Conclusion
Civelek et al. (2012)	Randomized, active-control trial	$N = 100$; patients with chronic LBP with failed conservative therapy	MBBB with LA and steroid	Conventional RFA at 80 °C for 120 seconds	1, 6, and 12 months	VNS, NASS patient satisfaction questionnaire, EQ-5D	MBBB in early post-op but RFA at 3,6, and 12 months showed better results on VNS ($p < 0.001$); NASS questionnaire results were significant only at 12 months between the two groups ($p = 0.04$), no difference in EQ-5D at any time	First choice for treatment of chronic facetogenic LBP should be MBBB; however, if the relief is short-lasting, then RFA should be used
Lakemeier et al. (2013)	Randomized, double-blind, active-control trial	$N = 56$; facetogenic LBP diagnosed with a single LA block	IA facet injection of LA and steroid	Conventional RFA at 80 °C for 90 seconds	6 months	RMQ, VAS, ODI, analgesic intake	No significant difference between control ($n = 29$) vs RFA group ($n = 27$) was observed in any of the end points at 6-month follow-up	Both IA facet joint injections and RFA are viable therapeutic options for facetogenic LBP
Cohen et al. (2018)	Randomized, controlled clinical trial	$N = 229$; axial LBP for 3 months or more, average score more than 3 out of 10 over the past week on NRS, failure to respond to more conservative therapy	MBBB with saline	Conventional RFA at 90 °C for 135 seconds after a negative outcome with IA facet steroid +bupivacaine, MBBB with steroid and bupivacaine and control	1, 3, and 6 months	NRS pain scores 1 month after the facet or saline blocks and 3 months after RFA	At 3 months, the proportion of positive responders that underwent RFA in the IA, medial branch block, and placebo groups were 51%, 56%, and 24%, respectively ($p = 0.005$)	IA facet injections or MBBB have no therapeutic efficacy but may have prognostic value to predict a positive outcome with RFA

LBP low back pain, *IA* intra-articular, *HA* hyaluronic acid, *LA* local anesthetic, *NRS* numeric rating scale, *MBBB* medial branch block, *VAS* visual analogue scale, *MPQ* Mcgill pain questionnaire, *MSIP* mean sickness impact profile, *RMQ* Roland-Morris questionnaire, *ODI* Oswestry Disability Index, *IPS* improvement percentage scale, *RFA* radiofrequency ablation, *VNS* visual numeric pain scale, *NASS* North American Spine Society, *EQ-5D* Euro-QOL in five dimensions were followed at 3, 6, 12, 18, and 24 months. Eighty-five percent of patients in group I and 90% of patients in group II showed significant improvement with significant pain relief of ≥50% and functional improvement of ≥40% at 2-year follow-up. Authors of the study concluded that therapeutic medial branch blocks, with or without steroids, may be a treatment option for patients with chronic facetogenic LBP. No significant difference was found in each group with addition of sarapin.

Ribeiro et al. first compared the effectiveness of facet joint injection over systemic steroids in patients with the diagnosis of facet joint syndrome in a randomized clinical trial. Sixty patients were randomized in the control group ($n = 29$) and experimental group ($n = 31$). The experimental group was administered intra-articular injection at six lumbar facet joints with triamcinolone hexacetonide; the control group was administered triamcinolone acetonide via intramuscular injection at six lumbar paravertebral points.

Follow-up was at 1, 4, 12, and 24 weeks after interventions. Outcome measures used were pain visual analogue scale (VAS), pain visual analogue scale during extension of the spine, Likert scale, improvement percentage scale, Roland-Morris questionnaire (RMQ), 36-Item Short-Form Health Survey, and accountability of medications taken. Regarding the evolution of pain, assessed by VAS for spontaneous pain and pain on extension, significant reductions occurred in both groups over time ($p < 0.001$), with no differences between the groups. In the analysis at each time point, RMQ showed superiority of facet injection over systemic steroids at week 12 ($p = 0.01$). The response to treatment assessed by Likert scale showed superiority of facet joint injections at week 1 ($p = 0.03$); however, no significant difference was seen at subsequent visits. Authors concluded both treatments are effective in the treatment of facet joint pain with slight superiority of IA facet injections over systemic steroids.

Civelek et al. published the results of a study comparing effectiveness of the medial branch block of the posterior primary ramus and RFA in chronic LBP patients. One hundred patients were randomized in 1:1 ratio in two groups. The first group received a medial branch block of the posterior primary ramus with 1 cc of methylprednisolone acetate (40 mg) combined with 2 cc bupivacaine hydrochloride. The second group of 50 patients was treated with radiofrequency denervation at 80 °C for 120 seconds. The patient follow-up interviews were conducted by telephone at 3, 6, and 12 months. The visual numeric pain scale (VNS), North American Spine Society (NASS) patient satisfaction questionnaire, and EQ-5D (Euro-Qol in five dimensions) were used as outcome measures. Medial branch block in early post-op but RFA at 3, 6, and 12 months showed better results on VNS ($p < 0.001$). On analysis of NASS questionnaire results, significant difference was only found in the 12th month between the two groups ($p = 0.04$). EQ-5D analysis showed no significant difference between either groups at any time. Authors of the study concluded that the first choice for treatment of chronic facetogenic LBP should be medial branch blocks; however, if the relief is short-lasting, then RFA should be used.

Lakemeier et al. conducted a randomized, controlled, double-blind trial comparing the therapeutic efficacy of lumbar facet IA injections and RFA. Fifty-six patients were randomized into an IA facet injection group ($n = 29$) and RFA group ($n = 27$). Twenty-four of 29 patients in the IA group and 26 of 27 patients in the RFA group completed the 6-month follow-up period. The inclusion criteria were based first on magnetic resonance imaging findings showing hypertrophy of the facet joints L3/L4–L5/S1 and a positive response to an IA test infiltration of the facet joints L3/L4–L5/S1 with local anesthetics. The primary end point was the RMQ, while the secondary end points were the VAS and ODS. Patients experienced improvement in all primary and secondary end point in both groups. On analysis of the results, no significant difference between both groups was observed in any of the end points at 6-month follow-up. Authors concluded that both IA facet joint injections and RFA are viable therapeutic options for facetogenic LBP.

Cohen et al. recently published results of the Facet Treatment Study (FACTS), a randomized, controlled clinical trial, to evaluate the effectiveness of lumbar facet joint blocks and their predictive value before RFA. Inclusion criteria were patients with predominantly axial low back pain for 3 months or more, average back pain score more than three out of ten over the past week on a numerical rating scale (NRS), failure to respond to more conservative therapy (e.g., physical therapy, integrative therapy, and pharmacotherapy), and paraspinal tenderness. A total of 229 participants were randomized in a 2:2:1 ratio into three groups to receive IA facet injections with bupivacaine and steroid, medial branch blocks with bupivacaine and steroid, or saline. Patients were followed up at 1, 3, and 6 months. Coprimary outcome measures were average NRS pain scores 1 month after the facet or saline blocks and 3 months after ablation. Patients with a positive 1-month outcome (≥2 point reduction on NRS) and score >3 on a 5-point satisfaction scale were followed up to 6 months. Patients in the IA and medial branch block groups with a positive diagnostic block (50% or more relief) who experienced a negative outcome proceeded to the second phase and underwent RFA, while all patients in the saline group underwent ablation. Mean reduction in average NRS pain score at 1 month was 0.7 ± 1.6 in the IA group, 0.7 ± 1.8 in the medial branch block group, and 0.7 ± 1.5 in the placebo group; $p = 0.993$. RFA was performed on 135 patients (45, 48, and 42 patients from the IA, medial branch, and saline groups, respectively). The average NRS pain score at 3 months was 3.0 ± 2.0 in the IA, 3.2 ± 2.5 in the medial branch, and 3.5 ± 1.9 in the control group ($p = 0.493$). At

3 months, the proportion of positive responders in the IA, medial branch block, and placebo groups were 51%, 56%, and 24%, respectively ($p = 0.005$). Authors of the study concluded that even though facet blocks, i.e., IA facet joint injections and medial branch blocks, are not therapeutic, they may provide a prognostic value to predict a positive outcome with RFA.

Pearls and Pitfalls

Both lumbar facet and medial branch blocks are important tools for the diagnosis and treatment of facetogenic pain. However, even in the hands of an experienced interventional pain specialist, there are chances of having a false-positive or false-negative diagnostic block. The rates of false-positive blocks have been reported by many studies to be as high as 25% to 45%, and the rates of false-negative blocks can range from 6% to 30%. Here are some considerations to be taken into account while performing these blocks to minimize inaccuracy:

- *Proper patient selection*: Patient selection is of paramount importance in the success of any interventional pain procedure. It is important to take into consideration the psychosocial pathology of the patient and secondary gains, before the patient is subjected to either of these blocks.
- *Careful review of patient's imaging*: A thorough and careful review of the patient's low back imaging is needed prior to the procedure to determine the desired target level of the block. This is also helpful in determining any ambiguity in the patient's anatomy that may be encountered during the procedure.
- *Limiting the volume of local anesthetic injected to <0.5 ml*: The posterior ramus of the nerve root also gives off lateral and intermediate branches along with the medial branch. The lateral branch provides innervation to the paraspinous muscles and sacroiliac joint, while the intermediate branch innervates the longissimus muscle. Hence with large injectate volumes, the intermediate and lateral branches are likely to be anesthetized, blocking sensation from the paraspinous musculature, sacroiliac joint, and the longissimus muscle. This may result in a false-positive diagnostic block if the source of pain is any of these anatomic structures.

A false-positive facet block can also occur if large volume is injected intra-articularly, as it can result in rupture of the joint capsule and the inadvertent spread of the local anesthetic into the intervertebral foramina or epidural space.

- *Avoiding or minimizing the use of sedation during or prior to the procedure*: Use of sedation, such as benzodiazepines, prior to or during the procedure can result in muscle relaxation and contribute to the analgesia experienced by the patient. By decreasing the myofascial pain that the patient may be experiencing, this can result in higher false-positive block rates.
- *Use of live fluoroscopy while injecting contrast in an intra-articular facet joint injection*: One of the principal causes of a false-negative facet block is considered to be vascular uptake of the injectate. Injection of the contrast under live fluoroscopic guidance can assist in identifying any potential intravascular contrast uptake.
- *Targeting a lower point on the transverse process for medial branch blocks*: Dreifuss et al. conducted a cadaveric study comparing the contrast spread in human subjects with various needle tip positions. It was found that there is a higher chance of epidural and foraminal spread when the needle tip is located high at the superomedial border of the transverse process. It is recommended to target a lower point midway between the upper border of transverse process and mamilloaccessory ligament to avoid a false-positive block.
- *Limiting the use of superficial skin anesthetic*: Excessive use of local anesthetic for skin anesthesia prior to the needle entry (especially in lean patients) can result in the inadvertent spread of the local anesthetic to the neural structures and the musculature of the back resulting in a false-positive block. A single needle technique for medial branch blocks has been described and used by some physicians to minimize the use of skin anesthesia; however, this is not an ideal technique to be used during radiofrequency ablation of the medial branches.
- *Patient education*: Properly educating patients about documentation of pain scores following the procedure is extremely important in analyzing the success of the procedure. A successful block is considered when the patient experiences a 50–80% decrease in pain following the procedure.

Recommended Reading

1. Bogduk N, Wilson AS, Tynan W. The human lumbar dorsal rami. J Anat. 1982;134(Pt 2):383–97.
2. Carette S, Marcoux S, Truchon R, Grondin C, Gagnon J, Allard Y, et al. A controlled trial of corticosteroid injections into facet joints for chronic low back pain. N Engl J Med. 1991;325(14):1002–7.
3. Cavanaugh JM, Ozaktay AC, Yamashita HT, King AI. Lumbar facet pain: biomechanics, neuroanatomy and neurophysiology. J Biomech. 1996;29(9):1117–29.
4. Civelek E, Cansever T, Kabatas S, Kircelli A, Yilmaz C, Musluman M, et al. Comparison of effectiveness of facet joint injection and radiofrequency denervation in chronic low back pain. Turk Neurosurg. 2012;22(2):200–6.
5. Cohen SP, Raja SN. Pathogenesis, diagnosis, and treatment of lumbar zygapophysial (facet) joint pain. Anesthesiology. 2007;106(3):591–614.

6. Cohen SP, Doshi TL, Constantinescu OC, Zhao Z, Kurihara C, Larkin TM, et al. Effectiveness of lumbar facet joint blocks and predictive value before radiofrequency denervation: The Facet Treatment Study (FACTS), a randomized, controlled clinical trial. Anesthesiology. 2018;129(3):517–35.
7. Dreyfuss P, Schwarzer AC, Lau P, Bogduk N. Specificity of lumbar medial branch and L5 dorsal ramus blocks. A computed tomography study. Spine (Phila Pa 1976). 1997;22(8):895–902.
8. Fuchs S, Erbe T, Fischer HL, Tibesku CO. Intraarticular hyaluronic acid versus glucocorticoid injections for nonradicular pain in the lumbar spine. J Vasc Interv Radiol. 2005;16(11):1493–8.
9. Lakemeier S, Lind M, Schultz W, Fuchs-Winkelmann S, Timmesfeld N, Foelsch C, et al. A comparison of intraarticular lumbar facet joint steroid injections and lumbar facet joint radiofrequency denervation in the treatment of low back pain: a randomized, controlled, double-blind trial. Anesth Analg. 2013;117(1):228–35.
10. Lau P, Mercer S, Govind J, Bogduk N. The surgical anatomy of lumbar medial branch neurotomy (facet denervation). Pain Med. 2004;5(3):289–98.
11. Lewin T, Moffett B, Vidik A. The morphology of the lumbar synovial intervertebral joints. Acta Morphol Neerl Scand. 1962;4:299–319.
12. Manchikanti L, Singh V, Pampati V, Smith HS, Hirsch JA. Analysis of growth of interventional techniques in managing chronic pain in the medicare population: a 10-year evaluation from 1997 to 2006. Pain Physician. 2009;12(1):9–34.
13. Manchikanti L, Singh V, Falco FJ, Cash KA, Pampati V. Evaluation of lumbar facet joint nerve blocks in managing chronic low back pain: a randomized, double-blind, controlled trial with a 2-year follow-up. Int J Med Sci. 2010;7(3):124–35.
14. Marks RC, Houston T, Thulbourne T. Facet joint injection and facet nerve block: a randomised comparison in 86 patients with chronic low back pain. Pain. 1992;49(3):325–8.
15. Revel ME, Listrat VM, Chevalier XJ, Dougados M, N'Guyen MP, Vallee C, et al. Facet joint block for low back pain: identifying predictors of a good response. Arch Phys Med Rehabil. 1992;73(9):824–8.
16. Ribeiro LH, Furtado RN, Konai MS, Andreo AB, Rosenfeld A, Natour J. Effect of facet joint injection versus systemic steroids in low back pain: a randomized controlled trial. Spine (Phila Pa 1976). 2013;38(23):1995–2002.
17. Stojanovic MP, Zhou Y, Hord ED, Vallejo R, Cohen SP. Single needle approach for multiple medial branch blocks: a new technique. Clin J Pain. 2003;19(2):134–7.
18. van Kleef M, Barendse GA, Kessels A, Voets HM, Weber WE, de Lange S. Randomized trial of radiofrequency lumbar facet denervation for chronic low back pain. Spine (Phila Pa 1976). 1999;24(18):1937–42.
19. Walker BF. The prevalence of low back pain: a systematic review of the literature from 1966 to 1998. J Spinal Disord. 2000;13(3):205–17.

52 Sacroiliac Joint Injection

Ioannis M. Skaribas, Bryan K. Lai, Eric V. Ngo, and Elena E. Skaribas

Introduction

The sacroiliac joint (SIJ) is a diarthrodial synovial joint located adjacent to the lumbosacral anatomical structures. Pain from the sacroiliac joint has been considered a common cause of low back pain, which affects 15–30% of individuals. Sacroiliac joint pain without any identifiable joint pathology has been termed sacroiliac joint dysfunction syndrome. The diagnosis of sacroiliac joint dysfunction syndrome can be challenging to evaluate. There is no pathognomonic physical examination or imaging feature that can reliably establish the SIJ as the source of chronic pain. Physical examination with provocative maneuvering of the SIJ inevitably stresses the axial structures of the lumbar spine as well as the hip joint. In the detection of early sacroiliitis, MRI appears to be a useful diagnostic test. Perhaps the most useful diagnostic and definitive evaluation is image-guided sacroiliac joint injections. Although many therapies are available, there is currently no primary treatment option.

Background and Historical Perspective

The sacroiliac joint and its contribution to chronic pain symptomatology have been surrounded with controversy for many years. Some consider the sacroiliac joint to be one of the major causes of low back pain found in adults, while others have debated against this notion. Some of the main factors that feed this debate are the sacroiliac joint's location adjacent to other anatomical structures that cause similar symptoms and also the lack of a specific pathognomonic clinical sign or diagnostic technique. Common causes of sacroiliac joint pain are sacroiliac ligament and joint strain. Osteoarthritis is one of the major causes of sacroiliac joint pain followed by rheumatoid arthritis and traumatic arthritis. Less common causes include ankylosing spondylitis and infectious diseases such as gonorrhea or Lyme's disease. Gout, malignancy, and fractures can also be considered causes. Pain from the sacroiliac joint can present as low back pain or localized sacroiliac pain with radiation to the buttock area or posterior thigh. Typically, the pain is unilateral and produced upon exertion, which is partially relieved with heat, rest, and massage. A thorough history and physical examination should be taken to rule out other possible causes of joint pain. The reported prevalence rates of sacroiliac joint pain vary but have been described as the cause in 15–30% of patients with low back pain.

Anatomy

Bernhard Siegfried Albinus (1697–1770) and William Hunter (1718–1783) first described the sacroiliac joints and its true synovial nature. These observations were confirmed by Meckel in 1816. The specific structure of the joint has been debated through the centuries, and the opinions differ. Von Luschka (1864) was the first to offer the opinion that the sacroiliac joint is a true diarthrodial joint, an opinion that is still widely supported. Braus (1921) and Gray's Anatomy (1944) described the joint as an amphiarthrosis. Testut-Latarjet (1949) described the sacroiliac joint as a diarthro-amphiarthrodial joint. The pelvis is comprised of the two iliac bones, with the sacrum in between. The sacroiliac joints are the areas where iliac bones join on either side to the sacrum and are designed to dissipate the load of the upper body structures to the lower extremities (Fig. 52.1). The sacroiliac joint's stability is maintained through a plexus of strong intrinsic and extrinsic ligaments. The sacroiliac ligament complex immobilizes the sacrum between the two ilia,

I. M. Skaribas (✉) · B. K. Lai · E. V. Ngo
Expert Pain P.A., Department of Anesthesiology, McGovern Medical School, The University of Texas Health Science Center at Houston, Houston, TX, USA
e-mail: skaribasmd@expertpaincare.com; Bryan.K.Lai@uth.tmc.edu; Eric.V.Ngo@uth.tmc.edu

E. E. Skaribas
Southern Methodist University, Dallas, TX, USA
e-mail: eskaribas@smu.edu

T. R. Deer et al. (eds.), *Deer's Treatment of Pain*, https://doi.org/10.1007/978-3-030-12281-2_52

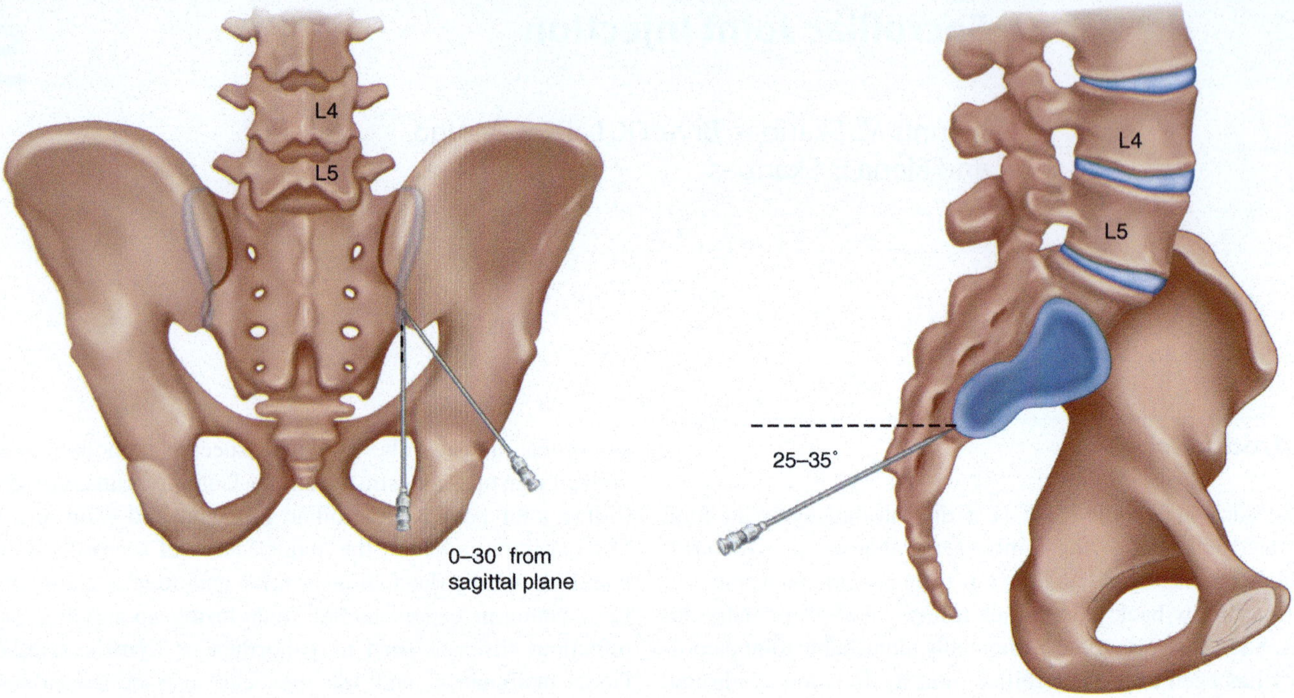

Fig. 52.1 This illustration depicts positioning of a needle for insertion and advancement to the sacroiliac (SI) joint. The cephalic angulation is necessary to bypass the posterior superior iliac spine (PSIS) and allow successful entry in to the SI joint

thus preventing excessive rotation. The sacroiliac joint (SIJ) contains a synovial joint in the anterior portion and interosseous ligaments in the posterior aspect of the joint. The joint capsule is absent posteriorly. The adult sacroiliac joint is auricular or C-shaped, and its size varies significantly between individuals. The sacroiliac joint's capacity is roughly 1.0–2.5 ml. The nerve supply to the SIJ varies between individuals, which may account for the variable patterns of referred pain from the SIJ. Posteriorly, the innervation of the sacroiliac joint arises from the lateral branches of the posterior primary rami of L4 to S3. The anterior aspect of the sacroiliac joint receives innervation from L2 to S2, L4 to S2, and L5 to S2 rami.

Patient Selection

The etiology of sacroiliac joint pain can be broadly divided into intra-articular and extra-articular. Intra-articular pain causes include arthritis and spondyloarthropathies. Extra-articular pain causes include those that pertain to the surround structures including adjacent ligaments and muscles. Risk factors to develop SIJ pain include leg length discrepancies, gait abnormalities, prolonged exercise, scoliosis, pregnancy, and lumbar or sacral spine surgery. Sacroiliac joint injections are utilized to diagnose and treat low back/buttock pain or sacroiliac joint localized pain. There are variable degrees of joint degeneration between different age groups and between men and women. Since sacroiliac joint pain is difficult to differentiate from other sources of low back pain, the performance of intra-articular image-guided sacroiliac joint injections is still considered the best diagnostic tool available.

Physical maneuvers utilized to provoke SI joint pain are not nearly specific enough to make a clear diagnosis. Also, there is no good imaging modality of the joint to determine a precise diagnosis. Typically, a diagnostic injection is done to determine if it will provide relief or not.

Some indications used in current practice to identify patient candidates for a sacroiliac joint injection are:

1. Pain on pressure of SI joint
2. Pain severity by history of greater than or equal to 4 out of 10 on the numeric rating scale
3. Positive Gaenslen's test and/or Patrick's test

Description of the Procedure

Fluoroscopy-Guided Sacroiliac Joint Injections

A sacroiliac joint injection can be done in an appropriately equipped clinical setting under fluoroscopic or ultrasound guidance. The most common facility utilized is an ambulatory surgical center where the procedure is performed in a sterile environment under monitored anesthesia care. The introduction of an intravenous line is mandatory regardless of the setting for resuscitation purposes. The administration of sedatives is optional based on the physician and patient preferences. Although this procedure can be performed under local anesthesia, most practitioners utilize mild sedatives with small doses of intravenous sedative and analgesic agents for patient comfort. Sterile conditions are utilized when performing these injections. The overlying skin is prepped with either chlorhexidine or iodine mixtures with isopropyl alcohol. In the operating room, the patient is placed in a prone position with the head resting comfortably to the side on a pillow or in a similar configuration to account for patient comfort and airway accessibility. A pillow placed under the pelvis can facilitate visualization of the sacroiliac joint regardless of imaging preference. Because of the lumbosacral anatomical variance as well as the variance of the sacroiliac joint size and orientation between patients, there is no one specific C-arm orientation. The C-arm should be positioned in a way so that fluoroscopy aligns the anterior and posterior sacroiliac joint spaces so they can overlap each other allowing for accurate needle placement into joint space (Fig. 52.2). A 20–30-degree caudal angulation of the fluoroscopic intensifier is initially used to place the iliac crest cephalad and away from the trajectory of the needle and project the posterior-inferior portion of the SI joint in a caudal direction. After the overlying skin is infiltrated with local anesthetic (2–5 cc of 1% lidocaine), a 22-gauge 3.5-inch spinal needle is utilized, inserted through the skin, and advanced coaxial to the x-ray beam until it enters the inferior-posterior aspect of the sacroiliac joint. Upon entry to the joint and penetration of the joint capsule, there is a tactile difference in needle advancement appreciated by the operator. After negative aspiration, a small amount of contrast dye, usually iohexol, is injected into the joint. Since the joint volume is rather small, 0.2–0.5 cc of nonionic contrast dye are sufficient to obtain a sacroiliac arthrogram (Figs. 52.3 and 52.4). Once an arthrogram is obtained, 2–3 cc of 0.25% bupivacaine or ropivacaine mixed with 40–80 mg of either triamcinolone (Kenalog) or methylprednisolone (Depo-Medrol) are slowly injected into the joint under fluoroscopy.

Ultrasound-Guided Sacroiliac Joint Injections

The sacroiliac joint is an attractive anatomical target for ultrasound utilization and blockade because of its rather superficial nature and the well-defined sonographic anatomy. An increasing number of pain medicine practitioners are utilizing this method because of its many advantages such as ease and accuracy of performance, as well as absence of radiation exposure for both patient and practitioner alike. Other favorable ultrasound properties are its easy portability and the low cost associated with its usage. Although some have argued that ultrasound-guided sacroiliac joint injections

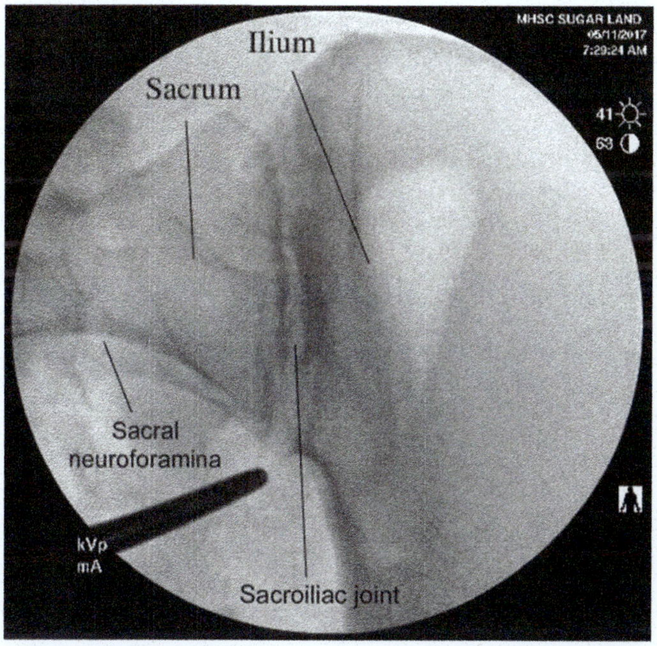

Fig. 52.2 Fluoroscopic image of right sacroiliac joint. Under correct fluoroscopic obliquity, the anterior and posterior portions of the joint are aligned so that they overlap projecting this diarthrodial joint as one. The surgical instrument points at the posterior-inferior aspect of the joint representing the target area where the needle will enter and advanced. This is further facilitated with a C-arm angulation of 20–30 ° caudad

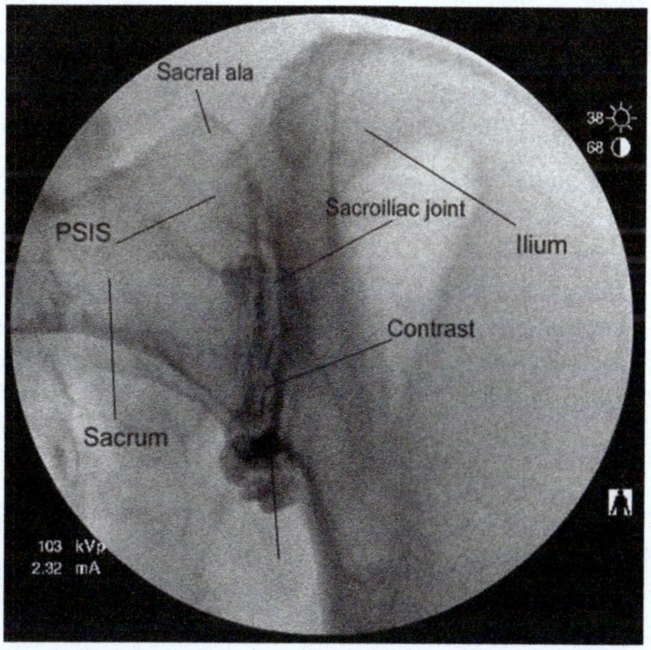

Fig. 52.3 Coaxial posterior-anterior fluoroscopic image of a spinal needle entering the posterior-inferior aspect of the right sacroiliac joint with contrast dye spread into the intra-articular joint space and capsule. The adjacent anatomy is described depicting the association of the iliac and sacral anatomical elements contributing to the configuration of the sacroiliac joint and affecting its percutaneous accessibility

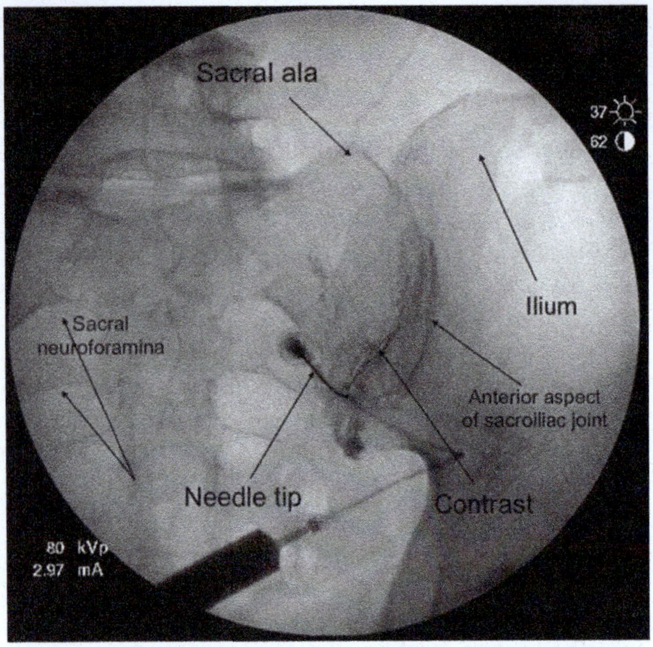

Fig. 52.4 Another fluoroscopic image of a right sacroiliac joint injection. The C-arm has been obliqued to demonstrate the spread of the contrast dye in to the anterior and posterior aspects of the joint

are associated with higher frequency of periarticular injections, the accuracy of the technique has been verified and reported in both cadaveric and human studies.

A curvilinear low-frequency ultrasound transducer is utilized for ultrasound-guided sacroiliac joint injections. The setting is the same as described in the fluoroscopic technique. The patient is placed prone with a wedge over the lower abdomen to reverse the lumbar lordosis. The operator is positioned to the left side of the patient regardless of the joint location with the ultrasound machine positioned on the same side of the operator, either to the left or right depending on the operator's dexterity. The ultrasound screen, keyboard, probe, and cords are all draped in a sterile fashion with commercially available products. The skin area is prepped and draped in a sterile fashion. After a layer of sterile gel has been placed between the ultrasound probe and the sterile sheath, another layer of gel is applied between the draped transducer and the skin. The curvilinear transducer is placed in a transverse orientation over the sacral hiatus to identify the sacral cornua. Moving the transducer laterally to the side of the joint to be injected and always in a transverse orientation, first the lateral edge of the sacrum is identified followed by a lateral-cephalad movement to identify the ileum. In a short-axis view of the sacroiliac joint, the posterior edge of the sacroiliac joint is seen as a cleft between the bony edges of the sacrum and ileum. The injection is performed with either a 22-gauge 3.5-inch spinal needle or a similar echogenically insulated gauge ultrasound needle advanced in a mediolateral "in-plane" orientation. After the skin is infiltrated with 2–5 cc of 1% lidocaine, the needle is inserted 1 cm away from the medial side of the probe and advanced under continuous ultrasound vision in-line until it is seen positioned into the sacroiliac joint.

Contraindications

Patient refusal
Local or systemic infection
Anticoagulation and bleeding disorders
Allergy to medications
Pregnancy (fluoroscopy)

Complications

Exacerbation of painful symptoms
Bleeding
Infection
Nerve injury

Recommended Reading

1. Calvillo O, Skaribas I, Turnipsed J. Anatomy and pathophysiology of the sacroiliac joint. Curr Rev Pain. 2000;4:356–61.
2. Narouze SN. Atlas of ultrasound –guided procedures in interventional pain management. New York: Springer; 2010. p. 185–7.
3. Rathmell JP. Atlas of image-guided intervention in regional anesthesia and pain medicine. Chapter 8, Sacroiliac joint injection. Philadelphia, USA: Lippincott, Williams and Wilkins; 2006. p. 93–100.
4. Schwarzer AC, April CN, Bogduk N. The sacroiliac joint in chronic low back pain. Spine. 1995;20:31–7.

Sacroiliac Joint Radiofrequency

53

Susan Lim and Christopher Gilligan

Introduction

The sacroiliac joint (SIJ) is the largest axial joint in the human body. It is a unique joint, with significantly decreased and unconventional motion compared to other synovial joints. This makes it a difficult joint to study. It is an important source of chronic low back pain, which is the number one cause of disability in the United States. An estimated 15–25% of patients may have SIJ pain as the cause of their symptoms. Furthermore, according to several sources, this may be an underestimate. The anatomy and physiology of SIJ is unique, which makes accurate diagnosis and management very challenging.

Background and Historical Perspective

Anatomy and Innervation of the Sacroiliac Joint

Historically, SIJs were thought to be mobile only during pregnancy in women. However, eighteenth-century studies revealed that they have a synovial membrane and are mobile in both men and women. The SIJ is the largest axial joint in the human body. It is formed by the articulation of the medial surfaces of the ilium and lateral sacral segments S1, S2, and S3. SIJs have a rigid structure with tight fibrous ligaments that are essential for load transfer between the spine and the legs. SIJ movements such as forward and backward tilting are not independent and directly influence lumbar joints such as L5–S1 and higher spinal levels.

The innervation of the SIJ is variable, complex, and controversial. This makes evaluation, diagnosis, and treatment challenging. The lumbosacral plexus provides sensory innervation for the SIJ. A recent cadaveric study found that the *posterior* SIJ is innervated by the lateral branches of the posterior rami of L5–S4. The lateral branches of S1 and S2 contribute to the innervation in 100% of specimens, S3 in 88%, L5 in 8%, and S4 in 4%. Lateral branches of S1–S4 exit the sacral foramina and traverse the sacrum in an unpredictable fashion. Other sources claim that medial branches of L4 and L5 may also provide innervation to the posterior SIJ. The S1 level likely provides the greatest innervation to the posterior SIJ.

The *anterior* SIJ is innervated by the posterior rami of L1–S2 and by the superior gluteal and obturator nerves. It is important to note that SIJ pain originating from the anterior SI joint line cannot be effectively targeted by radiofrequency ablation (RFA). There are no reliable and SIJ-specific RFA targets for the obturator and superior gluteal nerves. This may, in part, account for the ineffectiveness of some RFA interventions for SIJ pain. Although imaging findings do not necessarily correlate with pain, one study revealed 69% of joint pathology by computed tomography (CT) to be in the anterior/ventral aspect of the SIJ in 13 patients with block-confirmed SIJ pain.

Pathology, Clinical Symptoms, and Diagnosis of Sacroiliac Joint Pain

Acute and chronic axial or rotational overloading can lead to SIJ injury. In 40–50% of occurrences, SIJ pain is associated with a specific inciting event such as a motor vehicle collision or a fall onto the buttocks. Other causes include cumulative injuries from lifting and running. Intra-articular pathology, extra-articular ligamentous damage, and inflammation can cause pain. Common causes of SIJ pain include

Sections "Introduction", "Background and Historical Perspective", and "Uses and Indications" of this chapter are reproduced from Gilligan C., Malik O.S., Hirsch J.A. Radiofrequency Ablation for Sacroiliac Joint Pain. In: Marcia S., Saba L. (eds) *Radiofrequency Treatments on the Spine*. Switzerland. Springer International Publishing; 2017. With permission from Springer Nature.

S. Lim (✉) · C. Gilligan
Brigham and Women's Hospital, Boston, MA, USA
e-mail: Slim8@partners.org; cgilligan@bwh.harvard.edu

T. R. Deer et al. (eds.), *Deer's Treatment of Pain*, https://doi.org/10.1007/978-3-030-12281-2_53

osteoarthritis, repeated athletic endeavors leading to joint stress, HLA-B27 seronegative spondyloarthropathies such as psoriatic arthritis, and peri- or postpartum patients. Pain in gluteal or paraspinal regions below the fifth lumbar vertebrae is the most common complaint. SIJ pain may radiate to the thigh. Nearly one fourth of the patients may have referred pain distal to the knee. SIJ pain may be worsened during transitional movements such as rising from a sitting position.

Unique characteristics, which are typically not seen in other diarthrodial joints, make diagnosing SIJ pathology difficult and elusive. Anatomic abnormalities may not be present on imaging. Previous studies have shown that no single test can reliably identify SIJ pathology. Therefore, multiple studies have been done to improve the accuracy of SIJ pain diagnosis including local anesthetic blocks, combinations of physical maneuvers, and imaging techniques. Szadek et al. conducted a systematic review and concluded that three or more positive stressing tests, the compression test, and the thigh thrust have enough discriminative power that they can be used for diagnosing SIJ pain. However, Song et al. later reported that this is of limited value in establishing a diagnosis of sacroiliitis. Multiple Cochrane review publications indicate that there is moderate evidence for the accuracy and validity of local anesthetic injections to establish SIJ as the cause of pain. Other sources such as the Centre for Reviews and Dissemination of the University of York from the National Institute for Health Research cite a lack of evidence for diagnostic local anesthetic injections. Despite the differing opinions, clinicians typically diagnose SIJ pain by one or two intra-articular local anesthetic blocks with greater than 50 percent decrease in pain.

Uses and Indications

Radiofrequency ablation (RFA) is appropriate for patients with a positive diagnosis of SIJ pathology as the cause of their symptoms. Appropriate patient choice is of paramount importance. Typically, this consists of one or two intra-articular local anesthetic blocks. Establishing an accurate diagnosis of SIJ pain remains a point of controversy among practitioners. Contraindications to RFA include coagulopathies, ongoing sepsis, therapeutic anticoagulation, or presence of nearby invasive lesions such as tumor or infection. Relative contraindications include previous failed RFA to same target, psychopathology, unoptimized psychiatric conditions, target site deafferentation / neuropathic disorders, alteration of target anatomy with prior surgical intervention, and unrealistic expectations of pain relief. Patients with spinal cord stimulators and pacemakers need special care as RFA devices may interfere with their function. Grounding pad should be placed away from these devices so that current may be drawn away.

Interestingly, RFA is more effective for extra-articular rather than intra-articular joint pain. RFA for SIJ pain poses unique challenges to the practitioner. RF lesions are prolate ellipsoidal in shape. In conventional RFA, the bulk of the lesion's volume is spread circumferentially around the long axis of the uninsulated tip of the probe (Fig. 53.1). Therefore, optimal positioning of a conventional RFA probe lies parallel to the path of sensory nerves. Perpendicular positioning is not optimal and carries a higher probability of unsatisfactory nerve ablation. SIJ innervation is variable and includes nerves that travel laterally from the sacral foramina toward the SIJ. It is not practical to place the RFA probe parallel to the horizontal path of these nerves due to the flat posterior plane of the sacrum. Therefore, the location for proper RFA probe placement is unclear, and various techniques have been studied.

RFA after diagnostic SIJ local anesthetic blocks has inherent limitations. Not all patients with SIJ pathology as the true source of their pain and with >50% pain relief after diagnostic local anesthetic blocks will not benefit significantly from RFA. It is not possible to reproduce a local anesthetic block with RFA. RFA is limited to neurotomy of posterior SIJ innervation, but local anesthetic solution spreads within the joint and has the potential to block sensation from intra-articular surfaces and surfaces innervated by ventral nerves. Variations in SIJ anatomy due to the bony contours of the sacrum and varying paths of the sacral nerves make it technically challenging to perform RFA parallel to the target nerves. Consequently, it is impossible to denervate the entire nerve network that contributes to SIJ pain. In addition, guidelines for facet joint RFA are based on 100% pain relief with local anesthetic blocks. As a result, it may be difficult to replicate the results of facet joint RFA for SIJ pathology.

Larger gauge electrodes (size 14–16) have a higher likelihood of mechanical injury, bleeding, and deafferentation pain. However, SIJ RFA targets are not adjacent to major vessels or important functional nerves. Therefore, larger gauge electrodes may be used for SIJ RFA. In addition, SIJ RFA target sites are not excessively vascular, and they are well insulted by the bony structure of the sacrum. Dissipation of heat away from the contacted tissue (i.e., heat washout) is less of a concern. However, it is important to monitor the rate of temperature change because raising the tissue temperature too quickly risks unpredictable lesions and cavitations.

There is no absolute indication for SI joint ablation or diagnostic criteria for patient selection. In a 2013 review of the treatment of the SI joint, Cohen et al. stated that poor patient selection, inaccurate diagnosis, and technical failures are all causes of treatment failures. Future studies are necessary to determine selection criteria of optimal patients

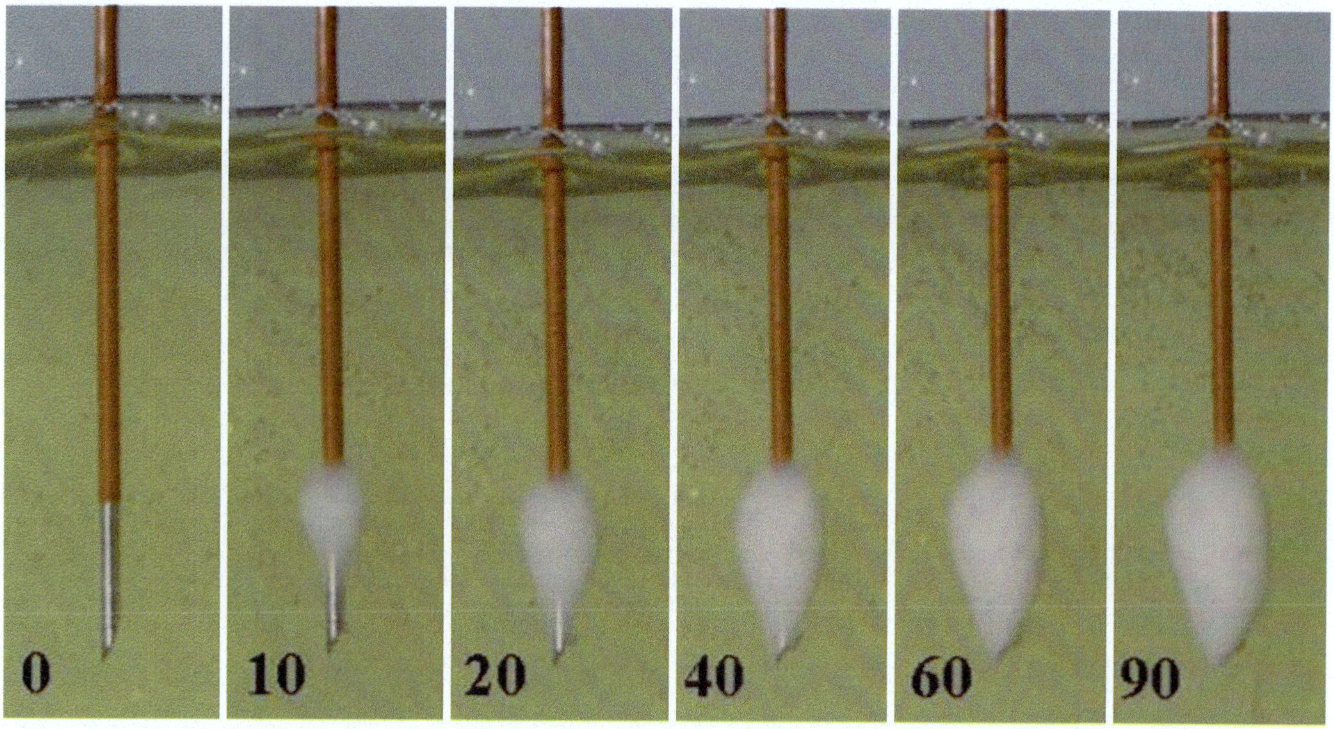

Fig. 53.1 A 22 gauge 10 cm SMK radiofrequency cannula with a 5 mm active tip is immersed in egg white and CRF applied at 80 °C for 90 seconds. The radial size of the lesion is maximal near the midportion of the active tip. Thus, for optimal application of CRF treatment, the shaft of the needle's active tip is optimally placed parallel to the target nerve. The size of the lesion is near maximal by 60 seconds of treatment. (Reproduced from James P. Rathmell MD, *Atlas of Image-Guided Intervention in Regional Anesthesia and Pain Medicine*, Wolters Kluwer, 2011. With permission from Wolters Kluwer)

for SI RFA. In a retrospective study comparing cooled vs. conventional radiofrequency ablation, Cohen et al. looked at demographic and clinical variables that could predict positive treatment outcome. It was shown that positive predictors of failure included pre-procedure pain intensity, age older than 65 years, and pain radiating below the knee. The only positive predictor of success they found was the use of cooled RFA. This outcome has not been replicated by other studies.

Evidence for Efficacy

There are various types of radiofrequency ablation that can be used for the sacroiliac joint. The forms of ablation can be categorized as monopolar or bipolar. Monopolar techniques include conventional, pulsed, and cooled ablation. Although there are multiple modalities for conducting radiofrequency ablation on the SI joint, there is limited data evaluating their effectiveness in treating sacroiliac joint pain. Randomized trials and retrospective or prospective studies for SI joint RFA and its effectiveness are summarized in Table 53.1. There are only two randomized controlled trials studying cooled versus sham technique and two retrospective studies comparing conventional vs. cooled ablation of the SI joint. No other studies compare different types of radiofrequency ablation directly to each other or compare ablation to other conservative methods of treating SI joint pain. The majority of the studies consist of small patient populations. It is difficult to compare the studies to one another because there are differences with selection criteria of patients, technique of the ablation performed, what primary outcomes were studied, and how they were defined. Larger, prospective, randomized controlled trials need to be needed to further evaluate the efficacy and usefulness of this intervention.

Conventional Radiofrequency Ablation for Sacroiliac Joint Pain

One of the first studies looking at the effectiveness of SI joint RFA was conducted in 2002 by Gervargez et al. The prospective study included 38 patients undergoing CT-guided conventional radiofrequency ablation with a primary outcome of pain at follow-up. For selection criteria, patients who underwent one to two facet joint injections and ethanol denervation in L3–L4, L4–L5, and L5–S1 levels and still experienced persistent lower back pain were included. These patients then underwent CT-guided diagnostic SI joint blocks. Thirty-eight patients reported only temporary

Table 53.1 Summary of sacroiliac joint radiofrequency ablation studies

Authors	Study design	# Patients	RF mode	Technique	% Patients with >50% relief at 3 or more months
Gevargez (2002)	Prospective observational	38	Conventional	CT-Guided CRF to L5 dorsal ramus and posterior interosseous SI ligaments. 23 ga electrodes with 5 mm active tips. Lesion time 90 seconds at 90 °C	66%
Schmidt (2014)	Retrospective	60	Conventional	Multi-lesion probe CRF lesions at 80–85 °C for 60–90 seconds. CRF to L5 dorsal ramus 80 °C, 90 seconds	71.4%
Mitchell (2015)	Prospective observational	215	Conventional	CRF to dorsal and lateral branches of S1–S3 and descending branch of L5. 18 ga electrodes with 1 cm active tips. Lesion time 90 seconds at 90 °C	Not applicable
Cohen (2008)	Randomized placebo controlled	28 (14 treatment, 14 control)	Cooled or sham	CRF to L4–L5 dorsal ramus and WCRF to S1–S3 lateral branches. 18 ga electrodes with 4 mm active tips (17 ga cannula). Lesion time 2.5 minutes at 60 °C probe temp	64%
Patel (2012)	Randomized placebo controlled	51 (34 treatment, 17 control)	Cooled versus sham	Cooled RFA to S1–S3 lateral branches and L5 dorsal ramus. 17 ga, 75 mm cooled electrode with 4 mm active tip. Lesion time 150 seconds at 60 °C	47% (treatment group)
Stelzer (2013)	Retrospective	126	Cooled	Cooled RFA to L5 dorsal ramus and lateral to S1, S2, and S3 posterior sacral foraminal apertures. Lesion time 2.5 minutes at 60 °C probe temp	86% (4–6 months)
Cohen (2009)	Retrospective	77	Conventional + cooled	CRF to L4–L5 dorsal ramus and WCRF to S1–S3 lateral branches. 18 ga electrodes with 4 mm active tips (17 ga cannula) spaced ~10 mm apart	52%
Cheng (2013)	Retrospective	88 (30 conventional, 58 cooled)	Conventional + cooled	Conventional RFA to L5 dorsal rami and S1–S3 lateral branches. 25 ga electrodes with 5 mm active tips. Lesion time 90 seconds at 80 °C. Cooled RFA with 17 ga, 75 mm electrodes with 4 mm active tips. Lesion time 150 seconds at 60 °C	50% (conventional) 60% (cooled)
Vallejo (2006)	Prospective observational	22	Pulsed	PRF to MB of L4, dorsal ramus of L5, lateral branches of S1 and S2. 22 ga electrodes with 10 mm active tips. PRF 42 °C at 45 V for 120 seconds	73%
Burnham (2007)	Prospective observational	9	Bipolar	L4–L5 dorsal ramus + BRF strip lesions to S1–S3. For BRF, 20 ga electrodes with 10 mm active tips spaced 4–6 mm apart. Lesion time 90 seconds at 80 °C	67%
Ferrante (2001)	Retrospective	33	Bipolar	Leapfrog technique along posterior SIJ. 20/22 ga cannula spaced <10 mm. Lesion time 90 seconds at 90 °C	36%
Buijs (2004)	Prospective observational	38	Conventional	L4–L5 dorsal ramus and "3 puncture technique" lateral upper quadrant of S1–S3 dorsal foramina. Lesion time 60 seconds at 80 °C	63%
Yin (2003)	Retrospective	14	Conventional	Sensory stimulation-guided CRF S1–S3 lateral branches. 20 ga electrodes with 10 mm active tips. Lesion time 90 seconds at 80 °C	64%
Cohen (2003)	Retrospective	9	Conventional	CRF to L4–L5 dorsal ramus and S1–S3 lateral branches. 22 ga electrodes with 5 mm active tips. Lesion time 90 seconds at 80 °C	89%
Kapural (2008)	Retrospective	26	Cooled	Lateral edges of S1–S3 sacral foramina. 18 ga electrodes with 4 mm active tips (17 ga cannula) spaced ~10 mm apart	50%

Table adapted from Paterno, J, Rathmell, J, Gilligan, C. Cryoanalgesia and Radiofrequency Ablation. Bajwa, Z, Wootton, R, Warfield C, editors. *Principles and Practice of Pain Medicine*. McGraw-Hill Education; 2017. With permission from McGraw-Hill Education
CRF Conventional radiofrequency, *WCRF* Water-cooled radiofrequency, *PRF* Pulsed radiofrequency, *MB* Medial branch, *BRF* Bipolar radiofrequency, *SIJ* Sacroiliac joint

pain relief and were included in the study. For the RF denervation, CT image guidance was used to find the best entry point to the posterior interosseous sacroiliac ligaments. 23 G insulated RF cannulae with a 5 mm uninsulated tip (Leibinger) were used. The monopolar electrode was then inserted into the cannula. Three steps of 90-degree temperature were used, and after each step of 90 seconds, the set was withdrawn by 5 mm. The dorsal branches of L5 were then targeted by CT images finding the upper part of the junction of the sacral ala and the superior articular process of S1. The same radiofrequency technique was then used. A patient questionnaire was used at 2 days, 7 days, 1 month, and 3 months after therapy. At 3 months 34.2% of patients still had complete relief of pain (n = 13), 31.6% of patients reported a substantial pain reduction (n = 12), 18.6% reported a slight reduction (n = 7), and 3% of patients (n = 3) reported no pain reduction. The study demonstrated that CT-guided conventional radiofrequency ablation could possibly be a successful technique in the treatment of SI joint pain.

The introduction of multi-lesion probes to the methods of radiofrequency ablation of the SI joint is a new development. They were designed to target the sacral lateral branches of the SI joint, creating a continuous strip lesion with only a single entry point. Currently two probes exist. The Simplicity III (Neurotherm, Middleton, MA) uses conventional radiofrequency ablation with a 17 gauge, multi-electrode, curved probe. The probe creates a strip lesion with three electrodes creating five lesions (Fig. 53.2). Three lesions are monopolar, and two are bipolar. Compared to the SInergy probe, the Simplicity III does not directly lesion the L5 dorsal ramus. The SInergy probe (Halyard) uses cooled radiofrequency ablation and can operate at a lower temperature, 60 °C versus 80–90 °C in the Simplicity III. It creates larger lesions than conventional RFA. The SInergy probe creates three lesions lateral to S1 and S2, two lesions lateral to S3, and a single lesion at the L5 dorsal ramus. Due to the variation in sacral structure among patients, targeting nerves by a single probe proves to be difficult. The SInergy probe has greater flexibility, and direct lesioning of the L5 dorsal ramus is possible. There are no studies that demonstrate the effectiveness of multi-lesion probes versus other methods of SI joint radiofrequency ablation. Only one retrospective case series has been conducted. A recent paper by Gilligan et al. [8] demonstrated a novel single-puncture approach for the Simplicity probe. Instead of using multiple needle placements along the placement of the ablation tract, a technique was described using a modified Seldinger approach (Fig. 53.3). This may reduce the potential complications of the multi-lesion probe technique including bowel perforation or probe insertion through a neural foramen. This new technique may also decrease procedure time and radiation exposure.

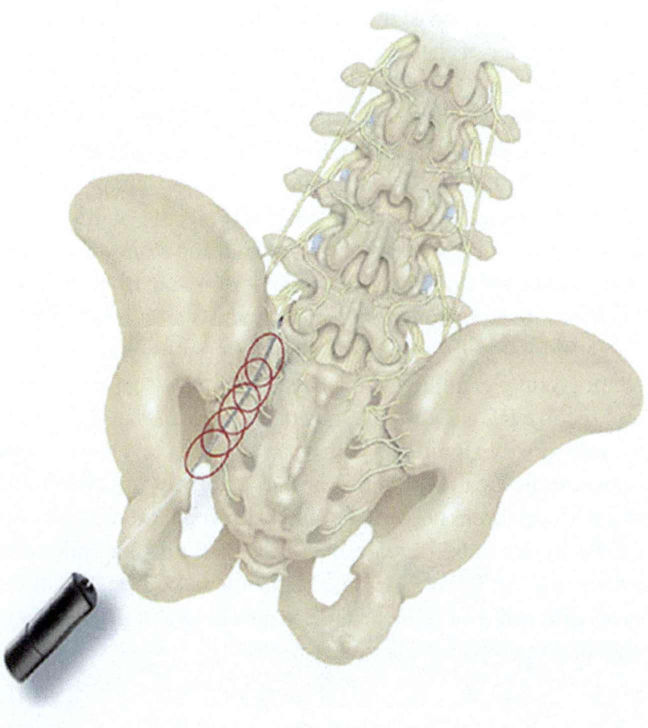

Fig. 53.2 Simplicity III electrode using NT1100 NeuroTherm generator's unique algorithm to create 5 lesions along its length. The electrode creates three monopolar and two bipolar lesions. (Simplicity and St. Jude Medical are trademarks of St. Jude Medical, LLC or its related companies. Reproduced with permission of St. Jude Medical, ©2018. All rights reserved)

In 2014, Schmidt et al. conducted a noncontrolled, retrospective trial using conventional technique with a multi-lesion probe. They demonstrated that results with the multi-lesion probe were comparable to both bipolar and cooled RFA at 6 months. The primary outcome was greater than 50% pain relief at various time points. The Simplicity III was the multi-lesion probe used for the patients in this study. No cannulae or introducers are needed, and a continuous strip lesion is created. The inclusion criteria consisted of patients with presumed SI joint pain who had >50% pain relief after fluoroscopically guided intra-articular injections. Seventy-seven radiofrequency treatments were thus included for study. These patients subsequently underwent conventional RF with the Simplicity III probe. Local anesthetics were used to anesthetize the area, and the probe was positioned over the posterior surface of the sacrum. Lesions were created at 80–85 °C for 60–90 seconds. RFA lesions were also performed separately at the L5 dorsal ramus and some also at the L4 ramus. Verbal pain scales were then used for patients to evaluate their pain relief at 6 weeks, 6 months, and 1 year after the procedure. Results demonstrated that 71.4% had >50% pain relief at 6 weeks, 54.5% at 6 months, and 15.6% at 1 year. It was determined that this technique provided similar results to both the leapfrog technique and cooled RFA.

Mitchell et al. [11] conducted a prospective observational study for traditional RFA. It demonstrated that this technique provided decreased average pain and analgesic use and increased employment capacity for those included in this study. Two hundred fifteen patients with SI joint pain confirmed by diagnosis with local anesthetic blocks under fluoroscopic guidance to the SIJ and deep interosseous ligament were selected. Pain was measured on an 11-point numerical rating scale, and patients with greater than 80% pain reduction 2 hours after injection were diagnosed as having SIJ pain. These patients

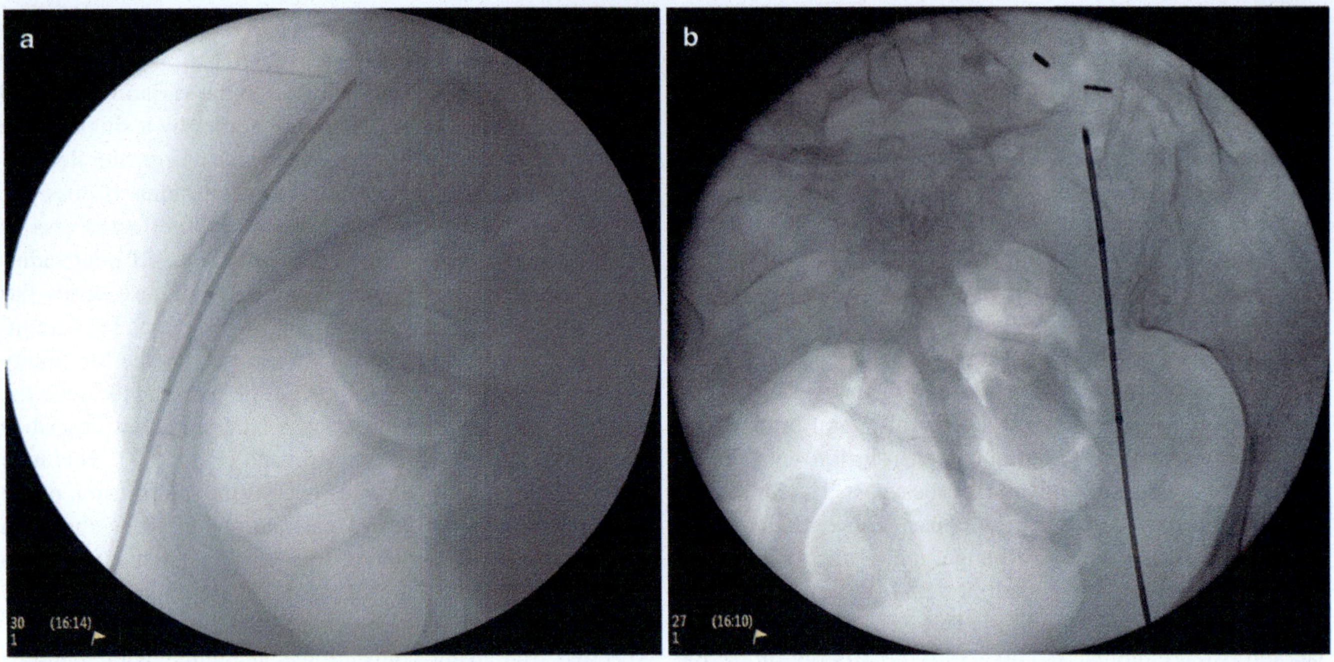

Fig. 53.3 Fluoroscopic image confirms adequate positioning of the Simplicity III RF Probe. (**a**) Lateral view. (**b**) AP view. (Image courtesy of Chris Gilligan, MD)

went on to have RFA at a single center. Conventional RFA was used targeting the S1–S3 foramen with 18 G RFN needles with a 1 cm active tip under fluoroscopic guidance. Needles were placed flat to the surface of the sacrum and were used at 90 °C for 90 seconds. The dorsal, lateral, and L5 descending branches were all targeted along with further lesions to capture the lateral branches of S1, S2, and S3. Patients were followed for a range of 6–49 months. Outcome measures included pain level measured on the 11-point NRS scale, changes in analgesic use, and capacity for paid employment. They found an average pain reduction of 2.3 +/− 2.1 points following RFN at a mean follow-up period of 14.9 +/− 10.9 months, and overall 42.2% of patients with reduced analgesic use, and 21 out of 82 patients stated improvement in employment capacity. Sixty-seven percent of patients were satisfied with the outcome. The study stated that RFN was an effective treatment for SI joint pain. Limitations to the study included its prospective nature, lack of control group, and patient population from only one clinic location.

van Tilburg et al. published the most recent randomized, controlled, double-blind trial in 2016 comparing the Simplicity III probe (Neurotherm, Wilmington, MA) versus sham procedure. The study included 60 patients with suggested SI joint pain diagnosed by medical history, physical exam, and a reduction of 2 or more points on the NRS scale after one SIJ injection. The primary outcome was reduction in pain using the NRS, and the secondary outcome was scored using the Global Perceived Effect. The test SI joint injection was performed using a 10 cm Sluijter-Mehta Kit needle under fluoroscopic guidance with an injection of 3 mL of 2% lidocaine. The Simplicity III probe was used for RF ablation. The location for the insertion of the probe was at the ipsilateral, lateral, inferior border of the sacrum, 1 cm lateral of the S4 foramen. The probe was advanced lateral to the sacral foramen and medial to the SI joint. Heat lesions at 85 °C were performed five times for 90 seconds each in order to capture the lateral branches of the S1–S4 nerve roots. The L5 dorsal root was ablated separately with a 10 cm SMK needle at 85 °C for 90 seconds. The sham group underwent the same procedure, but without RF ablation. Time points for evaluation included the day of first consultation, 1 month, and 3 months after treatment. Similar to the prior RCTs, after 3 months, patients in the sham group were allowed to cross over to the treatment group and receive RF ablation. Results demonstrated that there were no statistically significant differences in pain levels over time between the treatment and sham group. If the treatment and sham groups were pooled, the study showed there was a statistically significant difference in pain levels 1 and 3 months after treatment. van Tilburg concluded that the hypothesis that there is no difference in NRS or GPE scales between the treatment and sham groups could not be rejected.

Cooled Radiofrequency Ablation for Sacroiliac Joint Pain

A newer modality includes cooled radiofrequency ablation. In this technique, large-bore electrodes are cooled by irrigation.

Conceptually, this cooled ablation allows for less tissue damage surrounding the target area and creates a larger diameter of neuroablation. Studies demonstrate that compared to conventional methods, the diameter with cooled RFA can increase twofold and the area can thus increase eightfold (Fig. 53.4). Unlike conventional ablation, the probes can be placed in a slightly different manner. Due to the increased neuroablative area, the probes can be positioned perpendicularly versus parallel to the sacral foramina. This approach allows for decreased risk of complications due to inadvertent bowel perforation. Due to the increased area of the cooled radiofrequency probes, it is thought that this technique can create a contiguous lesion that would be more effective in targeting the multitude of nerves needing ablation for successful treatment of sacroiliac joint pain.

The only two prospective, randomized, controlled trials that have been conducted regarding SI joint ablation were with cooled radiofrequency ablation. Both Cohen et al. [4] and Patel et al. [14] looked at this technique. With a randomized placebo-controlled trial, Cohen et al. produced preliminary evidence that RFA may provide intermediate-term pain relief and functional benefit in patients with suspected SI joint pain. Of note, crossover patients received conventional ablation unlike the randomized group that initially received cooled RFA. It was shown that there was no difference between cooled and conventional ablation. The study consisted of 28 patients: 14 received cooled radiofrequency ablation at the L4 and L5 dorsal rami and S1–S3 lateral branches, and 14 patients received sham technique (Fig. 53.5). Patients who did not respond to the sham technique crossed over to the treatment arm but received conventional radiofrequency ablation instead of cooled due to availability of equipment. Patients included in the study responded to screening sacroiliac joint injections. The bottom one third of the joint was targeted using 22 G spinal needles. Enrollment in the study mandated that patients experienced >75% pain relief for at least 3 hours and returned to baseline within 3 months using a 10-point NRS scale. For the lesioning of L4 and L5 dorsal rami, 22 G SMK-C10 cannulae (Radionics, Burlington, MA) with 5 mm active tips were used. Electrostimulation at 50 Hz was used to confirm placement. Ninety seconds of 80 °C lesioning was used at each site. A 17 G, 75 mm cooled electrode with a 4 mm active tip was used for the S1–S3 lateral branches (Baylis Medical, Montreal, Quebec, Canada). An 8–10 mm lesion was created at 75 °C at each target site. The patients in the crossover arm received identical treatment described in the treatment group, using 22 G SMK-C10 (Radiontics)

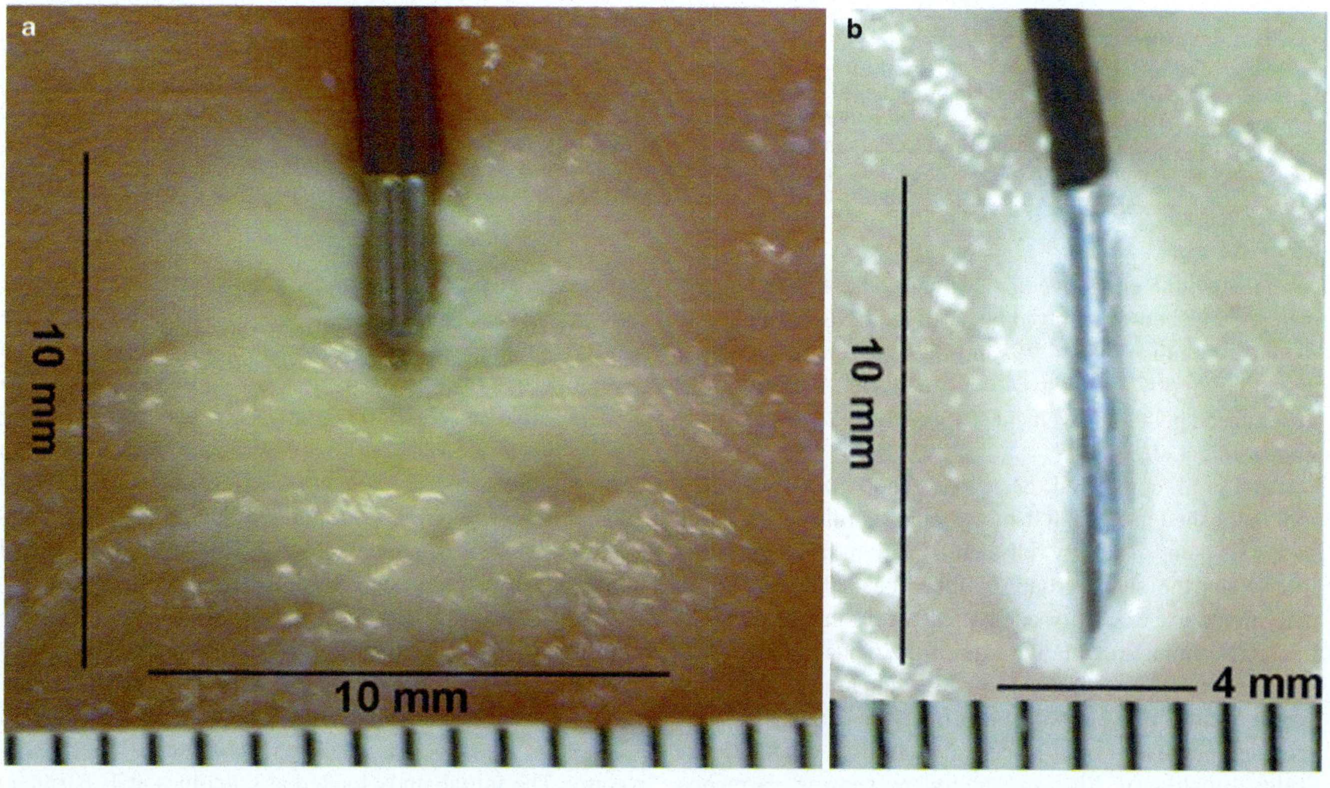

Fig. 53.4 Adjacent photographs demonstrating the difference in lesion size between cooled (**a**) and conventional (**b**) radiofrequency probes in chicken meat. Each small line represents a distance of 1 mm. (Reproduced from Cohen, Steven P.; Hurley, Robert W., Randomized Placebo-controlled Study Evaluating Lateral Branch Radiofrequency Denervation for Sacroiliac Joint Pain, *Anesthesiology*, Vol 109, Issue 2, 279–288. http://anesthesiology.pubs.asahq.org/article.aspx?articleid=1922283&resultClick=3. With permission from Wolters Kluwer Health, Inc.)

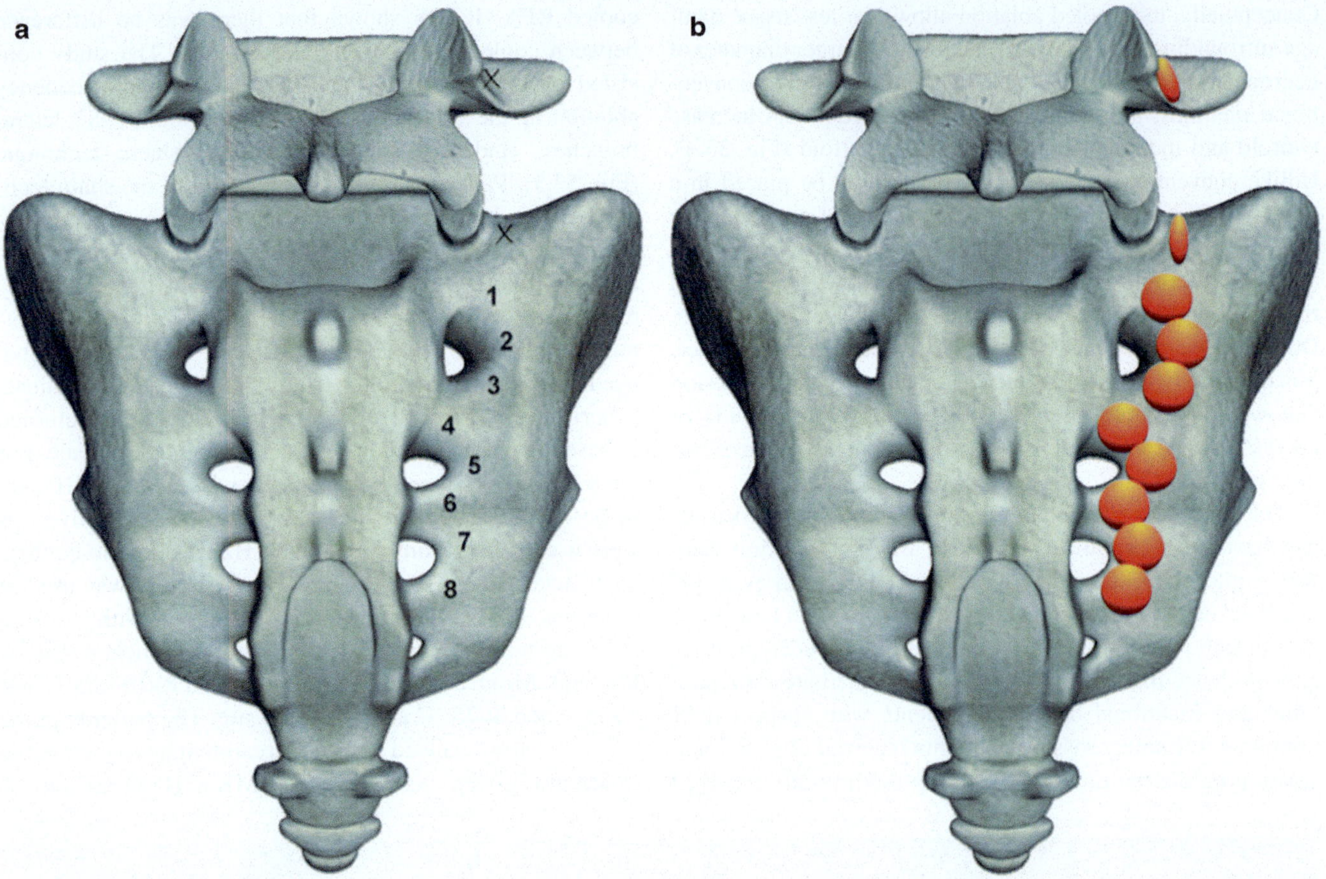

Fig. 53.5 Schematic diagram illustrating: (**a**) Target points for right-sided conventional (L4 and L5) and cooled (S1–S3) radiofrequency denervation at the junction of the L5 superior articular and transverse processes (L4 primary dorsal ramus), the sacral ala (L5 primary dorsal ramus), and S1–S3 foramina (lateral branches). (**b**) Typical lesion locations. (Reproduced from Cohen, Steven P.; Hurley, Robert W., Randomized Placebo-controlled Study Evaluating Lateral Branch Radiofrequency Denervation for Sacroiliac Joint Pain, *Anesthesiology*, Vol 109, Issue 2, 279–288. http://anesthesiology.pubs.asahq.org/article.aspx?articleid=1922283&resultClick=3. With permission from Wolters Kluwer Health, Inc.)

cannulae with 5 cm active tips. Primary outcome of average pain experienced was judged by a 10-point NRS scale. At 1, 3, and 6 months, 79%, 69%, and 57% of patients reported pain relief of 50% or greater. Two patients in the sham group experienced pain improvement at 1 month, and none reported improvement afterward.

Patel et al. conducted the second randomized controlled trial, published in 2012. It demonstrated significant improvements in pain, disability, physical function, and quality of life versus the sham group. Number needed to treat was determined to be 3. Fifty-one patients were included within the study, almost double the size of the Cohen study. They were split into a 2:1 ratio of cooled lateral branch neurotomy versus sham intervention. The primary outcome measures included pain rated on a NRS scale, physical function, disability, quality of life, and treatment success. Screened patients underwent two injections, one at the lateral branches of S1–S3 and the other at the dorsal ramus of L5. A positive response was defined as having greater than 75% pain relief between 4 hours and 7 days and had to achieve baseline pain levels before entry into the study. A cooled RF SInergy probe (Kimberly Clark Health Care, Roswell, GA) was used for the L5 dorsal ramus. RF energy was used for 150 seconds at a temperature of 60 °C. A 17 G, 75 mm, cooled electrode with a 4 mm active tip (Kimberly Clark Health Care) was used for the S1, S2, and S3 lateral branches. Again, RF energy at a temperature of 60 °C was delivered to the target sites for 150 seconds. The primary endpoint was at 3 months, demonstrating that 47% of patients and 12% of sham patients had treatment success with significant improvements in pain, disability, physical function, and quality of life.

Patel et al. published a follow-up to this randomized controlled trial in 2016, looking at all of the study subjects, specifically those patients defined as "treatment successes" 12 months after cooled radiofrequency lateral branch neurotomy. The initial study looked at outcomes at 1, 3, 6, and 9 months. The goal was to determine success rates at longer-term follow-up and the durability of the treatment. Sham subjects were unblinded at 3 months and were offered ablation at that time; therefore they were only at 3 months posttreatment at the end of the original study. The same outcomes were measured in the original study and in this follow-up study. To be labeled a treatment success or "responder," the subject had to have experienced a drop in the NRS score by greater than or equal to 50% and had to have a 10-point or greater increase in the 36-physical functioning assessment (SF-36BP) for disability or a reduction in the Oswestry Disability Index (ODI) score by 10 points or greater. In the cooled RFA group, at 12 months there was a mean 2.7 drop in NRS scores, a 15.8 increase in SF-36BP, and a 13.9 decrease in ODI. In the original sham group who elected for ablation, at 6 months there was a mean 2.5 drop in NRS scores, a 8.8 decrease in ODI, and a 11.9 increase in SF-36BP. Forty percent of the original RFA group were defined as treatment responders at 12 months, and 44% of crossover subjects were successes at 6 months. The authors concluded that cooled RFA was a durable and effective treatment for SI joint pain.

The other study looking at cooled RFA was by Stelzer et al. in 2013. It was a retrospective study consisting of 126 patients who underwent cooled RF of the L5 dorsal ramus and lateral to the S1, S2, and S3 posterior sacral foraminal apertures. The study followed patients for up to 20 months, one of the longest lengths of follow-up compared to subsequent studies. It demonstrated decreased pain scores, increased quality of life, and decreased or terminated opioid use. Patients included in the study needed to have greater than 50% pain relief from an intra-articular SI joint injection. Nine lesions were created during the cooled RF procedure, including the L5 dorsal root, three lateral to the S1 and S2 sacral foramina and two lateral to the S3 sacral foramen. The Pain Management SINergy system (Kimberly Clark Corporation, Roswell, GA) was used, and energy was delivered for 150 seconds at 60 °C. Follow-up was at 3–4 weeks after treatment and one between 4 and 20 months after treatment. Splitting time to follow-up between 4–6 months, 6–12 months, and greater than 12 months, 86%, 71%, and 48% of patients reported greater than 50% reduction in VAS pain scores; 96%, 93%, and 85% reported their quality of life as much improved or improved; and 100%, 62%, and 67% of opioid users either terminated or decreased use of opioids.

Conventional Versus Cooled Radiofrequency Ablation for Sacroiliac Joint Pain

Both Cohen et al. [5] and Cheng et al. [2] studied cooled versus conventional radiofrequency ablation with retrospective studies. The purpose of the Cohen et al. study was to evaluate any demographic or clinical variables that could predict SI joint RF denervation outcome. Results demonstrated that the use of cooled versus conventional ablation was associated with a higher percentage of positive outcomes. As discussed above, it was determined that significant predictors of negative outcomes included pre-procedure pain intensity, age older than 65 years, and pain radiating below the knee. Including 77 patients from 2 academic institutions, the study retrospectively defined a primary outcome of greater than 50% reduction in pain for at least 6 months and secondary outcomes of ODI scores, medication reduction, and retention of active duty soldiers. Patients included needed to have refractory injection-confirmed SI joint pain. This was by either one or two SI joint injections or prognostic lumbar medial branch blocks at the L4–L5 dorsal rami. The technique of the ablation consisted of lesioning of the L4 medial branches and L5 dorsal rami with 22 gauge cannulae parallel to the nerves with confirmation by electrostimulation at 50 Hz. For S1–S3 lateral branch denervation, 22 gauge conventional electrodes or 17 gauge cooled electrodes were used and inserted perpendicularly. Results showed that 52% of patients (n = 40) had a positive primary outcome, 65% of those who received cooled RF and 47% who received conventional. The only positive predictor variable found was the use of cooled RF. Other outcome predictors studied included physical examination, prior surgery, etiology, concomitant medical illness, disability claims, number of SI joint blocks, or previous prognostic lumbar medial branch block and were shown to not have predictive value.

Cheng et al., in 2013, published the other retrospective study that compared traditional vs. cooled techniques. Its objective was to determine if cooled RFA was superior to conventional in regard to length of pain relief. The results demonstrated that there was no evidence that cooled RFA provided longer relief than traditional RFA. The study looked at 88 patients retrospectively with the primary outcome being the length of time until pain relief was reported as <50% using NRS pain scores. The time periods were 1, 3, 6, and 12 months after the procedure, and the degree of pain relief was grouped as <50%, 50–80%, and >80%. Thirty of the patients underwent traditional RFA compared to 58 receiving cooled RFA. The study showed no significant relationship between type of RFA used and length of pain relief. It was determined that both techniques on average produced >50% pain relief for 3–6 months. Inclusion criteria included patients who underwent two SI joint blocks and reported >50% pain relief for under 1 month. For the traditional RFA technique, lesioning of the L5 dorsal rami was accomplished by placing a 22 G SM-C10 (Radionics, Burlington, MA) cannula with a 5 mm active tip in a parallel fashion. The cannulae were inserted perpendicularly to target the S1–S3 lateral branches. All sites were confirmed using electrostimulation at 50 Hz. Ninety-second, 80-degree Celsius lesions were created. Cooled RFA was accomplished by inserting 17 G electrodes with 4 mm active tips using a water-cooled heating system (Pain Management SInergy System, Baylis Medical Company,

Montreal, Canada). Similar technique and placements were used as the conventional method described. The results showed that 50–60% of patients in both groups achieved >50% pain relief for 3 months. Forty percent of patients continued to have relief at 6 months. Thirty percent of patients had >50% relief at 9 months. No significant relationship was found between cooled or conventional techniques and duration of pain relief achieved.

N Patel and SP Cohen both responded to this retrospective study. They commended the authors for demonstrating the effectiveness of both conventional and cooled radiofrequency ablation in producing >50% pain reduction in 50–60% of patients. In regard to the results showing no difference in outcomes between conventional and cooled techniques, they discussed the flaws of the study. It was retrospective in nature with a small patient population, had a difference in baseline characteristics such as two physicians performing the procedures, and had no functional outcome measure as a criterion for success. By comparing cooled versus conventional ablation, they state that one could logically deduce that the larger lesion size created by the cooled technique would create better outcomes. This again demonstrates the need for additional randomized controlled trials comparing the various ablation techniques.

Tinnirello et al. [20] were the first group to compare the two types of multi-lesion probes for RFA, Simplicity III (conventional) versus SInergy (cooled), in a retrospective observational study. The study included 43 patients, 21 of which received Simplicity III denervation and 22 of which underwent SInergy ablation. Patients included in this study were required to have pain relief by an intra-articular SI joint injection. This was defined as pain relief greater than or equal to 50% up to 5 hours after the test block. Primary outcomes included NRS and ODI scores at 12 months, and secondary outcomes included average time for the RF procedure and complications. Statistically significant results were lower average NRS and ODI scores in the SInergy probe cohort versus the Simplicity III group at 6 and 12 months. There was no difference found at 1 month between groups. The procedure for the Simplicity III probe was on average 2.5 times faster than with the SInergy probe. The Simplicity III RF intervention was accomplished by inserting the probe under the sacrum, about 1 cm lateral and 1 cm under S4, lateral to the sacral foramen and medial to the joint line. Placement was confirmed by sensory stimulation at 50 Hz. A strip lesion was created by three monopolar lesions and two bipolar lesions for 90 seconds at 85 °C. For the SInergy procedure, technique was as described for the Simplicity probe, but in this case cooled RF was performed at 60 °C for 150 seconds. This study is unique in that it compared the two multi-lesion probes on the market, but it was a retrospective study and there were baseline differences between the treatment groups.

Pulsed Radiofrequency Ablation for Sacroiliac Joint Pain

Unlike conventional, cooled, or bipolar radiofrequency ablation, pulsed RF creates an electrical field. It does not cause nerve destruction in contrast to the other techniques but inhibits transmission through pain fibers (A-delta and C). It is used more commonly for neuropathic pain. It delivers short bursts of current allowing for tissue cooling in between bursts and thus creates less tissue damage around the target sites. The needle used for pulsed RF has the most electrical field around the tip; thus perpendicular placement is preferred. Conventional RFA creates a field around the needle, having maximum effect with parallel placement.

Vallejo et al. conducted one of the only studies looking at pulsed radiofrequency denervation (PRFD). It was a prospective observational study evaluating 22 patients after receiving PRFD at the medial branch of L4, posterior primary rami of L5, and lateral branches of S1 and S2. Primary outcome measures included visual analog score (VAS) and quality of life (QOL) assessments before and after the procedure. Patients included experienced 75% or greater pain relief between 1 and 8 hours after two or more diagnostic blocks performed at 2-week intervals. They then underwent repeated SJ injections, and those who did not respond (n = 22) were included in the study. For the PRFD of the aforementioned sites, a 22 G 10-cm-long, 10 mm active tip RFK needle (Radionics, Burlington, MA) was used. Placement was confirmed by stimulation at 50 Hz. The pulsed RF was performed at 45 V for 120 seconds with temperatures between 39 and 42 °C. Results demonstrated that 16 patients (72.7%) experienced >50% reduction in VAS or >80% reduction in VAS after the treatment. Pain relief was 6–9 weeks in four patients, 10–16 weeks in five patients, and 17–32 weeks in seven patients. Six patients were treatment failures. They found that a high percentage of patients (73.9%) treated with PRFD have good/excellent pain relief for >3 months.

Bipolar Radiofrequency Ablation for Sacroiliac Joint Pain

Different from monopolar radiofrequency ablation, bipolar ablation uses two electrodes placed next to each other. Current flows between these two electrodes; thus the patient does not have to be grounded. Similar to the multi-lesion probes, this current forms a continuous lesion between the two points. Forming a continuous strip lesion increases the likelihood of targeting more of the sacral lateral branches than individual ablation sites (Fig. 53.6).

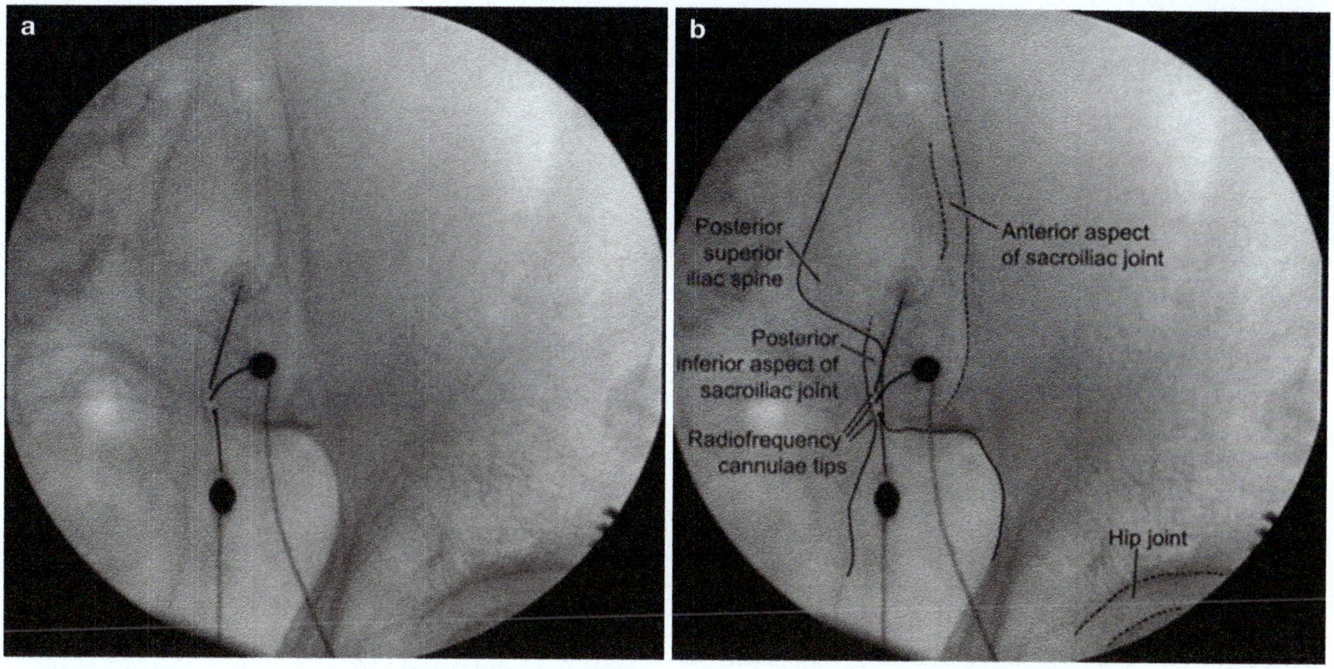

Fig. 53.6 (**a**) AP radiograph of SIJ during bipolar radiofrequency treatment. Three separate 22 gauge 10 cm SMK cannulae with 5 mm active tips are in position over the posterior-inferior aspect of the right SIJ. One cannula is attached to the active output from the RF generator and the other to the ground port. A third cannula is in position 6 mm cephalad to the second cannula. The superior limit of the treatment is limited by access to the SIJ, which is blocked by the posterior superior iliac spine. (**b**) Labeled image. (Reproduced from James P. Rathmell MD, *Atlas of Image-Guided Intervention in Regional Anesthesia and Pain Medicine*, Wolters Kluwer, 2011. With permission from Wolters Kluwer)

Burnham et al. conducted one of the only studies evaluating bipolar RFA. The prospective cohort study included nine patients. It reported a reduction of back and leg pain frequency and severity, analgesic intake, and dissatisfaction with current level of pain (1, 3, 6, 9, and 12 months after the procedure). Eight of the 9 patients were satisfied with the procedure. Patients included in the study had SI joint pain confirmed by one SI joint injection. The RF ablation consisted of strip lesions adjacent to the lateral dorsal foraminal aperture and conventional monopolar ablation at the L5 dorsal ramus. A 20 G, 10-cm-long, 10 mm exposed curved tip cannula (model PMC 20-100-10CS; Baylis Medical Company, Montreal, Quebec) with an active probe was used to ablate the L5 posterior ramus. Two 20 G 10 mm exposed RF cannulae were placed 4–6 mm apart to create bipolar strip lesions. They were perpendicularly placed 5 mm lateral to the edge of the lateral half of the dorsal sacral foraminal apertures of S1, S2, and S3 (site article here). Ninety seconds of 80 °C temperature was used to create each lesion. After the ablation, follow-up at 1, 3, 6, 9, and 12 months demonstrated a median improvement in pain intensity of 4.1 (NRS) and 17.8 reduction in disability (Oswestry disability scale). At 12 months, magnitude of these improvements was less than half.

New Radiofrequency Techniques for Sacroiliac Joint Pain

The vast majority of RFA is guided by fluoroscopy. New methods of achieving successful ablation of the SI joint have been created in the recent years, including both ultrasound-guided and endoscopic techniques.

Roberts et al. published a cadaveric study in 2017 evaluating ultrasound-guided RFA. The new method could have the potential to decrease radiation exposure and cost and increase the availability of the procedure. Bilateral sides of ten cadaveric specimens were included in the study. Ultrasound was used to identify key bony landmarks including the fourth posterior sacral foramen at the level of the sacral cornua and the first to third posterior sacral foramina and their correlating transverse sacral tubercles. Ultrasound guidance was then used to place 22 G spinal needles along the lateral sacral crest from the first to the third transverse sacral tubercles. Afterward, the posterior sacral network was exposed, and the proximity of the spinal needles was evaluated. It was determined that 18 out of 20 specimens had needles located along the lateral sacral crest and that 93% of the posterior sacral network would be captured if an RFA strip lesion was created. The results in this cadaveric study were promising, and there is an ongoing clinical study evaluating this technique.

Endoscopic RFA of the SI joint is another recent method devised for the treatment of SI joint pain. A retrospective study by Choi et al. reviewed 17 patients who underwent endoscope-guided RFA. The inclusion criteria consisted of patients whose signs and symptoms were consistent with SI joint pain, with failed conservative therapy, and who had persistent low back pain despite other pain procedures. If patients experienced 50% or greater pain relief after two diagnostic intra-articular injections performed 2 weeks apart or greater, they were included in the study. For the procedure, an 18 G needle was placed in the interosseous ligament surrounding the posterior sacroiliac joint. A guide wire was then placed through the needle, and a cannulated obturator was inserted alongside it. A 6.9 mm × 5.6 mm endoscope was then introduced through the cannula. A trigger-flex bipolar probe (Elman International, Inc.) was used to ablate the posterior sacroiliac ligament using endoscopic aid. Follow-up immediately after, and 1, 3, and 6 months post-procedure included visual analog scale and ODI. Both VAS and ODI scores decreased significantly at all time points, and 88.6% of patients reported they were satisfied with the procedure.

Pearls and Pitfalls

- The sacroiliac joint is the largest axial joint of the body with both anterior and posterior innervation. Posterior innervation is thought to be from the lateral branches of the S1, S2, and S3 dorsal rami along with the medial branches of the L4 and L5 dorsal rami. These are the targets of SI joint RFA, whereas anterior innervation is inaccessible.
- Diagnosis of SI joint pain is challenging with no definitive history or physical exam findings. Most use a positive response to joint injection as the standard for diagnosis.
- RFA for the SI joint is a treatment option for those with chronic and refractory SI joint pain.
- There are multiple modalities of RFA for the sacroiliac joint, including conventional, cooled, pulsed, and bipolar.
- Multi-lesion probes create continuous strip lesions with only a single entry point. The Simplicity III probe uses conventional RFA, whereas the SInergy probe uses cooled RFA.
- There is a large need for determining long-term outcomes of radiofrequency ablation of the sacroiliac joint and the type of RFA that provides the best pain relief for patients. Currently there are two prospective RCTs comparing cooled radiofrequency ablation vs. sham, and there are retrospective studies comparing cooled vs. conventional RFA. No gold standard for RFA of the SI joint exists.

Recommended Reading

1. Burnham RS, Yasui Y. An alternate method of radiofrequency neurotomy of the sacroiliac joint: a pilot study of the effect on pain, function, and satisfaction. Reg Anesth Pain Med. 2007;32(1):12–9.
2. Cheng J, Pope JE, Dalton JE, Cheng O, Bensitel A. Comparative outcomes of cooled versus traditional radiofrequency ablation of the lateral branches for sacroiliac joint pain. Clin J Pain. 2013;29:132–7.
3. Choi WS, Kim JS, Ryu KS, Hur JW, Seong JH, Cho HJ. Endoscopic radiofrequency ablation of the sacroiliac joint complex in the treatment of chronic low back pain: a preliminary study of feasibility and efficacy of a novel technique. Biomed Res Int. 2016. https://doi.org/10.1155/2016/2834259.
4. Cohen SP, Hurley RW, Buckenmaier CC 3rd, Kurihara C, Morlando B, Dragovich A. Randomized placebo-controlled study evaluating lateral branch radiofrequency denervation for sacroiliac joint pain. Anesthesiology. 2008;109(2):279–88.
5. Cohen SP, Strassels SA, Kurihara C, Crooks MT, Erdek MA, Forsythe A, Marcuson M. Outcome predictors for sacroiliac joint (lateral branch) radiofrequency denervation. Reg Anesth Pain Med. 2009;34(3):206–14.
6. Cohen SP, Chen Y, Neufeld NJ. Sacroiliac joint pain: a comprehensive review of epidemiology, diagnosis and treatment. Expert Rev Neurother. 2013;13:99–116.
7. Gevargez A, Groenemeyer D, Schirp S, Braun M. CT guided percutaneous radiofrequency denervation of the sacroiliac joint. Eur Radiol. 2002;12:1360–5.
8. Gilligan J, Shih JC, Cai VL, Hirsch JA, Rodrigues C, Irani ZD. Novel single puncture approach for simplicity 3 sacral plexus radiofrequency ablation: technical note. Pain Physician. 2016;19(4):E643–8.
9. Gilligan C, Malik OS, Hirsch JA. Radiofrequency ablation for sacroiliac joint pain. In: Marcia S, Saba L, editors. Radiofrequency treatments on the spine. Cham: Springer; 2017.
10. Hansen H, Manchikanti L, Simopoulous TT, Christo PJ, Gupta S, Smith HS, Hameed H, Cohen SP. A systematic evaluation of the therapeutic effectiveness of sacroiliac joint interventions. Pain Physician. 2012;15:E247–78.
11. Mitchell B, Macphail T, Vivian D, Verrills P, Barnard A. Radiofrequency neurotomy for sacroiliac joint pain: a prospective study. Surg Sci. 2015;06(07):265–72.
12. Patel N. Twelve-month follow-up of a randomized trial assessing cooled radiofrequency denervation as a treatment for sacroiliac region pain. Pain Pract. 2016;16(2):154–67.
13. Patel N, Cohen SP. Response to: Cheng et al Comparative outcomes of cooled versus traditional radiofrequency ablation of the lateral branches for sacroiliac joint pain. Clin J Pain. 2013;29:132–137. Clin J Pain. 29(12):1097–8.
14. Patel N, Gross A, Brown L, Gekht G. A randomized, placebo-controlled study to assess the efficacy of lateral branch neurotomy for chronic sacroiliac joint pain. Pain Med. 2012;13:383–98.
15. Roberts SL, Burnham RS, Agur AM, Loh EY. A cadaveric study evaluating the feasibility of an ultrasound-guided diagnostic block and radiofrequency ablation technique for sacroiliac joint pain. Reg Anesth Pain Med. 2017;42(1):69–74.
16. Rupert MP, Lee M, Manchikanti L, Datta S, Cohen SP. Evaluation of sacroiliac joint interventions: a systematic appraisal of the literature. Pain Physician. 2009;12(2):399–418.
17. Schmidt PC, Pino CA, Vorenkamp KE. Sacroiliac joint radiofrequency ablation with a multilesion probe: a case series of 60 patients. Anesth Analg. 2014;119:460–2.
18. Simopoulos TT, Manchikanti L, Gupta S, Aydin SM, Kim CH, Solanki D, Nampiaparampil DE, Singh V, Staats PS, Hirsch JA. Systematic review of the diagnostic accuracy and therapeu-

tic effectiveness of sacroiliac joint interventions. Pain Physician. 2015;18(5):E713–56.

19. Stelzer W, Aiglesberger M, Stelzer D, Stelzer V. Use of cooled radiofrequency lateral branch neurotomy for the treatment of sacroiliac joint-mediated low back pain: a large case series. Pain Med. 2013;14:29–35.
20. Tinnirello A, Barbieri S, Todeschini M, Marchesini M. Conventional (Simplicity III) and cooled (SInergy) radiofrequency for sacroiliac joint denervation: one-year retrospective study comparing two devices. Pain Med. 2017;0:1–14. https://doi.org/10.1093/pm/pnw333.
21. Vallejo R, Benyamin RM, Kramer J, Stanton G, Joseph NJ. Pulsed radiofrequency denervation for the treatment of sacroiliac joint syndrome. Pain Med. 2006;7(5):429–34.
22. van Tilburg CW, Schuurmans FA, Stronks DL, Groeneweg JG, Huygen FJ. Randomized sham-controlled double-blind multicenter clinical trial to ascertain the effect of percutaneous radiofrequency treatment for sacroiliac joint pain. Clin J Pain. 2016;32(11):921–6.

Sacroiliac Joint Fusion

54

Edna Gouveia, Daniel R. Denis, Taylor Brittan, Joshua Hanna, and Maged Guirguis

Introduction

Sacroiliac joint (SIJ) fusion is quickly becoming a prominent treatment modality for SIJ dysfunction, defined as "pain and disability resulting from abnormal function of the joint, and its effects on quality of life." Moreover, SIJ dysfunction is a common source of low back pain (LBP), and SIJ fusion in the proper surgical candidate can offer long-term relief when more conservative measures have failed. The lifetime incidence of LBP in the general population approaches 80 to 90%. LBP is the most common type of pain reported by adults, one of the top three causes of reduced quality-adjusted life years (QALYs), and the sixth most common cause of loss of global disability-adjusted life years (DALYs). As such, the epidemic of chronic LBP in modern society should not be understated, with an annual loss of approximately 83 million healthy life years.

In the recent past, it has been shown that the SIJ is a major pain generator implicated in the pathogenesis of LBP. The most recent study by Sembrano and Polly in 2009 attributes SIJ dysfunction to as much as 25% of patients diagnosed with low back pain. This picture is further complicated by the fact that up to 40% of patients with a prior history of lumbar fusion re-present with SIJ dysfunction. The management in LBP incurs significant economic burden at an estimated 3-year cost of $1.6 billion USD per 100,000 commercial covered lives and a 5-year estimated cost of $270 million USD for Medicare beneficiaries. Considering that as much as one-fourth of this burden may be attributable to SIJ dysfunction, very real consideration needs to be taken into the diagnosis and management of this condition.

Background and Historical Perspective

Historically, the treatment of choice for SIJ pain has been tenuously established, even despite decades of study. The earliest accounts of the anatomical and biomechanical complexity of SIJ anatomy and its derivative pathology was first described by Meckel in 1816 as an articulation with smooth surfaces in the young that became rough with age. Cohen et al. later expanded on this observation, stating that before the age of 50, the normal SIJ possesses smooth synovial surfaces, while those age greater than 50 displayed a higher incidence of coarsened and eroded joint spaces. Numerous research studies have been conducted to expand on the mobility of the joint, with various authors arriving at differing conclusions; however in 1940 the SIJ was first described by Kopsch as an intermediate-type joint possessing both synarthrotic and diarthrotic attributes. In 1949, the SIJ was more accurately described as a movement-limited diarthro-amphiarthrosis by Testut and Latarjet. In keeping with this more accurate description, the SIJ is largely restricted in movement, with the exception of pregnancy. Today, it continues to be widely accepted that the SIJ is an extremely limited range of motion with minor movements possessing the ability to destabilize and/or contribute to pain syndromes and degenerative changes.

E. Gouveia · T. Brittan · J. Hanna
Neurosurgery Department, Ochsner Health System, New Orleans, LA, USA
e-mail: v-egouveia@ochsner.org; v-tbrittan@ochsner.org

D. R. Denis (✉)
Ochsner Health System, Kenner, LA, USA

Neurosurgery Department, Ochsner Health System, New Orleans, LA, USA
e-mail: daniel.denis@ochsner.org

M. Guirguis
Interventional Pain Management, Department of Anesthesiology & Critical Care Medicine, Ochsner Health System, New Orleans, LA, USA

University of Queensland Ochsner Medical School, Brisbane, QLD, Australia

Louisiana State University School of Medicine, New Orleans, LA, USA
e-mail: mguirguis@ochsner.org

T. R. Deer et al. (eds.), *Deer's Treatment of Pain*, https://doi.org/10.1007/978-3-030-12281-2_54

Structurally, the SIJ possesses the unique quality of being characterized as both diarthrotic and amphiarthrotic. This distinction is attributed to the fact that the anterior-inferior two-thirds of the joint is a true synovial joint, while the posterior-superior third is a syndesmosis that is strongly attached to the surrounding stabilizing ligaments and muscles. The iliac side is convex at S2, whereas the sacral surface is concave, with numerous anatomically significant ridges and depressions. Biomechanically, the joint forms a C-shape with two lever arms that interlock at the level of S_2 and gives rise to the characteristic "keystone-like" shape. This shape is essential to the creation of a *form closure*—a term that describes the inherent stability of the joint due to the intrinsic anatomy of the joint and the friction created by surrounding structures. The combination of muscles, ligaments, fascia, and neurological innervation contribute to *force closure*, which is defined as the dynamic stabilization of the joint by extrinsic forces working across it. Cadaveric studies have demonstrated that most of the SIJ innervation comes from the lateral branches of S1, S2, and S3, with some additional contributions from L5 and S4 in less than 10% of the time. It should be noted that the complex biomechanical mechanisms working across this joint make it such that a disruption to any one of the forces contributing to the stability of the joint may cause dysfunction and pain generation. Therefore, it is necessary for the physician to appropriately identify the specific pain generator prior to proceeding to intervention.

Clinically, patients with LBP due to SIJ dysfunction often complain of pain below the L5 vertebral body. Pain from the SIJ localizes to the gluteal region in 94% of patients. Referred pain may be experienced in the lower lumbar region (72%), groin (14%), upper lumbar region (6%), abdomen (2%), or lower limb in 28% of patients with 12% experiencing pain in the foot. SIJ pain may also disturb a patient's sitting posture or sleep patterns. Patients with SIJ pain often present with a history of chronic LBP, trauma, arthritis, recent childbirth in women, or a previous long-standing lumbosacral fusion. Of note, the three symptoms most sensitive for SIJ dysfunction are (1) pain while sitting on the affected side, (2) ipsilateral pain standing on one leg, and (3) frequent stumbling due to "give way" of the affected leg.

Uses and Indications

The possible pain generators in the lumbosacral region in patients complaining of LBP include the spine, the hip joints, and the SIJ. There is no universally accepted "gold standard" for diagnosing SIJ dysfunction, and the use of imaging technologies has limited diagnostic value in localizing the major pain generators. Where medical imaging may not elucidate the source of LBP, it does have value in ruling out other pathologies in the presence of "red flag" symptoms such as weight loss, night pain, or recent trauma.

The following six clinical tests have been used to evaluate SIJ dysfunction:

1. Compression test (approximation test)
2. Distraction test (gapping test)
3. Patrick's sign (flexion abduction external rotation test)
4. Gaenslen test (pelvic torsion test)
5. Thigh thrust test (posterior shear test)
6. Fortin's finger test

A recent meta-analysis showed that if three or more of the above tests were positive, there exists significant positive predictive value in diagnosing pain originating from the SIJ. Dual comparative local anesthetic joint blocks with at least 70% pain relief are considered a validated diagnostic test for SI joint pain. A single SIJ diagnostic block with at least 75% pain relief has also been reported in multiple studies to measure the prevalence of SIJ pain.

Treatment of SIJ pain begins with a multidisciplinary approach, with conservative management being the first step in treatment with the major objective to address the underlying etiology. Options include anti-inflammatory pharmacological therapy, cognitive-behavioral therapy, physical therapy, exercise therapy, and rehabilitation, as well as psychiatric evaluation. Physical therapy can improve SI joint pain by increasing force closure. Pelvic stabilization with a pelvic belt, strengthening, and self-bracing exercises have been shown to improve force closure and may provide SI joint pain relief.

If pain persists beyond conservative therapeutic measures, then interventional pain management may be initiated. Up to now, the level of evidence for SIJ intraarticular or periarticular steroid injections is mainly limited to short-term outcome (3 months), and the effectiveness results are conflicting between different studies.

To provide longer-term pain relief, either SIJ radiofrequency neurotomy (RFN) or minimally invasive (MIS) SIJ fusion may be offered to patients with SIJ dysfunction who have failed conservative management. These patients must present without abnormal MRI finding to explain their pain. The diagnosis of SI joint dysfunction is supported by at least three positive provocative maneuvers during physical examination and more than 75% pain relief, sustained for at least 2 hours in a 10-hour period, after a single SIJ block using 2% lidocaine done under fluoroscopic guidance.

Evidence for Efficacy

SIJ Radiofrequency Neurotomy

The innervation pattern of the sacroiliac joint is complex. Innervation of the anterior SI joint is even more controversial. Early studies suggested the obturator nerve, the superior gluteal nerve, and the lumbosacral trunk; however, more recent studies show that the main sensory input of anterior SI joint is L2-S2 ventral rami. The posterior sacral innervation of the SIJ is mainly supplied by S1, S2, and S3 and the greatest concentration of fibers crossing the lateral sacral crest between S2 and S3.

Radiofrequency neurotomy (RFN, also called radiofrequency ablation) is a minimally invasive procedure in which radiofrequency currents are applied through an electrode to ablate the S1-S3 lateral branches and the L5 dorsal ramus. In doing so, a thermal lesion that interrupts the pain signal pathways to the brain is created. Currently, both conventional and cooled RFN are being used. Cooled radiofrequency ablation (C-RFA) is a more novel technique whereby the temperature of the probe is actively decreased by internal cold irrigation, thus allowing a higher energy that results in a larger lesion. When compared to conventional RFN, cooled RFN can ablate nerve endings in a larger territory and thus has the potential to be more effective. Two randomized controlled trials comparing cooled RFN vs placebo demonstrated a success rate varying between 38 and 57% at 6 months for cooled RFN. Observational studies also demonstrated success rate varying from 40% to 71% at 6 months for both conventional and cooled RFN. The effectiveness of conventional and cooled RFN at 9 and 12 months is more limited with some studies reporting loss of effectiveness at 12 months. Based on the available data, there is no enough evidence in the literature to support clinical superiority between traditional and cooled RFN. A retrospective study on 88 patients revealed comparable effectiveness between conventional and cool RFN with >50% pain reduction in the majority of patients between groups at 3 and 6 months. However, their two groups were not identical in baseline variables. The patients in C-RFA group were younger but had undergone more spine surgeries.

Minimally Invasive SIJ Fusion

Minimally invasive SIJ fusion is a surgical treatment aimed at stabilizing the SIJ to reduce pain and disability and improve quality of life. In a recent randomized controlled trial called Investigation of Sacroiliac Fusion Treatment (INSITE), minimally invasive SIJ fusion, using triangular titanium implants (iFuse Implant System, SI-BONE®, San Jose, CA), has been shown superior to nonsurgical treatments in managing SIJ dysfunction at 6 months (81.4% vs 26.1% success rate), and the results in the surgical group were sustained at 1 year and 2 years of follow-up. Similarly, a number of studies have shown favorable patient-reported to nonsurgical treatments in managing SIJ pain outcomes following SIJ fusion. In addition to MIS, the studies also included open approaches (see Table 54.1).

Technical Aspects of MIS SIJ Fusion

Prior to the procedure, radiology imaging is reviewed to identify potential SIJ anatomical abnormalities. Electromyography to nonsurgical treatments in managing SIJ neuromonitoring can be used as an adjunct to avoid nerve injury during implant placement. Under general anesthesia, the patient is positioned prone on a Jackson four-post table.

Using fluoroscopy in lateral projection, the incision is planned. The surgery is performed on the opposite site of the image intensifier to provide increased room for instrument manipulation by the operator to nonsurgical treatments in managing SIJ. For bilateral SIJ fusion, bilateral c-arms are used. The lateral view should include the L5 vertebra, the L5-S1 disc space, and the sacrum. The orientation of the fluoroscopy picture should mirror the prone position of the patient to facilitate the positioning of the k-wire and implant.

A vertically oriented line is drawn first using the anatomical alar line, while a second line, more horizontally oriented

Table 54.1 Pain outcomes after SIJ fusion

Study	Study design	Type of fusion	*N*	Age mean (SD or range)	Follow-up months (range)	Outcomes measure (VAS and/or ODI)	VAS mean difference	ODI mean difference
Duhon (2013)	Prospective	MIS	33	50.2 (12.6)	6	VAS/ODI	36.33, $p < 0.00001$	8.38, $p < 0.00001$
Khurana (2009)	Retrospective	Open	15	48.7 (37.3–62.6)	17 (9–39)	N/A		N/A
Ledonio (2014)	Retrospective	Open/MIS	22	51 (9.4)/47.9 (13.1)	13 (11–33)/15 (12–26)	ODI	N/A	2.53, $p < 0.00001$
Mason (2013)	Prospective	Open	55	57.9 (30–86)	36.2 (12–84)	VAS	26.74, $p < 0.00001$	N/A
Rudolf (2014)	Prospective	MIS	17	58.0 (13.6)	60	VAS	46.60, $p < 0.00001$	N/A
Sachs et al. (2014)	Prospective	MIS	244	57.7 (30–89)	16 (12–26)	VAS	49.15, $p < 0.00001$	N/A

Source: Lingutla et al. (2016)

MIS minimally invasive surgery, *N* number of subjects, *N/A* value not applicable to study, *ODI* Oswestry disability index, *SD* standard deviation, *VAS* visual analog scale

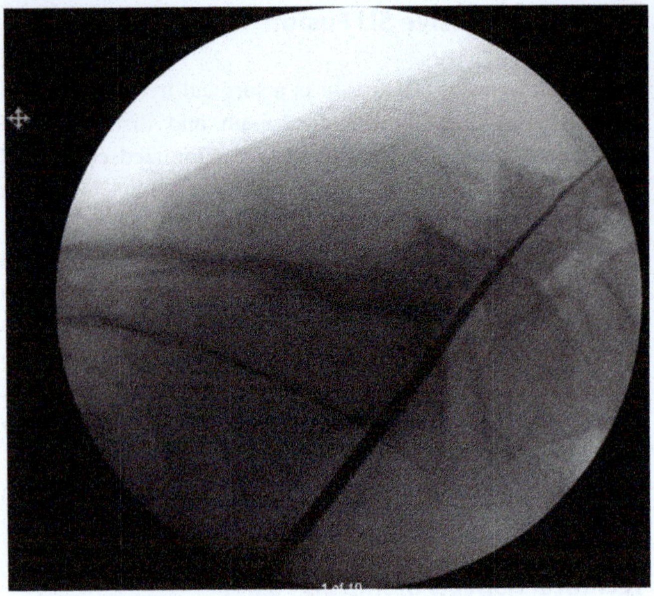

Fig. 54.1 Fluoroscopy in lateral view. A metallic marker is positioned in line with the alar line

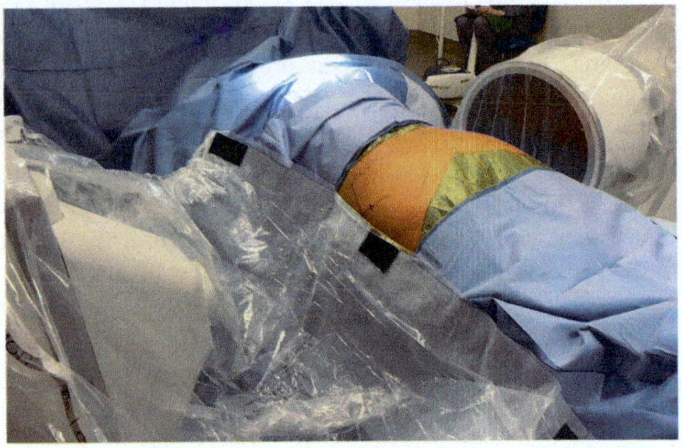

Fig. 54.2 The patient is positioned prone and skin marking has been done

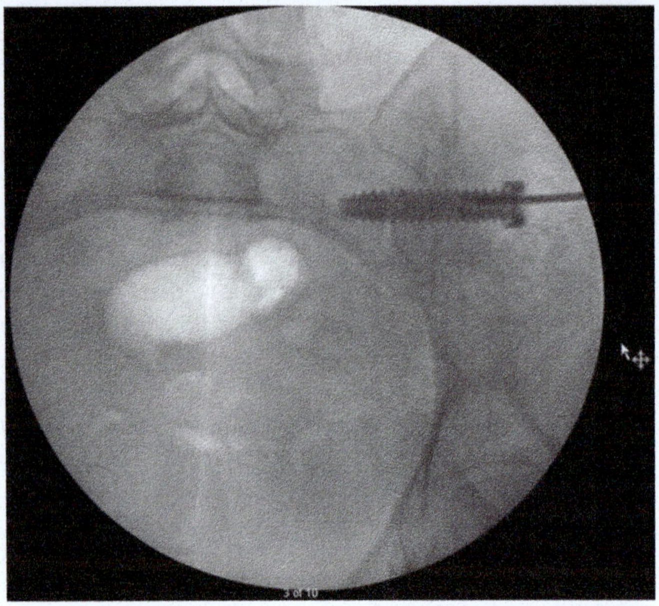

Fig. 54.3 Fluoroscopy in inlet view. This view is used to make sure that the trajectory will not violate the ventral sacral cortical surface. At the end of the surgery, the three implants should be superposed on this view. In this example one implant has already been installed

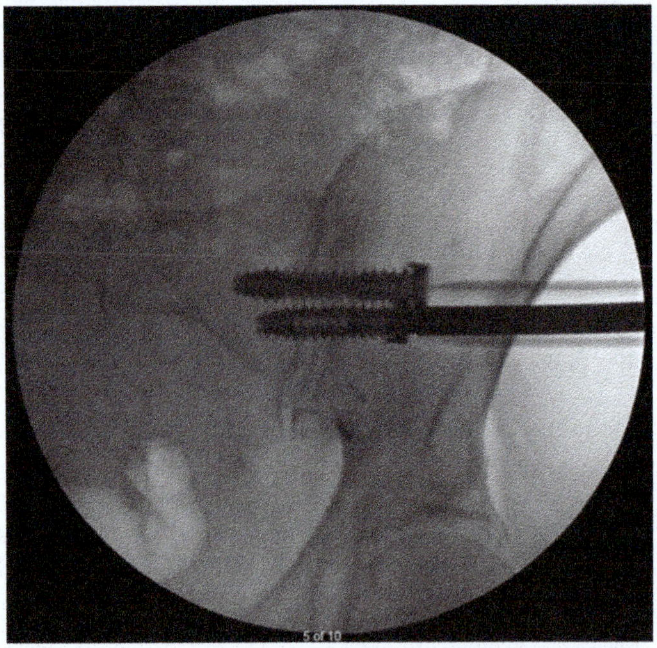

Fig. 54.4 Fluoroscopy in outlet view. Advancement of the k-wire through the SIJ, drilling, and placement of the implants is done using this view. The S1 and S2 foramen are well visualized. In this example a second implant is being installed

line to nonsurgical treatments in managing SIJ, is drawn based on the ventral aspect of the sacral cortical bone (Figs. 54.1 and 54.2). After local anesthesia, a 3–4 cm incision is carried along the horizontal line, caudal to the intersection of both lines.

An orthostatic retractor is placed and a sharp k-wire is driven through the gluteus fascia and muscle. On fluoroscopy, the tip of the k-wire is positioned just caudal to the alar line and superior to the ventral cortical to nonsurgical treatments in managing SIJ sacral line. Using the mallet, the k-wire is driven into the iliac bone to a depth of about 1 cm. The trajectory of the k-wire is then verified using first the inlet view to make sure that the implant will not violate to nonsurgical treatments in managing SIJ the pelvic surface (Fig. 54.3). The outlet view is then used to drive the k-wire across the SIJ using a mallet or a powered mini-driver (Figs. 54.4 and 54.5). Resistance is felt in most

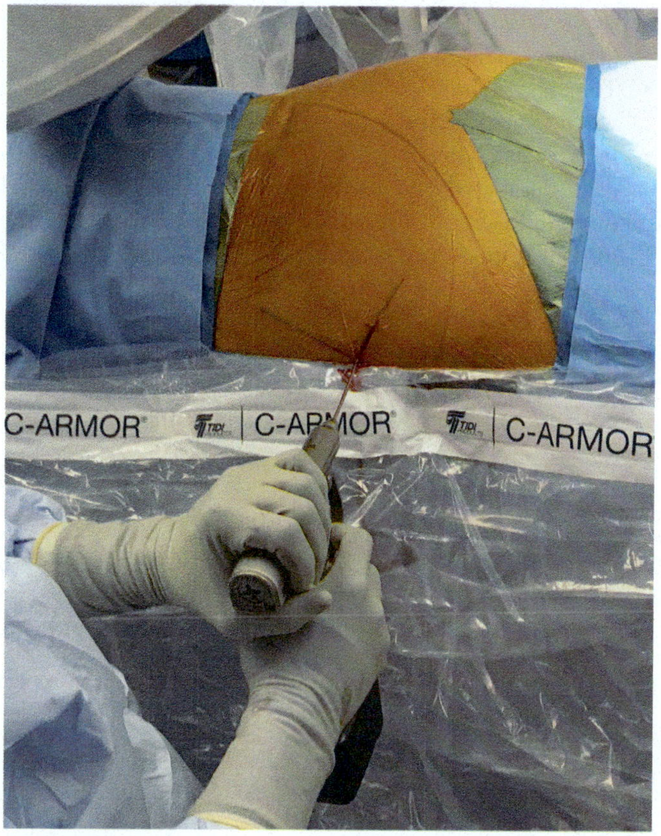

Fig. 54.5 The k-wire is driven through the SIJ with a powered mini-driver

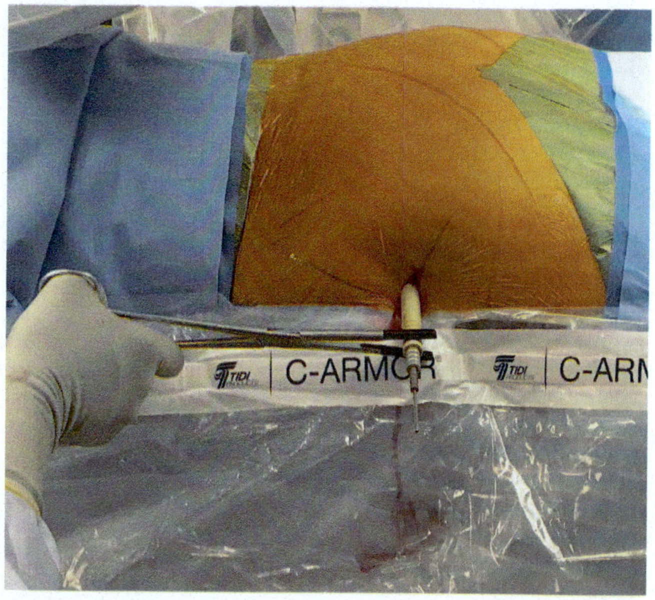

Fig. 54.6 Serial dilation of the gluteus muscle

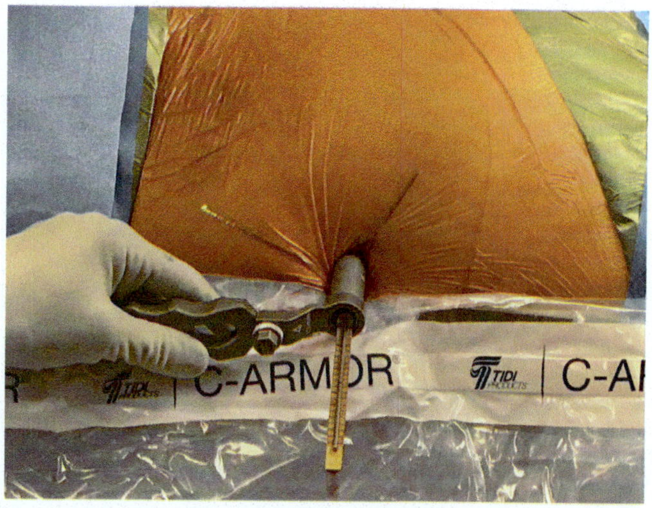

Fig. 54.7 Determination of implant length using the depth gauge

patients when the k-wire is driven through the SI joint. For the first implant, these authors recommend positioning the tip of the k-wire superolateral to the S1 foramen in the sacrum. The tip of the second k-wire will be positioned lateral to the S1 foramen, and the third k-wire will be inferolateral to the S1 foramen.

After placing the first k-wire, dilation tubes are inserted over the k-wire (Fig. 54.6), and a final handheld tubular retractor is maintained in position. A k-wire depth gauge is introduced over the k-wire, advanced until it reaches the iliac surface, and the length of the implant is determined (Fig. 54.7). Using the outlet view, a hole is created over the k-wire using a drill bit provided by the implant manufacturer. Care is taken to assure that the tip of the k-wire is not being driven deeper into the sacrum in order to avoid penetrating the S1 foramen or the spinal canal. Some bone autograft is harvested in the thread of the drill bit by maintaining gentle back pressure on the drill while keeping the drill bit rotating clockwise. By performing this maneuver, care must be taken so that the k-wire is not accidentally pulled out by the drill bit. To avoid this, a longer blunt k-wire may be gently pushed by the assistant through the drill and drill bit to keep the original k-wire immobile in the sacrum. If the k-wire is being accidentally pulled from the sacrum, it can be reintroduced into the hole using fluoroscopy or manual palpation. Finally, the hydroxyapatite-coated screw implant is loaded with the bone autograft and inserted over the k-wire in the proper position across the SIJ (Fig. 54.4). The same procedure is repeated just caudally to the first implant and again to place three implants (Figs. 54.8 and 54.9). The wound is irrigated; the gluteus fascia and the skin are closed with sutures.

SIJ fusions are generally performed in an outpatient setting. Patients are instructed to resume their normal physical activity as soon as postoperative day 3.

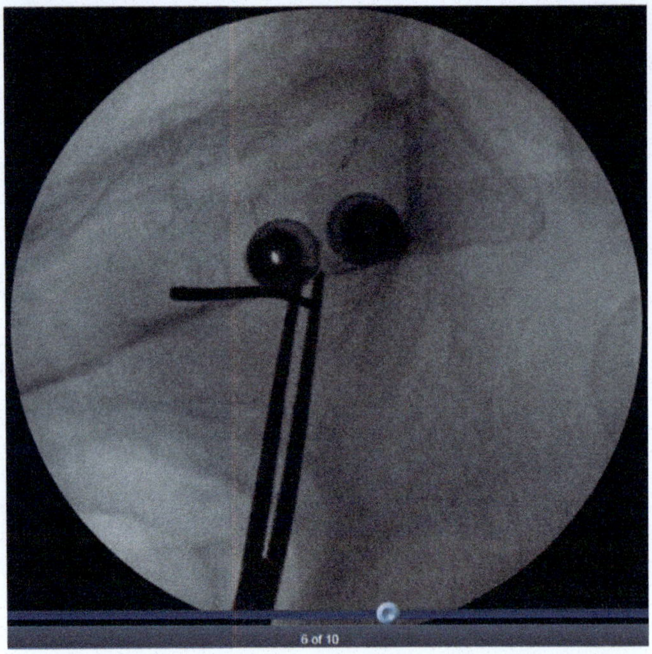

Fig. 54.8 Fluoroscopy in lateral view. A k-wire is positioned caudal to the second implant

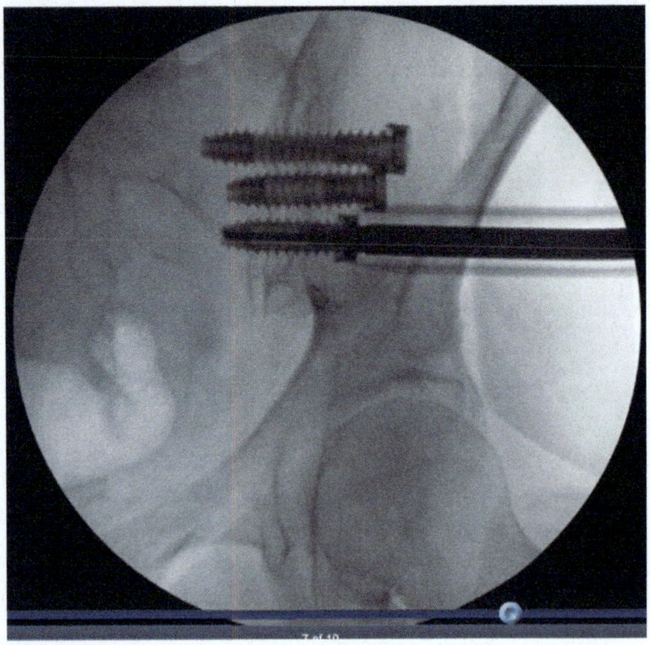

Fig. 54.9 Fluoroscopy in outlet view. Positioning of the third implant through the SI joint

Pearls and Pitfalls

- Adequate fluoroscopic images and consistency is required to position the implants appropriately.
- Vigilance must be taken when advancing the second k-wire as to not violate the S1 foramen. It is safer to keep a safe zone between the S1 foramen and the second k-wire knowing that a smaller implant will be used.
- The sharp k-wire can be exchanged with a blunt k-wire when the S1 foramen is at risk of being penetrated.
- In the lateral radiographic view, positioning the k-wires caudal to the alar line and just dorsal to the ventral cortical sacral line will ensure good positioning of the implants through the SI joint. A more dorsal entry point, i.e., in line with the sacral canal, will cause the implant to be dorsal to the SIJ.
- Although minimal blood loss is usually encountered, abnormal blood loss during the procedure can generally be controlled with manual pressure or hemostatic agent such as Gelfoam powder soaked in thrombin.

Recommended Reading

1. Ackerman SJ, Polly DW Jr, Knight T, Holt T, Cummings J. Management of sacroiliac joint disruption and degenerative sacroiliitis with nonoperative care is medical resource-intensive and costly in a United States commercial payer population. Clinicoecon Outcomes Res. 2014;6:63–74.
2. Bernard TN Jr, Kirkaldy-Willis WH. Recognizing specific characteristics of nonspecific low back pain. Clin Orthop Relat Res. 1987;217:266–80.
3. Cohen SP. Sacroiliac joint pain: a comprehensive review of anatomy, diagnosis, and treatment. Anesth Analg. 2005;101:1440–53.
4. Cohen SP, Hurley RW, Buckenmaier CC 3rd, Kurihara C, Morlando B, Dragovich A. Randomized placebo-controlled study evaluating lateral branch radiofrequency denervation for sacroiliac joint pain. Anesthesiology. 2008;109:279–88.
5. Dall BE, Eden SV. Outcomes of bilateral sacroiliac joint fusions and the importance of understanding potential coexisting lumbosacral pathology that might also require surgical treatment. Acta Orthop Belg. 2015;81:233–9.
6. DePalma MJ, Ketchum JM, Saullo TR. Etiology of chronic low back pain in patients having undergone lumbar fusion. Pain Med. 2011;12:732–9.
7. Deyo RA, Mirza SK, Martin BI. Back pain prevalence and visit rates: estimates from U.S. national surveys, 2002. Spine (Phila Pa 1976). 2006;31:2724–7.
8. Grob KR, Neuhuber WL, Kissling RO. Innervation of the sacroiliac joint of the human. Z Rheumatol. 1995;54:117–22.
9. Hogan DR, Zaslavsky AM, Hammitt JK, Salomon JA. Flexible epidemiological model for estimates and short-term projections in generalised HIV/AIDS epidemics. Sex Transm Infect. 2010;86(Suppl 2):ii84–92.
10. Liliang PC, Lu K, Liang CL, Tsai YD, Wang KW, Chen HJ. Sacroiliac joint pain after lumbar and lumbosacral fusion: findings using dual sacroiliac joint blocks. Pain Med. 2011;12:565–70.
11. Luukkainen R, Nissila M, Asikainen E, Sanila M, Lehtinen K, Alanaatu A, et al. Periarticular corticosteroid treatment of the sacroiliac joint in patients with seronegative spondylarthropathy. Clin Exp Rheumatol. 1999;17:88–90.
12. Luukkainen RK, Wennerstrand PV, Kautiainen HH, Sanila MT, Asikainen EL. Efficacy of periarticular corticosteroid treatment of the sacroiliac joint in non-spondylarthropathic patients with chronic low back pain in the region of the sacroiliac joint. Clin Exp Rheumatol. 2002;20:52–4.

13. Maigne JY, Aivaliklis A, Pfefer F. Results of sacroiliac joint double block and value of sacroiliac pain provocation tests in 54 patients with low back pain. Spine (Phila Pa 1976). 1996;21:1889–92.
14. Murray CJ, Vos T, Lozano R, Naghavi M, Flaxman AD, Michaud C, et al. Disability-adjusted life years (DALYs) for 291 diseases and injuries in 21 regions, 1990–2010: a systematic analysis for the Global Burden of Disease Study 2010. Lancet. 2012;380:2197–223.
15. Patel N, Gross A, Brown L, Gekht G. A randomized, placebo-controlled study to assess the efficacy of lateral branch neurotomy for chronic sacroiliac joint pain. Pain Med. 2012;13:383–98.
16. Roberts SL, Burnham RS, Ravichandiran K, Agur AM, Loh EY. Cadaveric study of sacroiliac joint innervation: implications for diagnostic blocks and radiofrequency ablation. Reg Anesth Pain Med. 2014;39:456–64.
17. Sachs D, Capobianco R, Cher D, Holt T, Gundanna M, Graven T, et al. One-year outcomes after minimally invasive sacroiliac joint fusion with a series of triangular implants: a multicenter, patient-level analysis. Med Devices (Auckl). 2014;7:299–304.
18. Sembrano JN, Polly DW Jr. How often is low back pain not coming from the back? Spine (Phila Pa 1976). 2009;34:E27–32.
19. Simopoulos TT, Manchikanti L, Gupta S, Aydin SM, Kim CH, Solanki D, et al. Systematic review of the diagnostic accuracy and therapeutic effectiveness of sacroiliac joint interventions. Pain Physician. 2015;18:E713–56.
20. Smith AG, Capobianco R, Cher D, Rudolf L, Sachs D, Gundanna M, et al. Open versus minimally invasive sacroiliac joint fusion: a multi-center comparison of perioperative measures and clinical outcomes. Ann Surg Innov Res. 2013;7:14.
21. Snijders CJ, Vleeming A, Stoeckart R. Transfer of lumbosacral load to iliac bones and legs Part 2: Loading of the sacroiliac joints when lifting in a stooped posture. Clin Biomech (Bristol, Avon). 1993;8:295–301.
22. Soisson O, Lube J, Germano A, Hammer KH, Josten C, Sichting F, et al. Pelvic belt effects on pelvic morphometry, muscle activity and body balance in patients with sacroiliac joint dysfunction. PLoS One. 2015;10:e0116739.
23. Szadek KM, van der Wurff P, van Tulder MW, Zuurmond WW, Perez RS. Diagnostic validity of criteria for sacroiliac joint pain: a systematic review. J Pain. 2009;10:354–68.
24. Vos T, Flaxman AD, Naghavi M, Lozano R, Michaud C, Ezzati M, et al. Years lived with disability (YLDs) for 1160 sequelae of 289 diseases and injuries 1990–2010: a systematic analysis for the Global Burden of Disease Study 2010. Lancet. 2012;380:2163–96.
25. Young S, Aprill C, Laslett M. Correlation of clinical examination characteristics with three sources of chronic low back pain. Spine J. 2003;3:460–5.
26. Zaidi HA, Montoure AJ, Dickman CA. Surgical and clinical efficacy of sacroiliac joint fusion: a systematic review of the literature. J Neurosurg Spine. 2015;23:59–66.

Caudal Epidural Injection

55

Atul A. Walia, Hiep Tran, and Dan DuBose

Introduction

Caudal epidural injections have been used in medicine for many years and extensively in pediatrics, obstetrics, and interventional pain medicine. Obstetric anesthesia has largely replaced this technique with lumbar epidural catheters for labor, but pediatric anesthesia and pain management still use it in daily practice. Pediatric anesthesiologists often use local anesthetics in caudal epidural nerve blocks for analgesia in surgeries below the umbilicus. Pain management physicians typically inject local anesthetics with or without corticosteroids in the caudal epidural space to treat pain from lumbar spinal stenosis, failed back surgery syndrome, lumbar radiculopathy, and other etiologies of low back pain.

Interventional pain management is a field that is rapidly advancing in technology and techniques. The caudal epidural injection is one of the oldest epidural injection techniques, and it continues to be used in pain management practices today. The physician must understand the anatomy, limitations, risks, and benefits before proceeding. Although the injection site is below the dural sac, inadvertent dural puncture and intrathecal injection are still a risk. Other risks include intravascular injection, bleeding, infection, epidural hematoma, and postdural puncture headache. Caudal epidural injections should not be performed in patients with an active infection, pilonidal cyst, or certain coagulopathies. There are situations where patients can discontinue their anticoagulation medications prior to caudal epidural injection.

The caudal approach to the epidural space offers several advantages compared to other epidural injections. It is considered safer because the injection occurs below the level of the dural sac, which makes intrathecal injection less likely. Well-defined landmarks make identifying the injection site possible without fluoroscopy, which is helpful for physicians who do not have fluoroscopy in their office or are traveling overseas for humanitarian work. Patients with previous back surgeries often have altered anatomy or implanted hardware that make epidural injections difficult to perform, and the caudal epidural injection provides a safe alternative for these patients.

Background and Historical Perspective

Caudal epidural injections have been used in medicine for many years. The technique was first described in the early 1900s for the treatment of sciatic pain and low back pain as well as in urologic procedures. The first anesthetic used was cocaine, which had some unpleasant side effects. Over time, newer local anesthetics were developed with improved side effect profiles. Corticosteroids were first administered through caudal epidural injections in the 1950s. Today, pain management physicians perform caudal epidural injections with local anesthetics with or without corticosteroids.

Multiple approaches to the epidural space are available. Interlaminar injections deliver the medication close to the presumed site of pathology. Transforaminal injections are considered to be target-specific and require the lowest volume of medication to reach the site of pathology. Caudal epidural injections are considered to be the safest and easiest, with the least likelihood of unintentional dural puncture. They require larger volumes of medication and can be performed without fluoroscopy if needed.

Chronic low back pain is one of the most common causes of pain in the United States. It is estimated that more than

A. A. Walia (✉)
Integris Pain Management, University of Oklahoma Health Sciences Center, Oklahoma City, OK, USA

H. Tran
Department of Anesthesiology, Baylor Scott and White Health, Temple, TX, USA

Texas A&M University College of Medicine, Killeen, TX, USA

D. DuBose
Department of Anesthesiology, Baylor Scott and White Health, Temple, TX, USA

T. R. Deer et al. (eds.), *Deer's Treatment of Pain*, https://doi.org/10.1007/978-3-030-12281-2_55

100 million people suffer from chronic low back pain. Billions of dollars are spent on the diagnosis and treatment of back pain every year. Physical therapy, chiropractors, massage therapy, exercise, medications, procedures, and surgical procedures are just a few of the many treatment modalities employed to tackle this problem. For many patients, a surgical procedure is the last resort after all conservative options have been exhausted. Caudal epidural injections can obviate the need for surgery, and for others, they are a bridge to a surgical intervention.

There has been an explosion in the number of epidural injections performed by physicians during the last 20 years. One of the earliest specialties to use caudal epidural injections was obstetrics. Initially, analgesia was obtained by a single injection into the epidural space through the sacral hiatus. In the 1930s, obstetricians began leaving a catheter in the epidural space, allowing them to give repeated doses of medication without performing multiple procedures. Over time, lumbar epidural catheters have become the predominant method to provide labor analgesia because they make it is easier to position patients for the procedure and allow physicians to use the catheter for cesarean sections if needed.

Caudal epidural nerve blocks were first used in pediatric surgery in the 1930s, and they continue to be a pillar of pediatric regional anesthesia. They were first used in urological surgeries but quickly expanded to other surgical procedures. Caudal anesthesia allows for excellent postoperative pain control as well as less opioid use intraoperatively. Today, pediatric anesthesiologists routinely perform caudal epidural nerve blocks for surgical procedures below the umbilicus.

Uses and Indications

Caudal epidural injections are one of the most commonly performed epidural injections. They have been used for many years to treat various conditions. They are used extensively in pediatric anesthesia and in interventional pain management. In pediatric anesthesia, caudal epidural nerve blocks are used for intraoperative and postoperative analgesia for surgical procedures below the umbilicus. Interventional pain physicians frequently perform caudal epidural injections of local anesthetics with or without steroids for lumbar spinal stenosis, failed back surgery syndrome, and lumbar radiculopathy. Other indications include pelvic pain syndromes, postherpetic neuralgia, chronic pain from rectal malignancies, or bony metastasis to the lumbar spine. Caudal epidural nerve blocks can also be used for adults undergoing surgical procedures below the umbilicus; however, they are used in adults less frequently than in pediatric patients. Acute pain management services also perform caudal epidural nerve blocks for postoperative pain as well as other acute pain crises.

Knowing anatomy is imperative for performing successful interventional procedures. The spinal cord ends at L1 to L2 in adults and L2 to L3 in neonates and infants. The dural sac continues caudally and terminates at S1 to S2 in adults and S2 to S3 in neonates and infants. The sacrum is the most caudal border of the spinal canal. It is a triangular-shaped bone that is made up of five fused vertebrae (see Fig. 55.1). It articulates with the fifth lumbar vertebra at the cephalad end and the coccyx on the caudad end. The sacral spinous processes make up the median crest. The sacral cornua and coccygeal cornua are palpable landmarks that help in identifying the sacral hiatus. The sacral hiatus is found on the posterior wall of the sacrum. It is an inverted U shape that is covered by the sacrococcygeal ligament and serves as the entry point for caudal epidural injections. Significant variations exist in the depth of the sacral canal and the distance from the entry point to the dural sac. This variability is one reason that some argue for using fluoroscopy to ensure a safe and successful injection. The anterior and posterior rami of S1-S4 exit the canal through the anterior and posterior sacral foramina, respectively. The S5 nerve roots and coccygeal nerves exit the canal through the sacral hiatus. The epidural space is filled with veins, arteries, fat, and lymphatics. The epidural venous plexus typically terminates around S4. It is mostly located against the anterolateral portion on the sacrum. The majority of the epidural space in the sacral canal is filled with fat, which decreases in density with aging. This decrease likely accounts for the unpredictable spread of medications in older patients.

In the perioperative setting, caudal epidural nerve blocks are used extensively in the pediatric population undergoing surgical procedures of the perineum and rectum, urologic procedures, femoral and inguinal herniorrhaphy, and other operations below the umbilicus. Due to potential postoperative motor blockade, these nerve blocks are most frequently performed in children who have not yet started walking. The landmarks are much easier to palpate in the pediatric population, which makes it easier to perform without fluoroscopy. The nerve block is typically performed under general anesthesia in the lateral position.

Caudal epidural nerve blocks can also be performed in adults for perioperative analgesia. They work well for surgical procedures involving the rectum and pelvis. Acute pain management services perform caudal epidural nerve blocks for postoperative pain management. Some of the common indications include pain from lower extremity trauma as well as pain due to pelvic, genital, and rectal malignancies and bony metastasis to the lumbar spine. Prolonged motor blockade can cause prolonged stays in the recovery room and is not ideal for outpatient surgical procedures. Several notable differences between adult and pediatric patients have been observed. In adults, caudal epidural nerve blocks are typically performed in the prone position, but the lateral position

Fig. 55.1 Sacrum

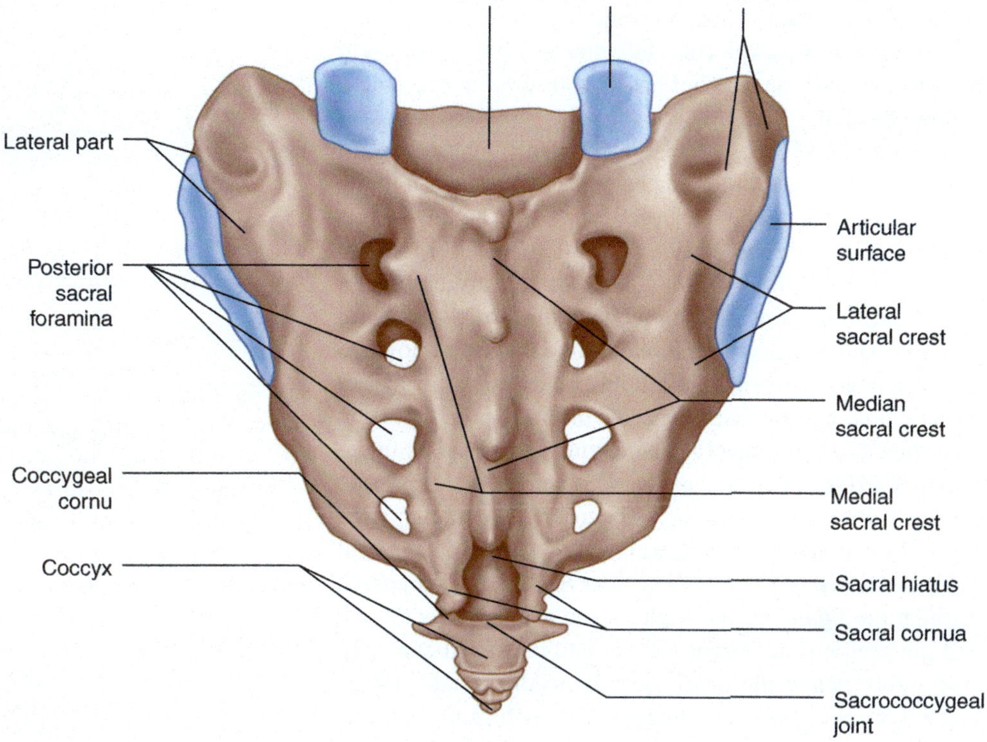

is possible if a patient cannot lie prone or if the physician prefers this position. Fluoroscopy is optional and used less frequently in the perioperative setting. Although some studies advocate for the use of fluoroscopy for more successful placement, it is not always available in these settings. The landmarks are the same in the adult population; however, they may be more difficult to feel due to body habitus. The sacrococcygeal ligament can undergo calcification as people age, which can be a barrier to this technique in the elderly population.

Pain management physicians frequently perform caudal epidural injections with local anesthetics with or without corticosteroids. Most commonly they are performed for lumbar spinal stenosis, failed back surgery syndrome, and lumbar radiculopathy. Other indications include pelvic pain syndromes, postherpetic neuralgia, chronic pain from rectal malignancies, or bony metastasis to the lumbar spine.

Failed back surgery syndrome is one of the common indications for caudal epidural injections. A potential mechanism for continued back pain following a surgical procedure seems to be epidural fibrosis and scar tissue that impinge on nerve roots. Other causes of persistent pain following back surgery include facet joint pain, sacroiliac joint pain, spinal stenosis, discogenic pain, herniated disc, and paraspinal muscle spasms. Patients with failed back surgery syndrome often have pathology that makes interlaminar and transforaminal epidural injections difficult. Pedicle screws used in spinal fusion can make the transforaminal approach difficult, and a patient who has had a laminectomy is no longer a candidate for the interlaminar epidural approach. The caudal approach allows the physician to avoid hardware while still reaching areas of the lumbar spine in patients that would otherwise be difficult to treat.

Severe spinal stenosis is another common indication for caudal epidural injections. Not surprisingly, spinal stenosis is also one of the most common indications for back surgery. Spinal stenosis is a narrowing of the spinal canal with compression of the neural structures by bone and soft tissue. The mechanism of pain from nerve compression with stenosis is not fully understood. However, inflammation and nerve compression might explain why corticosteroids are believed to be helpful. Another postulated mechanism is ischemic pain due to central canal narrowing. Lumbar extension reduces the cross-section area of the central canal, which compresses the vasculature supplying nerve roots and causes ischemic pain. This explains the reversible nature of spinal stenosis pain with flexion of the lumbar spine.

Caudal epidural injections performed by interventional pain physicians are typically done in the prone position with fluoroscopic guidance. The patient is positioned with a pillow under the head and another pillow under the hips. Abduction of the legs and heels prevents the patient from tightening gluteal muscles, which makes palpation of the landmarks easier. Wide preparation with an antiseptic solution is imperative, and a sterile drape is applied. The Center for Disease Control and Prevention Guideline for the Prevention of Surgical Site Infections recommends skin preparation with an alcohol-based antiseptic agent unless contraindicated.

The tip of the coccyx is palpated, identifying the sacral midline. The sacral cornua can be palpated just lateral to the midline. This should be the level of the sacral hiatus. At this point, the C-arm is positioned in the anteroposterior (AP) or lateral position. The sacral hiatus is difficult to identify in the AP position, so it is recommended to start in the lateral position. The posterior sacral plate can be followed down to its most inferior aspect. This should be the superior aspect of the sacral hiatus. Once the needle insertion point has been determined, a skin wheel is made with subcutaneous injection of 1% lidocaine. A 22 gauge, 1.5-inch needle is inserted at a 45-degree angle into the sacrococcygeal ligament (see Fig. 55.2). When the needle penetrates the sacrococcygeal ligament, a distinct pop is felt. After the needle has passed through the ligament, the angle of the needle is decreased, and the needle is advanced 1–2 cm into the spinal canal. To stay safely below the dural sac, the needle should not go beyond S3. AP and lateral images will confirm proper needle position in the sacral canal (see Fig. 55.3). Keep the needle midline in the sacral canal, and the needle bevel tip can be rotated to direct medications toward the patient's most symptomatic side if applicable. Once you are confidently in the sacral canal, gently aspirate to check for the return of cerebrospinal fluid or blood. If either is positive, the needle should be withdrawn slightly and repositioned. After negative aspiration, 1–1.5 ml of nonionic radiographic contrast should be injected under live fluoroscopy to rule out intravascular placement or intrathecal injection (see Fig. 55.4). Once proper caudal epidural needle placement has been confirmed, local anesthetic with or without

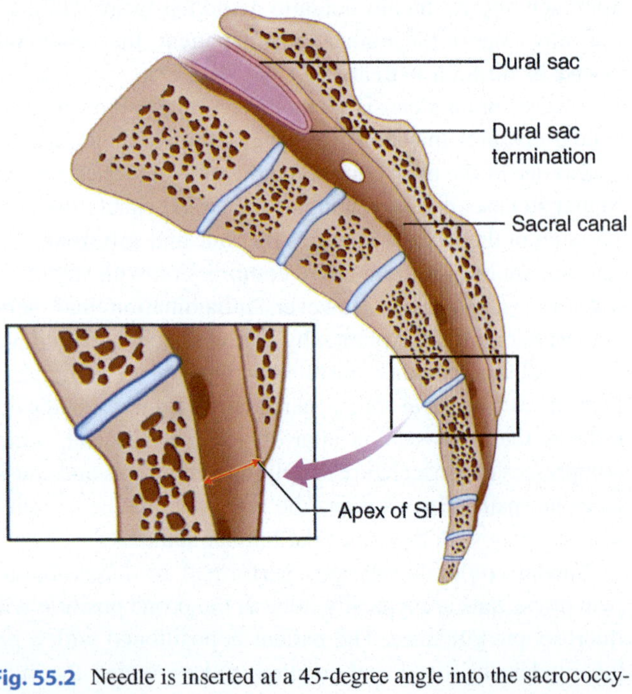

Fig. 55.2 Needle is inserted at a 45-degree angle into the sacrococcygeal ligament

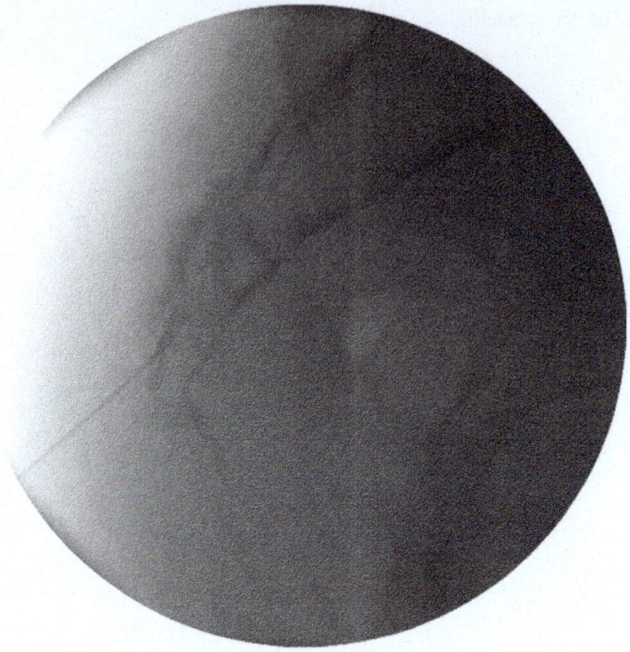

Fig. 55.3 Proper needle position in the sacral canal

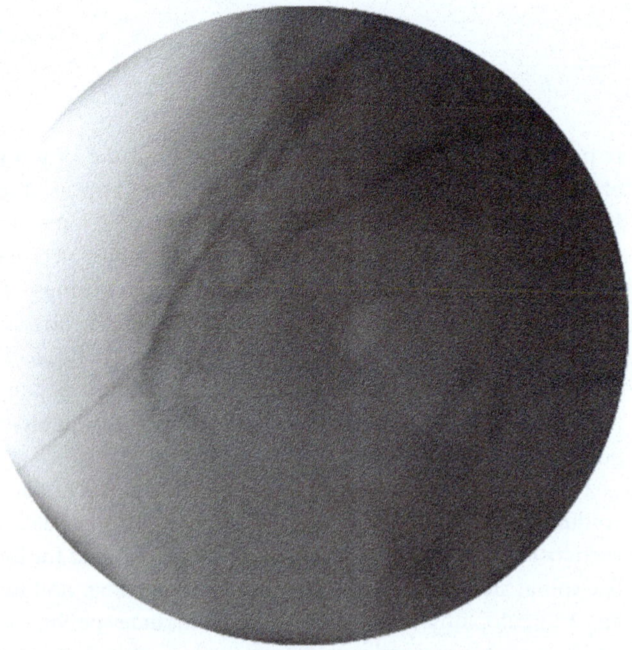

Fig. 55.4 Nonionic radiographic contrast confirming proper placement

corticosteroids is injected into the caudal epidural space. If a steroid is used, follow the injection with 2 ml of sodium chloride. Remove the needle and hold pressure until sufficient hemostasis is achieved.

Caudal epidural injections can be performed with local anesthetic with or without steroids. Recently much discussion has taken place about the type of steroid added to the injection. Steroids can be broken down into two broad categories: particulate and nonparticulate. Particulate steroids are typically poorly soluble in water and, therefore, may precipitate out of solution and crystalize in a hydrophilic environment. Examples of particulate steroids include triamcinolone acetonide, betamethasone acetate, methylprednisolone acetate, and prednisolone acetate. In contrast, nonparticulate steroids are freely water soluble. Dexamethasone sodium phosphate is an example of a nonparticulate steroid. Particulate steroids have generated some controversy. Serious complications have occurred following epidural injection of particulate steroids, including infarction of the cerebellum, brainstem, and thalamus as well as the cervical and lumbar spinal cord. Nonparticulate steroids have not been attributed to these same complications. However, the pathophysiology of paraplegia associated with epidural steroid injections is unclear. Studies have suggested that nonparticulate steroids are not as effective as particulate steroids for pain relief. These controversies should lead the administering physician to be aware of the risks and benefits of each steroid before choosing the type of steroid to be used.

The caudal epidural space can accommodate larger volumes of injectate. The volume of the sacral canal has been measured to roughly 30–34 mL in dried bone models. The range of injectate has been reported from as low as 5 mL to as high as 20 mL. The typical caudal epidural injection is 10 mL.

Several filling patterns that can result when contrast is injected under fluoroscopy are worth noting. An irregular or cotton-ball appearance is suggestive of an extra-epidural injection. Rapid filling and disappearance under live fluoroscopy is suggestive of an intravascular injection. Intrathecal injection will result in myelographic patterns, with contrast in the thecal sac and lumbar nerve roots appearing radiolucent as they are surrounded by contrast within the cerebrospinal fluid.

Ultrasound is being used more frequently for spine procedures including caudal epidural injections. It is excellent for visualizing soft tissues and real-time needle manipulation as well as major nerves and blood vessels. It can be used in situations when fluoroscopy is not available or when radiation should be avoided, such as in pregnancy. Ultrasound has several limitations. Deep structures can be difficult to visualize, and the bone obstructs visualization of objects beneath it. Accidental intravascular injection is better detected under fluoroscopy than ultrasound.

Table 55.1 Evidence for efficacy

	Local anesthetic	Local anesthetic + steroid
Lumbar disk herniation	fair	good
Axial pain	fair	fair
Spinal stenosis	fair	fair
Post-surgery syndrome	fair	fair

Evidence for Efficacy

The American Society of Interventional Pain Physicians publishes evidence-based guidelines for interventional techniques, as summarized in Table 55.1. They develop their recommendations by performing a systematic assessment of the most recent literature and classify them according to the US Preventive Services Task Force (USPSTF) criteria of good, fair, and poor.

The evidence is good for short-term and long-term relief in lumbar disc herniation with radiculitis treated with local anesthetics with steroids. The evidence is fair for short-term and long-term relief with local anesthetics only. The evidence is fair for discogenic or axial pain without disc herniation, radiculitis, sacroiliac joint pain, or facet joint pain. The evidence is fair for long-term relief in spinal stenosis treated with local anesthetic with or without steroids. The evidence is fair for post-lumbar surgery syndrome treated with local anesthetics with or without steroids.

Pearls and Pitfalls

- Caudal epidural injections provide a safe method of epidural injections in patients with lumbar hardware from previous back surgeries.
- Caudal epidural injections are safer and may be as efficacious as interlaminar and transforaminal epidural injections.
- Thorough and wide preparation with an alcohol-based antiseptic solution is imperative given the location of this injection.
- Caudal epidural injections can be with local anesthetic alone or with corticosteroids.
- In adults, to avoid inadvertent dural puncture and intrathecal injection, do not advance your needle past S3.
- Understand the risks associated with caudal epidural injections, including inadvertent dural puncture and intrathecal injection, intravascular injection, bleeding, infection, epidural hematoma, and postdural puncture headache.
- Absolute contraindications are active infection, pilonidal cyst, and certain coagulopathies. There are situations where patients can discontinue their anticoagulation medications prior to caudal epidural injection.

- Having the C-arm in the lateral position provides the best image of the location of the sacral hiatus.
- Abduction of the legs and heels prevents the patient from tightening their gluteal muscles, which makes palpation of the landmarks easier.
- The evidence is good for managing disk herniation or radiculitis with caudal epidural injections.
- The evidence is fair for managing axial or discogenic pain without disk herniation, radiculitis, or facet joint pain with caudal epidural injections.
- The evidence is fair for managing spinal stenosis with caudal epidural injections.
- The evidence is fair for managing failed back surgery syndrome with caudal epidural injections.

Recommended Reading

1. Brown TC. History of pediatric regional anesthesia. Paediatr Anaesth. 2012;22(1):3–9.
2. Conn A, Buenaventura RM, Datta S, Abdi S, Diwan S. Systematic review of caudal epidural injections in the management of chronic low back pain. Pain Physician. 2009;12(1):109–35.
3. Friedman JH, Dighe G. Systematic review of caudal epidural injections in the management of chronic back pain. R I Med J. 2013;96(1):12–6.
4. Karkera MM, Harrison DR, Aunspaugh JP, Martin TW. Assessing caudal block concentrations of bupivacaine with and without the addition of intravenous fentanyl on postoperative outcomes in pediatric patients: a retrospective review. Am J Ther. 2016;23(3):e792–8.
5. Kaye AD, Manchikanti L, Abdi S, et al. Efficacy of epidural injections in managing chronic spinal pain: a best evidence synthesis. Pain Physician. 2015;18(6):E939–1004.
6. Manchikanti L, Singh V, editors. Interventional techniques in chronic spinal pain. Paducah: American Society of Interventional Pain Physicians; 2007.
7. Manchikanti L, Cash KA, McManus CD, Pampati V, Abdi S. Preliminary results of a randomized, equivalence trial of fluoroscopic caudal epidural injections in managing chronic low back pain: part 4--spinal stenosis. Pain Physician. 2008;11(6):833–48.
8. Manchikanti L, Singh V, Cash KA, Pampati V, Damron KS, Boswell MV. A randomized, controlled, double-blind trial of fluoroscopic caudal epidural injections in the treatment of lumbar disc herniation and radiculitis. Spine (Phila Pa 1976). 2011;36(23):1897–905.
9. Manchikanti L, Cash KA, McManus CD, Pampati V, Fellows B. Results of 2-year follow-up of a randomized, double-blind, controlled trial of fluoroscopic caudal epidural injections in central spinal stenosis. Pain Physician. 2012a;15(5):371–84.
10. Manchikanti L, Singh V, Cash KA, Pampati V, Datta S. Fluoroscopic caudal epidural injections in managing post lumbar surgery syndrome: two-year results of a randomized, double-blind, active-control trial. Int J Med Sci. 2012b;9(7):582–91.
11. Manchikanti L, Falco FJ, Pampati V, Cash KA, Benyamin RM, Hirsch JA. Cost utility analysis of caudal epidural injections in the treatment of lumbar disc herniation, axial or discogenic low back pain, central spinal stenosis, and post lumbar surgery syndrome. Pain Physician. 2013a;16(3):E129–43.
12. Manchikanti L, Abdi S, Atluri S, et al. An update of comprehensive evidence-based guidelines for interventional techniques in chronic spinal pain. Part II: guidance and recommendations. Pain Physician. 2013b;16(suppl 2):S49–283.
13. Manchikanti L, Pampati V, Falco FJ, Hirsch JA. Assessment of the growth of epidural injections in the medicare population from 2000 to 2011. Pain Physician. 2013c;16(4):E349–64.
14. Manchikanti L, Benyamin RM, Falco FJ, Kaye AD, Hirsch JA. Do epidural injections provide short- and long-term relief for lumbar disc herniation? A systematic review. Clin Orthop Relat Res. 2015;473(6):1940–56.
15. Parr AT, Manchikanti L, Hameed H, et al. Caudal epidural injections in the management of chronic low back pain: a systematic appraisal of the literature. Pain Physician. 2012;15(3):E159–98.
16. Rathmell JP. Atlas of image-guided intervention in regional anesthesia and pain medicine. 2nd ed. Philadelphia: Lippincott Williams & Wilkins; 2012.
17. Rho ME, Tang CT. The efficacy of lumbar epidural steroid injections: transforaminal, interlaminar, and caudal approaches. Phys Med Rehabil Clin N Am. 2011;22(1):139–48.
18. Silva M, Halpern SH. Epidural analgesia for labor: current techniques. Local Reg Anesth. 2010;3:143–53.
19. Waldman SD. Atlas of interventional pain management. 3rd ed. Philadelphia: Saunders Elsevier; 2009.

Stellate Ganglion Block

56

Ioannis M. Skaribas, Aanchal Sharma, and Elena E. Skaribas

Introduction

Stellate ganglion block was first described in the 1930s by Fontaine and Leriche as a method to relieve reflex sympathetic dystrophy symptoms of the upper limbs. Since then it has been used for diagnosis and treatment of many sympathetically mediated pain states of the head, neck, and upper extremities such as CRPS-I (RSD) and CRPS-II (causalgia), postherpetic neuralgia, and vasospastic disorders. In addition to neuropathic pain, an increase in stellate ganglion activity has also been postulated to cause many ventricular arrhythmias including congenital QT prolongation, ventricular tachycardia, and ventricular fibrillation. The block has been used to treat life-threatening ventricular arrhythmia and congenital long QT syndrome. So far various techniques have been employed to successfully block the stellate ganglion including anatomical landmarks, fluoroscopic guidance, CT guidance, and most recently ultrasound guidance. As all the sympathetic supply of head and neck and most of the sympathetic supply of upper extremity either synapse or pass through stellate ganglion, this is considered as a complete sympathetic block.

In this chapter, we intend to discuss the anatomy of stellate ganglion, the technique of the ganglion block, its indications, its contraindications, and the complications associated with the block.

I. M. Skaribas (✉) · A. Sharma
Expert Pain P.A., Department of Anesthesiology, McGovern Medical School, The University of Texas Health Science Center at Houston, Houston, TX, USA
e-mail: skaribasmd@expertpaincare.com; aanchal.sharma@uth.tmc.edu

E. E. Skaribas
Southern Methodist University, Dallas, TX, USA
e-mail: eskaribas@smu.edu

Anatomy

Sympathetic supply to the head, neck, and upper extremity is derived from the preganglionic fibers arising from the cell bodies located in the anterolateral horn of T1 and T2 segments of the spinal cord. Some sympathetic innervation to the upper extremities originates from T2 to T3 via anatomically distinct nerves (Kuntz's nerves). Preganglionic fibers leave the spinal cord and enter their respective spinal nerves. They then pass through the white rami communicantes to enter the cervical sympathetic ganglia. The cervical sympathetic ganglia are located along the prevertebral fascia behind the cervical neurovascular bundle extending from the level of the transverse process of the second cervical vertebrae to the first rib where they transition to the thoracic sympathetic chain. They are divided to superior, middle, and inferior cervical sympathetic ganglia. In 80% of the population, the inferior cervical ganglion and the first thoracic ganglion are fused to create the cervicothoracic or stellate ganglion. In the remaining 20% of individuals, the first thoracic vertebral ganglion is called stellate ganglion. The postganglionic fibers from the stellate ganglion either pass upward to supply the head or join the gray rami communicantes to supply the neck and upper extremity. All the sympathetic supply to the head and neck and most of the upper extremity passes through the stellate ganglion. The stellate ganglion is oval or star shaped and measures approximately 2.5 cm in length and 1 cm in width and is 0.5 cm in thickness. Understanding its anatomy is important for an effective blockade and to avoid unnecessary complications. When fused, the ganglion lies against the C7 transverse process and the neck of the first rib. Anterior to the ganglion lies the subclavian and vertebral artery; posteromedial the longus colli muscle; laterally the carotid sheath, scalene muscles, and the brachial plexus; and medially the trachea, esophagus, and recurrent laryngeal nerve. Inferior to the ganglion is the pleura and the dome of the lung (Fig. 56.1).

T. R. Deer et al. (eds.), *Deer's Treatment of Pain*, https://doi.org/10.1007/978-3-030-12281-2_56

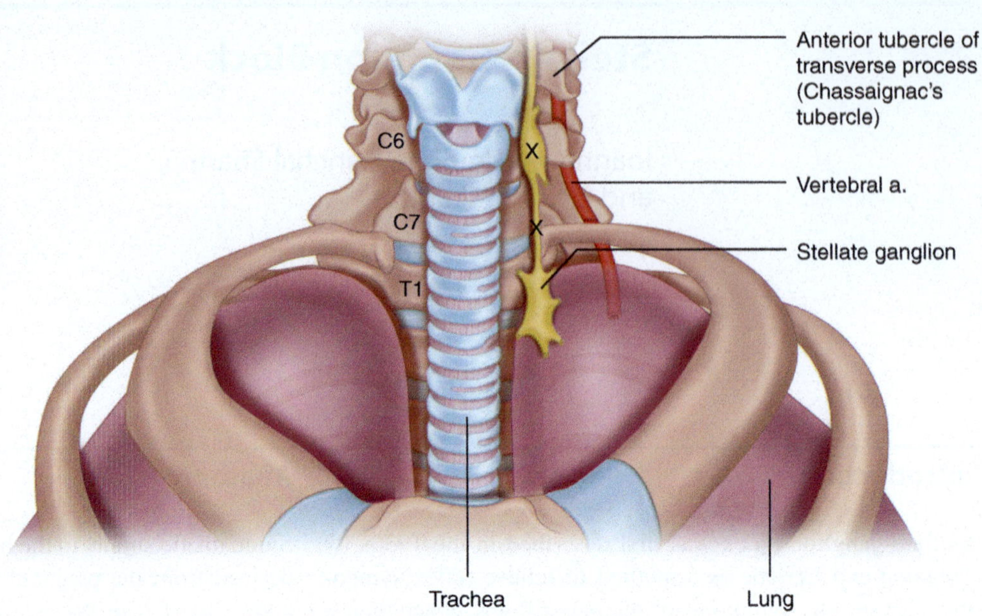

Fig. 56.1 Anatomy of the stellate ganglion. The location of the star(stellate) ganglion is appreciated on the left. The location of relevant adjacent anatomical structures is seen including the anterior tubercle of the C6 transverse process where the stellate ganglion block is performed, as well as the location of the first rib, cupola of the lung, and vertebral artery

Indications

The stellate ganglion has been successfully used in various pain syndromes as well as other conditions, including:

1. Complex regional pain syndrome type I (reflex sympathetic dystrophy/RSD) of the head and upper extremities
2. Complex regional pain syndrome type II (causalgia) of the head and upper extremities
3. Phantom limb pain
4. Postherpetic neuralgia
5. Orofacial pain syndromes including trigeminal neuralgia and orofacial neuropathic pain
6. Sympathetically maintained headaches, cluster headaches
7. Neuropathic cancer pain
8. Postradiation neuropathic pain
9. Postmastectomy pain
10. Vascular insufficiency
11. Raynaud's disease
12. Acute vasospasm following intra-arterial injection
13. Refractory anginal cardiac pain

In addition to the conditions outlined above, stellate ganglion blocks have been used successfully in the treatment of non-painful conditions such as cardiac arrhythmias, hyperhidrosis, and post-traumatic stress disorder (PTSD).

Contraindications

1. Patient refusal
2. Infection at the site of the needle insertion
3. Bilateral stellate ganglion blocks
4. Bleeding disorders
5. Patient on anticoagulation therapy
6. Unilateral recurrent laryngeal nerve palsy or phrenic nerve palsy
7. Pregnancy (fluoroscopy)

Fluoroscopic Technique

The most common approach to the stellate ganglion is the anterior paratracheal approach at the C6 transverse process level (Chassaignac's tubercle) where anatomical landmarks are easily palpable and identifiable by imaging. This approach significantly reduces the risk of pneumothorax and intravascular injection. Most stellate ganglion blocks in chronic pain medicine are performed with fluoroscopic guidance, although an ultrasound-guided technique has been developed.

After informed consent is obtained, the patient is taken to the operating room where he/she is positioned supine with a pillow under the shoulders to hyperextend the neck. This hyperextension serves two purposes: to stretch the esophagus away from the transverse process and to facilitate clarity of the osseous anatomical landmarks. Although this procedure can be performed with only local anesthesia, most physicians prefer to use mild sedation for patient comfort. The neck is prepped and draped in a sterile manner. A sterile draped C-arm is introduced and positioned over the cervical spine in a posterior-anterior orientation without oblique or cephalocaudal angulation to identify the vertebral bodies of the sixth and seventh cervical vertebral body (C6, C7). The stellate ganglion block is preferably performed at a C6 level. Macroscopically, this corresponds to the level of the cricoid cartilage. The transverse process of C6 is identified as well as the anterior tubercle of the transverse process (Chassaignac's tubercle), which is important if the procedure is to be performed blindly as it is an easily identifiable anatomical landmark by palpation. Fluoroscopic land marking for needle placement is the junction of the transverse process to the base of the corresponding uncinated process. The superimposed skin is infiltrated with 3–5 cc of 1% lidocaine. The patient is asked to refrain from talking or swallowing. A 22 gauge 3 ½ inch needle is inserted through the skin, and under fluoroscopic guidance utilizing a coaxial technique is advanced until periosteum is contacted at the previously mentioned anatomical target. Once in its final position, the needle should be situated firmly into the tissue layers. The depth from the skin to target varies between patients. After negative aspiration is performed for blood or cerebrospinal fluid (CSF), 1–2 ml of radiographic contrast dye (iohexol 180 or 240 mg/ml) is injected under real-time, continuous fluoroscopy to rule out any intravascular or intrathecal spread and to verify accurate cephalocaudal spread of the contrast material along the anterolateral surfaces of the corresponding vertebrae (Figs. 56.2 and 56.3). Both posterior-anterior (PA) and lateral fluoroscopic views are utilized for verification. This fluoroscopic confirmation illustrates the spread of the injectate in the prevertebral fascia where the stellate ganglion is located. A negative aspiration cannot exclude possible intravascular or intrathecal administration, so a high level of awareness is required when performing this procedure. A commonly used therapeutic injectate consists of a 10 ml

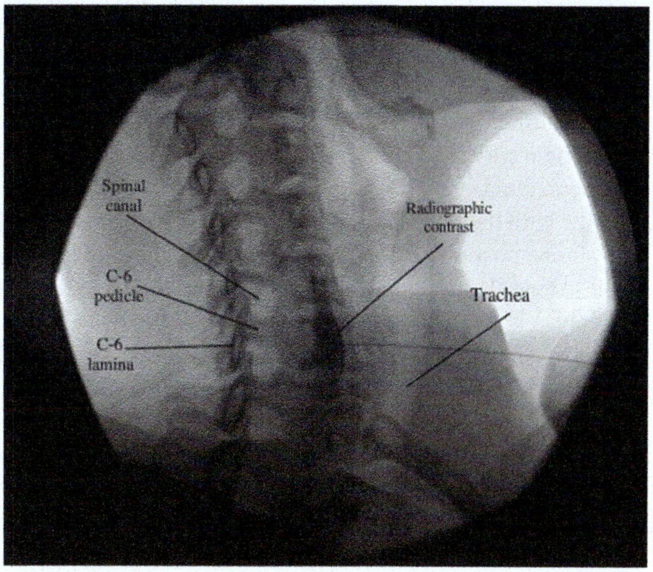

Fig. 56.3 This is a lateral fluoroscopic view of a C6 stellate ganglion block at C6 level. The spread of the contrast is appreciated at the anterolateral surface of C6

mixture of 0.25% ropivacaine with 40–80 mg of triamcinolone (Kenalog). A test dose of 1 ml is initially injected while observing for signs and symptoms of intravascular or intrathecal injection. If no abnormalities are noted, the test dose is followed by a slow injection of the remaining volume under intermittent or continuous fluoroscopy. If a C7 approach is desired, the anatomical considerations are important. At C7 level there is no anterior tubercle, and often there is no transverse foramen to protect the vertebral artery that is located anterior to the lateral C7 transverse process. Therefore, it is imperative to be constantly aware of the needle trajectory and to keep the needle at/or medial to a line connecting the uncinated processes to avoid accidental vertebral artery puncture and inadvertent intra-articular injection. At the end of the procedure, the patient is transferred to the recovery room and is observed for signs of a successful sympathetic block and for possible complications before discharged.

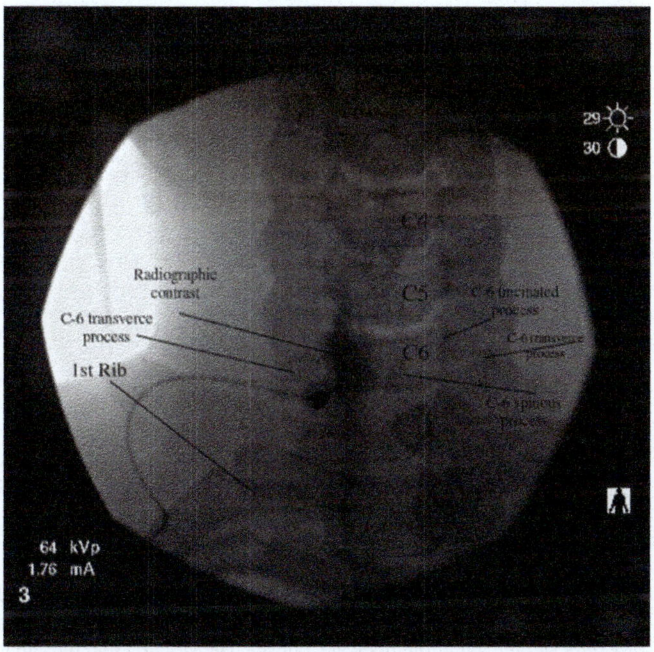

Fig. 56.2 Posterior-anterior fluoroscopic view depicts placement of the needle for the performance of fluoroscopy-guided right stellate ganglion block at C6 level. The needle is identified under fluoroscopy with the tip placed at the junction of the right C6 uncinated and transverse process. The contrast is identified spreading both cephalad and caudad

Ultrasound Technique

In the last 10 years, the utilization of ultrasound for regional anesthesia and analgesia has transferred over to the field of pain medicine. Stellate ganglion block is one of the procedures where ultrasound guidance is frequently performed. There are obvious advantages to the usage of ultrasound for stellate ganglion blockade including the real-time visualization of all anatomical structures and real-time advancement of the needle accounting for improved safety and avoidance of radiation exposure for both physician and patient alike. The utilization of ultrasound has confirmed the significant variability of the anatomical structures surrounding the stellate ganglion and the cervicothoracic sympathetic chain in general. Esophageal deviation from the midline is very common, and accidental penetration can result to severe complications such as mediastinitis. Vascular anatomical variations of the inferior thyroidal artery and other vessels can result in inadvertent vascular penetration with secondary formation of a hematoma.

Like with the fluoroscopic technique, the patient is placed in a supine position and with a pillow under the shoulders to hyperextend the neck. After the neck is prepared and draped sterilely, a linear ultrasound transducer (6–13 MHz) is introduced under sterile conditions. The transducer is positioned to contact skin in a transverse orientation to the axis of the neck and to the right or left of midline at the level of the cricoid cartilage, which corresponds to the level of C6. A cross-sectional scan is obtained, and all the anatomic structures are sonographically identified before the needle insertion (Fig. 56.4). Color Doppler can be utilized to further facilitate the identification of vessels such as the carotid artery or the inferior thyroid artery. Both an in-plane and an out-of-plane technique can be utilized (Fig. 56.5a, b). The in-plane technique is favored since it provides real-time "step-by-step" visualization of the needle tip as it travels through the different fascial planes. After the skin is infiltrated with 3–5 ml of 1% lidocaine, a 22 gauge 3.5 inch spinal needle or an echogenically insulated 22 gauge 80 mm regional block needle is inserted through the skin and advanced under real-time

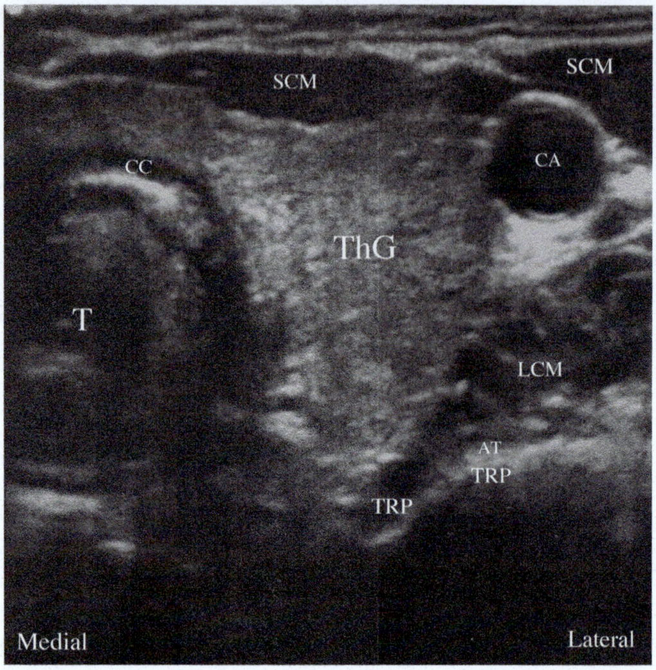

Fig. 56.4 Sonographic image of a cross-sectional scan at right C6 level. The relevant anatomical structures are clearly seen. From medial to lateral: T (trachea), CC (cricoid cartilage), SCM (sternocleidomastoid muscle), ThG (thyroid gland), TRP (transverse process of C6), AT TRP (anterior tubercle of C6 transverse process/Chassaignac's), LCM (longus coli muscle), CA (carotid artery)

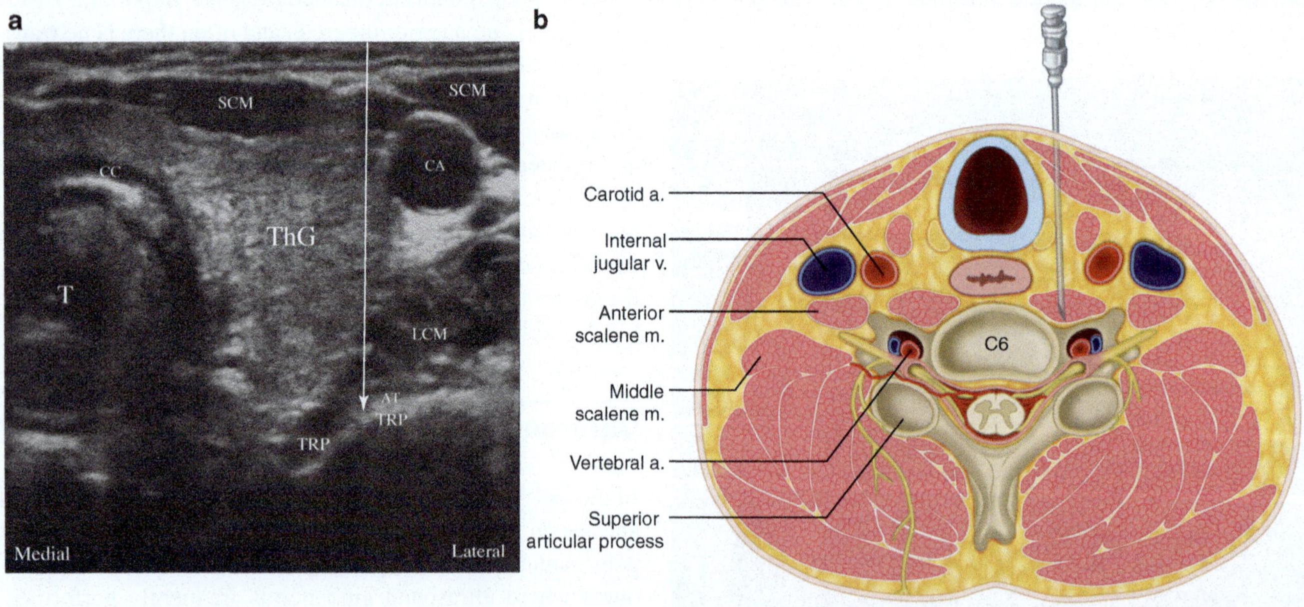

Fig. 56.5 (**a**) Sonographic depiction of an out-of-plane needle insertion for purposes of a right C6 stellate ganglion block. This sonographic image depicts the classic trajectory of the needle during fluoroscopy-guided stellate ganglion blocks and its relationship to the adjacent anatomical structures. The tip of the needle is located at Chassaignac's tubercle near the prevertebral fascia and the longus coli muscle. One can appreciate the location of both the carotid artery and the thyroid gland and their proximity to the needle. (**b**) Cross-sectional illustration of a right stellate ganglion block at C6 level. The vascular and muscular relevant anatomy is depicted as the needle advances toward Chassaignac's tubercle

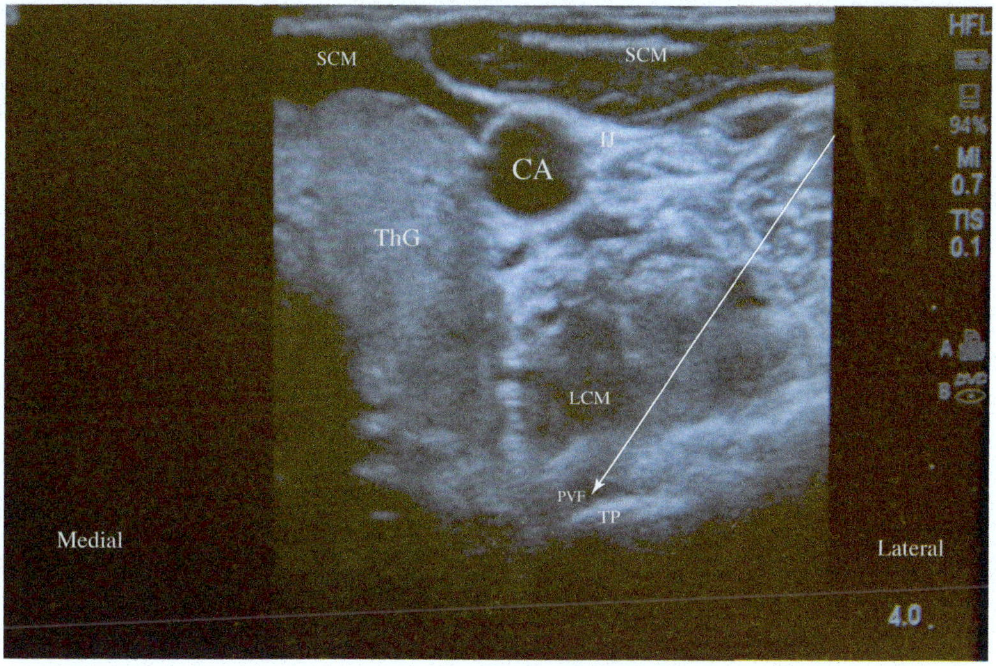

Fig. 56.6 Sonographic depiction of a right C6 ultrasound-guided stellate ganglion block using an in-plane technique. The needle is inserted through the skin and advanced under real-time ultrasound guidance in a latero-medial direction toward the prevertebral fascia and longus colli muscle traveling between the anterior tubercle and the carotid artery

ultrasound guidance in a latero-medial direction toward the prevertebral fascia and longus coli muscle traveling between the anterior tubercle and the carotid artery (Fig. 56.6). Once in position and after negative aspiration for blood or CSF is performed, a test dose of 1 ml is given sonographically observing spread in the prevertebral fascia. Lastly, the rest of the 5–10 ml volume is injected slowly under ultrasound.

Signs of Successful Stellate Ganglion Block

1. Horner's syndrome (ptosis, myosis, anhidrosis, enophthalmos, nasal congestion)
2. Ipsilateral conjunctival injection
3. Vasodilation of the ipsilateral upper extremity
4. Temperature elevation of the ipsilateral upper extremity by 1–3 °C

Complications

1. Related to the technique
   - (i) Injury to surrounding vascular structures (carotid artery, subclavian artery, vertebral artery, internal jugular vein).
   - (ii) Hematoma formation especially in patients on anticoagulants.
   - (iii) Intravascular injection.
   - (iv) Intrathecal injection.
   - (v) Cardiovascular collapse.
   - (vi) Injury to pleura leading to pneumothorax, esophageal perforation, and injury to thoracic duct leading to chylothorax.
   - (vii) Stellate ganglion block due to inhibition of sympathetic fibers can lead to profound bradycardia and even heart block.
   - (viii) Vasovagal attack.
2. Infection
   - (i) Cellulitis
   - (ii) Soft tissue infection
   - (iii) Osteitis of vertebral body and transverse process
   - (iv) Meningitis
3. Related to local anesthetic medication injected
   - (i) Spread of local anesthesia to recurrent laryngeal nerve and phrenic nerve
   - (ii) Hoarseness
   - (iii) Dyspnea
   - (iv) Intra-arterial injection of local anesthetic
   - (v) Seizures
   - (vi) Local anesthetic systemic toxicity
   - (vii) Neuro-blockade of the brachial plexus

Recommended Reading

1. Bonica JJ. Sympathetic nerve blocks for pain diagnosis and therapy. Technical considerations Vol. II. Block of stellate ganglion and cervicothoracic and thoracic chains. Winthrop. 1984; p. 61–77.
2. Deer TR. Treatment of chronic pain by interventional approaches: the American Academy of pain medicine textbook on patient management. New York: Springer; 2015.

3. Elias M. Cervical sympathetic and stellate ganglion blocks. Pain Physician. 2000;3(3):294–304.
4. Lofstrom B, Cousins M. Sympathetic neural blockade of the upper and lower extremity. In: Cousins M, Bridenbaugh PO, editors. Neural blockade in clinical anesthesia and management of pain, second edition. London: J.P. Lippincot; 1988.
5. Peng P, Narouze S. Ultrasound-guided interventional procedures in pain medicine: a review of anatomy, sonoanatomy, and procedures: part I: nonaxial structures. Reg Anesth Pain Med. 2009;34(5):458–74.
6. Rathmell JP. Atlas of image-guided intervention in regional anesthesia and pain medicine. 1st ed. Philadelphia, USA: Lippincott, Williams and Wilkins; 2011.

Lumbar Sympathetic Block

57

Sascha Qian, Vikram Sengupta, Ned Urbiztondo, and Nameer Haider

Introduction

The lumbar sympathetic block targets the sympathetic chain into the lower extremities with the objective of disrupting the nerve supply. This has been useful for the treatment of sympathetically mediated pain pathologies such as complex regional pain syndrome, peripheral vascular disease, vasospastic syndrome, frostbite, phantom limb pain, hyperhidrosis, and postherpetic neuralgia.

Background and Historical Perspective

While the anatomy of the sympathetic nervous system was delineated as early as the sixteenth century by Renaissance physician Vesalius, the functions of the sympathetic nervous system were not explored until the end of the nineteenth century with a series of surgical sympathectomies. In 1917, Rene Leriche, a military surgeon, performed the first periarterial sympathectomy on a patient with chronic hand pain and numbness after a gunshot wound to the axilla. After noting complete resolution of his patient's pain, Leriche successfully replicated his surgical technique for other syndromes with marked vasomotor dysregulation and conceived of the term "sympathetic neuritis"—a concept that emphasized the crucial role of the sympathetic nervous system in pathophysiology of neuropathic pain. With the goal of targeting the sympathetic ganglia, Royle and Hunter performed the world's first lumbar sympathectomy in 1923 on a young World War I veteran with spastic paralysis. They noted not only the anticipated result of reduced spasticity but also increased temperature and bright color of the affected limb—a seminal milestone that was quickly followed by Brown and Adson in 1925 who demonstrated the efficacy of lumbar sympathetic blockade for Raynaud's and obliterative arterial disease.

In 1924, Brunn and Mandl in Vienna described the first percutaneous lumbar sympathetic block, for which they initially used local anesthetic and later 70% alcohol. The original description outlined a paravertebral approach: (1) the spinous processes of the second through fourth lumbar vertebra were palpated, and three needles were placed 5–6 cm laterally to the spinous processes with a needle at each level, and (2) the needles were then advanced in a medial direction until contact with the anterolateral aspect of the vertebral body. In 1949, Haxon applied the same paravertebral technique in 220 patients with 1 important modification: he used phenol for sympathetic neurolysis rather than alcohol. The result was significant pain reduction for patients with hyperhidrosis, frostbite, and peripheral vascular disease; one patient even experienced 2 years of sympathetic denervation. Overall, the complications were noted to be minimal compared to the mortality and morbidity associated with open sympathectomy.

During World War II, lumbar sympathetic blockade rose in popularity as a treatment option for patients with lower extremity neuropathic pain and has continued to evolve over the past century as a commonly used interventional pain procedure. With the advent of fluoroscopy, CT, and ultrasound for visualization, lumbar sympathetic block has developed an improved safety profile, while the options for disrupting sympathetic innervations have expanded to include not only surgical ligation and local anesthetic infiltration but also various forms of chemical neurolysis and radiofrequency lesioning.

Uses and Indications

Lumbar sympathetic blocks are indicated for a multitude of sympathetically mediated pain disorder. These include the following (for full list, see Table 57.1):

S. Qian (✉) · V. Sengupta · N. Urbiztondo · N. Haider
Spinal & Skeletal Pain Medicine, Utica, NY, USA
e-mail: vsengupta@thrivewellinfusion.com; drhaider@killpain.com

T. R. Deer et al. (eds.), *Deer's Treatment of Pain*, https://doi.org/10.1007/978-3-030-12281-2_57

Table 57.1 Potential indications for lumbar sympathetic block

Complex regional pain syndrome I and II
Chronic occlusive arterial disease (includes critical limb ischemia)
Diabetic neuropathy
Phantom limb pain
Vasospastic disorders (Raynaud's phenomenon, acrocyanosis, livedo reticularis)
Thromboangiitis obliterans
Erythromelalgia
Cancer pain
Radiation neuritis
Frostbite
Acute herpes zoster, postherpetic neuralgia
Renal colic
Hyperhidrosis

I. *Complex regional pain syndrome (CRPS)* is a regional pain of complex pathophysiology involving disturbance of both central and autonomic nervous system. CRPS I is formerly known as reflex sympathetic dystrophy and entails presence of initiating noxious event or a cause of immobilization, while CRPS II is formerly known as causalgia and entails the presence of continuing pain after nerve injury. Patient typically endorses symptoms and exhibits signs of allodynia, hyperalgesia, vasomotor dysfunction, edema, and trophic changes of the affected limb.

The optimal management of CRPS involves early diagnosis and time-dependent, interdisciplinary treatment, which focuses on rehabilitation, pain management, and psychological therapy. Any delay can adversely affect response to treatment. Therefore, a minimally invasive interventional pain procedure, such as lumbar sympathetic block, should be considered earlier in the treatment algorithm, especially when a patient has reached a plateau in progress after intensive rehabilitation and aggressive pharmacotherapy. In providing an updated algorithm of the management of CRPS, a panel of experts meeting in 2002 recommended minimally invasive procedures such as sympathetic nerve block in conjunction with mainstay therapy within the first 12–16 weeks—after which, failure to progress should prompt consideration of more advanced techniques such as spinal cord stimulation and DRG stimulation. Positive response to sympathetic nerve block may also bode well for spinal cord stimulation; a study in 2003 showed that patients with a good response to sympathetic blocks were more likely to have pain relief during SCS trial and long-term pain relief after placement of permanent device.

While the sympathetic nervous system is traditionally implicated in the origin of CRPS, the terms sympathetically maintained pain and sympathetically independent pain have been employed to account for the inconsistent response to sympathetic blocking procedures.

II. *Chronic obstructive arterial disease (COAD)* is the reduction in blood flow in the arterial beds of the lower extremities, often manifesting as intermittent claudication when the obstruction of the vessel is greater than 50% and progressing onto severe persistent pain at rest when the collateral flow becomes insufficient, such as when COAD developed into critical limb ischemia (CLI). Because CLI is often associated with ulcers and gangrene, interventions such as bypass, endarterectomy, and stenting have to be undertaken. Lumbar sympathetic blockade is a viable treatment option for patients with painful COAD and CLI, for whom revascularization is not feasible, and should be considered prior to proceeding with amputation. Some vascular surgeons may even consider lumbar sympathetic neurolysis as a treatment for ulcers or as a bridge to revascularization. Lumbar sympathetic chemical neurolysis, a fairly safe and minimally invasive procedure, has similar short-term success rates compared to surgical sympathectomy and may be an effective strategy in avoiding or delaying surgical trauma.

The mechanism of pain control after sympathetic blockade is likely related to the transient abolishment of basal and reflex constriction of arterioles and precapillary sphincters leading to increased flow through the occluded vessel as well as increased perfusion through collateral circulation. The improvement in blood flow bears nutritive value for the capillary beds and may alleviate further tissue damage. Furthermore, the sympathetic blockade may directly interrupt or attenuate nociceptive transmission directly via decreasing tissue norepinephrine levels, which would account for analgesic relief in the patients with severe multilevel arterial occlusions who are still able to experience pain relief without improvement in distal perfusion. Clinically, patients will typically demonstrate significant increase in warmth of the affected extremity due to shunting through cutaneous arteriovenous anastomosis as well as increased filling of the veins and increase in arterial pulsations.

III. *Vasospastic disorders*, including Raynaud's phenomenon, acrocyanosis, and livedo reticularis, present with the hallmark symptom of episodic cyanosis of the extremities. Excessive spasm of the peripheral blood vessels in the lower extremities results in numbness as well as pain. Conservative treatment includes lifestyle modification and calcium channel blockers, which may be effective in only two thirds of the patients; refractory cases of vasospasm can lead to unremitting pain as well as digital ulceration. While there is a paucity of data on efficacy of lumbar sympathetic blockade in vasospastic disorders, there exist case reports of successful bilateral lumbar sympathetic blockade performed on patients with refractory Raynaud's phenomenon. The benefit of lumbar sympathectomy is likely due to its reduction of vasoconstrictor tone and improvement of circulation to the ischemic region.

IV. *Diabetic neuropathy* is a relatively common condition of microvascular dysfunction secondary to chronic hyperglycemia. Neuropathic pain can often occur as the presenting symptom, and patients may experience gradual onset of paresthesia, allodynia, and hyperalgesia. The pathophysiology of painful diabetic neuropathy is thought to involve increased cross talk between sympathetic fibers and peripheral sensory nerves, elevated circulation of norepinephrine and inflammatory mediators, and heightened dysregulation of sympathetic-mediated local circulation. When a newly diagnosed diabetic patient presented to Cleveland Clinic in 2012, Cheng recommended a series of lumbar sympathetic block over the course of 2 years. Each block resulted in 1–2 months of significant analgesic relief of the patient's painful diabetic neuropathy. The lumbar sympathetic block was hypothesized to decrease the patient's pain via reducing sympathetic outflow and improving circulation.

V. *Phantom limb pain* is the painful sensation of the amputated limb. Patients may often experience intermittent recurrence of the pre-amputation pain. Multiple mechanisms have been proposed for phantom pain, including peripheral consequences of amputation leading to the development of neuroma, loss of inhibitory control in the dorsal root ganglion, increased excitability of spinal cord neurons, as well as inappropriate central reorganization of the thalamus and cortex. Sympathetically maintained pain is hypothesized to occur when sympathetic nerve fibers secrete not only sympathetic neurotransmitters, such as norepinephrine, but also inflammatory mediators, which can directly stimulate and sensitize the peripheral nociceptive fibers. The sensitized peripheral fibers then release more neurotransmitters to sensitize other pain fibers and contribute to the overall inflammatory state. In amplifying the general inflammation with vasodilation, edema, and activation of white blood cells and other inflammatory cells, the sympathetic nervous system plays a key role in maintaining and exacerbating the chronic pain state. Successful lumbar sympathetic blockade for the treatment of phantom limb pain has been described in multiple case reports; however, the results are not consistent as there may be a subset of phantom limb pain which is sympathetically independent.

VI. *Plantar hyperhidrosis* is a functional disorder of excessive secretion of the sweat glands of the feet that is associated with an overacting sympathetic nervous system. Severe cases of plantar hyperhidrosis can be disabling and personally and professionally limiting. In patients who do not respond to conventional treatment, such as topical agents and botulinum toxin injections, percutaneous lumbar sympathetic neurolysis and radiofrequency ablation have been attempted with varying success. Since 2008, an endoscopic approach to lumbar sympathectomy, entailing clamping of the sympathetic chain at L3 or L4, has been gaining traction among surgeons as an outpatient procedure. Multiple prospective studies demonstrate at least a 95% success rate in achieving anhidrosis.

Anatomy

The sympathetic trunk, also known as the paravertebral ganglia for it lies alongside the vertebral column, is composed of bilateral sympathetic chain ganglia, extending from the cervical spine down to the coccyx. There are 3 pairs of ganglia in the cervical region, 11 pairs in the thoracic region, 4 pairs in the lumbar region, and 4 to 5 pairs in the sacral region. The lumbar portion of the sympathetic trunk lies along the anterolateral aspect of the first through fourth lumbar vertebra. Anterior to the chain on the right is the IVC; anterior to the chain on the left lies the abdominal aorta. Posterior and medial to the chain are the intervertebral foramina. Posterior and lateral to the chain is the psoas muscle, which separates the lumbar sympathetic chain from the somatic plexus and minimizes spread of local anesthetic or chemical neurolysis (see Fig. 57.1). The preganglionic neurons of the lumbar sympathetic trunk arise from the intermediolateral nucleus of the lateral gray column of the spinal cord at levels T10 to L3 and emerge via the white rami of the ventral roots of spinal nerves L1–L4 before synapsing at the paravertebral ganglia. The axons of the postganglionic neurons then extend distally and innervate specific sites in the pelvis, lower abdomen, and lower extremities.

Despite variability in anatomic locations, most cadaveric studies suggest lumbar sympathetic plexus is most dense at the level of the mid-body of the third lumbar vertebra and the discs above and below. Specifically, the ganglia is most frequently located 0–0.5 cm posterior the anterior body of the third lumbar vertebral and 1.8–3.0 cm laterally from the center of the vertebra. Studies of radiofrequency ablation of L3 ganglia are consistent with anatomic studies in showing that adequate block can often occur from blocking L3 ganglia alone, while studies of ganglionectomy show that resection at L2 and L3 is usually sufficient. Therefore, the best approach is to advance the needle paravertebrally to lower third of L2 or upper third to midpoint of the body of L3 (see Fig. 57.2).

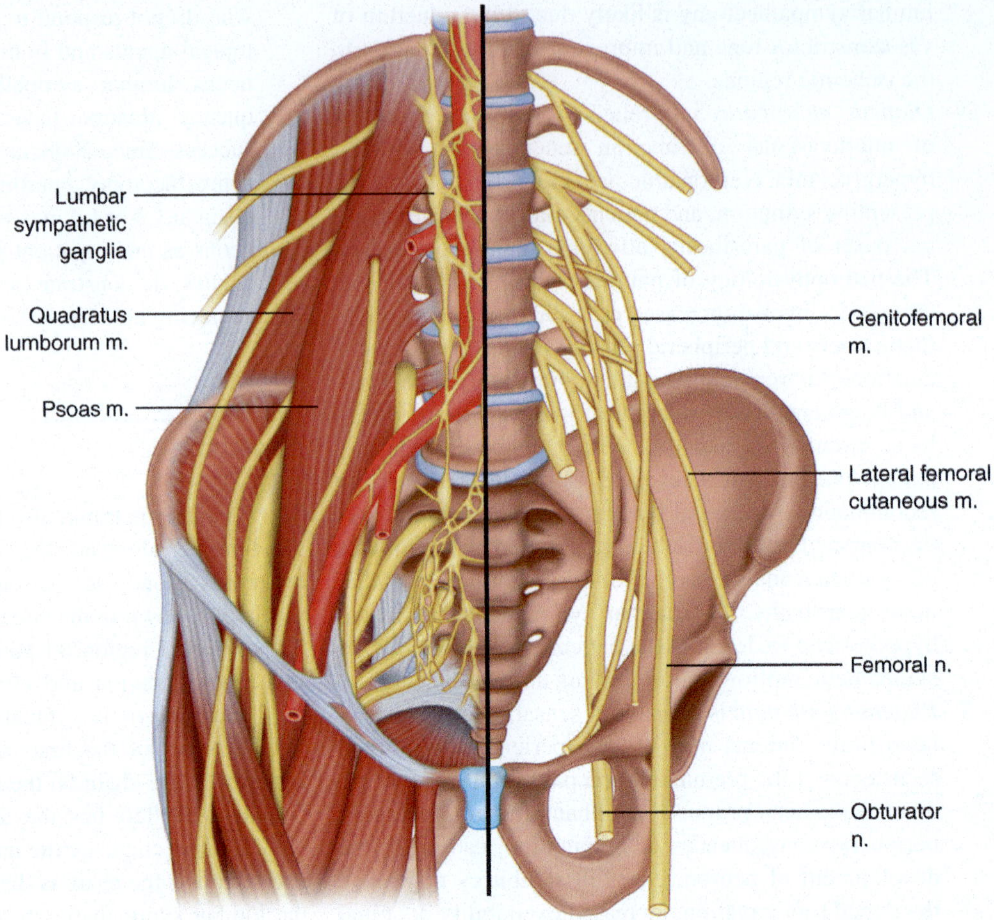

Fig. 57.1 Schematic of lumbar sympathetic ganglia located anterior to the psoas muscle, which separates the ganglia from the lumbar plexus

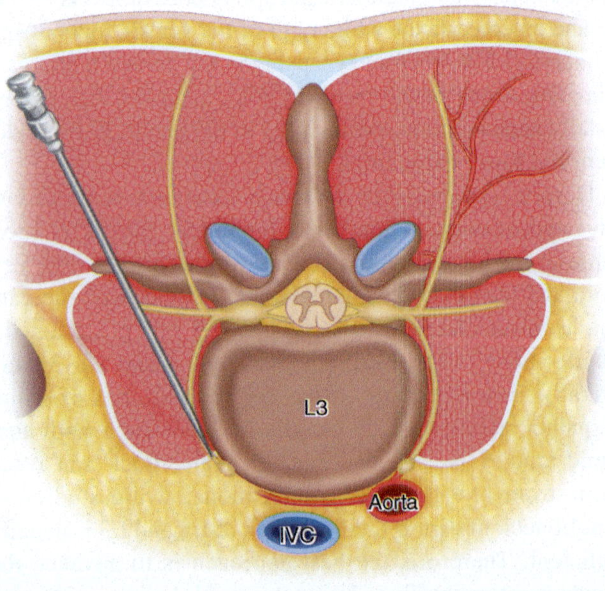

Fig. 57.2 Axial schematic of needle trajectory using paravertebral approach

Technique

Prior to positioning, the baseline temperature of bilateral lower extremities should be established and recorded. Continuous EKG, oxygen saturation, and intermittent blood pressure monitoring along with intravenous access are recommended. The patient is positioned prone with a cushion placed under the abdomen to reduce the lumbar lordosis. Fluoroscopic beam is adjusted until the superior end plates of L2–L3 are aligned. From there, the C-arm is rotated ipsilaterally until the tip of ipsilateral L2 or L3 transverse process is superimposed with the lateral border of the L2 or L3 vertebral body. The desired entry point is typically along the inferior third of the anterolateral border of the L2 vertebral body or superior to mid-third of the anterolateral border of the L3 vertebral body. In this oblique view, the needle is advanced until the needle tip contacts the anterolateral border of the vertebral body.

Lateral imaging is obtained to confirm that the needle tip is at the anterior vertebral line. An AP image is taken to verify that the needle tip remains within the medial border of the ipsilateral pedicle. 1–5 ml of contrast is injected. Appropriate spread of contrast typically appears "cloudy" and extends superiorly and inferiorly in front of the ipsilateral lumbar vertebra rather than laterally; ideally, there is sufficient spread from L1 to L3, and if not, a multi-needle technique should be considered. The contrast spread should not be "streaky" and extend caudally and laterally in outlining the psoas muscle. If the needle tip is still within the psoas muscle, the needle should be advanced slightly until repeat injection of contrast shows appropriate spread; failure to advance past the psoas muscle may result in blockage of the anterior rami of the upper lumbar region.

Digital subtraction angiography (DSA) can be used to confirm lack of vascular pattern as it is more sensitive than continuous fluoroscopy. Once appropriate contrast spread is demonstrated on fluoroscopy, 5–15 ml of local anesthetic, usually 1% lidocaine or 0.25% bupivacaine or 1:1 mixture, is injected in 1–2 ml increments after verifying negative aspiration for heme and CSF. If chemical neurolysis is desired, 2–3 ml of phenol (3%–6%) or alcohol (50%–100%) is injected. Failure to obtain appropriate contrast spread should prompt consideration of aborting the procedure.

A technically successful block is supported by post-procedural temperature rise of at least 3 °C in the ipsilateral lower extremity. Following the procedure, patient's pain is re-evaluated for any resolution or reduction of pain. EKG changes and any mental status changes should be closely observed. Of note, some protocols recommend maintaining patients in the prone position afterward with the needles in situ for 20–30 minutes to minimize posterior spread of the solutions into the psoas muscle, but this is usually considered when phenol is used rather than local anesthetic. Regardless, the patient should be monitored for at least 20 minutes post-procedure.

With minimal modification to the technique, conventional radiofrequency ablation could be undertaken. A 20 gauge 150-mm-long radiofrequency needle with a 10 mm non-insulated tip should be utilized. Two levels, i.e., L2 and L3, could be considered though one level has been shown to be adequate in many cases. After confirming appropriate position via contrast, electrical stimulation can be carried out using 50 Hz and 5 Hz to identify any proximity to sensory and motor nerves and to decrease the risk of ablating a segmental nerve root. 1 ml of 2% lidocaine is injected prior to lesioning at 80 ° for 1 minute. Pulsed radiofrequency ablation can similarly be performed over 3 cycles and 120 seconds/cycle per level at a temperature of 42 °C. The generator is usually set at a target voltage of 45 Volts with a pulse width of 20 ms and a pulse rate of 2 Hz though these parameters are usually automatically changed to maintain the temperature.

Efficacy

Evidence for efficacy of lumbar sympathetic blocks in the treatment of sympathetically mediated pain disorders comprise primarily of case studies and single-center randomized trials. There is a paucity of high-quality randomized control trials comparing treatment with placebo.

Evidence for Efficacy in Complex Regional Pain Syndrome

Lumbar Sympathetic Block Versus Placebo

Price in 1998 evaluated seven patients with complex regional pain syndrome in a double-blind, placebo-controlled cross-over study. Four patients underwent stellate ganglion block, while three underwent lumbar sympathetic block. Magnitude and duration of pain relief were monitored. There was no significant difference in the initial peak reduction of pain intensity, as measured by mechanical allodynia 30 minutes after the block, between patients who received saline and local anesthetic. However, there was a significant difference in duration of local anesthetic (90 hours) as compared to saline (19 hours) in all patients.

Cochrane review in 2016 concluded that there was insufficient evidence to support or refute the efficacy of lumbar sympathetic block for the treatment of CRPS. To date, the most rigorous trial of note is a double-blind, placebo, cross-over trial in 23 patients, age 10–18 years of age, with CRPS. Half of the patients were randomized to lumbar sympathetic blockade with lidocaine and an IV saline infusion, while the other half were randomized to a lumbar sympathetic blockade with saline and an IV lidocaine infusion. Patients who received lumbar sympathetic blockade with lidocaine demonstrated significant pain reduction and improvement in sensory dysfunction compared with placebo—this provided evidence that a portion of pain secondary to CRPS was mediated by abnormal sympathetic outflow.

Radiofrequency of Lumbar Plexus Versus Chemical Neurolysis

In a comparison study of radiofrequency denervation and phenol sympathetic blocks, 17 patients in 1991 underwent either lumbar sympathetic neurolysis with phenol or radiofrequency of the lumbar sympathetic plexus. Eighty-nine percent of patients in the phenol group were shown to have sympathetic blockade after 8 weeks whereas only 12% in the radiofrequency ablation group ($P < 0.05$). The radiofrequency ablation group was noted to have lower incidence of post-sympathetic neuralgia. A similar study was undertaken in 2008 with refinement of the radiofrequency ablation technique. In the ten patients randomized to conventional radiofrequency, the radiofrequency cannula was introduced lateral to L2, L3, and L4 with two sites lesioned at each level, whereas in the ten patients randomized to neurolysis, the cannula was similarly placed, but this was followed by 3 ml of 7% phenol at every level. The conclusion was that there was no statistical significant difference in efficacy in the days to 4 months following the procedure. Freitas in 2014 randomized 40 patients with CRPS Type I to pulsed radiofrequency ablation or sympathetic neurolysis. Pain scores and quality of life were recorded in follow-up of 1 day, a week, 2–4 months, and 6 months; based on these measures, pulsed radiofrequency was found to have comparable results to phenol neurolysis.

Lumbar Sympathetic Block with Botox Versus Conventional Lumbar Sympathetic Block

A preliminary study in patients with refractory complex regional pain syndrome (CRPS) by Carroll in 2009 showed the addition of botulinum toxin A to bupivacaine, a standard local anesthetic in lumbar sympathetic blocks, can significantly prolong the median analgesic period from 10 days to 71 days. One proposed mechanism of analgesia is the inhibition of release of acetylcholine from the cholinergic sympathetic ganglia.

Evidence for Efficacy in Peripheral Vascular Disease

Cohort Studies

The evidence for efficacy in peripheral vascular disease comprises of both cohort studies and early randomized trials. A retrospective study of 153 patients who underwent surgical lumbar sympathectomy showed that after 5 years, 67% of patients with claudication and 54% of patients with rest pain were able to avoid further surgery. A study of 385 patients after surgical lumbar sympathectomy by Matarazarro in 2002 reported improvement in pain, recovery of trophic lesions, and rise in skin temperature in 63% after 1 year.

In 1995, Mashiah described a prospective study of 373 patients with peripheral vascular disease who underwent a phenol lumbar neurolysis; over 1–10-year follow-up, it was found that 58% experienced pain relief and healing of gangrenous ulcers. The results were most notable in diabetic patients with rest pain and in nondiabetic patients with digital gangrene or ulcers, suggesting patient selection is key.

Chemical Neurolysis Versus Placebo

In 1975, Fyfe randomized 25 patients with claudication pain to phenol sympathectomy and local anesthetic control and found that there was no subjective improvement in pain or objective evidence in improvement with treadmill testing. In 1985, 41 patients with intermittent claudication were randomized to either phenol lumbar neurolysis or a placebo bupivacaine injection; 83% of patients in the treatment group reported decreased pain compared to the 23% of patients in the placebo group at 6 months. Updated Cochrane review in 2016 concluded that there was no high-quality randomized controlled trials that compared surgical or percutaneous lumbar sympathectomy with no treatment in patients with critical lower limb ischemia as there were only four randomized trials described in the literature to date and patient selection was not based on sufficiently objective criteria.

Pearls and Pitfalls

Lumbar sympathetic block is a minimally invasive and relatively safe pain reduction procedure. The most common complications include bleeding, swelling, and soreness at the injection site. However, the complications can span a full spectrum of categories, including neurologic, renal and ureteric, and vascular sequelae (see Table 57.2 for comprehensive list of pitfalls and pearls).

To minimize procedural complications, one must focus on both careful patient selection and precise needle advancement. Pre-procedure discussion with the patient should involve a discussion of anticoagulation; specifically, patient must hold anticoagulation for the same specified number of days as he or she would for a neuraxial procedure. To highlight the incompatibility of concurrent anticoagulation and lumbar sympathetic block, Hohf in 1953 presented a series of cases, which ultimately all resulted in death from massive retroperitoneal hematoma.

CT scans of cadavers suggest that the paravertebral distance of insertion of needles should not exceed 6, 7, and 10 cm lateral to the spinous processes of L2, L3, and L4, respectively, so as to avoid puncturing internal organs. Placement at the superior third of L2 is potentially challenging as the needle tip might approach the vertebral insertion of the diaphragm. The correct final needle position should be 0.5–0.8 cm dorsal to the anterior vertebral border, for if it were a right-sided lumbar sympathetic block, advancement toward the vertebral border might led to inadvertent IVC puncture in 20% of the cases. The optimal approach is to advance the needle paravertebrally through the fascia of the psoas muscle slightly cephalad to the midpoint of the body of L3; excessive anterior advancement of the needle will likely result in intravascular puncture, whereas insufficient advancement of the needle past the psoas muscle will likely result in partial block of the lumbar plexus, resulting in a temporary ipsilateral weakness post-procedurally.

Table 57.2 Complications following lumbar sympathetic block and tips

Complication	Description	Tips
Neuralgia	The most common neuralgia is that of genitofemoral nerve (incidence varies from 6 to 40% after chemical neurolysis); patient will typically present with dysesthesia in the anteromedial upper thigh, approximately 2–6 weeks in duration Depending on the extravasation to the psoas muscle, neurolysis may also spill over to the lateral cutaneous nerve of the thigh, resulting in transient meralgia paresthetica	Do not inject if the contrast spread suggest the needle tip is in the psoas muscle Use smaller volumes of neurolytic agent at levels above L4 to minimize spread to genitofemoral nerve Symptoms can be relieved with transcutaneous electric nerve stimulator and intravenous lidocaine infusion
Somatic nerve block	Patients may exhibit reduced strength in the myotomes of L1–L4, suggesting posterior spread of local anesthetic along tendinous arches which bridges the concave sides of lumbar vertebra, or reduced strength in the distribution of the femoral nerve, suggesting inadvertent injection of local anesthetic into the psoas muscle	Do not inject if the contrast spread suggest the needle tip is in the psoas muscle Use smaller volumes of local anesthetic to minimize extravasation
Subarachnoid injection	Death can result following lumbar sympathetic blockade, following inadvertent subarachnoid injection, leading to rapid motor block and hypotensive collapse seizures	Pre-procedural intravenous access and monitoring of vitals are recommended as safeguards All practitioners should have ready access to resuscitation equipment and be ready to administer cardiopulmonary resuscitation
Post-dural puncture headache (PDPH)	There have been cases of PDPH without signs of subarachnoid injection. Entry point for inadvertent dura puncture may be a dural root sleeve or other anatomical variants	Epidural blood patch may not be effective if there was puncture of anatomical variant
Paraplegia	While the risk for paraplegia is higher with thoracic paravertebral alcohol injection or celiac plexus neurolysis, there is one documented of a T10 myelopathy. The mechanism of injury is unclear and may be either due to an anterior spinal artery ischemia or a direct spinal cord injection. Inadvertent intrathecal injection of neurolysis may also cause paralysis but is more likely to be transient	Alcohol likely provides more intense neural destruction than phenol and diffuse more rapidly through tissue. While phenol provides a shorter duration compared to alcohol, phenol may be a safer choice though there is no controlled study comparing the two for lumbar sympathetic block
Aseptic meningitis	There have been 2 cases of self-limiting aseptic meningitis without any obvious signs of an intrathecal injection	
Epidural injection	Retrograde spread via communicating sympathetic rami into the epidural space can result depending on the volume of injectate. In one study, 5/6 patients were shown to have epidural spread when 5 ml of injectate was used at L2, whereas in another study, 3/5 patients were shown to have epidural spread extending to T10 when 10 ml of injectate was used	Use smaller volumes of injectate to minimize posterior extravasation Maintaining the patient in the prone position for 20–30 more minutes following the procedure may limit posterior spread
Renal and ureteric injuries	Patient may experience hematuria, which resolves spontaneously after 2–3 days, suggesting puncture injury to the kidney or ureter. Sequelae of renal puncture also include transient hematuria, renal colic, dysuria, and massive subcapsular hematoma	Use paravertebral technique with fluoroscopy or CT. The needle entry should not be too lateral Anatomical study using CT showed that insertion of needles in L2, L3, and L4 should not exceed 6, 7, and 10 cm from midline, respectively
Vascular complications	Multiple reports of retroperitoneal hematomas in patients who were concurrently on anticoagulation were described in the 1950s	Patients on anticoagulation should not undergo lumbar sympathetic blocks The pain practitioner should abide by the American Society of Regional Anesthesia (ASRA) guidelines for holding anticoagulation for neuraxial procedures
Hypotension	Hypotension may result immediately following the procedure due to vasodilation following sympathetic blockade and may also develop in the hours to days following the procedure due to an occult bleed	Limit injectate volume and perform unilateral lumbar sympathectomy rather than bilateral If large volumes of local anesthetic are desired, consider administering IV fluids prior to the procedure in healthy patients who can tolerate increased preload

(continued)

Table 57.2 (continued)

Complication	Description	Tips
Local anesthetic toxicity	Provided that the injection is not intravascular, there is low risk for local anesthetic toxicity as the lumbar sympathetic ganglion is not localized to a highly vascular area. The local anesthetic absorption is notably slow. In one study, patients who received lumbar sympathetic blocks with 20 ml of 0.25% bupivacaine did not demonstrate peak levels above the toxic threshold; the duration to peak plasma concentration was approximately 24–60 minutes later	Injectate volume of 20 ml of local anesthetic can be considered Consider test dose of lidocaine with 1:200 K epinephrine with pulse monitoring to assess if there's any intravascular spread Be ready to administer intralipid in an emergent situation. May require extracorporeal membrane oxygenation if bupivacaine is injected intravascularly.
Pneumothorax	Rare complications following lumbar sympathetic block include pneumothorax	Avoid placement of needle at the superior third of L2 as the needle tip will approach the vertebral insertion of the diaphragm If abnormal anatomy is anticipated, consider CT-guided lumbar sympathetic block or obtaining a CT prior to the procedure for planning the safest needle trajectory
Discitis	Discogenic pain may result from inadvertent intra-discal injection	Place needle tip at the level of mid-body of vertebrae
Sexual dysfunction	Retrograde ejaculation is a known risk following bilateral lumbar sympathetic block. Diabetes is a risk factor for retrograde ejaculation	Avoid bilateral lumbar sympathetic block

Recommended Reading

1. Brunn J, Mandl F. Die paravertebrale Injektion zur Bekampfung visceraler Schmerzen. Wien Lin Wochenschr. 1924;37:511–4.
2. Cheng J, Daftari A, Zhou L. Sympathetic blocks provided sustained pain relief in a patient with refractory painful diabetic neuropathy. Case Rep Anesthesiol. 2012;2012:285328.
3. Cohen SP, Gambel JM, Raja SN, et al. The contribution of sympathetic mechanisms to postamputation phantom and residual limb pain: a pilot study. J Pain. 2011;12(8):859–67.
4. Cross FW, Cotton LT. Chemical lumbar sympathectomy for ischemic rest pain. A randomized, prospective controlled clinical trial. Am J Surg. 1985;150(3):341–5.
5. Dick A, Gabbott D, Hardy P. Plasma concentrations of bupivacaine following a single needle lumbar sympathectomy using two volumes of 0.25% bupivacaine plain solution. Anaesthesia. 1996;51:750–1.
6. Evans J, Dobben G, Gay G. Peridural effusion of drugs following sympathetic blockade. JAMA. 1967;200:93–8.
7. Freitas TS, Deusdara R, Kessler I. Pulsed radiofrequency of sympathetic lumbar plexus versus sympathetic block in the management of lower limb complex regional pain syndrome type. Stereotact Funct Neurosurg. 2014;91:107.
8. Fyfe T, Quin RO. Phenol sympathectomy in the treatment of intermittent claudication: a controlled clinical trial. Br J Surg. 1975;62:68–71.
9. Garcia LA. Epidemiology and pathophysiology of lower extremity peripheral arterial disease. J Endovasc Ther. 2006;13:113–9.
10. Halbert J, Crotty M, Cameron ID. Evidence for the optimal management of acute and chronic phantom pain: a systematic review. Coin J Pain. 2002;18(2):84–92.
11. Haxton HA. Chemical sympathectomy. BMJ. 1949;1(4614):1026.
12. Haxton HA. Paravertebral block with aqueous phenol in the treatment of vascular disease. Angiology. 1953;4:268–80.
13. Haynsworth RF, Noe CE. Percutaneous lumbar sympathectomy: a comparison of radiofrequency denervation phenol neurolysis. Anesthesiology. 1991;74(3):459–63.
14. Hohf RP. Danger of lumbar sympathetic blocks during anticoagulant therapy. JAMA. 1953;152(5):399–400.
15. Holliday FA, et al. Lumbar sympathectomy in critical limb ischemia: surgical, chemical or not at all? Cardiovasc Surg. 1999;7:200–2.
16. Hord ED, Cohen SP, Cosgrove GR, et al. The predictive value of lumbar sympathetic block for success of spinal cord stimulation. Neurosurgery. 2003;53(3):626–32. discussion 632–3.
17. Katz J. The role of the sympathetic nervous system in phantom pain. In: Phantom pain. The Springer series in behavioral psychophysiology and medicine. Boston: Springer; 1997.
18. Manjunath PS. Management of lower limb complex regional pain syndrome type 1: an evaluation of percutaneous radiofrequency thermal lumbar sympathectomy versus phenol lumbar sympathetic neurolysis- A Pilot Study. Anesth Analg. 2008;106(2):647–9.
19. Mashiah A. Phenol lumbar sympathetic block in diabetic lower limb ischemia. J Cardiovasc Risk. 1995;2:467–9.
20. Matarazzo A, et al. Possibilities at present for the application of lumbar sympathectomy in chronic occlusive arterial disease of the lower limb. Minerva Cardioangiol. 2002;50:363–9.
21. Meier PM, et al. Lumbar sympathetic blockade in children with CRPS: a double blind placebo-controlled cross over trial. Anesthesiology. 2009;11(2):372–80.
22. Middleton W, Chan V. Lumbar sympathetic block: a review of complications. Tech Reg Anesth Pain Manag. 1998;2(3):137–46.
23. Neil EO, et al. Local anesthetic sympathetic blockade for CRPS. Cochrane Database Syst Rev. 2016;4:CD004598.
24. Nesargikar PN, et al. Lumbar chemical sympathectomy in peripheral vascular disease: does it still have a role? Int J Surg. 2009;7:145–9.
25. Price DD, Long S, Wilsey B, Raffi A. Analysis of peak magnitude and duration of analgesia produced by local anesthetics injected into the sympathetic ganglia of complex regional pain syndrome patients. Clin J Pain. 1998;14(3):216–26.
26. Repelaer van Driel OJ, et al. Lumbar sympathectomy for severe lower limb ischaemia: results and analysis of factors influencing the outcome. J Cardiovasc Surg. 1988;29:310–4.
27. Rieger R. Management of plantar hyperhidrosis with endoscopic lumbar sympathectomy. Thorac Surg Clin. 2016;26(4):465–9.
28. Rocco AG, Palombi D, Raeke D. Anatomy of the lumbar sympathetic chain. Reg Anesth. 1995;20:13–9.
29. Royle JP. A History of sympathectomy. Aust NZJ Surg. 1999;69:302–7.

30. Stanton-Hicks MD. Complex regional pain syndrome: manifestations and the role of neurostimulation in its management. J Pain Symptom Manag. 2006;31(4S):S20–4.
31. Stanton-Hicks MD, Burton AW, Bruehl SP, et al. An updated interdisciplinary clinical pathway for CRPS: report of an expert panel. Pain Pract. 2002;2:1–16.
32. Straube S, Derry S, Moore RA, McQuay HJ. Cervico-thoracic or lumbar sympathectomy for neuropathic pain and complex regional pain syndrome. Cochrane Database Syst Rev. 2010;7:1–15.
33. Tsigos PR, et al. Plasma norepinephrine in sensory diabetic polyneuropathy. Diabetes Care. 1993;16(5):722–7.
34. Verma YS, Thakur JR, Sodhi SS. Evaluation of chemical lumbar sympathectomy for chronic arterial ischaemia of lower limb(s). J Anaesthesiol Clin Pharmacol. 2007;23:391–4.
35. Wall PD, Gutnick M. Ongoing activity in peripheral nerves: the physiology and pharmacology of impulses originating from a neuroma. Exp Neurol. 1974;43(3):580–93.
36. West M, Wu H. Pulsed radiofrequency ablation for residual and phantom limb pain: a case series. Pain Pract. 2010;10(5):485–91.
37. Weyland A, Weyland W, Carduck H. Optimization of the intensifier-assisted technique of lumbar sympathetic block. Anaesthesist. 1993;42:710–8.

Celiac Plexus Block and Superior Hypogastric Plexus Block

58

Dawood Sayed, Patrick D. Grace,
and Brian H. Wetherington

Celiac Plexus Block

Introduction

The celiac plexus, also known as the coeliac or solar plexus, is situated on the anterolateral surface of the aorta next to the celiac trunk and superior mesenteric artery at the T12/L1 vertebral level. Lying posterior to the stomach and omental bursa, this plexus is composed of numerous fibers and individual celiac ganglia. The sympathetic innervation originates in the anterolateral horn within the T5 to T12 levels. Afferent fibers from the abdominal viscera carry pain signal along with the sympathetic nerves. Passing through the thoracic sympathetic chain, the presynaptic sympathetic fibers are grouped T5 to T9 as the greater splanchnic nerve, T10 and T11 as the lesser splanchnic nerve, and T12 as the least splanchnic nerve. The presynaptic splanchnic fibers synapse in the celiac ganglia, and the postsynaptic fibers from the celiac ganglia innervate the most in the abdominal viscera including the liver, stomach, spleen, diaphragm, kidneys, adrenal glands, small intestine, and colon up to the splenic flexure. Abdominal viscera excluded is the descending colon, sigmoid colon, rectum, and pelvic viscera.

Background and Historical Perspective

The celiac plexus block (CPB) is one of the oldest and most studied neurolytic blocks. Dating back to the early 1919, Max Kappis performed transcutaneous injections of prilocaine into the back of dogs and demonstrated that pain from the organs in the upper abdomen is carried by the splanchnic fibers. Even though this technique is not a celiac plexus block, his work highlighted a part of the neural network associated with pain in the upper abdomen. In the 1950s, JJ Bonica described and documented the percutaneous celiac plexus block, along with using alcohol-based neurolysis for intra-abdominal malignancies. Since that time, imaging techniques such as plain radiographs, fluoroscopy, ultrasound, and computed tomography (CT) have all been described as methods for successful needle placement during a CPB. Despite the diversity in imaging techniques, none of these have been proven to be safer or superior to the others.

Uses and Indications

Visceral abdominal pain from the stomach to the splenic flexure of the colon, liver, pancreas, gall bladder, omentum, and mesentery has all been targeted by the celiac plexus and splanchnic block. The primary indication for a neurolytic celiac plexus block is cancer-related pain, specifically pancreatic cancer. In patients with gastrointestinal malignancies, both the celiac plexus and splanchnic neurolysis have been shown to increase the quality of life, reduce pain, and, in some cases, reduce the need for oral medications. Bridenbaugh and colleagues reported that 40 out of 41 patients had meaningful improvement in pain without significant side effects after a neurolytic celiac plexus block. Several studies have highlighted the similarities in outcomes between the celiac plexus block and the splanchnic block. Amera and colleagues documented that a neurolytic celiac plexus block was comparable to a bilateral splanchnic block in regard to pain control in 60 patients with upper gastrointestinal tract tumors. As mentioned later in this chapter, the evidence strongly supports the use of these techniques for cancer-related pain; however, it is highly debatable for nonmalignant or benign visceral pain due to lack of supporting evidence. The use of the blocks for nonmalignant pain, particularly in chronic pancreatitis, is debated due to short-term relief and lack of evidence supporting long-term benefit.

D. Sayed (✉)
The University of Kansas Health System, Kansas City, KS, USA
e-mail: dsayed@kumc.edu

P. D. Grace · B. H. Wetherington
Department of Anesthesiology and Pain Medicine,
The University of Kansas Health System, Kansas City, KS, USA
e-mail: pgrace@kumc.edu

T. R. Deer et al. (eds.), *Deer's Treatment of Pain*, https://doi.org/10.1007/978-3-030-12281-2_58

Techniques/Approaches/Positioning

Celiac Plexus Block

Posterior Percutaneous Transcrural (Classic): Fluoroscopy

Positioning

Using fluoroscopy, this technique involves the patient lying in the prone position. The C-arm is obliquely turned 20–30° until the transverse process of L1 is in line with the contralateral facet joint or lies over the anterolateral margin of the L1 vertebral body. While positioned at the thoracolumbar junction, the tip of the transverse process at L1 should be "hidden" or "eliminated." If further adjustment is needed, cephalad or caudad tilt can be utilized to optimize the view. The final position of the needle is at the level of T12/L1 and beside the anterolateral surface of the aorta (See Figs. 58.1 and 58.2).

Technique

Subcutaneous 1% lidocaine is injected over the upper margin of the L1 vertebral body. Some providers use the middle margin of the vertebral body, while others recommend the superior margin as their starting location. A left-sided approach is recommended due to the probability of performing this block as a single-needle approach. Using a 22 gauge spinal needle, 5 inch for normal-size patients or 8 inch for obese, the provider advances the needle in a coaxial view inferior to the 12th rib and superior to the transverse process of L1 with the final location being anterior to the L1 vertebral body. As the needle advances, repeat imaging should be performed to confirm coaxial needle position. Once the needle is beside the anterolateral margin of the L1 vertebral body, the C-arm is rotated to the lateral position. The provider should use continuous aspiration as the needle advances 2–3 cm anteriorly beyond the margin of the L1 vertebral body. Using the lateral view, contrast dye is injected under live fluoroscopy. If an aortagram is observed, then advance the needle through the opposing aortic wall. Repeat the injection of radiographic contrast under live fluoroscopy to confirm that the needle is not intravascular. If blood is aspirated while advancing the needle in the lateral view, then the needle has entered the aorta, and the technique is now a transaortic approach. The needle should be advanced until blood is no longer aspirated and the needle has passed through the aorta. Once aspiration is negative for blood, then radiographic contrast is injected under live fluoroscopy to confirm that the needle is not intravascular. The final position of the needle is confirmed after 1–2 mL of radiographic contrast is injected with spread along the anterior surface of the aorta with a pulsatile-like effect, without signs of vascular uptake, and with negative aspiration of blood. The C-arm

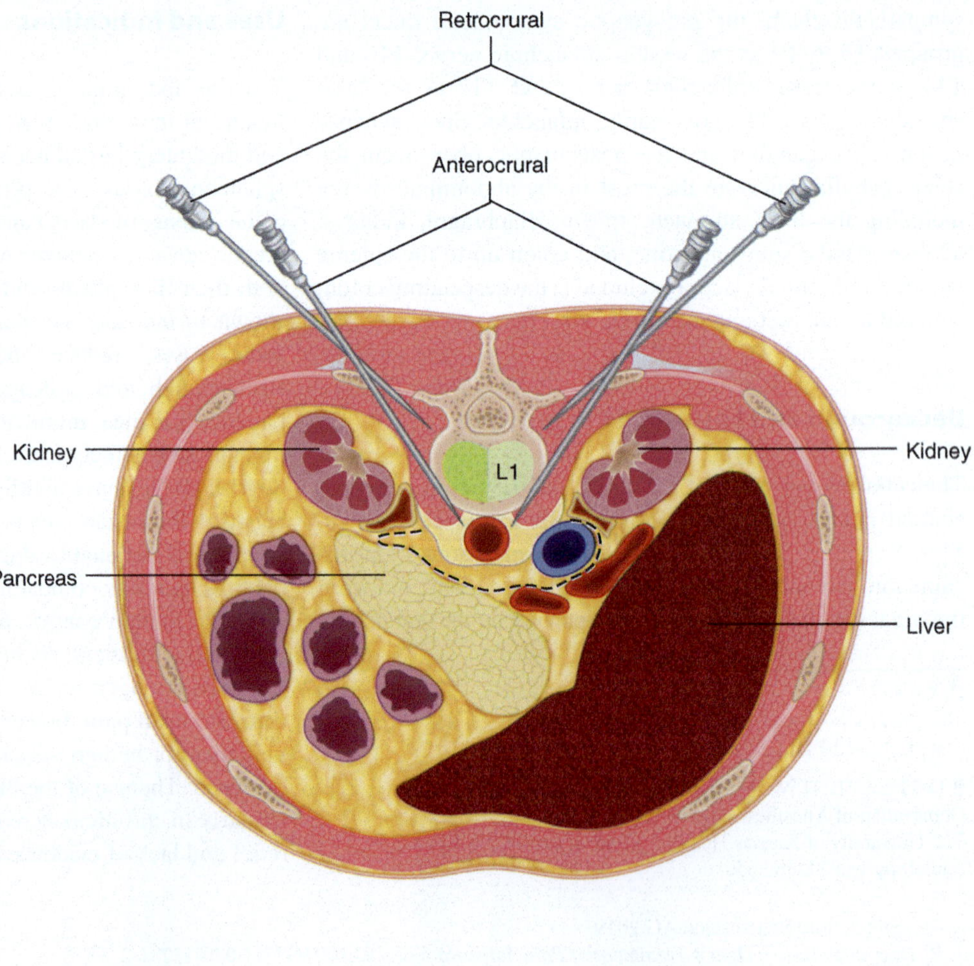

Fig. 58.1 Axial view of needle position for percutaneous celiac plexus block in anterocrural and retrocrural approach

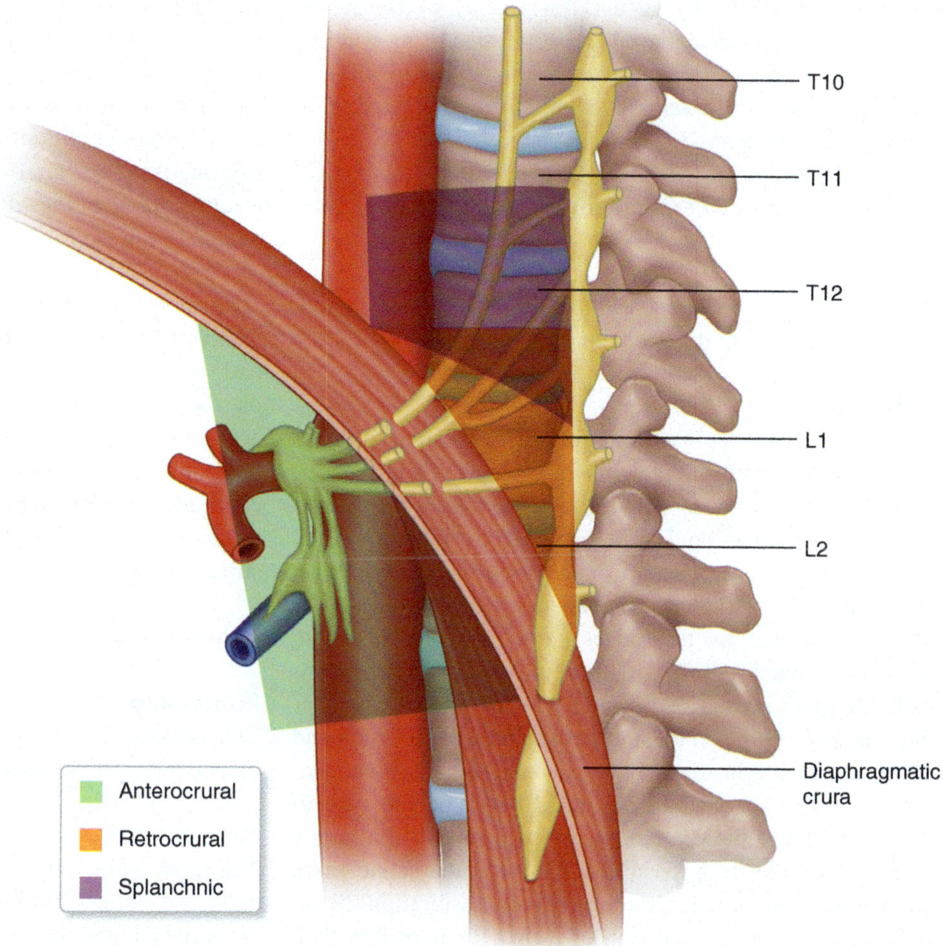

Fig. 58.2 Sagittal view of the target zone for the anterocrural, retrocrural, and splanchnic approach for celiac plexus blockade

is turned to an AP position, and the needle should be medial to the lateral margin of the vertebral body. If the radiographic contrast spread crosses midline to the contralateral side, then a single-needle approach is adequate. However, if the spread of contrast stays ipsilateral and does not cross midline, then a second needle is placed on the contralateral side, and the same technique is used. After confirmation of the final needle position and use of contrast dye, a diagnostic block can be achieved with 20–30 mL of 0.25% bupivacaine. If a bilateral approach is necessary, then the total dose is divided. Regardless, incremental injection followed by gentle aspiration is recommended to assess for intravascular involvement. The patient should be monitored for clinical signs of intravascular uptake or neuraxial blockade.

Posterior Percutaneous Transcrural: Computed Tomography Guided

Positioning

The patient is placed in the prone position, and the skin is anesthetized similarly to the fluoroscopy approach.

Technique

Three-dimensional reconstruction and cone beam guidance are the two modalities that are utilized for computed tomography-guided needle placement. With three-dimensional reconstruction, the initial CT scan determines the plane and depth for the needle placement. The patient is removed from the CT machine, and a needle is placed using the information gathered from the initial CT scan. The patient returns to the CT scanner for a follow-up image to verify the final needle position. If the needle is not optimally placed, then the imaging technique is repeated. Once the position is verified, contrast dye is injected, and the dispersion is confirmed with either repeated CT imaging or fluoroscopy. The three-dimensional reconstruction technique can take longer to perform than other techniques and can be linked to higher doses of radiation to both the patient and the provider. The cone beam guidance is a new technique that operates using 50–70% less radiation than traditional computed tomography machines. In addition to lower radiation exposure, the cone beam is a combination of CT and fluoroscopic imaging. Software enhances this combination of imaging and highlights the expected needle insertion point, direction, and depth. Using live fluoroscopy overlying the CT image, the needle is placed and confirmed using contrast dye. This method is theoretically superior to the former CT technique due its shorter procedure time, lower radiation exposure, and preserved accuracy.

Ultrasound-Guided Percutaneous

Positioning

The patient is placed supine and may need to control the rate of respiration during this technique.

Technique

Starting in the midepigastric region of the patient, a cured array 3–5 MHz transducer with low frequency is positioned in a transverse view to demonstrate the descending aorta, liver, and vertebral body. The celiac trunk is located and color Doppler flow is used to confirm vascular structures. With the celiac structure positioned in the middle of the ultrasound screen, the transducer is rotated longitudinally to both the celiac trunk and the superior mesenteric artery. Color Doppler is used again, and a 22 gauge, 10–15 cm needle is advanced toward the area between the celiac trunk and superior mesenteric artery. In plane versus out of plane, needle placement should be determined based on the type of needle used and the desired needle path toward the target. Once the needle tip is positioned between the celiac trunk and the superior mesenteric artery, negative aspiration should be done followed by injection of 3 mL 1% lidocaine with epinephrine to assess for intravascular spread. Diagnosed block can be performed after a negative response for intravascular uptake with 5 mL incremental injections. This technique is commonly described as a single-needle technique; however, a two-needle technique has been documented. With this technique, the celiac trunk is localized in the transverse view, and a needle is inserted laterally on both sides of the transducer. Proponents of this technique suggest enhanced demonstration of medication spread on injection.

Splanchnic Nerve Block (Retrocrural)

Positioning

In similar fashion to the classic approach, the patient lies prone, the C-arm is in position, and the skin is anesthetized with lidocaine.

Technique

This block requires bilateral needle placement. With the C-arm oblique in a similar fashion to the classic celiac plexus block approach, the C-arm is also tilted cephalad by a range of 20–30 °. A 22 gauge spinal needle (5 inch in most patients, 8 inch for obese) is introduced superior to the L1 transverse process and directed toward the anterolateral aspect of the T12 vertebral body. As the needle advances every few cm, a new fluoroscopic image should be taken. Once the needle contacts the T12 vertebral body, the C-arm is repositioned in the lateral view. The needle is advanced with repeat imaging every couple of cm until the needle tip rests along the anterior one-third portion of the T12 vertebral body. The C-arm is repositioned in the AP view, and the needle should be seen medial to the lateral aspect of the T12 body. Using live fluoroscopy, 1–2 cm of contrast media is injected. Appropriate contrast spread should highlight the anterior surface of the T12 vertebral body with most of the contrast on the ipsilateral side of the needle placement. This procedure is repeated on the contralateral side following the steps mentioned above. A diagnostic block is obtained by injecting a total dose of 10–15 mL of 0.25% bupivacaine divided evenly on each side. Incremental injection along with gentle aspiration to ensure that the needle has not advanced into a vascular structure should always be performed.

Celiac and Splanchnic Neurolysis

Positioning

The position for neurolysis is the same as the diagnostic blocks for each corresponding approach.

Medications

The most commonly used agents for neurolysis are phenol and ethyl alcohol. Phenol has local anesthetic and neurolytic properties depending on whether it is a low concentration or high concentration. Its anesthetic properties in higher dosages, 1000 mg or higher, can be seen clinically as generalized seizures or cardiovascular collapse if there is systemic uptake by intravascular injection. There is minimal if any pain on injection, but phenol can become viscous if mixed in a syringe with other solutions such as contrast media. Ethyl alcohol is used in concentrations greater or equal to 98%. It is easily injected; however, it causes pain on injection unless a local anesthetic is used prior to injection. Ethanol does not carry the local anesthetic properties of phenol; however, if a total dose of ethanol is mistakenly injected into a vascular structure, the blood alcohol level will rise above the legal driving limit. More pharmacological information regarding these two medications can be found in another chapter of this book (assuming there is a chapter on pharmacology, if not this section can be expanded).

Technique

Concentrations of phenol ranging from 10 to 12% can be mixed with contrast media (usually isohexol 180 mg/mL) to allow live fluoroscopy as the medication spreads on injection. For the celiac plexus neurolysis, a divided total volume of 20–30 mL is injected (10–15 mL per side). If ethanol is used, local anesthetic should be injected first to anesthetize the surrounding tissue. Like the classic approach for diagnostic block, if contrast spreads to the contralateral side of the vertebral body, then a single-needle approach can be used. The injection of the mixed solution should be stopped if spread is seen posteriorly due to the nerve root exiting the foramen. For the CT-guided approach, local anesthetic is first injected for a diagnostic block, followed by 20–40 mL of ethanol or phenol. For ultrasound-guided techniques, 10–50 mL of neurolytic solution has been reported. Finally, with the splanchnic approach, 10–15 mL total volume divided evenly on both sides should be used. Regardless of technique, needles should be flushed with normal saline or local anesthetic to prevent tracking neurolytic agent along the needle path as the needle is removed.

Evidence

A systemic review by Nagles looked at the efficacy of celiac plexus neurolysis for abdominal cancer. This systematic review assessed the effectiveness and side effects of celiac plexus neurolysis (CPN) in the treatment of upper abdominal cancer pain and evaluated whether there are any differences between the percutaneous and endoscopic ultrasound (EUS)-guided denervation techniques. The systematic review showed that percutaneous CPN significantly improves pain in patients with upper abdominal cancer, with a decrease in opioid consumption and side effects. It is unclear whether there is any change in quality of life. Case series suggest that EUS CPN improves pain. No conclusion can be made about EUS CPN's influence on opioid consumption. Although CPN is a safe procedure, side effects and complications can occur with both the percutaneous and EUS techniques.

Pearls and Pitfalls

(a) The most common side effect includes transient diarrhea (44%) and orthostatic hypotension (38%).
(b) Postprocedural pain is common (approx. 90%)and, however, should subside within 24–48 hours.
(c) Mechanism of action for common side effects is thought to be related to blockade of sympathetic fibers leaving unopposed parasympathetic signaling. Effects can last for several days.
(d) Rare complications (less than 1%) include retroperitoneal hematoma, intestinal injury, renal injury, pneumothorax, and spinal cord injury due to inadvertent injection of neurolytic agent into the artery of Adamkiewicz.
(e) Isolated reports with unknown incidence: superior mesenteric vein thrombosis after use of alcohol for neurolytic celiac plexus block.
(f) Intravascular injection of phenol can lead to signs of local anesthetic systemic toxicity with signs of central nervous system excitatory state with possible generalized seizures and potential cardiovascular collapse.
(g) Intravascular injection of ethanol can lead to blood alcohol levels that exceed the legal limit for driving.

Superior Hypogastric Plexus Block

Introduction

Overview

Visceral pelvic pain involving the bladder, uterus, rectum, vagina, and prostate can present as diffuse and vague-like pain that can be difficult to treat. Pathologies involving the distension, ischemia, and inflammation of affected tissues cause visceral pain and furthermore can be specifically targeted at the sympathetic level. While not as well studied as other sympathetic blocks, the superior hypogastric plexus block (SHGPB) has been shown to be an effective and safe method for visceral pelvic pain relief in observational and case series data.

Anatomy

Situated in the retroperitoneal space, the superior hypogastric plexus is a bilateral structure which extends from the anterior portion of the L4 and L5 vertebral bodies to the upper third of the S1 vertebral body. It lies anterior to the psoas muscle and within the fascia between the bifurcations of the common iliac arteries. The lumbar sympathetic chain supplies the afferent and postganglionic efferent fibers, while S2 to S4 supply the parasympathetic fibers. The superior hypogastric plexus travels caudally as the hypogastric nerves and eventually form the inferior hypogastric plexus.

Background and Historical Perspective

In 1990, Plancarte published a report involving the improvement or resolution in sympathetically mediated visceral pelvic cancer pain in 28 patients after a neurolytic superior hypogastric plexus block. Seven years later, he published a 3-year cohort study of 227 cancer patients (gynecological, colorectal, or genitourinary) with poor pain control (7–10/10 VAS) and suggested that 72% of the patients had a satisfactory response (<4/10 VAS), while 28% had a moderate response (4–7/10 VAS) after receiving a diagnostic and neurolytic superior hypogastric plexus block. However, this only represented 51% of the enrolled patients and was hypothesized to be related to the unknown spread of injected medication into a widely progressed disease area. Since Plancarte's initial study, others have documented the anatomy and technique of the superior hypogastric block using different imaging modalities.

Uses and Indications

Indications

Pain originating from the pelvic viscera is treated with a superior hypogastric plexus block (SHGPB). Neurolysis of the superior hypogastric plexus has demonstrated pain relief from those with malignant cancer pain that involves specifically pelvic structures such as the descending colon, uterus, proximal vagina, ovaries, prostate, and rectum. For nonmalignant cancer pain, diagnostic SHGP blocks are useful for diagnosing the source of pain.

Techniques/Approaches/Positioning

Classic Posterior Approach

Positioning

Using fluoroscopy, this technique involves the patient lying in the prone position. The posterior approach utilizes maneuvering the C-arm obliquely at roughly 25–35 ° and caudally with 25–35 ° of angulation to focus on lumbosacral junction. One study by Choi et al. found that the optimal oblique angle of fluoroscopy for the SHGPB was approximately 15 ° for males and 20 ° for females. These angle differences are associated with gender differences in pelvic anatomy where the pelvis of females tends to have a wider transverse diameter.

Technique

The target for a SHGPB involves the anterolateral border of the L5 vertebral body as the sympathetic ganglion is a retroperitoneal structure that extends bilaterally from the lower third of the L5 vertebral body to the upper third of the S1 vertebral body. The classic posterior approach originally described by Plancarte et al. in 1990 involved targeting the region where the hypogastric plexus has already divided into its right and left trunks and thus required two needles to reach both trunks. This approach was further modified by Waldman et al. who used computed tomography guidance to perform the block using a single needle and found bilateral spread of contrast. In the classic approach, the L5 spinous process is identified, and a mark is made about 5–7 cm lateral on either side from the midline. After 2–3 mL of 1% lidocaine is injected into the skin and subcutaneous tissue, a 22 gauge spinal needle, 5 inch for normal-size patients or 8 inch for obese, is advanced by using fluoroscopic guidance. Furthermore, there is a triangular window described by Dr. Rathmell that is bordered superiorly by the L5 transverse process, medially by the L5/S1 facet joint, and laterally by the iliac crest where the needle must pass through. The needle is at risk for making contact with the L5 spinal nerve root passing through this window to ultimately lie anterolateral to the L5/S1 intervertebral disc or the inferior third of the L5 vertebral body. Using the lateral view, aspiration should be applied to help exclude intravascular entry into one of the iliac vessels that lie in close proximity. In the rare case that blood is aspirated, the needle should be retracted slightly. Under live fluoroscopy, 2–3 mL of contrast is injected to confirm spread along the anterolateral surface of the lumbosacral junction. More specifically, there should be good linear spread over the anterior surface of the L5 vertebral body and the superior portion of the sacrum. The AP view can be used to confirm radiographic contrast spread crossing midline to the contralateral side in which case only a single-needle approach is necessary. However, if the spread of contrast remains ipsilateral and does not cross midline, then a second needle is placed on the contralateral side, and the same technique is performed. After confirming the final needle position with the use of contrast dye, a diagnostic block can be achieved with 8–10 mL of 0.25% bupivacaine. If a bilateral approach is necessary, then the total dose is divided. Regardless, incremental injection followed by gentle aspiration is recommended to assess for intravascular involvement. The patient should be monitored for clinical signs of intravascular uptake or neuraxial blockade. (See Fig. 58.3.)

Posteromedial Transdiscal Approach

Positioning

Using fluoroscopy, this technique involves the patient lying in the prone or lateral position.

Technique

The newer posteromedial transdiscal approach described by Turker et al. in 2005 involves identifying midline of the L5-S1 interlaminar space, and once 2–3 mL of 1% lidocaine has been injected into the skin and subcutaneous tissue, a 22 gauge spinal needle is advanced perpendicularly to the skin toward the intervertebral disc. The needle pierces the thecal sac from the lateral view and is advanced further only if there is absence of nerve injury or paresthesias until the needle exits the anterior surface of the intervertebral disc. As with all sympathetic blocks, contrast is used to identify and confirm correct positioning. The benefit of this newer approach was to overcome the technical challenges of the classic posterior approach which involved avoiding obstacles such as the large transverse processes of the L5 vertebral body, the high arch of the iliac crest, and the L5 spinal nerve roots. The transdiscal approach also has the added benefits of utilizing a single injection to provide an adequate block and allowing the patient the flexibility of being either in the prone or lateral

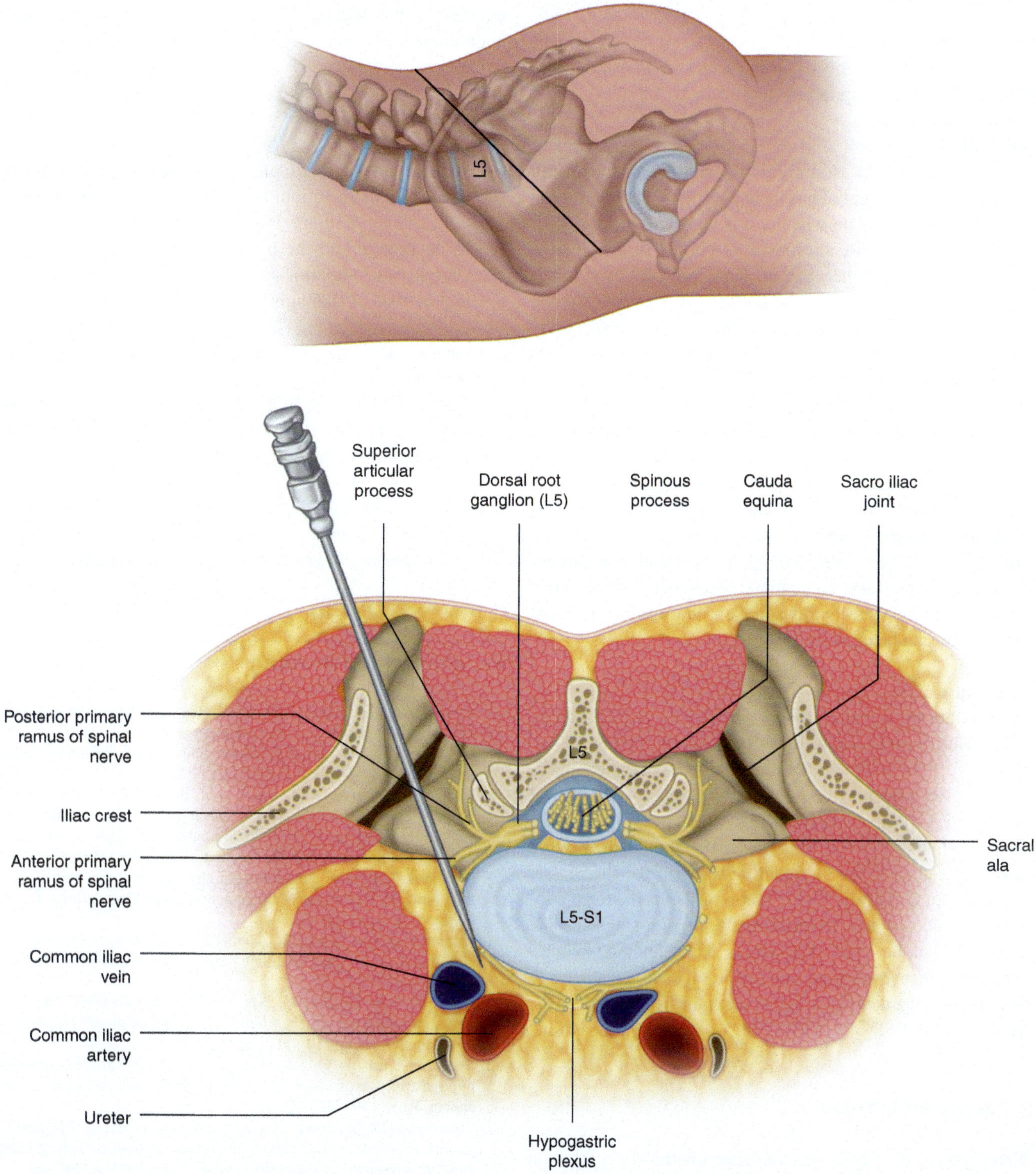

Fig. 58.3 Illustration of needle position and vital structures with percutaneous approach to superior hypogastric nerve block

position. Although the incidence is low at 1–2%, the transdiscal approach carries with it the serious risk of discitis. Overall, several studies have shown support of the transdiscal approach as an easier, safer, and more effective way to perform the SHGPB with less side effects and less anatomical obstructions than the classic approach.

Superior Hypogastric Plexus Neurolysis

Positioning

The position for neurolysis is the same as the diagnostic blocks for each corresponding approach.

Medications

The most commonly used agents for neurolysis are phenol and ethyl alcohol. Phenol has local anesthetic and neurolytic properties depending on whether it is a low concentration or high concentration. Its anesthetic properties in higher dosages, 1000 mg or higher, can be seen clinically as generalized seizures or cardiovascular collapse if there is systemic uptake by intravascular injection. There is minimal if any pain on injection, but phenol can become viscous if mixed in a syringe with other solutions such as contrast media. Ethyl alcohol is used in concentrations greater or equal to 98%. It is easily injected; however, it causes pain on injection unless a local anesthetic is used prior to injection. Ethanol does not carry the local anesthetic properties of phenol; however, if a total dose of ethanol is mistakenly injected into a vascular structure, the blood alcohol level will rise above the legal driving limit. More pharmacological information regarding these two medications can be found in another chapter of this book (assuming there is a chapter on pharmacology, if not this section can be expanded).

Technique

Concentrations of phenol ranging from 10% to 12% can be mixed with contrast media (usually isohexol 180 mg/mL) to allow live fluoroscopy as the medication spreads on injection. For the superior hypogastric plexus neurolysis, a total volume of 5–10 mL is injected (2.5–5 mL per side if necessary). If ethanol is used, local anesthetic should be injected first to anesthetize the surrounding tissue. Like the classic approach for diagnostic block, if contrast spreads to the contralateral side of the vertebral body, then a single-needle approach can be used. Regardless of technique, needles should be flushed with normal saline or local anesthetic to prevent tracking neurolytic agent along the needle path as the needle is removed.

Evidence for Efficacy

Neurolysis of the SHGP was associated with both significant reduction in pain severity scores and decreased opioid consumption. In fact one study by Plancarte et al. found a 43% reduction in opioid usage in roughly three-fourths of their patients. Another study by de Leon-Casasola found nearly 70% of patients had effective pain relief and 67% reported significant reduction of their mean opioid consumption at their 6-month follow-up. However, new prospective and better-designed studies are still needed to confirm the effectiveness of this therapy as this is a more recently developed intervention with similarly limited studies performed.

Pearls and Pitfalls

(a) With any sympathetic plexus injection, there is a risk of intravascular injection, hematoma, subarachnoid injection, and nerve injury. However, due to its close proximity to ureters and the bifurcation of the common iliac vessels, the superior hypogastric plexus block is at higher risk of damaging these important vascular and urologic structures. This further highlights the importance of accurate technique and proper needle entry approach.

(b) The success of the SHGPB is much less likely in cases of extensive retroperitoneal disease in close proximity to the sympathetic ganglion as there is poor spread of the neurolytic or local anesthetic.

(c) Success utilizing the classic posterior approach involves overcoming obstacles such as the iliac crest and the transverse processes of the fifth lumbar vertebral body.

Recommended Reading

1. Ahmed DG, Mohamed MF, Mohamed SA. Superior hypogastric plexus combined with ganglion impar neurolytic blocks for pelvic and/or perineal cancer pain relief. Pain Physician. 2015;18(1):E49–56.
2. Bhatnagar S, Gupta D, Mishra S, et al. Bedside ultrasound-guided celiac plexus neurolysis with bilateral paramedian needle entry technique can be an effective pain control technique in advanced upper abdominal cancer pain. J Palliat Med. 2008;11:1195–9.
3. Bonica JJ. The celiac plexus and ganglia and the splanchnic nerves. In: Bonica JJ, editor. The Management of Pain. Philadelphia: Lea & Febiger; 1953. p. 446–56.
4. Bridenbaugh LD, Moore DC, Campbell DD. Management of upper abdominal cancer pain: treatment with celiac plexus block. JAMA. 1964;190:877–80.
5. Choi JW, Kim WH, Lee CJ, Sim WS, Park S, Chae HB. The optimal approach for a superior hypogastric plexus block. Pain Pract. 2017. https://doi.org/10.1111/papr.12603
6. De Leon-Casasola OA, Kent E, Lema MJ. Neurolytic superior hypogastric plexus block for chronic pelvic pain associated with cancer. Pain. 1993;54:145–51.
7. Fitzgibbon DR, Schmiedl UP, Sinanan MN. Computed tomography-guided neurolytic celiac plexus block with alcohol complicated by superior mesenteric venous thrombosis. Pain. 2001;92:307–10.
8. Ischia S, Polati E, Finco G, et al. 1998 Labat lecture: the role of the neurolytic celiac plexus block in pancreatic cancer pain management: do we have the answers? Reg Anesth Pain Med. 1998;23:611–4.
9. Kappis M. Sensibilitat und lokale Anasthesie im chirurgischen Gebiet der Bauchhohle mit besonderer Berucksichtigung der splanchnicus-Aasthesie. Beitrage zur klinischen Chirurgie. 1919;115:161–75.

10. Plancarte R, Amescua C, Patt RB, et al. Superior hypogastric plexus block for pelvic cancer pain. Anesthesiology. 1990;73:236–9.
11. Plancarte R, de Leon-Casasola OA, El-Helaly M, Allende S, Lema MJ. Neurolytics superior hypogastric plexus block for chronic pelvic pain associated with cancer. Reg Anesth. 1997;22(6):562–8.
12. Rathmel JP. Atlas of image-guided intervention in regional anesthesia and pain medicine. Philadelphia: Lippincott Williams & Wilkins; 2012.
13. Shwita AH, Amr YM, Okab MI. Comparative study of the effects of the retrocrural celiac plexus vs splanchnic nerve block, C-arm guided, for upper gastrointestinal tract tumors on pain relief and the quality of life at six-month follow up. Korean J Pain. 2015;28(1):22–31.
14. Türker G, Basagan-Mogol E, Gurbet A, Ozturk C, Uckunkaya N, Sahin S. A new technique for superior hypogastric plexus block: the posteromedian transdiscal approach. Tohoku J Exp Med. 2005;206:277–81. https://doi.org/10.1620/tjem.206.277.

Ganglion Impar Block

59

Markus A. Bendel

Introduction

Chronic pelvic, perineal, and coccygeal pain has long been a difficult problem for patients who suffer from it and for providers who have limited options to intervene. The ganglion impar (ganglion of Walther) is a sympathetic ganglion formed by the convergence of the distal ends of the lumbosacral sympathetic chains. The ganglion provides sympathetic efferent fibers to and receives afferent sensory information from many pelvic structures. The distal rectum, anus, distal urethra, distal one-third of the vagina, vulva, and penis may send visceral input through the ganglion impar. Traditionally, the location of the ganglion is taught to be anterior to the sacrum at the level of the sacrococcygeal junction; however, recent studies show that this is accurate less than 20% of the time. Other sources describe its location variably along the anterior surface of the coccyx all the way to its tip. Fortunately, anatomic studies have sought to clarify this situation and have identified multiple different shapes, sizes, and locations of the ganglion. The most commonly identified location is approximately 1 cm distal to the sacrococcygeal joint at approximately the level of the first intercoccygeal joint. This certainly has important implications for proceduralists.

Ganglion impar blockade has been performed to alleviate certain pain syndromes of the perineum and pelvis. There have been many approaches and techniques described in the literature. The block is generally performed utilizing fluoroscopy, although computed tomography (CT) and ultrasound (US) guidance have also been described. There are many technical variations described below, but the ultimate goal is to successfully direct a needle to the anterior surface of the coccyx or sacrococcygeal junction to allow for the administration of local anesthetic, steroid, or neurolytic substance while avoiding injury to any pelvic organs. Radiopaque contrast medium is administered to identify proper retroperitoneal spread along the anterior surface of the coccyx, sometimes referred to as the "comma sign." Understanding and practicing a variety of techniques will allow for completion of the procedure in a vast number of clinical situations.

Background and Historical Perspective

Credit for the discovery of the ganglion impar is given to Dr. Augustin Walther. He described its location on the anterior surface of the coccyx in the 1720s. It was over 250 years later that the initial report of a ganglion impar block appeared in the medical literature in 1990. It was then that Dr. Plancarte described his technique of a neurolytic block for 16 patients with advanced cancer and related perineal pain that was resistant to other pain management modalities. The technique involved placing a pre-bent needle through the anococcygeal ligament toward the anterior surface of the coccyx with fluoroscopic guidance. Additionally, a finger would be placed in the rectum to detect an ill-placed needle. This case series described very positive results in regard to reduction in patient-reported pain scores.

Over the subsequent years, many additional techniques and modalities have been utilized in an attempt to improve the procedure and its outcomes. In 1995, Dr. Wemm and colleagues described the trans-sacrococcygeal technique in which a needle would traverse the sacrococcygeal disc directly from the posterior aspect (Figs. 59.1 and 59.2). This would limit the potential damage to pelvic organs and structures and potentially provide a more tolerable experience to the patient. Additionally, it was theorized that the increased distance between the needle entry point and the anus may decrease infectious risk. In 1997, Dr. Nebab and colleagues described a method similar to the approach of Dr. Plancarte but with a curved needle rather than an acutely bent one. It was proposed that would allow for easier placement, less tissue strain, and less chance for needle breakage. The following year, Dr. Loev and colleagues described the application

M. A. Bendel (✉)
Mayo Clinic, Rochester, MN, USA
e-mail: Bendel.markus@mayo.edu

T. R. Deer et al. (eds.), *Deer's Treatment of Pain*, https://doi.org/10.1007/978-3-030-12281-2_59

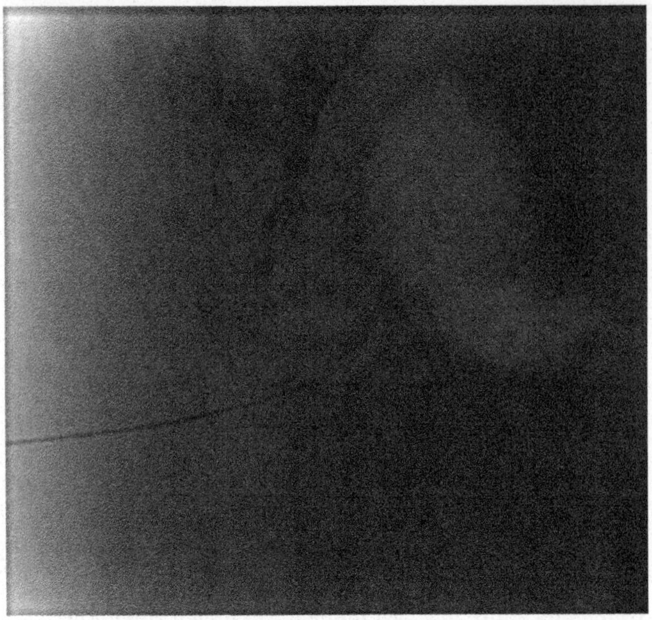

Fig. 59.1 A lateral fluoroscopic image showing needle placement through the sacrococcygeal junction

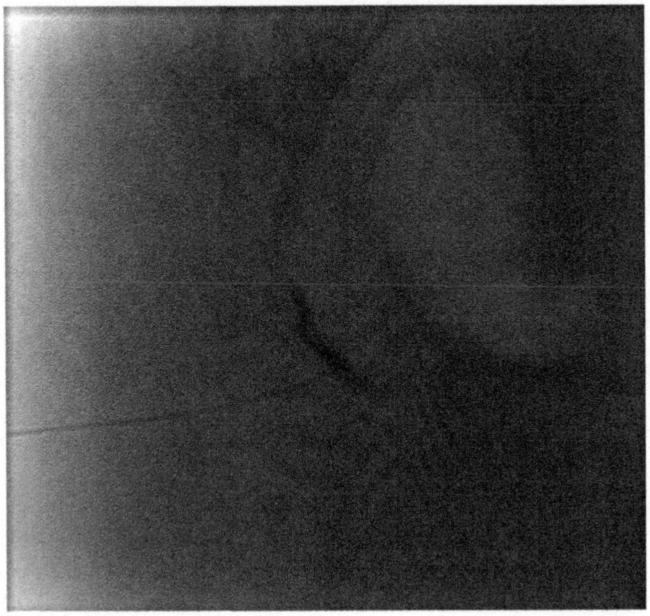

Fig. 59.2 A lateral fluoroscopic image demonstrating contrast spread anterior to the sacrococcygeal junction

of cryoablation to the ganglion impar. This was accomplished by introducing the cryoablation probe using the trans-sacrococcygeal route. In 2003, Dr. Huang described a paramedian approach in which the transverse process of the coccyx is identified and used as the primary anatomic landmark. A bent needle would be directed to the transverse process under fluoroscopic guidance and, after contacting the bone, would be walked to the anterior surface of the sacrococcygeal junction. This technique would allow for a shorter needle path than the anococcygeal ligament route and would still allow access in the situation of a calcified sacrococcygeal junction. A needle-inside-needle approach was described by Dr. Munir and his team in 2004. This approach involved the placement of a larger needle via the trans-sacrococcygeal route first, followed by the introduction of a second, smaller needle through the first. It was surmised that this may decrease the rate of needle breakage and possibly decrease the risk of rectal perforation. In 2006, Dr. Hong and colleagues described a ganglion impar blockade for cancer-related pain by approaching through the first intercoccygeal joint due to ossification of the sacrococcygeal disc. This technique produced good results in the case report and may allow for better coverage of the ganglion impar based on the more recent anatomic studies available. In 2009, another variation of the paramedian approach was described by Dr. Foye which de-emphasized the need to identify the coccygeal transverse process. This "corkscrew technique" involves a slightly lateral needle entry to allow the needle to contact the coccyx and then utilize the pre-bent needle to walk anterior and medially along the coccyx to the location of the ganglion impar.

The previously described techniques all rely on the utilization of fluoroscopy to confirm proper needle placement. There have been descriptions of non-fluoroscopic approaches to the ganglion impar as well. Dr. Ho and colleagues described the application of CT to complete a neurolytic blockade for recurrent vulvar cancer. This case report utilized two needles and a far lateral trajectory to accomplish the procedure. This offered debatable benefit over the traditional fluoroscopic technique as a much longer needle path is required. Dr. Agarwal-Kozlowski and team reported on 43 patients with perineal pain of varying etiologies who underwent CT-guided ganglion impar blockade and/or neurolysis with an average pain score decrease from 8.2 to 2.2. In 2010, Dr. Lin and colleagues described an ultrasound-guided technique which resulted in successful placement of a needle in the sacrococcygeal junction. However, fluoroscopy was still required to determine proper needle depth. In 2012, Drs. Johnston and Michalek added a loss of resistance technique to the ultrasound-guided needle placement to avoid any use of fluoroscopy. After seating the needle in the sacrococcygeal disc, loss of resistance to saline was applied to find the space just anterior to the disc where the ganglion traditionally lies. There is emphasis, however, that this technique should not be applied for neurolytic blockade where X-ray confirmation is likely still required for patient safety. Most recently, in 2016, a cadaveric study investigated the feasibility of utilizing magnetic resonance imaging (MRI) to guide the ganglion impar procedure. It was found to be technically feasible but, at this time, has not been evaluated clinically.

Uses and Indications

Blockade of the ganglion impar has been applied to patients suffering from chronic pain of the perineum and coccyx. Each of these conditions has a wide variety of etiologies. The complex innervation of the pelvic structures additionally adds a degree of difficulty in identifying the proper diagnosis and treatment plan in these clinical scenarios. Certainly, more randomized, controlled studies are needed to provide definitive clinical evidence on the efficacy of this block across differing etiologies. However, the literature provides many case reports and case series of successful ganglion impar blockade to help guide clinical application.

There have been many reports on the application of ganglion impar blockade for perineal pain related to advanced cancers of the pelvis. The block is also applied for nonmalignant indications, but the evidence is largely limited to individual case reports. Some of the conditions that have been reported with positive outcomes include sacral postherpetic neuralgia, tenesmoid pain, perianal sweating, vulvodynia, radiation induced cystitis, and several idiopathic cases. Coccydynia has been perhaps the most studied indication at this point in time, with mixed results among the available literature.

Evidence for Efficacy

As previously stated, the amount of randomized controlled literature is limited. A vast majority of the medical reports are case reports and case series which limit the current ability to analyze the potential benefits and harms of the procedure. A summary of the larger retrospective and prospective studies is undertaken below (Table 59.1).

In 2007, Toshniwal et al. published a prospective study investigating the trans-sacrococcygeal approach of ganglion impar blockade when applied to chronic perineal pain of differing etiologies. They were able to show a statistically significant reduction in VAS scores (from time of presentation) at all time points up to 2 months. No complications were reported. In 2010, Demircay et al. published a retrospective study of ten patients who underwent radiofrequency ablation of the ganglion impar for chronic coccydynia. This study showed a statistically significant decrease in pre- to post-procedure pain scores. When patients were evaluated at 6 months, 90% of the patients were deemed successful (>50% pain reduction). No complications were reported. Another 2010 publication examined the efficacy of CT-guided ganglion impar blockade. Eight patients were followed prospectively for 6 months. The study determined a 75% success rate among the patients at 6 months. Of the responders, the VAS score decreased from a mean of 8 to a mean of 2. No complications were reported.

In 2015, a retrospective pilot study was published that investigated the outcomes of 22 patients with chronic coccydynia who had received ganglion impar blockade. With success defined as a 50% reduction in VAS, this study reported an 82% success rate after a first injection. A median duration of relief of 6 months was achieved. In 2016, another retrospective review of radiofrequency ablation of the ganglion impar for chronic coccydynia was published by Adas et al. This reported a success rate over 90% with statistically significant reductions in the VAS between pre-procedure and 6-month time points. It should be pointed out that there have been negative studies published in the literature as well, resulting in an overall mixed picture. It would be important for well-designed trials to be undertaken to truly delineate which indications have the best response to ganglion impar interventions.

Pearls and Pitfalls

- The anatomic location of the ganglion impar has been discovered to be slightly more caudal along the coccyx than traditionally thought. There remains significant variation in anatomic localization.
- The sacrococcygeal disc can be ossified preventing direct access via the sacrococcygeal junction.

Table 59.1 Summary of literature related to ganglion impar interventions

Article	Condition	Design	Number of patients	Results
Toshniwal et al. (2007)	Chronic perineal pain	Prospective, observational	16	Significant reduction in VAS score for 2 months
Demircay et al. (2010)	Chronic coccydynia Radiofrequency ablation	Retrospective	10	Significant reduction in VAS at 6 months
Datir et al. (2010)	Chronic coccydynia CT guidance	Prospective, observational	8	75% responder rate at 6 months
Gunduz et al. (2015)	Chronic coccydynia	Retrospective	22	82% of patient obtained 50% benefit for a median time of 6 months
Adas et al. (2016)	Chronic coccydynia Radiofrequency ablation	Retrospective	41	90% success rate significant reduction in VAS at 6 months

- Consider a small volume (2–3 mL) for neurolytic procedures to prevent damage to the sacral nerve roots.
- Imaging guidance should be utilized to prevent needle trauma to the rectum or other pelvic structures.
- Administration of radiopaque contrast is important to identify proper retroperitoneal contrast pattern – "the comma sign."

Recommended Reading

1. Demircay E, et al. Radiofrequency thermocoagulation of ganglion impar in the management of coccydynia: preliminary results. Turk Neurosurg. 2010;20(3):328–33.
2. Gunduz OH, et al. Pain relief due to transsacrococcygeal ganglion impar block in chronic coccygodynia: a pilot study. Pain Med. 2015;16(7):1278–81.
3. Oh CS, et al. Clinical implications of topographic anatomy on the ganglion impar. Anesthesiology. 2004;101(1):249–50.
4. Scott-Warren JT, et al. Ganglion impar blockade: a review. Curr Pain Headache Rep. 2013;17(1):306.
5. Toshniwal GR, et al. Transsacrococcygeal approach to ganglion impar block for management of chronic perineal pain: a prospective observational study. Pain Physician. 2007;10(5):661–6.
6. Walters A, et al. One is the loneliest number: a review of the ganglion impar and its relation to pelvic pain syndromes. Clin Anat. 2013;26(7):855–61.

Large Joint Injections

60

Yasmine Hoydonckx and Philip Peng

Introduction

Pain originating from the musculoskeletal system is one of the major causes worldwide of disability. Osteoarthritis is the most common joint disorder in the United States and the leading cause of disability in the elderly.

Background and Historical Perspective

Osteoarthritis arises when the cartilage of a joint is damaged by a combination of mechanical stress and suboptimal repair response to this stress, leading to a chronic state of inflammation and pain. Corticosteroids are strong anti-inflammatory agents with established use in osteoarthritis treatment; however, evidence for effectiveness remains debatable. Conventionally, joint injections have been performed with landmark or fluoroscopy guidance. With emerging popularity of the application of ultrasound in pain medicine, joint injections under ultrasound guidance have become more popular and well established. The anatomy and sonoanatomy relevant to injections of shoulder, hip, and knee joint are described in this chapter, as well as the practical aspects.

Shoulder

Almost 16% of all musculoskeletal complaints concern the shoulder. It is the most important region for joint injection procedures because it is prone to injury and attrition. Pain can originate from several structures in the shoulder girdle: the scapula, clavicle, and proximal humerus.

The shoulder has three joints: the glenohumeral, acromioclavicular, and sternoclavicular joint. Commonly performed interventions focus on the subacromial bursa, glenohumeral joint, and acromioclavicular joint. In this chapter, we will focus on the glenohumeral joint.

Y. Hoydonckx (✉) · P. Peng
Department of Anesthesia, Toronto Western Hospital, Toronto, ON, Canada
e-mail: Philip.peng@uhn.ca

Anatomy

Glenohumeral Joint (GHJ)

The GHJ is a synovial ball-and-socket joint, formed by a round humeral head and a small, pear-shaped glenoid fossa. A fibrocartilaginous rim – the glenoid labrum – widens and deepens the glenoid cavity for optimal contact (Fig. 60.1). Because only one-third of the humeral head is covered by the glenoid cavity and the capsule is lax, it allows the shoulder the widest range of movement of all joints but creates at the same time inherent instability and high risk for subluxation and dislocation. More stability to this joint is given by ligaments, tendons, and the deltoid muscle. Three glenohumeral ligaments (GHL) – superior, middle, and inferior – strengthen the front of the capsule. The coracohumeral ligament (CHL) is a strong band arising from the coracoid process with insertion on the tuberosities (Fig. 60.1).

Rotator cuff interval is a triangular space, created between the tendons of the subscapularis and supraspinatus and the base of the coracoid process with the roof formed by the CHL (Fig. 60.2). It allows access to the GHJ.

Acromioclavicular Joint (ACJ)

This small diarthrodial joint is located between the medial end of the acromion and the lateral end of the clavicle. The articular surfaces are separated by a wedge-shaped fibrocartilaginous disc (Fig. 60.3). The capsule of the ACJ is attached to the articular margins. Extra stability to this joint is created by the acromioclavicular, coracoclavicular, and coracoacromial ligaments, as well as the deltoid and trapezius muscles.

This complex joint has limited range of motion but allows the shoulder gliding, hinge-like, and rotational movement. The accompanying shear stress and high compressive force from the surrounding muscles make this joint prone to degeneration. The inferior surface of the joint is in direct

T. R. Deer et al. (eds.), *Deer's Treatment of Pain*, https://doi.org/10.1007/978-3-030-12281-2_60

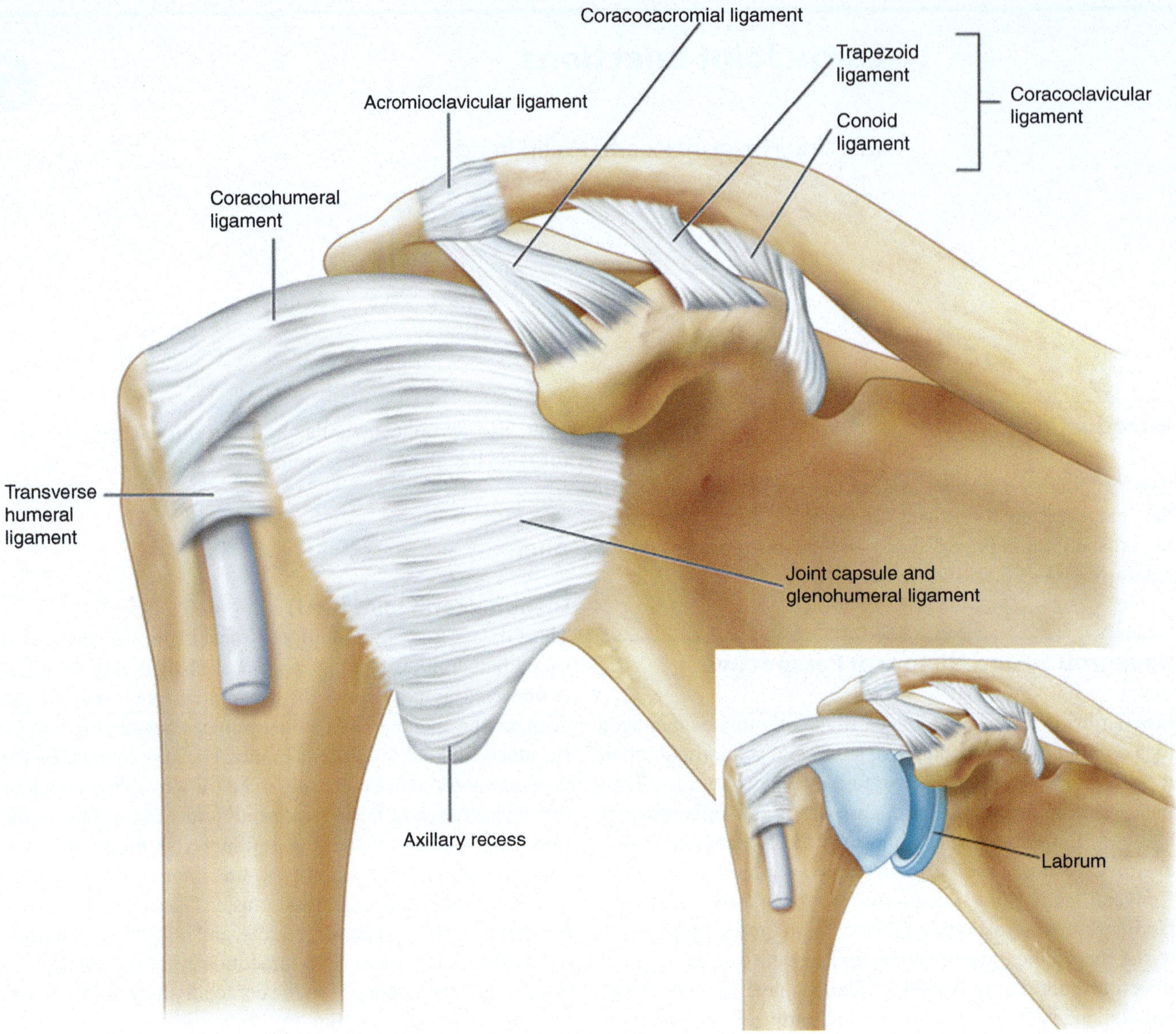

Fig. 60.1 Glenohumeral joint with various ligaments and the joint capsule. The anterior capsule is reinforced by the superior, middle, and inferior glenohumeral ligament. The insert shows the articular surface, the glenoid process, and the labrum. (Reprinted with permission from Philip Peng Educational Series)

contact with the subacromial bursa and rotator cuff. Therefore, this joint may play a role in the development of impingement syndrome.

Although a common source for shoulder pain, it is often neglected by clinicians because of higher prevalence of rotator cuff pathology. Diagnosis of ACJ osteoarthritis is made by thorough physical exam, radiography, and diagnostic local injection.

Indication

Glenohumeral Joint

The main indication for injection of GHJ is adhesive capsulitis (frozen shoulder), although it is also commonly used for glenohumeral arthrosis. Since the natural course of a frozen shoulder is usually self-limiting, the role of this injection is mainly symptom relief or improvement of rehabilitation.

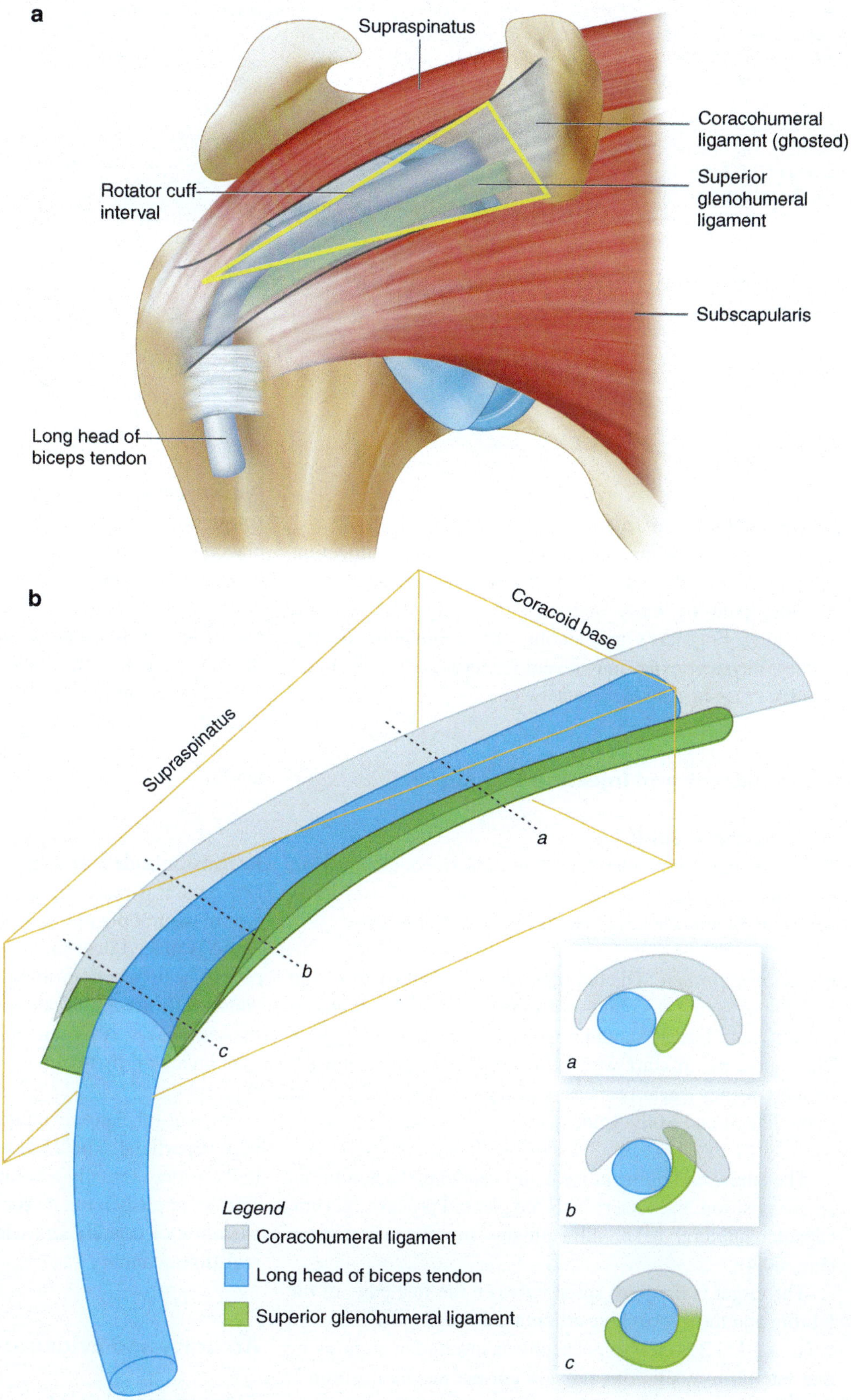

Fig. 60.2 (**a**) The anterosuperior view showing the rotator cuff interval, which is a triangular space between the tendons of subscapularis (anterior) and supraspinatus (posterior) muscles and the base of the coracoid process. The roof is the coracohumeral ligament (ghosted), and the contents are the long head of the biceps tendon (blue) and superior glenohumeral ligament (green). (**b**) The cutout of the rotator cuff interval to show the content. The superior glenohumeral ligament, a focal thickening of the glenohumeral joint capsule, runs anterior to the tendon of the long head of the biceps tendon initially (position a). The superior glenohumeral ligament maintains a close relationship with the long head of the biceps tendon and subsequently inserts into a small depression above the lesser tuberosity (position b), contributing to the biceps reflection pulley (position c) to prevent the dislocation of the LHB tendon. (Reprinted with permission from Philip Peng Educational Series)

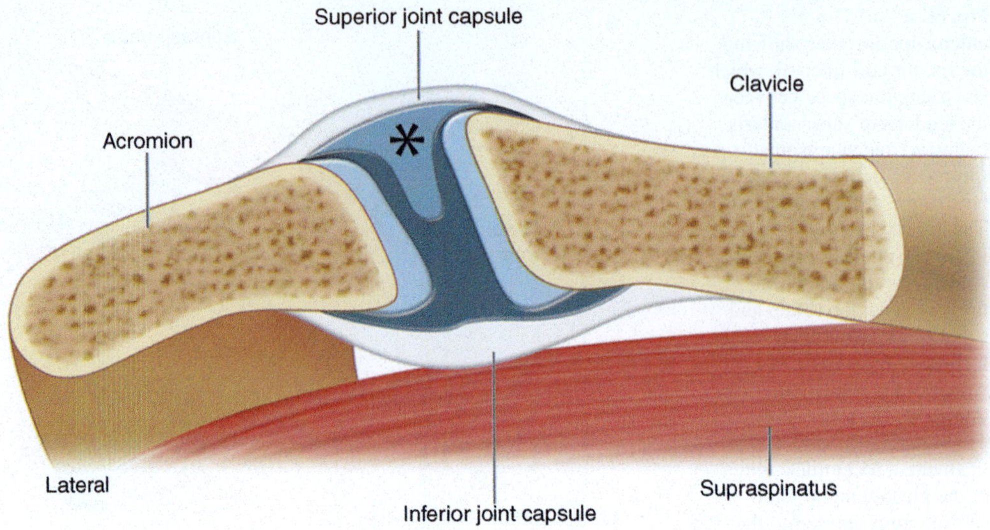

Fig. 60.3 The acromioclavicular joint is a synovial joint with the articular surfaces separated by a wedge-shaped fibrocartilaginous disc (asterisk). The inferior surface of the joint is in direct contact with the subacromial bursa and supraspinatus muscle and may play a role in the development of the impingement syndrome. (Reprinted with permission from Philip Peng Educational Series)

Acromioclavicular Joint

Osteoarthritis is the main therapeutic indication for injection of ACJ (acromioclavicular joint). Symptoms such as anterior shoulder pain by daily activities (reaching back pocket, unhooking brassiere) are among the complaints of the patient. Physical exam may reveal tenderness over ACJ and positive cross-arm adduction test.

Sonoanatomy and Injection Technique

Glenohumeral Joint

Three possible approaches have been described: the anterior, posterior, and rotator cuff interval. Only posterior and rotator cuff interval approach will be discussed in this chapter.

Posterior approach The optimal position is either in sitting position or lateral decubitus with the ipsilateral hand placed on the contralateral shoulder (to open up the GHJ space). The landmark to start with is the scapular spine, and the high-frequency linear probe is placed just caudal and parallel to the lateral end of the spine.

The lateral end of the probe is just caudal to the acromion. In this position, the scan reveals the glenoid process, labrum, capsule, humeral head, infraspinatus muscle, and tendon (Fig. 60.4).

The target is the joint space between the free edge of the labrum and the hypoechoic articular cartilage of the humeral head. A 22 G 3.5-inch spinal needle is inserted in an in-plane and lateral-to-medial direction. A correct needle position is confirmed when observing displacement of the posterior joint capsule upon injection of saline. An injectate volume of 4 mL (mixture of local anesthetic and steroid) is injected afterward.

Rotator cuff interval approach The patient is placed in a sitting or supine position. A high-frequency linear probe is placed – in a transverse position – over the long head of the biceps (LHB) tendon above the bicipital groove. This tendon is a hyperechoic oval structure, sandwiched between the supraspinatus tendon and the subscapularis tendon on the lateral and medial sides, respectively (Fig. 60.5). The CHL forms the roof of this interval. A 25 G needle is directed in a caudal-to-cephalad (out-of-plane) or lateral-to-medial (in-plane) direction on either side of the LHB tendon.

Acromioclavicular Joint

The patient is placed in a sitting or supine position, with the arm in neutral position as this opens the joint space. A linear probe is placed over the joint in the coronal plane. The scan reveals a hypoechoic joint space between the hyperechoic ends of the acromion and clavicle, which may not appear at the same level. A hyperechoic structure – the superior acromioclavicular ligament – covers the surface of the joint (Fig. 60.6).

An out-of-plane technique is preferred since the joint is very superficial. The 25 G needle is directed almost parallel to the probe. Usually a volume of 2 mL local anesthetic and steroid is sufficient. A successful injection is noticed by elevation of capsule and widening of the joint space during real-time scanning.

Accuracy and Evidence for Efficacy

Glenohumeral Joint

Although the GHJ is not a superficial joint, excellent accuracy (100%) has been published in validation studies for both fluoroscopy- and ultrasound-guided injections. Ultrasound-

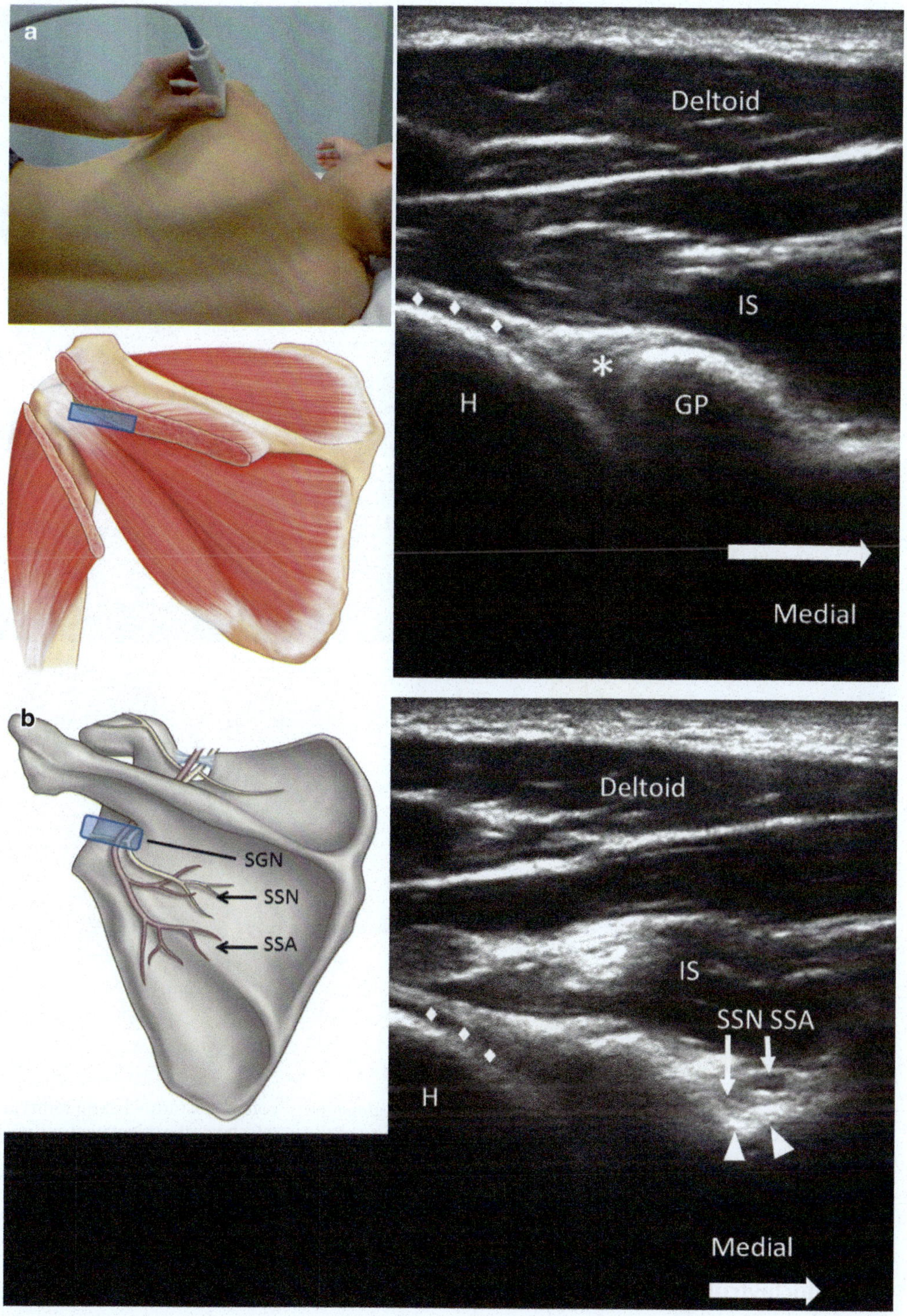

Fig. 60.4 (**a**) Ultrasound image of the posterior glenohumeral joint. The glenoid process (GP) and humeral head (H) both appear as hyperechoic structures with anechoic shadow. The insert on the top shows the position of the patient and the ultrasound probe, whereas the one below shows the probe position and the structures underneath. (**b**) Ultrasound image of the spinoglenoid notch by moving the ultrasound probe slightly medially. The insert shows the position of the probe and the spinoglenoid notch, as well as the suprascapular neurovascular bundle. H indicates humeral head, GP glenoid process, SSN and SSA suprascapular nerve and artery (line arrows in ultrasound image), SGN spinoglenoid notch (arrowheads), IS infraspinatus, *glenoid labrum, and ʋ articular cartilage of the humeral head. (Reprinted with permission from Philip Peng Educational Series)

guided technique achieved higher first-attempt rate, less time spent, and lower patient discomfort compared with landmark-guided technique, strongly supporting the use of this technique. Morbid obesity can however make this procedure more difficult.

The use of intra-articular steroid injections for shoulder pain has been investigated in multiple systematic reviews. A few high-quality studies showed indeed beneficial effect for use of multiple (up to three) steroid injections for adhesive capsulitis with pain reduction and improved function. The effect lasted until 16 weeks after the first injection.

In contrast to adhesive capsulitis, study investigating the efficacy of steroid injection in GHJ arthrosis is scant. Its role remains therefore unclear. Apart from steroid, there is some evidence for pain relief after injection of hyaluronic acid for GHJ osteoarthritis.

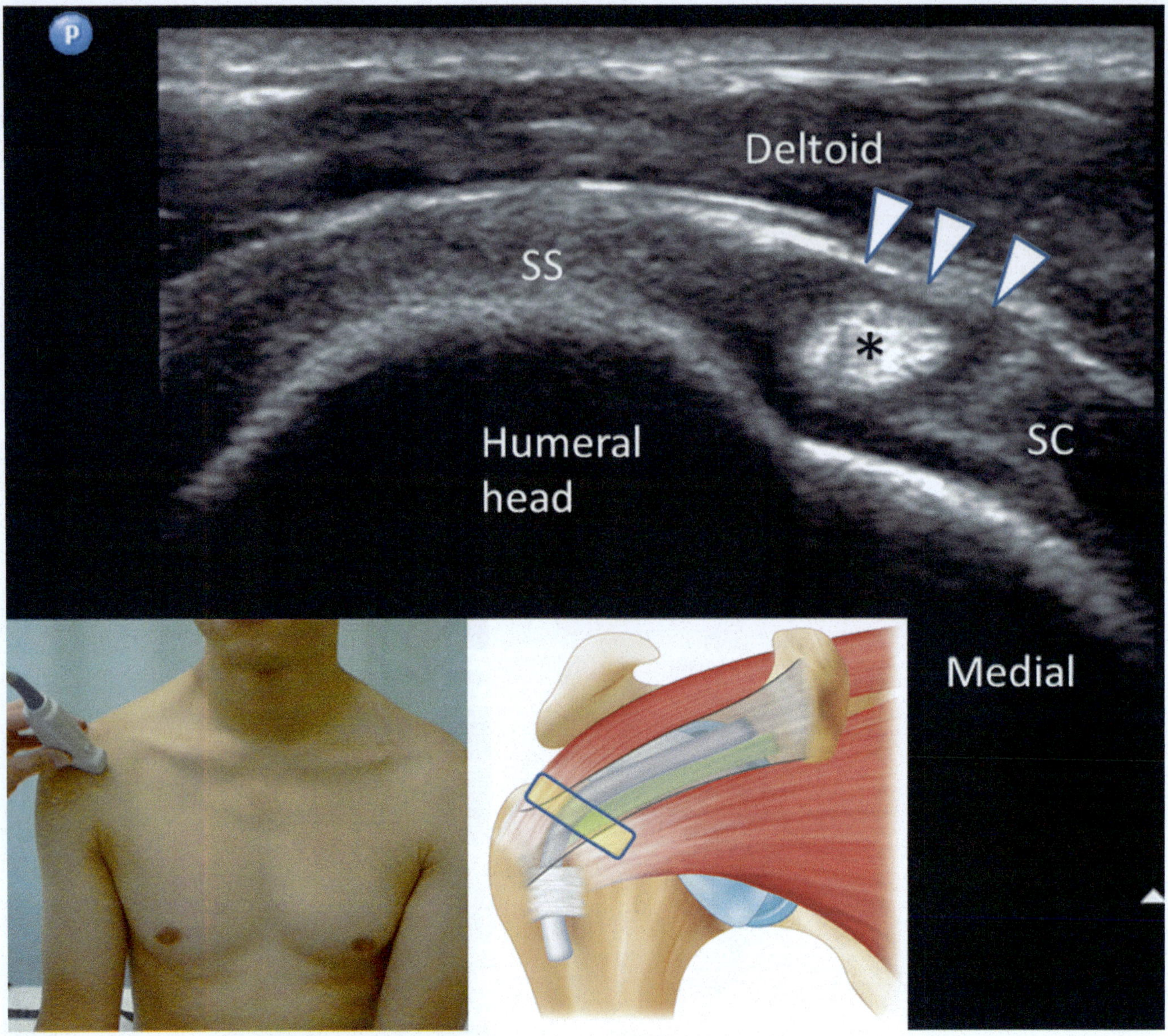

Fig. 60.5 By moving the ultrasound probe more proximally along the orientation of the long head of the biceps (LHB) tendon, a view of the rotator cuff interval is shown. The LHB tendon (asterisk) is always hyperechoic at this level and sandwiched between the supraspinatus (SS) tendon laterally and subscapularis (SC) tendon medially. The coracohumeral (arrowheads) forms the roof of the interval. The insert on the left shows the orientation and position of the probe, and the insert on the right shows the probe position and the structures underneath it. (Reprinted with permission from Philip Peng Educational Series)

Acromioclavicular Joint

The technique is highly accurate when performed with ultrasound and fluoroscopy. Where the diagnostic role for ACJ injection is widely accepted, no RCT have been published to confirm the effectiveness of steroid ACJ injection, though case series show improvement of pain and function up to 14 weeks.

Clinical Pearls

Glenohumeral Joint

- Avoid puncturing the glenoid labrum.
- If resistance is felt during injection, a slight manipulation of the needle tip is usually sufficient (turning 90°, slight withdrawal).

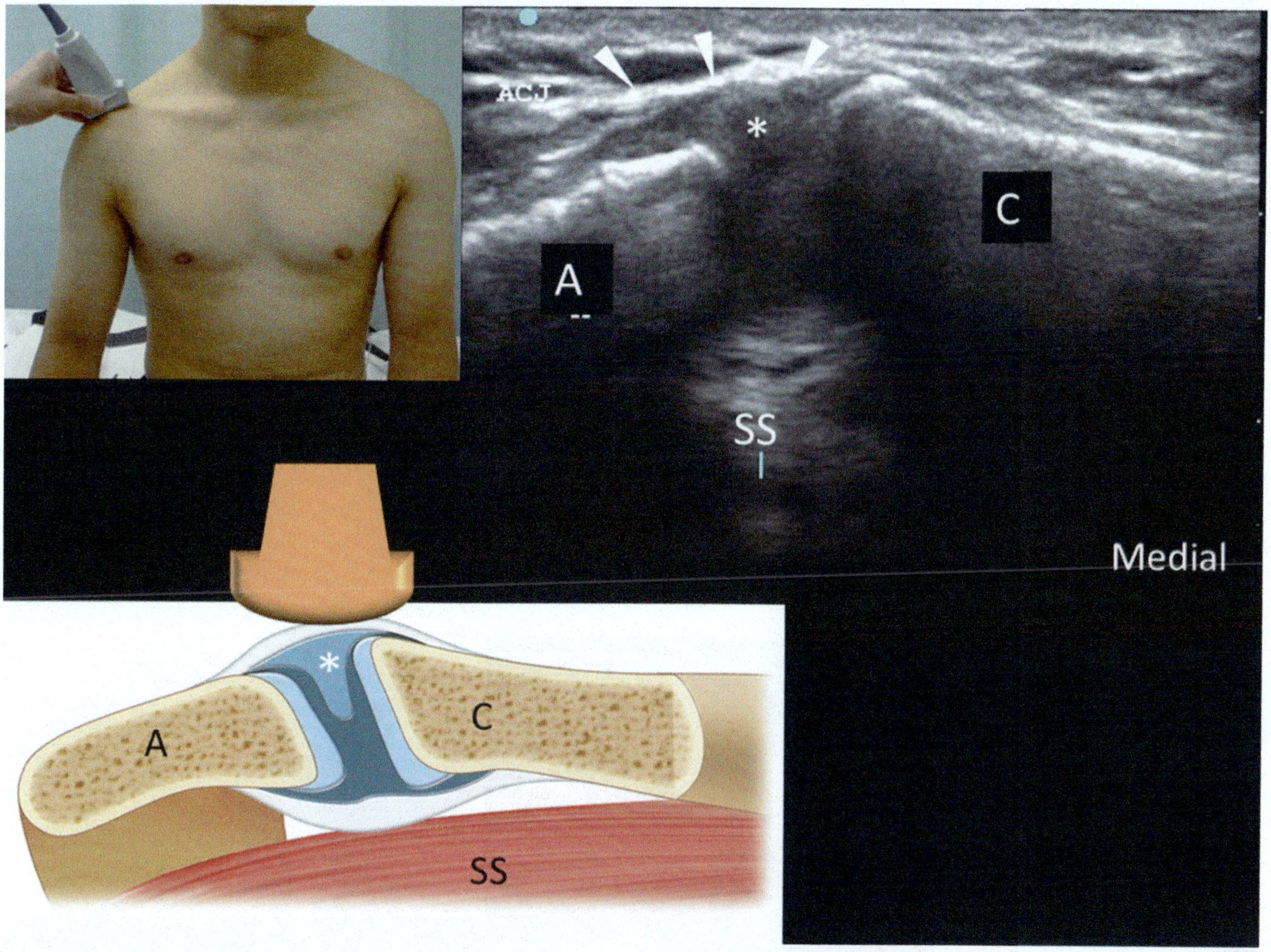

Fig. 60.6 Ultrasound image of the acromioclavicular joint (ACJ). The upper insert shows the position of the probe and the patient, and the lower insert shows the position of the probe and the structures underneath. A acromion process, C clavicle, SS supraspinatus muscle, *wedge-shaped fibrocartilaginous disc. Arrowheads point to the superior joint capsule. (Reprinted with permission from Philip Peng Educational Series)

- If the patient is nervous, lateral decubitus is a better position for the procedure because of the possibility of vasovagal response.

Acromioclavicular Joint

- To allow the precision of first needle insertion attempt, the needle can be placed parallel to the skin, right under the ultrasound probe until the anechoic shadow from the needle is seen right over the entrance of ACJ. The needle is then withdrawn to an angle ready for insertion.
- The needle should not be inserted more than 1.5 cm as it will pierce through the inferior capsule to enter the subacromial bursa or even the supraspinatus tendon.

Hip

Hip pain can be the consequence of a wide range of intra-articular or extra-articular pathologies. Osteoarthritis of the hip is the most common reason for referral for an intra-articular hip injection.

Anatomy

The hip is a ball-and-socket synovial joint, formed by the articulation of the femoral head and the acetabulum. The acetabular labrum, a fibrocartilaginous ring, attached directly to the rim of the acetabulum increased the depth and surface of the acetabular cavity, therefore optimizing the congruity between the acetabulum and femoral head (Fig. 60.7).

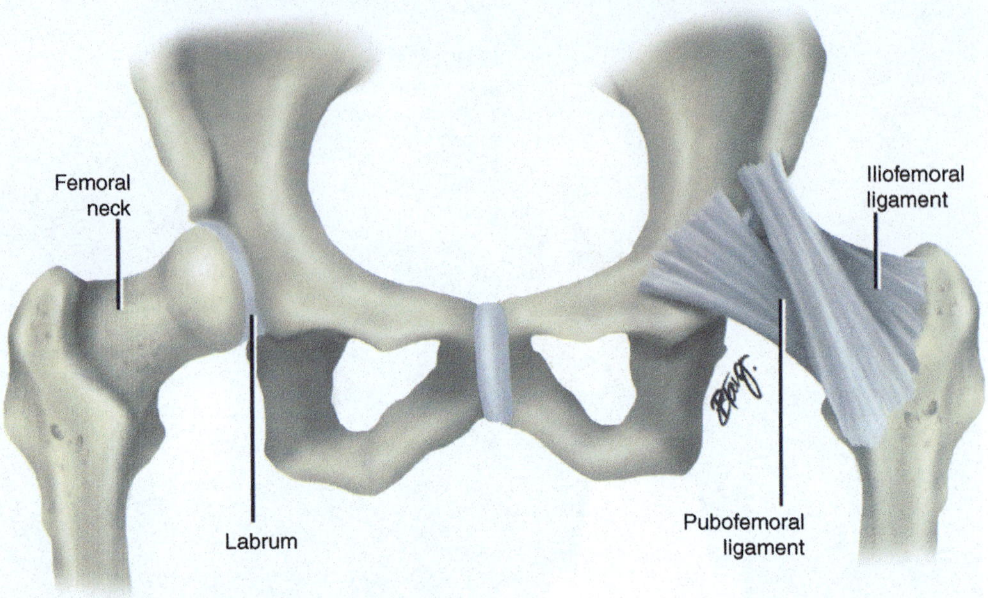

Fig. 60.7 Front view of the hip joint, the labrum (left), and the hip ligaments. The ischiofemoral ligament cannot be seen from this view because of the posterior location. (Reprinted with permission from Philip Peng Educational Series)

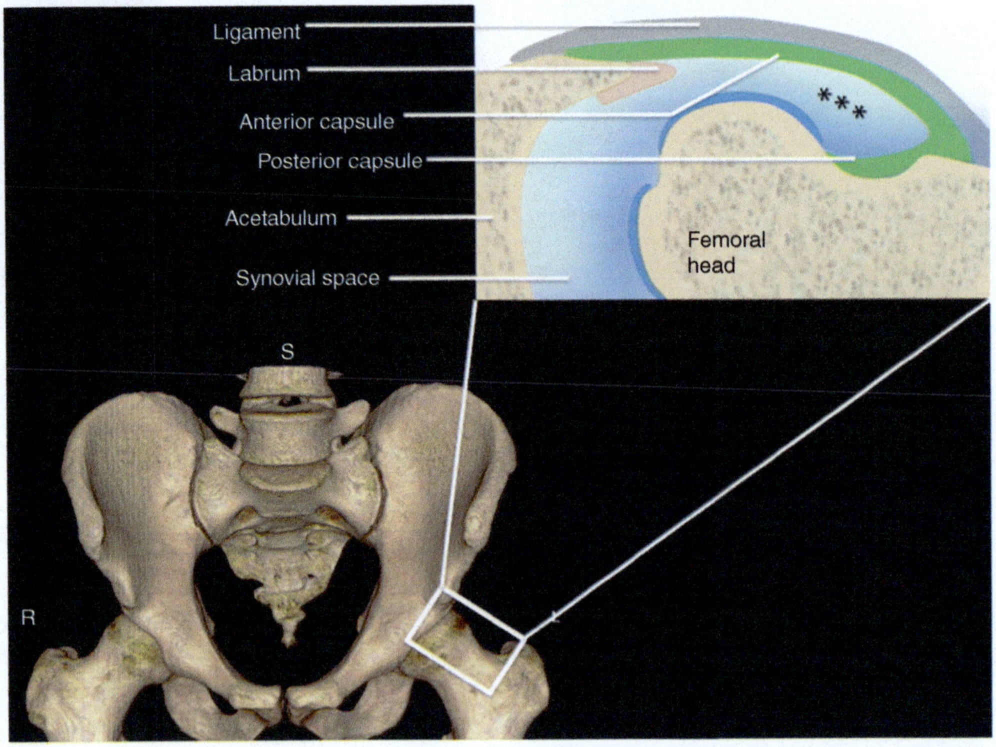

Fig. 60.8 Figure shows the anterior synovial recess (***). Under normal circumstances, the amount of synovial fluid in the recess is kept at a minimum. This figure shows a hip with effusion for demonstration. (Reprinted with permission from Philip Peng Educational Series)

With every movement of the hip, approximately 40% of the articular surface of the femoral head is covered by the acetabulum. Extra stability to the hip joint is brought by the strong joint capsule and several para-articular ligaments. This joint capsule covers the outer surface of the labrum and inserts distally to the intertrochanteric region and posterior aspect of the femoral neck. The anterior joint capsule is formed by two layers (anterior/posterior) that are separated by the anterior recess of the joint space. The anterior layer runs caudally and inserts on the intertrochanteric line, where it blends with the periosteum. The anterior recess is the common target for the intra-articular injection (Fig. 60.8).

In the anterior hip region, the structures, from medial to lateral, are the following: pectineus muscle, femoral neurovascular bundle, iliopsoas muscle and tendon, and sartorius and rectus femoris muscles.

Indication

Intra-articular hip injection is considered for the treatment of a wide variety of hip disorders, including osteoarthritis, rheumatoid arthritis, and acetabular labrum tears.

Osteoarthritis is the most common joint disorder. These patients typically complain of anterior or inguinal pain, which increases with joint movement and is (partially) relieved with rest. However, other causes such as tumors, infection, chronic inflammatory arthritis, or crystal-induced arthropathies have to be ruled out.

For patients with pain and poor response to conservative treatments or those that are not a surgical candidate because of age or comorbidity, this intra-articular injection can be considered.

Injected medications include corticosteroids, local anesthetics, and viscosupplements (VS).

Sonoanatomy and Injection Technique

These can be performed landmark based or with fluoroscopy or ultrasound guidance. The ultrasound-guided technique comes with higher accuracy and will be further discussed.

As stated before, the point of interest is the synovial anterior recess, underneath the joint capsule between the femoral head and neck. The patient is placed supine, with the hip in neutral position and groin exposed. A curvilinear probe is preferred for better panoramic view of the anterior recess and femoral neck and placed over the infrainguinal region with anterior oblique sagittal technique. First, the femoral neurovascular bundle is located. In this view, the femoral head and acetabulum can usually be seen underneath the iliopsoas muscle and its tendon (Fig. 60.9a). The probe is then rotated along with the axis of the femoral neck, thereby revealing the femoral head, neck, joint capsule, and anterior recess (Fig. 60.9b).

Before needle insertion, it is important to survey the needle path with Doppler scan for any suspected vessels. A 22-gauge, 3.5 inch spinal needle is inserted in-plane from lateral to medial direction to the junction between the femoral head and neck. The needle is inserted until the bone is contacted and then withdrawn 1–2 mm to avoid injection in the posterior capsule. The spread of the injected volume is monitored in real time to ensure spread within the joint space. A total volume of 5 mL of local anesthetic and steroid is sufficient.

Accuracy and Efficacy

The landmark-based technique has low accuracy and holds a high risk for damaging the femoral nerve. In contrast, the ultrasound-guided technique has very high accuracy (97–100%).

Five randomized controlled trials (RCT) examining the analgesic efficacy of intra-articular hip steroid injection have been published. All injections were performed under image guidance (fluoroscopy = 3, ultrasound = 2). Four out of five demonstrated improvement in pain and functions. In contrast, the evidence of analgesic efficacy of VS is weak.

Clinical Pearls

- When the needle is inserted from lateral to medial in-plane, it is in the proximity of the lateral circumflex femoral artery or its branch. Make sure to scan for the vessel in the needle path.
- When the tip of the needle is at the junction of the femoral neck and head, make sure the spread of the injectate is toward the hip joint. If not, withdraw the needle 1–2 mm. If the injectate spread is not ideal, move the needle tip toward the head, but pay attention to the labrum.

Knee

Anatomy

The knee joint consists of three components: the femorotibial, patellofemoral, and superior tibiofibular joints. Two menisci (medial, lateral) increase the surface of contact between the convex femoral condyles and flat tibia plateau.

The joint is reinforced by various surrounding structures: anteriorly, the quadriceps and patella tendons, the medial and lateral patellofemoral ligaments, and the retinaculum from the vastus medialis and lateralis protect the joint; medially, the medial collateral ligament; and on the lateral side, the iliotibial band, the lateral collateral ligament, and the biceps tendons and their fascial expansion.

There are many recesses to the femorotibial joint, but the widest one is the suprapatellar recess (SPR), which originates from the fusion of the subquadriceps bursa with the joint cavity and allows an access for injection into the joint cavity (Fig. 60.10).

Indication

The main indication for intra-articular knee injection is osteoarthritis.

Sonoanatomy and Injection Technique

The patient lies in a supine position, with the knee slightly flexed (20–30 °) and supported by a pillow. A high-frequency

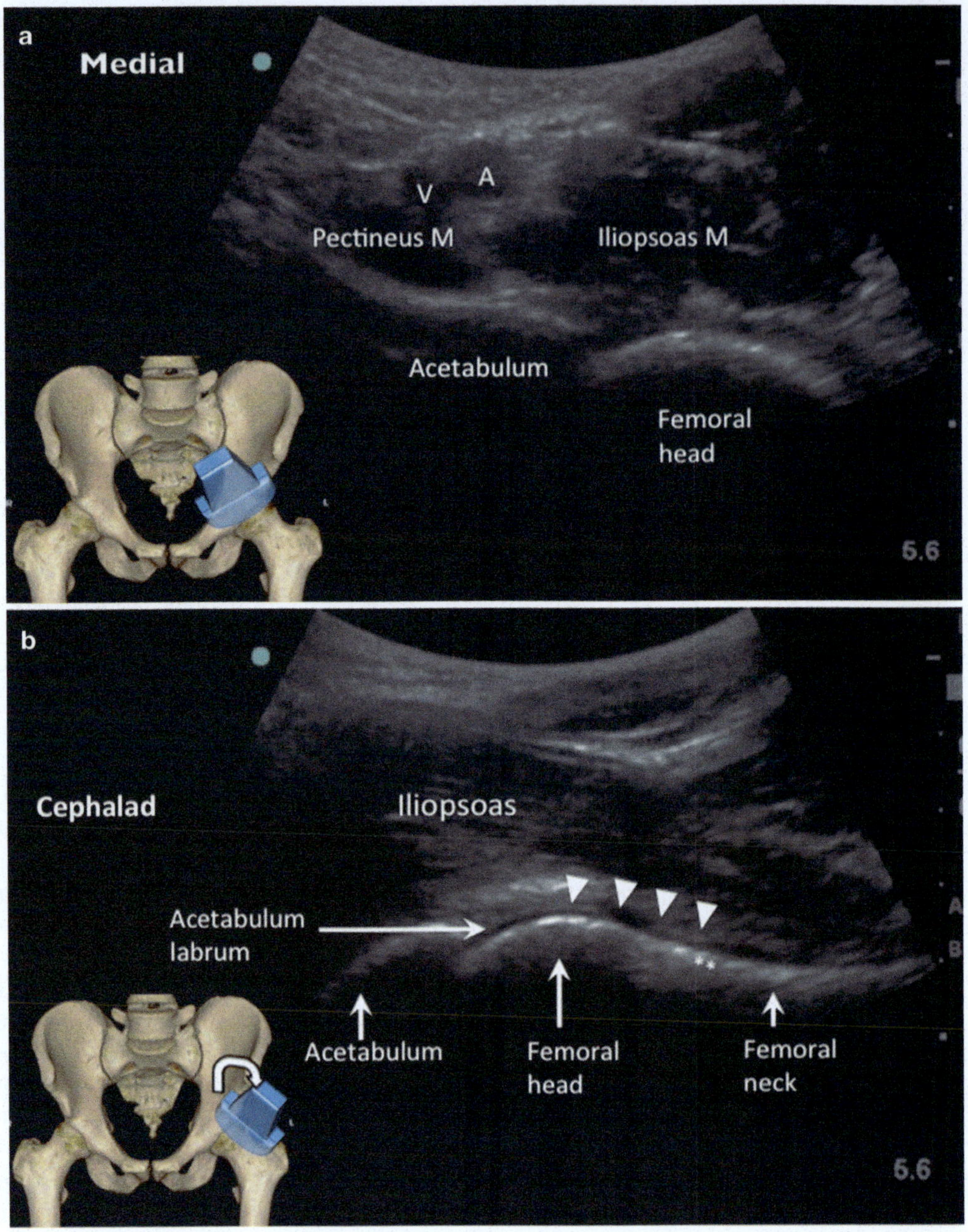

Fig. 60.9 (**a**) Sonoanatomy of the infrainguinal hip region. The position of the transducer is shown in the insert. A indicates femoral artery and V, femoral vein. (**b**) Sonoanatomy of the anterior hip region when the transducer is placed in the long axis of the femoral neck. The arrowheads indicate the anterior recess. The position of the transducer is shown in the insert. (Reprinted with permission from Philip Peng Educational Series)

linear probe is placed longitudinally just superior of the patella, visualizing the quadriceps femoris tendon. Just underneath, the suprapatellar fat pad is shown, and the prefemoral fat pad is seen in the depth, lying over the femur. The suprapatellar bursa appears as a thin hypoechoic line between these two fat pads. This is the commonly chosen site for knee joint injection (Fig. 60.11).

With the proper positioning, the suprapatellar recess between the suprapatellar and prefemoral fat pads can be visualized. Once the SPR is seen, the ultrasound probe is rotated 90 ° above the patella. A 22-gauge needle is inserted from lateral to medial in-plane technique toward the SPR (Fig. 60.12). Aspiration of synovial fluid should always be considered. A total volume of 5 mL including local anesthetic and steroid is used as an injectate.

Accuracy and Efficacy

Image-guided injection is superior to landmark-guided injection in literature (97% vs 81%). A recent Cochrane review evaluated the treatment of intra-articular corticosteroids for knee osteoarthritis. Use of intra-articular steroids was associated with slightly larger pain reduction than control, and this moderate benefit lasted up to 2 weeks after treatment. These findings are consistent with older literature guidelines. Some

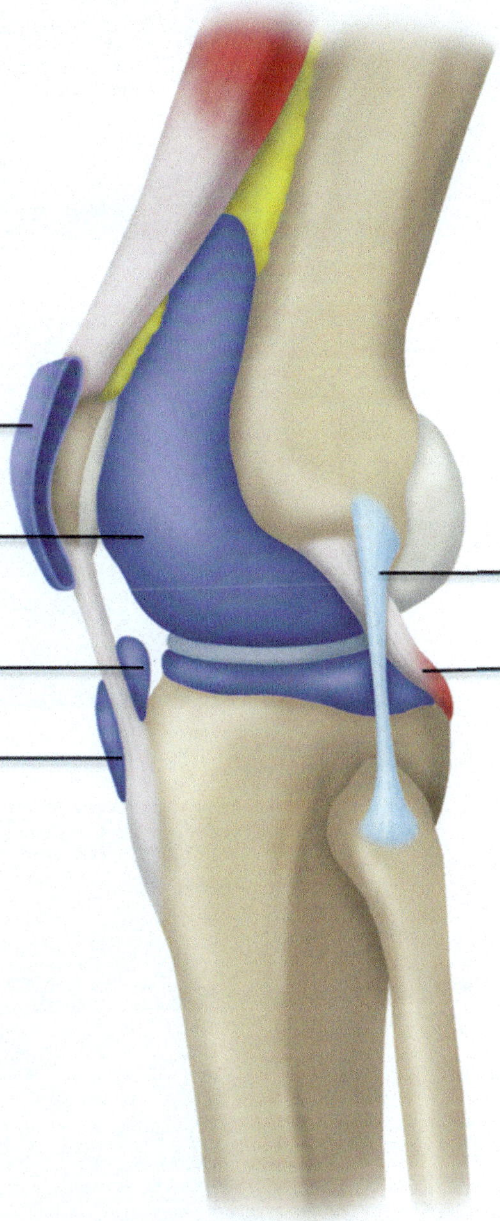

Fig. 60.10 Lateral view of the knee showing various bursas. (Reprinted with permission from Philip Peng Educational Series)

literature however reports substantially greater and longer benefit associated with high-dose steroid administration. Viscosupplement in general provides longer-lasting effect (3 months) but is not effective in advanced osteoarthritis ("bone on bone" in X-ray).

Clinical Pearls

- The reason to rotate the probe for needle insertion is to avoid the quadriceps tendon. Usually, upon rotation of 60°, the needle path is clear of the quadriceps tendon.
- It is important to visualize the spread of injectate toward the joint during injection. Pay attention to the fat pad since the commonest reason for failure of intra-articular spread is the needle tip inside the fat pad.

Conclusion

Ultrasonography is a very good tool allowing accurate localization and injection of various target structures of shoulder, hip, and knee injections. A good understanding of the anat-

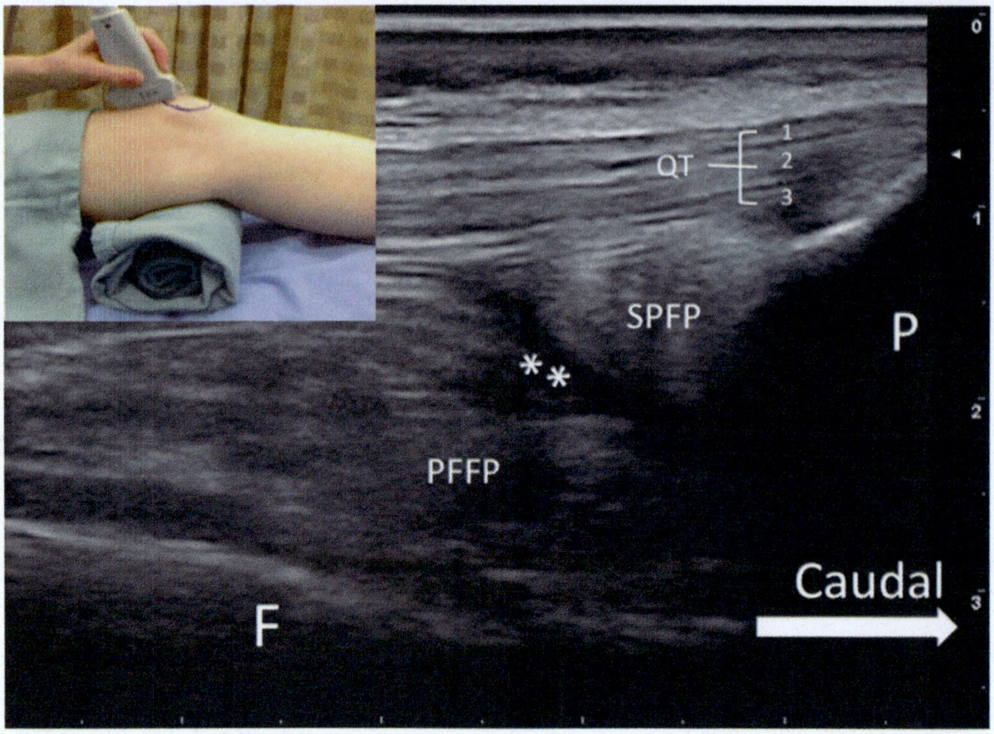

Fig. 60.11 Sonogram of the suprapatellar view of the normal knee. The insert showed the position of the patient and the ultrasound probe. SPFP suprapatellar fat pad, PFFP prefemoral fat pad, P patella, F femur, **suprapatellar recess. The trilaminar structure of the quadriceps tendon (QT) is also shown here. (Reprinted with permission from Dr. Philip Peng from Philip Peng Educational Series)

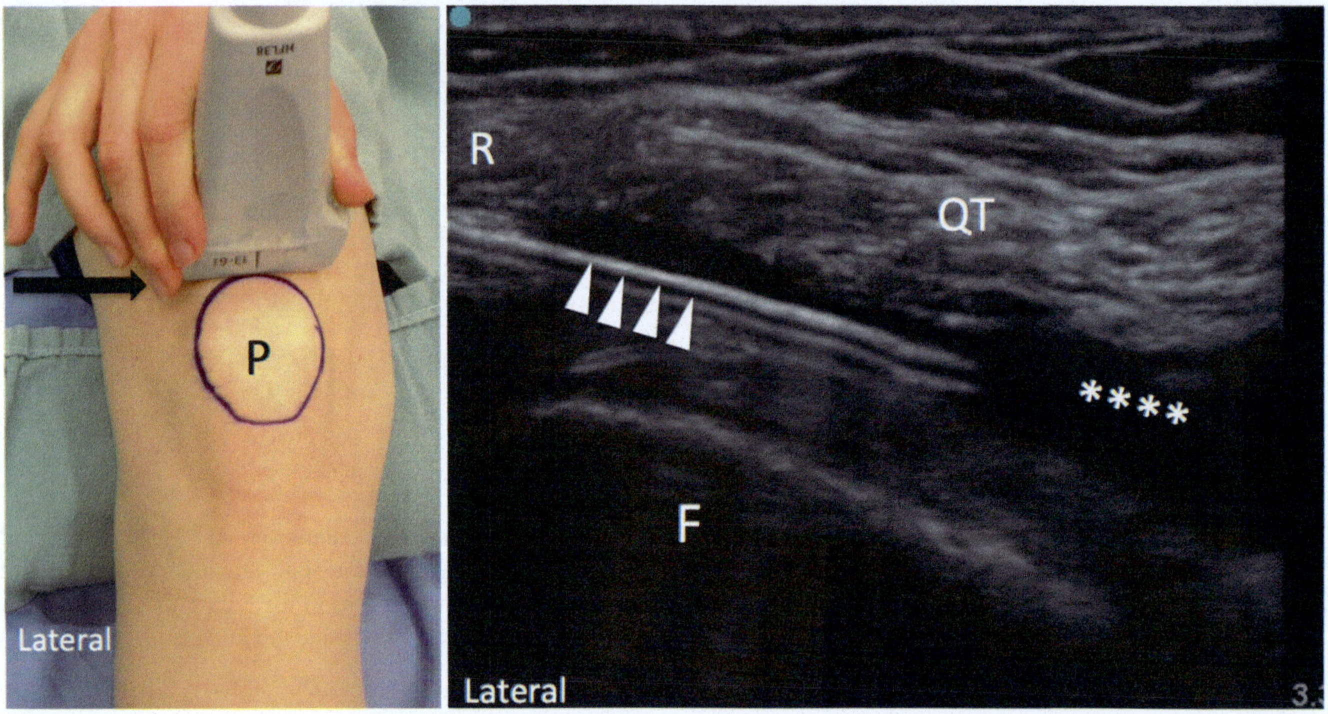

Fig. 60.12 Picture shows the injection technique. The ultrasound probe is placed between the patella and quadriceps tendon initially and then turned 90 ° upon visualization of the suprapatellar recess (SPR). The needle is then approached from lateral to medial to avoid puncturing the quadriceps tendon. The needle is indicated by the arrowheads and the SPR by asterisks (****). R retinaculum, QT quadriceps tendon, F femur. (Reprinted with permission from Philip Peng Educational Series)

omy and sonoanatomy is essential for successful procedure. Use of ultrasound for MSK interventions offers many advantages over traditional (landmark or fluoroscopy based) modalities: ultrasound avoids radiation and risks associated with use of contrast and augments accuracy by real-time visualization of soft tissue, vascular, and nerve structures.

Recommended Reading

1. Buttaci CJ, Stitik TP, Yonclas PP, Foye PM. Osteoarthritis of the acromioclavicular joint: a review of anatomy, biomechanics, diagnosis, and treatment. Am J Phys Med Rehabil. 2004;83(10):791–7.
2. Felson DT. Intra-articular corticosteroids and knee osteoarthritis: interpreting different meta-analyses. JAMA. 2016;316(24):2607–8.
3. Peng PW. Ultrasound-guided interventional procedures in pain medicine: a review of anatomy, sonoanatomy, and procedures. Part IV: hip. Reg Anesth Pain Med. 2013;38(4):264–73.
4. Peng PW. Ultrasound guided musculoskeletal injections – shoulder, hip and knee. In: Benzon, editor. Essentials of pain medicine. 4th ed. New York/Heidelberg/Dordrecht/London: Springer; 2017.
5. Peng PW, Cheng P. Ultrasound-guided interventional procedures in pain medicine: a review of anatomy, sonoanatomy, and procedures. Part III: shoulder. Reg Anesth Pain Med. 2011;36(6):592–605.
6. Peng PW, Shankar H. Ultrasound-guided interventional procedures in pain medicine: a review of anatomy, sonoanatomy, and procedures. Part V: knee joint. Reg Anesth Pain Med. 2014;39(5):368–80.
7. Shaffer BS. Painful conditions of the acromioclavicular joint. J Am Acad Orthop Surg. 1999;7(3):176–88.

Part VI

Neuromodulation

Deep Brain Stimulation

61

James Dierkes, Julie G. Pilitsis, and Steven Falowski

Abbreviations

ACC	Anterior cingulate cortex
CM-Pf	Center median-parafascicular complex
CT	Computed tomography
DBS	Deep brain stimulation
FBSS	Failed back surgery syndrome
FDA	Food and Drug Administration
GPi	Globus pallidus internus
MER	Microelectrode recording
MRI	Magnetic resonance imaging
PAG	Periaqueductal gray matter
PVG	Periventricular gray matter
SCS	Spinal cord stimulation
SF-36	Short-Form Health Survey
STN	Subthalamic nucleus
Vim	Ventral intermediate nucleus
VPL	Ventral posterolateral nucleus
VPM	Ventral posteromedial nucleus

Introduction

Deep brain stimulation (DBS) is a form of neuromodulation in which electrical current is delivered intracranially to stimulate the deep nuclei or structures of the brain. It has become a common neurosurgical procedure with an increasing number of indications. The major benefits of deep brain stimulation include its minimally invasive nature, a low adverse event profile, and reversibility as it is non-ablative. This low risk profile keeps morbidity low and mortality very rare.

J. Dierkes (✉)
Department of Anesthesiology, Duke University Medical Center, Durham, NC, USA

J. G. Pilitsis
Department of Neuroscience and Experimental Therapeutics, Neurosurgery, Albany Medical College, Albany, NY, USA
e-mail: PilitsJ@amc.edu

S. Falowski
Functional Neurosurgery, Neurosurgical Associates of Lancaster, Lancaster, PA, USA

The surgery itself involves the placement of a DBS lead into the target nucleus/region. The surgeon guides the lead through a burr hole to the target using magnetic resonance imaging (MRI), with stereotactic navigation. A lead is implanted at a precise location in the deep nuclei of the brain using microelectrode recording (MER) or MR guidance. The surgeon can confirm the placement through additional stimulation, that is, macrostimulation through the lead itself, therefore ensuring adjacent structures are not affected and causing undesirable side effects. The permanent lead is then placed with the extension wires connected to the lead externalized, similarly to what may be done in a spinal cord stimulator (SCS) trial. The surgery takes approximately 2–3 hours and is typically performed under intravenous sedation with local anesthesia. Intraoperative testing is performed to determine accurate coverage for stimulation per patient. A computed tomography (CT) scan or MRI is performed after the surgery to confirm lead placement and the absence of hemorrhage or other complications. After a 1–2-week trial period, the electrode leads are either removed if unsuccessful in treating the pain or internalized. If internalized, they are attached to a pulse generator, which is implanted subcutaneously, usually inferior to the clavicle. The generator is programmed initially during the surgery and then adjusted in follow-up outpatient visits as needed. Optimization of the device may take 3–6 months. Figure 61.1 shows the leads in place in the deep brain with the subcutaneous pulse generator in place on the right chest.

The most serious complications for DBS are intracranial hemorrhage with an incidence of 1.8–2.5% of cases. Fortunately, the majority of these cases are asymptomatic, and the permanent neurological deficit has an incidence of only 0–0.2%. More commonly, infection may occur in 3.3–13.3% of patients in some studies. The frequency of these complications varies among institutions and surgeons. For

T. R. Deer et al. (eds.), *Deer's Treatment of Pain*, https://doi.org/10.1007/978-3-030-12281-2_61

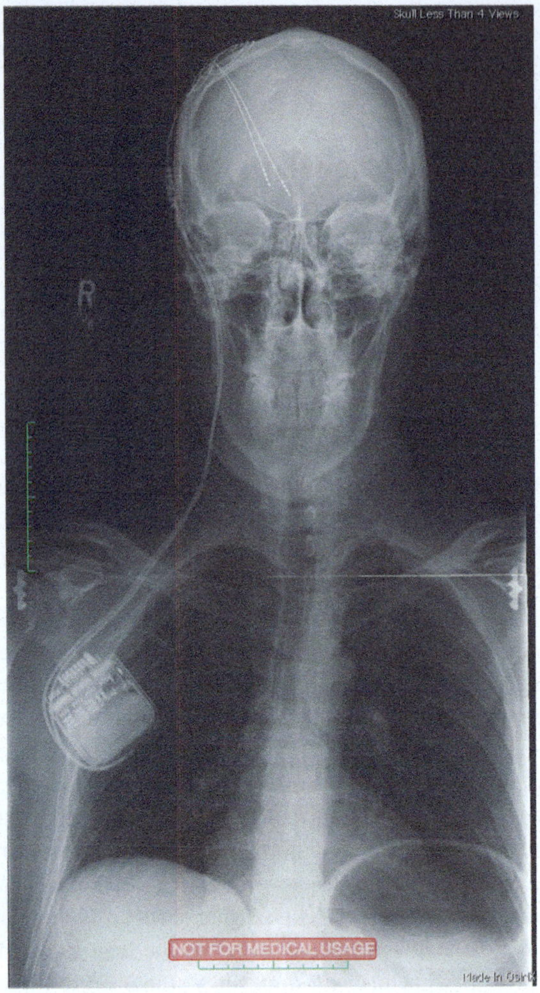

Fig. 61.1 X-ray image displaying a complete deep brain stimulation system implant with lead, extension, and subcutaneous pulse generator

example, techniques that involve isolating the implants from skin incisions have been identified to lower infection rates to 1.2%, while the use of simultaneous multichannel MER has shown to possibly lower the hemorrhage and repositioning rate.

Although the most common indication for DBS at this time is movement disorders, the treatment of chronic pain continues to be investigated. Chronic pain is becoming an increasingly prevalent and difficult to treat condition, with therapies for refractory pain syndromes in demand. Neuromodulation has a long history in assisting to manage refractory chronic pain, but more definitive research needs to be completed to compare its risk and benefit profiles. Older and more recent studies, mostly case series, have shown success in targeting various structures for many different painful conditions. This chapter will include sections on the background of DBS, indications for its use related to chronic pain, evidence of efficacy, and a review of relevant pearls and pitfalls.

Background and Historical Perspective

DBS has been used to successfully treat the symptoms of movement disorders such as Parkinson's disease, dystonia, and essential tremor. This treatment started in the 1990s when DBS was noted to be effective for tremors and safer than the thalamotomy or ablative procedures. Two of the first targets were the subthalamic nucleus (STN) for Parkinson's disease, which treated the bradykinesia, tremor, and rigidity, and the globus pallidus (GPi) for dystonia. These indications gained approval by the Food and Drug Administration (FDA) in 1997.

Although these are the most frequent indications for DBS currently, the first modern examples of therapeutic applications for brain stimulation included severe psychosis in 1938 and pain control in 1950. In the mid-1960s, Melzack and Wall developed the gate theory for pain that asserted non-painful stimuli could inhibit a painful stimulus from traveling through the nervous system. This theory allowed for the rise in neuromodulation as a proposed treatment for chronic pain by continuously delivering a stimulus capable of inhibiting pain processing through peripheral nerve stimulation, spinal cord stimulation, and eventually deep brain stimulation. By the early 1970s, there were some reports of chronic DBS systems implanted in the thalamus for the treatment of chronic pain. DBS was approved by the FDA for chronic pain in 1989 following a multicenter trial, but this approval was later retracted, indicating the need for more clinical trials. Although the current status for DBS for chronic pain is now only investigational, viable treatment plans for complex pain syndromes often include DBS. Indications have extended beyond chronic pain with DBS considered for Tourette syndrome and obsessive-compulsive disorder. Its use for depression, obesity, eating disorders, and drug-resistant hypertension remains under study.

Chronic pain has both physical and psychological components, which affect the patient's ability to function in daily life. Complications in daily living include overall health, sleep patterns, personal relationships, social interactions, employment status, and everyday activities. Treatment goals for DBS tend to be at least a 50% reduction in pain, but these elements make pain difficult to quantify and analyze. Studies have utilized different scales in order to determine changes in pain level and function after DBS, such as the Short-Form (36) Health Survey (SF-36). Analyses span eight areas including general physical health, general mental health, physical functioning, physical role limitations, bodily pain, feeling of vitality, social functioning, and emotional role limitations. A composite score is then calculated. Other methods for measurement also incorporate daily functioning with pain scores, allowing a more thorough determination of the effects of the surgery. A downside to this strategy as well as most pain questionnaires is that almost all information at this point is patient-reported.

Although the mechanism of action of DBS is still unknown, abnormal rhythmic activity in certain subcortical structures has been observed in patients with chronic pain. Targeting these structures, particularly the periventricular/periaqueductal gray area (PVG/PAG), the ventral posterolateral/medial nucleus (VPL/VPM), nuclei of the sensory thalamus, and the anterior cingulate cortex (ACC), has demonstrated success in alleviating different components of neuropathic pain. The dorsal medial lemniscus pathway, which carries sensory information, travels through the same region as the VPL/VPM nuclei. Both this target and the PVG/PAG can treat the sensory-discriminative (intensity) component of pain. The ACC is involved in psychological and motor functions, and targeting this structure treats the affective (unpleasantness) component.

Uses and Indications

Potential targets for DBS include the STN, ventral intermediate nucleus (Vim), GPi, PVG/PAG, VPL/VPM, ACC, posterior hypothalamus, center median-parafascicular (CM-Pf) complex, and internal capsule. These targets and their indications are shown in Table 61.1. The positions of these targets in relation to other brain structures and their accessory pathways are mapped in Fig. 61.2. For chronic pain relief specifically, the PVG/PAG, VPL/VPM, ACC, posterior hypothalamus, CM-Pf complex, and internal capsule have been investigated. The results of studies on DBS for chronic pain are presented in the "Evidence of Efficacy" section of this text in Table 61.2.

Table 61.1 Deep brain stimulation targets and the diseases that can be treated

Target	Diseases treated
Subthalamic nucleus (STN)	Parkinson's disease
Ventral intermediate nucleus (Vim)	Essential tremor
Globus pallidus (GPi)	Dystonia
Periventricular/periaqueductal gray area (PVG/PAG)	Postamputation phantom limb/brachial plexus injury, failed back surgery syndrome (FBSS), post-stroke pain, spinal cord injury, multiple sclerosis, other neuropathic pain
Ventral posterolateral/medial nucleus (VPL/VPM)	Postamputation phantom limb/brachial plexus injury, failed back surgery syndrome (FBSS), post-stroke pain, spinal cord injury, multiple sclerosis, other neuropathic pain
Anterior cingulate cortex (ACC)	Post-stroke pain, failed back surgery syndrome (FBSS), brachial plexus injury, spinal cord injury, other neuropathic pain
Posterior hypothalamus	Cephalgias, particularly cluster headaches
Center median-parafascicular complex (CM-Pf)	Thalamic pain syndrome, cephalgias, chronic neuropathic pain
Internal capsule	Post-stroke pain, thalamic pain syndrome, multiple sclerosis

Patient selection for DBS aimed at chronic pain is not standardized, and there are no universal inclusion or exclusion criteria. However, the patients that may benefit from DBS tend to suffer from complex chronic pain conditions that fail customary treatments including conservative measures, medications, and extracranial procedures. This situation arises usually from ineffective treatments or treatment with intolerable side effects. As these patients have failed multiple attempts for pain alleviation before the consideration of DBS, a multidisciplinary treatment team is usually involved, including a pain specialist, a neurosurgeon, and a neuro- or pain psychologist. The patients require a detailed history and physical exam with particular note of pain treatment history including medications, procedures, and prior surgeries. The pain itself needs proper classification including intensity and distribution. Psychological screening for psychiatric disorders and/or psychogenic pain should be utilized to rule those conditions out before surgery. Potential candidates have an identifiable organic origin of their pain, particularly high in the central nervous system, that is refractory to medications and/or previous surgery.

The lack of standardization in both patient and target selection is the result of the few developed clinical trials that have been published. Current studies lack randomized or case-controlled trials, creating limitations in the interpretation of data. Other difficulties include unblinded studies, heavy variations in targeting, parameters, and pain syndromes, as well as lack of detail in patient selection criteria. The initial basis for FDA approval included multicenter trials back in the 1980s that demonstrated success. However, the FDA removed that approval based on the need to expand experimentation to include clinical trials. Recently, more studies have begun incorporating randomized double-blind clinical trials which are increasingly being published. They achieve this goal by implanting all patients with DBS electrodes and having sham and active stimulation groups in a double-blinded fashion. A crossover design with a washout period is recommended.

As these pain syndromes are complex, the use of targets is variable, even among the same syndromes. For example, failed back surgery syndrome (FBSS) often has both nociceptive and neuropathic components, creating difficulty in determining a treatment plan. One meta-analysis noted the highest success with targeting PVG/PAG for long-term treatment of intractable low back pain, particularly nociceptive pain. A different study noted more clearly delineated intraoperative stimulation effects, less risk of side effects, and a strong connection to appendicular pain syndromes with

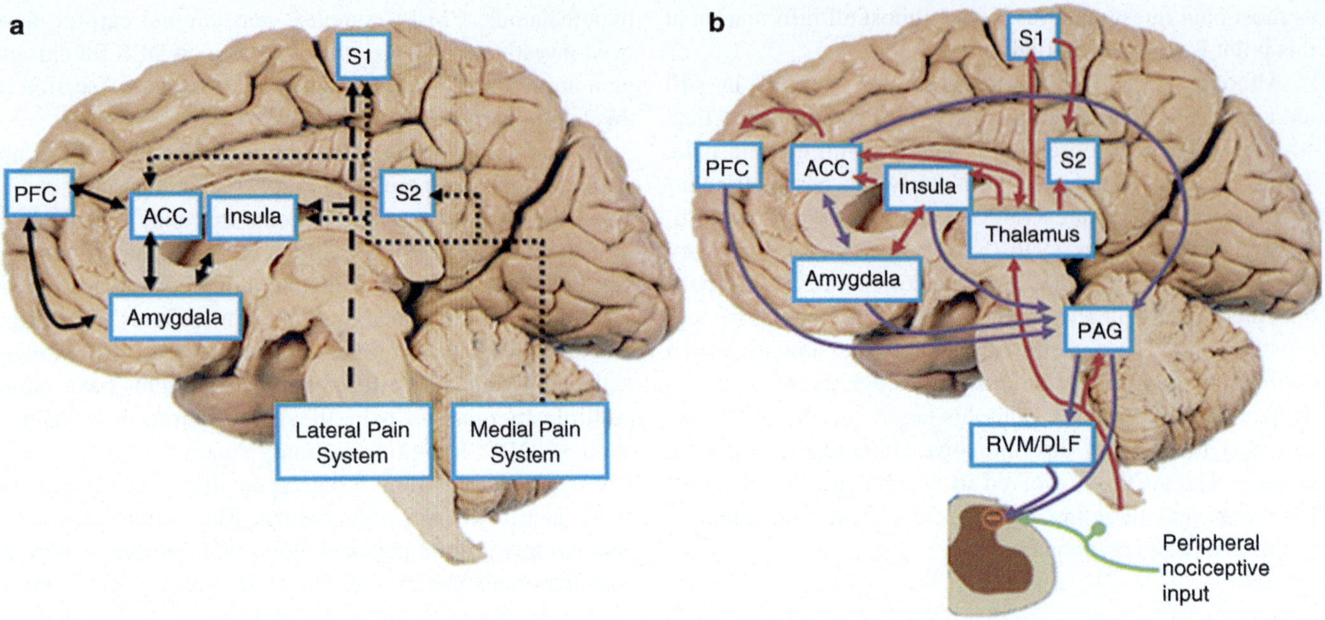

Fig. 61.2 The lateral and medial pain systems (**a**) carry the sensory-discriminative and affective-emotional components of pain, respectively. The lateral pain system consists of fibers from the neospinothalamic, neotrigeminothalamic, cervical bundle and dorsal horn to the lateral thalamus. The medial system consists of fibers from the paleospinothalamic, spinomesencephalic, spinoreticular, spinoparabrachial hypothalamic, and spinothalamic tracts to the medial thalamus. From the thalamus, information is projected to higher-order brain centers. There are ascending (red) and descending (purple) pathways of pain transmission (**b**). The periaqueductal gray receives projections from many supraspinal areas in the pain neuromatrix and influences peripheral nociceptive inputs at the spinal cord level through the rostral ventromedial medulla and dorsolateral funiculus. S1 primary somatosensory cortex, S2 secondary somatosensory cortex, ACC anterior cingulate cortex, PFC prefrontal cortex, PAG periaqueductal gray, RVM rostral ventromedial medulla, DLF dorsolateral funiculus. (This image is courtesy of Lucy Gee, PhD, from Albany Medical College)

the VPL as the target. Both of these targets are frequently utilized simultaneously to optimize an individual patient's pain treatment.

Commonly studied indications for DBS include postamputation limb pain, brachial plexus injury, and FBSS. One meta-analysis for pain relief of intractable low back pain from phantom limb pain, FBSS, and other neuropathies demonstrated long-term success of DBS, especially for nociceptive pain over neuropathic pain. Efficacies, in an otherwise refractory treatment group, have been reported at 47–71% for all neuropathic pain at 80 months follow-up.

Other indications frequently included in the literature are post-stroke pain, pain from multiple sclerosis, pain from spinal cord injury, and postherpetic neuralgia. A prospective double-blind randomized clinical trial of ten patients with post-stroke pain was negative for the primary endpoint of statistically significant pain relief overall but demonstrated statistically significant improvements in various measures that contribute to the negative impact of pain. A single study found post-stroke pain response to DBS to be 70%. A case report about a patient with spinal cord injury also noted improvement in pain from severe to minimal and overall reduction in the size of painful area with bilateral PAG stimulation. Postherpetic neuralgia of the trigeminal nerve has been treated with DBS targeting the PVG/PAG and/or the VPM with similarly successful results. Others, however, have found DBS for post-stroke pain and pain from spinal cord injury to be less successful than other indications.

Cephalgias have a high disease burden and prevalence that has been reported of in up to 3% of population. Groups have investigated these retractable diseases demonstrating very successful treatment with DBS. Cluster headaches in particular may carry the most significant success of cephalgias from targeting the posterior hypothalamus with efficacy rates being reported at 66% in a large case series of 90 patients.

Complex pain syndromes often can be treated most optimally with a combination of DBS and other interventional therapies such as spinal cord stimulation (SCS), peripheral nerve stimulation, and intrathecal therapy. A notable example includes treatment of FBSS which can include neuropathic leg pain and nociceptive back pain. SCS may be best equipped to treat the neuropathic pain, while DBS may treat the nociceptive pain. Cluster headaches may be best treated with a combination of supraorbital nerve stimulation and DBS.

Table 61.2 Evidence of efficacy for deep brain stimulation of various targets for the treatment of chronic pain

Study name	Type of study	Number of patients	Targets	Pain syndromes	Results
Yamamoto et al.	Case series	18	Thalamic nucleus ventralis caudalis	Phantom limb pain	All patients received DBS; 14/18 achieved favorable pain relief (78%)
Hamani et al.	Case series	21	Thalamic nucleus ventralis caudalis	Chronic neuropathic pain	13 received DBS at that target, 10 had successful trial, but only 2/10 achieved favorable pain relief (20%)
Pereira et al.	Case series	12	Sensory thalamus – VPL	Phantom limb pain or brachial plexus avulsion	All patients received DBS; 11/12 achieved favorable pain relief (92%)
Rasche et al.	Case series	56	Primarily PVG/PAG with VPL/VPM co-target	FBSS, anesthesia dolorosa, phantom limb pain, spinal cord injury, post-stroke pain, postherpetic pain	32 received DBS; 22/32 achieved favorable pain relief (69%)
Owen et al.	Case series	47	Primarily PVG/PAG with VPL/VPM co-target	Post-stroke, phantom limb, brachial plexus injury	38 received DBS with 6 lost to follow-up; 17/32 achieved favorable pain relief (53%)
Boccard et al.	Case series	85	Primarily PVG/PAG with VPL/VPM co-target	Phantom limb pain, brachial plexus injury, post-stroke pain, spinal cord injury, facial pain	74 received DBS with 15 lost to follow-up; 39/59 achieved favorable pain relief (66%)
Boccard et al.	Case series	24	Anterior cingulate cortex	Post-stroke pain, failed back surgery syndrome (FBSS), brachial plexus injury, spinal cord injury, other neuropathic pain	22 received DBS with 83% improvement at 6 months
Namba et al.	Case series	7	Posterior limb of internal capsule	Post-stroke pain, thalamic pain syndrome, multiple sclerosis	6 received DBS; 3 excellent response, 2 fair response, 1 poor response
Namba et al.	Case series	11	Posteromedial part of internal capsule	Post-stroke pain, thalamic pain syndrome, multiple sclerosis	11 received DBS; 8/11 achieved favorable pain relief (73%)
Franzini et al.	Case report	1	Internal capsule	Post-stroke pain	Favorable pain relief at 5 years
Lempka et al.	Clinical trial	10	Ventral striatum and anterior limb of internal capsule	Post-stroke pain	10 received active or sham DBS; elements of pain improved
Andy et al.	Case series	5	CM-Pf complex and related intralaminar nuclear structures	Thalamic pain syndrome, headache	5 received DBS; 5/5 achieved favorable pain relief
Krauss et al.	Case series	11	CM-Pf complex	Chronic neuropathic pain	10 received DBS; 10/10 achieved favorable pain relief
Krauss et al.	Case series	3	CM-Pf complex	Chronic neuropathic pain with concurrent movement disorder	3 received DBS; 3/3 achieved relief from movement disorder; 2/3 achieved favorable pain relief
Fontaine et al.	Clinical trial	11	Posterior hypothalamus	Chronic cluster headache	11 received sham or active DBS; 6 achieved favorable pain relief (all were switched to active at 1 month) with 3 being pain free
Seijo et al.	Case series	5	Posterolateral hypothalamus	Chronic cluster headache	5 received DBS; 5/5 achieved favorable pain relief with 2/5 being pain free
Leone et al.	Review	90	Posterior hypothalamus	Chronic Cluster headache	66% success rate
Abreu et al.	Case series	16	VPL	Phantom limb pain, brachial plexus injury	15 received DBS with 1 lost to follow-up; mean pain relief sustained over 36 months

Evidence of Efficacy

There is varying literature investigating different aspects of the treatment of chronic pain with DBS. Most of these studies are case series with a variety of patients and some new clinical trials with relatively small sample sizes. A summary of these studies including authors, diseases, targets, and results is displayed in Table 61.2, with explanations of the evidence following in this section. The publications of these studies are also included in the recommended reading section and can be referenced for additional information. Response rate is often identified in these cases as a 50% reduction in pain.

One of the most popular targets for DBS in the treatment of chronic pain is the sensory thalamus or VPL/VPM nuclei. Success rates in the literature for this target range from 50% to 92% for treatment of phantom limb pain, brachial plexus injury, and other neuropathic pain syndromes. These studies are case series with small populations of 12–21. Another popular target is the PVG/PAG, which has had literature success in treating many syndromes including post-stroke pain, phantom limb pain, anesthesia dolorosa, FBSS, and spinal cord injury. The PVG/PAG is often co-targeted with the VPL/VPM nuclei in cases where the surgeon wants broader coverage for potential stimulation. This target has had published success rates of 53–69% treating the varying diseases mentioned previously. These studies were case series with patient populations of 47–85, about half of whom received combination stimulation with both PVG/PAG and VPL/VPM. The best results have been in phantom limb pain and FBSS, and often both PVG and VPL electrodes are activated, leading to improved clinical symptoms. Generally, DBS surgeons place leads in both targets and during externalization determine whether one or both leads should be permanently implanted. In most clinical settings, two burr holes are necessary to accommodate such placement.

The third most popular target is the ACC for the treatment of neuropathic pain. This target can be utilized for a variety of syndromes, including post-stroke pain, brachial plexus injury, spinal cord injury, FBSS, other neuropathic pain. A recent case series shows a success rate of 83% at 6 months with a sample of 24 patients, with continued success at longer-term follow-up as far as 3 years out.

Far less commonly used are the other targets. The internal capsule can be targeted for treating post-stroke pain, thalamic pain syndrome, and multiple sclerosis. Studies on this target show success rates of 73–83% in case series with 7–11 patients. There was also a recent double-blind randomized clinical trial involving ten patients with post-stroke pain comparing sham and active stimulation to the anterior limb of the internal capsule and the ventral striatum. Although the primary endpoint was negative, there were statistically significant improvements in many of the factors that were demonstrated to contribute to pain.

More research is being conducted into targeting the center median-parafascicular complex for the treatment of chronic pain related to thalamic pain syndrome, headache, and other neuropathic pain disorders. Case series involving this target have demonstrated good to excellent pain relief in all their patients of small sample sizes from 3 to 11.

Patients with refractory cephalgias, particularly chronic cluster headaches, have benefited from DBS that targets the posterior hypothalamus. Success rates have been reported at 50–66% for posterior hypothalamus DBS of chronic cluster headaches, with studies of over 90 patients. There has also been a double-blind randomized control trial containing 11 patients who received sham or active stimulation. Initially in the first month, there was no statistically significant difference between the two groups. However, when they were all switched to active stimulation, six experienced a greater than 50% decrease in headache frequency, and three of those six were pain-free. For even greater results, the vagal nerve or supraorbital nerve stimulation may be used in combination with DBS. Of note, in the original publication, one of the patients died as a result of surgery. As this result occurred simultaneously with the development of peripheral nerve stimulation, enthusiasm for this target tempered.

There is evidence for some variations to typical treatment measures. Some groups advocate for coverage with a single electrode, as multiple electrodes may incur additional risk and are expensive. Another area for research includes pulse generators that can adapt to ongoing physiologic changes of the patient in order to deliver the appropriate amount of stimulation, that is, a closed-loop system.

As previously mentioned, the measurement of pain improvement is difficult due to the subjective nature of pain. One study utilizing the SF-36 methodology for improvement quantification found a significant improvement in the mental component of the score, particularly better scores in general health, social functioning, and bodily pain. However, there was no statistical improvement in the physical component score demonstrating that the absolute pain score is only one factor and not necessarily a marker of functionality. A different group that used the SF-36 noted improvements at 26% at the 1-year mark and 34% at the 4-year mark in one study. A different study showed no statistically significant changes, but certain categories greatly improved, such as physical functioning by 64.7% and bodily pain by 39.0%. A third group that utilized the SF-36 noted significant improvements in physical role limitations and mental role limitations and a continued elevation on all subscales relative to a normative sample.

The targets and indications in this section have been presented with their corresponding research studies. The two most popular targets are the PVG/PAG and VPL/VPM and are most successful in treating FBSS and postamputation phantom limb pain. These targets have also shown some success treating post-stroke pain, pain from spinal cord injury, pain from multiple sclerosis, and other neuropathic pain conditions. The internal capsule can also be targeted to treat the pain from these diseases. For cephalgias, the most effective targets are the posterior hypothalamus and the CM-Pf complex. The combination of multiple targets can increase the likelihood that the stimulation coverage will be adequate to relieve the patient's pain. DBS can also be combined with different modalities for pain relief, including spinal cord stimulation, peripheral nerve stimulation, and intrathecal therapy. These integrated therapies allow even more success in treating refractory pain syndromes.

Pearls and Pitfalls (Bullet Points)

- DBS is an essential consideration for the treatment of chronic pain that has failed conventional therapy. Success rates are higher than most interventions in this population of patients and should be considered in the context that these complex cases have already failed various treatment methods.
- DBS carries low morbidity and very low mortality. Rare, but serious, complications include intracranial hemorrhage, infection, and permanent neurological deficit.
- Although commonly used and FDA approved for movement disorders, DBS for chronic pain is now considered investigational by the FDA, although it is utilized by physicians and did carry an initial approval.
- Combination therapies with DBS have yielded high success rates, including spinal cord stimulation, peripheral nerve stimulation, and intrathecal therapy.
- The most promising results include treatment of phantom limb pain, facial neuropathic pain, FBSS, and nociceptive pain, with cephalgias having the best results of these diseases. The most frequent targets are the PAG/PVG and the sensory thalamus, often together.
- More basic and translational research is needed to understand the mechanism of action.
- More clinical trials are necessary to provide evidence of the effectiveness of DBS and to help determine the most appropriate target.
- According to the literature, around 60–75% of patients that undergo a successful DBS trial for chronic pain obtain sustained pain relief after permanent implantation.

Recommended Reading

1. Abreu V, Vaz R, Rebelo V, et al. Thalamic deep brain stimulation for neuropathic pain: efficacy at three years' follow-up. Neuromodulation. 2017;20. https://doi.org/10.1111/ner.12620.
2. Andy OJ. Thalamic stimulation for chronic pain. Appl Neurophysiol. 1983;46(1–4):116–23.
3. Bittar RG, Kar- Purkayastha I, Owen SL, Bear RE, Green A, Wang S, Aziz TZ. Deep brain stimulation for pain relief: a meta- analysis. J Clin Neurosci. 2005;12(5):515–9.
4. Boccard SG, Pereira EA, Moir L, Aziz TZ, Green AL. Long-term outcomes of deep brain stimulation for neuropathic pain. Neurosurgery. 2013;72(2):221–30; discussion 231.
5. Boccard SG, Fitzgerald JJ, Pereira EA, Moir L, Van Hartevelt TJ, Kringelbach ML, et al. Targeting the affective component of chronic pain: a case series of deep brain stimulation of the anterior cingulate cortex. Neurosurgery. 2014;74(6):628–35; discussion 635–7.
6. Boccard S, Prangnell S, Pycroft L, et al. Long-term results of deep brain stimulation of the anterior cingulate cortex for neuropathic pain. World Neurosurg. 2017. https://doi.org/10.1016/j.wneu.2017.06.173.
7. Chodakiewitz YG, Bicalho GV, Chodakiewitz JW. Multi-target neurostimulation for adequate long-term relief of neuropathic and nociceptive chronic pain components. Surg Neurol Int. 2013;4(Suppl 3):S170–5.
8. Deer TR, Mekhail N, Petersen E, Krames E, Staats P, Pope J, et al. The appropriate use of neurostimulation: stimulation of the intracranial and extracranial space and head for chronic pain. Neuromodulation Appropriateness Consensus Committee. Neuromodulation. 2014;17(6):551–70; discussion 570.
9. Falowski SM. Deep brain stimulation for chronic pain. Curr Pain Headache Rep. 2015;19(7):27. https://doi.org/10.1007/s11916-015-0504-1.
10. Falowski S, Dierkes J. An analysis of the use of multichannel microelectrode recording during deep brain stimulation surgeries at a single center. Oper Neurosurg. 2017;14. https://doi.org/10.1093/ons/opx139.
11. Falowski S, Ooi YC, Smith A, Verhargen Metman L, Bakay RA. An evaluation of hardware and surgical complications with deep brain stimulation based on diagnosis and lead location. Stereotact Funct Neurosurg. 2012;90(3):173–80.
12. Fine PG. Long-term consequences of chronic pain: mounting evidence for pain as a neurological disease and parallels with other chronic disease states. Pain Med. 2011;12(7):996–1004.
13. Fontaine D, Lazorthes Y, Mertens P, Blond S, Geraud G, Fabre N, et al. Safety and efficacy of deep brain stimulation in refractory cluster headache: a randomized placebo-controlled double-blind trial followed by a 1-year open extension. J Headache Pain. 2010;11(1):23–31.
14. Franzini A, Cordella R, Nazzi V, Broggi G. Long-term chronic stimulation of internal capsule in poststroke pain and spasticity. Case report, long-term results and review of the literature. Stereotact Funct Neurosurg. 2008;86(3):179–83.
15. Franzini A, Messina G, Cordella R, Marras C, Broggi G. Deep brain stimulation of the posteromedial hypothalamus: indications, long-term results, and neurophysiological considerations. Neurosurg Focus. 2010;29(2):E13.
16. Gray AM, Pounds-Cornish E, Eccles FJ, Aziz TZ, Green AL, Scott RB. Deep brain stimulation as a treatment for neuropathic pain: a longitudinal study addressing neuropsychological outcomes. J Pain. 2014;15(3):283–92.
17. Green AL, Nandi D, Armstrong G, Carter H, Aziz T. Post-herpetic trigeminal neuralgia treated with deep brain stimulation. J Clin Neurosci. 2003;10(4):512–4.
18. Hamani C, Schwalb JM, Rezai AR, Dostrovsky JO, Davis KD, Lozano AM. Deep brain stimulation for chronic neuropathic pain: long-term outcome and the incidence of insertional effect. Pain. 2006;125(1–2):188–96.
19. Hollingworth M, Sims-Williams HP, Pickering AE, et al. Single electrode deep brain stimulation with dual targeting at dual frequency for the treatment of chronic pain: a case series and review of the literature. Brain Sci. 2017;7(1). https://doi.org/10.3390/brainsci7010009.
20. Jenkins B, Tepper SJ. Neurostimulation for primary headache disorders: part 2, review of central neurostimulators for primary headache, overall therapeutic efficacy, safety, cost, patient selection, and future research in headache neuromodulation. Headache. 2011;51(9):1408–18.
21. Jermakowicz WJ, Hentall ID, Jagid JR, et al. Deep brain stimulation improved the symptoms and sensory signs of persistent central neruopathic pain from spinal cord injury: a case report. Front Hum Neurosci. 2017;11:177. https://doi.org/10.3389/fnhum.2017.00177.
22. Krauss JK, Pohle T, Weigel R, Kalbarzcyk A. Somatosensory thalamic stimulation versus center median-parafascicular complex stimulation in 11 patients with neuropathic pain. Stereotact Funct Neurosurg. 2001;77:194.

23. Krauss JK, Pohle T, Weigel R, Burgunder JM. Deep brain stimulation of the centre median-parafascicular complex in patients with movement disorders. J Neurol Neurosurg Psychiatry. 2002;72(4):546–8.
24. Lempka SF, Malone DA, Hu B, et al. Randomized clinical trial of deep brain stimulation for post-stroke pain. Ann Neurol. 2017;(5). https://doi.org/10.1002/ana.24927.
25. Leone M, Cecchini AP. Central and peripheral neural targets for neurostimulation of chronic headaches. Curr Pain Headache Rep. 2017;21(3):16. https://doi.org/10.1007/s11916-017-0616-x.
26. Leone M, Franzini A, Broggi G, Bussone G. Hypothalamic deep brain stimulation for intractable chronic cluster headache: a 3-year follow-up. Neurol Sci. 2003;24:S143–5.
27. Leone M, Franzini A, Proietti Cecchini A, Mea E, Broggi G, Bussone G. Deep brain stimulation in trigeminal autonomic cephalgias. Neurotherapeutics. 2010;7(2):220–8.
28. Levy RM, Lamb S, Adams JE. Treatment of chronic pain by deep brain stimulation: long term follow-up and review of the literature. Neurosurgery. 1987;21(6):885–93.
29. Levy R, Deer TR, Henderson J. Intracranial neurostimulation for pain control: a review. Pain Physician. 2010;13(2): 157–65.
30. Namba S, Nakao Y, Matsumoto Y, Ohmoto T, Nishimoto A. Electrical stimulation of the posterior limb of the internal capsule for treatment of thalamic pain. Appl Neurophysiol. 1984;47(3):137–48.
31. Namba S, Wani T, Shimizu Y, Fujiwara N, Namba Y, Nakamua S, et al. Sensory and motor responses to deep brain stimulation. Correlation with anatomical structures. J Neurosurg. 1985;63(2):224–34.
32. Owen SL, Green AL, Nandi DD, Bittar RG, Wang S, Aziz TZ. Deep brain stimulation for neuropathic pain. Acta Neurochir Suppl. 2007;97(Pt 2):111–6.
33. Parmar VK, Gee L, Smith H, Pilitsis JG. Supraspinal stimulation for treatment of refractory pain. Clin Neurol Neurosurg. 2014;123:155–63.
34. Pereira EA, Aziz TZ. Neuropathic pain and deep brain stimulation. Neurotherapeutics. 2014;11(3):496–507.
35. Pereira EA, Boccard SG, Linhares P, Chamadoira C, Rosas MJ, Abreu P, et al. Thalamic deep brain stimulation for neuropathic pain after amputation or brachial plexus avulsion. Neurosurg Focus. 2013;35(3):E7.
36. Rasche D, Rinaldi PC, Young RF, Tronnier VM. Deep brain stimulation for the treatment of various chronic pain syndromes. Neurosurg Focus. 2006;21(6):E8.
37. Seijo F, Saiz A, Lozano B, Santamarta E, Alvarez-Vega M, Seijo E, et al. Neuromodulation of the posterolateral hypothalamus for the treatment of chronic refractory cluster headache: experience in five patients with a modified anatomical target. Cephalalgia. 2011;31(16):1634–41.
38. Stadler JA 3rd, Ellens DJ, Rosenow JM. Deep brain stimulation and motor cortical stimulation for neuropathic pain. Curr Pain Headache Rep. 2011;15(1):8–13.
39. Thomas L, Bledsoe JM, Stead M, Sandroni P, Gorman D, Lee KH. Motor cortex and deep brain stimulation for the treatment of intractable neuropathic face pain. Curr Neurol Neurosci Rep. 2009;9(2):120–6.
40. Yamamoto T, Katayama Y, Obuchi T, Kano T, Kobayashi K, Oshima H, et al. Thalamic sensory relay nucleus stimulation for the treatment of peripheral deafferentation pain. Stereotact Funct Neurosurg. 2006;84(4):180–3.

Motor Cortex Stimulation

62

Kurt A. Yaeger and Brian Harris Kopell

Introduction

As discussed throughout this textbook, neuropathic pain is a difficult entity to treat. Diagnosis can be ambiguous, and treatment strategies are diverse, including medical, surgical, and psychological modalities. Regardless, chronic, neuropathic pain represents a growing public health concern, burdening both patients and clinicians and straining the economy of the medical system.

The surgical treatment of neuropathic pain is a relatively new concept, one that is intrinsically linked to evolving medical technologies. As a result, it is constantly being developed and refined, utilizing the latest technological advances in neuromodulation. Deep brain stimulation (DBS) and motor cortex stimulation (MCS) are two neuromodulatory techniques that are currently employed for neuropathic pain. DBS for pain is discussed elsewhere in this textbook. This chapter will present MCS as an alternative surgical strategy for neuropathic pain.

Background and Historical Perspective

Early Research

The first reported link between the human motor cortex and pain relief was described by Wilder Penfield and Herbert Jasper in 1954. In their textbook, *Epilepsy and the Functional Anatomy of the Human Brain*, Penfield and Jasper document a patient's relief of severe, neuropathic-type pain following resection of the primary motor cortex, albeit with significant comorbid complications. Throughout the 1970s and 1980s, research conducted at the University of California, San Francisco, focused mainly on stimulation of sensory pathways for pain control. Although deep, subcortical stimulation of thalamic somatosensory regions was found to provide relief from deafferentation or neuropathic pain, cortical stimulation of the primary somatosensory area has been proven ineffective.

In 1991, Tsubokawa and colleagues presented their preliminary experience with chronic motor cortex stimulation for the treatment of central pain. Based on the group's earlier experimental feline models, in which they illustrated inhibition of thalamic hyper-excitability with motor cortex stimulation, the group presented 12 patients who had intractable pain due to a central lesion such as thalamic infarct or hemorrhage, internal capsule mass, or multiple sclerosis. Of these patients, who had subsequently undergone surgical placement of epidural electrodes and intermittent motor cortex stimulation, ten patients achieved satisfactory pain relief during the first month. At 1 year, five patients reported complete pain relief, and a further three patients had considerable reduction of pain. Importantly, the group determined that precise lead placement over the motor cortex was essential in providing pain control, as the pain inhibition threshold was observed at a lower intensity than the threshold for muscle contraction.

The early work by Tsubokawa and colleagues paved the way for further research on motor cortex stimulation for chronic deafferentation or neuropathic pain. Throughout the 1990s and early 2000s, many studies assessed analgesic response of MCS on trigeminal neuralgia, atypical facial pain, poststroke pain, phantom limb pain, and various other neuropathic pain syndromes. Accounting for inherent biases of these small, nonrandomized surgical studies, the response to MCS ranged from 0% to 100%, with larger series averaging around a 50% analgesic response.

K. A. Yaeger
Department of Neurosurgery, Icahn School of Medicine, Mount Sinai Hospital, New York, NY, USA
e-mail: kurt.yaeger@mountsinai.org

B. H. Kopell (✉)
Center for Neuromodulation, Department of Neurosurgery, Mount Sinai Health System, New York, NY, USA
e-mail: brian.kopell@mountsinai.org

T. R. Deer et al. (eds.), *Deer's Treatment of Pain*, https://doi.org/10.1007/978-3-030-12281-2_62

Contemporary Analysis

As observed throughout the current literature, studies assessing efficacy of MCS are heterogeneous, both in surgical technique and in assessment of analgesic efficacy. Surgical strategies for MCS vary in approach (craniotomy versus burr hole), lead placement (epidural versus subdural), localization (neuronavigation versus intraoperative imaging versus intraoperative monitoring [somatosensory evoked potentials, SSEPs, or motor evoked potentials, MEPs]), and electrode positioning (perpendicular or parallel to precentral gyrus). Anesthetic strategy also varies, with some studies performed under general anesthesia, relying on direct cortical stimulation (SSEPs and MEPs) for localization, and some investigators performing awake craniotomies to assess the intraoperative therapeutic response to MCS. An in-depth assessment of the current literature follows in this chapter.

Pathophysiology

Deafferentation pain (anesthesia dolorosa) denotes pain referable to peripheral nerve or central afferent fibers. Accordingly, damage to peripheral nerves, spinal cord, thalamus, and cortical regions may contribute to the sensation of pain. The ventrocaudal nucleus (Vc) of the thalamic is the major relay site for ascending somatosensory information. The sensation of deafferentation pain has several proposed mechanisms, including (1) loss of low-threshold mechanoreceptive neurons such that nociceptive output predominates, (2) reduced tonic inhibition of thalamic or cortical nociceptive fibers, and (3) unmasking or strengthening of nociceptive pathways. Furthermore, in some patients with deafferentation pain, abnormal sensations of pain have been provoked by non-noxious stimuli, indicating some aberration of afferent neural connection. Taken together, it is evident that nociceptive output can be enhanced when afferent somatosensory signals are either diminished or misconnected or if thalamic hyperactivity is present.

The exact mechanism of analgesia from motor cortex stimulation remains uncertain. However, as hypothesized in early studies of MCS, it is likely that stimulation of motor efferent fibers modulate hyperactive thalamic relay nuclei, resulting in the negative feedback of nociceptive signals.

Uses and Indications

Patient Selection

According to the limited published literature, patients most likely to benefit from motor cortex stimulation (MCS) have deafferentation-type neuropathic pain, referable to a neurologic injury. Specific conditions include poststroke pain, trigeminal neuralgia, multiple sclerosis, postherpetic neuralgia, spinal cord injury, phantom limb pain, brachial plexus lesions, and complex regional pain syndrome. Importantly, patients have failed conservative management, including non-pharmacological and medical treatment modalities. Non-pharmacologic pain management strategies include physical therapy, behavioral therapy, and psychological evaluation. These patients are also typically unresponsive to both opioid and non-opioid analgesics.

Preoperative Evaluation

When the appropriate patient is selected for MCS therapy, preoperative medical and psychological evaluations must be completed prior to surgery. Given the inherent risks to surgery, as well as the added risks of implanting a medical device, the patient must be medically optimized preoperatively, with strict blood pressure control and blood glucose regulation. Some patients, such as those with advanced cardiopulmonary disease, may not be candidates for general anesthesia, and the operative plan should be adjusted accordingly. Patients should be psychologically screened for expected adherence and compliance, and their social support system should be assessed, given the need for strict postoperative follow-up and frequent programming sessions.

Furthermore, patients should be counseled on their expectations for pain control after surgery. The literature should be cited for rates of MCS efficacy on the patient's specific cause of pain (trigeminal neuralgia, poststroke pain, etc.). Given the wide range of efficacy, it is critical that the patient understand that his or her pain might respond suboptimally to MCS.

Surgical Technique

- Preoperative volumetric imaging is obtained and the motor cortex is localized using stereotactic guidance software (Fig. 62.1).
- The patient is brought into the operating room and moved onto the operating table in the supine position. Depending on surgeon preference, the patient is then either induced under general anesthesia and intubated or fully sedated. A Mayfield head holder is applied to the patients head and secured to the operating table. The head is turned to the contralateral side. Using intraoperative image guidance, the motor cortex is localized and skin incision is marked.
- The patient's head is shaved, prepped, and draped in the standard sterile fashion. Routine perioperative antibiotics are provided, depending on institutional practice. Skin incision is made. Again, depending on surgeon prefer-

ence, either a burr hole is drilled or a small craniotomy is performed over the motor cortex.

- The motor cortex is identified by the presence of phase reversal on somatosensory evoked potentials (SSEPs). A contact paddle (Fig. 62.2a, b) is placed either in the epidural or subdural space, and either parallel or perpendicular to the precentral gyrus, depending on surgeon preference. The lead is used to assess motor evoked potentials (MEPs) to confirm location. If the patient is awake, analgesic response to stimulation can be assessed. If seizure activity is induced during stimulation, iced saline should be used to bathe the subjacent cortex. When proper positioning is confirmed, the lead should be sutured to the dura. Craniotomy bone flap should be replaced if necessary. The distal lead should be tunneled and remotely externalized. The skin incision is then closed in layers, and a sterile dressing is applied.
- The patient is then woken and extubated if necessary. Imaging can be obtained to confirm electrode placement (Fig. 62.3). Consequently, a trial of stimulation is performed. Optimal pain relief is usually noted with fairly low frequency and high pulse width. Example initial stimulation parameters are 50 Hz with 450 msec pulse width and titrated accordingly.
- If patient receives benefit from stimulation trial, the patient is again brought to the operating room (typically several days later), where the leads are internalized and connected to an implantable pulse generator (IPG) (Fig. 62.4).

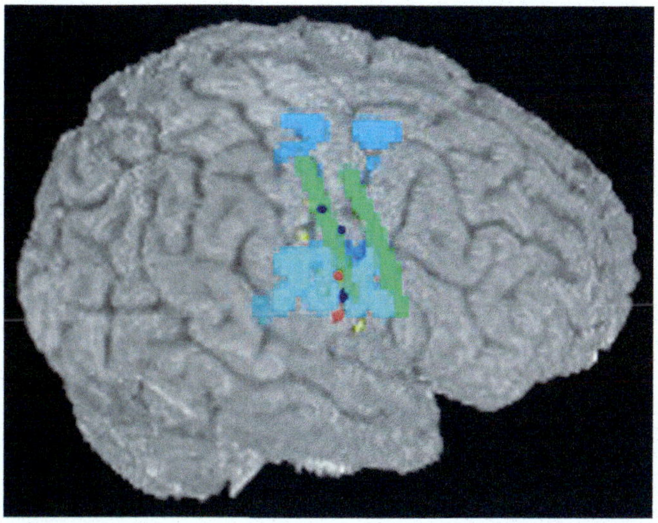

Fig. 62.1 Three-dimensional reconstructions of functional magnetic resonance image (fMRI), localizing precentral gyrus/motor cortex (blue) and planned electrode placement (green)

Evidence for Efficacy

Beginning in the early 1990s, many studies have investigated the effectiveness of motor cortex stimulation (MCS) for medically refractory neuropathic pain. Overall, these stud-

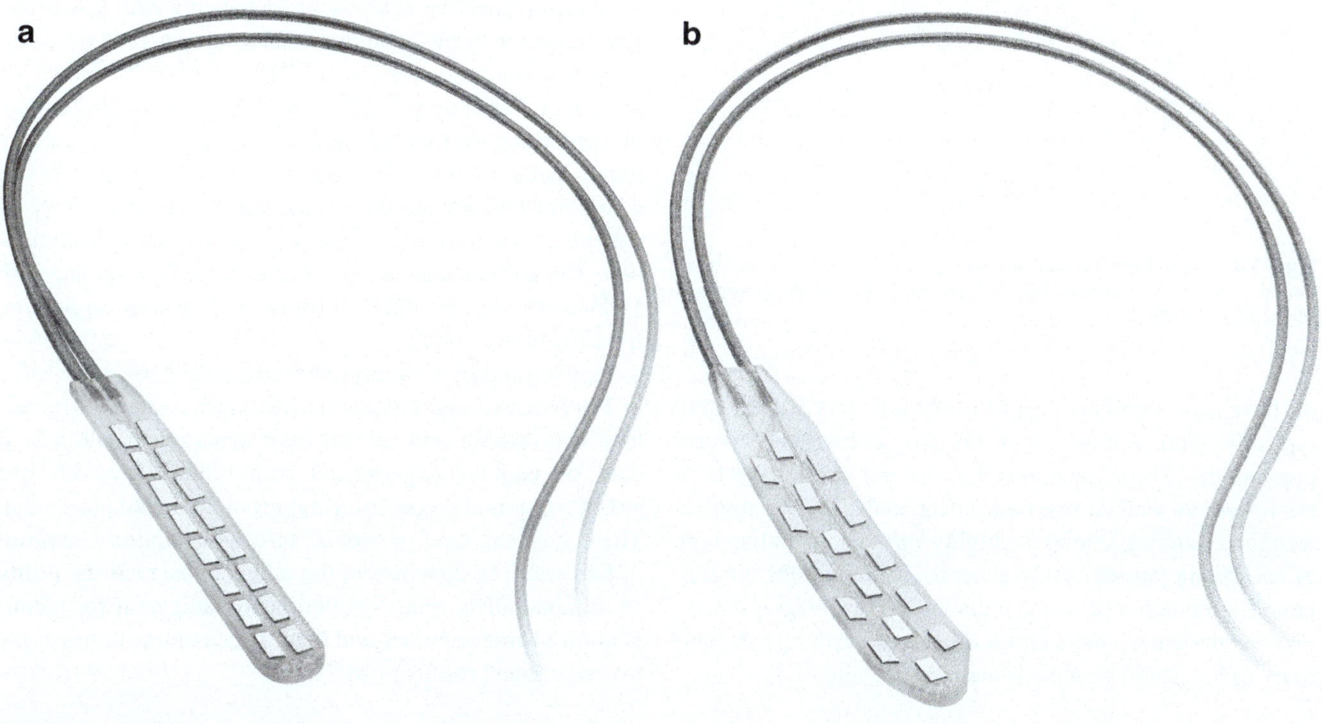

Fig. 62.2 Examples of implantable neurostimulator leads in varying configurations, Medtronic 8 × 2 lead (**a**) and Medtronic 5-6-5 lead (**b**). (Reprinted with the permission of Medtronic, Inc. ©)

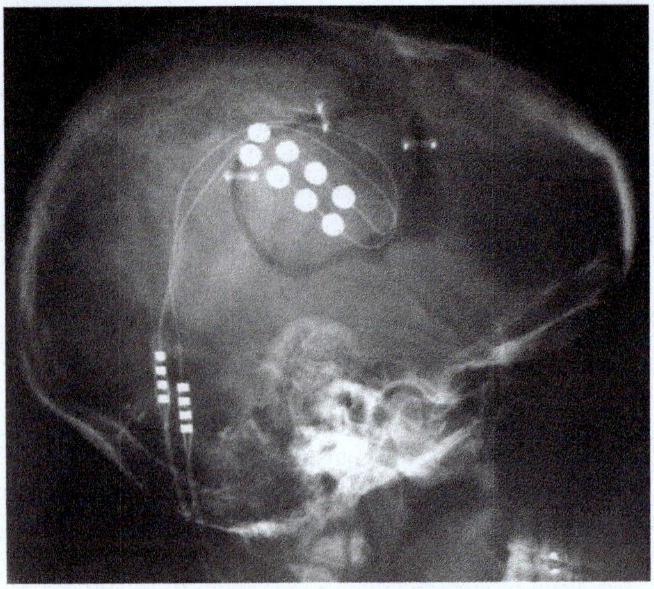

Fig. 62.3 Postoperative lateral skull X-ray showing a small frontoparietal craniotomy and 8-lead paddle (2 × 4) perpendicular to motor cortex. Leads tunneled remotely from skin incision

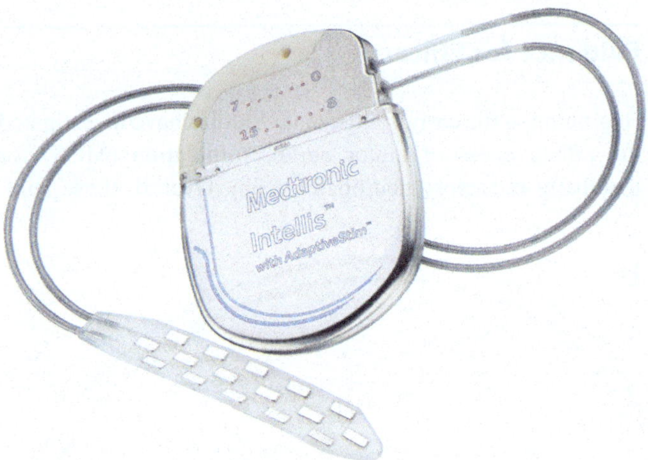

Fig. 62.4 Example of implantable pulse generator, with connection to implantable neurostimulator lead. (Reprinted with the permission of Medtronic, Inc. ©)

ies have been small case series (most less than 30 patients), typically nonrandomized, non-blinded, and without control populations. Three randomized, crossover trials have been published, as well as one large meta-analysis. The surgical techniques among studies are highly variable, including type of anesthesia (awake versus general), technique for intraoperative stimulation (direct stimulation versus image-guided), and electrode placement (epidural versus subdural). A summary of key studies can be visualized in Table 62.1.

Motor Cortex Stimulation (MCS)

In 1993, Tsubokawa and co-authors presented the first series of patients who underwent MCS for chronic deafferentation pain. They describe 8 of 11 patients (73%) with excellent results of trial stimulation following lead placement, resulting in internalization and generator implantation. Of these patients, five had sustained effects of stimulation at long-term follow-up. In this study, three patients required lead revision due to scar formation and resultant loss of clinical efficacy. Following this work, Meyerson and colleagues presented a series of ten patients who underwent MCS for intractable neuropathic pain. Although the three patients with poststroke pain did not experience relief with stimulation, the remaining seven patients (two with peripheral nerve injury, five with trigeminal neuralgia) had at least a 50% reduction in pain. The authors observed that most patients experienced brief generalized seizures during initial stimulation but that none experienced lasting motor deficits as a result.

Ebel and co-authors reported in 1996 on seven patients for whom they performed MCS for neuropathic facial pain. Six of these patients had immediate pain relief postoperatively. Three patients had sustained pain control at last follow-up, whereas the other three patients experienced decreasing efficacy over several months. One patient experienced a postoperative focal seizure, likely due to an "accidently increased stimulation intensity." No postoperative infection or other surgical morbidity was observed.

In a retrospective analysis of 31 patients with poststroke pain treated with MCS, study by Katayama in 1998 observed an immediate response rate in 74% of patients. However, the effect was only persistent in 48% at 2-year follow-up. In comparing responders and nonresponders, the authors found that pain relief was achieved in 70% of patients in whom muscle contraction was inducible, compared to 9% of patients in whom contractions were not elicited with stimulation. The authors concluded that an analgesic response with MCS might require intact corticospinal circuits originating from the motor cortex.

Nguyen and co-authors published their experience of MCS in 1999, describing 32 patients who were treated for refractory neuropathic and central pain syndromes. Ultimately, 75% of patients experienced pain relief. However, five patients required reoperation and revision of lead placement. There was one case of wound infection requiring removal of hardware. In conclusion, the authors observed the utility of intraoperative, image-guided neuronavigation for identification of motor cortex and lead placement to improve the overall clinical results of MCS.

Table 62.1 Summary of key studies assessing the efficacy of motor cortex stimulation

Study	Design	Patients	Efficacy	Adverse events
Tsubokawa et al., *JNS* 1993	Prospective	11, chronic deafferentation pain	73% with excellent initial pain relief, 45% with sustained effects	3 patients needing lead revision due to loss of effect
Meyerson et al., *Acta Neurochir* 1993	Retrospective	10, chronic neuropathic pain	70% with at least 50% reduction in pain	Most patients had seizures during test stimulation, but no lasting motor effects
Ebel et al., *Acta Neurochir* 1996	Retrospective	7, neuropathic trigeminal pain	6/7 patients with immediate pain relief, 3/6 with prolonged relief	1 post-op seizure
Katayama et al., *JNS* 1998	Retrospective	31, poststroke pain	74% with immediate pain relief, 48% with relief at follow-up	3 patients with stimulation-related seizures, 1 infection
Mertens et al., *Stereotact Funct Neurosurg* 1999	Prospective	20, poststroke pain	75% response rate, 25% with excellent pain relief	Not reported
Nguyen et al., *Pain* 1999	Retrospective	32, central and neuropathic pain	75% with pain relief at follow-up	1 post-op infection, req device removal; 1 asymptomatic epidural hematoma
Carroll et al., *Pain* 2000	Prospective	10, axial and facial pain	50% with immediate pain relief	3 post-op wound infections, 1 death due to pulmonary embolism
Sol et al., *Stereotact Funct Neurosurg* 2001	Retrospective	3, phantom limb pain	100% initial pain relief, sustained in 2 patients at long-term follow-up	None
Nandi et al., *J Clin Neurosci* 2002	Retrospective, DBS after MCS	6, poststroke pain	1/6 responded to MCS, 4 patients had DBS placement, 3 of 4 with pain relief	None
Saitoh et al., *Acta Neurochir* 2003	Prospective	19, chronic deafferentation pain	74% with reduction in pain (32% excellent results)	Not reported
Brown et al., *Neurosurgery* 2005	Prospective	10, neuropathic facial pain	80% with immediate pain relief, 100% at last follow-up	1 post-op wound infection, req device removal
Nuti et al., *Pain* 2005	Prospective	31, central and peripheral neuropathy	10% with excellent relief, 42% with good relief	3 partial seizures, 2 transient neuro deficits, 3 wound issues (no device removals)
Rasche et al., *Pain* 2006	Retrospective	17, trigeminal and poststroke pain	47% with long-term pain relief	7 with intraoperative seizure; 1 infection, req device removal
Lefaucheur et al., *Brain* 2009	Prospective, randomized	16, chronic peripheral neuropathy	60% with good or satisfactory pain relief on long-term follow-up	3 patients dropped out
Buchanan et al., *Neuro Report* 2014	Retrospective	8, trigeminal or thalamic pain	Significant reduction in pain at 3 mo	Not reported
Delavallée et al., *Acta Neurochir* 2014	Retrospective	18, chronic neuropathic pain	78% favorable outcome (>50% pain relief)	3 infections, req device removal
Sachs et al., *Neuromodulation* 2014	Retrospective	14, chronic neuropathic pain	5 patients with transient efficacy; of these patients, only 2 with long-term effect	2 infections, req device removal; 3 transient seizures
Son et al., *Stereotact Funct Neurosurg* 2014	Prospective, simultaneous MCS and DBS	9, chronic neuropathic pain	8 of 9 patients successful trial; MCS effective in 6 of 8, DBS in 2 of 8	None
Radic et al., *Can J Neurol Sci* 2015	Prospective, randomized	12, CRPS, phantom limb, brachial plexus avulsion, facial pain	6 patients withdrew from study, no change in remaining patients, trial terminated early	1 infection, 3 seizures
Kolodziej et al. J *Neurol Surg A Cent Eur Neurosurg* 2016	Retrospective	22, chronic neuropathic pain	50% complete pain relief, 36% good pain relief	2 lead revisions; 1 infection, req device removal; 1 asymptomatic epidural hematoma
Ivanishvili et al. *Neuromodulation* 2017	Prospective, randomized	6, chronic neuropathic pain	67% responders to "cyclical" stimulation	None

CRPS complex regional pain syndrome, *DBS* deep brain stimulation, *MCS* motor cortex stimulation

In 2000, Carroll and colleagues presented their series of ten patients who had prospectively undergone MCS for chronic neuropathic pain. In the study, the surgeons performed awake craniotomies and intraoperative motor cortex localization and had successfully localized motor cortex in all ten patients. Despite this, only five patients experienced pain relief postoperatively and at long-term follow-up. This study had a relatively high rate of complications, with three patients experiencing postoperative wound infections requiring debridement. One of these patients suffered a subdural hematoma after device removal, which necessitated further surgical evacuation. This patient ultimately died of a pulmonary embolus within 6 months.

Sol and co-authors published in 2001 their small series of three patients with phantom limb pain who underwent MCS. All three patients initially had complete pain relief. At long-term follow-up, two had sustained analgesia, but one patient had progressive loss of efficacy over 4 months.

In 2003, Saitoh et al. reported their results of 17 patients with chronic deafferentation pain who underwent MCS. For this study, patients initially underwent subdural grid placement to effectively localize the motor cortex. Fourteen patients (74%) experienced pain relief after lead placement, with six patients experiencing excellent results. The group concluded that lead placement within the central sulcus provided optimal stimulation results.

Brown and Pilitsis published a prospective analysis in 2005 of ten patients with neuropathic facial pain treated with MCS. The most common cause of pain was trigeminal neuralgia, refractory to both medications and prior invasive treatment such as microvascular decompression or rhizotomy. Immediately after surgery, eight patients (80%) had more than 50% relief of pain. At 10-month follow-up, all patients had pain relief, and four had discontinued pharmaceutical analgesia. One patient in the series developed a postoperative wound infection, requiring device removal and long-term parenteral antibiotics.

In 2005, Nuti and co-authors published their prospective experience with 32 patients for whom they performed MCS. At long-term follow-up, 10% continued to experience excellent pain relief, defined by >70% reduction in pain, whereas 42% had good results (40–69% pain relief). Although 26% had experienced a side effect, including partial seizures (3), temporary postoperative neurologic deficits (2), and wound issues (3), none led to stimulator device removal.

In 2006, Rasche et al. described their series of 17 patients with chronic poststroke or trigeminal neuralgia who underwent MCS. At long-term follow-up, 47% of patients experienced pain relief. Furthermore, the authors performed double-blinded placebo testing, which showed a non-response rate of 35%. In these patients, implantation of generator was not performed.

Accumulating the relevant data from across the literature, Fontaine and co-authors published an MCS meta-analysis in 2009, including 152 patients who underwent MCS for various types of chronic neuropathic pain syndromes. Overall, 55% of patients experience a good response (≥40% reduction in pain) after surgery, and 45% of patients have sustained results with follow-up at 1 year. The authors also observed various complications, including a 6% rate of infection, a 5% rate of hardware problem, and a 12% early seizure rate. No cases of chronic seizures were reported. To date, this meta-analysis represents the highest level of evidence supporting the use of MCS in chronic neuropathic pain.

Following this meta-analysis, several further case series have been published. In 2014, Sachs et al. reported on 14 patients who underwent MCS for chronic neuropathic pain, only 5 of which had therapeutic results. In contrast, Buchanan et al. reviewed their case series of MCS in eight patients, all of whom experienced varying degrees of pain relief. Similarly, in a 2014 study by Delavallée et al. of 18 patients who underwent subdural MCS lead placement, 78% experienced a good outcome, defined as at least a 50% reduction in pain. Another retrospective case series of 22 patients published in 2016 by Kolodziej and colleagues highlighted complete pain relief in 50% of patients and a total of 86% of patients with at least "good" pain relief. For these patients, leads were placed under local anesthesia via a single burr hole. Most recently, in 2017, Ivanishvili et al. published a small series of six patients who underwent randomization for a "cyclical" stimulation protocol. Of these patients, four had documented response to cyclical stimulation, at an optimized "dosage" of 15 minutes alternating on and off.

Two prospective, randomized crossover trials have been performed to assess MCS efficacy. In 2009, Lefaucheur and colleagues presented their trial of 16 patients with chronic peripheral neuropathy, who underwent MCS implantation. Two patients experienced good results immediately and refused to participate in the randomization, and one patient suffered a fall after her surgery and was excluded from the study after a complicated hospital course. Of the remaining patients, 60% ultimately experienced good or satisfactory pain relief after simulation. In 2015, Radic and co-authors published the results of their prospective, randomized, crossover trial, consisting of 12 patients with complex regional pain syndrome, neuropathic deafferentation facial pain, or neuropathic pain due to phantom limb or brachial plexus avulsion. Study participants all underwent surgical implantation of motor cortex simulator lead and were then randomized to either high or low stimulation and blinded to their protocol assignment. Six patients were withdrawn from the study due to adverse events, including one infection requiring device explantation and three partial seizures. Overall, there were no changes in efficacy between high and low stimulation, as well as compared to baseline. Furthermore, high stimulation had significant negative impact on physical and mental health scores, compared to low stimulation. Given these findings, the trial was halted early.

Deep Brain Stimulation (DBS) Versus MCS

Two trials assessing both DBS and MCS have been performed. In 2002, Nandi and co-authors presented a series of six patients who underwent MCS implantation. After long-term follow-up, only one patient had persistent pain relief (16%). Consequently, the authors implanted DBS in four patients in whom MCS failed, targeting the ventroposterolateral thalamic nucleus (VPL). Of these four patients, three experienced relief of pain during stimulation. Importantly, these patients had relief of hyperesthesia in addition to an analgesic response.

In 2014, Son et al. performed a prospective trial assessing the simultaneous implantation of MCS and ventrocaudal nucleus (Vc) thalamic DBS in nine patients with chronic neuropathic pain. In all, six patients responded to MCS, and two patients had pain relief with DBS. Efficacy of both modalities decreased over time, with only 40% of patients responding at long-term follow-up.

Summary of Evidence

Taken together, the body of evidence supporting the use of motor cortex stimulation for chronic neuropathic pain is highly variable, both in terms of study design and results. In the series presented, MCS seems to be modestly effective for up to 50–70% of the study population, in some cases with decreasing efficacy over time. However, when analyzing the studies with higher level of evidence (prospective randomized trials and meta-analysis), the results are mixed. Two of the randomized crossover studies show benefit to MCS, whereas one actually showed a harmful effect of surgery and stimulation. The meta-analysis of more than 150 patients showed that about half the patients benefit from MCS and yielded an overall complication rate of 25% (including 6% infection and 5% hardware malfunction). However, this meta-analysis does not include any studies after 2006.

Future Directions

Overall, the paucity of large volume trials limits definitive conclusions regarding the efficacy of MCS. Certainly, further study in this realm is required, specifically with prospective randomized, crossover trials to limit investigator bias and the inherent placebo effect with surgery.

Given the heterogeneity of historical study results, the ability to predict which patients benefit from MCS is of critical importance. A study by Lefaucheur and colleagues in 2011 assessed the predictive value of preoperative transcranial magnetic stimulation (TMS). After accounting for placebo effects, TMS was found to have a positive predictive value of 1.0 for response to MCS. Future studies can help identify patient characteristics associated with MCS response.

Conclusions

In September 2017, a European expert meeting was organized and consensus was gathered about the use of MCS in patients with chronic neuropathic pain. The authors made four conclusions:

- Patients who suffer from neuropathic pain that is caused by a neuroanatomic substrate are the only potential candidates for MCS.
- Multidisciplinary assessment before MCS should be carried out to prevent inclusion of patients with psychological or psychiatric disorders and/or substance abuse problems.
- In order to optimize the potential analgesic effect from MCS, sophisticated targeting of the primary motor cortex must be carried out.
- Pain intensity scores (i.e., VAS and NRS scales) alone are not meaningful enough to evaluate the effects of MCS. A multidimensional evaluation including pain intensity, pain medication intake, and quality of life must be implemented in future clinical trials.

These conclusions ultimately help create a new foundation for future research in this field. Novel studies are certainly warranted so that this technology may continue to benefit the appropriate patient population.

Pearls and Pitfalls

- Central and peripheral neuropathies are associated with deafferentation and can be due to loss of thalamic inhibitory circuits and unmasking of nociceptive fibers.
- In animal models, stimulating the motor cortex below the motor threshold inhibits thalamic hyper-excitability.
- Early human trials of motor cortex stimulation (MCS) proved successful in providing pain relief in a majority of patients.

- Over the past 25 years, many small series of MCS have been performed, with rates of efficacy ranging between 0% and 100%.
- Study protocols vary in many regards, including anesthesia strategy (awake vs. general), surgical approach (burr hole vs. craniotomy, subdural vs. epidural lead placement), and localization (image-guided vs. direct cortical stimulation).
- A key meta-analysis observed a long-term efficacy rate of 45% but an overall complication rate of 25%.
- Patients with deafferentation-type neuropathic pain (e.g., poststroke, phantom limb, trigeminal neuralgia) may benefit from MCS.
- An in-depth discussion with the patient preoperatively is essential; the patient must have reasonable expectations and must understand the uncertain benefit of surgery.

Recommended Reading

1. Fontaine D, Hamani C, Lozano A. Efficacy and safety of motor cortex stimulation for chronic neuropathic pain: critical review of the literature. J Neurosurg [Internet]. 2009 [cited 2017 Jul 16];110(2):251–6. Available from: http://thejns.org/doi/10.3171/2008.6.17602.
2. Honey CM, Tronnier VM, Honey CR. Deep brain stimulation versus motor cortex stimulation for neuropathic pain: a minireview of the literature and proposal for future research. Comput Struct Biotechnol J [Internet]. 2016 [cited 2017 Oct 1];14:234–7. Available from: http://www.ncbi.nlm.nih.gov/pubmed/27413477.
3. Kurt E, Henssen DJHA, Steegers M, Staal M, Beese U, Maarrawi J, et al. Motor cortex stimulation in patients suffering from chronic neuropathic pain: summary of an expert meeting and pre-meeting questionnaire, combined with a literature review. World Neurosurg [Internet]. 2017 [cited 2017 Oct 1];108:254–63. Available from: http://linkinghub.elsevier.com/retrieve/pii/S187887501731478X.
4. Ostergard T, Munyon C, Miller JP. Motor cortex stimulation for chronic pain. Neurosurg Clin N Am [Internet]. 2014 [cited 2017 Jul 15];25(4):693–8. Available from: http://www.ncbi.nlm.nih.gov/pubmed/25240657.
5. Tsubokawa T, Katayama Y, Yamamoto T, Hirayama T, Koyama S. Chronic motor cortex stimulation for the treatment of central pain. Acta Neurochir Suppl (Wien) [Internet]. 1991 [cited 2017 Sep 4];52:137–9. Available from: http://www.ncbi.nlm.nih.gov/pubmed/1792954.
6. Tsubokawa T, Katayama Y, Yamamoto T, Hirayama T, Koyama S. Chronic motor cortex stimulation in patients with thalamic pain. J Neurosurg [Internet]. 1993 [cited 2017 Oct 1];78(3):393–401. Available from: http://thejns.org/doi/10.3171/jns.1993.78.3.0393.

63 Occipital Nerve Stimulation

Lucas W. Campos

Introduction

Peripheral neuromodulation is the application of electrical current to areas outside the CNS for medical use. The first reported use of direct electrical stimulation to treat pain was in 1859 by Julius Althaus. He used direct electrical stimulation of a peripheral nerve to alleviate surgical pain in an extremity. Early work examining peripheral nerve stimulation in the treatment of chronic pain management was done by Dr. Campbell and Dr. Long at Johns Hopkins in 1976. Disorders of the peripheral nervous system often present a unique challenge to the clinician or surgeon, because the neuropathic pain associated with them can be extremely resistant to pharmacologic and surgical treatments. Painful peripheral nerve disorders require treatment that delivers targeted relief to the precise distribution of the pain. The ability to focus therapeutic stimulation onto a specific peripheral nerve without providing unwanted stimulation into other areas is the primary advantage of PNS. PNS has undergone several refinements in recent years, enabling the treatment of painful peripheral nerve problems that until fairly recently were either untreatable or poorly treated with traditional SCS techniques.

In peripheral nerve injury, ectopic discharges are transmitted by injured nerves. Low threshold Aβ and high threshold Aδ and C fibers all contribute to the generation of pain. It is postulated that PNS or direct non-painful electrical stimulation may alter ectopic discharge leading to decreased pain perception. It has also been hypothesized that PNS may affect local concentrations of biochemical mediators that enhance the pain response. Biochemical mediators of pain lead to lowered neural activity thresholds which contribute to the development of chronic pain. Studies have suggested that PNS may directly inhibit pain neurotransmission through alteration of local inflammatory mediators.

L. W. Campos (✉)
Interventional Pain Physicians, Chico, CA, USA

PNS is indicated when the pain is confined to the distribution of a single peripheral nerve or a limited number of individual peripheral nerves. One of the reasons it has grown in popularity is that placement of the electrode array along the desired peripheral nerve can be done easily. The use of PNS to treat craniofacial neuropathic pain has emerged in the last decade as a viable treatment modality for this disorder. PNS gives a new therapeutic alternative for patients suffering from a wide array of craniofacial pain syndromes such as postherpetic neuralgia involving the supraorbital nerve or occipital neuralgia following trauma or surgery. PNS treatment in these areas has also made it an excellent therapy for atypical and classic migraine as well as cluster headaches.

Background and Historical Perspective

Of the available headache treatments, neurostimulation is not a novel approach. In the first century, Emperor Claudius' doctor, Scribonius Largus, recommended application of a live electric fish (*Torpedo marmorata*) on the site of head pain. This was effective for many headaches that were not responsive to the usual botanical cocktails created by the physicians of that era. These first uses of medical electricity were also used as effective treatments for gout and other arthralgias. The Egyptians were also known to have used electric catfish for similar treatments.

Pain in the occiput that radiates cephalad or laterally is often secondary to abnormalities of the divisions of the occipital nerve. The occipital nerve pain syndromes are usually due to nerve trauma caused by myofascial spasm causing compression, cervicogenic disease, cervical spondylosis, posterior fossa surgery, and transformed migraine. Inflammation of the C2 nerve root will also cause severe pain in this region, consistent with cervical radiculitis. The transformed migraine begins with pain in the occipital nerve distribution and then evolves into a full migraine headache. Neurostimulation has also been employed in the treatment of chronic tension-type headache, hemicrania continua,

T. R. Deer et al. (eds.), *Deer's Treatment of Pain*, https://doi.org/10.1007/978-3-030-12281-2_63

short-lasting unilateral neuralgiform headaches, and cluster headaches. Treatment of these headache conditions may include direct stimulation of the greater and lesser occipital, supraorbital and supratrochlear, auriculotemporal, and infraorbital nerves.

The treatments of headache pain syndromes include oral medications, physical therapy, nerve blocks, and radiofrequency ablation. In the past, occipital neurectomy, which involved the destruction of the nerve, was performed by neurosurgery, but this fell out of favor because of the development of anesthesia dolorosa causing a worsening of the pain syndrome. Cryotherapy and radiofrequency procedures appear to have some efficacy but unfortunately are short lived in duration and require the patient to undergo multiple procedures over time. Stimulation of the occipital nerves has evolved over the past decade and has become a standard treatment of chronic headache pain that does not respond to these other conservative surgical interventions.

Uses and Indications

Stimulation of peripheral branches of the occipital nerves also has central nervous system effects. This is consistent with our current understanding of the trigeminocervical pain pathway, which plays an essential role in migraine and other headaches; see Fig. 63.1. Animal and human studies have shown that the trigeminocervical pathway projects to many areas of the brain involved in migraine headache. Thus, activation of one part of the system results in activation of other components. An illustrative example is the superior sagittal sinus: mechanical and electrical stimulation here activates cells that extend from the trigeminal nucleus caudalis to C1 and C2 dorsal horns. Greater occipital nerve stimulation has also been shown to increase metabolic activity in the dorsal horn at C1 and C2 as well as in the trigeminal nucleus caudalis. Positron emission tomography studies of eight patients with chronic migraine effectively treated with bilateral occipital nerve stimulation demonstrated changes in thalamic activation that correlated with improvement of the headache symptoms. Thus, pain modulation occipital nerve stimulation produces beneficial effects by activating both the peripheral and central nervous systems.

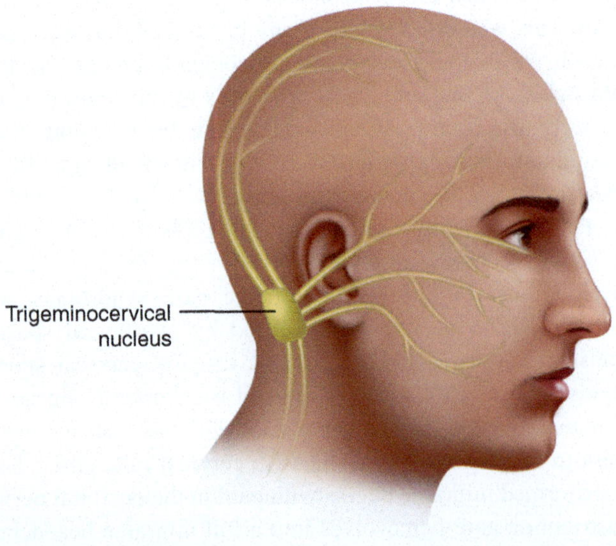

Fig. 63.1 The occipital nerve can generate multiple headache syndromes by activating the trigeminocervical complex

Indications

Current indications for PNS include neuropathic pain disorders such as postherpetic, occipital, inguinal, and genitofemoral neuralgia. PNS is also used off-label to treat migraine (chronic and transformed), hemicrania continua, and cluster headaches. To be considered for PNS of the occipital nerve, or occipital nerve stimulation (ONS), patients should have chronic, severe, disabling neuropathic pain or headache refractory to long-term treatments, including medications, nerve blocks, trigger point injections, and physical therapy. Local anesthetic block may confirm that the occipital nerve is affected, but is not predictive of ONS success.

A pretrial psychological screening is recommended to identify any psychosocial issues that may adversely impact the therapy. This screening includes assessment of any cognitive impairment or dementia, substance abuse, untreated anxiety or depression, or unrealistic expectations related to the stimulator. The success of the therapy hinges on appropriate candidate selection and optimal placement of the leads for most effective stimulation. Although ONS has a lower risk of complications than SCS, infection, lead erosion, and mechanical issues must be considered. Patients with suboptimal outcomes may have unrealistic expectations for the device. An ongoing dialogue between the provider and patient about the risks and benefits and their expectations for pain relief should be part of the patient preparation process.

Evidence for Efficacy

Migraine Headache

Transformed migraine is the most common cause of chronic daily headache and affects close to 5% of the population. Transformed migraines are chronic (more than 15 days per month) and are nonparoxysmal (lasting more than 4 hours). Transformed migraine most often develops in the setting of symptomatic medication overuse and becomes disabling, incapacitating, and refractory to most treatments.

Current treatment for transformed migraine may include hospitalization or intensive outpatient IV treatments. The goal is to interrupt the daily headache pattern with parenteral protocols and implement effective preventive and abortive treatment.

Applying ONS may dampen the severity of transformed migraines by reducing the chronic bombardment of sensory input to the trigeminocervical complex. Data from two small, retrospective, uncontrolled studies suggest that occipital nerve stimulation results in less frequent and less severe migraine headaches. Schwedt et al. retrospectively studied a mixed group of 15 patients with chronic headache for 19 months. Eight had chronic migraine and two suffered from hemicrania continua. Headache frequency was reduced from 89 to 64 days in each 90-day period. Headache severity on a visual analogue scale (VAS) decreased from 7.1 preoperatively to 4.7 postoperatively, and the Migraine Disability Assessment (MIDAS) was reduced by 39%. Popeney and Aló performed occipital nerve stimulation on 25 patients with medically refractory transformed migraine and retrospectively analyzed their data. At a mean follow-up of 18 months, they observed a reduction in headache frequency from 76 to 38 days in each 90-day period. Severity was 9.3 preoperatively and 5.7 postoperatively. The MIDAS score decreased by 89%.

In patients with chronic migraine, Silberstein and colleagues studied 268 patients who were enrolled from 15 investigational sites. Of these, 157 were implanted with a permanent system and randomized and followed over 3 months. The design of this study was interesting due to the control group receiving a sham device. Control group patients were implanted with the ONS system and given a sham programmer that did not communicate with the IPG, and therefore no stimulation was delivered. This randomized, double-blind, controlled clinical trial showed significant differences between each group. Pain was reduced by 30% on VAS, and the number of headache days and MIDAS scores were also significantly lower in the treatment group. Yet, the study failed to show a significant difference in the number of patients who achieved a 50% reduction on the VAS for headache pain. The 12-month follow-up showed almost 60% of patients achieved a 30% or greater reduction in headache days and pain intensity as measured by a VAS, and almost half of the patients achieved a 50% reduction.

In the sham-controlled PRISM study, 139 episodic and chronic migraine patients were enrolled and randomized in either an active bilateral ONS group or a sham group. After 12 weeks, the ONS did not produce any significant reduction of migraine days compared with sham. Heterogeneity of the cohort could account for these results (patients had migraine with or without aura, chronic migraine, and drug overuse headache), because patients who had overused medication, for example, had a less favorable outcome. This idea was also suggested in a retrospective study of various types of headaches treated with ONS.

Occipital Neuralgia

Occipital neuralgia is a disorder characterized by sharp, electrical, paroxysmal pain, occasionally throbbing in quality, originating from the occiput and extending along the posterior scalp, in the distribution of the greater, lesser, and/or third occipital nerve; see Fig. 63.2. Symptoms can be triggered or unprovoked and pain tends to be unilateral; however, bilateral pathology is not uncommon. Compression or trauma to one or more of the involved nerves may result in ON but there is often an unclear etiology. Medical management with neuropathic agents such as antiepileptic and/or antidepressant medications is the first line of treatment. Injections to the nerves with local anesthetic, steroids, or even botulinum toxin can be effective in transiently relieving symptoms. Lesioning procedures, including dorsal root entry zone lesioning, posterior partial rhizotomy, and neurolysis, as well as decompressive techniques are other common modalities, with variable benefit, poor longevity, and frequent side effects.

The initial rationale for use of occipital nerve stimulation in headache treatment is based on animal studies showing the convergence of cervical, somatic, and dural (trigeminovascular) afferents on second-order nociceptors in the trigeminocervical complex. In 1999, Weiner and Reed used occipital nerve stimulation to successfully treat drug-resistant occipital neuralgia. This work opened the way for observational studies of this non-harmful method of neurostimulation in various chronic primary headache disorders. Application of ONS for this condition is promising because it is reversible with minimal side effects and has shown continued efficacy with long-term follow-up. Although prospective, randomized, controlled studies demonstrating the effectiveness of ONS have been conducted, the patient populations evaluated in these studies were not specific to medically refractory occipital neuralgia patients. Prospective comparative studies are needed to fully determine the long-term utility of ONS to treat occipital neuralgia.

Kapural et al. published a small retrospective series of patients (n = 6) with a follow-up of 3 months. All patients underwent a preoperative pain psychology evaluation and an ONS trial with good results. Patients completed a Pain Disability Index questionnaire comprising eight subscales, including the VAS, before ONS implantation and again at 3 months post-implantation. The mean VAS score decreased from 8.7 to 2.5 and all six patients had significant reductions in their Pain Disability Index at 3 months. They reported that all patients who had a successful trial elected to have a permanent implantation. In a slightly larger retrospective study with

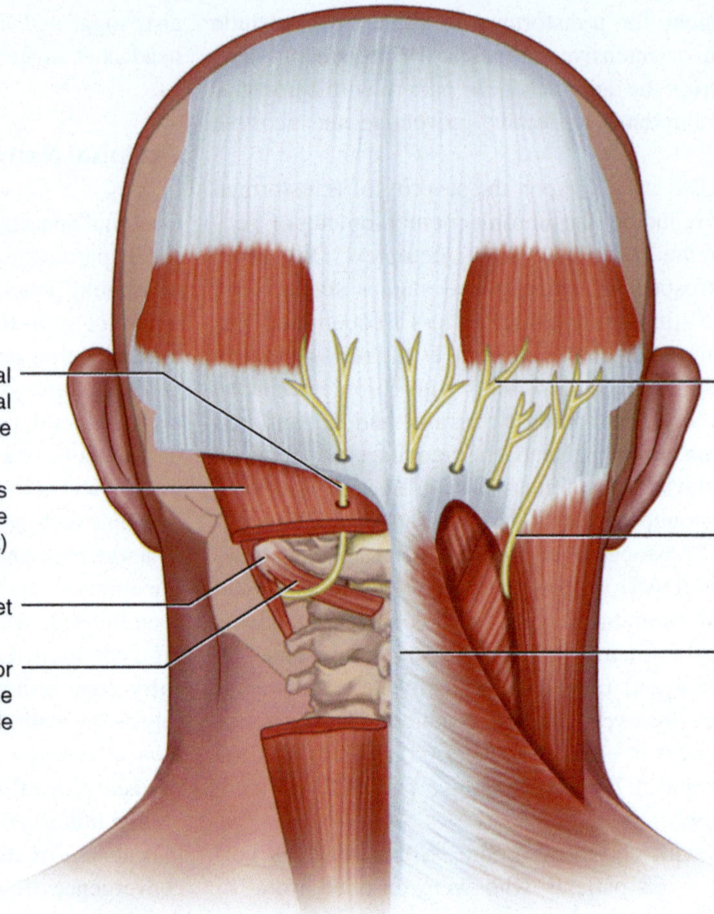

Fig. 63.2 Anatomy of the greater occipital nerve

a much longer follow-up, Johnstone and Sunderaj reported the outcomes of eight patients with a mean follow-up of 25 months. Seven of the eight patients had a successful trial of stimulation. Of the seven patients who underwent implantation, five (71%) had decreased VAS scores at last follow-up of 6–47 months (mean, 25 months; range, 6–47 months), and two patients (29%) acquired full-time employment.

In an even larger series, Slavin et al. performed occipital nerve stimulation on 14 patients with occipital neuralgia. This was a retrospective study with a mean follow-up of 22 months. Ten of the 14 patients had a successful trial and underwent implantation of a permanent system. At follow-up, seven of the ten patients continued to benefit significantly. Three patients were explanted – two due to complications (infection, neck tightness) and one due to complete resolution of pain. Reduced pain scores of 60–90% were documented in the remaining seven patients at follow-up.

Magown et al., in 2009, reported on seven patients with medically intractable ON. These patients did not have a trial of stimulation before permanent system implantation, but had experienced significant pain relief from a double-blinded C2 root block. Patients were assessed by a third party using VAS scores. In six of the seven patients (86%), the VAS score decreased to 0 postoperatively. The remaining patient (14%) experienced a 75% reduction in the VAS score.

It will be difficult to conduct blinded trials of ONS because the therapy depends on the production of paresthesia detected by the patient in the painful region. The closest alternative is the use of subthreshold stimulation, but there are some who believe that even subthreshold stimulation can result in a therapeutic effect. Research also needs to be conducted into the optimal region for lead placement and the optimal lead type.

Cluster Headache

Cluster headache is a neurological disorder characterized by recurrent, severe headaches on one side of the head, typically around the eye. There are often accompanying autonomic symptoms during the headache such as eye watering, nasal congestion, and swelling around the eye, typically confined to the side of the head with the pain. Individuals typically experience repeated attacks of excruciatingly severe unilateral headache pain. The cause of cluster headache has not been identified. While there is no known cure, cluster headaches can sometimes be prevented and acute attacks treated. Recommended treatments for acute attacks include oxygen or fast-acting triptans. Steroids may be used as a transitional treatment and may prevent attack recurrence until preventative treatments take effect. The condition affects approximately 0.2% of the general population, and men are more commonly affected than women, by a ratio of about 2.5:1–3.5:1.

Several groups have published safety and efficacy data on ONS for the treatment of cluster headache. Burns et al. and Magis et al. reported their findings with eight subjects in each of their series. Subjects were stimulated bilaterally in the series by Burns and unilaterally in the series by Magis. Burns had a median follow-up of 20 months and showed 90% relief by two patients, 50% relief by three patients, and 30% by one and no relief by two patients. Five of the eight patients continued to have daily cluster headache attaches, and six of the eight patients reported that they would recommend ONS to other similar patients. Magis had a mean follow-up of 15 months and showed two of eight patients were pain-free, three had approximately 90% reduction in headache frequency, two had an approximate 40% reduction, and one experienced no benefit. Magis followed up 15 cluster headache patients up to 36 months after ONS as well. Eighty percent of this group showed a 90% reduction in attack frequency, and 60% were pain-free for periods as long as months to years.

Pearls and Pitfalls

ONS is not without safety concerns and potential adverse events. Adverse events can be subdivided into hardware-related complications and biological complications. The commonest hardware-related complication is lead migration. Other lead-related complications such as failure or fracture have also been reported. Serious biological complications such as neurological damage are rarely observed. Stevanato et al. showed in 33% of their studies that lead migration was the most common complication of ONS. This was also further supported by reviews of data from the Neuromodulation Appropriateness Consensus Committee that showed that lead migration was the most common complication of spinal and peripheral nerve stimulation. In addition, minimal data regarding ONS in patients that are acutely and chronically anticoagulated presents an additional safety concern.

Using a widely spaced octipolar lead array, please see Fig. 63.3, the area of stimulation increases, covering the multiple branches of the occipital nerve. When two leads are placed, it is not uncommon to use one lead with primar-

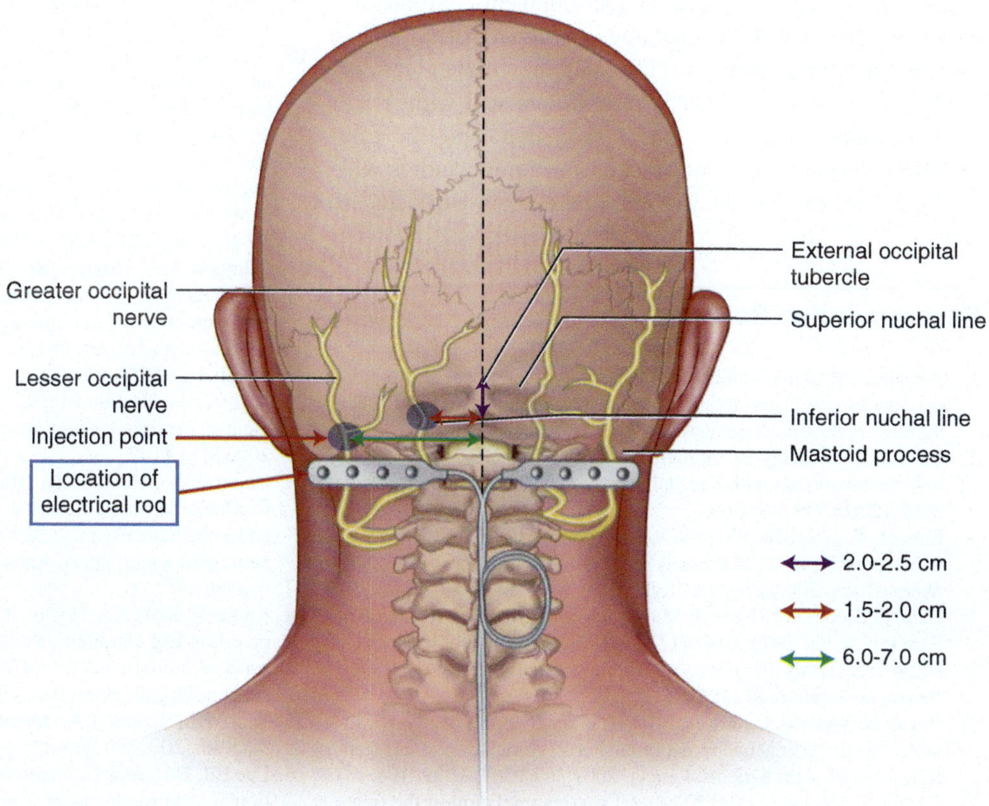

Fig. 63.3 Occipital nerve stimulator with cylindrical leads treats headaches effectively

ily anodes and the other with primarily cathodes to create a cross talk allowing wider coverage of the neuropathic pain. For permanent implants, the leads are anchored to the fascia with nonabsorbable suture. Pocketing options include the anterior chest wall in the subclavicular region, posterior axillary region, buttock, and flank. If pockets are made in more distal locations, it may be necessary to add lead extensions to reach the pocket which will increase the impedance and drain the battery faster. Postimplant, the patient's movement should be restricted for the first 6 weeks to prevent lead migration.

Conclusion

Current medicinal and nonpharmacological treatments for migraine and cluster headache are often inadequate for effectively and consistently treating attacks. Safe and effective methods of noninvasive neurostimulation might provide an adjunctive treatment option for these headache patients who are currently receiving suboptimal pharmacologic treatment. Percutaneous methods of neurostimulation clearly serve an important role in the treatment of patients with severe forms of migraine and cluster headache. The benefits of this procedure include reductions in headache intensity, the number of headache days per month, and the use of medications. The efficacy of ONS appears to be independent of the duration of or the type of headache. Development continues to target possible wireless modalities, external patch strategies, and miniaturization of IPGs. With the growing ease of implantation, it is anticipated that the field will witness an unprecedented growth in clinical data supporting the role of ONS. Standardization of outcomes in future studies will facilitate comparative analysis and future pooling of data.

Recommended Reading

1. Althaus J. A treatise on medical electricity: theoretical and practical and its use in the treatment of paralysis, neuralgia, and other diseases. London: Longmans; 1873.
2. Bartsch T, Goadsby PJ. Stimulation of the greater occipital nerve induces increased central excitability of dural afferent input. Brain. 2002;125(Pt 7):1496–509.
3. Bartsch T, Goadsby PJ. Increased responses in trigeminocervical nociceptive neurons to cervical input after stimulation of the dura mater. Brain. 2003;126(Pt 8):1801–13.
4. Beck E, Sieber WJ, Trejo R. Management of cluster headache. Am Fam Physician. 2005;71(4):717–24.
5. Bittar RG, Teddy PJ. Peripheral neuromodulation for pain. J Clin Neurosci. 2009;16(10):1259–61.
6. Burns B, Watkins L, Goadsby PJ. Treatment of medically intractable cluster headache by occipital nerve stimulation: long-term follow-up of eight patients. Lancet. 2007;369(9567):1099–106.
7. Campbell JN, Long DM. Peripheral nerve stimulation in the treatment of intractable pain. J Neurosurg. 1976;45(6):692–9.
8. Campbell CM, Jamison RN, Edwards RR. Psychological screening/phenotyping as predictors for spinal cord stimulation. Curr Pain Headache Rep. 2013;17(1):307.
9. Deer TR, Mekhail N, Provenzano D, et al. The appropriate use of neurostimulation: avoidance and treatment of complications of neurostimulation therapies for the treatment of chronic pain. Neuromodulation Appropriateness Consensus Committee. Neuromodulation. 2014;17(6):571–97; discussion 597–598.
10. Dodick DW, Silberstein SD, Reed KL, et al. Safety and efficacy of peripheral nerve stimulation of the occipital nerves for the management of chronic migraine: long-term results from a randomized, multicenter, double-blinded, controlled study. Cephalalgia. 2015;35(4):344–58.
11. Eldabe S, Buchser E, Duarte RV. Complications of spinal cord stimulation and peripheral nerve stimulation techniques: a review of the literature. Pain Med. 2016;17(2):325–36.
12. Falowski S, Wang D, Sabesan A, Sharan A. Occipital nerve stimulator systems: review of complications and surgical techniques. Neuromodulation. 2010;13(2):121–5.
13. Fumal A, Schoenen J. Current migraine management - patient acceptability and future approaches. Neuropsychiatr Dis Treat. 2008;4(6):1043–57.
14. Goadsby PJ, Knight YE, Hoskin KL. Stimulation of the greater occipital nerve increases metabolic activity in the trigeminal nucleus caudalis and cervical dorsal horn of the cat. Pain. 1997;73(1):23–8.
15. Goadsby PJ, Schoenen J, Ferrari MD, Silberstein SD, Dodick D. Towards a definition of intractable headache for use in clinical practice and trials. Cephalalgia. 2006;26(9):1168–70.
16. Goroszeniuk T, Pang D. Peripheral neuromodulation: a review. Curr Pain Headache Rep. 2014;18(5):412.
17. Headache Classification Committee of the International Headache Society (IHS). The international classification of headache disorders, 3rd edition (beta version). Cephalalgia. 2013;33(9):629–808.
18. Hoskin KL, Kaube H, Goadsby PJ. Sumatriptan can inhibit trigeminal afferents by an exclusively neural mechanism. Brain. 1996;119(Pt 5):1419–28.
19. Huntoon MA, Burgher AH. Ultrasound-guided permanent implantation of peripheral nerve stimulation (PNS) system for neuropathic pain of the extremities: original cases and outcomes. Pain Med. 2009;10(8):1369–77.
20. Huntoon MA, Huntoon EA, Obray JB, Lamer TJ. Feasibility of ultrasound-guided percutaneous placement of peripheral nerve stimulation electrodes in a cadaver model: part one, lower extremity. Reg Anesth Pain Med. 2008a;33(6):551–7.
21. Huntoon MA, Hoelzer BC, Burgher AH, Hurdle MFB, Huntoon EA. Feasibility of ultrasound-guided percutaneous placement of peripheral nerve stimulation electrodes and anchoring during simulated movement: part two, upper extremity. Reg Anesth Pain Med. 2008b;33(6):558–65.
22. Johnstone CSH, Sundaraj R. Occipital nerve stimulation for the treatment of occipital neuralgia-eight case studies. Neuromodulation. 2006;9(1):41–7.
23. Kapural L, Mekhail N, Hayek SM, Stanton-Hicks M, Malak O. Occipital nerve electrical stimulation via the midline approach and subcutaneous surgical leads for treatment of severe occipital neuralgia: a pilot study. Anesth Analg. 2005;101(1):171–4, table of contents.
24. Kaube H, Keay KA, Hoskin KL, Bandler R, Goadsby PJ. Expression of c-Fos-like immunoreactivity in the caudal medulla and upper cervical spinal cord following stimulation of the superior sagittal sinus in the cat. Brain Res. 1993;629(1):95–102.
25. Kidd BL, Urban LA. Mechanisms of inflammatory pain. Br J Anaesth. 2001;87(1):3–11.
26. Lee PB, Horazeck C, Nahm FS, Huh BK. Peripheral nerve stimulation for the treatment of chronic intractable headaches: long-term efficacy and safety study. Pain Physician. 2015;18(5):505–16.

27. Magis D, Allena M, Bolla M, De Pasqua V, Remacle J-M, Schoenen J. Occipital nerve stimulation for drug-resistant chronic cluster headache: a prospective pilot study. Lancet Neurol. 2007;6(4):314–21.
28. Magis D, Gerardy P-Y, Remacle J-M, Schoenen J. Sustained effectiveness of occipital nerve stimulation in drug-resistant chronic cluster headache. Headache. 2011;51(8):1191–201.
29. Magown P, Garcia R, Beauprie I, Mendez IM. Occipital nerve stimulation for intractable occipital neuralgia: an open surgical technique. Clin Neurosurg. 2009;56:119–24.
30. Matharu MS, Bartsch T, Ward N, Frackowiak RSJ, Weiner R, Goadsby PJ. Central neuromodulation in chronic migraine patients with suboccipital stimulators: a PET study. Brain. 2004;127(Pt 1):220–30.
31. Mathew NT. Transformed migraine, analgesic rebound, and other chronic daily headaches. Neurol Clin. 1997;15(1):167–86.
32. Nesbitt AD, Goadsby PJ. Cluster headache. BMJ. 2012;344:e2407.
33. Paemeleire K, Van Buyten J-P, Van Buynder M, et al. Phenotype of patients responsive to occipital nerve stimulation for refractory head pain. Cephalalgia. 2010;30(6):662–73.
34. Papuć E, Rejdak K. The role of neurostimulation in the treatment of neuropathic pain. Ann Agric Environ Med. 2013;Spec no. 1:14–7.
35. Petersen EA, Slavin KV. Peripheral nerve/field stimulation for chronic pain. Neurosurg Clin N Am. 2014;25(4):789–97.
36. Popeney CA, Aló KM. Peripheral neurostimulation for the treatment of chronic, disabling transformed migraine. Headache. 2003;43(4):369–75.
37. Reed KL, Black SB, Banta CJ 2nd, Will KR. Combined occipital and supraorbital neurostimulation for the treatment of chronic migraine headaches: initial experience. Cephalalgia. 2010;30(3):260–71.
38. Saper JR. Daily chronic headache. Compr Ther. 1992;18(5):6–10.
39. Schwedt TJ, Dodick DW, Hentz J, Trentman TL, Zimmerman RS. Occipital nerve stimulation for chronic headache--long-term safety and efficacy. Cephalalgia. 2007;27(2):153–7.
40. Siberstein SD, Lipton RB, Solomon S, Mathew NT. Classification of daily and near-daily headaches: proposed revisions to the IHS criteria. Headache. 1994;34(1):1–7.
41. Silberstein SD, Silberstein JR. Chronic daily headache: long-term prognosis following inpatient treatment with repetitive IV DHE. Headache. 1992;32(9):439–45.
42. Silberstein SD, Dodick DW, Saper J, et al. Safety and efficacy of peripheral nerve stimulation of the occipital nerves for the management of chronic migraine: results from a randomized, multicenter, double-blinded, controlled study. Cephalalgia. 2012;32(16):1165–79.
43. Slavin KV, Nersesyan H, Wess C. Peripheral neurostimulation for treatment of intractable occipital neuralgia. Neurosurgery. 2006;58(1):112–9; discussion 112–119.
44. Soin A, Fang Z-P, Velasco J. Peripheral neuromodulation to treat postamputation pain. Prog Neurol Surg. 2015;29:158–67.
45. Stevanato G, Devigili G, Eleopra R, et al. Chronic post-traumatic neuropathic pain of brachial plexus and upper limb: a new technique of peripheral nerve stimulation. Neurosurg Rev. 2014;37(3):473–9; discussion 479–480.
46. Stovner L, Hagen K, Jensen R, et al. The global burden of headache: a documentation of headache prevalence and disability worldwide. Cephalalgia. 2007;27(3):193–210.
47. Tavanaiepour D, Levy RM. Peripheral neuromodulation for treatment of chronic migraine headache. Neurosurg Clin N Am. 2014;25(1):11–4.
48. Tsoucalas G, Karamanou M, Lymperi M, Gennimata V, Androutsos G. The "torpedo" effect in medicine. Int Marit Health. 2014;65(2):65–7.
49. Weaver-Agostoni J. Cluster headache. Am Fam Physician. 2013;88(2):122–8.
50. Weiner RL, Reed KL. Peripheral neurostimulation for control of intractable occipital neuralgia. Neuromodulation. 1999;2(3):217–21.

Sphenopalatine Ganglion Block

64

Mark N. Malinowski and Nicholas J. Bremer

Introduction

The patient who presents with headaches and facial pain can prove to be very challenging from a diagnostic standpoint. Headaches may be intracranial or extracranial and result from a variety of pathologic, genetic, structural, inducible, or idiopathic causes. Because of the complexity of patient presentation, the physician must perform a thorough history and physical examination in order to correlate the symptoms to location, quality, frequency, duration, and other precipitating factors associated with the symptoms. The International Classification of Headache Disorders 3rd Edition (ICHD-3) provides a comprehensive system of hierarchical and phenotypical presentations. Headaches associated with the sphenopalatine ganglia (SPG) is now known as a primary headache as part of the trigeminal autonomic cephalgia (TAC) family, subtype cluster headache. Under certain circumstances, this headache may also be considered secondary or both primary and secondary. While this is beyond the scope of this chapter, the importance of patient history within this classification system is paramount to proper diagnosis.

A variety of diagnostic terms similar to SPG headache were previously used and include Vidian neuralgia, Sluder's neuralgia, and migrainous neuralgia of Harris among others. Agitation of this ganglia is implicated in "brain freeze" headaches. The presentation of these headaches is sudden, severe, and unilateral. They may not be daily but are present most days of the week. Severe cases may have many independent headaches in 1 day. Similarly, the headaches may demonstrate autonomic qualities such as nasal congestion, lacrimation, and rhinorrhea. Other autonomic qualities present involve pupillary and eyelid involvement and perspiration. While the disorder may involve bouts that last several weeks to month, patients may also experience periods of remission.

M. N. Malinowski (✉)
Adena Spine Center, Chillicothe, OH, USA

N. J. Bremer
Center for Pain Relief, Spine and Nerve Centers of the Virginias, Charleston, WV, USA
e-mail: Nicholas.Bremer@CenterforPainRelief.com

Background and Historical Perspective

The SPG is a cluster of cell bodies located within the pterygopalatine fossa and contains sensory and autonomic fibers of the head and is one of the largest ganglia outside of the brain. The fossa is bordered anteriorly by the posterior wall of the maxillary sinus and posteriorly by the pterygoid process; the floor is represented by the palatine bone, inferior aspect of the orbit, and laterally by the pterygomaxillary fissure (Figs. 64.1 and 64.2). The ganglion is one of four parasympathetic ganglia of the head. The ganglion receives parasympathetic input

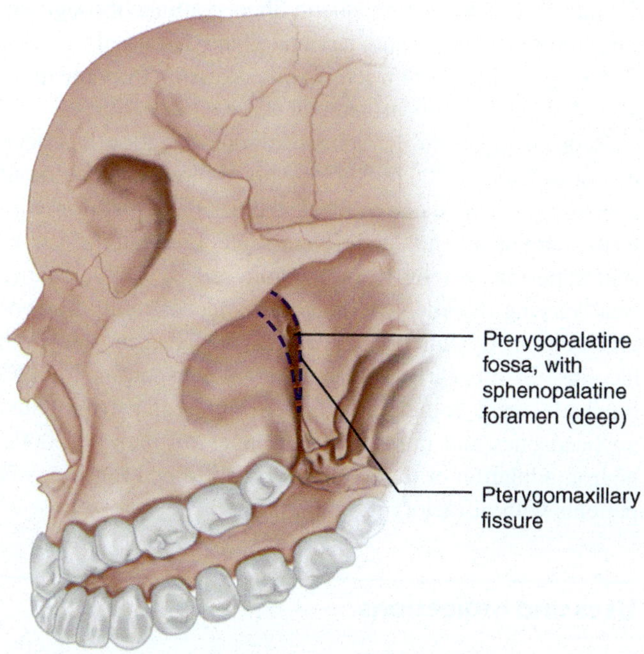

Fig. 64.1 Pterygomaxillary fissure (inferior/oblique view). The pterygomaxillary fissure is visualized medial to the zygomatic arch and is the opening to the pterygopalatine fossa

T. R. Deer et al. (eds.), *Deer's Treatment of Pain*, https://doi.org/10.1007/978-3-030-12281-2_64

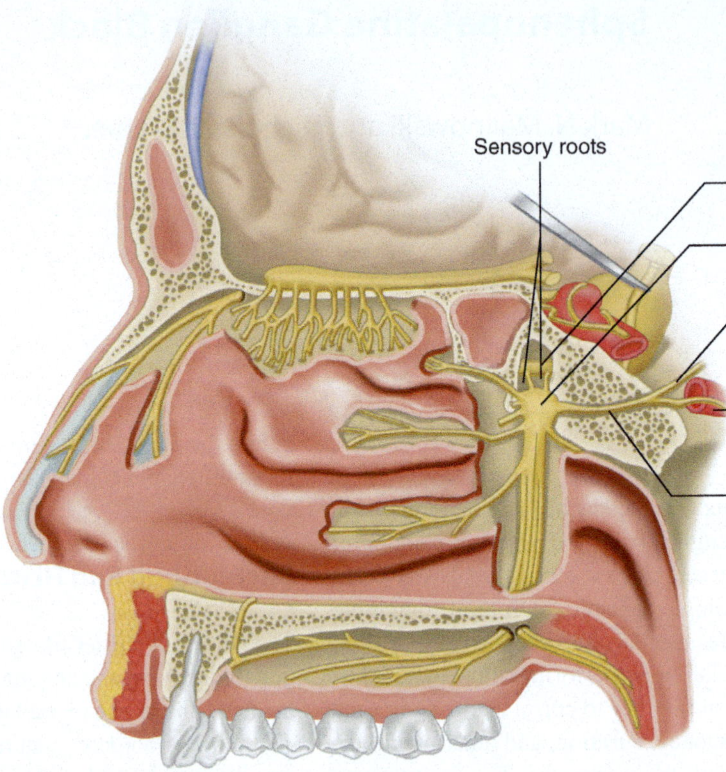

Fig. 64.2 The sphenopalatine ganglion input. The sphenopalatine ganglion is located posterior to the nasopharynx medial to the pterygomaxillary fissure

from the superior salivatory nucleus in the pons and input from the cranial nerve VII facial nerve (greater petrosal nerve) and sympathetic fibers arising from the superior cervical ganglion by way of the deep petrosal nerve and Vidian nerves of the pterygoid canal. Sympathetic fibers continue through the ganglion to synapse at the lacrimal gland and nasal mucosa. The ganglion hangs from sensory fibers arising from the maxillary branch V2 of the trigeminal nerve.

Pain arising from the sphenopalatine ganglion has been implicated since 1908 by Sluder who employed a trans-nasal approach using cocaine to block the SPG and ablation with formaldehyde, phenol, and silver nitrate. Later, in the 1970s, a literature review by Ruskin implicated SPG blockade to treat varying disorders to include headaches, temporomandibular joint dysfunction, neuralgias of the face, and even hiccups. In the early 1980s, favorable responses to SPG blockade were found in patients who suffer from cluster headaches and intractable migraines. In the late 2000s, neuromodulation of the SPG was found to be efficacious in patients with refractory migraines.

Uses and Indications

The use of SPG block is for the diagnosis and treatment of headache associated with the sphenopalatine ganglion. The common indications include trigeminal neuralgia, SPG neuralgia, cluster headaches, migraine headache, paroxysmal hemicranias, and trigeminal neuralgia, among others. There are other potential remote indications in the literature, but this is beyond the scope of this chapter.

Evidence for Efficacy

In addition to the early work of Sluder, there is a moderate amount of data supporting SPG blockade in the treatment of some forms of recurrent and/or chronic headache.

Devoghel (1980) performed a large trial of 120 patients with cluster headache. In the study, over 80% of the patients experienced complete relief of their symptoms following lateral approach and chemical ablation with alcohol. In some cases, symptom relief lasted more than 1 year. Other smaller studies supported significant relief with trans-nasal application of local anesthetic and/or radiofrequency ablation. Similarly, onabotulinumtoxin A has also demonstrated efficacy in treating SPG-mediated headaches using either a trans-nasal or lateral approach. The trans-nasal approach has been shown to be successful in performing SPG blockade, but some have criticized the accuracy of the technique. Emerging technologies have attempted to address this concern (Sphenocath®, Allevio®, others), but there is a paucity of clinical data in support of these devices.

Pearls and Pitfalls

There are two techniques associated with injection of the SPG ganglion. In either case, caution is used with preoperative preparation. In addition to a thorough history and physical, the physician must ensure that the patient demonstrates no evidence that would contraindicate performing the procedure. Systemic or local infection will prevent the safe completion of the procedure. Given the highly vascularized nature of the SPG and surrounding structures, the presence of an irreversible coagulopathy is an absolute contraindication. Reversible coagulopathies should be evaluated on a case by case basis that allows for a risk stratification versus benefit to the patient. Similarly, while there are no clear established guidelines for platelet concentration, appropriate levels and function are warranted to avert the risk of bleeding. The physician may use consensus guidelines recently published in 2018 by the American Society of Regional Anesthesia and Pain Medicine. Lastly, complications associated with the application of local anesthetic solution with potential vascular uptake are also possible to include, but not limited to, orthostasis, hypotension, seizure, and cardiovascular collapse. Similar to other interventional pain management procedures, intraoperative monitoring standards are recommended.

The physician should also be aware of structural or anatomical anomalies that may be incidental (neoplasm), invoked (trauma), or iatrogenic (surgical). Intraoperative complications may occur in the presence of traumatic or surgical deformity that may create a physical barrier to smooth needle passage. These anatomical situations may also involve neovascularization compounding risk. In some cases, advanced imaging may help identify potential issues prior to the injection.

Procedure

Three approaches are recognized to perform the SPG ganglion block, the trans-nasal approach, the greater palatine foramen approach, and the lateral approach. In all three, the patient is always lying supine, but the trans-nasal approach can be performed safely in the lateral position and is the only one that can be performed safely without the use of fluoroscopic guidance.

Trans-nasal Approach

The trans-nasal approach to the SPG block is performed traditionally with the patient in supine position as gravity can impact distribution of the solution and the outcomes of the block. The patient's nares are inspected for any potential obstruction. The liquid local anesthetic (typically 1–2 mL of lidocaine 1% or 2%) is delivered to the nares whereby the patient is asked to inhale through the nose. This provides anesthesia of the mucosa and allows for procedure comfort. Cotton-tipped applicators are then soaked with viscous anesthetic (e.g., viscous lidocaine 20 mg/mL). One or two applicators are then delivered through the nares gently in an anterior to posterior and slightly cephalad direction until the tip comes in contact with the posterior wall of the nasopharynx adjacent to the middle turbinate (Fig. 64.3). The physician may also dribble another milliliter more of local anesthetic along the route of the applicator. This wall is shared with the SPG. Passive diffusion across the membrane provides anesthetization of the SPG.

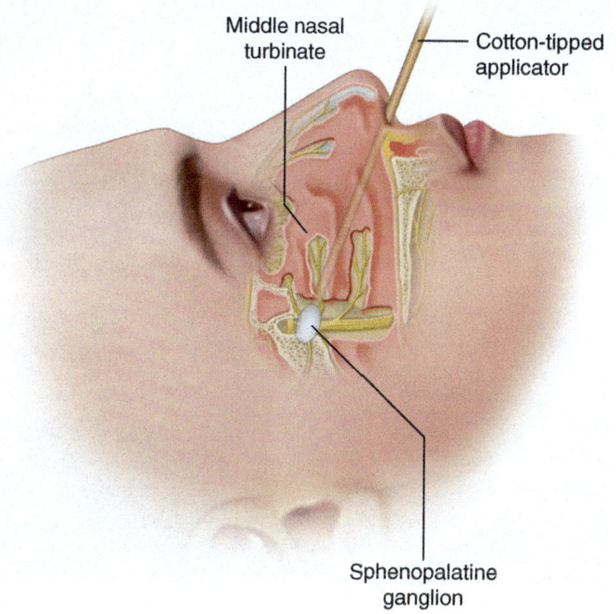

Fig. 64.3 The trans-nasal approach. The trans-nasal approach is performed with the patient supine. A cotton-tipped applicator is used to deliver local anesthetic posteriorly adjacent to the middle turbinate

Lateral Approach

The lateral approach is performed with fluoroscopic guidance. The patient is placed in a supine position, and the head is supported with an annular pillow allowing for rotation stability of the head. In some cases, the physician may immobilize the head into position using bandage tape or another means, but this can be somewhat distressing to the patient. Fluoroscopy is used to align the head and cervical spine in the neutral position. Under lateral

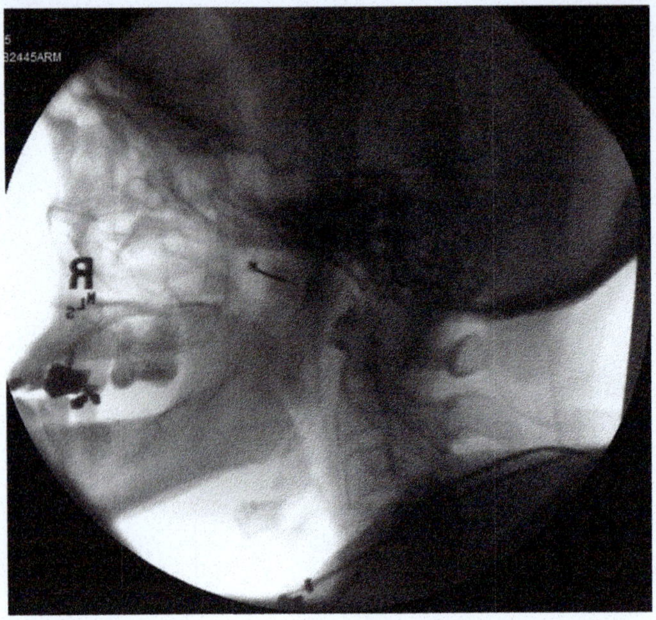

Fig. 64.4 The lateral approach. The mandibular notch denotes the skin entry point. The clivus, mandible, and pterygomaxillary fissure is aligned

view, the mandible, clivus, and pterygomaxillary fissure are aligned, and the mandibular notch is noted (Fig. 64.4). The patient should be asked to slightly relax the jaw to aid in visualization, but opening the mouth too far will inappropriately change the skin entry point. Once the midpoint of the coronoid notch is identified, the skin overlying this area is anesthetized with local anesthetic such as lidocaine 2%. Typical skin entry is anterior (and sometimes also slightly inferior) to the tragus. Under certain circumstances, the entry point can be over the coronoid process unless the coronoid process overlaps the shadow of the pterygomaxillary fissure. This author will use a blunt needle technique, and an 18-gauge angiocatheter is used as an introducer for a 22-gauge blunt nerve block needle. The angiocatheter is advanced through the skin and subcutaneous tissue until the mandibular notch is reached. Once the notch is contacted, this author removes the needle leaving the catheter in place and inserts the 22-gauge blunt nerve block needle into the catheter and advances in over the middle of the coronoid notch. The needle is then guided anterior, cephalad, and medial taking care not to run into the posterior portion of the maxillary sinus. Once positioned within the fissure, a small amount of nonionic contrast is administered to ensure proper distribution and localized any potential vascular uptake. If the distribution of contrast is appropriate, 1 mL of ropivacaine 0.2% is delivered into the area. Frequently, ropivacaine is combined with a non-particulate glucocorticoid such as dexamethasone. Once complete, the needle and introducer catheter are removed.

Greater Palatine Approach

The greater palatine approach is used commonly in dental anesthesia. The greater palatine foramen is located in the posterior hard palate and is the avenue for passage of the greater palatine nerve and associated vasculature. The foramen is located adjacent to the second or third molars in most cases, but it can also be present posterior to the molars. With the patient placed supine and in cervical flexion, the patient is asked to open the mouth. A cotton-tipped applicator is used to probe for the depression of the foramen. The area is then anesthetized with 1 mL of lidocaine 2% solution. A straight or angled needle is then inserted through the foramen and advanced approximately 1–2 cm. If the needle advanced too far, the patient will experience uncomfortable paresthesia in the maxilla. After aspiration, contrast may be injected under lateral view to demonstrate cephalad spread, followed by ropivacaine 0.2% (or analogous) with or without dexamethasone. In addition to the bacteria of the oral cavity, this area is highly vascularized, and therefore, this approach is not preferred by the author.

Key Points

1. The SPG is one of four parasympathetic ganglia of the head.
2. Given the extensive neurological input and output that spans several organs, SPG blockade may provide a solution to many pathologies of the head and face.
3. Ample preoperative planning must be performed prior to blockade of the SPG.
4. The trans-nasal approach may be used to determine whether the lateral approach is worthy of performing when the trans-nasal approach provides short-term diagnostic or therapeutic benefit.
5. Competency in fluoroscopic anatomy is critical to safely perform the lateral approach.

Recommended Reading

1. Costa A, Pucci E, Antonaci A, Sances G, Granella F, Broich G, Nappi G. The effect of intranasal cocaine and lidocaine on nitroglycerin – induced attacks in cluster headache. Cephalalgia. 2000;20(2):85–91.

2. Devoghel J. Cluster headache and sphenopalatine ganglion block. Acta Anaesthaesthiol Belg. 1980;32(1):101–7.
3. Mojica J, Mo B, Ng A. Sphenopalatine ganglion block in the management of chronic headaches. Curr Pain Headache Rep. 2017;21(27):1–8.
4. Robbins M, Robertson C, Kaplan E, Ailani J, Charlston L, Kuruvilla D, Blumenfeld A, Berliner R, Rosen N, Duarte R, Vidwan J, Halker R, Gill N, Ashkenazi A. The sphenopalatine ganglion: anatomy, pathophysiology and therapeutic targeting in headache. Headache. 2016;56:240–58.
5. Ruskin A. Sphenopalatine (nasal) ganglion: remote effects including "psychosomatic" symptoms, rage reaction, pain and spasm. Arch Phys Med Rehabil. 1979;60:353–9.
6. Sluder G. The anatomical and clinical relations of the sphenopalatine ganglion to the nose. NY State J Med. 1908;90:293–8.
7. Tepper S, Caparso A. Sphenopalatine ganglion (SPG): stimulation mechanism, safety and efficacy. Headache. 2017;57:14–28.

Percutaneous Cervical Spinal Cord Stimulation

65

Jeffery Rowe and Dawood Sayed

Introduction

Due to the demonstrated benefit of thoracolumbar spinal cord stimulation (SCS) in improved pain management, safety, and cost-effectiveness, exploration into cervical spinal cord stimulation has dramatically increased over time. Spine and extremity pathology is not limited to the thoracolumbar region so as neuromodulation studies, interventional techniques, and safety grow, effort is being made to extend the success of thoracolumbar spinal cord stimulation to the cervical spine.

Background and Historical Perspective

Historically, cervical spinal cord stimulation for the management of pain has not been as extensively studied compared to thoracolumbar SCS, and thus, reimbursement to perform cervical SCS has not been as widely supported. Cervical SCS is underutilized and occupies significantly less neuromodulation volume compared to thoracolumbar SCS. In a study by Rosenow et al. evaluating over 500 spinal cord stimulators, only 36% were cervical.

Placement of cervical leads poses more serious risk and technical difficulties compared to thoracic SCS due to the increased challenges of accessing the upper thoracic interspaces and tunneling the leads farther distances to reach the typical location for battery placement. Lead migration is a particular problem for thoracic SCS where lead migration is the most common adverse complication reported at a rate of about 13–23%. Displacement of cervical leads is twice as likely at that of thoracic leads due to the enhanced mobility of the cervical spine. Not surprisingly, cervical leads have a higher likelihood of surgical revision. Although paddle leads with their size and shape are prone to less migration than percutaneous leads, it is their larger size that also lends to more complications in the cervical spine where the spinal canal diameter is narrower. Serious adverse complications include spinal cord injury and cord compression with associated cervical myelopathy due to the fibrous scar tissue formation that can occur. However despite these challenges, the risk of infection of cervical leads tends to be less than that of thoracic leads. As the field of neuromodulation progresses, more pain physicians will become more comfortable adopting cervical SCS in their practice especially as new indications and uses for the therapy are available through research.

Uses and Indications

Cervical SCS is an important treatment option in the management of chronic and refractory head, neck, and upper extremity pain. Although, not as commonly studied as thoracolumbar spinal cord stimulation, cervical spinal cord stimulation continues to emerge as a safe and viable treatment modality for many patients with chronic pain. Cervical spinal cord stimulation is currently being used to treat failed back surgery syndrome (also known as failed neck surgery syndrome), cervical radiculopathy, cervical degenerative disc disease, complex regional pain syndrome, brachial plexopathy, ischemic pain, Raynaud's disease, chronic migraine, trigeminal neuralgias, postherpetic neuralgia, and occipital neuralgia.

Complex Regional Pain Syndrome

Complex regional pain syndrome (CRPS) is a chronic neurological condition involving the limbs that is characterized by severe pain along with sensory, autonomic, motor, and trophic impairment. This condition may be induced by surgery, trauma, or minor injury. The disease has a varying course,

J. Rowe (✉)
Main Line Spine & Main Line Spine Surgery Center, King of Prussia, PA, USA

D. Sayed
The University of Kansas Health System, Kansas City, KS, USA

T. R. Deer et al. (eds.), *Deer's Treatment of Pain*, https://doi.org/10.1007/978-3-030-12281-2_65

ranging from mild and self-limiting to chronic disease. When severe, it can impair activities of daily living and health-related quality of life. CRPS can be classified in two types, CRPS type I and type II. CRPS type I, formerly reflex sympathetic dystrophy, is characterized by the absence of identifiable nerve injury. Whereas CRPS type II, formerly causalgia, is characterized by the presence of identifiable nerve injury. CRPS is diagnosed based upon the Budapest Clinical Diagnostic Criteria. The incidence rate of both CRPS type I and II is reportedly 6.28 per 100,000 person-years. However, newer studies have shown the incidence to be as high as 26.2 per 100,000 person-years. CRPS most frequently occurs in females between the ages of 61 and 70 years old and appears to have an increased preponderance for the upper limbs with a 3:2 ratio when compared to the lower limbs. One significant risk factor for the development of CRPS is upper extremity orthopedic surgery, specifically shoulder surgery. After shoulder surgery, the incidence of CRPS has been reportedly as high as 11%.

The cause and mechanism of CRPS is unknown, but sympathetic dysregulation, inflammation, tissue hypoxia, small fiber damage, central sensitization, and cortical deregulation are all implicated with this condition. It is speculated that SCS not only controls the neuropathic pain of CRPS, but may also modulate the sympathetically mediated pain (Figs. 65.1 and 65.2).

In 1989, Robaina et al. evaluated the effect of cervical SCS on 11 patients with reflex sympathetic dystrophy or Raynaud's disease. In this study, they showed that greater than 90% of patients received excellent pain relief. This study also showed cervical SCS improved blood flow and temperature to affected extremities. In 1998, Cavillo et al. reported the results of 36 patients who underwent cervical SCS for CRPS of one upper extremity. This study compared cervical SCS to peripheral nerve stimulation (PNS) with a combination of both cervical SCS and PNS. The study evaluated 36 patients. Twenty-four patients underwent cervical SCS only, five patients underwent PNS only, and seven patients underwent both cervical SCS and PNS. The results showed a decrease in the visual analog scale (VAS) of 45.3% for the cervical SCS only group, 51.3% for the PNS only group, and 63.5% for the cervical SCS and PNS group. The study also showed a significant decrease in opioid consumption and the number of patients who returned to work after stimulator implantation. In 2004, Forouzanfar et al. performed a prospective observational study of 36 patients with CRPS type I. In this study, they compared cervical SCS to thoracolumbar SCS. Patients were followed for 24 months after SCS implantation, and it was determined that there was no statistical difference in outcome between cervical and thoracolumbar SCS.

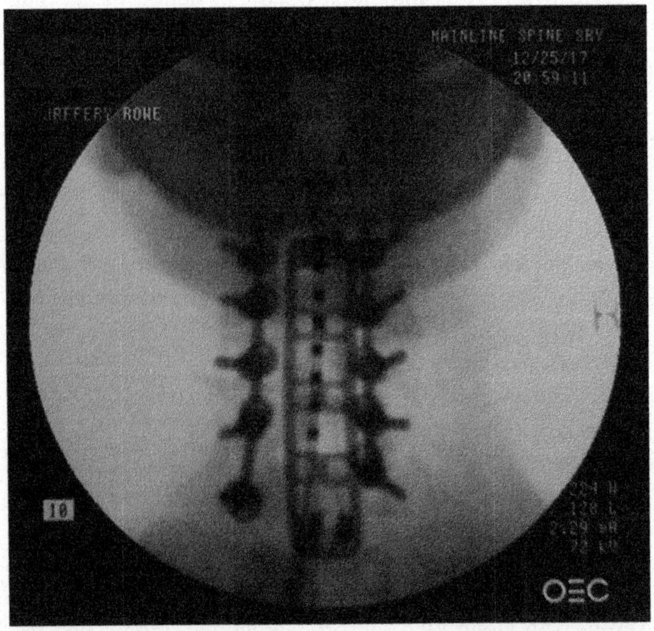

Fig. 65.1 A/P view of two 12 contact percutaneous leads placed in the cervical spine

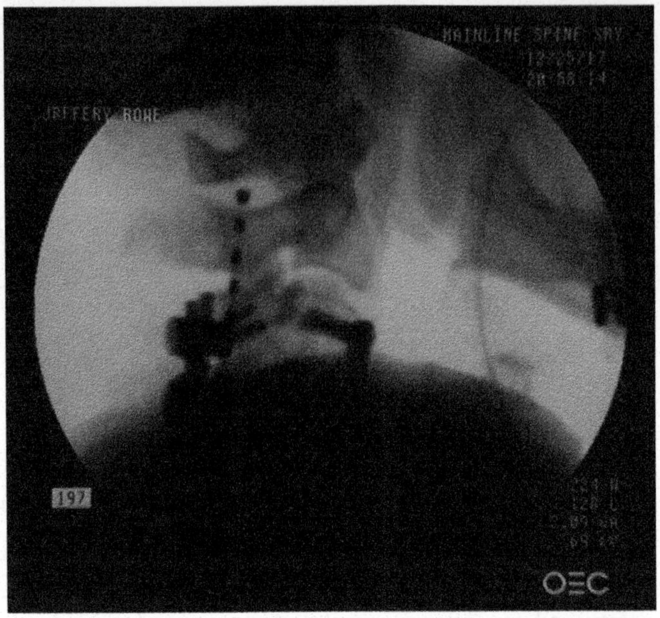

Fig. 65.2 Lateral view of two 12 contact percutaneous leads placed in the cervical spine

Failed Neck Surgery Syndrome and Cervical Axial Neck Pain

Although cervical SCS is approved to treat upper extremity pain, it has no indication to treat cervical axial pain. Currently, there is a study underway utilizing high-frequency therapy at 10,000 Hz to treat this challenging condition (Figs. 65.3, 65.4, and 65.5).

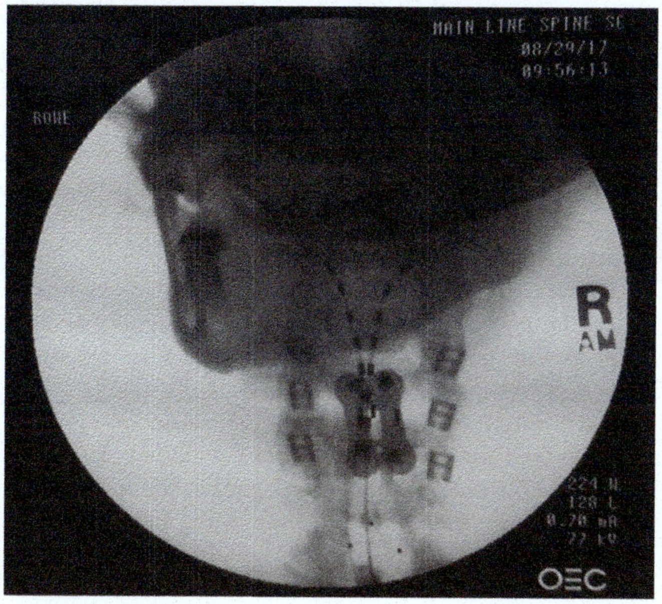

Fig. 65.3 A/P view of two 8 contact percutaneous leads placed after an anterior cervical fusion

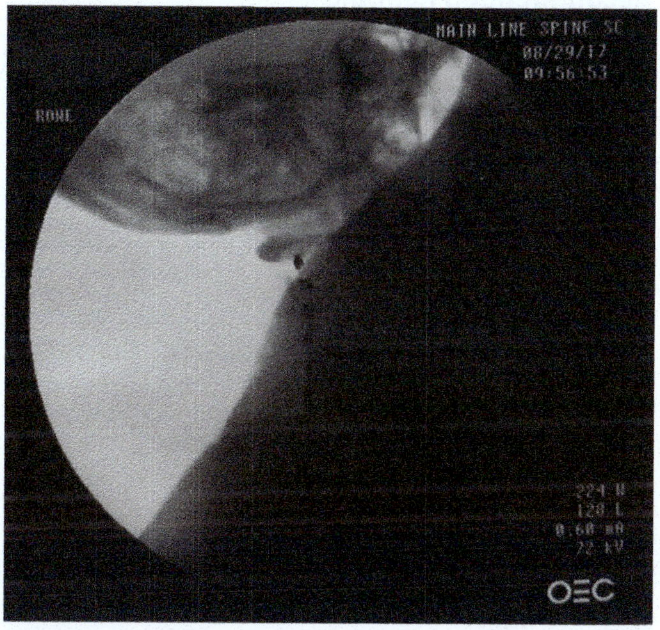

Fig. 65.4 A/P view of two 12 contact percutaneous leads placed after an anterior and posterior cervical fusion

Head and Face

At lower cervical levels (C3–C6), SCS induces increased blood flow in the upper extremities. In the upper cervical spine (C1–C2), SCS induces increased cerebral blood flow, which is associated with a decrease in sympathetic activity and an increase in vasomotor center activity and a release of neurohumoral factors (10). At the cervicomedullary junction (CMJ), SCS has been shown to interact with the nucleus caudalis, which contains the cell bodies of second-order neurons carrying pain and temperature sensation from the ipsilateral face. The nucleus caudalis also receives extra-trigeminal pain input from the head via cranial nerves VII, IX, and X, combining to form the spinal trigeminal tract (8). Interaction with this pathway has been the proposed mechanism with which SCS has been used to treat head and face pathology (Figs. 65.1 and 65.2).

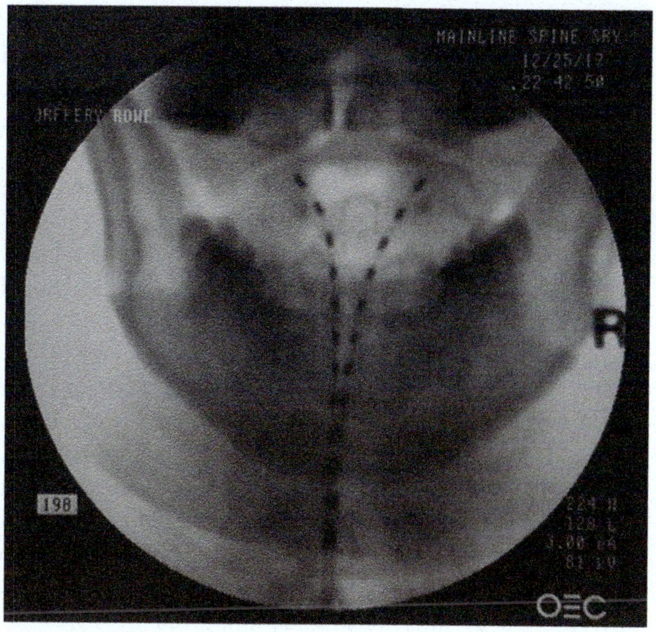

Fig. 65.5 Lateral view of two 12 contact percutaneous leads after an anterior and posterior cervical fusion

Evidence and Efficacy with Table

The effectiveness of cervical spinal cord stimulation for the management of chronic pain has been studied over the years as the use of cervical spinal cord stimulation for the treatment of chronic pain has become more prevalent. A study first published in the *Journal of Neuromodulation*, April 17, 2014, titled Effectiveness of cervical spinal cord stimulation for the management of chronic pain demonstrated scientific evidence which supports spinal cord stimulation as a cost-effective treatment option that, for many disease states, should be employed earlier in the treatment continual. The study also suggests that the use of SCS in the cervical spine is a medically effective method of pain management that satisfies and improves the quality of life of most patients and can reduce the high cost of direct medical treatment of pain, as well as increase in the productivity of patients, and therefore should be reimbursed in appropriately selected patients.

Data was collected as part of an institutional review board-approved, postoperative, multicenter, international registry: pain relief, Pain and Disability Index (PDI) score, quality of life (QoL), and satisfaction at 3, 6, and 12 months postimplantation. Descriptive statistics were provided for all measures. Changes from baseline in the PDI scores were analyzed using Tukey's pairwise comparisons.

In this study 38 patients underwent implantation of SCS leads in the cervical spine at 16 study sites in the United States and 3 international study sites. Direct patient report of percentage of pain relief was 54.2%, 16.2%, and 66.8% at 3, 6, and 12 month postimplantation, respectively. Pain relief was categorized as excellent/good by 61.6% of patients at 3 months, with similar results observed at 6 and 12 months. PDI scores were significantly reduced at all time points. At 3 months postimplantation, 92.4% of patients indicated that they were very satisfied/satisfied with the SCS device. No patients indicated that they were dissatisfied. Overall QoL was reported as improved/greatly improved by 73.1% of patients at 3 months. Similar results for QoL and satisfaction were reported at 6 and 12 months.

Pearls and Pitfalls

- Sterile technique utilized during trial and permanent implant is of utmost importance as this is a device implant procedure.
- Percutaneous cervical intralaminar approach at C7-T1, T1-2, and T2-3 can provide a wide intralaminar for access while maintaining a shallow needle angle of approach to reduce risk of dural puncture while reducing motion at the lead anchor location in the upper thoracic region.
- Placing the lower three contacts just left and right of midline while separating the upper contacts transitioned to approximately the top of C2 allows for occipital coverage with the upper two to three contacts, neck coverage with the middle two to three contacts, and coverage within the upper extremities with the lower two to three contacts. See Figs. 65.1, 65.2, 65.3, 65.4, and 65.5.
- Positioning the patient's head to the right and left during implant to ensure leads stay to the right and left with ranging during trial and permanent implant ensures that range of motion post trial/permanent implant does not create loss of coverage/benefit on one side or the other.
- Anchoring leads for permanent implant in close proximity to the lamina below the level of epidural access to the deep periosteal structures just lateral to the spinous process reduce lead migration rate when combined with upper thoracic access to limited motion at the lead anchor location.

Recommended Reading

1. Dam-Hieu P, Magro E, Seizeur R, Simon A, Quinio B. Cervical cord compression due to delayed scarring around epidural electrodes used in spinal cord stimulation. J Neurosurg Spine. 2010;12(4):409–12.
2. Deer TR, et al. Effectiveness of cervical spinal cord stimulation for the management of chronic pain. Neuromodulation. 2014;17:265–71.
3. Eldabe S, Buchser E, Duarte RV. Complications of spinal cord stimulation and peripheral nerve stimulation techniques: a review of the literature. Pain Med. 2016;17(2):325–30.
4. Wolter T. Spinal cord stimulation for neuropathic pain: current perspectives. J Pain Res. 2014;7:651–63. https://doi.org/10.2147/JPR.S37589.

Surgical Leads for the Cervical Spine

66

Roger Strachan and Sam Eldabe

Introduction

The prevalence of chronic pain in the United Kingdom is around one third to one half of the population amounting to almost 28 million adults. Estimates for chronic neuropathic pain are around 9.7% of the female adult population and 7.3% in males (Fayaz et al.). The economic burden of chronic pain is therefore considerable in the developed world, not just in relation to immediate health-care costs but in also with regard to the social costs of lost employment, welfare benefits, impact on family well-being and even lost revenue through income taxation. There has been significantly less research into chronic neck pain than low back pain, yet globally it is still within the top 25 of chronic conditions with the most disability-adjusted life years (DALYs) and has increased in its prevalence by 21% between 2005 and 2015 (GBD 2015). The application of neuromodulation therapies to conditions affecting the neck and upper limbs has been measurably lower than the lower back and lower limbs, and more effort and research in this area are required.

Background and Historical Perspectives

The early history for spinal cord stimulation (SCS) capitalizing on Melzack and Wall's Gate Theory of Pain is well known to most readers, its first application attributed to Shealy and colleagues in 1967. Traditionally, neuromodulation therapies for low back and lower limb conditions have been more popular and more universally adopted than those for the cervical spine and upper limb. However, the use of surgically implanted electrodes in the neck is not new – Wycis and Gildenberg, pioneers in functional neurosurgery, used SCS to treat spasmodic torticollis in 1969 inserting electrodes into the epidural space at C2. With the introduction of percutaneous electrodes, surgical electrodes lost their popularity as percutaneous electrodes could be inserted by non-surgeons and were inherently less invasive and safer. However, with the improvements in technology and electrode design and the realization that percutaneous electrodes cannot always provide a solution in all patients, there is clearly a need for surgically implanted paddle electrodes.

There is still a reluctance among neuromodulation practitioners to use stimulation techniques in the cervical spine, many practitioners put off by the higher variability of paraesthesia sensation as a result of the inherent mobility of the neck and, for the surgeons, the realization that the risks are potentially higher with cervical electrodes than thoracic placement and the consequences of getting it wrong are greater. Although some newer electrode designs with smaller more flexible paddles and better training help to overcome some of these barriers, there is equally a tendency for larger, broader and more rigid electrode design to embrace the philosophy that more is better for coverage. These have proved useful in the thoracic spine, but to our knowledge, no device company has attempted to design a bespoke cervical electrode, perhaps because the market for these would be much smaller. The application of paddle electrodes in the cervical spine raises concerns regarding their bulk in a narrower part of the spine and the consequences of this with advancing age. It also gives rise to the need for wider exposures, more bone removal and more sophisticated techniques to prevent migration (e.g. Armani). The authors have therefore tended to restrict themselves to using smaller electrodes in a paramedian or lateral position.

Uses and Indications

The debate between the benefits and risks of percutaneous versus paddle surgical electrodes has continued for many years. Several studies have concluded that paddle electrodes

R. Strachan (✉)
Department of Neurosurgery, James Cook University Hospital, Middlesbrough, UK

S. Eldabe
Department of Pain and Anaesthesia, James Cook University Hospital, Middlesbrough, UK

T. R. Deer et al. (eds.), *Deer's Treatment of Pain*, https://doi.org/10.1007/978-3-030-12281-2_66

are more likely to provide more consistent coverage of the painful area with lower risks of migration and positional side effects and achieve similar levels of stimulation at lower voltages with reduced energy requirements (North et al. 1997, 2002, 2005). It has always been the philosophy of the authors that there is a need for both, and despite the perceived benefits of surgical over percutaneous electrodes, percutaneous electrodes remain the mainstay for trials of SCS, and, in patients who achieve an excellent response from their percutaneous electrode, there seems little justification in always replacing it with a surgical paddle electrode. There are some indications where a surgical electrode is essential: where the anatomy prevents the insertion of a percutaneous electrode (e.g. scarring or previous spinal injury); repeated lead revisions as a result of recurrent lead migration or fracture; or where percutaneous lead revision is just not able to recapture the effective coverage that the patient enjoyed before.

Surgical electrodes do seem to benefit from lower migration and dislodgement rates and because of their relative bulk reduce the size of the CSF space between electrode and cord so allowing similar levels of stimulation at a lower voltage, with reduced pulse width and amplitude and therefore a lower current and energy requirement. They are therefore potentially a better choice in patients with high current requirements or who use their stimulators continuously, despite the introduction of rechargeable systems. Although the authors traditionally used percutaneous electrodes in the cervical spine (and still do for trials), the apparent variation in paraesthesia with neck movement altered our protocol, and now, even after a successful trial, many patients undergoing cervical SCS will have a surgical paddle electrode inserted at the second stage. Where percutaneous stimulation seems particularly effective, then the decision may be to persist with this, and if migration or failure of adequate stimulation occurs, a surgical electrode is inserted rather than attempt a percutaneous revision. It may be that the use of paraesthesia-free systems, subject to a better understanding and rationale for their target location on the spinal cord, will provide a paradigm shift away from the need for stable targeted sensations from paddle electrodes. Limited electrode migration may therefore become less of an issue.

Technique

Our choice has been to undertake a percutaneous trial under local anaesthetic and, if successful, undertake the second stage under general anaesthesia, which may include the insertion of a surgical electrode. If it is the reader's preference to do trials with a surgical electrode, then the choice of anaesthetic may be up to the practitioner's preference and of course patient preference and comfort. For obvious reason, insertion under spinal anaesthesia, while potentially suitable for thoracic implantation, cannot be used for cervical implantation. Some authors describe using local anaesthesia and conscious sedation (e.g. Pahapill). Unlike the thoracic spine, the depth of the exposure and the amount of muscle stripping are greater in the neck, making adequate local anaesthesia more difficult. Also, head position is crucial. Expecting a patient to maintain a prone position with the head in neutral alignment without movement (particularly at a crucial part of the electrode insertion) is more problematic and increases the risk. General anaesthesia allows good patient compliance, the maintenance of good neck and head alignment without any movement and even the application of a pin headrest in patients where their size or condition does not permit even some flexion of the cervical spine without it.

Given the need for general anaesthesia in the placement of paddle electrodes, particularly in the cervical spine, there is significant trend towards intraoperative neuromonitoring in these cases, particularly in the United States. Electrophysiological monitoring is not new in spinal surgery (Stecker), and the role of electromyographic studies (EMGs) and somatosensory evoked potentials (SSEPs) is gaining acceptance in facilitating lateralization of the stimulation (Mammis and Mogilner; Air et al.; Tamkus et al.; Falowski and Dianna). EMGs have some advantages over SSEPs because of their relative simplicity and the instantaneous neurophysiological feedback (Air et al.). With regard to SSEPs, SCS is known to reduce short- and mid-latency SSEPs and therefore has the potential to assist in correct lateralization of the stimulation and optimize electrode position. Neuromonitoring also offers a degree of neuroprotection with advanced warning of potential neurological injury during SCS paddle electrode implantation (Tamkus et al.; Falowski et al.). Efforts to lateralize and localize the stimulation are particularly appropriate if larger surgical paddle electrodes are being placed in the midline or paramedian position under general anaesthesia, either for a trial or as a single-stage procedure. The authors have not used neuromonitoring in their cases because the trials have usually been percutaneous and the final stage placements targeted in a lateral position using imaging alone.

Prior to any electrode insertion, it is essential that the patient has had suitable imaging carried out, usually an MR scan, so that cervical stenosis or any evidence of cord compromise at the anticipated level of electrode insertion is identified. In patients with a congenitally narrow spinal canal, it may not be appropriate to consider surgical paddle electrodes, particularly those of a larger design or where midline placement is anticipated. In these patients, progressive degenerative change and advancing years may lead to neurological problems from the mass effect of the electrode. Where MR scan is contraindicated, spiral CT scanning with 1.5 mm axial slices and sagittal reconstructions is adequate to visualize the dimensions of the cord and its spatial relationship to the discs and vertebrae. It has the added advantage of better identifying osteophytes or calcified (hard) discs that may make surgical electrode insertion too risky.

The percutaneous trial is undertaken in a prone position or sitting. A 14G Tuohy needle is inserted at the best place determined by the practitioner, usually the T4/5 or T3/4 interspace. This is normally approached from the left paramedian position, and the epidural space located in the normal fashion using a loss-of-resistance syringe or a hanging drop method. Access to the spine and insertion of the percutaneous lead are guided by image intensification. Depending on the pathology being treated and the anticipated stimulation algorithm that will be used, the lead tip is positioned in a paramedian or lateral position at the C4/5 disc level or in the midline at C2 (for HF10 therapy). Single-dose peroperative antibiotics are administered, ceftriaxone 1 g (or teicoplanin 400–600 mg in case of penicillin allergy), but no further antibiotic treatment is given during the trial. The trial insertion is concluded when appropriate paraesthesia is obtained that covers the painful area or, in the case of paraesthesia-free stimulation, the anatomical target area has been reached. The advent of paraesthesia-free stimulation makes targeting paraesthesias less of a crucial issue than has been the case in the past.

Most implanters of cervical electrodes, whether these are percutaneous or paddle electrodes, choose to insert these in a midline or paramedian position. In treating neuropathic conditions of the upper limb, the electrodes are positioned higher in the cervical spine to target the sensory pathways where they have become anatomically established within the spinal cord. Given that the spinothalamic tracts that subserve pain show the same laminar representation as other tracts within the spinal cord and that these cross within the spinal cord and ascend on the contralateral side, the fibres representing the upper limbs will be closer to the midline. Accepting that the site of action of SCS is not clearly understood and that a simplistic anatomical concept does not explain its action, there is at least some rationale why midline or paramedian electrodes will provide coverage of the upper limbs. Midline or paramedian placement is reported to produce effective results in treating neuropathic conditions affecting the upper limbs and therefore is an acceptable alternative to lateral placement. However, it has been the authors' experience that unwanted stimulation caudal to the neck and upper limbs was troublesome in some patients, coverage particularly of the hand was variable, and even limited migration caused a loss of effective coverage. This has not necessarily been the experience of other practitioners who use cervical electrodes. Nevertheless, we have preferred to use paraforaminal placement for conventional stimulation to reduce the occurrence of unwanted paraesthesia in the thorax or lower limbs and the positional variability of the stimulation seen particularly with midline placements. This means that rather than true SCS, it could be stimulation of the dorsal root entry zones (DREZ) or even the dorsal sensory roots themselves that is achieving the desired effect.

The trial period is variable but usually about 7–10 days. X-rays are taken after the procedure. If the trial is successful and the patient subsequently undergoes the placement of a permanent surgical paddle insertion or at any time their percutaneous lead is replaced by a surgical lead, then these x-rays (particularly the AP view) are used as a template to position the surgical electrode in exactly the same position. Most device companies now produce a range of surgical electrodes that are of an adequate length and configuration to cover from C5 to C7 or C8, depending on their length and placement. Octapolar leads can be positioned at the C4/5 disc space, thus allowing stimulation of the C5–C8 roots which is adequate to cover most of the upper limb (Fig. 66.1a, b).

Surgical paddle electrode insertion for most indications is performed under general anaesthesia, but local anaesthetic wound infiltration is still used to reduce the surgical stimulus. The patient is positioned prone with the neck slightly flexed in a foam block and the head in a straight alignment. A Mayfield pin headrest can be used to optimize the alignment and avoid any complications from pressure on the face or eyes. If the use of a pin headrest is anticipated, the patient should be advised about this beforehand to avoid any later explanations as to the presence of temporal or parietal puncture wounds.

The level of surgical access is decided using image intensification. Even though the spinous processes of C6 and C7 are larger and can usually be identified by palpation alone, image intensification allows you to accurately define the position of your wound to minimize the size of the surgical access and limit the amount of muscle stripping required. Entry is usually planned at C7/T1. Skin preparation is usually two Betadine washes followed by two chlorhexidine in spirit washes. The skin wash is left to dry for at least a minute. After muscle stripping, image intensification is used to confirm the proposed surgical entry point to the epidural space.

Insertion of the surgical electrode is carried out using a unilateral muscle strip and laminotomy on the affected side (Fig. 66.2a, b). It is important that the caudal end of the paddle electrode after placement is just visible at the top of the laminotomy to enable easy removal and revision – a laminotomy at C7/T1 allows the lowest electrode to be adjacent close to C8 and will certainly allow stimulation of C7 (C6/7) as well as C6 and C5. The first author undertakes the laminotomy under direct vision without a microscope, but it is important to appreciate that the lamina in the cervical spine can be much thinner than in the thoracic spine, so although access can be straightforward, extra care is needed. Where a midline placement is anticipated, it is better to undertake a midline laminotomy, and this is essential if a larger sur-

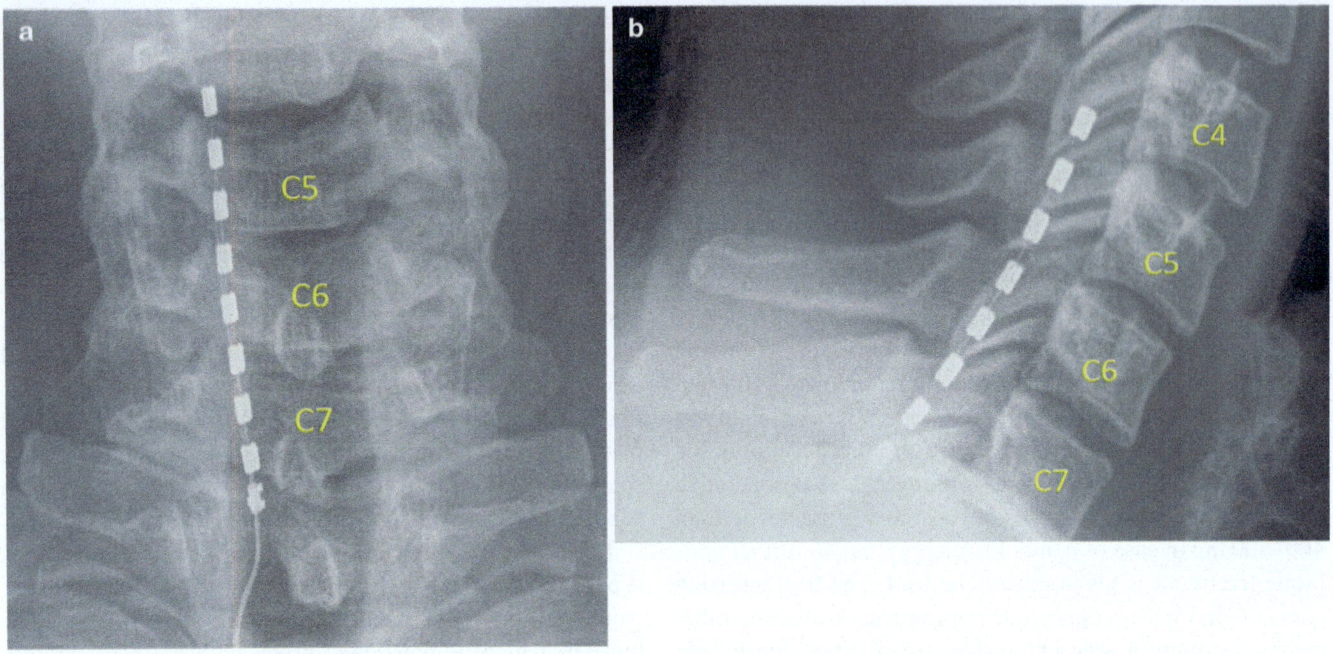

Fig. 66.1 (**a**) AP view of a right lateral octapolar electrode for CRPS (Lamitrode-S8); (**b**) lateral view

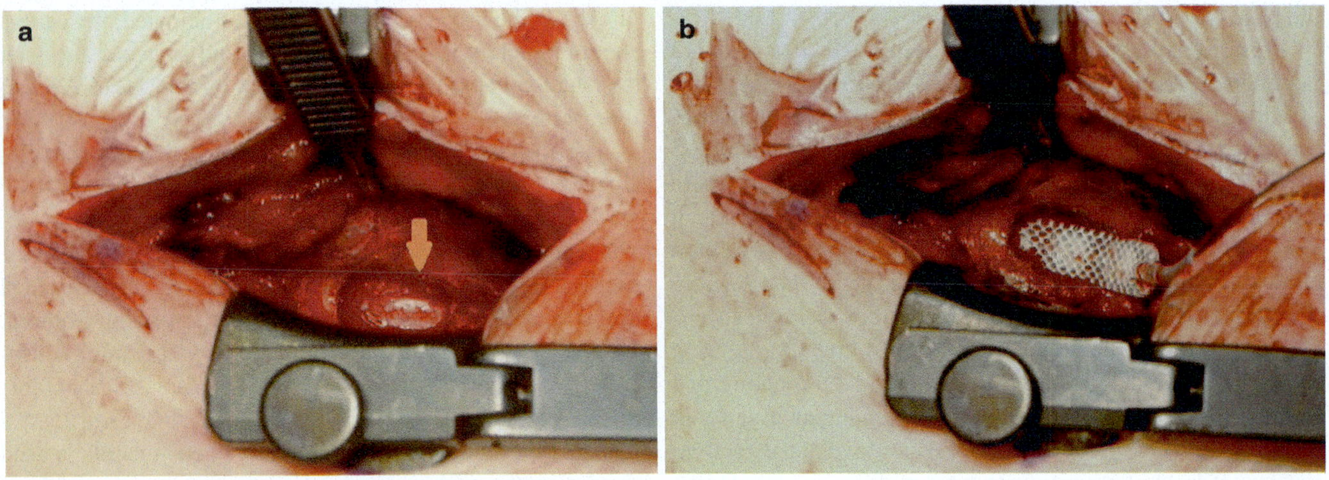

Fig. 66.2 (**a**) Laminotomy (arrowed); (**b**) insertion of the electrode (Resume-TL)

gical paddle is to be inserted. The cervical cord is larger or expanded when compared to the thoracic cord, with a smaller CSF layer around it, so extra care is required when inserting surgical electrodes. Under no circumstances should the insertion be forced.

Once the electrode position is confirmed by image intensification, it is anchored in the conventional way. Some authors have described insertion without anchoring and no increase in the migration rate (e.g. Pahapill). If there is a lack of good fascia or muscle to which the anchor can be secured, it can be glued to the spinous process using cyanoacrylate glue (Histoacryl® – B. Braun Medical).

The position of the battery will depend on the surgeon's and patient's preference, the length of the electrode and the need for extension leads. The authors have used thoracic (mid-axillary), abdominal and buttock implantations but tend to use standard abdominal placement where possible. Buttock implantation is convenient as the patient will not have to be repositioned, but this requires long subcutaneous extension leads, and it has been our experience that these have a higher incidence of chronic discomfort related to the pulse generator. The development of smaller pulse generators has allowed a wider choice of implantation sites with a lower complication rate.

The wounds and implanted hardware are washed frequently throughout the procedure with aqueous chlorhexidine solution. Chlorhexidine is known to have greater antistaphylococcal activity than iodine-containing solutions. The wounds are closed in layers, and skin closure will depend on the surgeon's preference, but the authors have always used subcuticular Vicryl and steristrips to achieve a clean and cosmetically good scar without the need for suture or clip removal.

Indications

There have been many studies undertaken regarding thoracic SCS with greater numbers of patients, more indications and, in recent years, several different programming algorithms or paradigms. The use of cervical electrodes has been more limited with fewer indications and so far limited to conventional stimulation paradigms, although there is currently at least one study underway utilizing high-frequency (HF10) therapy. In this respect, good studies relating to the use of cervical cord stimulation are lacking, and most publications are either limited to case series or cover heterogeneous groups of patients, of which the minority have conditions affecting the upper limb. The best indication remains chronic neuropathic pain affecting the upper limbs, particularly complex regional pain syndrome (CRPS).

CRPS

CRPS type 1 is a neuropathic condition that develops after an injury, sometimes even minor, with symptoms of pain, allodynia and hyperalgesia in the affected limb or limbs, usually non-dermatomal and disproportionate to the level of injury. CRPS type 2 occurs as the result of an obvious nerve injury. In a significant minority of patients, CRPS is difficult to treat and in many patients does not respond to the four pillars of treatment of conventional pain management, physical therapy, psychological interventions and patient education. In these patients, SCS is of proven value (Kemler et al. 2000), and where CRPS affects the upper limb or limbs, cervical electrode placement is mandatory. Although most studies describe thoracic SCS for treating the lower limbs, it is reasonable to assume that similar efficacy can be achieved with cervical SCS for upper limb CRPS. Again, it is our experience that lateral or paraforaminal electrode placement seems to produce the best results avoiding the complications associated with larger midline electrodes such as buckling and migration as a result of neck flexion or unwanted stimulation of the trunk and lower limbs. However, it remains common practice that many practitioners use a midline or paramedian position. Efficacy is known to wane with time in many patients, but these patients often report that they would still have undergone the treatment (Kemler et al. 2008).

Neck Pain and Chronic Radicular Neuropathic Pain

The treatment of chronic axial back pain has proved more difficult to treat than neuropathic leg pain, although advancements in electrode design and stimulation paradigms such as high frequency and burst stimulation have allegedly resulted in improved results. Similarly, the treatment of axial neck pain is not a good indication for SCS, and in most reports, it is difficult to isolate patients with neck pain that is not also associated with radicular shoulder or arm pain. The authors have used cervical surgical electrodes to treat neuropathic arm pain from cervical degenerative disc disease usually where cervical surgery has failed to address this. Anecdotally, we have noticed in one or two patients who have reported improvements in their arm pain have also reported improvements in their neck pain. It is intriguing to postulate that because the neck muscles are supplied by branches of the posterior cervical rami and nerves arising from the brachial plexus, SCS or nerve root stimulation may be modulating the activity of these nerves to alleviate some aspects of the neck pain. There are reports of improvements in neck pain after cervical SCS, although the numbers even in multicentre studies remain small and most involve neuropathic limb pain and percutaneous leads rather than paddle leads (Deer et al.).

Despite technically successful anterior cervical surgery, many patients continue to complain of neck and neuropathic arm pain, and a few may suffer a cervical nerve root injury as a result of surgery. Medical treatments are rarely effective in this group of patients. Some may be offered posterior cervical foraminotomy in an effort to relieve their radicular pain. This provides an opportunity to consider placing a paddle electrode at the same time as the foraminotomy, particularly if the surgeon is not optimistic that further decompressive surgery will help. The electrode can be left buried, and if the foraminotomy fails and the patient's pain persists, then the patient can easily be subsequently trialled and offered SCS (Fig. 66.3a, b).

Brachial Plexus Injury

High cervical SCS has been used for brachial plexus injuries (BPI). The incidence of chronic pain after BPI is as high as 80% (Abdul-Aziz and Ghaleb, Bertelli and Ghizoni). It is difficult to treat. Direct surgery, such as dorsal root entry zone (DREZ) lesioning and autologous nerve grafting, has been used with mixed results. DREZ lesioning can be associated with significant complications such as lower limb weakness and bladder dysfunction, and although it can be effective initially, there is a high failure rate in the long term (Sindou). SCS with cervical paddle electrodes usually around C3–C6 is reported (Lai et al.; Bennett and Tai), and high cervical stimulation has been used successfully after failed DREZ lesioning (Lai et al.). Many papers are restricted to small numbers and case reports, but most report encourag-

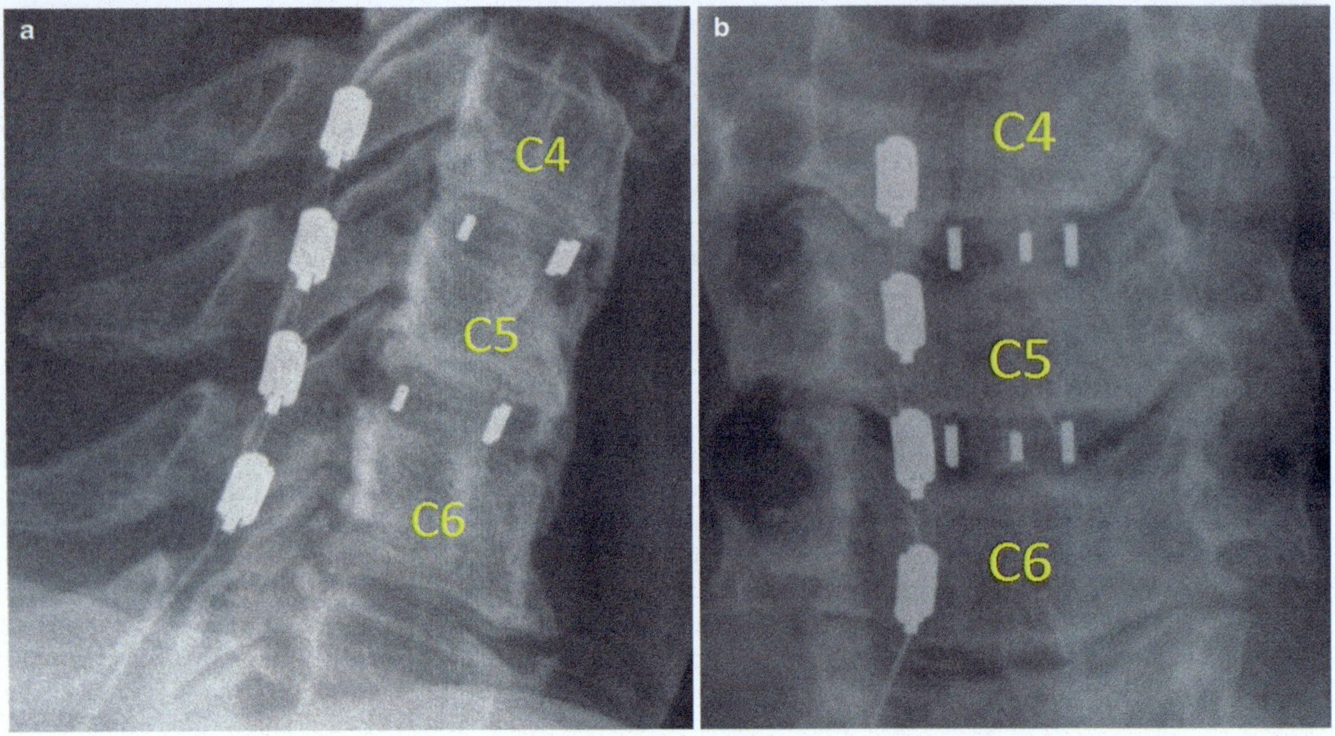

Fig. 66.3 (**a**) Cervical electrode left in situ after a two-level foraminotomy for persistent cervical radiculopathy after an anterior fusion. (**b**) lateral view. The patient had persistent radicular pain despite the foraminotomies (seen at the far left of the picture). After 3 months, a trial of SCS was successful using the previously implanted electrode

ing results (Bennett and Tai, Piva et al.; Brill and Aryeh). Treatment has involved percutaneous and paddle electrodes, usually placed in a midline position from C3 to C6.

Postamputation Pain

Postamputation pain, either from phantom limb pain or postsurgical neuropathic pain from the stump, is difficult to treat, and although SCS has proven to be of use, the degree of treatment success has been very variable. The incidence of upper limb amputation is proportionately much smaller than lower limb amputation, and studies that have looked at the effectiveness of SCS in treating amputation pain have either involved exclusively lower limb amputees or very few upper limb amputees. However, it is reasonable to expect that the results with lower limb amputation can be expected to be similar in upper limb amputees. Treatment with cervical paddle electrodes in these patients has been confounded by high migration rates and unwanted stimulation in the trunk and lower limbs (e.g. McAuley et al.). There is probably a need to do further studies in these patients using laterally placed electrodes which are less likely to be affected by buckling or migration with flexion movements of the spine.

Chronic Headache

High cervical cord stimulation has been used for both cluster headache and chronic migraine (Wolter et al.; Wolter and Kaube; De Agostino et al.). These studies report using bilateral high cervical percutaneous leads, but the placement of thin cervical paddle electrodes, perhaps where percutaneous leads have failed as a result of migration, may have similar but potentially more enduring results. SCS has also been used to treat chronic cervicogenic headache (Vallejo et al.; Dario et al.).

Evidence for Efficacy

CRPS and Chronic Neck/Arm Pain

Studies that review the application of SCS in CRPS and other chronic neuropathic conditions affecting the limbs rarely consider only patients that have conditions affecting the neck and upper limbs, and most studies largely involve the application of percutaneous electrodes rather than paddle electrodes. Many studies are retrospective or are case reports (e.g. Bennett et al.; Canlas et al.; Vallego et al.). Krishna et al. reported on 12 patients with CRPS, in 5 of whom it affected the upper limbs. The authors inserted 15 percutaneous quadripolar leads and 3 surgical leads via laminotomies. It is assumed that all were midline placements and it is not clear on which patients the three paddle leads were used (i.e. cervical or thoracic). All patients reported good (50–75%)

or excellent pain relief (75–100%) and a mean follow-up of 41 months. Bennett and Cameron reviewed ten studies and concluded that there was an overall success rate of 82%. Simpson et al. reported on 41 patients that were exclusively fitted with cervical paddle electrodes, and overall two thirds achieved a sustained benefit. This study included a heterogeneous group of patients with several pain conditions affecting the neck and upper limbs, but it is notable that in the 15 patients with CRPS, 10 achieved significant or moderate benefit, and in the 4 cases with failed neck surgery, all achieved significant or moderate benefit.

Kemler et al.'s landmark study in 2000 randomized 54 patients with CRPS into two groups: SCS plus physical therapy (PT) (36 patients) and PT alone (18 patients). This study used percutaneous electrode stimulation. It is notable that 61% of the SCS + PT group had CRPS affecting the upper limbs. In those treated with SCS, there was a 3.6 point reduction in the visual analogue scale (VAS) at 6 months compared with a marginal increase in the PT group (0.2). The global perceived effect (GPE) was much higher in the treated group compared to the control group (39% versus 6%). The same group reported on 5-year results in 2008. The VAS score in the implant group remained lower by 2.5 points which almost reached significance ($p = 0.06$), but the only statistically significant benefit that persisted was the GPE ($p = 0.02$).

Vallejo et al. reported on five patients who continued to have intractable neck and arm pain following previous anterior cervical surgery and were treated with high cervical cord stimulation (C2-4) using single 8-contact (three patients) or dual 8-contact (two patients) percutaneous electrodes. Four out of the five patients (80%) reported significant pain relief, and two patients had relief of their cervicogenic headaches. It is interesting that the radiology was unremarkable in all cases with no evidence of ongoing stenosis. It is also notable that the electrodes were placed in a midline position and three of the patients reported distal paraesthesias affecting their back, legs or feet. There were no lead migrations in this series. The use of cervical SCS in treating cervicogenic headache has also been reported elsewhere (e.g. Dario et al.).

A retrospective study of 20 patients who all had insertion of high cervical paddle electrodes included 7 patients with CRPS, 1 patient with neck pain and 5 patients with neuropathic pain (Whitworth and Feler). (There were also three patients with brachial plexus injuries.) The authors had a similar approach to the technique as described in this article: 16 patients had a percutaneous trial (the remaining four being trialled with a surgical lead), and all had their surgical lead or leads inserted under a GA with the neck stabilized using three-point fixation of the head. The leads were passed in a caudal direction via C0/1 and C1/2 laminotomies. The mean follow-up was 26 months with 18 of the 20 patients achieving a significant benefit, the mean VAS scores falling from 8.2 to 3. Overall, 70% had an excellent or good outcome. The best results seemed to be with CRPS (mean VAS scores falling from 8.7 to 2.3). The authors pointed out that there is more space in the upper cervical spine at the craniocervical junction making insertion of paddle leads at this level safer. Moens et al. have also described a similar retrograde insertion technique via the C0/1 interlaminar space to treat six patients with chronic neck and arm pain, reporting significant pain reduction in all patients.

Sears et al. reported a retrospective review of 35 patients with CRPS and failed back surgery syndrome, all treated with paddle electrodes; 18 patients had CRPS, but only 6 with CRPS affecting the upper limb. In the CRPS group, 55.6% achieved a greater than 50% reduction in pain after a mean follow-up of 5 years. There is reported evidence indicating no difference between the efficacy of SCS for the treatment of upper or lower limb CRPS (Forouzanfar et al.).

Brachial Plexus Injury

Most studies have been case reports or small numbers of patients. Abdul-Aziz and Ghaleb reported a good result in one patient using a midline paddle electrode at C3–C5 following right-sided nerve root avulsions from C6 to T1, with a 50% reduction in pain at follow-up, but it is unclear if this response was enduring. Lai et al. in another case report noted a good result with high cervical stimulation after failed DREZ lesions. Three other series, with a total of 11 patients treated with cervical SCS, all reported significant improvement in pain or good to excellent results (Bennett and Tai; Piva et al.; Brill and Aryeh). Bennett and Tai reported a mean reduction in the VAS of four points at an average follow-up of 13.5 months using percutaneous leads implanted at C5–C7. Piva et al. used specifically designed 7-contact percutaneous electrodes that could stimulate from C2 to T1-2, with three-point reduction in the VAS score at 6 months in four patients. The evidence for any additional benefit that might be obtained from cervical paddle electrodes is lacking.

Postamputation Pain

A multicentre study involving 363 patients noted that the subgroup of 26 patients who had phantom limb pain seem to derive the greatest benefit from SCS even over time (Servello et al.). Miles and Lipton in another much smaller study found that 5 out of 12 amputees had excellent pain relief, while Krainick et al. in a larger series of 64 patients found that effective pain relief had fallen to only 39% at 5 years. These studies relate more to lower limb amputees, and although it could be expected that similar results would be achieved in upper limb amputees, one study noted poor results in all four arm amputees who had brachial plexus lesions combined with cervical root avulsions (Krainick and Thoden). Because the number of upper limb amputees is proportionally much smaller than lower limb amputees, it is difficult to draw firm conclusions about the effectiveness of SCS in this small subgroup. In a small study of 12 post-amputees treated with paddle electrodes which reported on 5 of the patients, only 2 of these were upper limb amputees (McAuley et al.). These two patients reported 90% and 50% reduction in their pain. However, this paper is also interesting with regard to cervical paddle electrode placement: in addition to arm stimulation, both these patients had stimulation affecting their trunk, legs and feet, and right leg stimulation was troublesome in one of the patients. In addition to the problems with migration related to midline paddle electrodes, this is some vindication for using laterally positioned electrodes in treating these patients.

Headache

The benefits of high cervical spinal cord stimulation in the treatment of cluster headaches were reported in a paper by Wolter et al. (2011) in which seven patients were implanted with bilateral percutaneous high cervical electrodes. The authors concluded that SCS achieved results that were comparable or better than occipital nerve stimulation, with a reduction in frequency (84%), strength (41%) and duration (56%) of attacks. The study however was confounded by high rate of lead breakages and dislocations. The use of small bilateral cervical paddle electrodes in this scenario may reduce such complications and provide a more robust and enduring solution. A recent study reported on the benefits of high cervical stimulation in the treatment of medically intractable chronic migraine (De Agostino et al.). This study involved 17 patients with a median follow-up of 15 months. Mean pain intensity was reduced by 60% with 71% of patients experiencing a decrease of 50% or more. However, the infection rate was 13% (three patients, all explanted and not included in the final analysis) and lead dislocation rate 17.6%. The authors used bilateral quadripolar percutaneous leads. Again, it may be that small bilateral quadripolar surgical leads would reduce the lead migration or dislocation rate, but there are no current studies to support this assumption.

In summary, given there is still a reluctance to use cervical paddle electrodes in preference to percutaneous electrodes and the number of patients with upper limb neuropathic conditions is much smaller than those with low back pain and neuropathic conditions affecting the lower limbs, the number of published studies and reports that relate specifically to the use of cervical paddle electrodes for SCS is limited.

Pearls and Pitfalls

It is important that prior to any electrode insertion, adequate imaging of the insertion site and the proposed trajectory and final position of the electrode is carried out to exclude any possible structural or degenerative abnormalities that might make the insertion unsafe. In younger patients with a congenital stenosis, larger midline electrodes may be subject to neurological risks if in time progressive degenerative change narrows the canal further. In such patients, SCS should either be avoided or percutaneous electrodes may be preferable. If a single limb is the target for treatment, then lateral placement of the electrode is in our opinion safer and less likely to suffer from migration or buckling as a result of movements of the neck. If access to the spine is limited to a small hemilaminotomy, surgical injury is less and recovery faster. Even where both upper limbs are affected, bilateral electrodes may be more effective than a single midline electrode. Midline paddle electrodes can be subject to migration and buckling, and others have tried techniques such as multiple level laminotomies, suturing to the dura and sub-laminar sutures to secure the electrode. While these methods will reduce the migration rate, they add complexity to the operation and additional risks. Midline electrodes can also cause unwanted paraesthesias affecting the trunk, back and lower limbs. In some cases, such as treating brachial plexus injuries, midline or paramedian electrodes higher in the spine may be more appropriate because of nerve root avulsion and a loss of efficacy if lateral and lower electrodes were to stimulate at the site of injury. In patients who require a posterior foraminotomy to decompress a nerve root or roots, it is worthwhile considering the simultaneous insertion of a "sleeping" paddle electrode especially if the surgeon is not optimistic that the root decompression will be of significant benefit in relieving the neuropathic pain due to prior injury from degenerative stenosis or surgery. This allows subsequent SCS without the need for reoperation on the spine and the difficulties of inserting a surgical electrode when scarring from the foraminotomy is already established.

Complications of surgical paddle electrodes such as infection, loss of efficacy with time and device failure are in the main similar to other invasive neuromodulation procedures. Although the perception is that they carry additional risks of neurological injury because of their size and the need for insertion by open surgery, Petraglia et al. looking retrospectively at 8326 patients did not confirm this. Indeed, spinal cord injury (SCI) was higher in the percutaneous electrode-implanted patients than the surgical paddle electrode-implanted patients (2.35% versus 1.71%) which almost reached significance. This was attributed to the fact that percutaneous insertion is a blind procedure. However, the study did not clarify what the nature and extent of the cord injuries were in the two groups. These findings were contrary to an earlier study that suggested the incidence of neurological injury from paddle electrodes was less than 0.6% (Levy et al.), but this difference is probably attributable to the different data sources interrogated in each study. There is no published evidence to suggest that cervical paddle electrodes carry a higher risk than those inserted in the thoracic spine, but the consequences of injury are clearly greater; the cervical spinal cord has significantly greater axial dimensions than the thoracic cord with a relatively smaller epidural space.

It is important to leave the most proximal part of the paddle adjacent or close to the laminotomy so that this can be identified and freed to allow easy revision of the electrode. As long as revision involves replacing like with like, the original electrode can be easily withdrawn and the new electrode inserted into the same space. Revision of one electrode for a different type will require a greater surgical exposure and may involve further bone removal and laminotomies at multiple levels. In patients who have previously had a percutaneous lead removed for infection, and the intention is to replace this with a surgical electrode after a suitable time has passed, the surgeon should expect significant epidural scarring and be prepared for a longer procedure with greater exposure of the dura and painstaking division of adhesions. The technique of using a bone scalpel or diamond burr to cut a narrow 3–4 mm trench through the midline of the lamina at the level of electrode placement is to be commended, allowing the dura to be mobilized by blunt dissection while retaining enough bone to hold the electrode in place.

Pearls

- Ensure that the patients have been adequately imaged before implantation. Fine axial CT with sagittal reconstructions is a suitable alternative in patients who cannot undergo MR scanning.
- Following a successful trial with a percutaneous lead, x-ray the patient. If insertion of a paddle electrode is anticipated or the percutaneous lead requires revision to a surgical lead, its position can match exactly the position of the percutaneous lead.
- Consider laterally placed electrodes to treat upper limb neuropathic pain rather than midline electrodes.
- Always use image intensification in theatre, both for targeting the skin wound and the proposed laminotomy site.
- Where possible limit the surgical approach and laminotomy to reduce surgical trauma, and preserve bone to maintain the paddle electrode in place.
- Ensure the laminotomy is appropriately positioned so that the lower end of the electrode is just within the laminotomy site. This enables easier removal or revision of the electrode.
- Consider simultaneous placement of an electrode in patients who are offered posterior foraminotomy and cervical nerve root decompression for persistent neuropathic pain as a result of degenerative foraminal stenosis and failed anterior cervical fusion surgery.

Pitfalls

- Inserting paddle electrodes without prior imaging to exclude structural abnormalities is dangerous.
- Insertion of large paddle electrodes in patients with a significant congenital canal stenosis increases the risk of injury or may cause cord compression over time with advancing degenerative change.
- The cervical lamina is thinner than in the thoracic spine and the epidural space smaller because of the anatomical expansion of the cervical cord.
- Some patients will fail permanent implantation even after a successful trial, and efficacy can diminish with time.
- In patients who have had long-term prior percutaneous electrodes and particularly in patients who have had previous infection, epidural scarring can be considerable, and more extensive surgery, even at multiple levels, may be required.
- Midline electrode placement can lead to unwanted paraesthesias in the trunk, back and lower limbs.
- Large paddle electrodes placed in the midline can be subject to buckling with extension of the neck.

Recommended Reading

1. Abdul-Aziz S, Ghaleb H. Cervical spinal cord simulation for the management of pain from brachial plexus avulsion. Letters to the Editor. Pain Med. 2014;15(4):712–4.
2. Air EL, Toczyl GR, Mandybur GT. Electrophysiologic monitoring for placement of laminectomy leads for spinal cord stimulation under general anesthesia. Neuromodulation. 2012;15:573–80.
3. Armani J. A novel technique for the implantation of paddle leads in the cervical spine. Neuromodulation. 2013;16:546–50.
4. Bennett DS, Alo K, Oakley J, Feler C. Spinal cord stimulation for complex regional pain syndrome I: a retrospective multicentre experience from 1995 to 1998 in 101 patients. Neuromodulation. 1999;2:202–10.
5. Bennett DS, Cameron TL. Spinal cord stimulation for complex regional pain syndromes. In: Simpson B, editor. Electrical stimula-

tion and the relief of pain. Pain research and clinical management. Amsterdam: Elsevier; 2003. p. 111–29.
6. Bennett MI, Tai YM. Cervical dorsal column stimulation relieves pain of brachial plexus avulsion. J R Soc Med. 1994;87:5–6.
7. Bertelli JA, Ghizoni MF. Use of clinical signs and computed tomography myelography findings in detecting and excluding nerve root avulsion in complete brachial plexus palsy. J Neurosurg. 2006;105:835–42.
8. Brill S, Aryeh I. Neuromodulation in the management of pain from brachial plexus injury. Pain Physician. 2008;11:81–5.
9. Canlas B, Drake T, Gabriel E. A severe case of complex regional pain syndrome 1 (reflex sympathetic dystrophy) managed with spinal cord stimulation. Pain Pract. 2010;10(1):78–83.
10. Dario A, Scamoni C, Peron S, Tomei G. A case of post-traumatic cervicogenic headache treated by cervical cord stimulation. J Headache Pain. 2005;6:473.
11. De Agostino R, Federspiel B, Cesnulis E, Sandor PS. High-cervical spinal cord stimulation for medically intractable chronic migraine. Neuromodulation. 2015;18:289–96.
12. Deer TR, Skaribas IM, Haider N, Salmon J, Kim C, Nelson C, et al. Effectiveness of cervical spinal cord stimulation for the management of chronic pain. Neuromodulation. 2014;17:265–71.
13. Falowski S, Dianna A. Neuromonitoring protocol for spinal cord stimulator cases with case descriptions. Int J Acad Med. 2016;2:132–44.
14. Falowski SM, Celii A, Sestokas AK, Schwartz DM, Matsumato C, Sharan A. Awake versus asleep placement of spinal cord stimulators: a cohort analysis of complications associated with placement. Neuromodulation. 2011;14:130–5.
15. Fayaz A, Croft P, Langford RM, Donaldson LJ, Jones GT. Prevalence of chronic pain in the UK: a systematic review and meta-analysis of population studies. BMJ Open Access. 2016;6:e010364.
16. Forouzanfar T, Kemler MA, Weber WEJ, Kessels AGH, van Kleef M. Spinal cord stimulation in complex regional pain syndrome: cervical and lumbar devices are comparably effective. Br J Anaesth. 2004;92(3):348–53.
17. GBD 2015 Disease and Injury Incidence and Prevalence Collaborators. Global, regional, and national incidence, prevalence and years lived with disability for 310 diseases and injuries, 1990 – 2015: a systematic analysis for the global burden of disease study 2015. Lancet. 2016;388:1545–602.
18. Kemler MA, Barendse GA, van Kleef M, de Vet HC, Rijks CP, Furnée CA, van den Wildenberg FA. Spinal cord stimulation in patients with chronic reflex sympathetic dystrophy. N Engl J Med. 2000;343(9):618–24.
19. Kemler MA, de Vet HC, Barendse GA, van den Wildenberg FA, Van KM. Effect of spinal cord stimulation for chronic complex regional pain syndrome type I: five-year final follow-up of patients in a randomized controlled trial. J Neurosurg. 2008a;108(2):292–8.
20. Kemler MA, De Vet H, Barendse G, van den Wildenberg FAJM, van Kleef M. Effect of spinal cord stimulation for complex regional pain syndrome type 1: five year follow-up of patients in a randomised clinical trial. J Neurosurg. 2008b;108:292–8.
21. Krainick JU, Thoden U. Spinal cord stimulation in postamputation pain. In: Siegfried J, Zimmerman M, editors. Phantom and stump pain. Berlin/Heidelberg: Springer; 1981. p. 163–6.
22. Krainick JU, Thoden U, Riechert T. Pain reduction in amputees by long-term spinal cord stimulation. Long-term follow-up study over 5 years. J Neurosurg. 1980;52:346–50.
23. Krishna K, Nath RK, Toth C. Spinal cord stimulation is effective in the Management of reflex sympathetic dystrophy. Neurosurgery. 1997;40(3):503–9.
24. Lai HY, Lee CY, Lee ST. High cervical spinal cord stimulation after failed dorsal root entry zone surgery for brachial plexus avulsion pain. Surg Neurol. 2009;72(3):286–9.
25. Levy R, Henderson J, Slavin K, Simpson BA, Barolat G, Shipley J, North R. Incidence and avoidance of neurologic complications with paddle type spinal cord stimulation leads. Neuromodulation. 2011;14:412–22.
26. Mammis A, Mogilner AY. The use of intraoperative electrophysiology for placement of spinal cord stimulator paddle leads under general anesthesia. Neurosurgery. 2012;70(ONS supple 2):230–6.
27. McAuley J, van Gröningen R, Green C. Spinal cord stimulation for intractable pain following limb amputation. Neuromodulation. 2013;16:530–6.
28. Melzack R, Wall PD. Pain mechanisms: a new theory. Science. 1965;150(3699):971–9.
29. Miles J, Lipton S. Phantom limb pain treated by electrical stimulation. Pain. 1978;5:373–82.
30. Moens M, De Smedt A, Brouns R, Spapen H, Droogmans S, Duerinck J, et al. Retrograde C0-C1 insertion of cervical plate electrode for chronic intractable neck and arm pain. World Neurosurg. 2011;76(3–4):352–4.
31. North RB, Lanning A, Hessels R, Cutchis PN. Spinal cord stimulation with percutaneous and plate electrodes: side effects and quantitative comparisons. Neurosurg Focus. 1997;2:e3.
32. North RB, Kidd DH, Olin JC, Sieracki JM. Spinal cord stimulation electrode design: prospective, randomized, controlled trial comparing percutaneous and laminectomy electrodes-part I: technical outcomes. Neurosurgery. 2002;51:381–9.
33. North RB, Kidd DH, Petrucci L, Dorsi MJ. Spinal cord stimulation electrode design: a prospective, randomized, controlled trial comparing percutaneous with laminectomy electrodes: part II-clinical outcomes. Neurosurgery. 2005;57:990–6.
34. Pahapill PA. A novel nonanchoring technique for implantation of paddle leads in the cervical spine under conscious sedation. Neuromodulation. 2015;18:472–7.
35. Petraglia FW III, Farber SH, Gramer R, Verla T, Wang F, Thomas S, et al. The incidence of spinal cord injury in implantation of percutaneous and paddle electrodes for spinal cord stimulation. Neuromodulation. 2016;19(1):85–90.
36. Piva B, Shaladi A, Saltari R, Gilli G. Spinal cord stimulation in the management of pain from brachial plexus avulsion. Neuromodulation. 2003;6:27–31.
37. Sears NC, Machado AG, Nagel SJ, Deogaonkar M, Stanton-Hicks M, Rezai AR, Henderson JM. Long term outcomes of spinal cord stimulation with paddle leads in the treatment of complex regional pain syndrome and failed back surgery syndrome. Neuromodulation. 2011;14:312–8.
38. Servello D, Dones I, Carbone G, Broggi G. Italian multicentric study on pain treatment with epidural spinal cord stimulation. Stereotact Funct Neurosurg. 1994;62:273–8.
39. Shealy CN, Mortimer JT, Reswick JB. Electrical inhibition of pain by stimulation of the dorsal columns: preliminary clinical report. Anesth Analg. 1967;46(4):489–91.
40. Simpson BA, Bassett G, Davies K, Herbert C, Pierri M. Cervical spinal cord stimulation for pain: a report on 41 patients. Neuromodulation. 2003;6(1):20–6.
41. Sindou MP. Microsurgical lesioning in the dorsal root entry zone for pain due to brachial plexus avulsion: a prospective series of 55 patients. J Neurosurg. 2005;102:1018–28.
42. Stecker MM. A review of intraoperative monitoring for spinal surgery. Surg Neurol Int. 2012;3:S174–87.
43. Tamkus AA, Scott AF, Khan FR. Neurophysiological monitoring during spinal cord stimulator placement surgery. Neuromodulation. 2015;18:460–4.
44. Vallejo R, Kramer J, Benyamin R. Neuromodulation of the cervical spinal cord in the treatment of chronic intractable neck and upper extremity pain: a case series and review of the literature. Pain Physician. 2007;10:305–11.

45. Whitworth LA, Feler CA. C1-C2 sublaminar insertion of paddle leads for the management of chronic painful conditions of the upper extremity. Neuromodulation. 2003;6(3):153–7.
46. Wolter T, Kaube H. Neurostimulation for chronic cluster headache. Ther Adv Neurol Disord. 2012;5(3):175–80.
47. Wolter T, Kieman A, Kaube H. High cervical spinal cord stimulation for chronic cluster headache. Cephalalgia. 2011;31:1170–80.
48. Wycis HT, Gildenberg PL. Long-range evaluation of the surgical treatment of spasmodic torticollis. Excerpta Med Int Congr Ser. 1969;193:97.

Dorsal Root Ganglion Stimulation: Cervical Spine

67

G. Baranidharan, Corey W. Hunter, and Jason E. Pope

Introduction

Spinal cord stimulation (SCS) has been used for the treatment of complex, neuropathic pain since 1967. It is a well-established treatment modality with good clinical and cost-effectiveness data currently available. Most often, SCS is used to treat trunk and/or limb pain. One of the key difficulties encountered when one attempts to utilize tSCS in cervical level is the inability to reliably and predictably deliver a smooth, consistent stimulation to the area(s) of need due to positional changes in the neck with paraesthesia inducing systems. This can lead to an unsatisfactory experience for the patient and possibly explant. DRGS is a relatively new innovation that was approved in Europe in 2011 and in the United States in 2016. The key feature of DRGS is the ability to provide focal stimulation to precise areas of the body without the worry of positional-related changes in stimulation.

While DRGS is not in and of itself "paresthesia-free," the lack of paresthesias perceived by the patient is a by-product of programming and the anatomy of the DRG, itself. In a sub-analysis, The ACCURATE study demonstrated that patients reported pain relief when the stimulator was programmed at sub-perception settings, unlike the control SCS cohort. Additionally, there is paucity of cerebrospinal fluid (CSF) around the DRG which means less energy is required to activate the neural tissue being targeted. Consequently, paresthesias are not part of the treatment algorithm with DRGS and are therefore not an issue with positional changes, or otherwise. Further, the patient's potential for pain relief is independent of the classic paresthesia-mapping inherent to tSCS leading to a better patient experience overall in cases where neurostimulation of the cervical spine is being considered.

G. Baranidharan (✉)
Leeds Pain and Neuromodulation Centre, Leeds, UK
e-mail: g.baranidharan@nhs.net

C. W. Hunter
Department of Rehabilitation Medicine, Icahn School of Medicine at Mount Sinai, New York, NY, USA

Ainsworth Institute of Pain Management, New York, NY, USA
e-mail: chunter@ainpain.com

J. E. Pope
Evolve Restorative Center, Santa Rosa, CA, USA

Anatomy

The DRG forms a gateway or interface between the peripheral and central nervous system and is reliably located immediately inferior to the pedicles. The DRG is not only a communicator between the two parts of the nervous system but also has a key role in the up- and downregulation of pain pathways which play a key role in the development of chronic pain conditions. The DRG is a collection of cell bodies whose neurons have pseudo-unipolar morphology with T-junctions that act as a filter function for cell transduction. The cell bodies contained within the DRG have somatotopically arranged neurons that allow one to target even smaller areas of the body.

There is some variation with regard to the location of the DRG in relation to the pedicle from one level to the next, especially in the cervical region. The distance from the thecal sac to the nerve root increases as one moves inferiorly from C4 (~4.3 cc) to C8 (~7.1 cc) (Yabuki et al). This means as one descends in the cervical spine, the DRG will be positioned more laterally than the level above.

It is not recommended to consider placing the therapy above C5. More cephalad placement carries an increased risk of vascular and neurologic injury.

Physiology

Initially, the DRG were thought to be passive structures with the sole purpose of facilitating communication between the peripheral and central nervous systems. It plays an active part in controlling the nociception through

T. R. Deer et al. (eds.), *Deer's Treatment of Pain*, https://doi.org/10.1007/978-3-030-12281-2_67

detection and production of relevant chemical modulations within the dorsal root ganglion. As stated above, the neurons of the DRG have T-junctions that play a significant role in the propagation of action potentials and also act as a filter in assimilating information from peripheral to central and vice versa. There is evidence to suggest the DRG are directly involved in the development of neuropathic pain through hyper-excitability and spontaneous ectopic firing. These factors have crucial implications on central sensitization and clinical changes in the patient such as allodynia and hyperalgesia.

There are interconnections between the DRG allowing them to communicate at adjacent levels which can be quite useful when utilizing them a target for neurostimulation in the treatment chronic pain conditions. These connections are evidenced in the study and subsequent documentation of ganglionectomies where multiple levels had to be removed to obtain relief in a single dermatome. This intercommunication is especially important when performing DRG in the cervical spine. Upper levels tend to be harder to safely target with DRGS due to the relatively small diameter of the central canal as one ascends in the cervical spine. Therefore, in a patient who has pain in the C5 and C6 distribution, one may only need to place a lead at C6 rather than assume additional risk by navigating the delivery apparatus in a far narrower region of the spine to gain access to C5 as well.

Patient Selection

As with any type of neuromodulation, patient selection is key. DRGS requires a multidisciplinary approach to selecting the right patient. In addition, patient expectations and clear understanding of the pros and cons of having an implanted device, as well as the potential complications, are vital. DRGS, specifically, is particularly useful for focal neuropathic pain; thus the patient being considered for this particular modality should fit a clear set of criteria to justify the added complexity inherent to DRGS as opposed to tSCS. Potential diagnoses include:

- Complex regional pain syndrome (CRPS), types I and II (aka reflex sympathetic dystrophy/RSD and causalgia)
- Peripheral neuropathy secondary to nerve damage
- Mononeuropathy
- Diabetic peripheral polyneuropathy
- Brachial plexopathy

Preoperatively, one should obtain imaging (i.e. MRI or CT myelogram) to assess the epidural space and foramen to ensure there is adequate space to safely accommodate the sheath and lead – this can either be done personally or with the assistance of radiologist.

DRG Level Selection

The most common levels to be targeted in the cervical spine are C8 and C7, respectively. In the majority of instances, one can cover most of the hand due to the cross-communication, as described above, between the DRG. While leads can theoretically be placed anywhere in the cervical spine, it is *not recommended to place leads higher than C5*. There is a significant risk for complication in the upper part of the cervical spine (i.e. epidural hematoma). Therefore, when choosing a patient for cervical DRGS, one should consider that the only levels that can be safely targeted are C6, C7 and C8 and should therefore pick patients accordingly whose pain distribution can be reasonably captured at one of those levels – C5 should only be attempted in extremely skilled hands and if a more inferior level was unsuccessful.

Technique

Patient Positioning

- The patient is placed in a prone position.
- The table should be adjusted such that the arms will rest below shoulder level or at the patient's sides with armrest. Most patients being considered for cervical DRGS will have neuropathic pain in the hands – thus, keeping their arms at or above the level of the shoulders might be uncomfortable.
- We would recommend a table that allows the head to be positioned face down and in the midline with the hands resting on a stool in front (Fig. 67.1). This would help

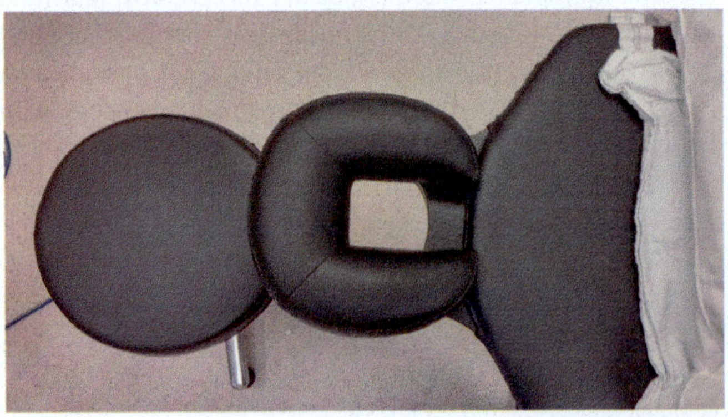

Fig. 67.1 Table. The operating table with a headrest to give a neutral position to the neck. This enables easy access for epidural and more convenience for the patients. The stool in front can be used to place the hands

keep the neck in a neutral position and prevent any pain in the shoulder or upper extremity.

- The neck should be positioned in slight flexion to allow a smooth and straight pathway for the sheath through the cervical spine. Moreover, this positioning will open the foramen making it easier to pass the sheath through and out the foramen. If flexion is not possible, extension in the neck should be limited as much as possible as any bend in the neck will cause the sheath to bend thus creating force/pressure against the dorsal aspect of the cervical spinal cord.

Needle Entry

- The epidural entry for cervical space is more challenging than the thoracic and lumbar regions and should not be attempted above C7/T1.
- The entry should be as flat as possible to get reasonable access to the dorsal root and allow the sheath to safely pass through the epidural space by minimizing the force being exerted by the sheath against the dorsal aspect of the spinal cord.
  - A more perpendicular entry will make it more difficult to navigate the sheath as well as increase the likelihood of lead fracture and more importantly the possibility of causing damage to the spinal cord.
- The authors recommend entering the epidural space 2–3 pedicles below the target, utilizing a paraspinal approach (Fig. 67.2).
  - Figure 67.2 illustrates where the target point will be for epidural access and the corresponding skin entry point for this level – note the entry point is several pedicles below which is contrary to the lumbar technique for DRGS.
- Under AP view, the C-arm is then adjusted to show an inferior oblique view where a small slit can be seen between the C7/T1 and T1/T2 levels (Fig. 67.3).
- The needle is then advanced from the entry point onto the lamina directly inferior to the target level (i.e. T1 in the case of epidural access at C7/T1) (Fig. 67.4).
- Once the lamina is contacted, one can now gauge the general depth – the needle is then withdrawn slightly and adjusted to now target the superior lamina (Fig. 67.5).
- The needle is then advanced to contact the superior lamina – at this point the needle tip is now positioned roughly over the interspace being targeted.
- The needle is now repositioned and angled downward toward the epidural space with the bevel up.
- An inferior oblique (foraminal) view suggested at this juncture as it will allow the implanter to visualize where the needle tip is.
  - A lateral fluoroscopic view is not advisable as it will likely be more difficult to see at the cervical level.

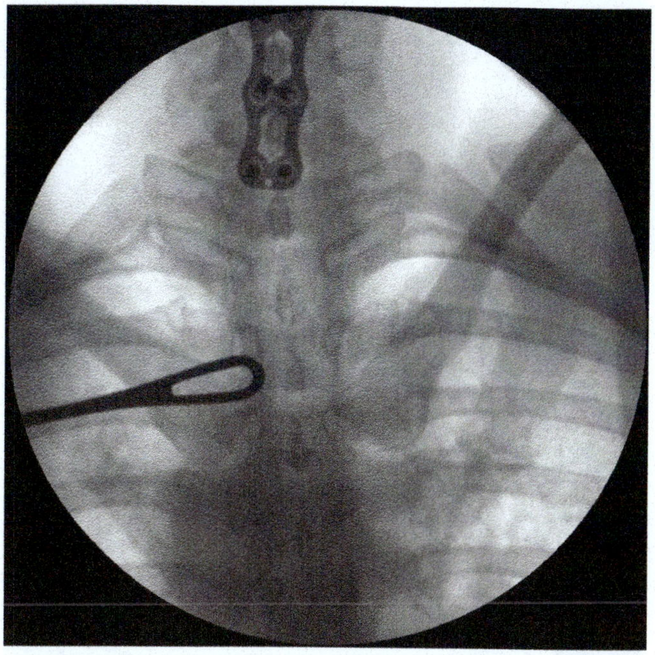

Fig. 67.2 Skin entry point 3–4 pedicles below which will enable a shallow entry to the epidural space

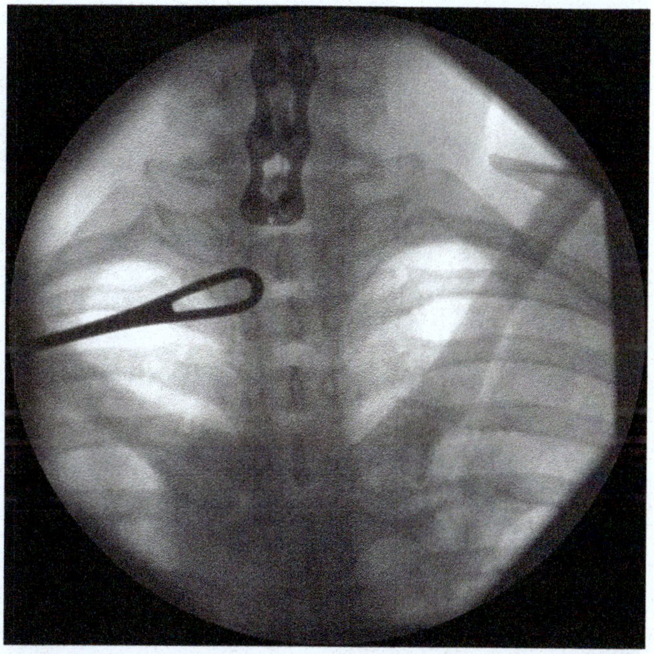

Fig. 67.3 The x-ray beam is then tilted inferior oblique to get a gun barrel approach to the space

- Epidural access is obtained using the classic "loss of resistance" technique.
  - Saline can be utilized as well as air, depending on the implanter's preference; however one should keep in mind that if saline is used, the impedances will be lower than expected until the saline is reabsorbed by

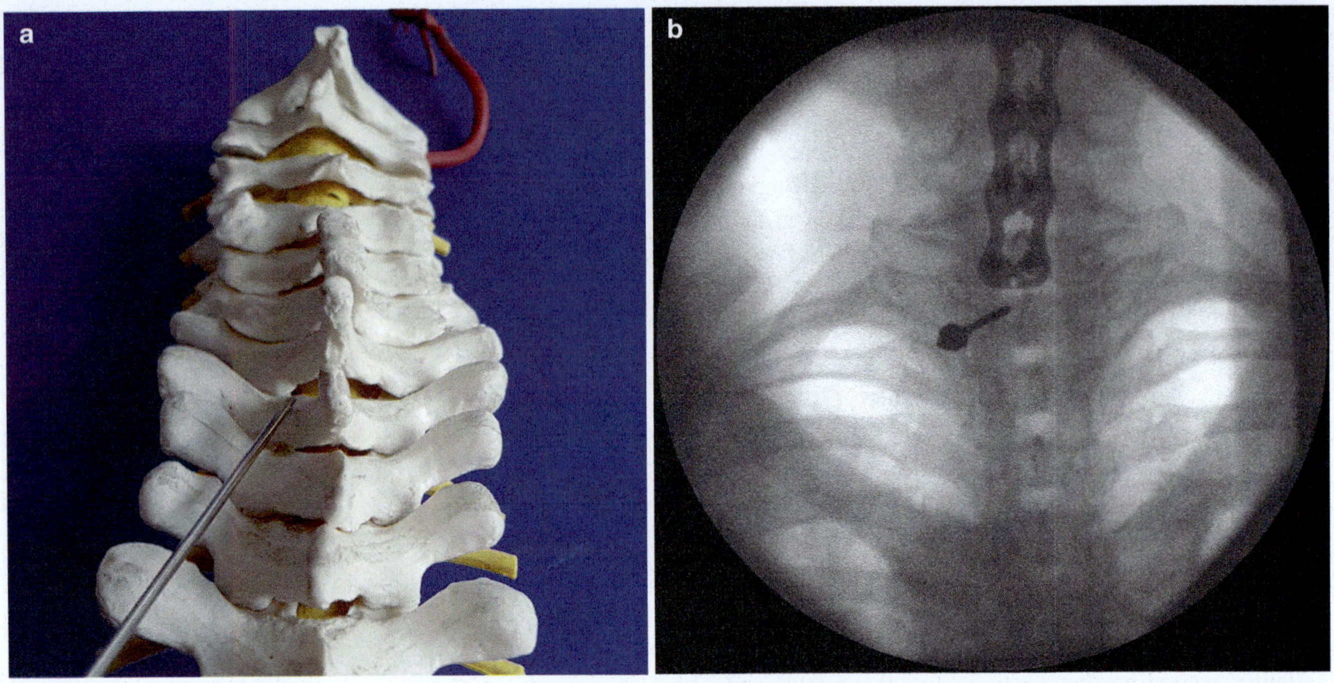

Fig. 67.4 (a, b) Epidural needle touching the lamina of the vertebra below the level of epidural entry

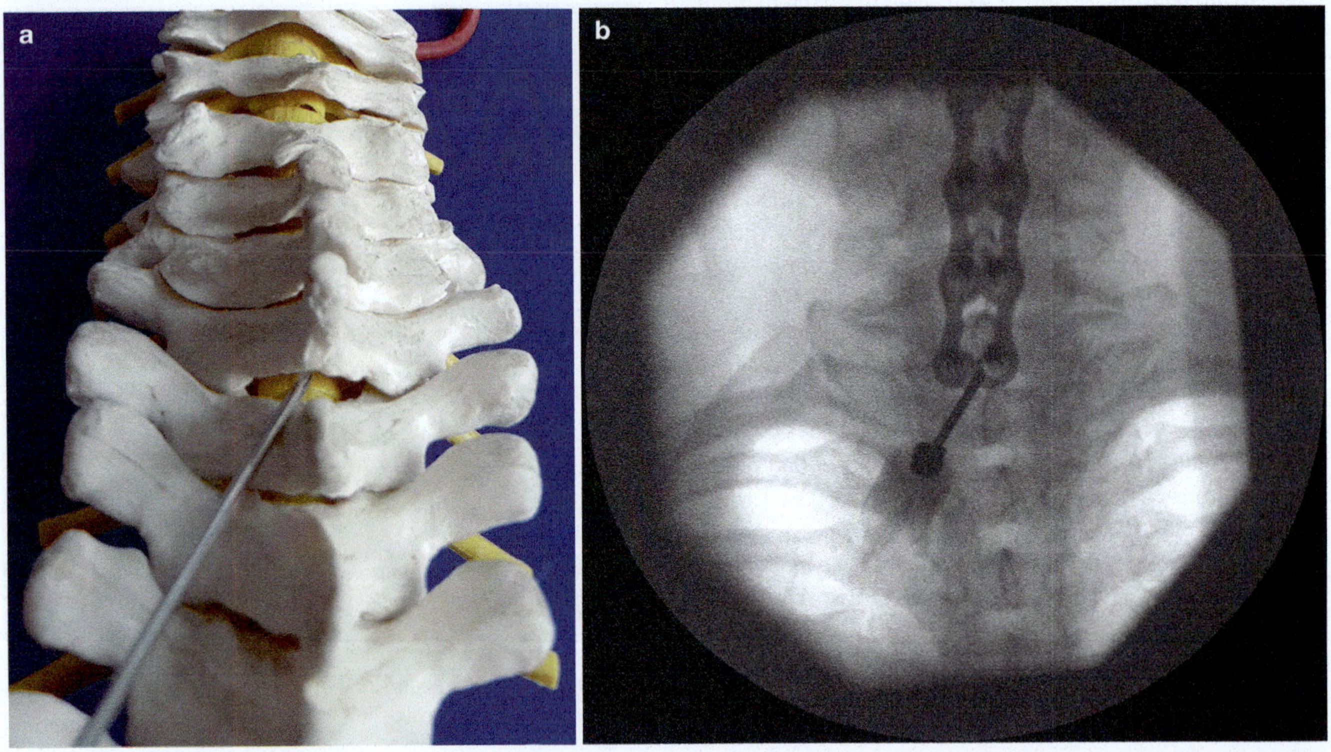

Fig. 67.5 (a, b) Epidural needle in contact with the lamina above the level of the epidural entry

the patient. Thus programming in the postoperative time period may be a challenge.

- The goal should be for the needle tip to enter the epidural space as close to midline as possible with a shallow angle (Fig. 67.6) – this will minimize the potential for a dural puncture and aid easy access to the DRG.

Sheath and Lead Placement

- The epidural space is accessed with the bevel facing up/dorsally.
- The lead will come preloaded into the sheath with the larger curve – either sheath is suitable depending on the

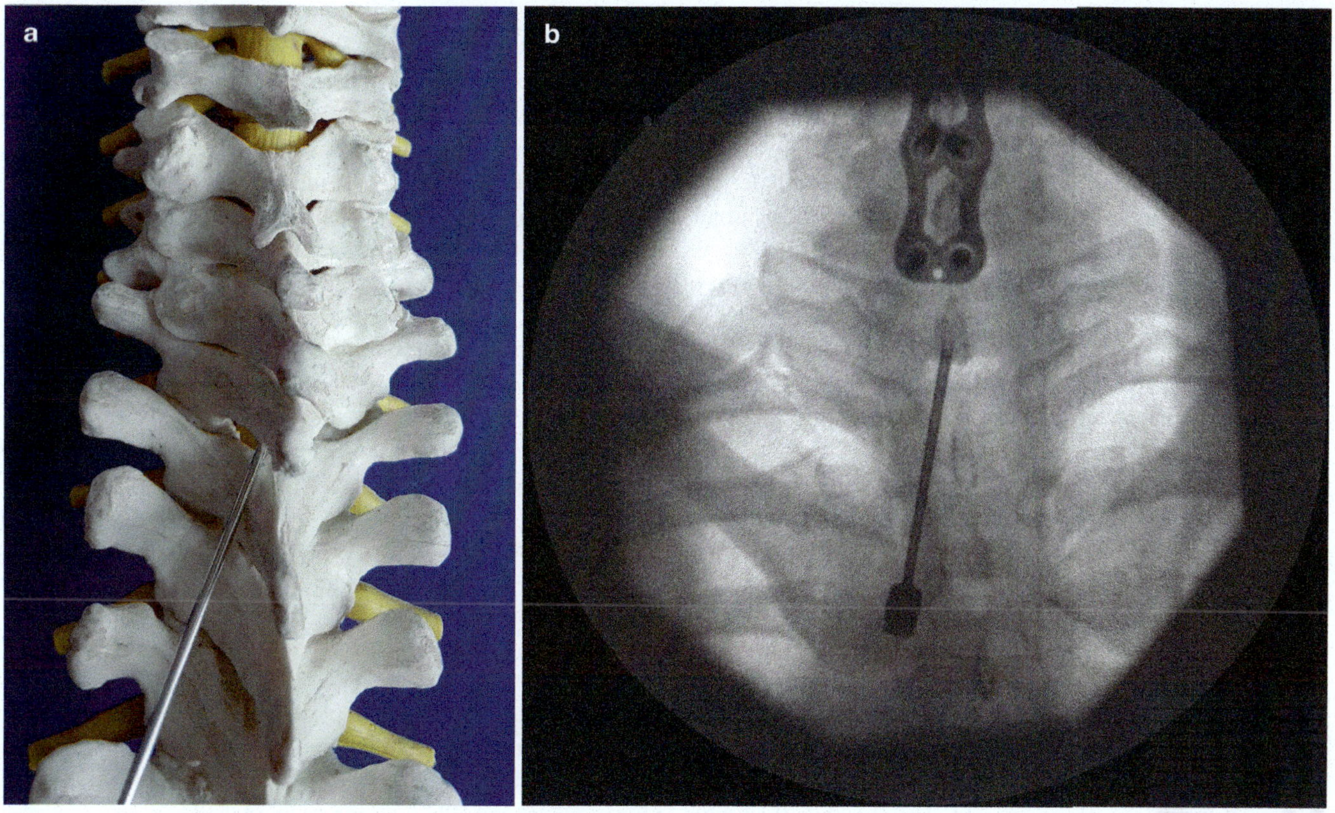

Fig. 67.6 (**a**, **b**) Epidural entry at a shallow angle shown with a model and an x-ray

angle of the needle in relation to the target and the intended path for the sheath.

- The larger curve will be preferable when targeting lower levels like C7 and C8 as there is less distance to traverse and the implanter will likely need to make an acute turn in either direction to get the sheath out the needle and under the pedicle.
- The smaller curve will be preferable when targeting higher levels like C5 or C6, as there is more distance for the sheath to traverse. Given the entry point into the epidural space will never be above C7/T1, the sheath will need to travel two vertebral levels to reach the C6 DRG. The larger curve will cause the sheath to veer off to the side rather than advance higher. Additionally, the smaller curve will exert less force when it is rotated from side to side for the purposes of steering – this is particularly important in the more superior level given there is less overall space in the central canal as opposed to the lower levels.

- The sheath and lead within are inserted through needle with the curve facing up, which should be the same direction as the bevel.
- Once the sheath is felt to have entered the epidural space, it should be withdrawn slightly until only 1–2 mm of the sheath/lead is extending beyond the needle.
- At this point the needle/bevel is rotated 90° to ipsilateral side of the foramen/DRG being targeted – this should also rotate the sheath as well.
- The sheath is then gently advanced toward the target DRG.
  - One should attempt to minimize rotating of the sheath back and forth as much as possible – each time the sheath rotates, the curve will rotate commensurately. The curve, while slight, does exert some force on the neural tissue and should therefore be minimized wherever possible.
- If the sheath appears to "overshoot" the target level, one can swap out the lead for the guide wire at this point.
  - By gently inserting the guide wire beyond the sheath, one can attempt to make contact with the target level. Once the guide wire has contacted or entered the desired level, the sheath can then be advanced over the guide wire into the desired location. The guide wire will act as a conduit for the sheath thus steering it farther laterally than it wanted to go previously
- Once the tip of the sheath is within the desired foramen, GENTLE pressure should be applied to advance the tip out the foramen.
  - If the sheath cannot be advanced with gently pressure, DO NOT ATTEMPT TO USE FORCE. This will cause the sheath to bow and may cause neural injury.
  - One can use the guide wire at this point – not to give the sheath more force but to attempt to "poke" through the obstruction or find a weak spot between the ligaments located within the foramen. Using a gentle tapping motion, the guide wire will find the path of least

resistance and advance out the foramen. At this point, one can attempt to advance the sheath over the guide wire. If force is again encountered, switch back to the lead, and advance the lead into the path just made by the guide wire.

- The sheath is then withdrawn over the lead, under live fluoro, making sure the lead stays properly positioned under the pedicle.
- Once the tip of the sheath is positioned within the tip of the needle, the stylet within the lead is withdrawn several cm to give the lead a more "floppy" feel.
- The needle and sheath are collectively rotated 90° upward such that the bevel of the needle and the curve of the sheath are now facing dorsally, once again.
- The superior loop in the cervical spine will take on a different shape in the cervical spine due to the anatomy – it will appear more horizontal than leads placed in the lumbar or thoracic spine. There are two techniques to create the superior loop:
  1. With the sheath now facing dorsally, simply advancing the lead may create a superior loop.
  2. If #1 is attempted and the loop is either not possible or it is not taking the desired shape, one can attempt to advance the sheath, superiorly, thus dragging the lead upward to the desired height. The sheath is then withdrawn over the lead, leaving it in position.

The inferior loops are made in the same fashion as a lumbar DRGS (Fig. 67.7).

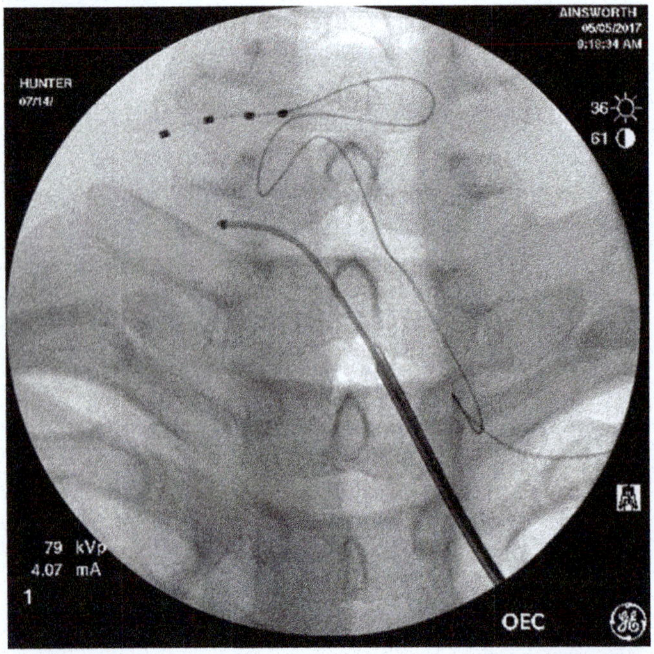

Fig. 67.7 DRG in the cervical space with a "S" loop for strain relief

Anchoring

Anchoring is a personal preference – the kit does include an anchoring device; however it may not be necessary in the presence of well-formed strain relief loops. Having a strain relief loop in the epidural space acts as a "soft anchor" thus nullifying the need for a proper anchor in the underlying tissue and thus saving time during the implant procedure.

- Before removing the needle, a small incision is made on either side of the needle, approximately 2–3 cm in diameter.
- Blunt dissection is performed to create a very small pocket.
- The lead is then coiled two times and then gently placed within the pocket using bayonet forceps.
- Using 2–0 silk suture, the coil is then secured to the underlying tissue.
- Once the lead is secured, tunnelling is then performed.

The battery can either be placed in the chest wall, buttock or abdomen. The tunnelling should occur more in the midline as far down as possible before it traverses towards the place where the IPG is going to be placed.

Temporary Trial Versus Tunnelled Trial (Permanent Trial)

The high trial/permanent ratio with DRGS has led some to perform "tunnelled trials" in anticipation of the likely and impending implant. In this model, the trial leads will stay in and simply be connected to the battery upon conclusion of the trial period. The advantages are preservation of the trial experience as it ensures the leads are in exactly the same position. While the placement of DRG leads is percutaneous and do not expose the central canal in any way, the manoeuvring of the sheath and creation of the loops within the epidural space during the trial can create scar tissue that will make it harder to place the leads a second during the trial. Therefore, many prefer to place the leads once and preserve their placement in such a way that the implanter only need connect those original leads to a battery to complete the implantation of a permanent system. The disadvantage of a tunnelled trial is an increased risk for infection and an unwanted scar at the tunnel site should the trial fail. The pros and cons should be weighed by the implanter and the patient when deciding which method will best benefit the patient.

The placement of the leads is the same; however a few extra steps are performed to tunnel the trial leads to allow them to be used in the permanent implant:

- Once the lead(s) is(are) placed and the needle(s) is(are) removed, a small secondary site is created away from the original skin entry site(s). A small incision is made along with blunt dissection to create a small pocket large enough to contain the lead(s), lead extension(s) and several coils.
- The lead is then tunnelled away from the original skin entry site to a secondary site.
  - If there are additional leads, they should all be tunnelled in a similar fashion to the same secondary site.
- The original trial leads are now connected to lead extensions. The end of the original trial lead (now connected to the extensions) should be tucked into the secondary pocket thus preventing any part of the lead from being exposed.
- The extension leads are now coiled several times and then exposed from this secondary site.
- The secondary site is then closed and dressed according to the implanter's preference.

Evidence

There is little evidence to support the use of cervical DRG other than a few case reports (Huygen, & Vesper). Cervical DRG is technically much more challenging than lumbar DRG and should only be attempted by experienced neuromodulators. It is recommended that one not attempt cervical DRG until at least 100 lumbar leads have been successfully placed. Additionally, one should ensure neurosurgical support is present in the event of complication.

Pearls and Pitfalls

- Reducing the angle between the skin and the epidural entry will make the access to DRG easier and reduces complications.
- DRG leads should not be placed above the C5 level, and the epidural needle entry should be at the level C7/T1 or below.

Conclusion

DRGS offers a number of advantages over tSCS – most notably consistent stimulation that is independent of movement or position and the ability to provide focal, concentrated stimulation to specific body parts. These two factors are crucial in the cervical spine as two common complaints are stimulation that varies and the inability to consistently capture the arms/hands. However, the operator should be extremely experienced lumbar DRG before attempting placement in the cervical spine. One must be cautious, as the margin for error in this portion of the spine is much smaller. Current evidence consists only few case reports; however further studies should help in establishing this therapy for this region of the spine.

Recommended Reading

1. Deer TR, Levy RM, Kramer J, et al. Dorsal root ganglion stimulation yielded higher treatment success rate for complex regional pain syndrome and causalgia at 3 and 12 months: a randomized comparative trial. Pain. 2017;158(4):669–81.
2. Devor M. Unexplained peculiarities of the dorsal root ganglion. Pain. 1999;82(6 suppl):S27–35.
3. Huygen F, Baranidharan G, Simpson K, et al. An upper limb neuropathic pain cohort treated with stimulation of dorsal root ganglia (DRG): pooled data from four prospective European studies (256). Neuromodulation. 18(2):86.
4. Krames ES. The dorsal root ganglion in chronic pain and as a target for neuromodulation: a review. Neuromodulation. 2015;18:24–32.
5. Van Buyten JP, Smet I, Liem L, Russo M, Huygen F. Stimulation of dorsal root ganglia for the management of complex regional pain syndrome: a prospective case series. Pain Pract. 2015;15(3):208–16.
6. Vesper J, Schu S, Slotty P, et al. Cervical and high-thoracic dorsal root ganglion stimulation (DRG) in chronic pain (10317). Neuromodulation. 2016;19(3):388.
7. Yabuki S, Kikuchi S. Positions of dorsal root ganglia in the cervical spine. An anatomic and clinical study. Spine. 1996;21(13):1513–7.

Percutaneous Thoracic Neurostimulation for Chronic Pain

68

Tory L. McJunkin, Paul J. Lynch, and Edward L. Swing

Introduction

Chronic pain affects close to 100 million Americans each year. The treatment of chronic pain typically begins with some forms of conservative care, such as rest, physical modalities (e.g., physical therapy, chiropractic care), and over-the-counter or non-opioid medications (e.g., NSAIDs, muscle relaxants, membrane stabilizers, and topical creams). In many cases, these treatments are sufficient to alleviate pain. In some cases, patients continue to experience moderate to severe pain despite these treatments, requiring more advanced treatments such as injection therapies (e.g., nerve blocks, epidural steroid injections, radiofrequency denervation, or regenerative treatments) and/or opioid medications. Some of these treatments, particularly opioids, carry a substantial risk of addiction or death. Patients may also undergo more invasive surgery of the spine or joints, which are costly and, in many cases, may not be effective.

Many patients with moderate to severe chronic pain who have failed conservative, interventional, and/or surgical treatments can get significant pain relief through neuromodulation – the use of electrical pulses delivered to the nerves as a treatment, primarily for relieving pain. These therapies offer substantial pain relief and allow some patients to forgo high-risk medications or repeated injections or surgeries. The efficacy of neuromodulation devices and their advantages compared to existing treatments have led to an expanding role for these devices in the treatment of chronic pain and particularly low back pain.

Background and Historical Perspective

The potential for electrical energy delivered to the body to alleviate pain has been noticed as far back as the first century CE, when the electricity-producing torpedo fish were used in Rome to treat arthritis. In 47 CE, a Roman court physician wrote of the accidental discovery of this potential treatment by a man walking on the beach. Use of torpedo fish was subsequently investigated and recommended for conditions such as cephalalgia and arthralgia by other writers throughout the Middle Ages. The seventeenth century saw the first artificial production of electricity with the electrostatic sulfur sphere, combined with the Leyden jar condensers. These tools enabled further applications of neuromodulation for pain relief. In the early 1800s, J. B. Sarlandiere experimented in combining electrical stimulation with the Eastern practice of acupuncture needling. He found that this enhanced the pain relief produced by acupuncture. Numerous cases were reported throughout the 1800s of chronic pain, particularly neuralgias, being relieved with electrical stimulation. Despite this extensive period of successfully treating pain with neuromodulation on a small scale, attention to the therapy declined in the first half of the twentieth century.

The modern interest in neuromodulation as a potential pain treatment was revived in 1965 with Wall and Melczak's gate control theory of pain. Gate control theory suggests that neural structures in the spine act as a kind of gate for sensations passing to the brain. In certain circumstances, such as when a large amount of sensory stimulation is experienced in a specific part of the body, the sensation is gated, meaning the perceived intensity of stimulation is reduced. This provided an explanation for the analgesic effect of electrical stimulation. The electrical stimulation forces the gate closed, leading to the perception of decreased or eliminated pain.

In 1967, Shealy and colleagues published the first report describing a case involving electrical stimulation of the spinal cord providing successful pain relief. In the years since, a number of commercial devices (e.g., spinal cord stimulators [SCS], transcutaneous electrical nerve stimulators [TENS], peripheral nerve stimulators, dorsal root ganglion stimulators, deep brain or motor cortex stimulators) that use electrical stimulation to relieve pain have been developed. These treatments are now widely used and are part of the standard of care for treating many types of chronic pain.

T. L. McJunkin · P. J. Lynch · E. L. Swing (✉)
Arizona Pain Specialists, Scottsdale, AZ, USA
e-mail: DrMcJunkin@PainDoctor.com; DrLynch@PainDoctor.com; TedS@PainDoctor.com

T. R. Deer et al. (eds.), *Deer's Treatment of Pain*, https://doi.org/10.1007/978-3-030-12281-2_68

Uses and Indications

The most widely used implanted neurostimulation device is the spinal cord stimulator (see Figs. 68.1 and 68.2). This device consists of one or more leads, often inserted percutaneously into the spinal canal parallel to the dorsal column in the epidural space. Desired lead placement depends on the targeted areas of pain, but for low back and/or leg pain, placement is typically in the thoracic and/or lumbar spine. These leads are attached to an implanted battery that generates pulses transmitted to specific electrodes located along the ends of the leads.

Percutaneous spinal cord stimulation leads are routinely used for the SCS trial and are commonly used for the permanent implant as well. On the other hand, paddle SCS leads can be placed by a surgeon for the permanent implant and are rarely used for open SCS trials. There are advantages and disadvantages for each that should be discussed. Percutaneous leads are less invasive, don't change the bony spinal anatomy (as paddle leads typically require a laminotomy to place), and are simpler to remove. Paddle leads are more energy efficient as they are unidirectional. Paddle leads also have a much lower incidence of lead migration than percutaneous leads, which remains the largest complication from SCS therapy. Some therapies initially were only available in percutaneous format like HF-10, and some are still currently only available in percutaneous format, like DRG therapy and Stimwave wireless stimulation (Figs. 68.3, 68.4, and 68.5).

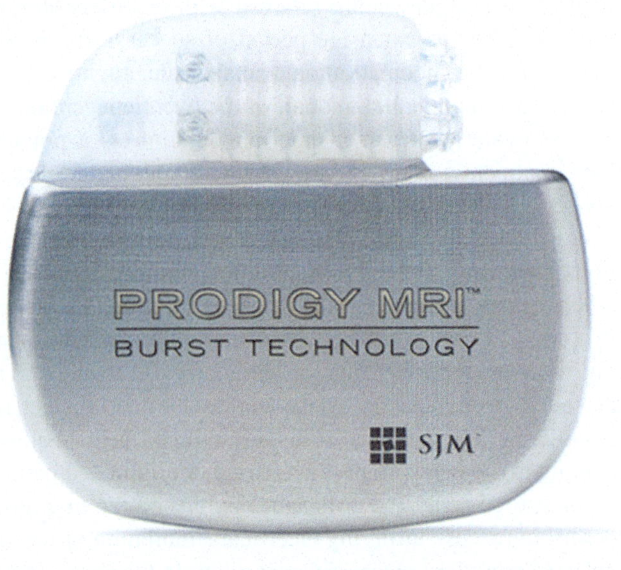

Fig. 68.1 The Abbott Prodigy MRI™ Implantable Pulse Generator (IPG). (Prodigy MRI is a trademark of Abbott or its related companies. Reproduced with permission of Abbott, © 2018. All rights reserved)

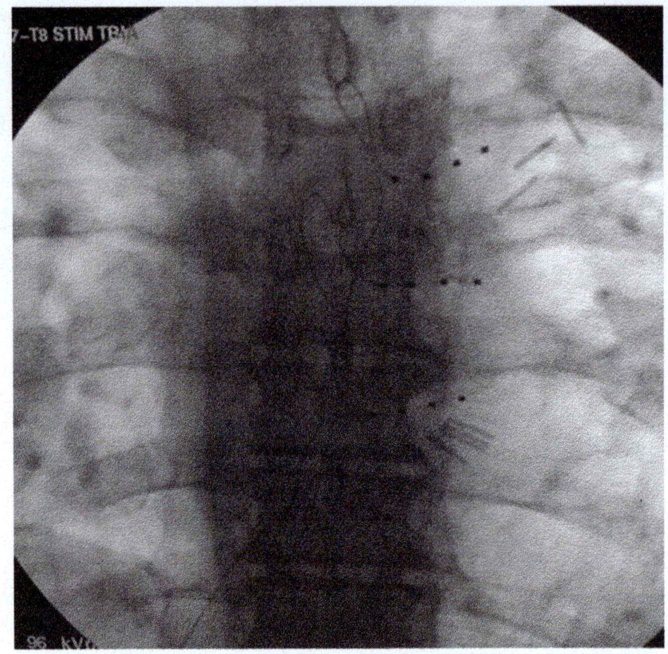

Fig. 68.2 Abbott Medical thoracic DRG lead placement. (Image courtesy of Tim Davis, MD)

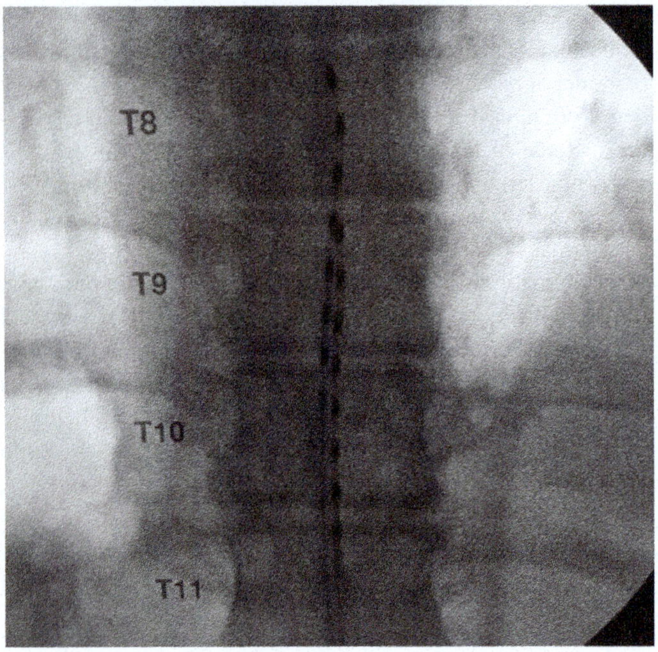

Fig. 68.3 Nevro percutaneous leads with staggered placement at T8/9 and T9/10 with the T9/10 disc "sweet spot" overlapped

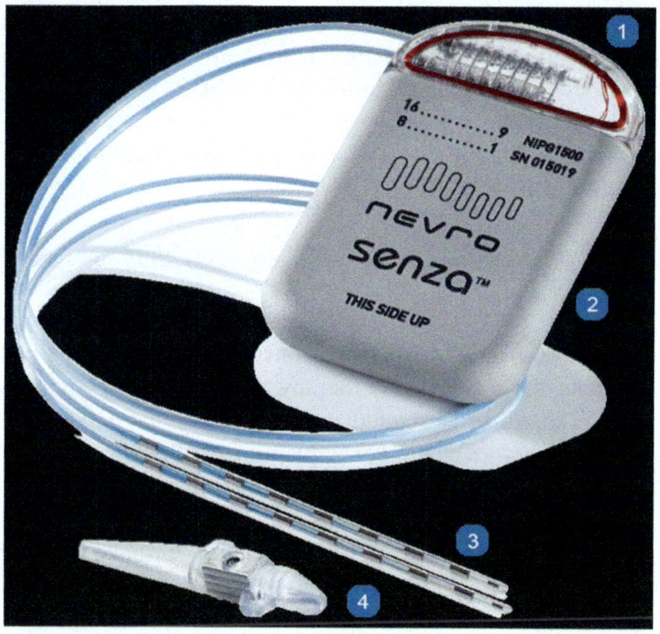

Fig. 68.4 Nevro Senza High Frequency IPG charge coil in header permits rapid charging without additional heat (**1**), Senza IPG (**2**), 8-contact percutaneous leads (**3**), and locking anchors (**4**). (Image courtesy of Nevro. SENZA, HF10, Nevro, and the Nevro logo are trademarks of Nevro Corp)

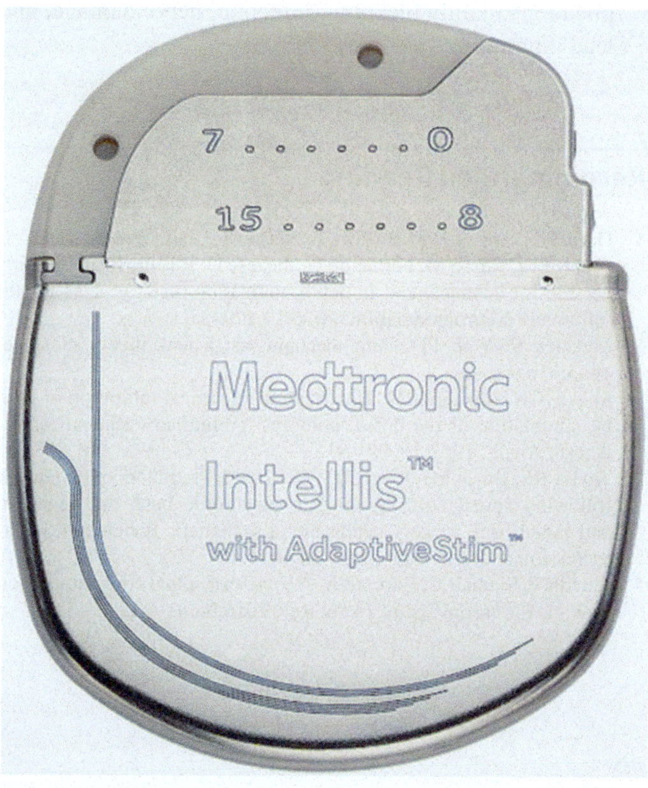

Fig. 68.5 Medtronic Intellis IPG. (Image courtesy of Medtronic. Reproduced with permission from Medtronic)

Waveforms

Traditionally stimulation parameters are programmed to keep stimulation within an appropriate range (high enough to produce pain-relieving paresthesias, but not so high that the electrical stimulation becomes unpleasant or painful), and patients are given a remote to make adjustments to the stimulation within that range. New "pulse trains" or "waveforms" like high frequency stimulation (HF-10), Burst-DR, and high dose (high density) have introduced paresthesia-free stimulation in which a patient does not feel the paresthesias of stimulation but only pain relief. Some technologies also utilize subthreshold stimulation in which electrical energy is programmed just below the patient's ability to perceive it. Upcoming modalities are being studied that adjust paresthesia-based stimulation waveforms in real time based on movements that occur at the level of the spinal cord (Saluda Medical).

New Neural Targets

Dorsal root ganglion (DRG) stimulation is a new type of stimulation that directly stimulates the dorsal root ganglion in precise fashion. Much has been learned about focal neuropathic pain conditions as the therapy has evolved and expanded. The therapy has been FDA approved for type I CRPS and type II CRPS or causalgia. The DRG acts as a clearing house of neurological activity from the peripheral nervous system to the central nervous system. The peripheral nerve cell bodies are located in the DRG, and it is these cell bodies which appear to be damaged and become activated with non-painful stimuli in CRPS and likely other neuropathic pain conditions. DRG stimulation therapy is sub-perception therapy during which the patient does not feel stimulation, but the hyperactive damaged nerves are stimulated and pain sensations are reduced. The ACCURATE study provided Level I evidence that DRG stimulation is superior to conventional stimulation for CRPS.

Additionally, new therapies such as HF-10 have introduced new neural targets or "sweet spots" for certain conditions that have been previously treated. Currently HF-10 focuses on the T9-10 disc space for low back pain which is traditionally lower than conventional stimulation which has primarily focused from T7 to T9. Additionally the HF-10 therapy is being used at C2 for axial neck pain which is higher than has been traditionally used with conventional SCS.

Indications

The traditional teaching is that neurostimulation therapies tend to be most effective for neuropathic pain (as opposed to nociceptive pain) although some are beginning to challenge this assumption. The most common indication and best studied use of spinal cord stimulation is failed back surgery syndrome or post-laminectomy syndrome – patients who have had some type of spine surgery (e.g., discectomy, laminectomy, fusion) and continue to have chronic pain in the back and/or legs. Other common indications for spinal cord stimulation include radicular leg pain, axial low back pain, peripheral neuropathy, complex regional pain syndrome (CRPS), as well as other neuropathic pain conditions. For most of these conditions, SCS is reserved for cases that are not adequately treated by conservative care, advanced medication regiments, and/or minimally invasive interventions. In the cases of FBSS and CRPS, treatment outcomes appear to be better when SCS therapy is delivered sooner after onset of the disease.

Evidence for Efficacy

Spinal cord stimulation has strong evidence of efficacy for several types of pain. A recent meta-analysis identified 74 studies of SCS for treating chronic back and leg pain. Of 63 studies with available data (including 3025 patients), patients received a mean level of 58% pain relief from SCS. A randomized controlled trial (RCT) demonstrated that, among patients with failed back surgery syndrome, patients receiving SCS were more likely to have significant pain relief than those receiving another spine surgery. Other meta-analyses have found that SCS also has Level I evidence for its efficacy in treating neuropathy and complex regional pain syndrome. We also now have Level I evidence in the Nevro Senza Study for treating those with primarily low back pain only.

In the cases of some other types of pain, the evidence for SCS is less clear. For example, some rare conditions (e.g., phantom limb pain, postherpetic neuralgia) have some supportive evidence but have not yet been studied in an RCT. Further, though SCS has demonstrated effectiveness in treating neuropathic pain, some specific types of neuropathies (e.g., diabetic peripheral neuropathy, small fiber neuropathy, idiopathic neuropathy) have not been fully studied as specific indications of SCS.

Pearls and Pitfalls

- Patient selection is probably the most important pearl and/or pitfall for success or failure with an implantable device.
- It is best to have realistic conversations with a patient about the goals of the therapy and specifically areas of pain that may be treated and those areas that may not be treated before trialing or implanting the therapy.
- Because we now have multiple and different unique therapy options, one must truly understand a patient's pain pattern and their overall health picture to make the best decision for a patient.
- It is imperative for doctors to understand the various therapies, their specific pros and cons, and the research that supports them: MRI compatibility, IPG upgradability, targeted focus, paresthesia-based, paresthesia-free, recharge ability, and IPG size are all important to consider.
- One must have a preoperative, intraoperative, and postoperative plan to timely identify and prevent potential complications mainly bleeding, infection, nerve damage, and lead migration.

Recommended Reading

1. Deer T, Skaribas I, McJunkin T, Nelson C, Salmon J, Darnule A, Braswell J, Russo M, Fernando Gomezese O. Results from the partnership for advancement in neuromodulation registry: a 24-month follow-up. Neuromodulation. 2016;19:179–87.
2. Melzack R, Wall PD. Pain mechanisms: a new theory. Science. 1965;150:971–9.
3. Shealy CN, Mortimer JT, Reswick JB. Electrical inhibition of pain by stimulation of the dorsal columns: preliminary clinical report. Anesth Analg. 1967;46:489–91.
4. Taylor RS, Desai MJ, Rigoard P, Taylor RJ. Predictors of pain relief following spinal cord stimulation in chronic back and leg pain and failed back surgery syndrome: a systematic review and meta-regression analysis. Pain Pract. 2014;14:489–505.
5. Verrills P, Sinclair C, Barnard A. A review of spinal cord stimulation systems for chronic pain. J Pain Res. 2016;9:481–92.

Surgical Lead for the Thoracic Spine

69

Geoffrey Stricsek and Steven Falowski

Introduction

Chronic pain impacts more than 100 million people. The direct costs of medical care and the indirect costs of lost productivity have been estimated at $560–635 billion, clearly making this a health crisis. Technology in the field of neuromodulation has been rapidly evolving leading to changes in operative technique for the placement of thoracic spinal cord stimulators.

Background

Historical Perspective

The first use of spinal cord stimulation (SCS) for the treatment of pain was in 1967 when Shealy and colleagues produced stimulation through a Vitallium electrode placed along the dorsal columns of a patient's spine, yielding resolution of his malignancy-induced chest and abdominal pain. The theoretical basis of the results seen in 1967 is rooted in the gate control mechanism of Melzack and Wall which states that activity in large-diameter type Aβ fibers inhibits transmission of noxious information to the brain by small C and Ad fibers. Exogenous stimulation of the larger fibers is believed to inhibit transmission of painful sensation by the smaller fibers. Combining this principle with Barolat's somatotopic mapping, symptom relief can be achieved by generating paresthesias concordant with the distribution of pain. However, newer technology is also able to provide pain relief without generating paresthesias.

G. Stricsek
Neurological Surgery, Thomas Jefferson University, Philadelphia, PA, USA
e-mail: Geoffrey.Stricsek@Jefferson.edu

S. Falowski (✉)
Functional Neurosurgery, Neurosurgical Associates of Lancaster, Lancaster, PA, USA

Stimulation Options

Conventional SCS

Conventional SCS relies on the generation of paresthesias in somatotopic distributions overlapping a patient's pain. Leads are placed in the extradural space over the posterior columns and are connected to an implanted pulse generator which delivers tonic stimulation at a frequency between 40 and 100 Hz. Randomized, controlled studies have demonstrated significant improvement in neuropathic radicular pain and health-related quality of life (HRQOL) metrics when comparing conventional SCS with best medical therapy and even repeat lumbar spine surgery. Where early SCS systems delivered the same current across all the electrodes, recent advances have enabled current adjustment at the level of each contact within an electrode. Fractionalization of current across individual contacts allows the electric field to be directed toward a specific region based on patient feedback, thereby improving paresthesia coverage.

High-Frequency SCS

Modification of conventional SCS hardware and software permitted investigation of a new form of tonic stimulation: high-frequency stimulation at 10,000 Hz (HF10 ® Nevro, Redwood City, CA). High-frequency stimulation provides paresthesia-free pain relief and therefore does not rely on the generation of paresthesias in a distribution overlapping with a patient's pain which allows leads to be placed anatomically without direct patient feedback. Randomized, controlled data has demonstrated significant benefits in pain control when compared with conventional SCS.

Burst SCS

The most recent waveform to receive FDA approval is BurstDR stimulation (Abbott). With the discovery that sensory information may be transmitted by parallel systems where one employs a tonic pattern of neuron firing and the other employs a burst pattern, translational work in an animal model demonstrated that burst firing is a more potent

T. R. Deer et al. (eds.), *Deer's Treatment of Pain*, https://doi.org/10.1007/978-3-030-12281-2_69

activator of the cerebral cortex than tonic firing. Two early studies investigated the effect of exogenously applied burst stimulation in patients with chronic low back and leg pain utilizing 40 Hz bursts with five spikes at 500 Hz per burst: results demonstrated a significant improvement in pain control versus placebo. Burst stimulation was found to be superior to conventional SCS with patient preference for this waveform.

High-Density (HD) Simulation

As conventional SCS pulse generators improved through successive iterations, their programming now permits stimulation frequencies up to 1200 Hz, even though standard programming paradigms remained in the 40–60 Hz range. Recognizing the benefit of a higher rate of energy delivery in burst and high-frequency stimulation for the treatment of chronic pain, the question arose whether maximizing energy utilization from a conventional SCS generator would yield similar results. Standardized programming has led to utilization of PW90 and a rate of 1000 Hz. Data is limited but suggests there may be some clinical benefit.

Technique

SCS therapy begins with placement of trial stimulator leads. The goals of a stimulation trial include identification of patients who may derive a clinically significant benefit from spinal cord stimulation, minimizing patient risk by reducing permanent implantation in those who do not derive significant relief, and minimizing medical waste by reducing the number of unsuccessful permanent implants. While there is no consensus, it is reasonable to obtain an MRI prior to implantation of any spinal cord stimulator lead. The rate of spinal cord injury (SCI) following SCS placement is cited at 0.6–2.35%, and it has been suggested that preoperative MRI can reduce the incidence of SCS-associated SCI.

Paresthesias-Generating SCS

For trial stimulator implantation, patients are often positioned prone on chest roles and sedated with monitored anesthesia care (MAC); alternatively, it may also be performed with the patient awake using only local anesthesia. Most trials utilize percutaneous implantation of cylindrical electrodes into the epidural space. A Tuohy needle is inserted into the skin at the level of the L3 pedicle for entrance into the epidural space at the L1-L2 interspace or the L4 pedicle level on the skin for entrance at the L2-L3 interspace. Entry and target points are localized using a C-arm or a biplanar fluoroscopy suite. A loss of resistance syringe is used to demonstrate entry into the epidural space; once accomplished, an electrode is guided through the needle, navigated to the desired spinal level, and connected to an external pulse generator. When performed under MAC, anesthesia is decreased, and the electrode positioning is adjusted until the patient confirms generation of paresthesias in a distribution overlapping with their pain; this step is unnecessary for procedures conducted with only local anesthesia. If desired, a second Tuohy needle can be inserted for placement of an additional trial lead. Once lead positioning is completed, a final radiograph is taken to document the final location. Trial duration can be variable, usually lasting 7–14 days; however, longer trials are not necessarily associated with an increased likelihood of a positive result.

Typically, a patient is eligible for a permanent implant if they experienced at least a 50% reduction in pain during the trial period. Permanent implants can be a cylindrical lead, similar to those used for the trial, or a paddle lead. While the surgical procedure for paddle implantation can have a slightly higher morbidity since it requires a laminotomy, research has shown that paddle implants offer better clinical results and improved efficiency in terms of battery life when compared to cylindrical percutaneous leads. However, recent advancements in battery technology may have mitigated some of these differences.

Permanent paddle lead implantation can be done with MAC or general anesthesia. Historically, MAC was used so patients could participate in awake testing, but the practice has shifted toward general anesthesia as data have suggested improved outcomes compared with MAC when utilizing neuromonitoring for both cord protection and confirmation of lead placement. When using general anesthesia, patients are sedated with total intravenous anesthesia (TIVA), and neuromuscular blockade is limited to pre-intubation. Following induction of anesthesia, the patient is positioned prone on the operating room table; if the generator is to be implanted in the abdomen, the patient may need to be in the lateral decubitus position. The implant level is determined from the trial and localized on the patient using fluoroscopy; it is important to keep the spinous processes centered between the pedicles and the endplates aligned in order to accurately localize the appropriate level. Laminotomy should be performed as close to the desired level of stimulation as possible to facilitate lead placement; accordingly, the incision is planned one or two levels below the targeted level depending on the paddle length and amount of dead space (Fig. 69.1). Once localized, the patient is prepped and draped in standard fashion with antibiotics administered prior to making incision. Subperiosteal

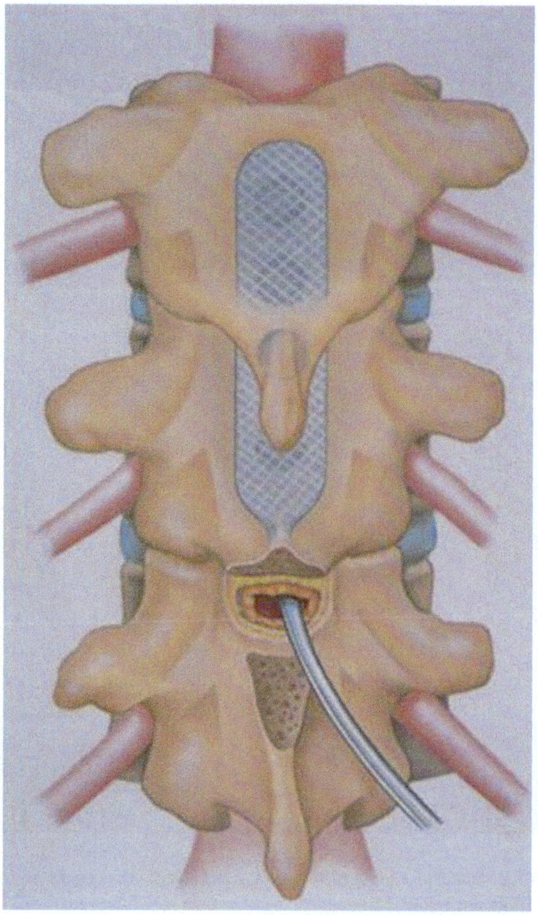

Fig. 69.1 Schematic of dorsal epidural spinal cord stimulator paddle with entry to epidural space planned below the level targeted for stimulation

dissection is performed down to the level of the lamina at which point fluoroscopy can be brought into the field to confirm the appropriate levels. Laminotomy is performed according to surgeon preference and may include the use of a high-speed drill and Leksell and/or Kerrison rongeurs; the ligamentum flavum is removed to expose the thecal sac. There have been reports of paddle placement via a unilateral laminotomy or tubular retractor and decreased length of hospital stay; however, the best procedure for placement is the one a surgeon can do most safely. The epidural space beneath the lamina can be probed with a Woodson tool or Penfield #3 to identify and break up any adhesions. The laminotomy should be wide enough to accommodate the paddle and large enough to allow the paddle to be advanced into the epidural space using a force vector directed parallel to the spinal cord. Dorsal adhesions, ligamentum infolding, or bony spurs may prevent smooth passage of the lead or cause the lead to not lay flat on the dural. If this occurs, additional bony removal may be required at the level of entry or higher levels; however, it is desirable to leave some lamina spanning the thecal sac at each level exposed to prevent the lead from floating away from the cord which could reduce its efficacy. It is generally recommended to place the base of the paddle just superior or at the lamina entry site which can aid in exposure if a revision procedure is ever necessary. This makes the level of entry very important in your preoperative planning.

Once safely in the epidural space, an x-ray is obtained to confirm placement of the lead in anatomic midline at the correct level (Fig. 69.2). At this point the lead can be connected to an external generator to guide any redirection to the physiologic midline and propagation of signal to targeted distributions. Since electrode positioning cannot be guided by patient feedback in the asleep patient, initial positioning is based on lead location from the trial, but intraoperative neuromonitoring (ION) is used to guide final lead placement. Monitoring modalities include somatosensory-evoked potentials (SSEPs), electromyography (EMG), and transcranial motor-evoked potentials. Retrospective and prospective data has shown that compound motor action potentials (CMAPs) generated from spinal cord stimulation can be used to effectively determine paddle position in relation to physiologic midline with paresthesia coverage overlapping painful dermatomes in greater than 90% of patients. ION can also be helpful in determining if a lead is lying flat on the dura by comparing the amplitudes at which a response is generated across

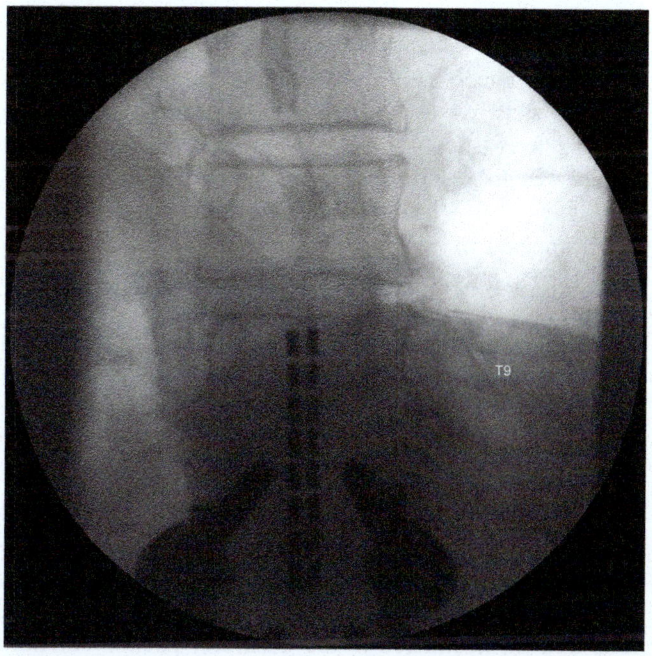

Fig. 69.2 Radiograph confirming midline placement of spinal cord stimulator paddle

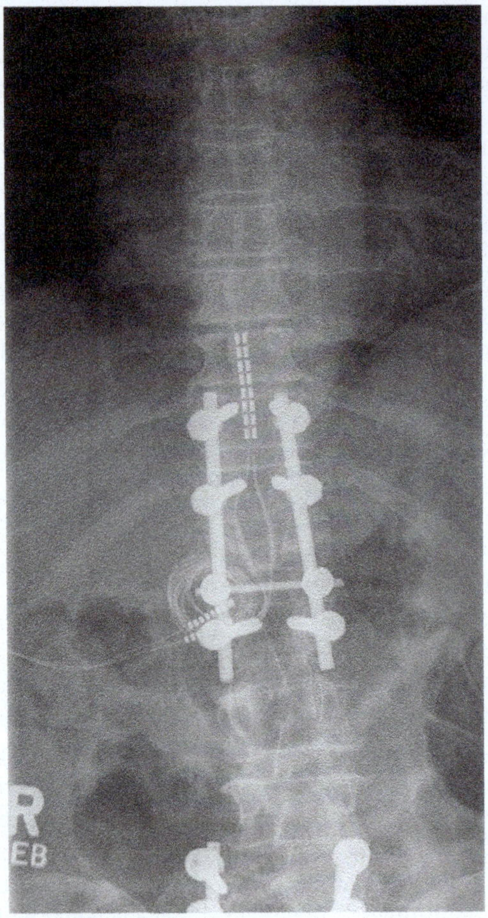

Fig. 69.3 AP radiograph showing paddle placement and strain relief loop with connectors

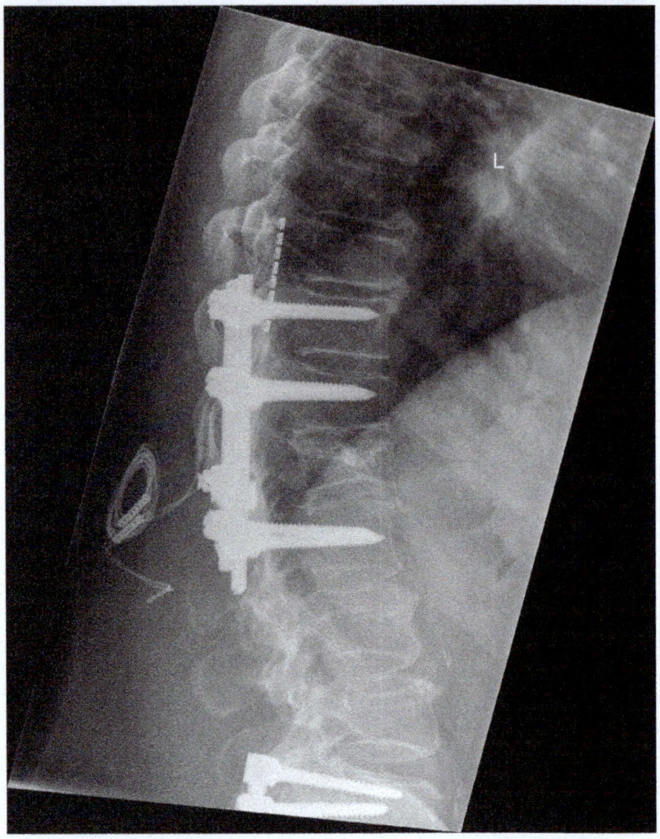

Fig. 69.4 Lateral radiograph showing paddle placement with strain relief loop with connectors

contacts. Prospectively collected data confirmed the therapeutic benefit observed with ION-assisted placement as patients were shown to have significant improvement in pain scores at 12 months, more accurate paresthesia coverage, less adverse events, and decreased operative times. EMG appears to be more effective in lead lateralization than SSEPs, 89% vs. 69%, an important point as anatomic midline does not always correlate with physiologic midline. Despite the success that is possible with ION-guided SCS placement, adequate paresthesia coverage does not guarantee pain relief; long-term data for SCS efficacy is discussed below. After satisfactory positioning is obtained, a strain relief loop is created and anchored to the paraspinal muscles (Figs. 69.3 and 69.4), and then the connectors are tunneled to the subcutaneous pocket where the generator will be implanted. For percutaneously placed leads, the leads are anchored to the fascia utilizing a strain relief loop and then tunneled to the generator pocket. Anchors are supplied with each manufacturer's kit. It is imperative that if an anchor is used, it should traverse the fascia but should not be overtightened to the point that it creates a fracture in the lead.

Non-paresthesia-Generating SCS

Similar to conventional SCS, trial implantation is an important part of patient evaluation. However, unlike conventional SCS, the therapeutic foundation of non-paresthesia-generating SCS does not rely on the generation of overlapping paresthesias. Trial and permanent implantation can be conducted based on individual patient need and clinician preference. Lead placement is solely anatomic and can be determined intraoperatively utilizing fluoroscopy. Buried trials can be inserted with tunneled connectors according to clinician preference and patient need. At the time of writing, paddle leads have recently been introduced for high-frequency stimulation, although in addition to the established cylinder percutaneous leads for this therapy.

Implantation for Non-pain Etiologies

The procedure when implanting a patient for other indications such as angina or ischemic limb pain is similar to above with electrode placement for ischemic limb pain typically between localized T9-L1 and placement for angina usually in upper thoracic spine.

Open Trial Implantation

Open trial implants can be done for patients with a history of prior thoracic and/or lumbar spine surgery where successful percutaneous lead placement would otherwise not be possible due to scar tissue formation and can also be performed with MAC or general anesthesia. Open trial implantation involves creating a laminotomy or laminectomy for placement of paddle stimulators. The benefit is that in a patient with a successful trial, only the generator needs to be implanted; however, for the negative trial, the patient must return to the operating room for removal of leads as opposed to cylindrical leads which can be removed in the office.

Uses and Indications

In the United States, spinal cord stimulation is FDA approved for the treatment of chronic pain. The chronic pain symptom complex encompasses many conditions, including persistent and/or recurrent lower extremity radicular pain following lumbar spine decompression (otherwise known as post-laminectomy syndrome or failed back surgery syndrome); persistent or recurrent axial low back pain; diabetic neuropathy; chronic regional pain syndrome (CRPS); postherpetic neuralgia; pain from severe peripheral vascular disease; pain from intractable angina; and abdominal and pelvic visceral pain.

Evidence for Efficacy

Chronic Pain

Conventional SCS

Kumar et al. observed that nearly 50% of patients derived at least a 50% improvement in lower extremity neuropathic pain after SCS implantation compared with only 9% of patients undergoing medical management at 6 months. This treatment effect was found to be durable at 12 months and even out to 24 months; however, other research has shown that there is a subset of SCS patients who experience decreasing efficacy of stimulation over time. Similar benefits were observed in a randomized, controlled study comparing SCS with reoperation in patients with signs of recurrent neural compression: nearly 50% of subjects had a minimum of 50% pain relief at 6 months with SCS compared with only 12% in the reoperation group. Conventional SCS has also been shown to be an effective treatment for diabetic neuropathy with patients deriving significant reduction in pain compared with medical therapy. Trial data suggested good response to steerable current with 75% of patients undergoing permanent implant after having received at least 50% pain relief. Unfortunately, long-term data from that study is limited owing to receipt of FDA premarket approval; however, 38 of the 49 implanted patients demonstrated an average of 60% pain relief at 3 months, decreasing slightly to an average of 53% pain relief in 34 patients followed out to 6 months.

High-Frequency Stimulation

An early prospective cohort study focusing on chronic low back pain in 25 patients observed greater improvement in VAS scores with high-frequency stimulation as compared with conventional SCS while also demonstrating the ability to achieve paresthesia-free pain relief, thereby challenging the previous paradigm of paresthesia-dependent pain control. Larger prospective trials demonstrated significant improvement of pain scores in 74% of patients with chronic, predominantly low back pain at 6 months and in 60% of patients at 24 months; significant improvements in leg pain were also noted. The observed efficacy of high-frequency stimulation led to a prospective, randomized controlled trial (SENZA-RCT) comparing it with conventional SCS. Results of the SENZA-RCT showed significantly more patients treated with 10,000 Hz stimulation derived a significant improvement in both back and leg pain at 3 and 12 months compared with traditional SCS. These findings were found to be durable with significant differences remaining for both back and leg pain with patients followed to 24 months. Recently released data at a large national meeting demonstrated efficacy of high-frequency stimulation for treatment of chronic neck and upper extremity pain as well. The stimulation frequency of 10,000 Hz may hold particular significance as another study found no difference when comparing sham to high-frequency stimulation at 5000 Hz in a patient population stabilized on conventional SCS.

Burst Stimulation

Early burst studies: Results were found to be equivocal in terms of pain control compared with conventional tonic SCS but did demonstrate a significant improvement versus placebo and an overwhelming patient preference for burst compared with SCS, possibly related to its limited incidence of paresthesias. The initial burst studies looked at differences in pain relief during a 28-day trial period, but subsequent studies have evaluated the impact of burst stimulation in patients who already had a conventional SCS implanted and had received treatment for at least 6 months. In follow-up, burst was shown to significantly reduce foot pain in patients with diabetic neuropathy, back and leg pain in patients with failed back surgery syndrome, and even further decrease leg and back pain in patients who had reduced efficacy of their conventional SCS. Given the positive results, a prospective, randomized controlled trial was undertaken to further evaluate burst versus tonic stimulation: SUNBurst IDE. Specifically designed as a crossover study, patients with medically refractory, chronic back and/or limb pain underwent a trial with conventional SCS and then were randomized to either a burst or conventional SCS treatment arm. Following 12 weeks of treatment, each patient would then be switched to the other therapy form so that each patient would serve as their own control. Final data has not yet been published, but preliminary results and presentations at large society meetings indicate a significant improvement in back, leg, and overall pain scores when comparing burst with conventional SCS. Similar to previous studies, a significant proportion of patients preferred burst stimulation to conventional tonic stimulation. These findings have led to an FDA approval with superiority labeling.

High-Density Stimulation

One study did show a significant improvement in back and leg pain following transition to HD stimulation from SCS; however, their sample size was small and only followed prospectively for 8 weeks. This has subsequently been followed up with a multicenter pivotal trial in which the results have not been published but are promising. This further demonstrates that patients may need to have options and a single waveform may not be universal for patients.

CRPS

Data also supports the efficacy of SCS for the treatment of CRPS. The degree of relief observed has been variable; early studies suggested pain relief in 43–100% of patients with durability of benefit out to 41 months. Follow-up data, however, has been mixed. One randomized, controlled study comparing SCS and physical therapy (PT) with PT alone demonstrated a significant benefit of SCS at 2 years, while this difference disappeared by 5 years. Another retrospective study showed significant improvement in VAS scores at an average of 88 months of follow-up, while a prospective cohort study observed at least a 30% improvement in VAS scores in 41% of patients at 11 years.

Angina

In Europe, SCS has approval for the treatment of refractory angina, in addition to chronic pain. Multiple studies have demonstrated significant improvement in angina pain and health-related quality of life metrics. SCS has also been shown to decrease the incidence of angina attacks and ischemic episodes, as determined by EKG. Efficacy in certain patients with coronary stenosis has even been shown to be comparable to coronary artery bypass grafting (CABG) in terms of mortality, percentage of cardiac deaths, reduction of angina attacks, and consumption of nitrates, while patients undergoing CABG had significantly more cerebrovascular events. Although a recent randomized controlled trial (RCT) was unable to meet recruitment goals for a comparison of SCS with standard of care for the treatment of refractory angina in patients otherwise ineligible for coronary revascularization procedures, a meta-analysis of seven RCTs looking at refractory angina found similar outcomes when comparing SCS with both open and percutaneous cardiac revascularization procedures.

Limb Ischemia

SCS has also been approved for ischemic pain resulting from peripheral vascular disease in Europe. Data from unmatched cohorts consistently demonstrate significant pain relief, increased skin temperature, improved blood flow, and improved healing of ulcers less than 3 cm^2. Evidence from randomized, controlled studies comparing SCS with medical therapy is mixed, with studies showing both a significant difference and no difference in pain relief. A Cochrane review drawing from six studies comparing SCS with conservative treatment found no significant difference in pain relief between groups but did see a significantly higher rate of limb salvage at 12 months in the SCS-treated group.

Abdominal and Visceral Pain

Several case series have demonstrated a benefit of SCS in the treatment of abdominal visceral pain attributed to various pathologies including mesenteric ischemia, irritable bowel syndrome, nonalcoholic pancreatitis, and postoperative abdominal wall neuroma formation. SCS has also been shown to provide improvement in VAS scores in women with a history of endometriosis and chronic visceral pelvic pain.

Pearls and Pitfalls (Table 69.1)

Fortunately, SCS implantation tends to be a well-tolerated procedure. The most common complication is lead migration and can occur in approximately 13% of patients followed by lead breakage in 9%. The risk of infection is slightly higher than 3%; at many institutions, patients with trial implants remain on oral antibiotics throughout the duration of their trial.

Traditional spinal cord stimulation relies on the generation of paresthesias overlapping the area of pain. Successful stimulation with a traditional waveform will deliver paresthesias to the full area of a patient's pain. However, it is also important to avoid paresthesia generation in any non-painful dermatome as it can be uncomfortable for patients and

Table 69.1 Pearls and Pitfalls

Pearls	Pitfalls
Successful opiate alternative	Some patients will have declining efficacy
Consider changing stimulation modalities for patients who have decreasing efficacy	A positive trial does not guarantee effective relief with stimulator implant
Limiting laminotomy size will preserve bone which can help keep the paddle in contact with the dorsal dura	An overtightened anchor can fracture the wires connecting the lead to the generator
Plan surgical incision and laminotomy close to the desired level of stimulation in order to limit the size of the exposure and the amount of epidural dissection	Rechargeable batteries may be an inconvenience for some patients
Preoperative MRI may reduce the risk of placement-induced adverse events	Poor fluoroscopy technique can hamper effective localization and placement
Utilize multiple strain relief loops when anchoring leads to limit the risk of lead migration and fracture	Laminotomies or laminectomies may need to be performed at multiple levels for patients with extensive epidural scarring who are undergoing paddle implantation

potentially negate the otherwise beneficial effects of spinal cord stimulation; this is not a concern in high-frequency stimulation as it is paresthesia-free. Prior to surgery, it is also important to review with patients the different types of pulse generators available for implantation: rechargeable and non-rechargeable. The rechargeable systems have a longer lifetime but require regular charging which can be an inconvenience for some. The high-frequency system only uses a rechargeable battery given its high energy requirement and must be charged daily. Stimulator coverage from both paresthesia- and non-paresthesia-generating SCS can change over time but often can be mitigated with changes in programming. The research behind each form of stimulation has shown they can all provide significant clinical improvement, but there are some patients that do not obtain relief or experience decreasing relief over time. Despite this, it is also clear that different stimulation modalities may provide a benefit where others have failed. While the phenomenon of pain is still poorly understood, it is clear that a single form of spinal cord stimulation will not treat everyone's pain; different forms of pain require different therapeutic modalities.

Percutaneous Lumbar Stimulation

70

Lucas W. Campos and Eric T. Lee

Introduction

Acutely, pain is a signal that tissue damage is occurring and activates a pathway to the brain. Eventually some chronic pain syndromes give those same high intensity neural signals without actual harm occurring. It is estimated that in the United States approximately 100 million people suffer from chronic pain and that 80% of Americans will suffer from back pain at some point in their lives. This can lead to chronic pain that limits activities of daily living and even workplace productivity. Pharmacological treatments, including opiates, physical therapy, or highly invasive spine surgeries, have been used to some degrees of varying success. As SCS became more thoroughly researched, the evidence not only demonstrated the efficacy of SCS but also the cost-effectiveness. Today, current evidence strongly suggests SCS may be used before invasive spinal surgery to treat axial and radicular lumbar spine pain. New SCS strategies employing new frequencies, waveforms, software, and hardware are under development. This chapter will examine the indications and evidence for the use of SCS as well as discuss best methods for lead placement in the lumbar epidural space.

Background and Historical Perspective

Pain has a long history of study as represented in works by Socrates, Aristotle, and Descartes. The word "pain" is derived from the name of the Greek goddess of revenge, Poine, who was sent to punish the mortals who had angered the gods. In more modern times, the nature and evaluation of pain was the subjects of controversy. In the late 1800s, there were at least two well-known opposing theories on the processing of pain: specificity theory and pattern theory. Specificity theory held that pain is a specific modality like vision or hearing, "with its own central and peripheral apparatus." Pattern theory maintained that the nerve impulse pattern of pain is produced by intense stimulation of nonspecific receptors since "there are no specific fibers and no specific endings." These were derived from original theories by von Frey and Goldscheider. These dogmatic theories were well in place when Melzack and Wall published their new theory on the transmission of pain signals in the journal *Science* in 1965. Their new posit was called gate control theory, and it imagined nerve impulses entering the spinal cord through large cutaneous nerve fibers where they came under the influence of a "control mechanism." These impulses were still in the "terminal arborization of the afferent fiber." This gate control mechanism determined the effectiveness of entering pain impulses on central spinal cord cells in the substantia gelatinosa (Fig. 70.1).

It was based on this theory that the neurosurgeon C. Norman Shealy applied stimulating electrodes to the dorsal columns of the spinal cord, where the large fibers were compactly arranged. He claimed that his approach could induce an "electronarcosis." When a pulsed DC of 2 milliamps at 0.3 volts programmed at 50 cycles per second was applied to a dorsal column electrode over the cervical cord, animals could be awake and tolerate forceful tail pinching or intense heat applied to their ears with no apparent distress. Later research suggests that in the absence of the large A-beta fibers, the small unmyelinated C fibers start firing spontaneously in a burst pattern or a series of rapid action potentials followed by a period of quiescence. Thus, without the inhibitory presence of the A-beta fibers, the spontaneous firing of the C fibers produced hyperalgesia leading to the development of neuropathic pain. Therefore by activating these A-beta fibers, as with spinal cord stimulation, the pain-generating activity of the C fibers could be overpowered resulting in analgesia. Electrical stimulation is needed as these A-beta fibers are normally inactive at baseline.

L. W. Campos
Interventional Pain Physicians, Chico, CA, USA

E. T. Lee (✉)
Musculoskeletal Care and Regenerative Medicine,
St Charles Spine Institute, Thousand Oaks, CA, USA

T. R. Deer et al. (eds.), *Deer's Treatment of Pain*, https://doi.org/10.1007/978-3-030-12281-2_70

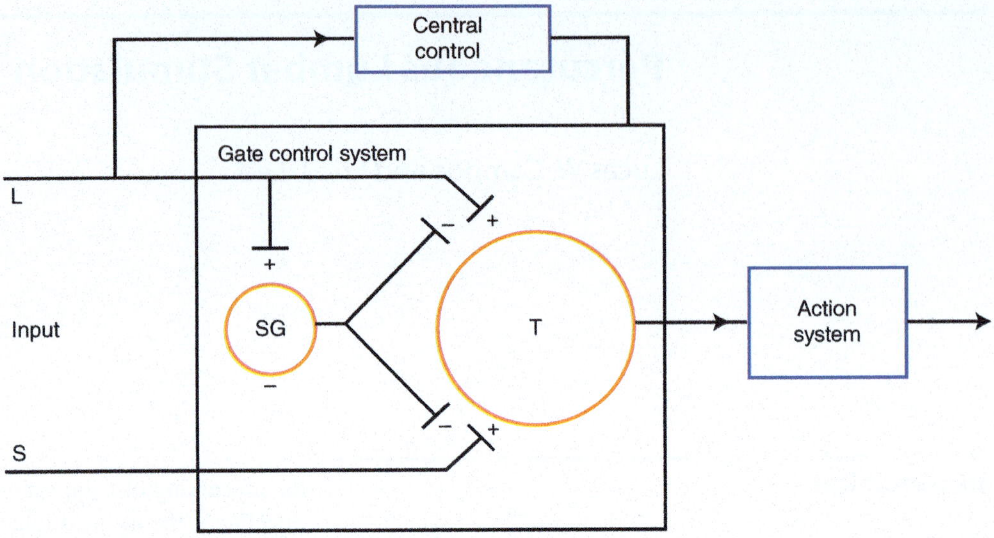

Fig. 70.1 Schematic of the original gate control theory proposed by Melzack and Wall

Uses and Indications

FDA-approved indications for SCS include treatment of pain due to FBSS, chronic painful peripheral neuropathy, multiple sclerosis, and complex regional pain syndrome. Treating FBSS with SCS starts by first excluding the presence of a causative lesion that can be treated surgically. The neuropathic pain component of FBSS is more likely to respond to SCS. The neuropathic component of SCS can manifest as radiculopathy or polyradiculopathy, and causes include epidural fibrosis, arachnoiditis, and intrinsic nerve root damage (radiculitis). The differential diagnosis may exclude entrapment neuropathies and referred pain patterns that may not be amenable to dorsal column treatment. Treatable causes of peripheral neuropathy must be excluded using blood work, electrodiagnostic studies, and, if necessary, nerve biopsy.

Although peripheral vascular disease (PVD) and refractory angina have literature support for treatment by SCS, they are not yet FDA approved. SCS does have a profound effect on sympathetic vascular tone and promotes local blood flow. Improved local blood flow by SCS has been demonstrated to improve ischemic ulcer healing in patients with PVD. As such, many US insurers now cover SCS treatment for this indication. Other conditions that are not FDA approved but have responded well to SCS in the literature include postherpetic neuralgia, post-thoracotomy pain, and phantom limb pain.

The mechanism of SCS treatment is still not well understood but seems to involve a combination of local spinal and supraspinal mechanisms. At the spinal level, the ascending dorsal column fibers, as well as the descending opioidergic and serotonergic pain modulatory systems, might be implicated in the pain-suppressing effect. SCS is also associated with enhanced gamma-aminobutyric acid and acetylcholine release and reduced glutamate transmission in the dorsal horn. For SCS to be effective, factors such as configuration of active electrodes, the stimulation frequency, pulse width, and pulse amplitude are adjusted to fit patient's pain treatment threshold. Electrical stimulation of the large-diameter fibers in the dorsal columns elicits tingling sensations (paresthesias) in most patients. These paresthesia perceptions vary among patients and tolerance varies as well. Some patients reject the device based on these paresthesias, and others prefer to feel them so they know their pain is being covered.

Evidence for Efficacy

As with any medical treatment, there exist some evidence gaps for SCS in the treatment of low back pain which have yet to be filled. So far, several randomized control trials exist which have examined the efficacy of SCS. All three of these trials clearly demonstrated the effectiveness of SCS for lumbar FBSS. With the advent of paresthesia-free SCS, as seen in HF10 and burst, placebo-controlled trials may now be conducted. Pulse shape is one factor that determines nerve fiber response to SCS. Another essential factor is the frequency of the pulse used to activate the large fibers in the dorsal columns. The frequencies of the SCS impulses used in conventional SCS are usually around 50 Hz but can vary between 30 and 120 Hz. New types of stimulation paradigms for SCS have used HF10, burst stimulation, and high-density (HD) stimulation.

HF10

Clinical evidence strongly supports the efficacy and safety of 10 kHz, high-frequency therapy in treating chronic neuropathic lumbar spine and limb pain. Kapural et al. conducted the largest RCT ever completed involving dorsal column stimulation. This study demonstrated clear superiority of HF10 over traditional tonic stimulation and followed patients for 24 months. Later, Grider et al. performed a methodological, systematic review of RCTs which evaluated SCS treatment of chronic pain. The HF10 study by Kapural received the highest quality score among all evaluated RCTs. Despite this initial strong evidence for HF10, evidence gaps continue to exist regarding optimal frequency use in SCS. Shechter et al. demonstrated no additional analgesic benefit when comparing 1000 Hz with 10,000 Hz in an animal study.

It has been shown that stimulation frequencies higher than 50 Hz demonstrated earlier onset of effect and require a lower intensity in order to therapeutically activate A-beta fibers that attenuate pain signals in the central nervous system. Perruchoud et al. did not find any additional benefit of 5000 Hz frequency treatment, as compared with sham, in individuals with previous successful traditional SCS. Factors that confound the evidence used in examining the effectiveness of various frequencies include waveform, programming, and lead placement. In a study examining higher frequencies in the range of 200 to 1000 Hz vs traditional SCS, the higher frequencies significantly altered mechanical pain thresholds as well as vibratory detection. Two small studies have also suggested that traditional SCS at higher frequencies (1000–1200 Hz range) can restore therapy in individuals previously thought to have become refractory to dorsal column stimulation. Some animal and clinical studies suggest that there could be a frequency range, below 10,000 Hz, which may provide analgesia at sub-perception threshold levels. The mechanism of action of HF10 and how it differs from traditional SCS is currently under intense investigation.

Burst

Burst stimulation delivers 5 consecutive 500 Hz bursts 40 times per second with a quiescent interspike interval (Fig. 70.2). Burst stimulation mirrors some of the neuronal firing patterns in the spinal cord associated with pain. These neurons fire in groups of action potentials followed by periods of quiescence. Other neurons at the same stage of sensory processing fire in a tonic or continuous manner. These transmitted neuronal languages allow communication from the spinal cord to the brain. To intervene effectively, an SCS device should speak these same languages. Laboratory and clinical studies suggest that both bursting and tonically firing neurons efficiently transmit information to the thalamus and brain. Laboratory animal studies suggest that burst firing is more powerful than tonic firing in activating the cerebral cortex. These studies have been interpreted as showing that burst activation requires less temporal integration and may activate dormant neurons not activated by tonic stimulation.

Burst SCS therapy has paresthesia-reduced or paresthesia-free programming parameters. A recent systematic review evaluating five studies of burst SCS use in chronic back and limb pain demonstrated limited evidence of efficacy. Studies involving burst have mainly consisted of short-duration, trial phase studies from 1 hour to 3 weeks and involved patients with existing SCS systems. The data reported shows that burst stimulation may result in an improvement in pain control when compared with traditional stimulation. The reduced and paresthesia-free stimulation parameters that can be used with burst are preferred by a substantial portion of patients. In a recent prospective randomized, double-blind, placebo-controlled study examining burst treatment of FBSS syndrome, burst was compared with 500 Hz tonic stimulation and placebo stimulation. In 1 week, this resulted in significantly better pain relief and improved quality of life compared with 500 Hz or placebo stimulation.

Burst stimulation seems to have an effect on the attention paid to pain and pain changes, analogous to cingulotomy. This observation suggests a novel mechanism of action for burst SCS through activation of the dorsal anterior cingulate and the right dorsolateral prefrontal cortex and has been substantiated using electroencephalogram studies. The idea that burst can modulate the affective and attentional pain pathways may give it a unique indication for chronic pain treatment. Traditional SCS is thought to

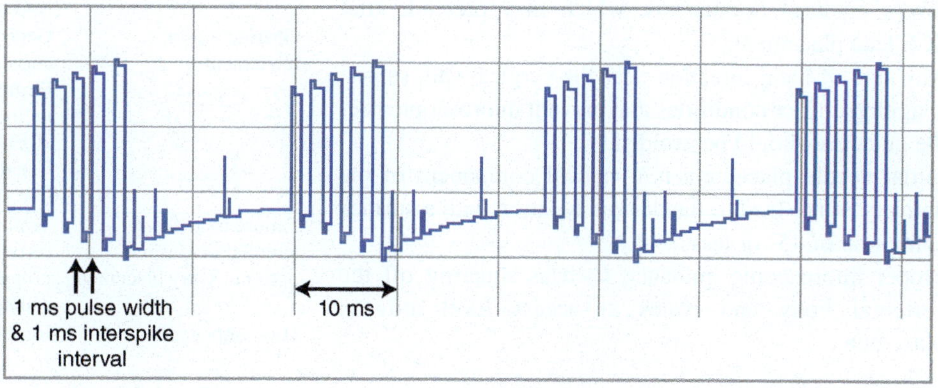

Fig. 70.2 Constant current burst mode (mA) showing 500 Hz spike mode and a 5 ms charge balance at 40 Hz

mainly treat the lateral, discriminatory pain pathways; however, a recent functional magnetic resonance imaging (fMRI) study demonstrated that traditional SCS also affects the medial pain system as well as regions of the brain thought to be involved with negative emotional pain processing centers.

Pearls and Pitfalls

- Accurate diagnosis is important to maximize the appropriateness of SCS therapy.
- Differential diagnosis of axial neuropathic back pain, not associated with prior surgery, is extensive and includes vertebral body compression fracture, discogenic pain, facet arthropathy, and sacroiliac joint arthropathy. Less common causes of chronic low back pain include spinal stenosis, spondylolisthesis, and myofascial pain syndrome.
- Realistic goals and expectations must be established with the patient regarding SCS treatment. The patient should understand that success with SCS is typically defined as a significant reduction in their pain and improvement in function.
- Patients must possess the cognitive ability to understand the device's purpose and how to manage the various stimulation patterns and settings available.
- Psychological factors such as untreated depression, anxiety, and addiction can predict a poor response even when the procedure is clinically indicated and the procedure is performed perfectly.
- Physical characteristics must be considered prior to electrode implantation.
- Patients should have thoracic imaging to ensure that there is adequate space to accommodate trial leads without producing iatrogenic spinal cord compression. These may include flexion and extension X-rays and CT and MRI study examination for possible need of corrective spine surgery instead of SCS.
- MRI helps determine the presence of severe soft tissue disturbances such as ligamentum flavum hypertrophy or severe epidural lipomatosis, which may preclude trial SCS lead placement.
- Any sign of local infection near the surgical site, sepsis, coagulopathy, or conditions that prevent fluoroscopic needle guidance should be avoided.
- Initial needle placement is a critical component of the delivery of the lead to the desired location with a surface entry goal of 45° or less.
- Proper fluoroscopic guidance such as squaring off the vertebral body end plates at access level aids in placement.
- Practitioners should have a low threshold for using multiple views such as lateral and oblique as well as withdrawing and readvancing if the lead encounters resistance.
- Physiologic midline does not always correlate with anatomic midline.
- Minimal sedation may provide a higher safety margin.
- Securing the leads for the duration of the trial is imperative to maintain efficacy.

Procedural and Technical Considerations

After proper patient selection and preoperative evaluation, one should plan what region of the spinal cord will be target for stimulation. In doing so, one will also need to develop a strategy for the needle placement to achieve this end. This should include the level of entry, angle, side, and method of identifying the epidural space. In many cases, guiding the lead may be simple. Easily identifiable landmarks coupled with good anatomy, an easily placed needle at the proper angle, and little to no obstructions in the posterior epidural space, and one may find this aspect to be simple from a technical perspective. However, not every case will afford such ease; many patients in need of a spinal cord stimulator may also have pathologies that can make lead guidance quite difficult. Many of these pathologies (Table 70.1) go hand in hand with their pain (i.e., epidural fibrosis and scarring resulting from previous surgery), which may facilitate some predictability prior

Table 70.1 Typical causes of obstructions encountered while steering the lead

Problem	Suggestion
Tight exit for lead	Lower the needle angle and approach at 45° or less on the axis of the ligamentum flavum
Paresthesia	Immediately remove the lead and/or needle; replace once the symptoms dissipate
Lateral lead movement	Rotate the hub of the needle or rotate the lead using the curved stylet
Obstruction to movement	Gently reposition the lead alternating the curved and straight stylet Gently tap the lead against the obstruction on multiple rapid attempts, withdrawing slightly each time Use the wire coil to pass the obstruction (use caution, and stop if pain occurs)
Failure to achieve stimulation despite optimal X-ray placement	Troll with the lead to find an area responsive to stimulation; try different programming arrays including a guarded cathode
High impedance	Reposition the lead cephalad or caudad

to beginning the procedure. As with any medical procedure, one must be prepared to make the proper adjustments when presented with unexpected difficulties to ensure a good outcome.

Needle placement into the epidural space with the goal to facilitate the placement of a percutaneous lead for spinal cord stimulation can present a unique set of variance and challenge. Needle placement should be viewed as a critical portion of the procedure – carefully planned and executed. In the case of a patient with history of spinal surgery involving a laminectomy, the ligamentum flavum will not be available at a particular level. This will in turn prevent loss of resistance as a viable technique into the epidural space so an alternative level must be chosen. Additionally, if a particular region of the spine is known to have severe scar tissue, adhesions, or stenosis, lead passage may be difficult or even impossible. Considerations such as these emphasize the importance of needle placement and preoperative planning.

Once the lead has exited the needle and entered the epidural space, the next component to give careful consideration is the stylet; this is the mechanism with which the lead will be guided through epidural space. Steering the lead requires patience, a gentle approach, and finesse as an improperly advanced lead can cause trauma or dural tearing. Once the lead is driven to the desired target, handheld computer testing can be used to assure that the patient has the desired response. In the event the response is not optimal, additional modifications may be needed. When the clinician is satisfied with the placement, a fluoroscopic image should be taken on lateral and anterior–posterior views and saved for future comparisons if there are any concerns about lead migration.

Cord or Nerve Root Injury

The risk of nerve injury should be considered when guiding a lead to the target zone. The lead is likely to contact a nerve root or dorsal root ganglion while being advanced if it strays laterally. If an excessive amount of force is used, the lead may cause injury when it makes contact. There are cases where a lead was advanced into the subdural space, unbeknown to the implanter, with the tip ultimately entering into the mass of the spinal cord causing paralysis (Fig. 70.3). In this particular case, the patient was under heavy sedation and unable to converse. These complications were only discovered when the patient was unable to wake up during recovery.

To avoid injury, the patient should be kept alert and conversant during lead placement. In the event the lead were to cause a paresthesia, the patient would be able to relay their discomfort, and the physician can adjust their trajectory accordingly.

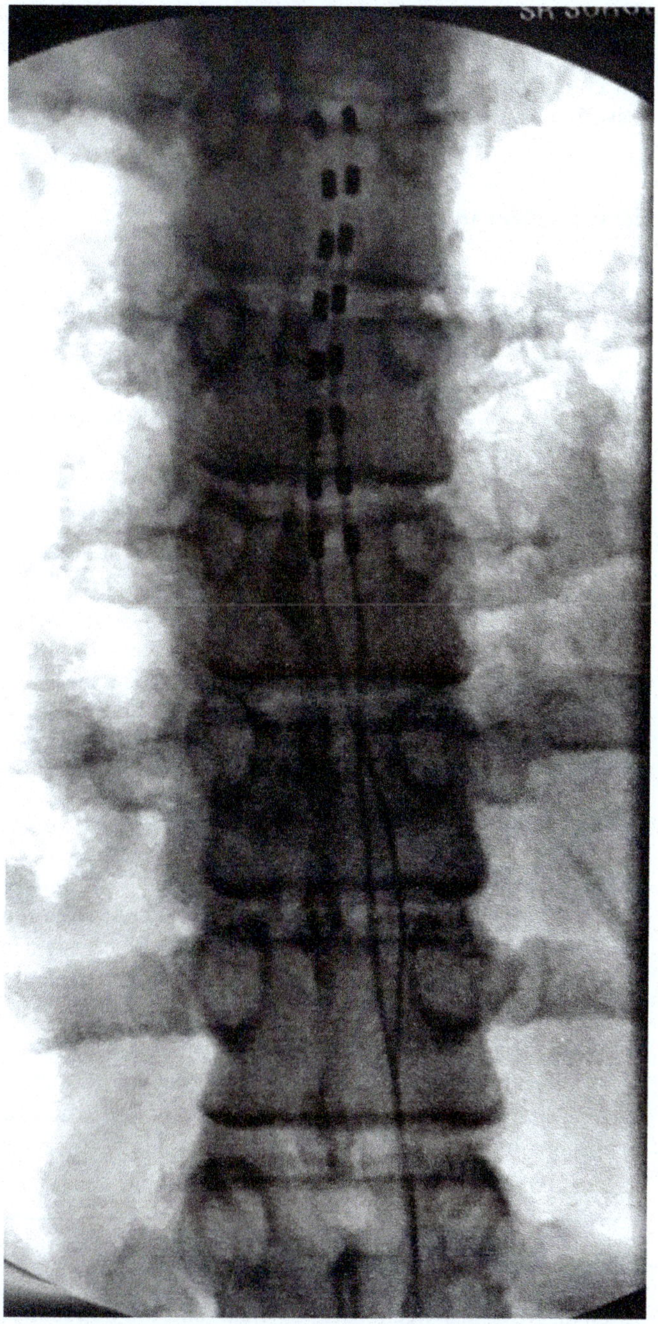

Fig. 70.3 Fluoroscopic image of a stimulator lead placement during a spinal cord stimulator trial. Octrode lead tips are at the top of T7

Dural Tear

Despite having a blunted tip, the lead can still cause a rent in the dura. If the lead is forcefully advanced thereafter, a dural tear may result and possibly lead to chronic leakage of the cerebrospinal fluid (CSF) and a post-dural puncture headache. The overall incidence of CSF leakage from a dural tear caused in the course of implanting a percutaneous lead has been reported at 0.3–7%. In the event an obstruction is encountered, one should be wary of a dural tear as a potential complication. The lead should only be advanced when resistance is minimal.

Epidural Hematoma

The epidural space is rich with fat and vessels. These vessels make epidural bleeding and anticoagulation status a concern. The lead has the potential to dissect an epidural vessel and cause a bleed potentially resulting in an epidural hematoma. The incidence of an epidural hematoma from a spinal cord stimulator lead has been reported at 0.19% and is considered by some to be underreported as many are asymptomatic. One should take careful stock of any medications that could potentially alter a patient's bleeding function, thus leading to this complication. The decision to stop Coumadin, Plavix (Clopidogrel), and other such drugs should be made by the prescribing physician. Laboratory values such as a complete blood count (CBC), comprehensive metabolic panel (CMP), and PT/INR should be considered prior to moving forward.

Motor Stimulation

If a lead strays too far laterally from midline, it has the potential to slide into the "gutter" of the epidural canal and even venture into the anterior epidural space. When activated in either the far lateral or anterior position, the lead may cause motor nerve stimulation that can be very painful and stressful to the patient. To avoid this, the lead should be advanced as proximal to the midline as possible in the anterior/posterior view, and a lateral image should be taken to assure the lead is not positioned ventrally.

Conclusion

Lumbar SCS has been used to treat chronic intractable pain for 40 years by dorsal horn neurons. SCS may work by inhibiting the conduction of pain signals to the brain according to the gate control theory proposed by Melzack and Wall in 1965. FBSS is defined as persistent back and/or leg pain after spine surgery. FBSS implies a constellation of different symptoms and etiologies including recurrent herniation, arachnoiditis, and epidural fibrosis. Since a significant percentage of FBSS patients experience some form of neuropathic pain, many of them may be good candidates for SCS. Although recent advances in SCS technology have improved pain coverage in many neuropathic conditions using burst, HF10, and HD, individuals with FBSS are still widely acknowledged to be the best candidates for this treatment. While SCS may reduce pain, it will not eliminate pain and this must be expected by the patient. The number and type of leads (unipolar, bipolar, or multipolar) and the parameters of stimulation (amplitude, pulse width, frequency) may vary depending on the nerve roots involved and the intensity of the pain being experienced by the patient. Appreciation for the technical difficulty of lumbar SCS lead placement is very important as is the psychological state of a prospective patient. Further evidence of effectiveness and safety of SCS is needed. Nonindustry-supported studies will provide patients and physicians with further unbiased clarity and provide a better understanding of lumbar spine neuromodulation as a valuable treatment.

Recommended Reading

1. Al-Kaisy A, Van Buyten J-P, Smet I, Palmisani S, Pang D, Smith T. Sustained effectiveness of 10 kHz high-frequency spinal cord stimulation for patients with chronic, low back pain: 24-month results of a prospective multicenter study. Pain Med. 2014;15:347–54.
2. Al-Kaisy A, Palmisani S, Smith T. The use of 10-kilohertz spinal cord stimulation in a cohort of patients with chronic neuropathic limb pain refractory to medical management. Neuromodulation Technol Neural Interface. 2015;18(1):18–23.
3. Amirdelfan K, McRoberts P, Deer TR. The differential diagnosis of low back pain: a primer on the evolving paradigm. Neuromodulation. 2014;17(Suppl 2):11–7.
4. Arle JE, Mei L, Carlson KW. High-frequency stimulation of dorsal column axons: potential underlying mechanism of paresthesia-free neuropathic pain relief. Neuromodulation Technol Neural Interface. 2016;19(4):385–97.
5. Atkinson L, Sundaraj SR, Brooker C, O'Callaghan J, Teddy P, Salmon J, Semple T, Majedi PM. Recommendations for patient selection in spinal cord stimulation. J Clin Neurosci. 2011;18:1295–302.
6. Bala MM, Riemsma RP, Nixon J, Kleijnen J. Systematic review of the (cost-)effectiveness of spinal cord stimulation for people with failed back surgery syndrome. Clin J Pain. 2008;24:741–56.
7. Beltrutti D, Lamberto A, Barolat G, et al. The psychological assessment of candidates for spinal cord stimulation for chronic pain management. Pain Pract. 2004;4:204–21.
8. Chou R, Baisden J, Carragee EJ, Resnick DK, Shaffer WO, Loeser JD. Surgery for low back pain: a review of the evidence for an American Pain Society Clinical Practice Guideline. Spine. 2009;34:1094–109.
9. Cohen RA, Kaplan RF, Moser DJ, Jenkins MA, Wilkinson H. Impairments of attention after cingulotomy. Neurology. 1999;53:819–24.
10. De Ridder D, Vanneste S, Plazier M, van der Loo E, Menovsky T. Burst spinal cord stimulation: toward paresthesia-free pain suppression. Neurosurgery. 2010;66:986–90.
11. De Ridder D, Plazier M, Kamerling N, Menovsky T, Vanneste S. Burst spinal cord stimulation for limb and back pain. World Neurosurg. 2013;80:642–649.e1.
12. De Ridder D, Vancamp T, Lenders MWPM, De Vos CC, Vanneste S. Is preoperative pain duration important in spinal cord stimulation? A comparison between tonic and burst stimulation. Neuromodulation. 2015;18:13–7; discussion 17.
13. De Ridder D, Lenders MWPM, De Vos CC, Dijkstra-Scholten C, Wolters R, Vancamp T, Van Looy P, Van Havenbergh T, Vanneste

S. A 2-center comparative study on tonic versus burst spinal cord stimulation: amount of responders and amount of pain suppression. Clin J Pain. 2015;31:433–7.
14. Deer T, Pope J, Hayek S, Narouze S, Patil P, Foreman R, Sharan A, Levy R. Neurostimulation for the treatment of axial back pain: a review of mechanisms, techniques, outcomes, and future advances. Neuromodulation. 2014;17(Suppl 2):52–68.
15. Deer TR, Narouze S, Provenzano DA, et al. The Neurostimulation Appropriateness Consensus Committee (NACC): Recommendations on bleeding and coagulation management in neurostimulation devices. Neuromodulation. 2017;20:51–62.
16. Deogaonkar M, Sharma M, Oluigbo C, et al. Spinal cord stimulation (SCS) and functional magnetic resonance imaging (fMRI): modulation of cortical connectivity with therapeutic SCS. Neuromodulation. 2016;19:142–53.
17. Flacco ME, Manzoli L, Boccia S, et al. Head-to-head randomized trials are mostly industry sponsored and almost always favor the industry sponsor. J Clin Epidemiol. 2015;68:811–20.
18. Frot M, Mauguière F, Magnin M, Garcia-Larrea L. Parallel processing of nociceptive A-delta inputs in SII and midcingulate cortex in humans. J Neurosci. 2008;28:944–52.
19. Grider JS, Manchikanti L, Carayannopoulos A, et al. Effectiveness of spinal cord stimulation in chronic spinal pain: a systematic review. Pain Physician. 2016;19:E33–54.
20. Guido W, Sherman SM. Response latencies of cells in the cat's lateral geniculate nucleus are less variable during burst than tonic firing. Vis Neurosci. 1998;15:231–7.
21. Gybels J, Erdine S, Maeyaert J, et al. Neuromodulation of pain. A consensus statement prepared in Brussels 16–18 January 1998 by the following task force of the European Federation of IASP Chapters (EFIC). Eur J Pain. 1998;2:203–9.
22. Haider S, Owusu-Sarpong S, Peris Celda M, Wilock M, Prusik J, Youn Y, Pilitsis JG. A single center prospective observational study of outcomes with tonic cervical spinal cord stimulation. Neuromodulation. 2017;20:263–8.
23. Hayek SM, Veizi E, Hanes M. Treatment-limiting complications of percutaneous spinal cord stimulator implants: a review of eight years of experience from an academic center database. Neuromodulation Technol Neural Interface. 2015;*18*(7):603–9.
24. Holsheimer J, Buitenweg JR. Review: bioelectrical mechanisms in spinal cord stimulation. Neuromodulation. 2015;18:161–70; discussion 170.
25. Hou S, Kemp K, Grabois M. A systematic evaluation of burst spinal cord stimulation for chronic back and limb pain. Neuromodulation. 2016;19:398–405.
26. Kapural L, Yu C, Doust MW, et al. Novel 10-kHz High-Frequency Therapy (HF10 Therapy) is superior to traditional low-frequency spinal cord stimulation for the treatment of chronic back and leg pain: The SENZA-RCT randomized controlled trial. Anesthesiology. 2015;123:851–60.
27. Kapural L, Yu C, Doust MW, et al. Comparison of 10-kHz High-Frequency and Traditional Low-Frequency Spinal Cord Stimulation for the Treatment of Chronic Back and Leg Pain: 24-Month Results From a Multicenter, Randomized, Controlled Pivotal Trial. Neurosurgery. 2016;79:667–77.
28. Krames ES, Oakley JC, Foster AM, Henderson J, Prager JP, Rashbaum RR, Stamatos J, Weiner RL. Spinal cord stimulation has comparable efficacy in common pain etiologies. Neuromodulation. 2008;11:171–81.
29. Kreis PG, Fishman S. Spinal cord stimulation: percutaneous implantation techniques: Oxford University Press; 2009.
30. Kulkarni B, Bentley DE, Elliott R, Youell P, Watson A, Derbyshire SWG, Frackowiak RSJ, Friston KJ, Jones AKP. Attention to pain localization and unpleasantness discriminates the functions of the medial and lateral pain systems. Eur J Neurosci. 2005;21:3133–42.
31. Kumar K, Wilson JR. Factors affecting spinal cord stimulation outcome in chronic benign pain with suggestions to improve success rate. Acta Neurochir Suppl. 2007;97:91–9.
32. Kumar K, Taylor RS, Jacques L, et al. Spinal cord stimulation versus conventional medical management for neuropathic pain: a multicentre randomised controlled trial in patients with failed back surgery syndrome. Pain. 2007;132:179–88.
33. Kumar K, Taylor RS, Jacques L, et al. The effects of spinal cord stimulation in neuropathic pain are sustained: a 24-month follow-up of the prospective randomized controlled multicenter trial of the effectiveness of spinal cord stimulation. Neurosurgery. 2008;63:762–70; discussion 770.
34. Kumar K, Caraway DL, Rizvi S, Bishop S. Current challenges in spinal cord stimulation. Neuromodulation. 2014;17(Suppl 1):22–35.
35. Lopez-Garcia JA, King AE. Membrane properties of physiologically classified rat dorsal horn neurons in vitro: correlation with cutaneous sensory afferent input. Eur J Neurosci. 1994;6:998–1007.
36. Manchikanti L, Manchikanti KN, Pampati V, Brandon DE, Giordano J. The prevalence of facet-joint-related chronic neck pain in postsurgical and nonpostsurgical patients: a comparative evaluation. Pain Pract. 2008;8:5–10.
37. Mekhail NA, Cheng J, Narouze S, Kapural L, Mekhail MN, Deer T. Clinical applications of neurostimulation: forty years later. Pain Pract. 2010;10:103–12.
38. Mekhail N, Wentzel DL, Freeman R, Quadri H. Counting the costs: case management implications of spinal cord stimulation treatment for failed back surgery syndrome. Prof Case Manag. 2011;16:27–36.
39. Melzack R, Wall PD. Pain mechanisms: a new theory. Science. 1965;150:971–9.
40. Moayedi M, Davis KD. Theories of pain: from specificity to gate control. J Neurophysiol. 2013;109:5–12.
41. Nelson DV, Kennington M, Novy DM, Squitieri P. Psychological selection criteria for implantable spinal cord stimulators. Pain Forum. 1996;5:93–103.
42. Nielson DM, Yang X, Vera-Portocarrero L, Molnar GF. Spinal cord stimulation (SCS) and functional magnetic resonance imaging (fMRI): modulation of cortical connectivity with therapeutic SCS. utd.edu.
43. North JM, Hong K, Cho PY. Clinical outcomes of 1 kHz subperception spinal cord stimulation in implanted patients with failed paresthesia-based stimulation: results of a prospective randomized controlled trial. Neuromodulation Technol Neural Interface. 2016;*19*(7):731–7.
44. Oswald A-MM, Chacron MJ, Doiron B, Bastian J, Maler L. Parallel processing of sensory input by bursts and isolated spikes. J Neurosci. 2004;24:4351–62.
45. Pai S, Sundaram LJ. Low back pain: an economic assessment in the United States. Orthop Clin North Am. 2004;35:1–5.
46. Perruchoud C, Eldabe S, Batterham AM, et al. Analgesic efficacy of high-frequency spinal cord stimulation: a randomized double-blind placebo-controlled study. Neuromodulation. 2013;16:363–9; discussion 369.
47. Pope JE, Falowski S, Deer TR. Advanced waveforms and frequency with spinal cord stimulation: burst and high-frequency energy delivery. Expert Rev Med Devices. 2015;12:431–7.
48. Price DD. Psychological and neural mechanisms of the affective dimension of pain. Science. 2000;288:1769–72.
49. Evans C. Relieving pain in America: a blueprint for transforming prevention, care, education, and research. Washington, DC: National Academies Press (US); 2012.
50. Rinaldi PC, Young RF, Albe-Fessard D, Chodakiewitz J. Spontaneous neuronal hyperactivity in the medial and intralaminar thalamic nuclei of patients with deafferentation pain. J Neurosurg. 1991;74:415–21.

51. Rupert MP, Lee M, Manchikanti L, Datta S, Cohen SP. Evaluation of sacroiliac joint interventions: a systematic appraisal of the literature. Pain Physician. 2009;12:399–418.
52. Russo M, Van Buyten J-P. 10-kHz high-frequency SCS therapy: a clinical summary. Pain Med. 2015;16:934–42.
53. Russo M, Verrills P, Mitchell B, Salmon J, Barnard A, Santarelli D. High frequency spinal cord stimulation at 10 kHz for the treatment of chronic pain: 6-month Australian clinical experience. Pain Physician. 2016;19:267–80.
54. Saadé NE, Jabbur SJ. Nociceptive behavior in animal models for peripheral neuropathy: spinal and supraspinal mechanisms. Prog Neurobiol. 2008;86:22–47.
55. Shealy CN, Taslitz N, Mortimer JT, Becker DP. Electrical inhibition of pain: experimental evaluation. Anesth Analg. 1967a;46:299–305.
56. Shealy CN, Mortimer JT, Reswick JB. Electrical inhibition of pain by stimulation of the dorsal columns: preliminary clinical report. Anesth Analg. 1967b;46:489–91.
57. Shechter R, Yang F, Xu Q, et al. Conventional and kilohertz-frequency spinal cord stimulation produces intensity-and frequency-dependent inhibition of mechanical hypersensitivity in a rat model of neuropathic pain. J Am Soc Anesthesiol. 2013;119:422–32.
58. Smith H, Youn Y, Pilitsis JG. Successful use of high-frequency spinal cord stimulation following traditional treatment failure. Stereotact Funct Neurosurg. 2015;93:190–3.
59. Song Z, Ultenius C, Meyerson BA, Linderoth B. Pain relief by spinal cord stimulation involves serotonergic mechanisms: an experimental study in a rat model of mononeuropathy. Pain. 2009;147:241–8.
60. Song Z, Viisanen H, Meyerson BA, Pertovaara A, Linderoth B. Efficacy of kilohertz-frequency and conventional spinal cord stimulation in rat models of different pain conditions. Neuromodulation. 2014;17:226–34; discussion 234–5.
61. Stancák A, Kozák J, Vrba I, Tintera J, Vrána J, Polácek H, Stancák M. Functional magnetic resonance imaging of cerebral activation during spinal cord stimulation in failed back surgery syndrome patients. Eur J Pain. 2008;12:137–48.
62. Swadlow HA, Gusev AG. The impact of "bursting" thalamic impulses at a neocortical synapse. Nat Neurosci. 2001;4:402–8.
63. Sweet J, Badjatiya A, Tan D. Paresthesia-free high-density spinal cord stimulation for postlaminectomy syndrome in a prescreened population: a prospective case series. Neuromodulation Technol Neural Interface. 2016;19(3):260–7.
64. Tiede J, Brown L, Gekht G, Vallejo R, Yearwood T, Morgan D. Novel spinal cord stimulation parameters in patients with predominant back pain. Neuromodulation. 2013;16:370–5.
65. Van Havenbergh T, Vancamp T, Van Looy P, Vanneste S, De Ridder D. Spinal cord stimulation for the treatment of chronic back pain patients: 500-Hz vs. 1000-Hz burst stimulation. Neuromodulation. 2015;18:9–12; discussion 12.
66. de Vos CC, Bom MJ, Vanneste S, Lenders MWPM, de Ridder D. Burst spinal cord stimulation evaluated in patients with failed back surgery syndrome and painful diabetic neuropathy. Neuromodulation. 2014;17:152–9.
67. Washburn S, Catlin R, Bethel K, Canlas B. Patient-perceived differences between constant current and constant voltage spinal cord stimulation systems. Neuromodulation. 2014;17:28–35; discussion 35–6.
68. Wille F, Breel JS, Bakker EWP, Hollmann MW. Altering conventional to high density spinal cord stimulation: an energy dose-response relationship in neuropathic pain therapy. Neuromodulation. 2017;20:71–80.
69. Wu G, Ringkamp M, Hartke TV, Murinson BB, Campbell JN, Griffin JW, Meyer RA. Early onset of spontaneous activity in uninjured C-fiber nociceptors after injury to neighboring nerve fibers. J Neurosci. 2001;21:RC140.
70. Youn Y, Smith H, Morris B, Argoff C. The effect of high-frequency stimulation on sensory thresholds in chronic pain patients. Stereotact Funct Neurosurg. 2015;93(5):355–9.

Thoracic and Lumbar Dorsal Root Ganglion Spinal Stimulation

71

Denis G. Patterson, Pankaj Mehta, Javid Baksh, Mathew Roberts, Maged Guirguis, Corey W. Hunter, Jason E. Pope, Jeffery Rowe, Dawood Sayed, and Jonathan D. Carlson

Introduction and History

Current epidemiological estimates place the prevalence of chronic pain at 25–30%, a healthcare burden that costs $600 billion annually in the United States alone [7]. Yet, many current treatments offer limited relief for those who suffer from it. In recent years, however, dorsal root ganglion (DRG) stimulation has emerged as a novel therapeutic technology with promising results for the treatment of chronic pain.

The dorsal root ganglion contains afferent cell bodies of sensory neurons that relay all incoming nociceptive information from a given spinal nerve before it ascends to the brain via the anterolateral system (ALS). The DRG has been targeted for therapeutic purposes since the late 1800s, when ganglionectomies and dorsal root rhizotomies were performed as a last resort option for refractory pain syndromes. Despite its limited efficacy at the time [4], this procedure is still performed today by surgical excision, radiofrequency ablation, and pulsed radiofrequency for patients with chronic or neuropathic pain unresponsive to conservative medical management (CMM). Additionally, the DRG has also been targeted for less invasive procedures such as corticosteroid injection to treat lumbosacral and cervical radiculopathy.

The nature and location of the DRG inherently make it an ideal candidate for neurostimulation in the treatment of intractable chronic pain. Its location in the intervertebral foramina also makes the DRG clinically accessible both externally through the neuroforamina and internally through the epidural space. Once implanted, the bony foramina provide innate physical protection against lead migration. Additionally, because the DRG lies outside the blood-brain barrier, there is both a significantly reduced risk of granuloma formation due to electrode placement and decreased current requirement due to lack of surrounding CSF which allows for subthreshold stimulation decreasing sensation of paresthesia. Recent evidence suggests that cell bodies contained within the DRG are not merely passive transmitters of pain but rather appear to play an active role in the pathophysiologic generation of neuropathic pain itself. Furthermore, the DRG has a second role as an active regulator of afferent nociceptive signaling to the ALS. Both of these aspects are leveraged in DRG stimulation to alleviate the conscious perception of pain.

D. G. Patterson
Nevada Advanced Pain Specialists, Reno, NV, USA
e-mail: patterson@nvadvancedpain.com

P. Mehta (✉)
Pain Specialists of Austin, Killeen, TX, USA

J. Baksh
Premier Pain Solutions, Asheville, NC, USA

M. Roberts
Medical University of South Carolina, Charleston, SC, USA

M. Guirguis
Interventional Pain Management, Department of Anesthesiology & Critical Care Medicine, Ochsner Health System, New Orleans, LA, USA

University of Queensland Ochsner Medical School, Brisbane, QLD, Australia

Louisiana State University School of Medicine, New Orleans, LA, USA
e-mail: mguirguis@ochsner.org

C. W. Hunter
Department of Rehabilitation Medicine, Icahn School of Medicine at Mount Sinai, New York, NY, USA

Ainsworth Institute of Pain Management, New York, NY, USA
e-mail: chunter@ainpain.com

J. E. Pope
Evolve Restorative Center, Santa Rosa, CA, USA

J. Rowe
Main Line Spine & Main Line Spine Surgery Center, King of Prussia, PA, USA

D. Sayed
The University of Kansas Health System, Kansas City, KS, USA
e-mail: dsayed@kumc.edu

J. D. Carlson
Hawaii Pain & Spine, Kailua, HI, USA

Midwestern Medical School, Glendale, AZ, USA

Hawaii Pain & Spine, Arizona Pain, Kailua, HI, USA

T. R. Deer et al. (eds.), *Deer's Treatment of Pain*, https://doi.org/10.1007/978-3-030-12281-2_71

Taken together with the strong theoretical framework supporting the use of DRG stimulation, early clinical studies paved the way for approval in the European Union and Australia in 2011. It was not until after the completion of the landmark multicenter ACCURATE study (*A Safety and Effectiveness Trial of Spinal Cord Stimulation of the DRG for Chronic Lower Limb Pain*) in 2016 that the FDA approved DRG stimulation for the treatment of chronic pain due to complex regional pain syndrome (CRPS) and/or causalgia. Also patients have been shown to have reduced other forms of chronic pain (i.e., postherpetic neuralgia, phantom limb pain, failed back surgery syndrome (FBSS), and post-herniorrhaphy groin pain) with DRG stimulation in case studies and in a small series of patients.

Background and Historical Perspective

Currently, the Food and Drug Administration (FDA) only approves DRG stimulation for use in the United States for complex regional pain syndrome (CRPS), types I and II. Additionally, the platform is approved for use from T10 to S2. However, a number of manuscripts have been published describing efficacy with a variety of other pain syndromes and leads placed at levels above and below the approved levels. While the indications for DRG stimulation do overlap with traditional SCS, the former has demonstrated consistent superiority rendering it the modality of choice when applicable.

True utility of DRG stimulation is twofold: (1) the capacity to provide focal stimulation to select regions of the body and (2) its ability to treat conditions and/or body parts that were previously difficult with traditional SCS (Table 71.1).

Targeting/Choosing Levels

An obvious advantage of DRG stimulation is the ability to selectively treat individual levels or a combination of up to four to focus treatment on defined regions/body parts. This is a stark contrast from traditional SCS where the operator is not typically required to do much preoperative planning insofar as deciding what level to place the lead(s) as T8/9 tends to be the most commonly targeted level. It is this level of "choice" that tends to give neuromodulators pause when utilizing DRG stimulation as there are many levels to choose from Tables 71.2 and 71.3 outline the suggested target levels based on diagnosis and by body part of interest.

Table 71.1 Indications for thoracic and lumbar DRG stimulation

Thoracic	Lumbar
Post-thoracotomy syndrome	Complex regional pain syndrome (CRPS), types I and II
Postmastectomy syndrome	Post-amputee syndrome/phantom limb pain
Postherpetic neuralgia	Chronic pelvic pain
Failed back surgery syndrome	Lumbar radiculopathy
	Discogenic pain
Intercostal neuralgia	Post-herniorrhaphy syndrome
	Postsurgical pain
	Post knee/hip replacement syndrome
	Failed back surgery syndrome
	Peripheral neuropathy (i.e., diabetic)
	Meralgia paresthetica
	Pudendal neuralgia
	Nerve injury

Relevant Anatomy

The dorsal root ganglion (DRG) is a neural structure located in or near the neural foramen between the medial and lateral aspects of the pedicle (Fig. 71.1). The DRG is responsible for transducing and modulating the bulk of sensory information from peripheral nerves and transmitting that information to the central nervous system. Nerve cells of the DRG include larger type A neurons (handling proprioception, touch, and vibration) as well as smaller type B neurons (handling nociception). The DRG is also involved as a primary pain processing point, especially with neuropathic pain. Chronic pain has been shown to lead to structural changes in the DRG in animal models. This includes changes in the electrophysiological membrane, integral membrane proteins, and genetic changes causing neuronal hyperexcitability. The DRG can act as

Table 71.2 Suggested levels for stimulations and means for choosing levels based on diagnosis

Diagnosis	Level
Amputee pain	Map-affected levels beforehand using either radiofrequency sensory testing or selective nerve root blocks
Discogenic pain	Above and below affected disc, bilaterally
Meralgia paresthetica	L2 and L3
Post-knee replacement syndrome	L3 and L4
Pelvic pain (including pudendal neuralgia)	L1 and S2 per side
Postherpetic neuralgia	Above and below affected dermatome/level but not the actual infected DRG (may require pre-trial testing as described above for amputees)
Post-thoracotomy syndrome	At the affected level(s)
Post-herniorrhaphy syndrome	T12, L1, and L2

Table 71.3 Suggested levels for stimulation based on body part

Body part	Level(s)
Back	T12, L1, and L2
Buttock	T12, L1, and L2 or L5 and S1
Groin	T12, L1, and L2
Pelvis	L1 and S2 (bilaterally if pain is bilateral)
Knee	L3 and L4
Foot	L5 and S1, add L4 if ankle pain present as well

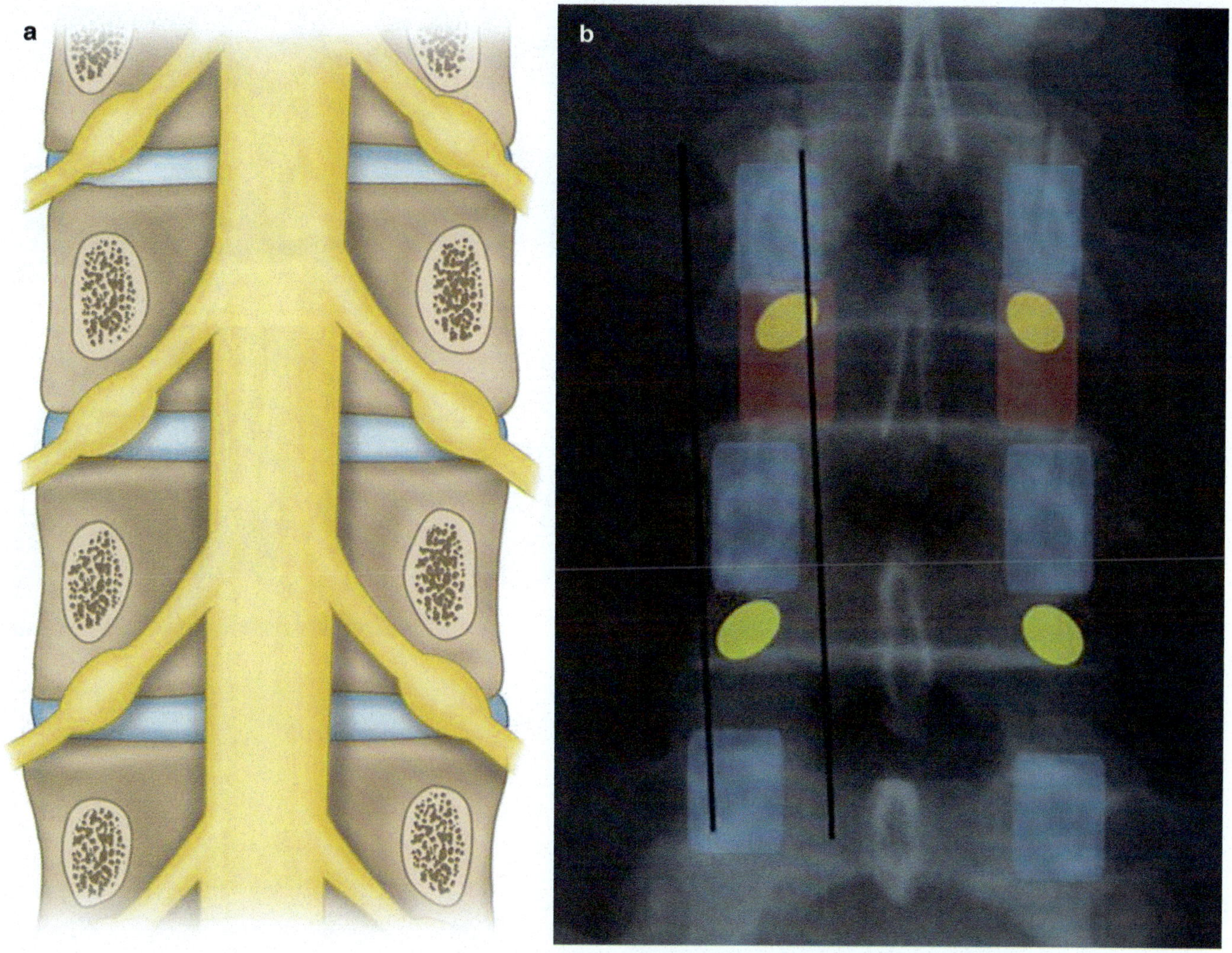

Fig. 71.1 (**a**) Location of the dorsal root ganglion (DRG) as compared to the pedicle. (**b**) Radiographic of DRG location. *Blue* indicates pedicle; *red* indicates neuroforamen; *yellow* indicates DRG. (Reproduced from Bara GA, Deer TR. Spinal cord stimulation of the dorsal root ganglion for the treatment of pain. In: Deer TR and Pope JE, editors. *Atlas of Implantable Therapies for Pain Management*. New York. Springer Science+Business Media: 2016)

a low-pass filter when neuromodulation is implemented causing a decrease in action potentials with the pain signals primarily at the respective level. It is important to note, for reasons not completely understood, there can also be a redundancy in pain relief at levels above or below the level of DRG stimulation. For example, if a DRG is stimulated at the left L5 level, there may also be pain relief noted at the dermatomal distribution of the left L4, L3, and L2 levels.

Surgical Approach

The DRG is accessible either from the epidural space outside through the neural foramen or from outside the neural foramen through to the epidural space. Medical interventions targeting the DRG include anti-inflammatory steroid injections, surgical ablation, radiofrequency ablation, and neuromodulation. Neurostimulator leads for DRG stimulation are typically inserted percutaneously at levels between T10 and S2 (depending on the dermatomal region of pain), with electrodes positioned in the lateral epidural space near the DRG.

Ligaments

Lead insertion for DRG stimulation can be obstructed by several transforaminal and extraforaminal ligaments (see Fig. 71.2). These include the superior and inferior corporopedicular ligaments, the superior, mid-transforaminal, and inferior transforaminal ligaments, and the superior and inferior cotransverse ligaments. The superior corporopedicular ligament attaches the superior pedicle (obliquely, anteriorly, inferiorly) to the posterolateral vertebral body. The inferior corporopedicular ligament attaches the inferior pedicle (obliquely, anteriorly, superiorly) to the posterolateral vertebral body. The superior transforaminal ligament attaches

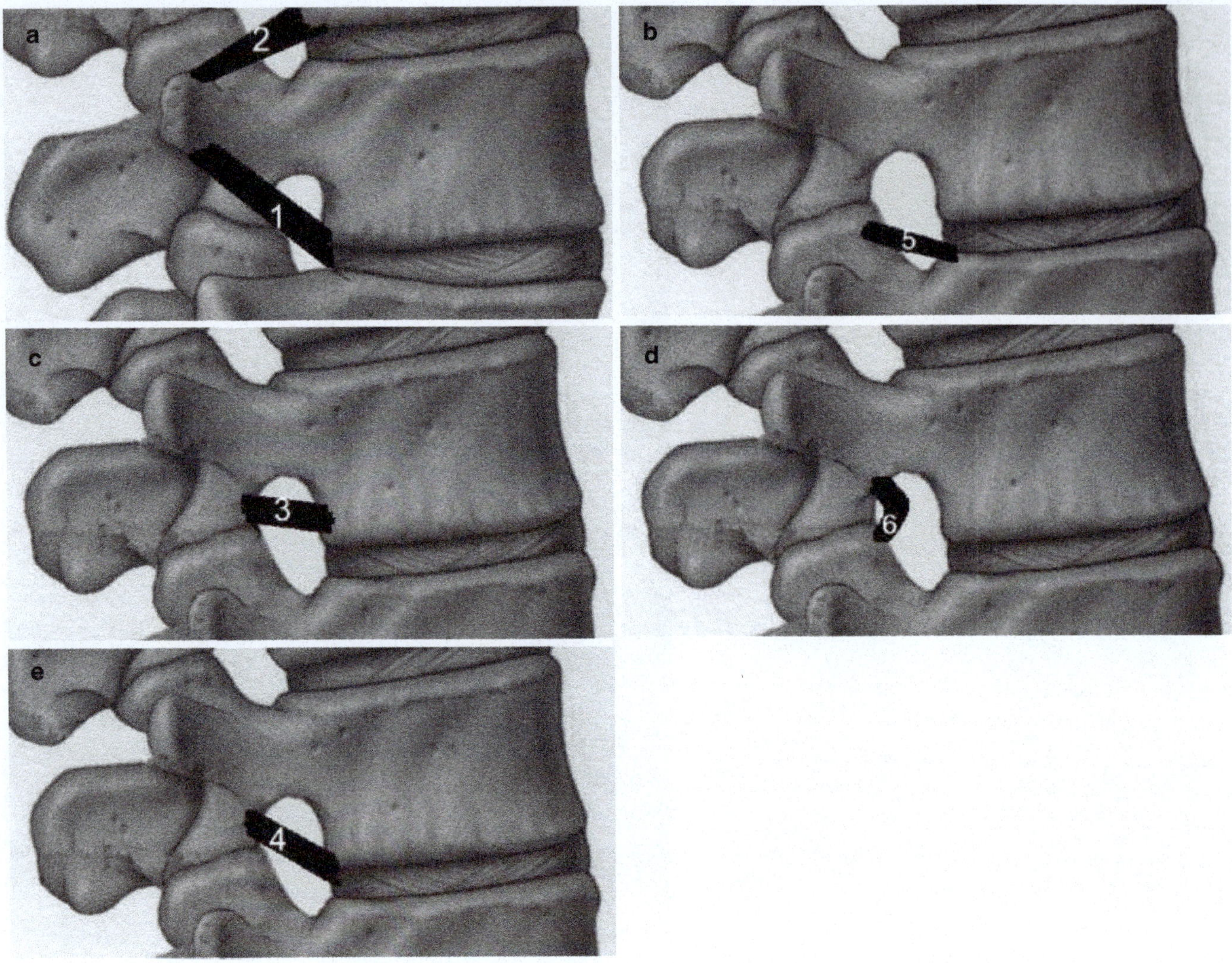

Fig. 71.2 (**a**) Corporotransverse superior (*1*) and inferior (*2*) ligament. (**b**) Superior transforaminal (*3*) ligament. (**c**) Mid-transforaminal (*4*) ligament. (**d**) Inferior transforaminal (*5*) ligament. (**e**) Posterior transforaminal (*6*) ligament. (Reproduced from Park HK, Rudrappa S, Dujovny M, Diaz FG. Intervertebral foraminal ligaments of the lumbar spine: anatomy and biomechanics. *Child's Nervous System*, May 2001, Volume 17, Issue 4–5. © Springer-Verlag Berlin Heidelberg 2001)

the arches of the inferior and superior vertebral notches to the superior pedicle at the articular capsule. The mid-transforaminal ligament attaches the annulus fibrosus and superior and inferior corporopedicular ligaments to the articular capsule. The inferior transforaminal ligament connects the junction of the annulus fibrosus and posterior vertebral body to the superior articular facet.

Efficacy and Indications

Inclusion Criteria

1. Primary research assessing treatment efficacy of dorsal root ganglion stimulation on humans.
2. Only manuscripts written in English and published in peer-reviewed journals were considered.

Exclusion Criteria

1. Single case studies

Across every study analyzed, dorsal root ganglion (DRG) stimulation offers significant efficacy in reduction of pain relative to conservative pain management strategies. The extent of mean pain reduction between studies varied from 52% to 93% across indications including, but not limited to, radiculopathy, postsurgical neuropathy, phantom limb pain, complex regional pain syndrome, and failed back surgery syndrome. Notably, participants in each considered study suffered from intractable chronic pain, that, regardless of etiology, had persisted for more than 6 months and had failed one or more conservative treatment regimens. The regions targeted for therapy covered the spectrum from cervical to sacral, typically involving 1–4 leads (Table 71.4).

Table 71.4 Studies demonstrating that DRG stimulation offers significant efficacy in reducing pain compared to conservative pain management strategies

Author and year	Implanted sample size	Study design	Indications	Study duration	Lead placement	Summary of key efficacy findings
Deer et al. (2013)	10	Prospective case series	Limb radiculopathy or neuropathic chest pain	3–7 days	2–4 leads in thoracic, lumbar, and sacral sites	Mean reduction in VAS pain across all participants was 70% compared to baseline 80% of patients had a pain reduction greater than 50%. 77% of participants reduced pain medication as a result of treatment
Liem et al. (2013)	32	Prospective case series	CRPS, FBSS, postsurgical neuropathy, radiculopathy, disc-related pain, and others	6 months	1–4 leads in thoracic, lumbar, and sacral sites	Mean reduction in VAS pain across all participants was 58% compared to baseline The percentage of patients with a greater than 50% reduction in pain for back, leg, and foot pain was 57%, 70%, and 89%, respectively
Zuidama et al. (2014)	3	Retrospective case series	Postsurgical neuropathy and meralgia paresthetica	2–3 months	1–2 leads at T11, T12, or L2	Cases 1 and 2 both saw 100% VAS pain reductions, while case 3 had a 90% VAS pain reduction compared to baseline
Liem et al. (2015)[a]	32	Prospective case series	CRPS, FBSS, postsurgical neuropathy, radiculopathy, disc-related pain, and others	12 months	1–4 leads in thoracic, lumbar, and sacral sites	Mean reduction in VAS pain across all participants was 56% compared to baseline Quality of life as measured by EQ-5D VAS improved by 64% compared to baseline across all participants
Eldabe et al. (2015)	8	Retrospective case series	Phantom limb pain	14.4 months (average)	1–2 leads in cervical, lumbar, and sacral sites	Mean reduction in VAS pain across all participants was 52% compared to baseline 88% of patients reduced pain medications as a result of treatment
Schu et al. (2015)	23	Retrospective case series	Postsurgical neuropathy of the back, groin, and thighs	27.8 weeks (average)	1–3 leads in thoracic and lumbar sites	Mean reduction in VAS pain across all participants was 71% compared to baseline 83% of patients had a pain reduction greater than 50% Patients with post-herniorrhaphy pain had the greatest reduction in VAS pain (78%, $N = 11$)
Van Buyten et al. (2015)	8	Prospective case series	CRPS of the leg and foot	12 months	Not reported	Mean reduction in VAS pain across all participants was 65% compared to baseline 75% of patients had a pain reduction greater than 50% Quality of life as measured by EQ-5D VAS improved by 74% compared to baseline across all participants
Weiner et al. (2016)	11	Prospective case series	FBSS	45 days	1 lead at L1–L5	Mean reduction in VAS pain across all participants was 63% compared to baseline

(continued)

Table 71.4 (continued)

Author and year	Implanted sample size	Study design	Indications	Study duration	Lead placement	Summary of key efficacy findings
Deer et al. (2017)	152 (76 DRG vs. 76 SCS)	Randomized controlled prospective study comparing SCS and DRG	CRPS of the buttocks and lower limb	12 months	1–4 leads at T7–T12 for SCS and T11-S1 for DRG	Mean reduction in VAS pain was 74% compared to baseline in the DRG group vs. 53% in the SCS group Paresthesia confinement to only the primary pain area was 95% in the DRG group vs. 61% in the SCS group 86% of patients had a pain reduction greater than 50% in the DRG group vs. 72% in the SCS group DRG therapy demonstrated both non-inferiority and superiority over SCS therapy for CRPS SCS patients were 7.1 times more likely to report paresthesia in nonpainful areas as DRG patients There was a twofold increase in postural pain (supine – upright) in the SCS group compared to none in the DRG group

[a]This 2014 study by Liem et al. was a continuation of the same participants from the 2013 study by the same authors

Key Advantages of DRG Efficacy

From a therapeutic standpoint, DRG stimulation offers several key advantages over traditional spinal cord stimulation (SCS):

- DRG stimulation offers discrete dermatomal coverage of areas that are difficult to treat by SCS (e.g., the feet).
- Unlike SCS, DRG stimulation is associated with little to no postural effects associated with inferior pain relief in certain positions.
- Decreased current levels are required for DRG versus SCS, which translates to greater battery life and application of rechargeable pulse generators, alone responsible for an estimated $100,000–$300,000 savings over a patient's lifetime.
- Relative to SCS, lead migration (and corresponding adverse events or unwanted paresthesia) is less common in DRG.
- In the only study directly comparing DRG to SCS, DRG was found to be both non-inferior and superior to SCS in reducing neuropathic pain.

Pearls and Pitfalls

- DRG stimulation requires a mindful understanding of the relevant anatomy to determine device accommodation.
- DRG is FDA on label from T10-S2.
- The sheath can be driven with either the lead or the guidewire in place, depending on operator preference. The guidewire makes the system more rigid.
- The complication rate for SCS and DRG stimulation is very similar and not statistically significantly different.
- Like any procedure around the spine, it is important to mitigate nerve injury. If sedation is used, it is important that they can detect nerve injury by movement or neuro-monitoring should be employed with or without general anesthesia.
- Lead placement validation can be performed with sensory testing, creating a paresthesia overlying the painful area, or absence of motor recruitment with high-amplitude stimulation, or impedance testing, or placement in the posterior foramen by not violating the posterior border of the vertebral body and with contacts 2–3 underneath the pedicle on the AP.
- Bilateral pain should be trialed with bilateral lead placement.

Recommended Reading

1. Deer TR, Pope JE. Dorsal root ganglion stimulation approval by the food and drug administration: advice on evolving the process. Expert Rev Neurother. 2016;16:1123–5.
2. Deer TR, et al. Dorsal root ganglion stimulation yielded higher treatment success rate for complex regional pain syndrome and causalgia at 3 and 12 months: a randomized comparative trial. Pain. 2017;158:669–81.

3. Devor M. Unexplained peculiarities of the dorsal root ganglion. Pain. 1999;Suppl 6:S27–35.
4. Echols DH. Sensory rhizotomy following operation for ruptured intervertebral disc. J Neurosurg. 1969;31:335–8.
5. Gemes G, et al. Failure of action potential propagation in sensory neurons: mechanisms and loss of afferent filtering in C-type units after painful nerve injury. J Physiol. 2013;591:1111–31.
6. Grigsby E, Deer T, Weiner R, Wilcosky B, Kramer J. Prospective, multicenter clinical trial studying dorsal root ganglion stimulation in the treatment of back pain. Neuromodulation. 2013;16(1):67–71; discussion 71-2. https://doi.org/10.1111/ner.12013. Epub 2012 Dec 14.
7. Hasegawa T, Mikawa Y, Watanabe R, An HS. Morphometric analysis of the lumbosacral nerve roots and dorsal root ganglia by magnetic resonance imaging. Spine. 1996;21:1005–9.
8. Institute of Medicine (US) Committee on Advancing Pain Research, Care, and Education. Relieving pain in America: a blueprint for transforming prevention, care, education, and research. Washington (DC): National Academies Press (US); 2011.
9. Johannes CB, Le TK, Zhou X, Johnston JA, Dworkin RH. The prevalence of chronic pain in United States adults: results of an internet-based survey. J Pain. 2010;11:1230–9.
10. Kandel ER. Principles of neural science. 5th ed. New York: McGraw Hill Professional; 2013.
11. Krames ES. The role of the dorsal root ganglion in the development of neuropathic pain. Pain Med Malden Mass. 2014;15:1669–85.
12. Liem L, et al. A multicenter, prospective trial to assess the safety and performance of the spinal modulation dorsal root ganglion neurostimulator system in the treatment of chronic pain. Neuromodulation J Int Neuromodulation Soc. 2013;16:471–82. discussion 482.
13. Macfarlane GJ. The epidemiology of chronic pain. Pain. 2016;157:2158–9.
14. Manchikanti L. Transforaminal lumbar epidural steroid injections. Pain Physician. 2000;3:374–98.
15. Nagda JV, Davis CW, Bajwa ZH, Simopoulos TT. Retrospective review of the efficacy and safety of repeated pulsed and continuous radiofrequency lesioning of the dorsal root ganglion/segmental nerve for lumbar radicular pain. Pain Physician. 2011;14:371–6.
16. Panjabi MM, Duranceau J, Goel V, Oxland T, Takata K. Cervical human vertebrae. Quantitative three-dimensional anatomy of the middle and lower regions. Spine. 1991;16:861–9.
17. Panjabi MM, et al. Thoracic human vertebrae. Quantitative three-dimensional anatomy. Spine. 1991;16:888–901.
18. Pope JE, Deer TR, Kramer J. A systematic review: current and future directions of dorsal root ganglion therapeutics to treat chronic pain. Pain Med Malden Mass. 2013;14:1477–96.
19. Sapunar D, Kostic S, Banozic A, Puljak L. Dorsal root ganglion - a potential new therapeutic target for neuropathic pain. J Pain Res. 2012;5:31–8.
20. Shanthanna H, Chan P, McChesney J, Thabane L, Paul J. Pulsed radiofrequency treatment of the lumbar dorsal root ganglion in patients with chronic lumbar radicular pain: a randomized, placebo-controlled pilot study. J Pain Res. 2014;7:47–55.
21. Shaw RC. A study of intractable pain relative to rhizotomy and spinal section. Br J Surg. 1924;11:648–75.
22. Struijk JJ, Holsheimer J, Boom HB. Excitation of dorsal root fibers in spinal cord stimulation: a theoretical study. IEEE Trans Biomed Eng. 1993;40:632–9.
23. Vad VB, Bhat AL, Lutz GE, Cammisa F. Transforaminal epidural steroid injections in lumbosacral radiculopathy: a prospective randomized study. Spine. 2002;27:11–6.
24. Weigel R, Capelle HH, Schmelz M, Krauss JK. Selective thoracic ganglionectomy for the treatment of segmental neuropathic pain. Eur J Pain Lond Engl. 2012;16:1398–402.

Percutaneous Sacral Nerve Stimulation

72

Corey W. Hunter and Dipan Patel

Introduction

Chronic pelvic pain (CPP) is a disabling and poorly understood syndrome that causes social, psychological, and physical distress. Like many suffering from poor pain control, these patients experience a progressively diminishing quality of life and decreasing daily function leading to lost wages and an increasing burden on the healthcare system. CPP is particularly difficult to treat, largely due to how poorly understood it is. Typically, these patients fail conservative therapy; while the exact pathophysiology is generally unknown, CPP frequently has a striking resemblance to other chronic neuropathic pain syndromes [i.e., complex regional pain syndrome (CRPS) or sympathetically driven pain] known to respond favorably to spinal cord stimulation (SCS). The use of SCS to treat CPP, however, has been frustrating for neuromodulators due to the difficulty in obtaining appropriate and/or adequate coverage over the area(s) of pain. Not surprisingly, CPP has the highest rate of explant of all diagnoses treated with SCS at 33.3%; the most common reason being a loss of therapeutic effect (39%). The difficulty in procuring and maintaining coverage is likely due in large part to the complex innervation of the pelvic viscera.

Many of the sentinel publications on the use of SCS in CPP focused on targeting the sacral region of the spinal cord. Intuitively, this made the most sense given the predominance of sacral innervation for syndromes like pudendal neuralgia, vulvodynia, and the like. While sacral fibers are obviously present throughout the length of the spinal cord, they are extremely difficult to recruit with conventional lead placement over the dorsal columns in the thoracic spine due to their size and position relative to other nearby fibers. Placing leads directly over the sacral roots within the sacral canal is an effective strategy for isolating the area of need while avoiding collateral stimulation to unwanted areas. The purpose of this chapter will be to elucidate the current role of percutaneous sacral nerve stimulation (SNS) in the long-term management of CPP.

Background and Historical Perspective

CPP can be nociceptive, neuropathic, or a combination of both – the most common being neuropathic. Typically, neuropathic pain (NP) is the result of central sensitization: a dysfunction in the central nervous system where the brain continues to receive pain signals even after removal of the underlying lesion. The main clinical symptoms of central sensitization are cutaneous hyperalgesia and allodynia; both of which are significantly higher in patients with CPP. The first-line treatment for NP typically includes medications such as gabapentin, pregabalin, amitriptyline, and the like; when used with CPP, efficacy has been extremely limited with most cases being refractory. Nerve blocks and sympathetic blocks have also been described in the literature for persistent cases of NP; however the relief in CPP tends to be limited and temporary rendering these treatments largely ineffectual. The next treatment typically considered for recalcitrant NP is neuromodulation.

The primary challenge with utilizing SCS for CPP relates to the complexity of the neuroanatomy of the pelvic region and successfully navigating it. The pelvic viscera contains lumbar and sacral innervation making it potentially difficult to capture all areas of pain simultaneously. In a patient with bladder, inguinal, and perineal pain, one would need to provide stimulation in the distribution of the ilioinguinal, iliohypogastric, genitofemoral, pudendal, and inferior rectal nerves all at the same time. The dermatomal distribution of the area coincides with T12, L1, and L2 and then skips to S2 and S3 (Table 72.1). Choosing the appropriate area of the

C. W. Hunter (✉)
Ainsworth Institute of Pain Management, New York, NY, USA
e-mail: chunter@ainpain.com

D. Patel
Garden State Pain Control Center, Clifton, NJ, USA

Residents & Fellows Society, North American Neuromodulation Society (NANS), Jersey City, NJ, USA

T. R. Deer et al. (eds.), *Deer's Treatment of Pain*, https://doi.org/10.1007/978-3-030-12281-2_72

Table 72.1 Relevant peripheral nerves of the pelvis and spinal nerve segments they are derived from

Nerve	T12	L1	L2	L3	L4	S1	S2	S3	S4	S5
Iliohypogastric	■	■								
Ilioinguinal		■								
Genitofemoral		■	■							
Obturator			■	■	■					
Posterior femoral cutaneous						■	■	■	■	
Inferior Rectal							■	■	■	
Pudendal							■	■	■	
Coccygeal									■	■

cord to target for stimulation presents an obvious challenge given the diversity of innervation.

Recruiting sacral fibers is an obvious necessity when utilizing SCS to treat CPP given the predominance of sacral innervation to the pelvic region. Unfortunately, sacral fibers are notoriously difficult to recruit with traditional stimulation due to their size and position within the dorsal columns (Fig. 72.1). Sacral fibers are smaller than lumbar thus requiring more energy to stimulate. If one were to increase the amplitude or pulse width in an attempt to recruit the sacral fibers, the patient would likely begin to experience unwanted or even uncomfortable stimulation in potentially unaffected areas. In addition, sacral fibers are located at the medial-most portion of each dorsal column – meaning a lead would need to be placed precisely over the anatomical midline should one hope to stimulate them first.

Given the discernible obstacles one would need to overcome, placing a lead in the sacral canal where only sacral fibers exist is obvious choice.

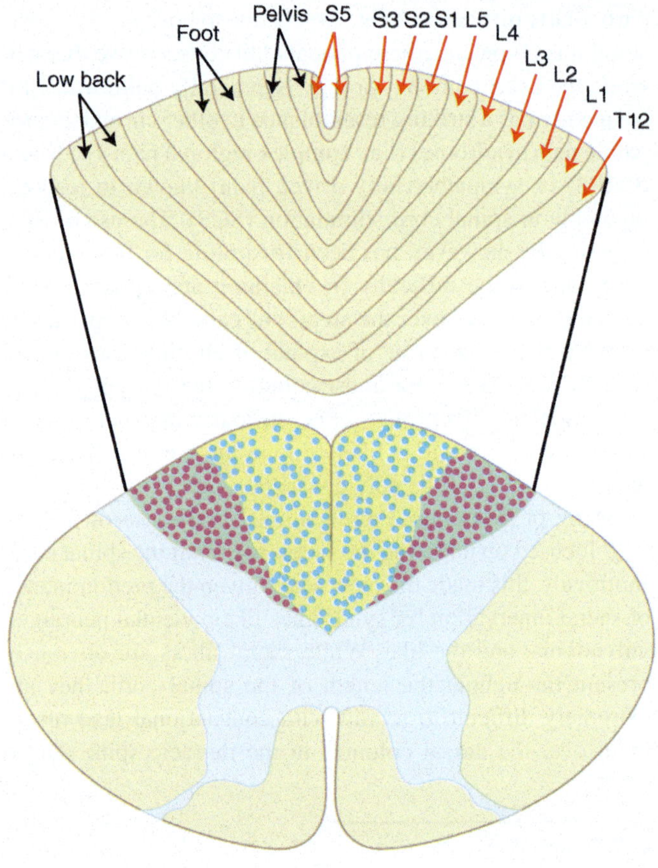

Fig. 72.1 Cross-sectional illustration of the dorsal columns showing the position of the sacral fibers with respect to the spinal cord

Anatomy

The sacral spine consists of five pairs of spinal nerves that exit the sacrum through their respective sacral foramen. The sacral nerve roots originate below the conus medullaris at the L1/2 region forming part of the cauda equine. These nerve roots then descend through the lumbar spine into the sacral canal – a continuation of the vertebral canal running through the posterior portion of the sacrum. The rostral portion of the canal is well formed and triangular-shaped, while the caudal aspect is oblong with an incomplete dorsal/posterior wall (Fig. 72.2).

There are typically four, sometimes five, pairs of sacral foramen on both the ventral and dorsal aspects of the sacrum, providing exit points for each of the sacral

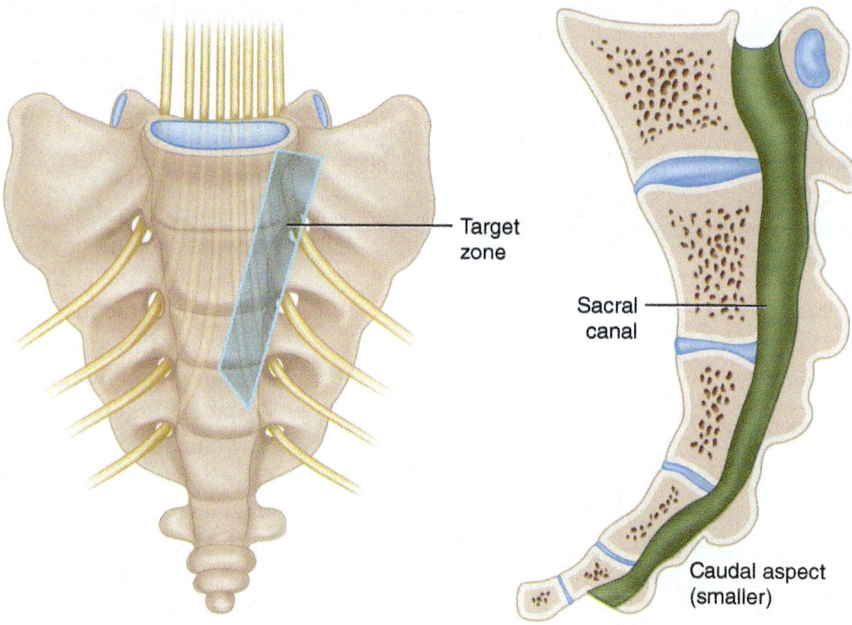

Fig. 72.2 Image on the left illustrates sacral nerves within the sacrum and their path of exit through the corresponding foramen, as well as target zone of potential lead placement to ensure the nerve is still present within canal and has not exited; image on the right illustrates the shape of the sacral canal and its variation at the rostral vs. the caudal aspects

nerves (Figs. 72.2 and 72.3). Sacral nerve roots exiting through the anterior foramen combine to form the sacral plexus and ultimately larger nerves such as the pudendal nerve or inferior rectal nerve (Fig. 72.4). The sacral nerves exiting posteriorly provide innervation to the sacroiliac joint.

Like nerves from the other regions of the spinal cord, sacral nerves contain both afferent and efferent fibers providing sensory and motor innervation to various organs including the descending colon, rectum, urinary bladder, and genitalia (6). The sacral dorsal root ganglia (DRG) are variably located in different regions of the sacrum. An anatomic study was performed to determine location and dimensions of the S1–4 DRG's (Fig. 72.3):

- S1: intraforaminal, 55–60%; intracanalar, 40–45%
- S2: intraforaminal, 15–50%; intracanalar, 50–85%
- S3 and S4: intraforaminal, 0%; intracanalar, 100%
- *None of the sacral DRGs were extraforaminal*

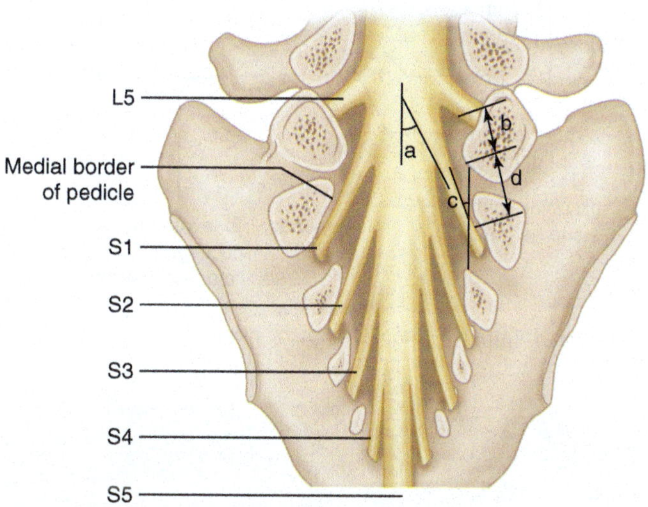

Fig. 72.3 Illustration of the anatomy of the sacrum and the location of the sacral DRG. (a) Angle of the sacral nerve root relative to the midline; (b) proximal length of the nerve root; (c) width of the sacral DRG; (d) length of the sacral DRG (7)

The S1 DRG is relatively larger, and its intracanalar position, relative to the other sacral DRGs, may be susceptible to compression by L5-S1 disc herniation. Sacral dorsal root ganglion stimulation will be covered later in this text (see Chap. 73).

The most common and simplest technique for gaining percutaneous access to the sacral canal is via the sacral hiatus. To locate the sacral hiatus, one must identify the following:

- Sacral and coccygeal cornua – both of which can be palpated to obtain a general frame of reference to compare to the imaging (Figs. 72.5 and 72.6).
- Sacrococcygeal junction (SCJ).
- Coccyx.
- Sacral foramina – lining these up on imaging will provide for a proper assessment of an anterior-posterior (AP) image.
- *The hiatus is easier to identify in a lateral image* (Fig. 72.7).

The sacral cornua (the roof of the hiatus) can be palpated by placing one's index finger over the intergluteal cleft with the tip of the digit aligned with the edge of the coccyx – the sacral cornua will typically lie beneath the proximal interphalangeal joint.

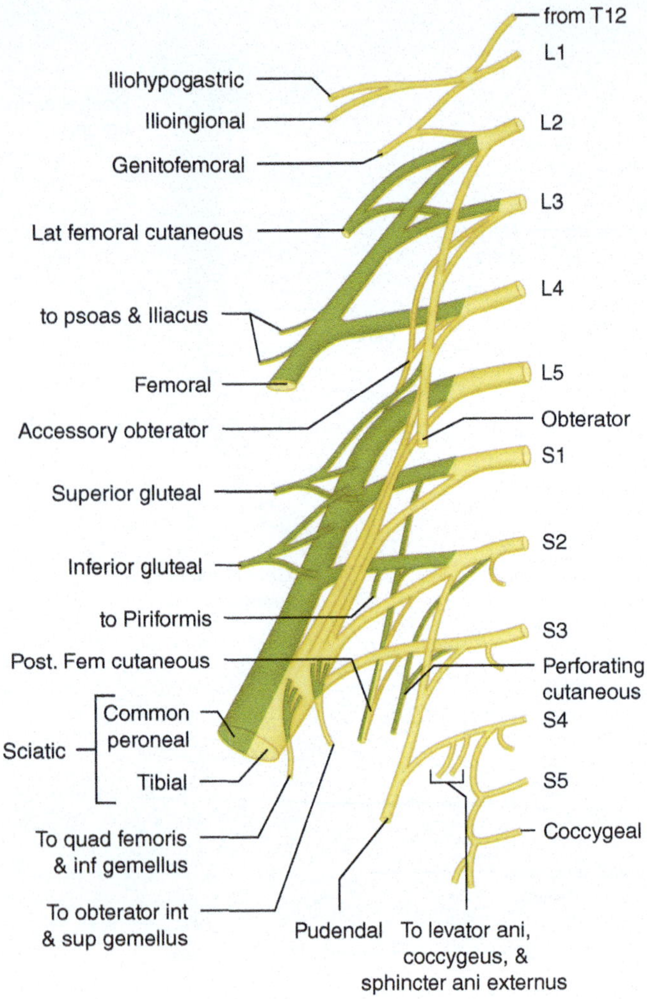

Fig. 72.4 Illustration of the lumbosacral plexus

Uses and Indications

Indications should include syndromes with a purely sacral distribution:

- Pudendal neuralgia
- Obturator neuralgia
- Vulvitis and vulvodynia
- Prostadynia and chronic prostatitis
- Anal pain (proctitis) and perianal pain
- Proctalgia fugax
- Radiation proctitis
- Distal urethral pain
- Scrotal and penile pain
- Coccygodynia
- Vaginal pain involving the distal 1/3
- Suspected CRPS or sympathetically maintained pain of the pelvic region
- Postsurgical pain
- Endometriosis or pelvic adhesions
- Pelvic floor dysfunction
- Postherpetic neuralgia
- Urgency-related pain

Other non-pain-related uses for SNS include:

- Urinary/urge incontinence
- Urinary retention
- Increased urinary frequency
- Fecal incontinence
- Spinal cord infarction

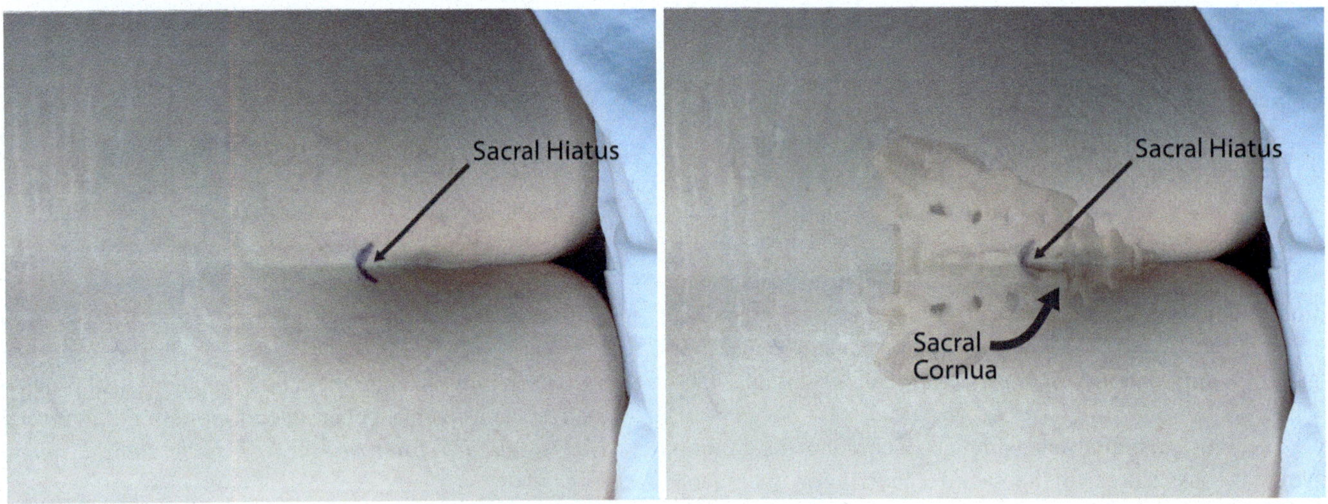

Fig. 72.5 Image on the left shows the skin marked for injection. Image on the right demonstrates a representation of the underlying bony anatomy. (Reproduced from Hunter CW, Chen GH. Sacral stimulation for pelvic pain. In: Diwan S and Deer TR, editors. *Advanced procedures for pain management: a step-by-step Atlas*. New York, Springer; 2018)

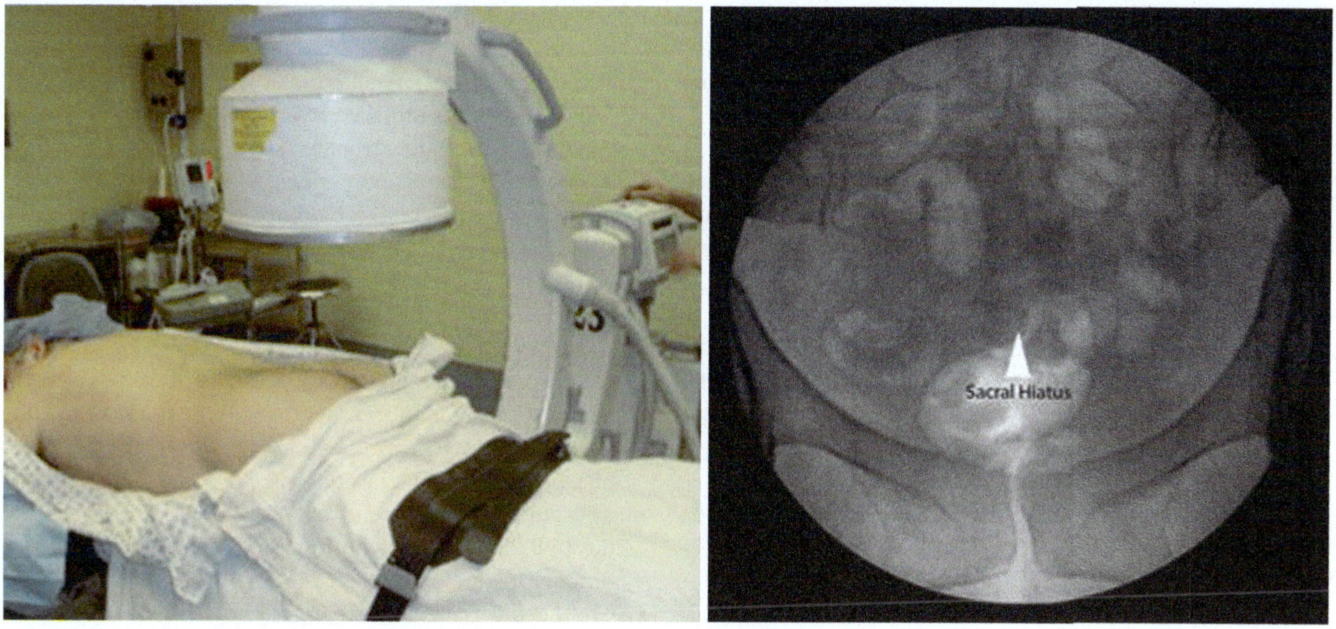

Fig. 72.6 Image on the left demonstrates the initial positioning of the C-arm over the patient for an AP view. The image on the right is the corresponding fluoroscopic view in AP. (Reproduced from Hunter CW, Chen GH. Sacral stimulation for pelvic pain. In: Diwan S and Deer TR, editors. *Advanced procedures for pain management: a step-by-step Atlas*. New York, Springer; 2018)

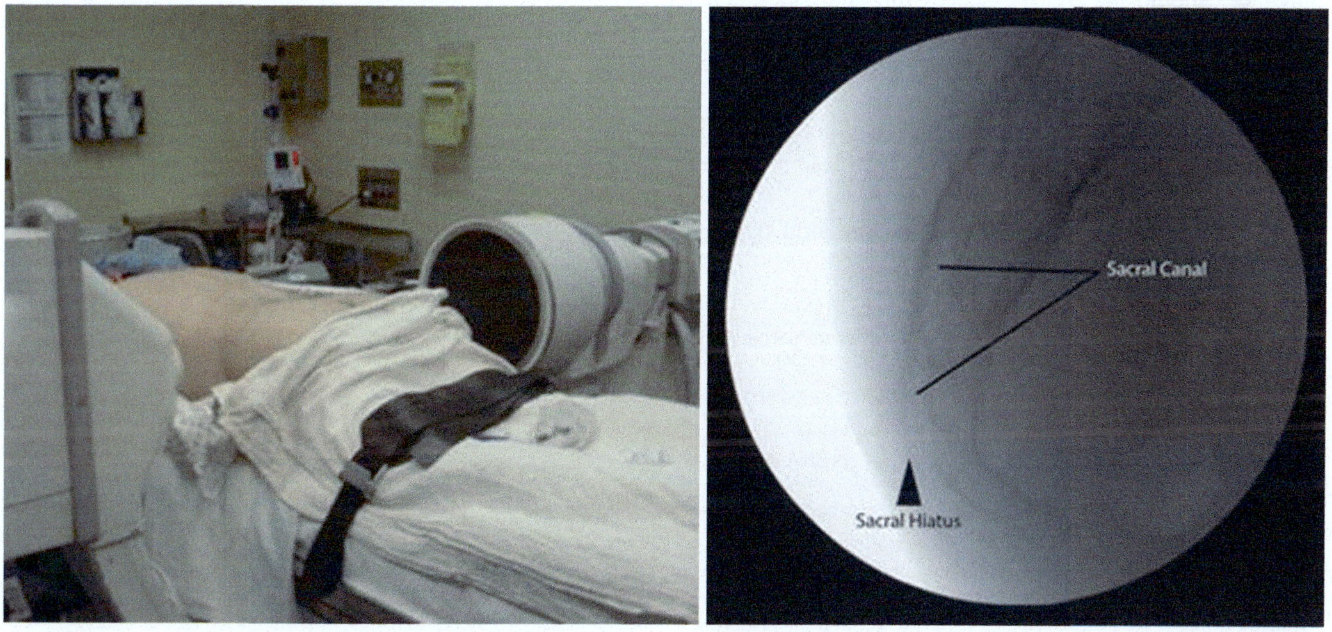

Fig. 72.7 Image on the left demonstrates the C-arm positioned about the patient for a lateral view. The image on the right is the corresponding fluoroscopic view. (Reproduced from Hunter CW, Chen GH. Sacral stimulation for pelvic pain. In: Diwan S and Deer TR, editors. *Advanced procedures for pain management: a step-by-step Atlas*. New York, Springer; 2018)

Procedural Techniques

A variety of techniques have been described in the literature for SNS (Table 72.2):

- Anterograde trans-hiatus technique – caudal approach with needle placed through the sacral hiatus and leads advanced cephalad
- Retrograde technique – epidural access is achieved in the lumbar spine and the lead is advanced caudally
- Transforaminal approach – needle is placed through the posterior sacral foramen and the lead advanced ventrally out the anterior sacral foramen (InterStim™ neurostimulator, Medtronic)
- Laminotomy with paddle lead placement
- Percutaneous retrograde peripheral nerve stimulation (PNS)

Each technique/approach is distinctly different with particular advantages and disadvantages (Table 72.3). When trialing SNS, we advocate the anterograde/trans-hiatus approach due to the ease with which the sacral nerves are able to be accessed as well as the low incidence of dural puncture. Should the trial be successful, and a permanent implant be considered, other options may be contemplated as the anchoring the leads can be difficult with this technique.

- The patient is placed in a prone position with padding and positioning typical of a conventional SCS lead placement (Fig. 72.8).
- The sacral cornua are identified and the skin over the sacral hiatus is marked (Fig. 72.5).

Table 72.2 A comparison of the various approaches for percutaneous sacral stimulation

Approach	Description
Anterograde trans-hiatus	Access via the sacral hiatus and the leads are advanced cephalad through the sacral canal
Retrograde	Access via the lumbar epidural space and the leads are advanced in reverse, through the lumbar spine and into the sacrum
Transforaminal	Needle is placed through the posterior sacral foramen, and lead is advanced out/through the anterior foramen (InterStim®)
Epidural technique with laminotomy	Surgical lead placement with paddle lead placed retrograde via laminotomy at L5/S1
Percutaneous cephalocaudal/retrograde peripheral nerve stimulation	Lead placed over the dorsal sacral foramina stimulating the sacral nerves exiting the posterior sacral foramen

- The position of the hiatus is confirmed with a lateral fluoroscopic image.
- The skin is prepared in a typical, sterile fashion.
- The skin is then infiltrated with 1% lidocaine with epinephrine to provide adequate skin analgesia.
- A small "stab" incision is made to one side of the sacral hiatus with either a #15 blade or an 18-gauge needle to aid in the entry of the spinal needle – this also helps prevent the transmission skin flora into the underlying tissue.
- A 14-gauge Coudé or Tuohy needle is inserted under lateral fluoroscopic imaging into one side of the hiatus, ipsilateral to the side of the sacral canal the lead is targeting (be certain to leave enough room within the hiatus to place another needle beside it).
- The authors recommend against injecting contrast dye through the needle to confirm epidural access as this may obscure the image.
- The needle is then rotated to the ipsilateral side of the sacrum to which the lead is to end up.
- Using the curve stylet, the lead is inserted through the needle with the bend of the lead concordant to the bend of the needle.

Table 72.3 Pros and cons of anterograde vs. retrograde techniques

Technique	Advantages	Disadvantages
Anterograde Trans-Hiatus	Less challenging technically	Increased difficulty in securing lead trial and maintaining site integrity during trial due to location in the intergluteal cleft
	Decreased risk of dural puncture or intrathecal lead placement	
	Shorter distance for leads to travel	Leads are difficult to steer
		Difficulty anchoring due to lack of surrounding tissue
		Increased risk of skin erosion over lead
		Increased risk of infection due to proximity to rectum
		Potentially close to or within painful area
Retrograde	Simple lead steering	More challenging technically
	Standard lead anchoring	Increased risk of dural puncture
	Lower migration risk	Increased risk of dural or intrathecal lead placement
	Decreased risk of wound dehiscence with implant	
	Away from potentially painful region	

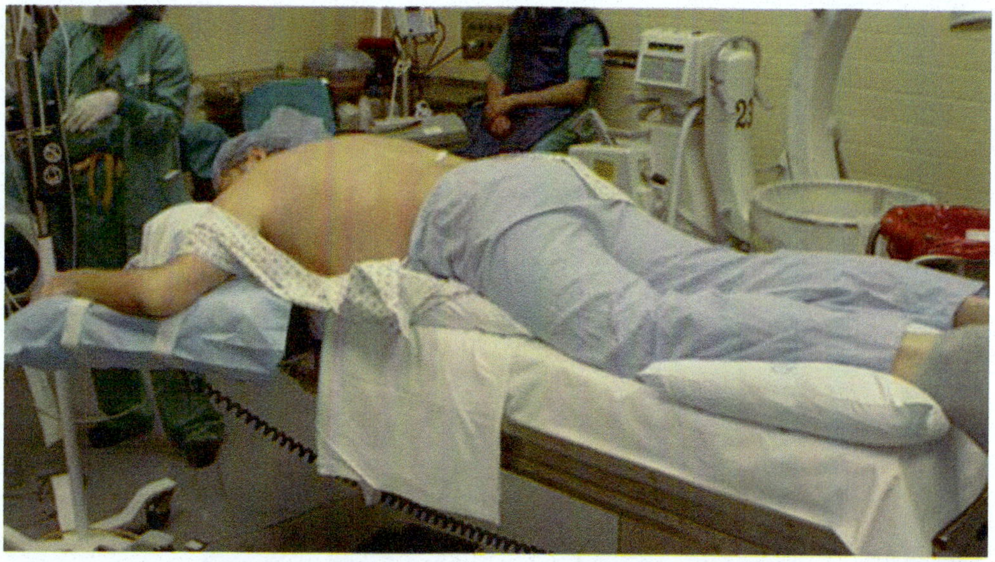

Fig. 72.8 Patient positioned in the prone position with pillow under the abdomen. (Reproduced from Hunter CW, Chen GH. Sacral stimulation for pelvic pain. In: Diwan S and Deer TR, editors. *Advanced procedures for pain management: a step-by-step Atlas*. New York, Springer; 2018)

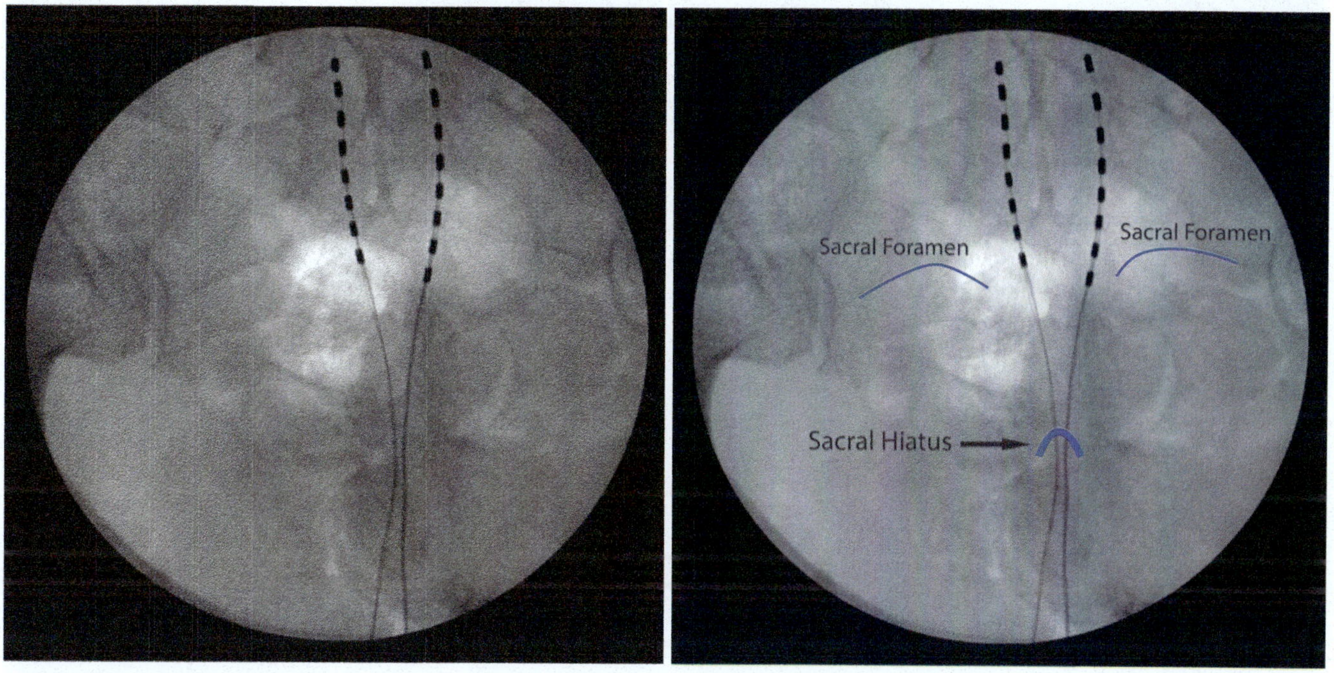

Fig. 72.9 AP fluoroscopic image of bilateral eight contact leads within the sacral canal; leads are placed medial to the sacral foramen. (Reproduced from Hunter CW, Chen GH. Sacral stimulation for pelvic pain. In: Diwan S and Deer TR, editors. *Advanced procedures for pain management: a step-by-step Atlas*. New York, Springer; 2018)

- The lead should be inserted through the needle in lateral until the first few contacts can be seen just beyond the tip of the needle – this is to ensure the lead is contained within the sacral canal.
- Using an AP view, the lead is then advanced to the ipsilateral side of the sacral canal, at the medial border of the sacral foramen (adjust the cephalocaudal tilt of the C-arm to better visualize the foramen) (Fig. 72.9).
- The distance of the lead within the sacral canal should correspond to which sacral nerves are being targeted – this should be verified in a lateral image (Fig. 72.10).

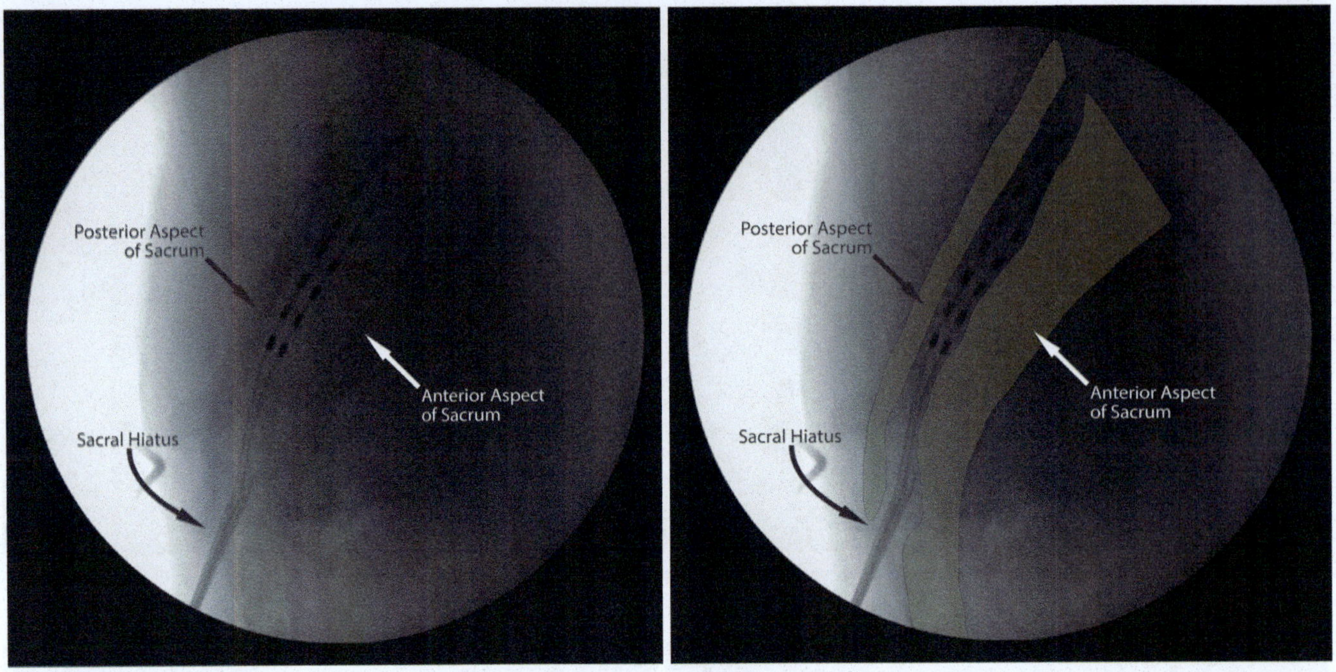

Fig. 72.10 Lateral fluoroscopic image with tip of leads positioned at S1. (Reproduced from Hunter CW, Chen GH. Sacral stimulation for pelvic pain. In: Diwan S and Deer TR, editors. *Advanced procedures for pain management: a step-by-step Atlas*. New York, Springer; 2018)

Evidence and Efficacy

Most of the early publications supporting the use of SCS in patients with CPP were authored by Kapural and Aló – the latter of which was among the first to describe SNS.

The rationale for treating CPP with SNS was founded when the relationship between visceral signal transmission in the pelvic region and pelvic pain was established (Kapural and Palecek). There is no true consensus on what region of the spinal cord should be targeted to yield the best pain relief in CPP. There have been a number of publications describing a variety of techniques ranging from mid-thoracic leads to "trolling" an active lead caudally. While all have merit, SNS appears to be more consistent with regard to obtaining adequate paresthetic coverage over the area(s) of need.

In 2001, Martellucci et al. presented the results of 27 patients treated with SNS. The authors reported a 59% trial/permanent ratio with significant decreases in pain. The mean preoperative VAS was 8.1 and decreased to 2.1 ± 1.2 at 6-month follow-up ($p < 0.0001$), to 2.1 ± 1.1 at 12 months (16 patients), to 2.0 ± 1.2 at 24 months (13 patients), to 2.3 ± 1.4 at 36 months (9 patients), to 2.1 ± 1.5 at 48 months (5 patients), and to 1.9 ± 1.3 at 60 months (3 patients). The study confirmed that SNS was an effective treatment option for carefully selected male and female patients affected by CPP. Of note, the authors also stated that patients who responded positively to gabapentin or pregabalin were the strongest predictors of success to SNS therapy for CPP.

Table 72.4 Conditions known to benefit from sacral stimulation and the potential targets

Conditions	Sacral targets
Sacroiliac joint	S1
Post laminectomy syndrome	S1, S2, S3, S4
Urgency-frequency disorders	S2/3
Vulvodynia	S2 and S3
Pudendal neuralgia	S2 and S3
Interstitial cystitis	S2 and S3
Urge incontinence	S3
Fecal incontinence	S4
Coccydynia	S4 and S5

Over time, the popularity of SNS grew and the potential indications grew along with it. Interstitial cystitis became an established diagnosis for treatment with SNS due to a number of publications by authors like Feler, Brookoff, Aló, and several others (Table 72.4). Eventually, the indications were expanded to pudendal neuralgia, vulvodynia, coccydynia, sacroiliitis, and even failed back surgery syndrome.

While no large randomized trials exist on the use of SNS for the treatment of CPP, there are several large studies in publication that support its use. Gajewski and Al-Zahrani reported on a larger case series of 78 patients with bladder pain syndrome, 46 of whom underwent permanent SNS implantation. Success was defined as a minimum 50% improvement on a Global Response Assessment scale, both during the testing period and after implantation. With an average follow-up of 5 years, the success rate of the patients receiving implants was 72%, and the overall success rate was

43% (the long-term efficacy of sacral neuromodulation in the management of intractable cases of bladder pain syndrome: 14 years of experience in one center).

Pearls and Pitfalls

Basic considerations should be implemented prior to performing SNS.

- While the trans-hiatus approach is technically the least challenging with regard to access and lead placement, it may not be the optimal technique for implant. Anchoring the lead is extremely difficult, and there is a high incidence of lead erosion due to the lack of tissue to guard the lead in and around the sacral hiatus. Also, patients suffering from pudendal neuralgia or perianal pain may be unable to tolerate a procedure in such close proximity to their primary area of preexisting pain.
- The retrograde approach is considerable more challenging and carries a higher risk of dural puncture. However, once the epidural space is accessed, lead steering should present less of a problem as is it performed in the same manner as dorsal column SCS, simply backward. Additionally, anchoring and tunneling is a non-factor as this is accomplished the same as any other standard SCS implant.
- During the trial procedure, bacitracin ointment should be applied to the skin in and around the lead(s) with a stay-fixe dressing used to secure the lead(s) in place. This should be practiced for trans-hiatus, retrograde, and transforaminal approaches.
- CPP tends to have a stronger psychologic component to their pain than most other SCS indications – be sure to utilize a particularly stringent therapist when seeking clearance prior to the procedure.
- CPP tends to have the highest explant rate of all indications treated with SCS. It is important to spend extra time discussing expectations prior to initiating SNS.

Recommended Reading

1. Alo K, Yland M, Redko V, Feler C, Naumann C. Lumbar and sacral nerve root stimulation (NRS) in the treatment of chronic pain: a novel anatomic approach and neuro stimulation technique. Neuromodulation. 1999;2(1):23–31.
2. Alo` KM, McKay E. Selective nerve root stimulation (SNRS) for the treatment of intractable pelvic pain and motor dysfunction: a case report. Neuromodulation. 2001;4(1):19–23.
3. Alo` KM, Yland MJ, Redko V, Feler C, Naumann C. Lumbar and sacral nerve root stimulation (NRS) in the treatment of chronic pain: a novel anatomic approach and neurostimulation technique. Neuromodulation. 1999;2:23–31.
4. Brookoff D, Bennett D. Neuromodulation in intractable interstitial cystitis and related pelvic pain syndromes. Pain Med. 2006;7(suppl 1):S166–84.
5. Deer T, Lamer T, Pope J, Falowski S, Provenzano D, Slavin K, Golovac S, Arle J, Rosenow J, Williams K, McRoberts P, Narouze S, Eldabe S, Lad S, De Andrés J, Buchser E, Rigoard P, Levy R, Simpson B, Mekhail N. The neurostimulation appropriateness consensus committee (NACC) safety guidelines for the reduction of severe neurological injury. Neuromodulation Technol Neural Interface. 2017;20(1):15–30.
6. Deer T, et al. The neurostimulation appropriateness consensus committee (NACC) recommendations for infection prevention and management. Neuromodulation Technol Neural Interface. 2017;20(5):516.
7. Deer T, et al. The neurostimulation appropriateness consensus committee (NACC): recommendations on bleeding and coagulation management in neurostimulation devices. Neuromodulation Technol Neural Interface. 2017;20(4):407.
8. Ebraheim N, Lu J. Morphometric evaluation of the sacral dorsal root ganglia: A cadaveric study. Surg Radiol Anat. 1998;20(2):105–8.
9. Feler C, Whitworth L, Brookoff D, Powell R. Recent advances: sacral nerve root stimulation using a retrograde method of lead insertion for the treatment of pelvic pain due to interstitial cystitis. Neuromodulation. 1999;2(3):211–6.
10. Gajewski J, Al-Zahrani A. The long-term efficacy of sacral neuromodulation in the management of intractable cases of bladder pain syndrome: 14 years of experience in one centre. BJU Int. 2010;107(8):1258–64.
11. Hayek SM, Veizi E, Hanes M. Treatment-limiting complications of percutaneous spinal cord stimulator implants: a review of eight years of experience from an academic center database. Neuromodulation Technol Neural Interface. 2015;18(7):603–9.
12. Hunter C, Davé N, Diwan S, Deer T. Neuromodulation of pelvic visceral pain: review of the literature and case series of potential novel targets for treatment. Pain Pract. 2012;13(1):3–17.
13. Kapural L, Narouze S, Janicki T, Mekhail N. Spinal cord stimulation is an effective treatment for the chronic intractable visceral pelvic pain. Pain Med. 2006;7(5):440–3.
14. Lavano A, Volpentesta G, Piragine G, Iofrida G, De Rose M, Abbate F, et al. Sacral nerve stimulation with percutaneous dorsal transforamenal approach in treatment of isolated pelvic pain syndromes. Neuromodulation Technol Neural Interface. 2006;9(3):229–33.
15. Martellucci J, Naldini G, Carriero A. Sacral nerve modulation in the treatment of chronic pelvic pain. Int J Color Dis. 2011;27(7):921–6.
16. McDonald JS, Alo KM. Bonica's Management of Pain, 3rd Edition. In: Loeser J, editor. Section E: Pain in Pelvis, Perineum, and Genitalia: Chapter 73, Pain of Urogenital Origin. Philadelphia, PA: Lippinncott, Williams & Wilkins; 2001. p. 1448–61.
17. Nair A, Klapper A, Kushnerik V, Margulis I, Del Priore G. Spinal cord stimulator for the treatment of a woman with vulvovaginal burning and deep pelvic pain. Obstet Gynecol. 2008;111(2, Part 2):545–7.
18. Paleček J. The role of dorsal columns pathway in visceral pain. Physiol Res. 2004;53(Supp. 1):S125–30.
19. Role of lumbosacral retrograde neuromodulation in the treatment of painful disorders. Pain Physician. 2013;16(2):145–53.
20. Sakas D, Krames E, Simpson B. Operative neuromodulation. Vienna: Springer; 2007.
21. Sator-Katzenschlager S, Scharbert G, Kress H, Frickey N, Ellend A, Gleiss A, et al. Chronic pelvic pain treated with gabapentin and amitriptyline: a randomized controlled pilot study. Wien Klin Wochenschr. 2005;117(21–22):761–8.

22. Stones R, Selfe S, Fransman S, Horn S. Psychosocial and economic impact of chronic pelvic pain. Best Pract Res Clin Obstet Gynaecol. 2000;14(3):415–31.
23. Stratton P, Khachikyan I, Sinaii N, Ortiz R, Shah J. Association of chronic pelvic pain and endometriosis with signs of sensitization and myofascial pain. Obstet Gynecol. 2015;125(3):719–28.
24. Woolf CJ. Central sensitization: Implications for the diagnosis and treatmentof pain. Pain. 2011;152:S2–15.
25. Yang C. Neuromodulation in male chronic pelvic pain syndrome: rationale and practice. World J Urol. 2013;31(4):767–72.
26. Zuidema X, Breel J, Wille F. S3 dorsal root ganglion/nerve root stimulation for refractory postsurgical perineal pain: technical aspects of anchorless sacral transforaminal lead placement. Case Rep Neurol Med. 2016;2016:1–3.

Sacral Dorsal Root Ganglion Spinal Stimulation

73

Jeffery Rowe, Timothy R. Deer, Pankaj Mehta, Jason E. Pope, Denis G. Patterson, Javid Baksh, and Maged Guirguis

Introduction and History

Based on current and available epidemiology, the estimate is that the prevalence of chronic pain is at 25–30% with healthcare cost in the United States alone of $600 billion annually. A considerable number of patients with chronic pain have involvement of the foot (S1) and pelvis (S2) due to a variety of chronic pain processes commonly postsurgical in nature. Until the recent addition of dorsal root ganglion (DRG) stimulation, there has been limited ability to target specifically the foot and ankle or pelvis.

The dorsal root ganglion contains afferent and cell bodies of these sensory neurons that related all incoming nociceptive information from the S1 and S2 spinal nerves through the anterior lateral system (ALS) to the brain. The location and the fact that the nerve cell bodies are contained within the dorsal root ganglion make this an ideal candidate for dorsal root ganglion stimulation at the S1 and S2 level to treat chronic intractable pain within the foot (S1) and pelvis (S2).

Historically it was somewhat problematic to anchor or prevent the migration of leads placed for S1 and S2 DRG targets. This is a technique developed and refined that allows for consistent and reproducible lead deployment and anchoring. Once the lead is deployed within or through the neuroforamina the epidural space and bony architecture of the sacrum is utilized to stabilize the lead with properly placed anchoring S-curves. Proper placement with ½-1 contact of the 4 contacts on the dorsal root ganglion lead placed ventral to the sacrum with anchoring S-curves provides targeted, reproducible, non-positional, and paresthesia-free stimulation.

Background and Historical Perspective

Currently, the Food and Drug Administration (FDA) has approved dorsal root ganglion (DRG) stimulation for use in the United States for complex regional pain syndrome Type I (formerly reflex sympathetic dystrophy) and causalgia (variants of complex regional pain syndrome Type II). The levels that are labeled for implant range from T10 to S2. The use of this valuable tool, however, ranges from C6 to S3. The use of DRG at the S3 level has been used for the treatment of some chronic pelvic pain syndromes as well as rectal pain generators.

Utilization of DRG stimulation within the sacrum provides (1) the ability to provide focal paresthesia-free stimulation to a painful region supplied by S1, S2, and S3 spinal nerves and (2) the ability to treat conditions (i.e., diabetic/nondiabetic peripheral neuropathy) previously considered difficult to treat with traditional SCS.

The table below contains indications for sacral DRG stimulation (Table 73.1).

Targeting the Correct DRG and Choosing Levels

DRG stimulation can be used to selectively target 1–4 dorsal root ganglions suspected to be contributing to the pain associated with a focal region of the body. Animal mod-

J. Rowe (✉)
Main Line Spine & Main Line Spine Surgery Center, King of Prussia, PA, USA

T. R. Deer
The Spine and Nerve Center of the Virginias, Charleston, WV, USA

P. Mehta
Pain Specialists of Austin, Killeen, TX, USA

J. E. Pope
Evolve Restorative Center, Santa Rosa, CA, USA

D. G. Patterson
Nevada Advanced Pain Specialists, Reno, NV, USA
e-mail: patterson@nvadvancedpain.com

J. Baksh
Premier Pain Solutions, Asheville, NC, USA

M. Guirguis
Ochsner Medical Center, Jefferson, LA, USA
e-mail: mguirguis@ochsner.org

T. R. Deer et al. (eds.), *Deer's Treatment of Pain*, https://doi.org/10.1007/978-3-030-12281-2_73

els and prospective studies have shown that stimulation of the DRG can dramatically enhance pain reduction in focal neuropathic distributions. Targeting these focal areas has been previously considered difficult to achieve adequate coverage with traditional SCS and often has led to long-term failure of devices and in some cases even to explant. The adequate focal treatment of neuropathic pain with DRG stimulation requires considerable preoperative symptom consideration/mapping when planning lead placement. Optimization of lead placement during both the trial and permanent implant dramatically enhances outcome and patient satisfaction.

The table below contains suggested targets based on diagnosis and body part affected by chronic pain (Table 73.2).

Table 73.1 Indications for sacral DRG stimulation

Sacral DRG stimulation
Complex regional pain syndrome (CRPS), Type I and II of the foot and ankle
Post-amputee syndrome/phantom lower limb pain
Chronic pelvic pain (L1 and S2) or (S1 and S2)
Lumbar radiculopathy
Discogenic pain
Postsurgical pain of the foot and ankle
Failed back surgery syndrome (S1 usually bilaterally)
Peripheral neuropathy (i.e., diabetic)
Pudendal neuralgia (S2 and S3)
Nerve injury (S1 and S2 on the affected side)

Table 73.2 Suggested sacral level for stimulations based on diagnosis

Diagnosis	Level
Amputee pain (S1and S2)	Map affected levels beforehand using either radiofrequency sensory testing or selective nerve root blocks (S1 usually with L5, L4 and L3 for BKA or AKA)
Discogenic pain	Above and below affected disc, bilaterally at L1 or 2, or bilaterally at L2 and S1
Pelvic pain (including pudendal neuralgia)	L1 and S2 per side or S2 and S3 per side
Neuropathic pain due to peripheral neuropathy	S1 (usually with L5), bilaterally
Foot pain (i.e., chronic plantar fasciitis)	L5 and S1 (add L4 if medial ankle pain present as well)
Chronic postsurgical pain of the foot and ankle	S1 (usually with L5), on affected side
Chronic pain associated with S1/S2 radiculopathy	S1 and/or S2 per affected side
Low back and buttock pain	T12 +/- T11 on affected side or bilaterally

Technique for Sacral Lead Placement and Anchoring with S-Curve Placement

The S1, S2, and S3 lead placement technique is used for the transforaminal placement of S1, S2, and S3 dorsal root ganglion (DRG) leads utilizing a specific sequence of steps to allow for the accurate deployment of the lead adjacent to the S1, S2, and S3 DRG on the right or left followed by the steps necessary to place epidural strain relief S-curves to anchor.

1. The patient is placed on the OR x-ray table in the prone position. Fluoroscopic imaging of the patient's lumbosacral spine is obtained in an AP view appropriately angled to best visualize the S1 foramen. The patient is then prepped and draped utilizing a standard surgical prep and drape technique.
2. With S1 DRG lead placement utilizing a transforaminal approach on the right, the 5 o'clock position on the bony perimeter of the right S1 foramen is identified fluoroscopically. With S1 DRG lead placement utilizing a transforaminal approach on the left, the 7 o'clock position on the bony perimeter of the left S1 foramen is identified fluoroscopically (Fig. 73.1).
3. The skin and subcutaneous tissue overlying the right and/or left S1 foramen is anesthetized utilizing 1–2 cc of 1% lidocaine.
4. The straight introducer needle supplied within the DRG kit supplied is then used to penetrate the skin perpendicular to the skin with the bevel of the needle facing in

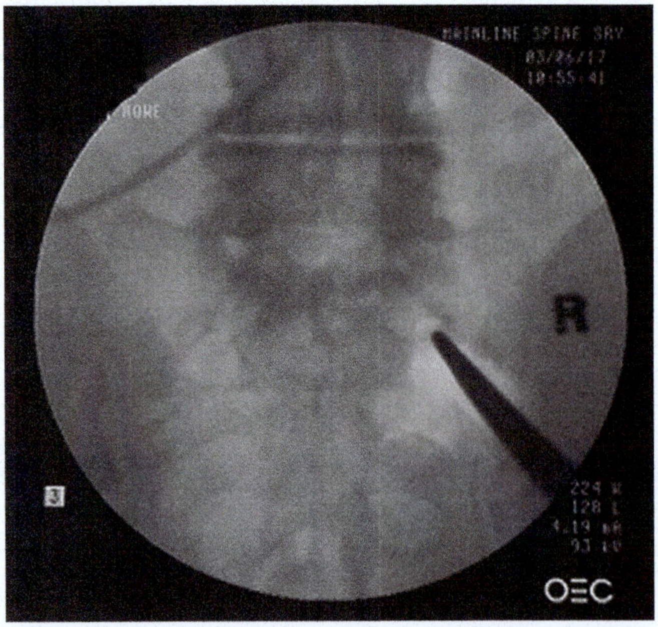

Fig. 73.1 Right S1 foramen is identified fluoroscopically

a caudal direction and is then advanced through the subcutaneous tissues to contact the bony edge of the right S1 foramen at the 5 o'clock position to determine accurately S1 foraminal depth. If the foramen to be accessed is the left S1 foramen, a straight introducer needle would be utilized to penetrate the skin perpendicular to the skin with the bevel of the needle facing in a caudal direction and would be advanced through the subcutaneous tissues to contact the bony edge of the left S1 foramen at the 7 o'clock position to determine accurately the S1 foraminal depth.

5. With the bevel of the needle maintained in a caudal direction, the needle is stepped off the bone edge from the 5 o'clock position of the right S1 foramen, and the hub end of the introducer needle is angled 10–15° in a caudal direction and 10–15° to the right when accessing the right S1 foramen. When accessing the left S1 foramen, the hub of the introducer needle is angled 10–15° in a caudal direction and 10–15° to the left after stepping off the bone edge from the 7 o'clock position.
6. Prior to advancing the needle into the S1 foramen on the right or left, the bevel of the needle requires repositioning angled medially by 45° turned clockwise when accessing the right S1 foramen and turned counterclockwise when accessing the left S1 foramen.
7. The straight introducer needle is then advanced through the S1 foramen on the right or left approximately 1 cm to 1.5 cm (Fig. 73.2 a, b).
8. The DRG introducer sheath with the large curve is then loaded with the DRG lead with approximately 1 mm of the lead tip exposed beyond the blunt edge of the introducer sheath. The DRG introducer sheath hub should be snugly locked around the DRG lead to maintain proper positioning of the lead within the introducer sheath displaying 1 mm of the lead tip exposed to be on the blunt edge of the introducer sheath.
9. The stylette is now removed from the introducer needle positioned appropriately within the S1 foramen ensuring the depth and positioning of the needle is maintained throughout the stylette removal process. The DRG introducer sheath containing the DRG lead appropriately locked into position is then advanced through the introducer needle ensuring that the introducer sheath injection port is pointing caudal and inferior while maintaining the introducer needle's position and depth during the process of advancing to sheath through the introducer needle.
10. When the introducer sheath reaches a depth where the first white band on the introducer sheath enters the hub of the introducer needle, the lead should be exiting the introducer needle into the S1 foramen.
11. The sheath containing the DRG lead with the injection port in a downward direction should be advanced into the S1 foramen while fluoroscopically imaging the advancing lead live and in a lateral view. The sheath and DRG lead should be advanced through the S1 foramen until ½-1 DRG contact is positioned ventral to the sacrum when imaged laterally (Fig. 73.3 a–c).
12. The DRG lead sheath hub is then loosened to allow the sheath to be back off the lead until the radiopaque marker at the distal end of the sheath is contained within the intro-

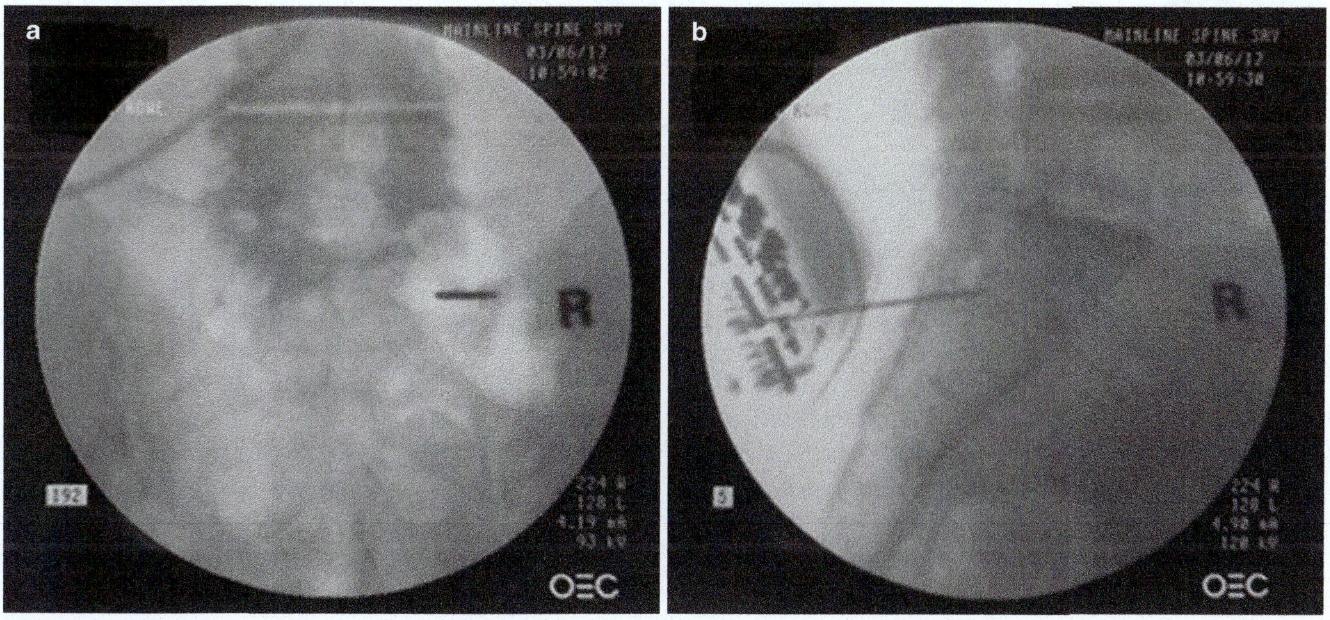

Fig. 73.2 **a**, **b**. Accurately determine right S1 foraminal depth

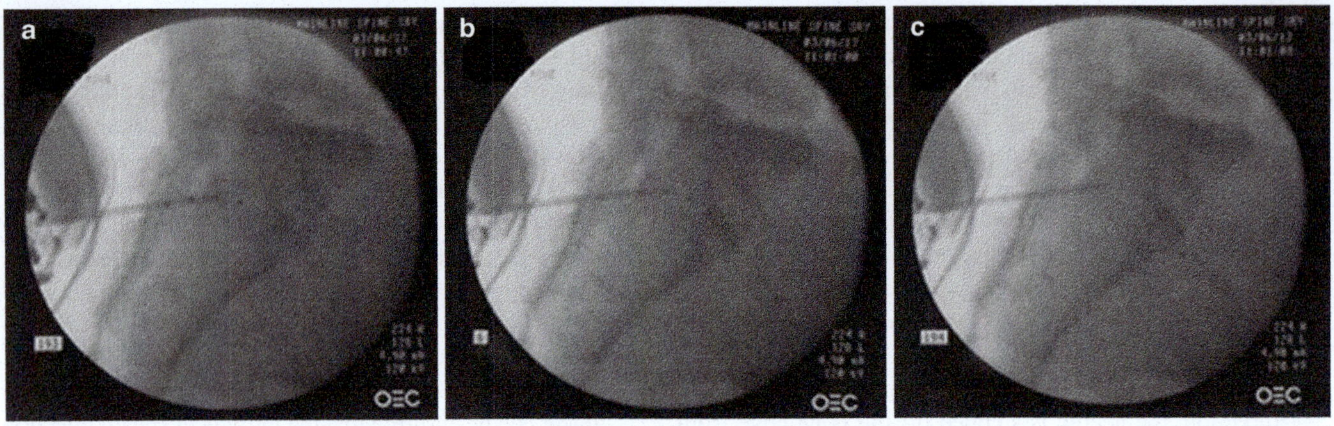

Fig. 73.3 **a–c**. DRG lead ½-1 DRG contact is positioned ventral to the sacrum

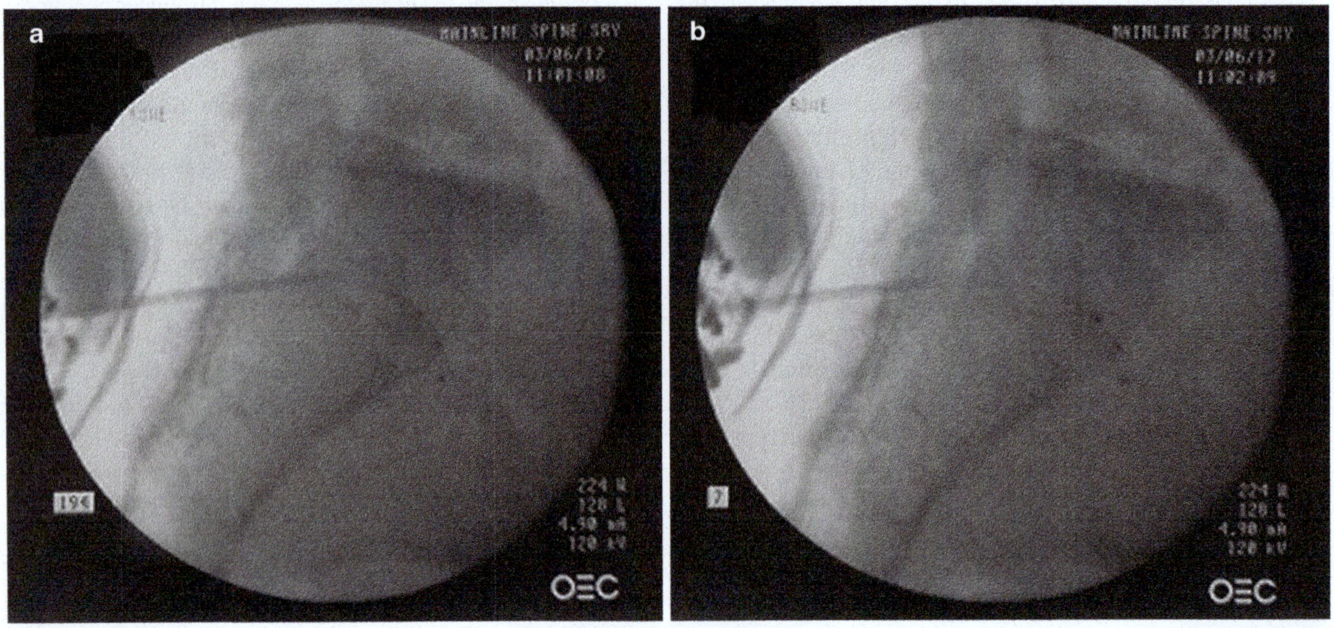

Fig. 73.4 **a**, **b**. Needle withdrawn to lie just inside the epidural space

ducer needle well maintaining the depth of the DRG lead with one contact ventral to the sacrum visualized with live fluoroscopy during the sheath retraction process.

13. Once the sheath radiopaque marker is within the introducer needle to protect the sheath from shearing, testing of the DRG lead position can begin utilizing the expertise of the St. Jude Medical DRG stimulator representative to facilitate programming and optimization of programming for adequate testing of lead position.
14. After verifying appropriate lead depth and position through intraoperative testing, the introducer needle is withdrawn under live fluoroscopy to lie just inside the epidural space (Fig. 73.4 a, b).
15. As a unit the sheath contained within the introducer needle and the introducer needle itself are rotated 180° to position the bevel and injection port cranial in an upward facing position.
16. Using the mechanical advantage of the large curved sheath, the lead and sheath are advanced through the epidural space to form the upper part of the epidural anchoring S-curve. Once an S-curve of adequate size, not advanced beyond the S1 and plate, is formed, the lead is maintained in position while retracting the sheath off the lead to allow the radiopaque marker to lie protected within the introducer needle (Fig. 73.5 a, b).

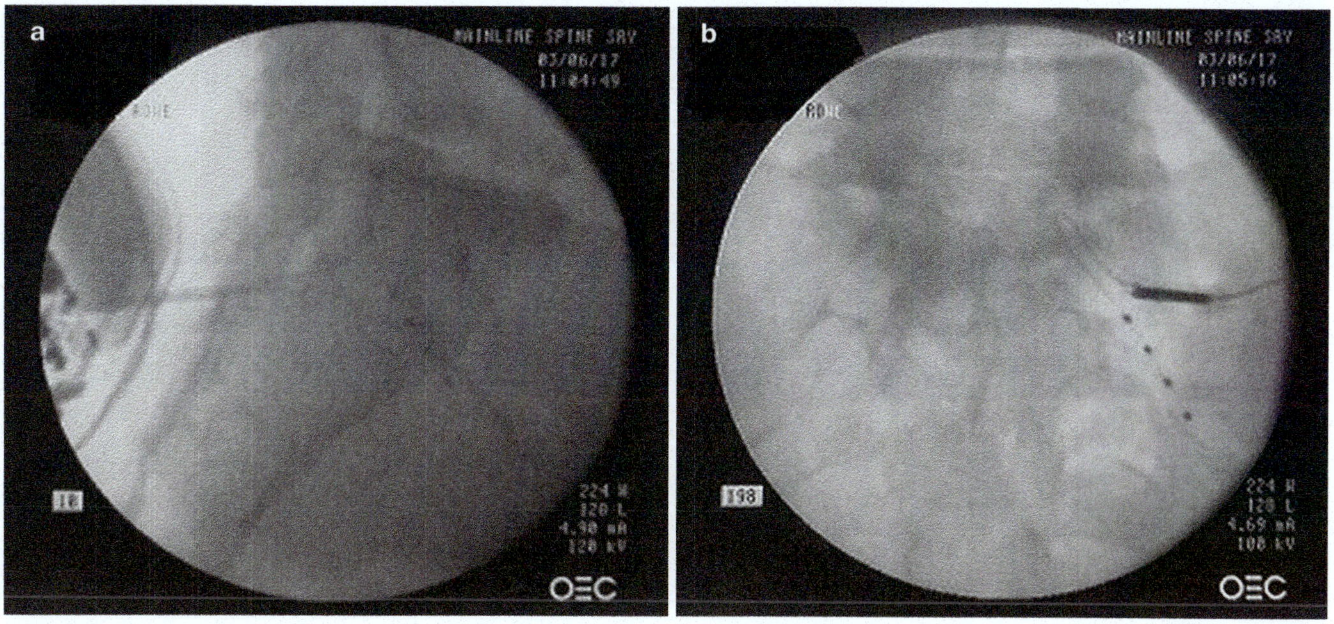

Fig. 73.5 **a**, **b**. Upper part of the epidural anchoring S-curve

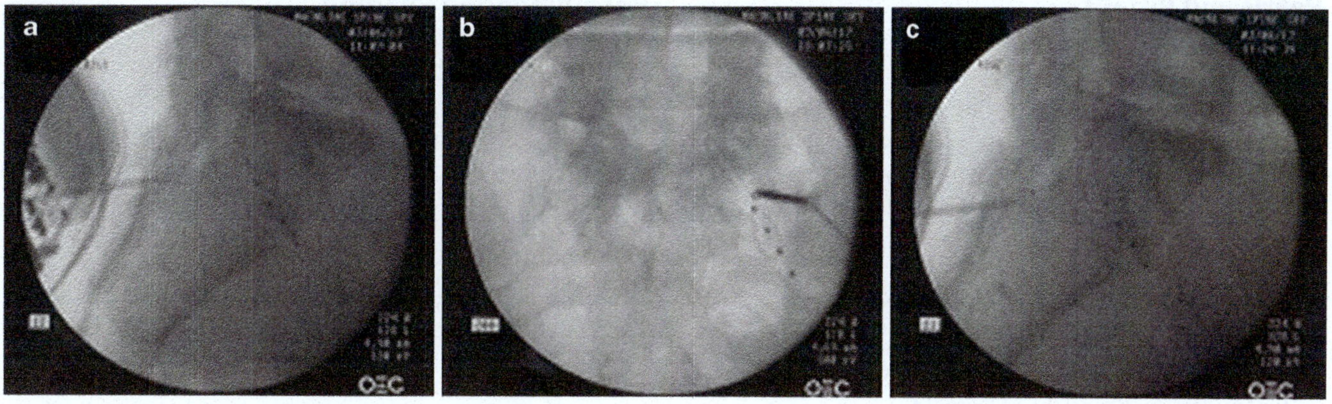

Fig. 73.6 **a**–**c**. Lower part of the epidural anchoring S-curve

17. Once the sheath radiopaque marker is within the introducer needle to protect the sheath from shearing, the introducer sheath and introducer needle are rotated 180° as a unit to allow the bevel of the introducer needle and injection port of the large curved sheath to lie in a downward facing position.
18. Using the mechanical advantage of the large curved sheath, the lead and sheath are advanced through the epidural space to form the lower part of the epidural anchoring S-curve. Once an S-curve of adequate size is formed, the lead is maintained in position while retracting the sheath off the lead to allow the radial opaque marker to lie protected within the introducer needle (Fig. 73.6 a–c).
19. Once appropriate lead depth is verified in the lateral and AP view, the sheath can be retracted off the lead well maintaining lead position. After full removal of the DRG lead introducer sheath, the introducer needle is removed off the lead well ensuring maintenance of lead positioning. Note ½-1 of a contact distance only ventral to the sacrum for optimum programming and effectiveness (Fig. 73.7 a, b).
20. The steps utilized to place needles and leads at the S1 level on the right and left can be used to place leads through a transforaminal approach at the S2 level on the right or left.

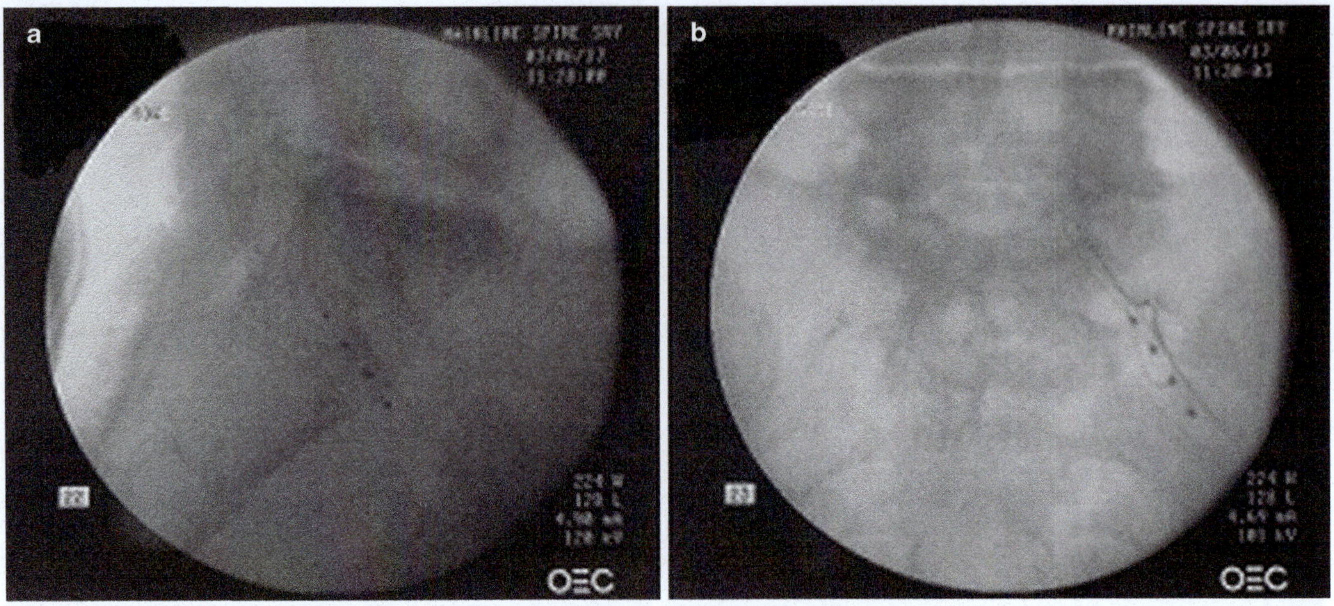

Fig. 73.7 **a**, **b**. Note ½-1 of a contact distance only ventral to the sacrum

Pearls and Pitfalls

- DRG stimulation performed at sacral levels requires the ability to three-dimensionally visualize the space accommodating the leads and deployment system.
- Sacral DRG leads are FDA approved to be placed at S1 and S2 only, but it is within the standard of care to implant S3 if indicated.
- The large curved sheath is usually required at all times during sacral lead placement. Unlike many levels above, the lead may give sufficient rigidity without the need for the guidewire during the placement.
- The sheath should always be protected within the needle prior to turning the needle 180° to be bevel up or bevel down.
- The most critical step in sacral lead placement is the change in needle depth required prior to placing anchoring S-curves.
- To protect all anchoring S-curves within the epidural space during system removal, the order should be:
  1. Needle removal back to the hub of the sheath.
  2. Sheath removal with needle removal as one unit.
  3. Stylette removal from the lead.

**Note that permanent implant requires a #11 blade stab incision performed prior to initial needle placement to provide adequate depth when tunneling from the skin incision into the pocket. At sacral levels no further loops or anchoring is required if adequate superior (cranial) and inferior (caudal) S-curves are created within the epidural space.

Recommended Reading

1. Deer TR, Pope JE. Dorsal root ganglion stimulation approval by the Food and Drug Administration: advice on evolving the process. Expert Rev Neurother. 2016;16:1123–5.
2. Deer TR, et al. Dorsal root ganglion stimulation yielded higher treatment success rate for complex regional pain syndrome and causalgia at 3 and 12 months: a randomized comparative trial. Pain. 2017;158:669–81.
3. Devor M. Unexplained peculiarities of the dorsal root ganglion. Pain. 1999;(Suppl 6):S27–35.
4. Gemes G, et al. Failure of action potential propagation in sensory neurons: mechanisms and loss of afferent filtering in C-type units after painful nerve injury. J Physiol. 2013;591:1111–31.
5. Grigsby E, Deer T, Weiner R, Wilcosky B, Kramer J. Prospective, multicenter clinical trial studying dorsal root ganglion stimulation in the treatment of back pain. 2010.
6. Hasegawa T, Mikawa Y, Watanabe R, An HS. Morphometric analysis of the lumbosacral nerve roots and dorsal root ganglia by magnetic resonance imaging. Spine. 1996;21:1005–9.
7. Institute of Medicine (US) Committee on Advancing Pain Research, Care, and Education. Relieving pain in America: a blueprint for transforming prevention, care, education, and research: National Academies Press (US); 2011.
8. Kandel ER. Principles of Neural Science, Fifth Edition: McGraw Hill Professional; 2013.
9. Krames ES. The role of the dorsal root ganglion in the development of neuropathic pain. Pain Med. Malden Mass. 2014;15:1669–85.
10. Liem L, et al. A multicenter, prospective trial to assess the safety and performance of the spinal modulation dorsal root ganglion neurostimulator system in the treatment of chronic pain. Neuromodulation. 2013;16:471–82; discussion 482.
11. Macfarlane GJ. The epidemiology of chronic pain. Pain. 2016;157:2158–9.
12. Panjabi MM, Duranceau J, Goel V, Oxland T, Takata K. Cervical human vertebrae. Quantitative three-dimensional anatomy of the middle and lower regions. Spine. 1991;16:861–9.

13. Panjabi MM, et al. Thoracic human vertebrae. Quantitative three-dimensional anatomy. Spine. 1991;16:888–901.
14. Pope JE, Deer TR, Kramer J. A systematic review: current and future directions of dorsal root ganglion therapeutics to treat chronic pain. Pain Med. Malden Mass. 2013;14:1477–96.
15. Sapunar D, Kostic S, Banozic A, Puljak L. Dorsal root ganglion - a potential new therapeutic target for neuropathic pain. J Pain Res. 2012;5:31–8.
16. Struijk JJ, Holsheimer J, Boom HB. Excitation of dorsal root fibers in spinal cord stimulation: a theoretical study. IEEE Trans Biomed Eng. 1993;40:632–9.

Peripheral Nerve Stimulation

74

Pankaj Mehta

Introduction

Prevalence of neuropathic pain stemming from peripheral nerves contributes to nearly 8–10% of adults with chronic neuropathic pain syndrome. Despite being an integral part of the interventional pain algorithm, spinal cord stimulation may not cover peripheral areas of pain. Stimulation of a peripheral nerve in these cases may lead to pain relief in the area supplied by that nerve. Peripheral nerve stimulation (PNS) or peripheral neuromodulation has been an effective neuromodulation therapy for many decades now. PNS therapies target nerve fibers either directly or sufficiently near to a peripheral nerve with the concept haven evolved over years from being a very invasive therapy to a much more advanced and percutaneously deployable stimulator systems.

Occasionally when the nerve may be inaccessible, a broader area covered by a known nerve may be stimulated (peripheral nerve field stimulation, PNfS). Previously termed as peripheral electrical nerve stimulation by early neuromodulators, it involves placing electrodes subcutaneously in area of maximal pain presumably within the catchment area of the peripheral nerve.

Background

PNS was introduced by Wall and Sweet in the 1960s for craniofacial neuropathic pain. The first peripheral nerve leads were implanted percutaneously in 1999 to manage intractable headaches. Since then it has been used for multiple mononeuropathic pain syndromes resulting from trauma, infection, or other etiologies. The initial electrode placement used to be a highly invasive technique involving a surgical cut down of the nerve under direct vision and placement of a paddle electrode system adjacent to the nerve fibers. This required a high level of surgical expertise, and the low-frequency direct stimulation sometimes caused more pain leading to inefficacious stimulation due to buildup of impedance.

Like other neuromodulation therapies, the evolution of PNS has seen miniaturization of systems and introduction of multiple therapies and delivery mechanisms. The use of ultrasound also has helped accurate placement of electrodes by direct visualization of the nerve (see Fig. 74.1).

Mechanism of Peripheral Neuromodulation

Pain modulation in the peripheral nervous system is mainly controlled by the nociceptive system. Multiple theories have been proposed, but the gate control theory provides the basis for understanding peripheral neuromodulation. Orthodromic stimulation of nociceptive A beta fibers results in excitation of the target dorsal horn interneurons specifically in the superficial lamina of the dorsal horn. These neurons are also involved in processing

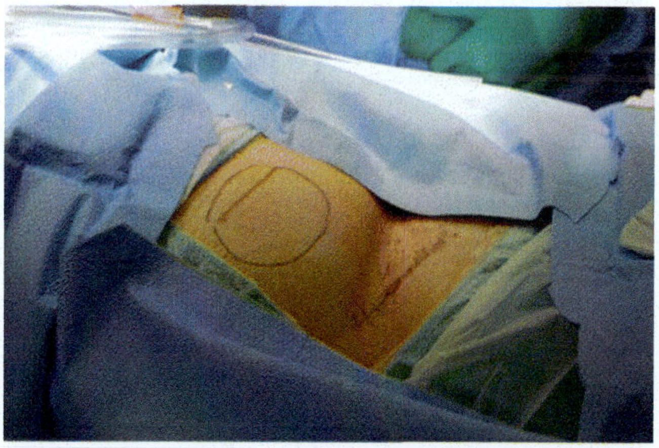

Fig. 74.1 Patient marking for the peripheral nerve stimulation (PNS) device pocket and lead target. (Reprinted from McRoberts WP, Deer TR, Abejón D, Barolat G. Stimulation of the extraspinal peripheral nervous system. In: Deer TR, Pope JE, editors. *Atlas of implantable therapies for pain management*. New York. Springer Science+Business Media; 2016)

P. Mehta (✉)
Pain Specialists of Austin, Killeen, TX, USA

T. R. Deer et al. (eds.), *Deer's Treatment of Pain*, https://doi.org/10.1007/978-3-030-12281-2_74

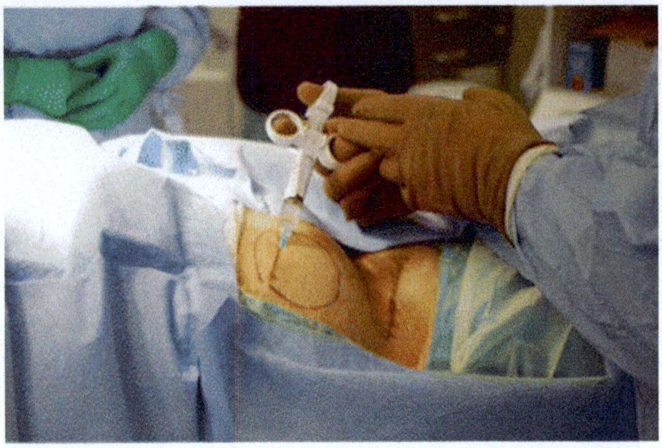

Fig. 74.2 Local anesthetic placement. (Reprinted from McRoberts WP, Deer TR, Abejón D, Barolat G. Stimulation of the extraspinal peripheral nervous system. In: Deer TR, Pope JE, editors. *Atlas of implantable therapies for pain management*. New York. Springer Science+Business Media; 2016)

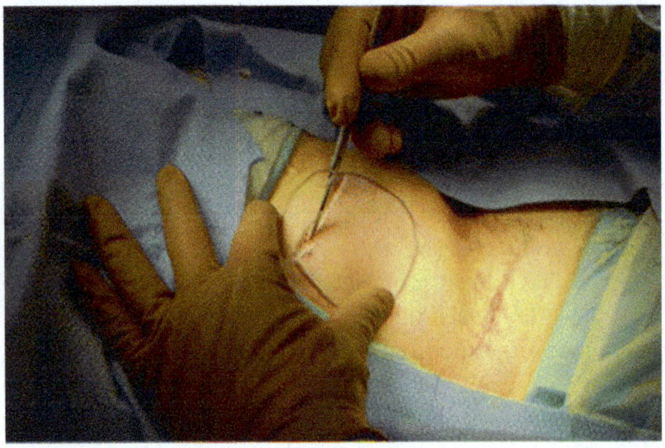

Fig. 74.3 Creation of a pocket for a PNS device. (Reprinted from McRoberts WP, Deer TR, Abejón D, Barolat G. Stimulation of the extraspinal peripheral nervous system. In: Deer TR, Pope JE, editors. *Atlas of implantable therapies for pain management*. New York. Springer Science+Business Media; 2016)

and transmitting nociceptive information via peripheral C fibers, and their activation results in decreased excitability, increased electrical threshold, and slowed conductivity (see Figs. 74.2 and 74.3).

This non-painful stimulation perceived as pleasant paresthesia ultimately results in decreased pain signals. Other mechanisms studied involve direct inhibition of nociceptive neurotransmitters and endorphin system activation.

Uses and Indications of PNS and PNfS (See Table 74.1)

Any peripheral nerve fiber when stimulated directly or indirectly could produce meaningful paresthesia and pain relief in the area supplied by that nerve. The commonly targeted neural structures by PNS and PNfS are the following.

Table 74.1 Commonly targeted peripheral neural structures

Peripheral neural targets	Common indications
Craniofacial *Greater and lesser occipital nerves*	Cervicogenic headache syndromes, C2 radiculitis, greater and lesser occipital neuritis
Trigeminal nervous system Ophthalmic, maxillary, and mandibular divisions	Post-herpetic neuralgia (PHN), Auriculotemporal neuritis after TMJ or parotid surgery, facial neuralgia, trigeminal neuralgia
Supraorbital and infraorbital nerves Auriculotemporal nerves *Superficial cervical plexus*	Postradiation or traumatic neuritis
Upper torso and extremity *Intercostal and subcostal nerves* *Radial, ulnar, and median nerves* *Axillary and suprascapular nerves*	[a]Post-herpetic neuralgia, trauma, postradiation neuritis, post-thoracotomy syndrome
Lower torso and extremity *Paravertebral and cluneal nerves*	Causalgia syndrome from carpel tunnel or ulnar transposition surgery, metabolic neuritis, trauma Shoulder pain
Ilioinguinal, iliohypogastric, and genitofemoral nerves	Axial lumbar pain, failed back surgery syndrome [a]Post-surgical neuritis or injury, e.g., hernia surgery
Lateral femoral cutaneous nerve *Saphenous nerve* *Sciatic, posterior tibial, and common peroneal nerve*	[a]Meralgia paresthetica [a]Medial knee neuropathic pain [a]Lateral knee neuropathic pain, neuralgia from trauma or surgery in foot and ankle

[a]DRG stimulation maybe a more efficacious and first choice therapy. PNS may be undertaken if DRG access has risks or is anatomically not possible

Craniofacial (See Figs. 74.4, 74.5, 74.6, and 74.7)

Occipital Nerves

Commonly targeted for neuritis of the greater and lesser occipital nerves, C2 radiculitis, certain migraine syndromes, and cervicogenic headaches. Modern consensus is to place leads via a midline incision near the nuchal line superiorly as this is a more sustainable system with less chances of migration.

The Trigeminal Nervous System (TNS)

- *Main divisions of the TNS*: The three trigeminal divisions (ophthalmic, maxillary, and mandibular) are commonly involved in trigeminal neuralgia and may be targeted either by peripheral leads, by high cervical SCS leads (lower divisions mostly), or even by a hybrid setup to cross talk the energy from central to peripheral.
- *Supraorbital nerve*: A common target for frontal neuropathic pain superior to the eyebrow from nerve trauma or infection, e.G., herpes zoster. Leads are commonly placed laterally within a cm of the brow. Allodynia over the area precludes lead placement.

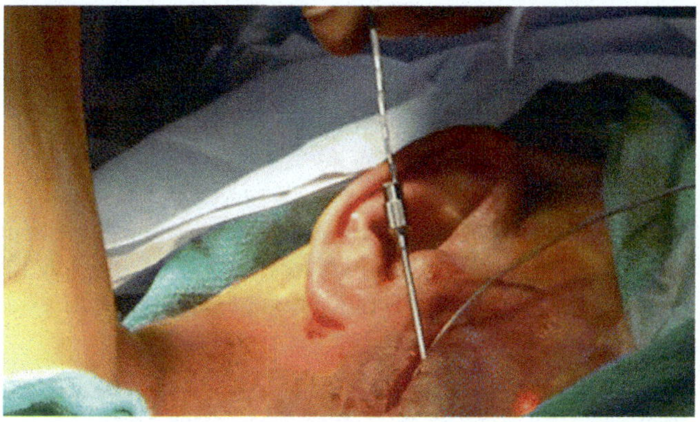

Fig. 74.4 Needle orientation and targeting is an essential part of head and neck implantation. (Reprinted from McRoberts WP, Deer TR, Abejón D, Barolat G. Stimulation of the extraspinal peripheral nervous system. In: Deer TR, Pope JE, editors. *Atlas of implantable therapies for pain management*. New York. Springer Science+Business Media; 2016)

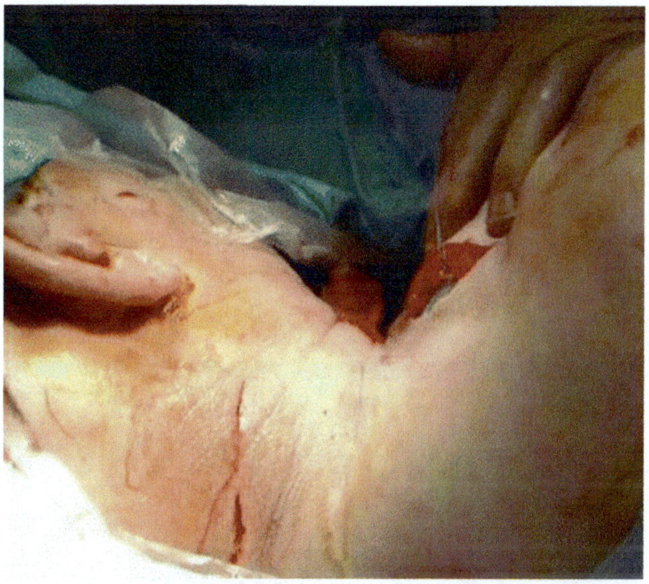

Fig. 74.5 Pectoral pocketing for head and neck implants is often desirable to reduce the risks of lead migration. (Reprinted from McRoberts WP, Deer TR, Abejón D, Barolat G. Stimulation of the extraspinal peripheral nervous system. In: Deer TR, Pope JE, editors. *Atlas of implantable therapies for pain management*. New York. Springer Science+Business Media; 2016)

- *Infraorbital nerve*: May be stimulated for neuropathic pain below the eye, with the leads placed a cm below the eye after preoperative skin mapping.
- *Auriculotemporal nerve*: A branch of mandibular nerve, it may be injured during TMJ or parotid surgery. Placement is like any other facial leads and relies upon pre-procedure topographical mapping of pain.

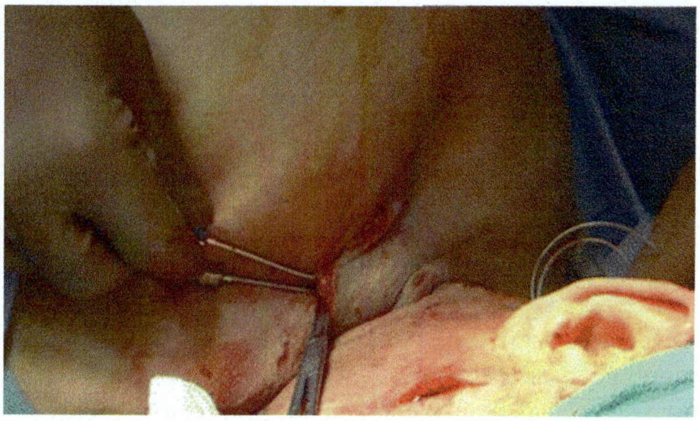

Fig. 74.6 Tunneling of the peripheral lead in the head and neck must be performed with caution to avoid the vessels in the area of the implant. (Reprinted from McRoberts WP, Deer TR, Abejón D, Barolat G. Stimulation of the extraspinal peripheral nervous system. In: Deer TR, Pope JE, editors. *Atlas of implantable therapies for pain management*. New York. Springer Science+Business Media; 2016)

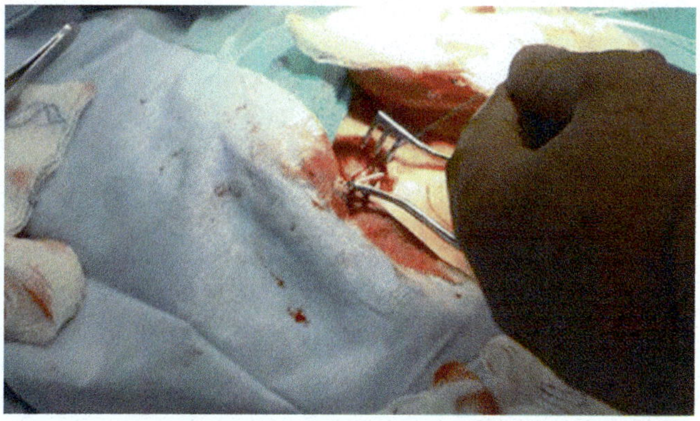

Fig. 74.7 Anchoring of the leads to the fascia behind the ear can lend extra stability to the system and can be cosmetically desirable (Reprinted from McRoberts WP, Deer TR, Abejón D, Barolat G. Stimulation of the extraspinal peripheral nervous system. In: Deer TR, Pope JE, editors. *Atlas of implantable therapies for pain management*. New York. Springer Science+Business Media; 2016)

Superficial Cervical Plexus

Affected mainly by trauma, post radiation or surgery the plexus maybe targeted by a peripheral lead with placement based on pain topographical mapping.

Upper Torso and Extremity

Intercostal and Subcostal Nerves

Neuropathic pain of the chest wall can occur because of infection (post-herpetic neuralgia), local nerve trauma, and postsurgical neuritis (post-thoracotomy). Even though a new stimulation therapy which involves modulating the dorsal root ganglion (DRG) within the spinal column has gained popularity, direct intercostal nerve and field stimulation could still be offered when DRG access is difficult or not possible. Hybrid models (dorsal column and peripheral) have been also been used for chest wall neuropathic pain.

Nerves to the Forearm (Ulnar, Median, and Radial)

Since peripheral nerves distal to the elbow are superficial at multiple locations during their course, they are easy targets to be stimulated in painful mono-neuropathic syndromes involving these nerves, e.g., persistent pain after carpel tunnel surgery, ulnar transposition surgery, or even long bone fractures. There is growing interest in peripheral modulation of these nerves, especially when access to the posterior epidural space to place a cervical dorsal column stimulator is limited (see Fig. 74.8).

Axillary and Suprascapular Nerves (Mixed Nerves)

One of the advantages of stimulating a mixed nerve (sensory and motor fibers) is the ability to provide pain relief while restoring myofascial function specific to that nerve. The axillary or suprascapular nerve stimulation in post stroke or post shoulder arthroplasty chronic pain thus may provide pain relief with the added benefit of restoring muscle tonicity.

Lower Torso and Extremities

Cluneal Nerves

Branches of the cluneal nerves specifically the superior cluneal nerves are often responsible for neuropathic lumbosacral pain specially after lumbar surgery. This is important because these are commonly missed even after successful spinal cord stimulation with epidural electrodes. Peripheral field stimulation helps cover the often missed rim of the axial lumbosacral area innervated by these nerves.

Ilioinguinal, Genitofemoral, and Iliohypogastric Nerves (The Groin Pain Syndrome)

Peripheral nerve trauma either from surgery or postsurgical scar entrapment is very common and equally distressing. Because of their location and course placement of peripheral, leads may be anatomically challenging. DRG stimulation upstream is a much efficacious way to target painful neuropathies related to these nerves. The *lateral femoral cutaneous nerve* is another such nerve which commonly gets affected by local trauma, ischemic insult from entrapment, or metabolic syndromes such as DM leading to meralgia paresthetica. Even though DRG stimulation is now the preferred therapy for this syndrome, in cases where the DRG access may be difficult, direct peripheral nerve stimulation may be offered. The leads are placed based on topographical mapping within the fascia with the generator implanted in close approximation to the leads (see Figs. 74.9 and 74.10).

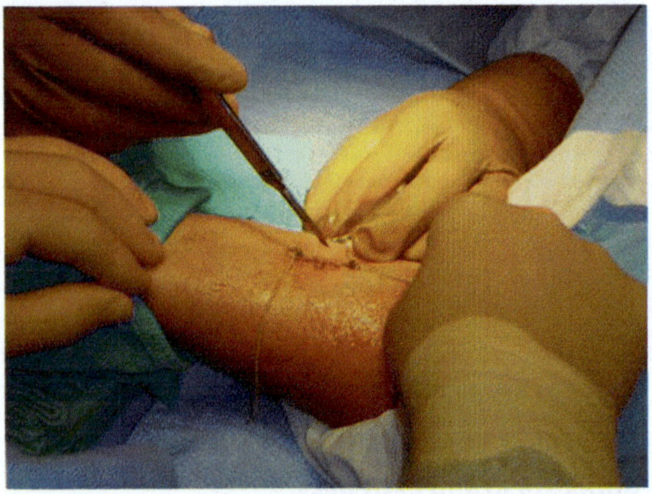

Fig. 74.8 Insertion of percutaneous leads in the area of the median nerve. (Reprinted from McRoberts WP, Deer TR, Abejón D, Barolat G. Stimulation of the extraspinal peripheral nervous system. In: Deer TR, Pope JE, editors. *Atlas of implantable therapies for pain management*. New York. Springer Science+Business Media; 2016)

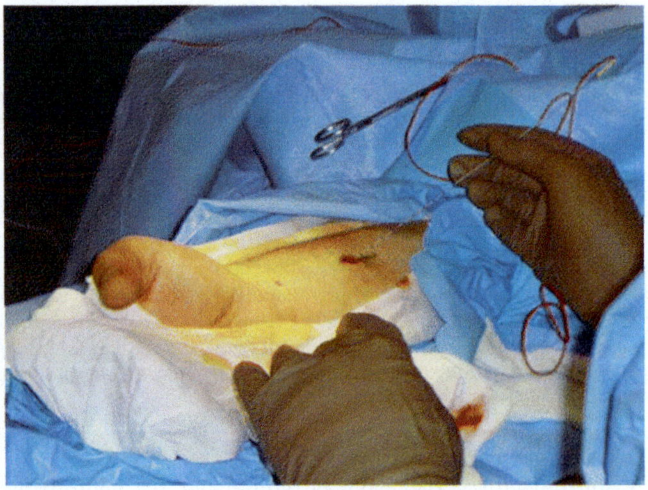

Fig. 74.9 PNS can be facilitated by identifying the nerve with a nerve stimulator, which can be used to guide the final lead placement. (Reprinted from McRoberts WP, Deer TR, Abejón D, Barolat G. Stimulation of the extraspinal peripheral nervous system. In: Deer TR, Pope JE, editors. *Atlas of implantable therapies for pain management*. New York. Springer Science+Business Media; 2016)

Saphenous Nerve and the Sciatic Nerve Complex

These nerves commonly fall victim to direct surgical trauma or neuritis from metabolic syndromes and certain drugs. With their distal anatomical course being superficial and accessible by ultrasound, they may be stimulated for specific mono-neuropathies, e.g., the patellar branch of the saphenous nerve for postsurgical anterior/medial neuropathic knee pain (see Figs. 74.11, 74.12, and 74.13). As the evidence for DRG stimulation for causalgia pain syndromes around the knee mounts, DRG modulation may become the therapy of choice for painful mono-neuropathic syndromes in the lower extremity.

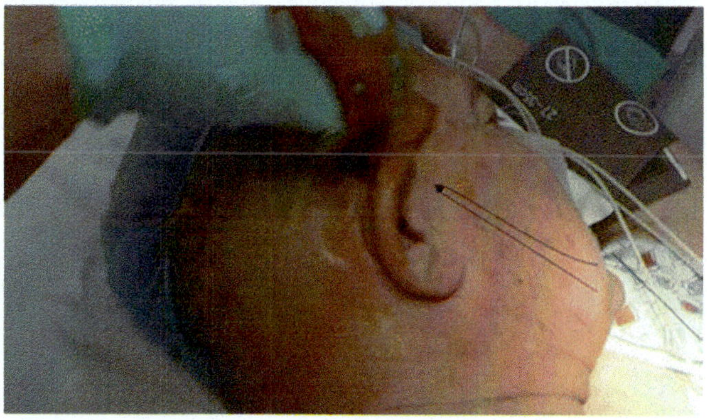

Fig. 74.10 Mapping of the neuropathic pain is helpful prior to implantation of the PNS device. (Reprinted from McRoberts WP, Deer TR, Abejón D, Barolat G. Stimulation of the extraspinal peripheral nervous system. In: Deer TR, Pope JE, editors. *Atlas of implantable therapies for pain management*. New York. Springer Science+Business Media; 2016)

Peripheral Nerve Field Stimulation (PNfS)

PNfS encompasses applying electrodes subcutaneously within the area of maximal pain that is within the catchment area of a peripheral nerve. The aim is to target the terminal sensory fibers deep to the basal skin layer within the deep dermis. Mechanistically it is presumed to activate antinociceptive neuromodulators up and downstream from the painful area (**see** Fig. 74.14). Large painful areas may need multiple leads to cross talk. Some of the pitfalls of this therapy are:

- Technically the depth of electrode placement must be carefully gauged. Too deep placement may lead to a higher electrical resistance. Too superficial placement may subject the lead to erode out and migrate.
- Hyperalgesic areas or allodynic areas do not respond well to direct lead placement but instead when the area is sandwiched between leads and energy made to cross talk between them.
- Pain outside the field of stimulation will not be relieved.

Advancements in PNS

StimRouter

Over the last decade, PNS systems have evolved with a focus on simplicity, miniaturization, and efficacious energy delivery. Some of the limitations in considering a conventional

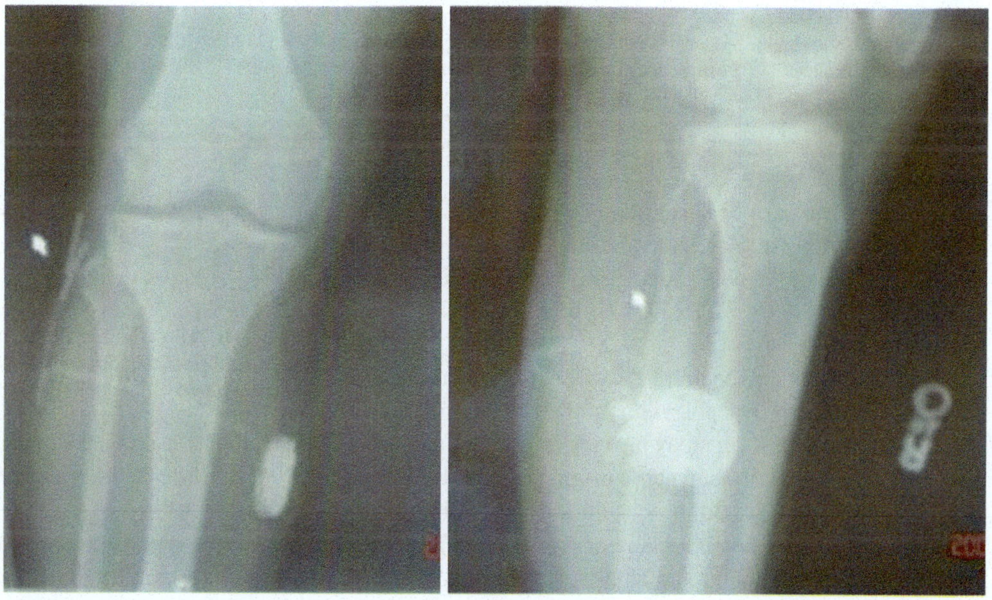

Fig. 74.11 Pocketing in an extremity. (Reprinted from McRoberts WP, Deer TR, Abejón D, Barolat G. Stimulation of the extraspinal peripheral nervous system. In: Deer TR, Pope JE, editors. *Atlas of implantable therapies for pain management*. New York. Springer Science+Business Media; 2016)

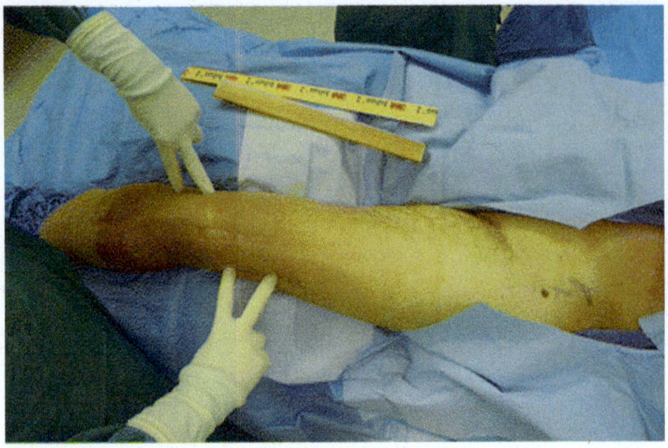

Fig. 74.12 Lead location for chronic postoperative knee pain. (Reprinted from McRoberts WP, Deer TR, Abejón D, Barolat G. Stimulation of the extraspinal peripheral nervous system. In: Deer TR, Pope JE, editors. *Atlas of implantable therapies for pain management*. New York. Springer Science+Business Media; 2016)

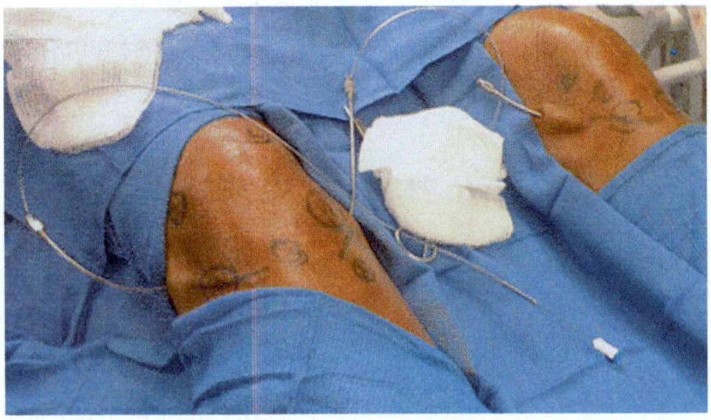

Fig. 74.13 Trialing lead location (with associated dermatographic marking) for bilateral knee pain. (Reprinted from McRoberts WP, Deer TR, Abejón D, Barolat G. Stimulation of the extraspinal peripheral nervous system. In: Deer TR, Pope JE, editors. *Atlas of implantable therapies for pain management*. New York. Springer Science+Business Media; 2016)

SCS system for peripheral implantation of leads has been the size of the pulse generator and the inability to implant proximal to the target nerve, frequently requiring lead extensions (**see** Figs. 74.15, 74.16, 74.17, 74.18, 74.19, 74.20, and 74.21).

Recently a design-specific PNS system was commercialized after FDA approval following a prospective multicenter double-blinded crossover study proving its efficacy and safety in chronic pain of peripheral nerve origin. This well-designed double-blinded trial tested the system for chronic intractable pain associated with posttraumatic or postsurgical peripheral neuralgia excluding the craniofacial area. This novel system called StimRouter is an inductively powered system and consists of one percutaneously implanted lead (length 15 cm and diameter 1.2 mm) with an inbuilt receiver at one end and three tight spaced contacts at the other. It can be implanted using nerve stimulation with or without imaging guidance. Once deployed, an external power transmitter is utilized to power the therapy. A RF signaling-based programmer-communicator enables patient control of the therapy.

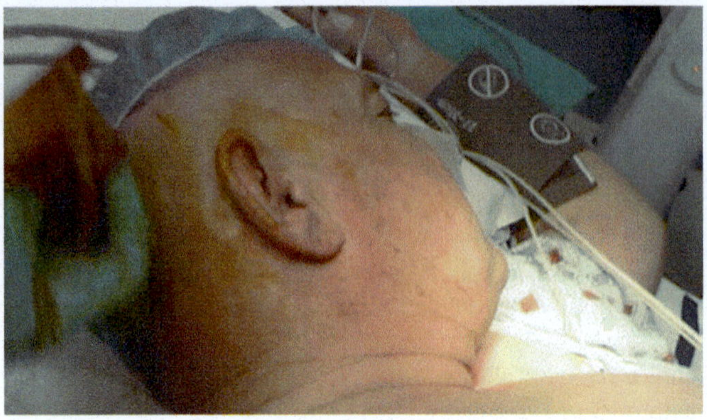

Fig. 74.14 Prepping should be well outside of the target area for implantation of the PNS device. (Reprinted from McRoberts WP, Deer TR, Abejón D, Barolat G. Stimulation of the extraspinal peripheral nervous system. In: Deer TR, Pope JE, editors. *Atlas of implantable therapies for pain management*. New York. Springer Science+Business Media; 2016)

a

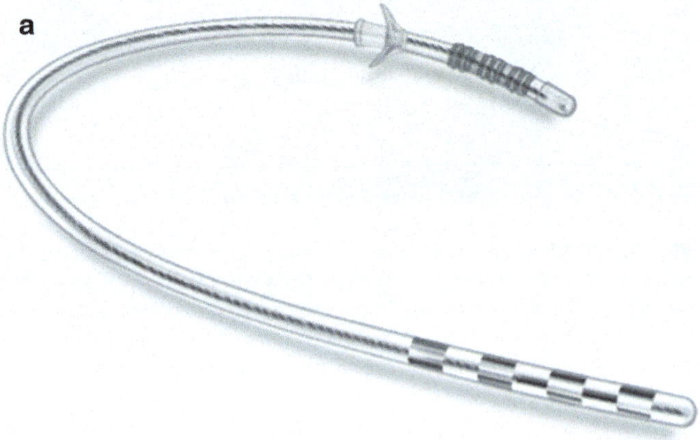

b

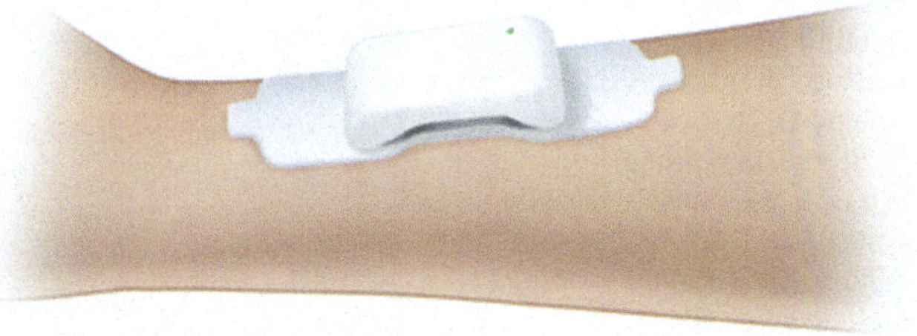

Fig. 74.15 (**a**) The Bioness StimRouter peripheral neurostimulator lead. For investigational use only. Not approved for sale in the United States. (**b**) The Bioness StimRouter peripheral neurostimulator EPT and electrode patch. For investigational use only. Not approved for sale in the United States. (Reprinted from McJunkin T, Lynch P, Deer TR. Peripheral nerve stimulation miniaturization. In: Deer TR, Pope JE, editors. *Atlas of implantable therapies for pain management*. New York. Springer Science+Business Media; 2016)

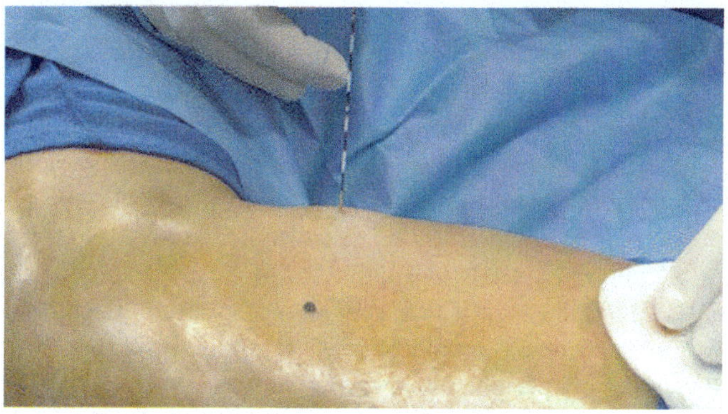

Fig. 74.16 Inserting the stimulation probe for Bioness StimRouter placement. (Reprinted from McJunkin T, Lynch P, Deer TR. Peripheral nerve stimulation miniaturization. In: Deer TR, Pope JE, editors. *Atlas of implantable therapies for pain management*. New York. Springer Science+Business Media; 2016)

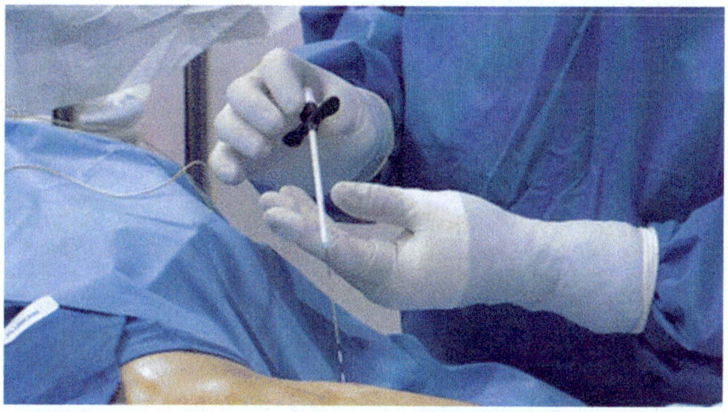

Fig. 74.17 Inserting the loader for Bioness StimRouter placement. (Reprinted from McJunkin T, Lynch P, Deer TR. Peripheral nerve stimulation miniaturization. In: Deer TR, Pope JE, editors. *Atlas of implantable therapies for pain management*. New York. Springer Science+Business Media; 2016)

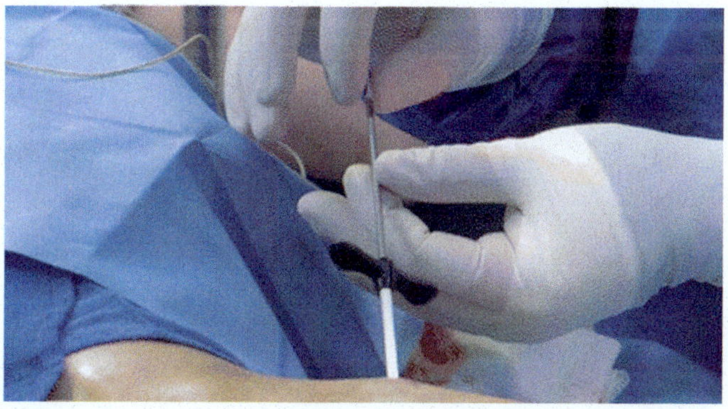

Fig. 74.18 Inserting the lead into loader for Bioness StimRouter placement. (Reprinted from McJunkin T, Lynch P, Deer TR. Peripheral nerve stimulation miniaturization. In: Deer TR, Pope JE, editors. *Atlas of implantable therapies for pain management*. New York. Springer Science+Business Media; 2016)

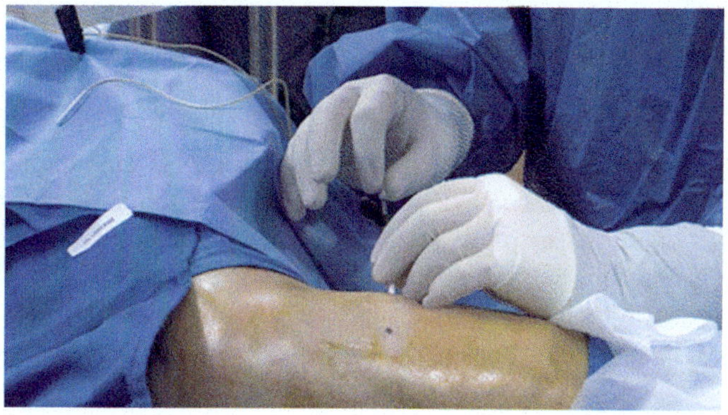

Fig. 74.19 Deploying lead anchor for Bioness StimRouter placement. (Reprinted from McJunkin T, Lynch P, Deer TR. Peripheral nerve stimulation miniaturization. In: Deer TR, Pope JE, editors. *Atlas of implantable therapies for pain management*. New York. Springer Science+Business Media; 2016)

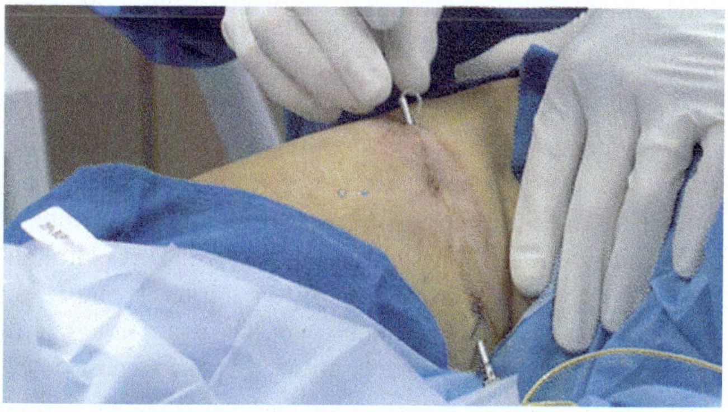

Fig. 74.20 Inserting tunneling device for Bioness StimRouter placement. (Reprinted from McJunkin T, Lynch P, Deer TR. Peripheral nerve stimulation miniaturization. In: Deer TR, Pope JE, editors. *Atlas of implantable therapies for pain management*. New York. Springer Science+Business Media; 2016)

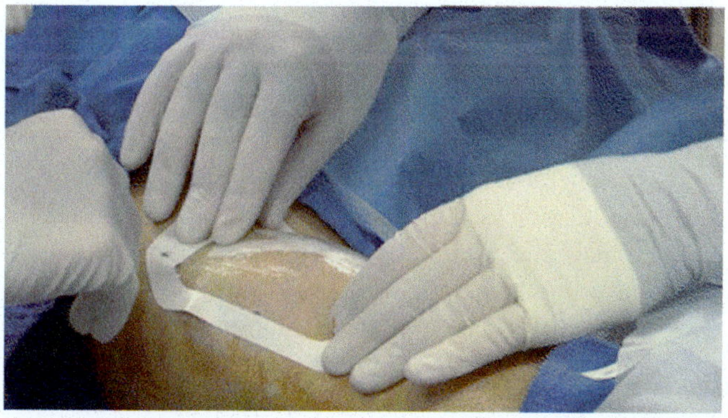

Fig. 74.21 Skin closure for Bioness StimRouter placement. (Reprinted from McJunkin T, Lynch P, Deer TR. Peripheral nerve stimulation miniaturization. In: Deer TR, Pope JE, editors. *Atlas of implantable therapies for pain management*. New York. Springer Science+Business Media; 2016)

- *Neuros Altius*: This device uses high-frequency alternating current (HFAC) to block nerve conduction. A cuff electrode is wrapped around a peripheral nerve to directly block conduction of pain signals within the peripheral nervous system. In a study done for post amputation nerve pain, the device was placed on the sciatic nerve or one of its main divisions. At least four sessions of therapy per week were completed by patients over a period of 3–12 months. Each session of HFAC lasting 10–30 min resulted in relief lasting up to a few hours. Further randomized trials are warranted to draw more conclusions.

Future of Peripheral Nerve Stimulation

The popularity of PNS has witnessed an upward trajectory since the advent of modern and technically simple delivery systems. The dorsal root ganglion (DRG), a structure in the path of the dorsal root of a spinal nerve, is also now a well-proven target for stimulation or neuromodulation therapy for peripheral neuropathic pain. It contains the cell bodies of the primary sensory neurons responsible for transducing and modulating sensory information from an injured peripheral nerve and transmitting it to the spinal cord. DRG stimulation is practiced worldwide safely for the truck and lower extremity peripheral neuropathic pain. The use is not as common for upper extremity and craniofacial pain because of the risks associated with access to the cervical DRG sites. Both PNS and DRG remain options for peripheral neuropathic pain, and the choice of a therapy is based on the target site, mechanism of nerve injury, and ease of implantation.

Main Points

- Neuropathic pain of peripheral origin is responsible for 8–10% of adult chronic neuropathic pain syndromes.
- If the area of pain is localized to a peripheral nerve, peripheral nerve stimulation or peripheral neuromodulation is the choice of therapy. Conventional spinal cord stimulation may not be successful in covering the painful area.
- Dorsal root ganglion stimulation is a new therapy targeting focal neuropathic pain and has become the therapy of choice for many peripheral nerve pain syndromes. It has anatomical challenges in certain areas of the spinal column where PNS remains the therapy of choice.
- Occipital nerve is a common neural target for cervicogenic headaches and has been well proven for intractable headache syndromes.
- PNfS is an alternative to PNS when the peripheral nerve is inaccessible or too deep to stimulate.
- A new device called StimRouter is now FDA approved for PNS and has met efficacy and safety parameters in a first ever prospective, multicenter randomized double-blinded, partial crossover trial for any peripheral nerve stimulating system.

Recommended Reading

1. Chakravarthy K, Nava A, Christo PJ, Williams K. Review of recent advances in peripheral nerve stimulation (PNS). Curr Pain Headache Rep. 2016;20(11):60. Review.
2. Deer TR. Stimulation of the extra spinal peripheral nervous system, Chapter 26. In: Atlas of implantable therapies for pain management. New York: Springer; 2015.
3. Verrills P, Russo M. Peripheral nerve stimulation for back pain. Prog Neurol Surg. 2015;29:127–38. https://doi.org/10.1159/000434666. Epub 2015 Sept 4.
4. Pope JE, Carlson JD, Rosenberg WS, Slavin KV, Deer TR. Peripheral nerve stimulation for pain in extremities: an update. Prog Neurol Surg. 2015;29:139–57.
5. Deer T, Pope J. Prospective, multicenter, randomized, double-blinded, partial crossover study to assess the safety and efficacy of the novel neuromodulation system in the treatment of patients with chronic pain of peripheral nerve origin. Neuromodulation. 2016;19:91–100.
6. Krames ES. The dorsal root ganglion in chronic pain and as a target for neuromodulation: a review. Neuromodulation Technol Neural Interface. 2015;18(1):24–32.

Stimulation Methods and Device Choices: Dorsal Root Ganglion Stimulation, Spinal Cord Stimulation, and Peripheral Nerve Stimulation

75

Seth Christian, Vafi Salmasi, and Michael S. Leong

Introduction

Neurostimulation was introduced as a concept shortly after the proposal of the gate control theory by Melzack and Wall in 1965. The first spinal cord stimulator was implanted directly on the spinal cord by Shealy in 1968; the leads were placed intradurally and directly on the dorsal column. Neurostimulation was applied to various areas in the body, including deep brain stimulation, spinal cord stimulation, and peripheral nerve stimulation. Early on, the practicality and widespread application of implantable neurostimulators was limited by a lack of processing power and battery technology. In the last 30 years, the processing power of portable devices has grown exponentially, as evidenced by the fact that a single personal cell phone now has several times more computing power than the 1985 Cray-2 supercomputer. The evolution of implantable neurostimulators has progressed at a similar rate.

Background and Historical Perspective

One of the early contenders in the field, Medtronic, used existing pacemaker technology and applied it to neurostimulation. In 1980, Medtronic released its first FDA-approved spinal cord stimulator. Other initial competitors like Cordis and Avery Labs were not as successful and could not continue in the field. Another company that used pacemaker technology in the field was Advanced Neuromodulation Systems (ANS) which was later acquired by St. Jude Medical and then Abbott. In following years Advanced Bionics (which was later acquired by Boston Scientific) became the third major provider of spinal cord stimulators.

From 1968 to 2015, the field of neuromodulation saw the introduction of percutaneous leads, primary cell batteries, more efficient rechargeable batteries, dual systems, dual trial systems, MRI compatibility, and independently programmable electrodes. During this time, devices were capable of traditional or tonic stimulation. With traditional tonic spinal cord stimulators, the lead placement is ultimately determined by mapping the paresthesia to the painful area, and the intensity, coverage area, and character of the paresthesia are further manipulated by adjusting amplitude, pulse width, and frequency, respectively, for maximal comfort.

Device manufacturers began exploring ways to improve the coverage and effectiveness of stimulation. Accelerometers were added to account for positional changes in the intensity of stimulation. After introduction of cochlear implant technology to the field of neurostimulation, newer devices allowed for partial anode and cathode arrangements at different contacts which allowed the current to be steered and intensified at the anode or point of stimulation. This allows number of possible configurations available for programming to be almost infinite and improved the ability to generate appropriate coverage areas.

Recent interest in manipulating the waveform to optimize pain relief led to the introduction of new energy delivery parameters in neuromodulation, such as high-frequency stimulation and burst stimulation parameters. Traditionally, the basic unit of electrical stimulation has been the pulse. Narrow pulse widths require high amplitudes to activate a neuron or axon, and wide pulse widths require lower amplitudes to activate a neuron or axon. Axon characteristics such as size, myelination, and distance from stimulus will influence activation.

High-frequency stimulation specifically uses a frequency more than 1000 Hz with much lower amplitude and pulse width less than traditional tonic stimulation, resulting in a

S. Christian
Paradigm Orthopedics and Sports Medicine, Slidell, LA, USA

V. Salmasi
Department of Anesthesiology, Perioperative and Pain Medicine, Systems Neuroscience and Pain Laboratory, Stanford University School of Medicine, Redwood City, CA, USA
e-mail: vsalmasi@stanford.edu

M. S. Leong (✉)
Stanford Pain Management Center, Redwood City, CA, USA
e-mail: msleong@stanford.edu

T. R. Deer et al. (eds.), *Deer's Treatment of Pain*, https://doi.org/10.1007/978-3-030-12281-2_75

Table 75.1 Comparison of tonic, HF10™, and BurstDR™, DRG, and peripheral nerve stimulation parameters

	Amplitude	Pulse width	Frequency	Charge per pulse	Charge per second	Paresthesia
Traditional or tonic stimulation	3.5–8.5 mA	100–400 μs	40–100 Hz	0.35–3.4 μC	14–340 μC/s	Yes
HF10™	1.6–3.8 mA	30 μs	10,000 Hz	0.05–0.11 μC	500–1100 μC/s	No
BurstDR™[a]	0.25–1.6 mA	1000 μs	200 Hz (5 * 40 Hz)	0.25–1.6 μC	50–320 μC/s	No
DRG stimulation	0.35–0.9 mA	40 μs	20 Hz	0.014–0.036 μC	0.28–0.72 μC/s	No
Peripheral nerve stimulation	0–30 mA	70–500 μs	1–200 Hz	0–15 μC	0–3000 μC/s	Yes

[a]Parameters reported in De Ridder et al. (2010)

lower charge per pulse. The low charge per pulse is unlikely to activate fibers or neurons, and the stimulation generally does not result in a paresthesia to the patient. In a large, multicenter randomized controlled pivotal trial, HF10™ therapy or 10,000 Hz therapy has been proven to be superior to traditional tonic stimulation for back and leg pain. Various hypotheses exist about the proposed mechanism of neuromodulation, including temporal summation, depolarization blockade, and desynchronization. In addition, there is relatively little known about the frequencies between 1000 Hz and 10,000 Hz; there is ongoing research investigating the efficacy of these intermediate frequencies.

Burst stimulation utilizes a very low-amplitude, longer pulse width and delivers energy in bursts of pulses with a period of inactivity between bursts. The "burst" pattern was arbitrarily chosen as a series of five 1000 μs pulses at a frequency of 500 Hz followed by a single repolarization pulse. Burst stimulation is proposed to provide a signal that is more similar and relevant to endogenous activation patterns in the nervous system, which has been reported in peripheral neurons and the thalamus. The hypothesis, however, does not explain how the stimulation pattern alters activity in the pain pathways. There are innumerable combinations of burst stimulation parameters, but BurstDR™ has been described in the SUNBURST trial as utilizing an amplitude of 0.25–1 mA, with a pulse width of 1000 μs and a burst frequency of 40 Hz with an intraburst frequency of 500 Hz. Burst stimulation also has a much lower charge per pulse and is generally a paresthesia-free therapy.

Both 10 kHz and burst stimulation patterns have been reported to produce pain relief without paresthesia in most patients. Paresthesia is the sensation that results from activation of sensory-specific dorsal column fibers, so the absence of paresthesia suggests that stimulation is not activating dorsal column Aβ fibers. Asynchronous firing is thought to occur once frequencies exceed the ability of neurons to entrain the stimulation. One hypothesis is that high-frequency SCS evokes an asynchronous firing mechanism, which leads to a change of perceived sensation. Typical hypotheses explaining the effects of 10 kHz and burst rely on neuronal activation, and the hypothesis of 10 kHz induced conduction block has been criticized.

While the mechanisms are unclear, both 10 kHz and burst stimulation both increase the overall charge delivered to the spinal cord. Burst stimulation uses low amplitudes and bursts which are functionally equivalent to a very long pulse width to deliver charge per second 2.5–3 times higher than that achievable using conventional patterns. High-frequency 10 kHz stimulation also uses very low amplitude but very high frequency to deliver 10 times more charge per second compared to conventional programming parameters. See Table 75.1 for comparison of tonic versus high-frequency and burst stimulation.

Currently, electrical stimulation is defined by the basic elements of amplitude, pulse width, and frequency, but variation in these parameters alone can generate near countless stimulation patterns. With the introduction of high-frequency and burst stimulation, much attention has been paid to the overall charge delivery, but there are still other parameters that are being considered, such as stimulation pattern, pulse shape, polarity, and neuronal targets. The concept of charge per second has been recently introduced and allows for consideration that the charge delivery may be a more appropriate measure of the effective dose of therapy. Feedback loops, advances in programming algorithms, and continued clinical trials will help further identify the most effective neural dose.

More recent technology has also allowed for specific systems to apply stimulation to either peripheral nerves or dorsal root ganglia (DRG). Currently, these two systems apply conventional energy delivery to these targets. However, for stimulation of DRG, much less energy is required which has made it sub-perception despite delivering tonic stimulation (Table 75.1).

Uses and Indications

Prior to stimulation many patients have undergone multiple interventional treatment options depending on the area of pain. Patients with pain in the head and neck as well as low back and legs usually have undergone epidural steroid injections or radiofrequency ablation procedures, which may have been ineffective or gradually lost efficacy. Patients with pain in the chest and abdomen may have undergone intercostal nerve blocks or paravertebral blocks, which are frequently diagnostic, but not therapeutic due to the limited duration of effect. Similarly, patients with peripheral nerve injuries may have undergone a variety of peripheral nerve blocks, including but not limited to radial, median, ulnar, supraclavicular, ilioinguinal, lateral femoral cutaneous, saphenous, tibial, and sural nerves. Peripheral nerve blocks are also frequently diagnostic, but not therapeutic due to the limited duration of effect.

If the aforementioned procedures either lost efficacy or simply did not provide prolonged relief, targeted neuromodulation is a logical next step. Pulsed radiofrequency neuromodulation can be considered prior to implantable therapies. Pulsed radiofrequency neuromodulation of peripheral nerves has been shown to be effective for variety of neuropathic pain syndromes. If pulsed radiofrequency neuromodulation is either ineffective or not possible, various implantable therapies are now available for targeted treatment which we have categorized anatomically in Fig. 75.1.

Conventional spinal cord stimulation indications include chronic intractable pain of the trunk and/or limbs including unilateral or bilateral pain associated with failed back surgical syndrome, complex regional pain syndrome, diabetic neuropathy, peripheral vascular disease, or chronic intractable angina pectoris. Dorsal root ganglion stimulation is indicated for CRPS I and II, ilioinguinal and genitofemoral neuropathy, phantom limb pain, and discogenic back pain. Of note, not all these applications are approved in the United States by Food and Drug Administration. Peripheral nerve stimulators are approved for conditions in the upper or lower limbs, entrapment syndromes, intercostal neuralgias, and other peripheral injuries or diseases; however, they are not intended to treat pain in the craniofacial region.

This chapter summarizes currently offered therapies and attempts to provide some structure for selecting therapy by optimizing neural targeting and programming parameters while taking into consideration unique features such as MRI compatibility, paresthesia preferences, battery life, recharging burden, and other technological innovations such as miniature stimulators and more convenient trial and advance programming options.

Pain in the Distribution of a Single Nerve

If the painful area is in the distribution of a single or possibly two nerves and has responded to peripheral nerve block, it is reasonable to next consider peripheral nerve or peripheral nerve field stimulation options due to the less invasive nature of the procedure and presumed decreased risk to the patient with respect to infection and bleeding, especially in those patients requiring long-term anticoagulation. These areas include but are not limited to peripheral stimulation of radial, median, ulnar, suprascapular, ilioinguinal, lateral femoral cutaneous, pudendal, saphenous, tibial, and sural nerves. In the past, traditional spinal cord stimulator systems were implanted on peripheral nerves, but the devices were not intended for this application. Recently two manufacturers

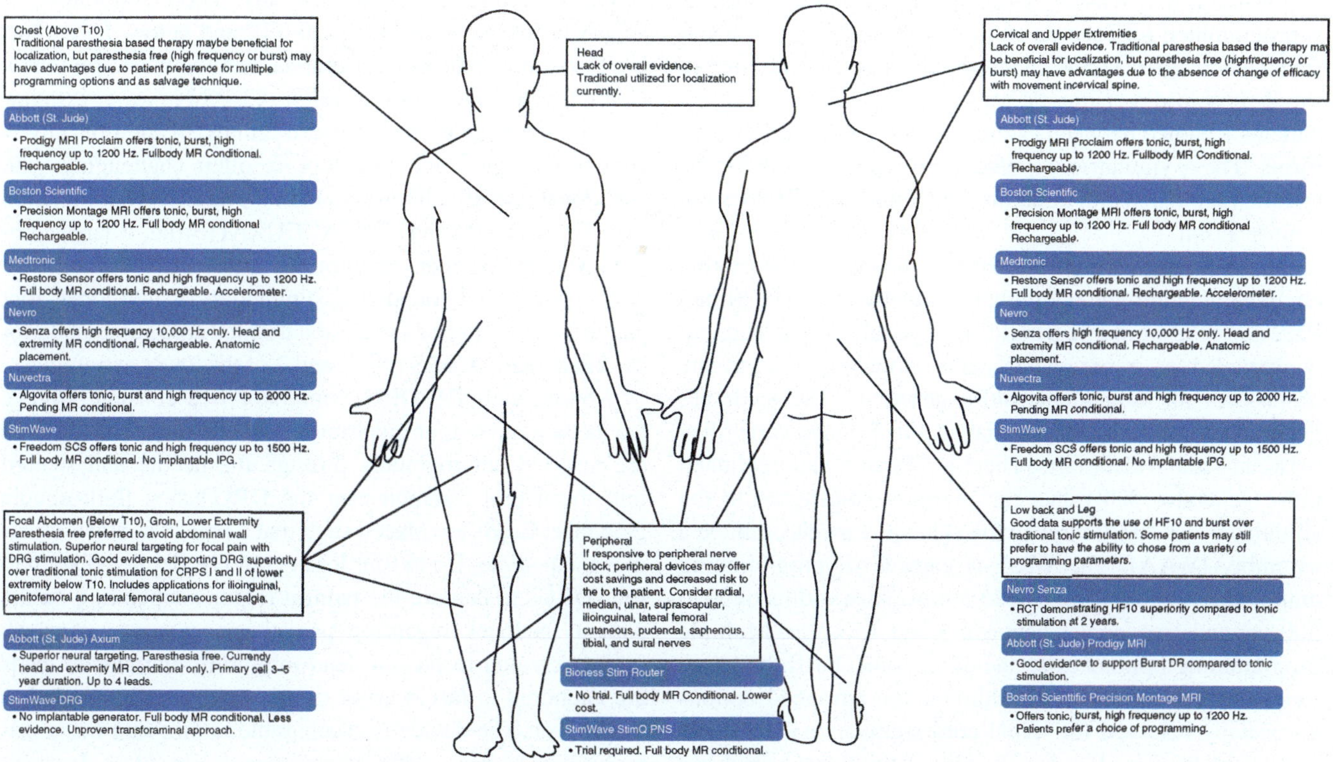

Fig. 75.1 Summary of neuromodulation targets and therapies organized by body map

Table 75.2 Comparison of peripheral nerve stimulator device parameters

Model	Technical placement	Battery life	Amplitude (mA)	Pulse width (μs)	Frequency (Hz)	Leads electrodes	Weight (g) Volume (cc)	MR conditional
Stimwave StimQ PNS	Less invasive Peripheral lead placement No implanted batteries Trial required	Rechargeable External generator Easily replaced	0–25.4 mA	50–500 μs	5–1500 Hz	4–8 electrodes per lead	45 cm 1.3 mm diameter	1.5 T full body
Bioness StimRouter™	Less invasive Peripheral lead placement No implanted batteries No trial	Rechargeable External generator Easily replaced	0–30 mA peak	70–500 μs	1–200 Hz	3 electrodes Monopolar	15 cm lenth 1.5–2 mm diameter	1.5 T full body

produce devices intended to be utilized specifically for peripheral nerve stimulation. Note that both devices are contraindicated in patients who have any active implanted device such as an implanted cardiac pacemaker or defibrillator, or any metallic implant in the *immediate area intended for implant*. It is recommended to maintain a minimum safe separation distance of 6 inches between the electrode and all other active implanted devices and metallic implants. Both devices are full-body MR conditional, although the Bioness StimRouter™ external pulse generator is not.

StimRouter™ is a small, flexible, 15-cm-long monopolar lead with three electrodes and a diameter of 1.5–2 mm that is implanted and tunneled beneath the skin. A small external pulse generator is applied over the proximal end of the lead to transmit power wirelessly through the skin. StimRouter™ is programmed for paresthesia using 100 μs pulse width and frequency of 120 Hz and an amplitude generally <20 mA to avoid muscle direct muscle stimulation. The device offers patients a choice between symmetric and asymmetric waveforms. The asymmetric waveform has a pulse width 4x the symmetric pulse width duration. The StimRouter™ does not require a trial.

Stimwave developed miniaturized neurostimulators that are integrated into the traditional stimulator lead. The StimQ PNS device is similar to a traditional dorsal column lead, but is marketed as a peripheral nerve stimulator due to the absence of an implantable pulse generator. The leads are generally 45-cm-long, have a diameter of 1.3 mm, and utilize between 4 and 8 electrodes. There is no traditional implanted pulse generator, but rather the power is transferred to the stimulator wirelessly through the skin via a wireless antenna assembly (WAA). The WAA is capable of programming amplitudes ranging from 0 to 25.5 mA, pulse widths of 50 to 500 μs, and frequencies between 5 and 1500 Hz. Multiple programming options exist, including tonic, burst, and high frequency (up to 1500 Hz), although the advanced options are usually reserved for spinal cord stimulation. The distal end of the lead is placed at the site of the target peripheral nerve, while the proximal end is simply anchored and buried in the soft tissue.

Sprint PNS offers a product similar to the StimRouter™, but the device utilizes an externalized lead that is only approved for short-term (<30 day) application and is not approved for MRI use. Please see Table 75.2 for comparison of permanent peripheral nerve stimulator parameters.

Focal Pain Located in the Lower Abdomen, Groin, or Lower Extremity

Stimulation of the dorsal root ganglion should be considered for focal pain that is either unilateral or isolated to the lower abdomen, groin, or lower extremity. DRG stimulation is approved for use at the levels of T10 and below. It has thus been used for ilioinguinal neuralgia, genitofemoral neuralgia, lateral femoral cutaneous neuralgia, CRPS I of lower extremities, and nerve injury of lower extremities. In addition, coverage of the lower leg and foot is often challenging with traditional dorsal column stimulation, and DRG stimulation may be more effective. The ACCURATE trial, a large, prospective, multicenter randomized controlled comparative effectiveness trial found that stimulation of the dorsal root ganglion was superior to traditional spinal cord stimulation for the treatment of CRPS type 1 and 2 of the lower extremities.

Abbott Axium™ DRG Stimulator is a constant-voltage device with up to four quadripolar percutaneous leads. Leads are inserted anterogradely through the needle and steered into the neural foramen near the DRG using fluoroscopic guidance. Leads are placed such that a pair of contacts straddles the pedicle. Up to four leads could be deployed at up to four DRGs to capture the painful regions depending on the patient feedback regarding paresthesia coverage. A slack loop is created to prevent lead migration. Permanent leads are anchored to fascia using tissue anchors and tunneled to the pocket. The device is comparable in size and has a primary cell battery with an estimated life of 3–5 years.

Currently, the Axium™ is MR conditional only for head and extremity, but a full-body MR-conditional version is being released.

The same Stimwave devices described in the peripheral nerve stimulation section also have an approval for dorsal root ganglion stimulation from T7 and below. While the Abbott Axium™ recommends an antegrade approach that steers the lead out of the neural foramen to target lead placement on the dorsal root ganglion, the Stimwave device advocates a transforaminal approach that utilizes lead with tines that guard against migration. There is less evidence describing this approach, as the ACCURATE trial utilized the Abbott device. After placement of the distal end of the 45-cm-long lead at the final target location, the proximal end is tunneled and buried under the skin using a microincision. Again, there is no traditional implanted pulse generator, but rather the power is transferred to the stimulator wirelessly through the skin via a wireless antenna assembly (WAA). The WAA is capable of programming amplitudes ranging from 0 to 25.5 mA, pulse widths of 50 to 500 μs, and frequencies between 5 and 1500 Hz. Multiple programming options exist, including tonic, burst, and high frequency (up to 1500 Hz), although the advanced options are usually reserved for traditional dorsal column stimulation.

In summary, the Abbott Axium™ dorsal root stimulator has been proven to be effective for focal pain of the lower trunk and lower extremities, but the device is a primary cell stimulator with a battery life of 3–5 years. Currently, Stimwave™ is full-body MR conditional, while the Abbott device is head and extremity only. Abbott will release a full-body MR-conditional device in the near future. The Stimwave device may offer advantages, because the absence of an implantable pulse generator would eliminate the need for revision and replacement and may reduce risks during implantation. However, better evidence is needed to establish the clinical efficacy of the device and approach in clinical practice. Please see Table 75.3 for a comparison of dorsal root ganglion stimulator parameters.

Pain Located in the Neck and Upper Extremities

For pain located in the neck and upper extremities, high-frequency stimulation has not been extensively studied yet. High-frequency stimulation has been used to treat head and neck pain, but without the ability to generate paresthesia, mapping to the painful area is not possible. Senza high-frequency clinical trial has completed enrollment to evaluate the utility and efficacy of 10,000 Hz stimulation for upper limb and neck pain. Another feasibility clinical trial to evaluate high-frequency spinal cord stimulation for the treatment of patients with chronic migraine is also completed, but the results have not been published yet. Currently, for this area, we first consider devices that can provide both a variety of programming options, including traditional tonic, burst, and high frequency (1000–1200 Hz). With these devices, tonic stimulation is used to generate paresthesias and map to the painful area, and then patients may choose to change the programming from tonic to burst or high-frequency parameters.

Boston Scientific has multiple devices in their product line, three rechargeable options, and a primary cell. The Precision Montage™ MRI, Spectra™, and Novi™ all offer multiple programming options including traditional tonic with anodal intensification, high frequency up to 1200 Hz, and burst (40 Hz bursts with interburst frequency of 200 Hz). All three devices have multiple independent current control (MICC) which has a dedicated power source for each contact to allow for precise neural targeting. Montage™ MRI and Spectra™ are rechargeable and require recharging either daily for minutes or weekly for hours and have an estimated battery life of 5 years. Precision Montage™ is full-body MR conditional, while Spectra™ and Novi™ are MR conditional for head only. Spectra™ is capable of accommodating up to 4 leads with 8 contacts each for a total of 32 contacts with 32 dedicated power sources to expand the coverage area. Precision Novi™ is the company's primary cell option, which has a volume of 33 cc and an estimated battery life of

Table 75.3 Comparison of dorsal root ganglion stimulator device parameters

Model	Technical placement	Battery life	Amplitude (mA)	Pulse width (μs)	Frequency (Hz)	Leads electrodes	Weight (g) Volume (cc)	MR conditional
Abbott Axium™ *DRG	Anatomic Antegrade	3–5 years Primary cell	0.35–0.9 mA But capable of 2 mA	40 μs	20 Hz	4 leads 8 electrodes per lead	32 cm^3	1.5 T head and extremity
Stimwave Freedom SCS	Traditional dorsal epidural or transforaminal needle placement targeting the DRG from levels T7–S1. Microincision to bury lead tip	Rechargeable External generator Easily replaced	0–25.4 mA	50–500 μs	5–1500 Hz	4–8 electrodes per lead May place multiple leads	45 cm long 1.3 mm diameter No implantable pulse generator	1.5 T full body

5 years, although this is based on nominal use and may be significantly decreased with alternative programming.

Abbott Prodigy™ MRI and Proclaim™ both feature multiple programming options including tonic stimulation, BurstDR, and high frequency (up to 1200 Hz). The Prodigy™ MRI is full-body MR conditional and is one of the smallest rechargeable generators at 17.7 cc and 29 g. The Proclaim™ Elite Recharge-Free SCS System is the primary cell offering which comes in two sizes: 48.9 g and 30.4 cm^3 or 58.3 g and 38.6 cm^3, respectively. BurstDR is the only specific burst programming that has been compared to traditional tonic stimulation the SUNBURST trial, which has not formally been published.

Nuvectra Algovita™ SCS offers 24-channel implantable pulse generators that offer two header configurations allow for choice of one to three leads, wireless programming, and compliant, stretchable leads that may decrease lead migration. Currently, Nuvectra is awaiting approval for full-body MR conditionality. The device specifications indicate the device is capable of programming parameters with higher pulse width (up to 1500 μs) and frequency (up to 2000 Hz) than many devices, but there is little evidence at this time to support the clinical utility of pulse widths greater than 1000 μs or frequencies between 1000 and 2000 Hz.

Medtronic offers four devices (Restore Sensor™, Restore Ultra™, Restore Advanced™, and Prime Advanced™), and all of their products are full-body MRI compatible and can accommodate two leads. Restore Sensor™ incorporates a three-dimensional accelerometer to automatically adjusts amplitude, pulse width, and electrode configurations to maintain optimal therapy energy with respect to changes in position. All of the devices are rechargeable (every 2 weeks) and have an estimated battery life of 9 years, except for Prime Advanced™ which is primary cell which has an estimated life of 3–5 years depending on programming. Medtronic devices are not capable of burst programming, but do provide traditional tonic stimulation in either high-density or low-density settings. Restore Sensor™ and Restore Ultra™ are capable of high-frequency stimulation up to 1200 Hz, but Restore Advanced™ and Prime Advanced™ are limited to 130 Hz.

The Nevro Senza™ can accommodate two eight contacts leads and utilizes anatomic placement at the top of T8 and mid-body of T9 for leads one and two, respectively. The device only offers HF10™ stimulation, which simplifies placement but does not allow for paresthesia mapping. The generator has an advertised duration of 10 years and requires daily charging. The Senza™ is MR conditional for 1.5 and 3 Tesla MRIs but for head and extremities only. Please see Table 75.4 for comparison of dorsal column stimulator device parameters.

Pain Located in the Back and Legs

For pain located in the back and legs, high-frequency stimulation has been shown to be superior to traditional tonic stimulation at 2-year follow-up in a large, multicenter, randomized controlled trial. Burst stimulation has promising data to support its efficacy compared to traditional tonic stimulation, but large, multicenter randomized controlled trial data has not yet been published. At the current time, HF10™ stimulation has the best evidence for back and leg pain usually secondary to failed back surgery syndrome (FBSS).

However, the Nevro Senza™ does not offer burst or traditional tonic programming and may not be preferable for patients who prefer paresthesia based therapy. In addition, the Nevro Senza™ is currently MR conditional for head and extremities only. Taking this into consideration, the same devices considered for neck, upper extremity, and upper thoracic pain should also be considered for low back and leg pain.

The Boston Scientific Montage™ MRI and Abbott Prodigy™ MRI offer the most flexible programming including tonic, burst, and high frequency up to 1200 Hz while being full-body MR conditional. BurstDR™ is the most extensively studied burst waveform and is only offered on Abbott devices.

See Table 75.5 for a summary of the specifications and programming parameters of the most commonly used devices in the market today. Some newer devices are skipped in this table because of lack of extensive clinical evidence with these devices.

Pearls and Pitfalls

The field of neuromodulation is rapidly evolving. Since 2015, disruptive innovations including 10 kHz stimulation, high-frequency and burst sub-perception stimulation, closed-loop feedback systems (ECAPS), dorsal root ganglion stimulation, and peripheral nerve stimulation made huge impacts on the field.

This chapter summarizes currently offered therapies and attempts to provide some structure for selecting therapy by optimizing neural targeting and programming parameters while taking into consideration unique features such as MRI compatibility, paresthesia preferences, battery life, recharging burden, and other technological innovations such as miniature stimulators. Highlights of the chapter can be summarized in Fig. 75.1. Cost is often a consideration for many providers, but it was not included in the clinical decision-making included in this chapter. However, implant costs are negotiable, and the ability to choose between vendors often comes at a high price, since vendors often provide

Table 75.4 Comparison of dorsal column stimulator device parameters

Model	Technical placement	Battery life	Amplitude (mA)	Pulse width (μs)	Frequency (Hz)	Leads electrodes	Weight (g) Volume (cm³)	MRI conditional
Nevro Senza™	Anatomic	10 years Rechargeable Daily x 45 minutes	1–5 mA	30 μs	10,000 Hz	2 leads 16 electrodes	59 g 37 cm³	1.5 and 3 T Head and extremities only
Medtronic restore Sensor Surescan™	Mapping	9 years Rechargeable Every 2 weeks (17 d)	0–10.5 V 41.7 mA	60–1000 μs	2–1200 Hz	2 leads 16 electrodes	45 g 22 cm³	1.5 T full body
Medtronic restore ultra Surescan™	Mapping	9 years Rechargeable Every 2 weeks (17 d)	0–10.5 V	60–1000 μs	2–1200 Hz	2 leads 16 electrodes	45 g 22 cm³	1.5 T full body
Medtronic restore Advanced Surescan™	Mapping	9 years Rechargeable Every 2 weeks (17 d)	0–10.5 V	60–450 μs	2–130 Hz	2 leads 16 electrodes	72 g 47 cm³	1.5 T full body
Medtronic prime advanced Surescan™	Mapping	3–5 years Primary cell battery Non-rechargeable	0–10.5 V	60–450 μs	2–130 Hz	2 leads 16 electrodes	67 g	1.5 T full body
Boston scientific Precision montage™ MRI	Mapping	5 years Rechargeable Daily for minutes or weekly for hours Every 1–4 weeks	0.–25.5 mA	20–1000 μs	2–1200 Hz	2 leads 16 electrodes	19.8 cm³	1.5 T full body
Boston scientific Precision Novi™	Mapping	5 years Primary cell	0–25.5 mA	20–1000 μs	2–1200 Hz	2 lead 16 electrodes	33 cm³	1.5 T head only
Boston scientific Precision spectra™	Mapping	5 years Daily for minutes or weekly for hours Every 1–4 weeks	0–25.5 mA	20–1000 μs	2–1200 Hz	4 leads 32 electrodes	21.2 cm³	1.5 T head only
Nuvectra Algovita™	Mapping	10 years Rechargeable 3–4 days, encourage daily for HF	Up to 30 mA	<=1500 μs	2–2000 Hz	Up to 24 electrodes	40 g 20 cm³	Under review FDA for full-body conditional
Abbott prodigy™ *Burst	Mapping	10 years	2.36 mA 0.05–4 mA	<= 1000 μs 1000 μs	Burst 40 hz Intra burst 500 Hz 1200 hz tonic	2 leads 16 electrode	29 g 17.7 cm³	1.5 T full body
Abbott proclaim™ *Burst	Mapping		2.36 mA 0.05–4 mA	1000 μs	Burst 40 hz Intra burst 500 hz 1200 hz tonic			1.5 T full body
Stimwave Freedom SCS	Traditional dorsal epidural or transforaminal needle placement targeting the DRG from levels T7-S1 Microincision to bury lead tip	Rechargeable External generator Easily replaced	0–25.4 mA	50–500 μs	5–1500 Hz	4–8 electrodes per lead May place multiple leads	45 cm long 1.3 mm diameter No implantable pulse generator	1.5 T full body

*BurstDR

Table 75.5 Comparison of properties of most common available systems

	Medtronic	Abbott	Boston Scientific	Nevro
Tonic stimulation	Yes	Yes	Yes	No
Burst stimulation	No	Yes (burst DR™)	Yes	No
High-frequency stimulation	Yes (up to 1200 Hz)	Yes (up to 1200 Hz)	Yes (up to 1200 Hz)	Yes (up to 10,000 Hz)
Primary cell battery	Yes	Yes	Yes	No
Rechargeable battery	Yes	Yes	Yes (wireless)	Yes (daily)
Unique features	Adaptive stimulation	Invisible trial system	Anodal intensification	Anatomical placement
MRI compatibility	Full body	Full body (except DRG)	Full body	Head and extremities

Table 75.6 Evidence for efficacy

Study	Author	Design	Key findings
PROCESS	Kumar et al.	Prospective randomized controlled trial	Spinal cord stimulation is superior to medical management in leg pain with 48% success rate in SCS group vs. 9% success rate in medical management group
	North et al.	Prospective randomized controlled trial with crossover	Spinal cord stimulation is superior to reoperation in back and leg pain with 47% success rate in SCS group vs. 12% success in reoperation group; moreover, SCS is more cost-effective than reoperation either before or after crossover
ACCURATE	Deer et al.	Pivotal, prospective, multicenter, randomized comparative effectiveness trial	For the treatment of CRPS type 1 or causalgia of the lower extremities, the proportion of subjects who received treatment success (>50% pain relief) at 12 months in the DRG arm (74.2%) was greater than that in the SCS arm (53%) which demonstrated both non-inferiority ($P < 0.0001$) and superiority ($P < 0.0004$)
SENZA 2	Kapural et al.	Pivotal, prospective, multicenter, randomized controlled trial	At 24 months, more subjects were responders to HF10™ therapy than traditional SCS therapy (back pain,76.5% vs 49.3%, $p < 0.001$ for non-inferiority and superiority; leg pain, 72.9% vs 49.3% $p < 0.001$ for non-inferiority and $p < 0.003$ for superiority)
Sunburst™	Slavin et al.	Prospective, multicenter, randomized controlled trial	Success using neuromodulation with BURST Study. 173 patients enrolled comparing Burst DR stimulation to traditional tonic stimulation. Completed January 2017. Results not yet published

lower rates for exclusive contracts. In general, peripheral nerve stimulator devices range from $4000–5000 (StimRouter™ and Sprint PNS) to $15,000 (StimQ PNS), while traditional implantable dorsal column and dorsal root ganglion stimulators range between $35,000 and $40,000.

New programming parameters have proven to be more effective than traditional tonic stimulation, but more clinical studies are needed to determine the optimal parameters and to establish durability over prior stimulation treatments. Recent data has been presented at the International Neuromodulation Society annual meeting exploring the efficacy of high-frequency stimulation between 1000 and 10,000 Hz and to evaluate the long-term safety and performance of a feedback-controlled, closed-loop spinal cord system using ECAPS to treat chronic pain of the trunk and or limbs. Table 75.6 summarizes some of the most important clinical trials showing efficacy of spinal cord stimulation systems. The future of stimulation technologies seems very exciting and could help more patients dealing with chronic pain, beyond low back pain and complex regional pain syndromes.

Recommended Reading

1. Al-Kaisy A, Van Buyten J, Smet I, Palmisani S, Pang D, Smith T. (2014) sustained effectiveness of 10 kHz high-frequency spinal cord stimulation for patients with chronic, low Back pain: 24-month results of a prospective multicenter study. Pain Med. 2014;15c:347–54.
2. Courtney P, Espinet A, Mitchell B, Russo M, Muir A, Verrills P, Davis K. Improved pain relief with burst spinal cord stimulation for two weeks in patients using tonic stimulation: results from a small clinical study. Neuromodulation; E-pub ahead of print. 2015; https://doi.org/10.1111/ner.12294.
3. Crosby N, Keiser M, Smith J, Zeemean M, Winkelstein B. Stimulation parameters define the effectiveness of burst spinal cord stimulation in rat model of neuropathic pain. Neuromodulation. 2015;18:1–8.
4. De Ridder D, Plazier M, Kamerling N, Menovsky T, Vanneste S. Burst spinal cord stimulation for limb and Back pain. World Neurosurg. 2013;80(5):642–9.
5. Deer TR, Mekhail N, Provenzano D, Pope J, Krames E, Leong M, et al. The appropriate use of neurostimulation of the spinal cord and peripheral nervous system for the treatment of chronic pain and ischemic diseases: the neuromodulation appropriateness consensus committee. Neuromodulation. 2014;17(6):515–50.
6. Deer T, Levy R, Kramer J, et al. Dorsal root ganglion stimulation yielded higher treatment success rate for complex regional pain

syndrome and causalgia at 3 and 12 months: a randomized comparative trial. Pain. 2017;158:669–81.
7. DeRidder D, Vanneste S, Plazier M, van der Loo E, Menovsky T. Burst spinal cord stimulation: toward paresthesia-free pain suppression. Neurosurgery. 2010;66(5):986–90.
8. Holsheimer J, den Boer A, Struijk JJ, Rozeboom AR. MR assessment of the normal position of the spinal cord in the spinal canal. Am J Neuroradiol. 1994;15(5):951–9.
9. Kapura L, et al. Novel 10-kHz high frequency (HF10™ therapy) is superior to traditional low-frequency spinal cord stimulation for the treatment of chronic back and leg pain: the SENZA-RCT. Anesthesiology. 2015;123(4):851–60.
10. Kapura L, et al. Comparison of 10-kHz high frequency and traditional low-frequency spinal cord stimulation for the treatment of chronic back and leg pain: 24-month results from a multicenter, randomized, controlled pivotal trial. Neurosurgery. 2016;79(5):667–77.
11. Kumar K, Taylor RS, Jacques L, et al. Spinal cord stimulation versus conventional medical management for neuropathic pain: a multicenter randomized controlled trial in patients with failed back surgery syndrome. Pain. 2007;132:179.
12. Kumar K, Taylor RS, Jacques L, et al. The effects of spinal cord stimulation in neuropathic pain are sustained: a 24-month follow-up of the prospective randomized controlled multicenter trial of the effectiveness of spinal cord stimulation. Neurosurgery. 2008;63:762–70.
13. Liem L, Russo M, huygen F, Van Buyten J, et al. One-year outcomes of spinal cord stimulation of the dorsal root ganglion in the treatment of chronic neuropathic pain. Neuromodulation. 2015;18:41–9.
14. Miller JP, Eldabe S, Buchser E, Johanek LM, Guan Y, Linderoth B. Parameters of spinal cord and their role in electrical charge delivery: a review. Neuromodulation. 2016;19:373–84.
15. Muhammad S, Roeske S, Chaudhry SR, Kinfe TM. Burst or high-frequency (10kHz) spinal cord stimulation in failed Back surgery syndrome in patients with predominant back pain: 1 year comparative data. Neuromodulation. 2017; E-pub ahead of print.
16. North RB, Kidd DH, Farrokhi F, Piantadosi SA. Spinal cord stimulation versus repeated lumbosacral spine surgery for chronic pain: a randomized, controlled trial. Neurosurgery. 2005;56:98–106.
17. Oakley J, Krames E, et al. A new spinal cord stimulation system effectively relieves chronic, intractable pain: a multicenter prospective clinical study. Neuromodulation. 2007;10., Number 3:262.
18. Provenzano D, Rebman J, Kuhel C, Trenz H, Kilgore J. The efficacy of high-density spinal cord stimulation among trial, implant, and conversion patients: a retrospective case series. Neuromodulation. 2017.; E-pub ahead of print;20:654. https://doi.org/10.1111/ner.12612.
19. De Ridder D, Vanneste S, Plazier M, Vancampt T. Mimicking the brain: evaluation of St. Jude Medical's prodigy chronic pain system with burst technology. Expert Rev Med Devices. 2015;12(2):143–50.
20. Schultz D, Webster L, et al. Sensor-driven position-adaptive spinal cord stimulation for chronic pain. Pain Physician. 2012;15:1–12.
21. Slavin K, North R, Deer T, Staats P, Davis K, Diaz R. Tonic and burst spinal cord stimulation waveforms for the treatment of chronic intractable pain: study protocol for a randomized controlled trial. Trials. 2016;17:569.
22. Tiede J, Brown L, Gekht G, Vallejo R, Yearwood T, Morgan D. Novel spinal cord stimulation parameters in patients with predominant back pain. Neuromodulation. 2013;16:370–5.
23. Weiner RL, Yeung A, Montes GC, Perryman TL, Speck B. Treatment of FBSS low back pain with a novel percutaneous DRG wireless stimulator: pilot and feasibility study. Pain Med. 2016;17(10):1911–6.

Patient Selection

76

Sean Li

Introduction

Selecting the appropriate candidate for neuromodulation therapy may be one of the most challenging aspects of treating chronic pain patients with this modality. There are increasing body of evidence to support the current approved indications for spinal cord stimulation (SCS) combined with emerging technologies that have been proven effective for increasing number of disease states. The individual patient with the disease state that presents with intangible variables that make patient selection both an art and a science. This section attempts to outline the process in which a neuromodulator identifies and selects the appropriate chronic pain patient for neuromodulation therapy.

FDA-Approved Indication for SCS Therapy

Managing chronic, intractable pain of the trunk of limbs, including unilateral or bilateral pain associated with failed back surgery syndrome (FBSS), intractable low back pain, and leg pain [1].

Common Indications

- Radiculopathy
- Failed back surgery syndrome (FBSS)
- Complex regional pain syndrome (CRPS)
- Postherpetic neuralgia

S. Li (✉)
Premier Pain Centers, An Affiliate of National Spine and Pain Centers, Shrewsbury, NJ, USA
e-mail: Sli@treatingpain.com

Investigational Indications

- Abdominal/pelvic pain
- Diabetic or peripheral neuropathy
- Postsurgical pain syndromes
- Chronic refractory angina
- Ischemic pain syndromes

Timing of SCS Therapy

Neuromodulation Appropriateness Consensus Committee (NACC) recommends that SCS be considered earlier (within the first 2 years) in the treatment algorithm when conservative therapy has failed [4]. There is evidence that the longer delay from diagnosis of chronic pain to SCS therapy may result in increased healthcare utilization. In this same study, the average pain to SCS time was 1.39 years [8].

Patient Expectations and Treatment Goals

- Sustained chronic pain relief
- Improvement of functional status
- Improvement of sleep, mood, and quality of life
- Psychological preparation
- Establishing treatment goals

Neuropsychological Evaluation

Chronic pain is a subjective phenomenon that is deeply associated with the patient's sensory and emotional experiences. There are biopsychosocial factors such as treatment expectations, mood, depression, and anxiety that shape the overall success of SCS therapy. The physician must clearly outline the treatment goals and understand the expectations of the

T. R. Deer et al. (eds.), *Deer's Treatment of Pain*, https://doi.org/10.1007/978-3-030-12281-2_76

patient. Most insurance carriers require neuropsychological clearance from a certified mental health specialist prior to SCS trial and implantation. NACC recommends such evaluation within 1 year of initiating SCS therapy.

Documentation: Establishing Medical Necessity

In the United States, a clinician must establish medical necessity for spinal cord stimulation prior to obtaining prior authorization or reimbursement for services. Medicare rules require the presence of chronic pain syndrome (ICD-10: G89.4) complemented by a secondary diagnosis of an approved SCS indication such as lumbar radiculopathy (ICD-10: M54.16). Additional variations may exist among commercial carriers depending on geographical region of service.

Definition of Successful Trial

Chronic pain patients exhibit a combination of biopsychosocial and neuropathological findings. The success of SCS trial must be determined with both objective and subjective metrics. One must first differentiate the difference between technical success and clinical or therapeutic success.

Key criteria include:

1. Coverage of stimulation with respect to the affected body part(s)
   *This may not apply to paresthesia-free SCS trial
2. Degree of pain relief, often described in VAS score change (>50%)
3. Opioid dosage during trial
4. Functional status
5. Sleep, mood, and overall quality of life

Providers should consider these factors when facilitating the decision to proceed with permanent implantation. Patients should be given adequate time to reflect and discuss this decision with family. The return of usual chronic pain after the removal of temporary leads will help patients confirm their decision.

Selection of Treatment Options: Paddle Versus Percutaneous, Rechargeable Versus Non-rechargeable

Decision to select percutaneous versus paddle lead options should be based on the individual patient needs, and information obtained during the temporary trial should be included in this process. When choosing between rechargeable and primary cell implantable generator, one must understand the power demands of the effective waveform and patient's ability to recharge. Additional considerations include the actual size of the generator, longevity of the power source, and MRI compatibility (Table 76.1).

Principles of Effective Communication with the Patient

Discussion of SCS therapy should begin early in the treatment of chronic pain. Patients with appropriate indications should be introduced to the concept and given information. Once conservative and less invasive options have been explored, the subject of SCS therapy will not be a foreign concept for the patient. Throughout the treatment course the physician must remain responsive to any questions regarding the therapy. This includes having the latest information regarding clinical data that support this modality. Physicians must serve as patient advocates and help patients make the appropriate decision in choosing specific SCS treatment options.

Table 76.1 MRI conditional status of various spinal cord stimulation systems[a]

	Boston Scientific	Medtronic	Nevro	Nuvectra	Stimwave	Abbott St. Jude
MR conditional system (rechargeable)	Precision Montage	RestoreSensor SureScan	Senza I and II	Algovita	Freedom-8A	Prodigy MRI
MRI scan compatibility	Full body	Full body	Full body	No	Full body	Full body
Max number of contacts	16	16	16	N/A	64	16
Magnet strength	1.5 T	1.5 T	1.5 T, (3.0 T head/ extremity)	N/A	1.5 T, 3.0 T	1.5 T
Coil requirement	None	None	Yes	N/A	None	None
Lead tip location requirement	Full spine	Full spine	Full spine	N/A	Full spine	T7–T12
MR conditional system (primary cell)	Precision Novi	Prime advanced SureScan	N/A	N/A	Freedom-8A	Proclaim elite
MRI scan compatibility	No	Full body	N/A	N/A	Full body	Full body
Max number of contacts	N/A	16	N/A	N/A	64	16
Magnet strength	N/A	1.5 T	N/A		1.5 T, 3.0 T	1.5 T
Coil requirement	N/A	None	N/A	N/A	None	None
Lead tip location requirement	N/A	Full spine	N/A	N/A	Full spine	T7–T12

[a]This list was compiled from vendor website information and package insert documentation

Checklist for Spinal Cord Stimulation (Table 76.2)

Contraindications

- Anatomical limitation to lead placement
- Medical comorbidities
- Surgical risk
- Coagulopathy
- Infection risk
- Psychological comorbidities

Table 76.2 Suggested checklist for performing spinal cord stimulation therapy*

Preoperative medical issues
Check for evidence of active dermal, dental, urologic, or other infections and treat as necessary
Order urinalysis before procedure
Address prior history of infection and make a plan for prophylaxis
Review MRI imaging of the spine in the past 12 months depending on diagnosis and planned placement of stimulator tip
Discontinue anticoagulation with approval of treating physician for a length of time prior to procedure that is appropriate for the specific anticoagulant and surgical bleeding risk
If patient was on warfarin, order prothrombin time testing on or before the morning of the procedure
Review psychological evaluation
Obtain cardiac clearance in patients at risk
Review trial films and operative notes in preparation for permanent implant
Examine the potential sites of implantation and battery pocket for infection or inflammatory process
If there are any potential, technical, or patient-specific concerns, communicate with the treating physician and/or the anesthesiologist prior to implant
Educate the patient/caregiver(s)
Obtain insurance coverage and document medical necessity
Surgical considerations
Assess health status on the day of surgery
Have patient empty bladder preoperatively
Review postoperative instruction sheet with patient/caregiver preoperatively
Check that adult driver has been arranged to take patient home, if necessary
Order preoperative antibiotics and administer 30–60 minutes before incision
Plan wound closure
Arrange for family to stay in postoperative area to observe programming and learn about recharging
Confirm follow-up appointment before discharge
Write prescriptions for postoperative antibiotics and analgesics if needed

Reprinted from Deer TR. The appropriate use of neurostimulation of the spinal cord and peripheral nervous system for the treatment of chronic pain and ischemic diseases: the Neuromodulation Appropriateness Consensus Committee. *Neuromodulation; Technology at the Neural Interface*. 2014;17(6):515–550. With permission from Robert M. Levy, Editor in Chief, © International Neuromodulation Society

*Element of this checklist (intended for patients scheduled for SCS) should be considered during patient selection process to avoid unnecessary trials or poor outcomes.

Informed Consent

The practice of SCS trial and permanent implant requires invasive procedures that may result in surgical risk. Thorough written informed consent must be obtained. It is recommended that the consent should be obtained by the physician performing the procedure rather than assistants. Key elements of the informed consent include indications, risks, benefits, and alternatives. Specific risks may include but not limited to lack of efficacy, post-procedural pain/discomfort, bleeding, infection (including meningitis), adverse response to anesthetics, spinal cord or nerve injury, equipment failure, and reduced efficacy over time.

The physician must clearly define:

- Indications
- Risks
- Benefits
- Alternatives
- Various SCS platforms including MRI compatibility

Tracking and Improving Outcomes

There are several landmark prospective studies that help support the efficacy of SCS therapy. Large-scale comprehensive tracking of SCS outcomes does not exist. Individual practices may have to soon adopt tracking databases in order to comply with eminent fee for quality- and merit-based payment models.

Summary

Long-term treatment success of spinal cord stimulation begins with identifying the appropriate candidate for this therapy. Appropriate patient selection is critical in the treatment process. One must understand the indications and limitations of this therapy and maintain clear lines of communication with patients on achieving realistic treatment goals. Standardization of the "workup" process will ensure consistent results. The provider must resist the temptation to rush through the steps despite patient urgency or productivity commitments. By maintaining clear treatment goals while upholding the fundamental principles of neuromodulation, we can ensure the best patient outcomes.

Recommended Reading

1. Deer TR, et al. Neuromodulation appropriateness consensus committee (NACC) recommendations on SCS and PNS for the treatment of chronic pain. Neuromodulation. 2014;17:515–50.
2. Deer TR, et al. Neuromodulation appropriateness consensus committee (NACC) recommendations on SCS and PNS for the treatment of chronic pain. Neuromodulation. 2014;17:515–50.

3. Kapural L, et al. Randomized controlled trial (2 years)Comparison of 10-kHz high frequency stimulation and traditional SCS for the treatment of chronic back and leg pain. Neurosurgery. 2016;0(0):1–10.
4. Kemler MA, De Vet HC, Barendse GA, Van Den Wildenberg FA, Van Kleef M. Randomized controlled trial (5 years). SCS in the treatment of complex regional pain syndrome. J Neurosurg. 2008;108(1):292–8.
5. Kreis PG, Fishman SM. Spinal cord stimulation: percutaneous implantation techniques. Oxford University Press; 2009: Chapter 2.
6. Kumar K, Taylor RS, Jacques L, et al. Randomized controlled trial: SCS versus conventional medical therapy in FBSS. Pain. 2007;132(1–2):179–88.
7. Lad, et al. Longer delay from chronic pain to spinal cord stimulation results in higher healthcare resource utilization. Neuromodulation. 2016;19:469–78.
8. North RB, Kidd DH, Farrokhi F, Piantadosi SA. Randomized controlled trial: SCS versus repeat spine surgery. Neurosurgery. 2005;56(1):98–1067.
9. Pope J, et al. Multi-center retrospective study of spinal cord stimulation failure with exit of therapy by explant. Neuromodulation. 2017;20:543–52.

Wound Closure and Surgical Healing

77

Stephen D. Coleman, Vafi Salmasi, and Michael S. Leong

Introduction

Surgical technique and wound healing are some of the most important factors in durability of neuromodulation. Many implanters have not trained in a surgical residency. Limited number of surgical procedures in most pain fellowship programs as well as limited number of weekend cadaver courses that the fellows can attend is usually not sufficient to prepare them as independent implanters. Moreover, more standardized guidelines are necessary in the field to help standardize the practice. This chapter will summarize our proposed guidelines and relate the protocols to optimize surgical outcomes.

Preoperative Considerations

Preoperative Assessment

Preoperative assessments are important in identifying risks associated with implanting spinal cord stimulators. Once identified, some risks may be modifiable, given sufficient time. Non-modifiable risk may be mitigated or if the risk remains unacceptable the procedure may be deferred. In addition, this is an opportunity for education and expectation management, which can reduce patient anxiety and improve patient satisfaction.

S. D. Coleman
Anesthesia, Perioperative and Pain Medicine, Stanford University, Stanford, CA, USA
e-mail: scoleman@stanford.edu

V. Salmasi
Department of Anesthesiology, Perioperative and Pain Medicine, Systems Neuroscience and Pain Laboratory, Stanford University School of Medicine, Redwood City, CA, USA
e-mail: vsalmasi@stanford.edu

M. S. Leong (✉)
Stanford Pain Management Center, Redwood City, CA, USA
e-mail: msleong@stanford.edu

Medical History and Physical Examination

Detailed history and physical examination will assist in the identification of comorbidities. These identified comorbidities may require additional laboratory studies, other testing, or consultation to fully assess the patient's risks. Modifiable risks and a plan to address these should be discussed with the patient. For these reasons the preoperative assessment should occur well in advance of the procedure.

History should include detailed information regarding current medications, including supplements, allergies, and intolerances. In patients who have regular medical care, this information will help identify active comorbidities. Surgical history obtained should include prior procedures, incision locations, as well as adverse surgical experiences, such as bleeding, poor wound healing, or perioperative infections. The medical history will include an assessment of the patient's integumentary, neurologic, cardiovascular, pulmonary, renal, hepatic, immunologic, and endocrine systems.

Physical examination will assess the organ systems reviewed during the medical history. Examination of neurologic status including history of headaches as well as chronic neck or back pain and radicular symptoms and gait should be documented. Examination of the skin may reveal surgical scars at the intended site of implantation which can cause problems with surgical closure as well as skin infections or rashes. Any other site of implanted devices, such as pacemakers/defibrillators, percutaneous vascular access, and suprapubic bladder catheter, should also be evaluated for possible chronic infection.

The conclusion of the history and physical examination and relevant comorbidities can be discussed with the patient. If the comorbidities are modifiable such as out-of-control diabetes, tobacco use active infections, or anticoagulation, a plan can be set out to minimize the risk of these comorbidities for the implantation of spinal cord stimulator (Tables 77.1 and 77.2).

T. R. Deer et al. (eds.), *Deer's Treatment of Pain*, https://doi.org/10.1007/978-3-030-12281-2_77

Table 77.1 History

Allergies
Medications: prescribed and supplements
Medical:
Coagulation, diabetes, and tobacco
Surgical:
Prior sites and locations
Bleeding
Wound healing/infections

Table 77.2 Physical

Neurologic status: headaches, neck or back pain, including gait and radicular symptoms
Skin: prior surgical scars that cause problems with surgical closure
Prior implanted devices:
Pacemakers
Vascular access
Suprapubic bladder catheters

Comorbidities

Diabetes Mellitus Diabetes mellitus has been identified in a number of clinical studies as a risk factor for developing perioperative infections. Yet multiple studies in patients undergoing orthopedic surgery or cardiac surgery have noted increased risk of infection when HbgA1c is elevated. A study including 3341 patients undergoing cervical discectomy and fusion were stratified by HgbA1c levels and evaluated for perioperative infection. The analysis determined that the inflection point for HgbA1c where the risk of infection increased was HgbA1c level above than 7.5 mg/dL. In another study patients undergoing coronary artery bypass were stratified by HgbA1c levels and evaluated for risk of deep sternal wound infection and respiratory complications. Overall HgbA1c level above 6.5% was associated with increased rate of sternal dehiscence (odds ratio 2.16). In another study of patients undergoing single-level lumbar decompression with diabetes mellitus, a total of 5194 patients were evaluated. After controlling for patient comorbidities, overall HgbA1c level above 7.5 mg/dL resulted in significantly higher risk for deep infection (odds ratio 2.9).

There is no one agreed-upon level of HgbA1c above which surgery should be postponed. However it is recommended that the patient consult with the physician controlling diabetic management to optimize diabetic control.

The Center for Disease Control and Prevention recommends maintaining perioperative blood glucose level target of less than 200 mg/dL. Elevated glucose levels where the patient is developing acidosis or hyperosmolar state may require medical care to improve diabetic management and postponing the surgery.

Tobacco Use Tobacco use has been associated with surgical site infections. In a large study including 40,465 patients undergoing plastic surgery, 15.7% were current smokers. Smokers had statistically higher likelihood of developing wound complications and wound dehiscence. In another study of total joint arthroplasty patients, smokers and nonsmokers were stratified. A total of 1251 smokers were included. These patients had a statistically significant higher rate of deep surgical site infection as well as a greater chance of readmission and other surgical complications.

In a study of 78 patients, smokers were randomized to continue smoking or abstinence with transdermal patch. Patients who continued smoking had statistically increased rate of wound infection compared to those who were nonsmokers. Smokers who abstained from smoking for 4 weeks had wound infection rate similar to nonsmokers.

Smoking cessation for at least 4 weeks before the procedure is recommended. This may include the use of transdermal nicotine patch, and the patients' primary provider may be helpful. Nicotine and replacement can attenuate inflammation, but the effect seems to be marginal.

Steroid Use In a population of 635, 265 surgical patients, 20,434 used steroids preoperatively. Superficial surgical site infections were more likely in the steroid use group (odds ratio 1.7), deep SSI odds ratio 2.35 and dehiscence increased by threefold. In collaboration with the prescribing physician, perioperative steroid use can be optimized.

Chemo and Radiation Therapy Patients who are undergoing chemotherapy for malignancies may be at increased risk for infection. The chemotherapies may reduce one's ability to fight infections as well as reduce platelet count. In addition, patients with malignancies may be nutritionally depleted increasing the risk for surgical site infections. These patients may have undergone radiation therapy or are being considered for radiation therapy. Wound healing may be compromised at sites of radiation. If there is additional chemotherapy or radiation planned, the treatment plan for the patient should be addressed with treating physicians.

Antiplatelet and Anticoagulant Therapy The use of antiplatelet and anticoagulation therapy has become increasingly more prevalent as the number of medications and indications has increased. Bleeding complications may result in neural compression as well as hematoma which provides a medium for bacterial growth and possible infection. A careful review of the patient's history and medications including prescribed and over-the-counter as well as supplements is necessary to assess the patient's bleeding risks. Understanding the circumstances of bleeding complications associated with prior procedures may be helpful in avoiding similar situation. If the risk is not understood, a referral to a hematologist for evaluation may be necessary.

Management of periprocedural anticoagulation therapy may require discontinuation of the medication and/or supplements. These medication changes to reduce the risk of periprocedural bleeding may increase the patient's risk of thrombotic events. The appropriateness and duration of holding these medications should be determined with input from the prescribing physician.

The American Society of Regional Anesthesia and Pain Medicine classify procedures into one of three groups by the potential risk for serious bleeding. Spinal cord stimulator trial and implantation are classified as high-risk procedures.

Non-aspirin NSAIDs

Non-aspirin NSAIDs are used for analgesia rather than for cardiac or cerebral protection; consequently these medications can be held without the risks associated with holding aspirin when used as secondary prevention. These may be started 24 h after the procedure (Table 77.3).

Aspirin

In individuals who are not taking aspirin for secondary prevention, the discontinuation time is 6 days if the dose is less than 1 g per day; otherwise the discontinuation time is 1 week. In individuals who are taking aspirin for secondary prevention, aspirin should be discontinued for a minimum of 6 days and the duration of the spinal cord stimulator trial be minimized. Aspirin can be resumed in 24 h after the procedure.

Table 77.3 Nonsteroidal Anti-inflammatory Drugs

	Half-life, h	Discontinuation time	
Agent	5 Half-lives, h	Discontinuation time, d	Recommended
Diclofenac	1–2	5–10	1
Etodolac	6–8	30–40	2
Ibuprofen	2–4	10–20	1
Indomethacin	5–10	25–50	2
Ketorolac	5–6	25–30	1
Meloxicam	15–20	75–100	4
Nabumetone	22–30	110–150	6
Naproxen	12–17	60–85	4
Oxaprozin	40–60	200–240	10
Piroxicam	45–50	225–250	10

Reprinted from Narouze S, Benzon H, Provenzano D, et al. Interventional Spine and Pain Procedures in Patients on Antiplatelet and Anticoagulant Medications: Guidelines From the American Society of Regional Anesthesia and Pain Medicine, the European Society of Regional Anaesthesia and Pain Therapy, the American Academy of Pain Medicine, the International Neuromodulation Society, the North American Neuromodulation Society, and the World Institute of Pain. *Regional Anesthesia and Pain Medicine*. 2015;40(3)

Clopidogrel and Prasugrel

Spinal cord stimulator trial or implantation in patients who are receiving clopidogrel requires consultation with the treating physician before stopping the medication. Recommendation is to be off clopidogrel for a minimum of 7 days before SCS trial or implantation. Similarly, prasugrel should be stopped for 7 to 10 days. Clopidogrel daily dose can be reinstituted 12 h after the procedure; prasugrel can be restarted 24 h after the procedure.

Warfarin

Changes in warfarin therapy should be done in consultation with prescribing physician. It should be stopped for 5 days and INR normalized before the procedure. Warfarin can be reinitiated the day following the procedure. If at high risk of thromboembolic events, these patients may require bridge therapy with low-molecular-weight heparin.

Procedural Concerns

Surgical procedures for implantation of neuromodulation devices can be associated with numerous complications including surgical site infection, lead migration, wound dehiscence, seroma formation, bleeding, neuraxial hematomas, dural puncture headaches, etc. Some of these complications can be minimized by optimization of surgical techniques and certain procedural considerations.

Surgical Site Infection Control

Currently, the incidence of surgical site infection after spinal cord stimulator implant is higher than other implantable devices including pacemaker implants. Therefore, it is essential to optimize best practice procedures for the field to decrease the risk of infection.

The first intraoperative step for minimizing infection is appropriate antimicrobial prophylaxis. Based on Neuromodulation Appropriateness Consensus Committee (NACC) guidelines, one single dose of antibiotic prior to skin incision is sufficient. However, timing of this single dose has to be optimized based on the choice of antibiotic. The antimicrobial agent of choice should have appropriate coverage for most common pathogens including *Staphylococcus aureus* and *Staphylococcus epidermidis*. Therefore, a first-generation cephalosporin is usually the best choice which can be substituted by clindamycin in patients with increased risk of allergic reaction to cephalosporins. It is also important to consider local community and hospital organisms and resistance patterns.

Limiting antimicrobial prophylaxis to one dose is supported by 2016 World Health Organization (WHO) guidelines. It is also shown in patients undergoing spine surgery that a shorter course of antibiotic administration after the surgery is associated with lower risk of surgical site infection. Cardiac and orthopedic surgery randomized controlled trials have demonstrated benefit in continuing the antimicrobial prophylaxis for 24 h. Same trials did not show any benefit in prolonging the duration of prophylaxis to more than 24 h.

The next step is skin preparation. Hair removal is only acceptable using a clipper if necessary. No hair removal is ideal if possible. Shaving has been shown to be associated with increased risk of infection. WHO guidelines recommend application of an alcohol-based chlorhexidine gluconate solution as choice of antiseptic solution for the skin. This has been shown to be superior to alcohol-based povidone-iodine solutions and water-based solutions. Chlorhexidine gluconate is not approved by the US Food and Drug Administration for surgical procedures accessing neuraxial structures secondary to absence of prospective clinical data.

However, a large retrospective study evaluating more than 12,000 spinal anesthetics using chlorhexidine gluconate antiseptic solution did not reveal any increase in neurological complications.

Positive pressure ventilation is recommended for operating room environment to decrease contamination with airborne pathogens. There is not enough clinical evidence to support addition of laminar airflow ventilation systems though. The other important factor in operating room environment is the number of people present in the operating room as well as the traffic of the operating room. Higher number of personnel as well as traffic flow rate in the operating room is positively correlated with airborne contamination. It is therefore essential to implement appropriate education and preoperative planning to decrease traffic flow. Limiting surgical time is another factor that can decrease operating room traffic flow. In addition, shorter surgical time is independently associated with decreased risk of surgical site infection.

Double-gloving is another controversial issue. Some studies suggest that addition of a pair of gloves can decrease the risk of perforation of the innermost gloves. They recommended the practice when consequences of contamination may be serious. An international survey of spinal cord stimulator implanters showed that less than 50% of proceduralists comply with this recommendation. Of note, WHO did not find the evidence sufficient to make a recommendation about this issue.

WHO guidelines for minimizing surgical site infection suggests that intraoperatively, maintenance of appropriate oxygenation, normothermia, normovolemia, and strict glucose control can decrease surgical site infection.

Appropriate tissue handling also plays a role in decreasing risk of surgical site infection. Gentle tissue handling, limiting surgical trauma, appropriate control of bleeding, and appropriate use of electrocautery are recommended to decrease infection risk. However, it is important to avoid excessive electrocautery, which can prolong the process of tissue healing by creating more necrotic tissue and can also increase risk of seroma formation.

Application of wound irrigation and antibiotic powder is another controversial topic. While, WHO guidelines for minimizing surgical site infection does not support routine irrigation of incisional wound, NACC guidelines advocates for saline irrigation with a bulb syringe. There is no guideline available for volume of irrigation even though animal data shows that larger volumes of irrigation are usually associated with lower risk of infection. Some practitioners consider irrigation with antibiotic solutions, but there is no clinical evidence to support such practice. Moreover, concentrations of antiseptic or antibiotic solutions used for wound irrigation can be toxic for fibroblasts and keratinocytes and thus inhibit healing. Current evidence in neuromodulation field does not support application of antimicrobial powder, pouches, or dressings in order to decrease risk of surgical site infection. Practitioners who consider application of vancomycin powder in the generator pocket usually extrapolate from spine surgery data; limited clinical evidence shows that application of vancomycin powder decreased risk of surgical site infection in patients undergoing spinal instrumentation. The other antibiotic powder considered is tobramycin. Its efficacy was shown in animal study investigating spinal instrumentation in rabbits. All surgical sites were inoculated with tobramycin-sensitive *Escherichia coli*. In animals whose wounds were treated with tobramycin powder, none of the bacterial cultures were positive, while all bacterial cultures were positive in control group. More clinical data is required for efficacy of this treatment though.

In 2008, an absorbable antimicrobial envelope was initially approved by the US Food and Drug Administration for implantable defibrillators. A similar envelope was approved for neuromodulation implants in 2013. Cardiology literature shows decreased risk of implantable cardiovascular defibrillator infection with application of these antibacterial envelopes; however, clinical data is absent for spinal cord stimulator implants. NACC guidelines recommend that surgeons consider these antimicrobial devices especially for high-risk patients considering the high level of evidence present in cardiology literature. There is currently an active recall by the US Food and Drug Association on this device. The recall was issued on August 15, 2016, to address issues with process control of the production.

Application of an occlusive dressing is recommended for 24–48 h postoperatively. This practice is being respected by around 80% of spinal cord stimulator implanters who responded to an international survey. However, application of advanced dressings does not have sufficient clinical evidence. An ideal dressing should be capable of:

- Providing mechanical and bacterial protection
- Maintaining a moist environment
- Not adhering to the wound
- Being nontoxic and non-allergenic
- Absorbing wound odor
- Remaining sterile

It also has to be cost-effective and easy to use.

Suture Material for Anchoring and Closure

Lead migration is one of more common complications of implantable devices. Manufacturers of different devices have been continuously trying to improve their anchoring devices. However, correct choice of suture material and knot tying technique are still very important in stability of leads. There are two major classifications of suture material:

1. Absorbable versus nonabsorbable
2. Monofilament versus multi-ligament

Initially, absorbable sutures were derived from animal intestines. These suture materials usually were broken down enzymatically between 1 and 12 weeks. However, synthetic absorbable sutures are broken down via hydrolysis and therefore cause less tissue reaction. These types of sutures are usually preferred for closure of more superficial fascial layers, whereas nonabsorbable sutures are preferred for closure of abdominal fascial layers.

Monofilament sutures consist of a single small strand of suture material, while multifilament sutures consist of multiple fibers appointment together. Multifilament sutures are easier to handle and tie and at times are less likely to slip. However, these types of sutures are more traumatic and cause more friction as they are passing through tissue planes. Multifilament sutures usually are secured with only three knots, whereas monofilament sutures usually need six knots. The first throw of the knot should be doubled for more stability; each successive knot will be laid down parallel to the previous one.

Nonabsorbable multifilament sutures are usually the best options for anchoring. Silk and braided polyester (Ethibond) are the two most commonly used suture materials. A study of ten different suture materials demonstrated that Ethibond has more tensile strength than silk; and moreover, it retains its mechanical properties even after 6 weeks in tissue. Braided polyester is thus recommended for anchoring leads.

Wound Closure

Appropriate wound closure is important to improve wound healing and decrease risk of complications including surgical site infection. The goals of optimal wound closure are:

- Ensuring hemostasis
- Closing dead space
- Maximizing blood flow
- Minimize bacterial contamination

Blood and foreign material can contribute to bacterial contamination and infection. Therefore, all foreign debris has to be judiciously removed or irrigated out, and appropriate hemostasis has to be achieved prior to closing the wound.

Layered closure can minimize the dead space present. Also, a layered closure decreases tension on each layer. Lower tension on tissue planes can improve healing process. Deeper layers can be better approximated using interrupted sutures. Interrupted sutures provide greater tensile strength with lower rate of tissue strangulation and edema formation. If deeper layers are appropriately closed and the skin tension is minimal, simple running subcuticular suturing technique can be then used to approximate skin edges. If the tension on skin edges is not minimal, alternative closure techniques including simple interrupted sutures, vertical mattress sutures, or staples have to be considered for the skin layer (Tables 77.4 and 77.5).

Postoperative Follow-Up

The main goal for postoperative follow-up is to maximize the success for surgical wound healing, identifying any surgical site infections or other problems, such as epidural hematoma, as early as possible. At the end of the operative

Table 77.4 Suggested choice of sutures for different stages of procedure

Procedure	Recommended sutures
Anchoring	Ethibond (0 or 2–0) Silk (0 or 2–0)
Deep layers	Vicryl (2–0 or 3–0)
Skin	Monocryl (3–0 or 4–0) Nylon (3–0 or 4–0) Staples

Table 77.5 Summary of steps during an implant. Please note that the order of some steps can be changed

Steps of procedure (intraoperative)	
Positioning	
Skin preparation	Hair removal Application of antiseptic Draping
Antibiotic prophylaxis	
Access	Incision Dissection Epidural access Lead/catheter placement
Anchoring	
Pocket creation	Incision Dissection
Hemostasis	
Irrigation	
Battery/pump implant	
Closure	Deep fascia layers Skin
Application of dressing	

procedure, most US practitioners apply occlusive dressings for spinal cord stimulator trials and implants (80% and 70%). Currently, the NACC recommendations are to discontinue antibiotic treatment within 24 h. Cardiac, orthopedic, and plastic surgery did not decrease infection rate with continuing beyond 24 h. In spine surgery, intravenous antibiotics greater than 48 h actually prolonged hospital stay by delaying normalization of body temperature and CRP levels. Nevertheless, not continuing antibiotics is controversial with historic practice, and on Dr. Provenzano's international survey, in general 50% of the practitioners surveyed continued antibiotics beyond the 24-hour period for both trials and implants.

For incision and wound care, sterile dressing and washing hands is advised. Glucose monitoring for diabetic patients is important for infection control. Any nonabsorbable sutures or staples should be evaluated and removed within 10 to 14 days. Some patients have questioned whether sutures or staples are the same for closure. Typically, we have not considered one closure technique to be superior and consider that staples may be advantageous to decrease operating room closure time (http://journals.plos.org/plosone/article?id=10.1371/journal.pone.0075132). One recent publication on the use of sutures vs staples for cesarean section closure suggests that staples can be associated with an increase in wound complications and sutures may be better.

Many of our patients referred to our institution can come from a distance. Some have requested that they have a local provider assess the wound and take out the sutures or staples. Although NACC recommendations include educating the family and patient about potential surgical site infections, the authors believe that early and direct observation can detect superficial infections that can be managed without surgical removal of the implanted device.

Table 77.6 Spinal or epidural abscess

1. Backache and local tenderness
2. Radicular symptoms and fever in 48–72 h
3. Motor and sensory dysfunction, reflex depression 3 to 4 days
4. Paralysis

Two recently published papers deserve some mention due to the number of patient data collected. Bendel published in Neuromodulation 2017 a retrospective analysis of 2737 SCS implant infections. He and his colleagues found that localized incisional pain and wound erythema were the most common presenting signs. The most common organism was *Staphylococcus aureus* at the IPG pocket. Seventy-eight percent of the patients had their SCS systems explanted, while 24 patients tried non-explantation therapy with 15 patients (63% of this subgroup) retaining their SCS systems. The other manuscript by Yusuf discussed a single center infection control bundle to reduce SCS infections. This bundle consisted of five items: (1) showering and decolonization for 5 days prior to surgery and showering in the hospital on the morning of surgery, (2) performing the SCS implantation as the first case in the daily operating room, (3) maintaining a minimal number of people in the OR, (4) providing home care nurses with a folder on SCS wound care instructions including pictures, and (5) giving oral specific wound care instruction to patients. For this institution with 410 SCS surgeries, there was a reduction in the number of infections. It remains to be seen if this five-part bundle can be applied to other settings (academic and community) to reduce infections.

Spinal or epidural abscess is one of the main concerns of any postsurgical evaluation or any implant and has an incidence of 2 per 10,000 requiring a hospital admission. In general, spine imaging (MRI or CT scan) and possible infectious disease consultation are required if any of the following signs or symptoms are present (Table 77.6).

Recovery is unlikely if paralysis is greater than 12 h, so surgical irrigation and debridement is urgent. If an abscess is greater than 36 h without being treated medically or surgically, full neurologic recovery is unlikely.

Conclusions

Spinal cord stimulator implantation and other implantable devices: intrathecal drug delivery systems have a higher risk of infection compared to other advanced interventional pain management procedures. Recommendations are often experiential and have conflicting evidence. Our chapter hopes to

Table 77.7 Summary of recommendations for decreasing the risk of infection based on the benefit they yield versus the amount of effort they require

Effort		
Benefit	Low	High
High	Preoperative bathing Chlorhexidine wipes Perioperative antibiotics Clipping hair (vs shaving) Skin preparation with alcohol-based solution Irrigation with saline Occlusive dressing	MRSA treatment Positive pressure ventilation in OR Proper surgical technique Normothermia Intraoperative glucose control Proper closure Appropriate follow-up
Questionable or low	Double-gloving Vancomycin powder Tobramycin powder	MRSA screening Laminar flow in OR Proper oxygenation
Potential harm	Irrigation with antibiotic solution Irrigation with betadine	

offer some direct and simple guidelines with Table 77.7 and highlight many of the discussion areas that are ongoing at this time.

Recommended Reading

1. Bendel M, O'Brien T, et al. Spinal cord stimulator related infections: findings from a multicenter retrospective analysis of 2737 implants. Neuromodulation. 2017;20:553–7.
2. Berrios-Torres C. For disease control and prevention guideline for the prevention of surgical site infection, 2017. JAMA Surg. 2017;152(8):784–91.
3. Cancienne J. The Association of Perioperative Glycemic Control with deep postoperative infection after anterior cervical discectomy and fusion in patients with diabetes. World Neurosurg. 2017a;102:13–7.
4. Cancienne J. Perioperative hemoglobin AC as a predictor of deep infection following single level lumbar decompression in patients with diabetes. Spine J. 2017b;17:1100–5.
5. Deer T. The Neurostimulation Appropriateness Consensus Committee (NACC) recommendations for infection prevention and management. Neuromodulation.
6. Goltsman D. The association between smoking and plastic surgery outcome in 40,465 patients: an analysis of the American College of Surgeons National Surgical Quality Improvement Program Data Sets. Plast Reconstr Surg. 2017;139:503.
7. Ismael H. Adverse effects of preoperative steroid use on surgical outcomes. Am J Surg. 2011;201:305–9.
8. Narayan P. Preoperative glycosylated hemoglobin: a risk factor for patients undergoing coronary artery bypass. Ann Thorac Surg. 2017;104:606–12.
9. Narouze S. Interventional spine and pain procedures in patients on antiplatelet and anticoagulation medications. Reg Anesth Pain Med. 2015;40:182–212.
10. Sahota S. The effect of smoking on thirty-day postoperative complication after total joint arthroplasty: a propensity score-matched analysis. J Arthroplasty. 2017 (in press).
11. Sorensen L. Abstinence from smoking reduces incisional wound infection: a randomized controlled trial. Ann Surg. 2003;238:1–5.
12. Yusuf E, Bamps S, et al. A multidisciplinary infection control bundle to reduce the number of spinal cord stimulator infections. Neuromodulation. 2017;20:563–6.

Complications of Neuromodulation

78

Tim J. Lamer

Introduction

Complications of neurostimulation and their avoidance have received much attention and, along with this, an improvement in outcomes and reduction in the frequency of many of the reported adverse events over time.

Table 78.1 Neurological complications associated with neurostimulation

Complication	Published frequency
Spinal cord injury with SCS	0–2.35%
Major motor deficit with SCS	0–0.25%
Major sensory deficit with SCS	0–0.1%
Symptomatic dural puncture with SCS	0.05–3%
Surgical site infection	2.5%
Hemorrhage/major bleeding with SCS	0–0.71%
Hemorrhage w DBS/MCS	1.8–3.1%

Neurological Complications

Neurological complications and adverse events associated with neurostimulation occur most commonly as a result of one of the following mechanisms: direct neural trauma related to the device placement, infection leading to neural injury, bleeding/hematoma leading to neural injury, or an adverse reaction to the device causing neural injury. Table 78.1 lists the frequency of neurological complications associated with the most common neurostimulation techniques/devices.

Percutaneous Spinal Stimulation

The frequency of neural injury from percutaneous spinal stimulator lead placement has been examined in several large series. Two large retrospective reviews, one series of over 2900 patients by Cameron and colleagues and the other series of over 700 patients by Mekhail and colleagues, did not identify any cases of direct spinal cord injury (SCI). On the other hand, Petraglia and colleagues reported the incidence of SCI in over 5400 patients who underwent percutaneous SCS to be 2.35%. Injury may occur from direct needle/introducer trauma or lead placement and manipulation. The 2017 Neurostimulation Appropriateness Consensus Committee (NACC) published a series of recommendations to reduce the risk of neurological injury in the setting of percutaneous spinal stimulation. The key findings in this evidence-based set of practice recommendations are:

1. Advanced imaging (MRI preferred, CT if MRI is contraindicated) should be obtained and personally reviewed prior to proceeding with implant. The implanting physician should be able to read the imaging study to be able to identify any potential anatomic barriers or concerns.
2. If a patient is on coagulation-altering medications/therapy, this must be actively managed in partnership with the patient and the patients' prescribing provider. Coagulation status should be optimized in accordance with recently published guidelines (see [2, 8]). It is important to recognize and understand that there is risk of bleeding, not only during lead placement but also during manipulation and removal.
3. During lead placement, current published guidelines recommend that if sedation/anesthesia is used, it must be sufficiently light sedation such that the patient is fully conversant enough to accurately report a paresthesia that could be a sign of impending nerve/cord trauma. Alternatively, if deep sedation or anesthesia is used, it is recommended that intraoperative neurophysiological monitoring be performed.
4. Infection remains a significant concern with SCS implantation. The incidence of infection is approximately 2.5% according to a recently published large multi-site study by Hoelzer and colleagues (Bendel et al. [1]). The

T. J. Lamer (✉)
Division of Pain Medicine, Department of Anesthesiology and Perioperative Medicine, Mayo Clinic, Rochester, MN, USA
e-mail: Lamer.tim@mayo.edu

T. R. Deer et al. (eds.), *Deer's Treatment of Pain*, https://doi.org/10.1007/978-3-030-12281-2_78

implanting physicians should follow recently published guidelines for managing and minimizing the risk of infection (see [3]).

5. Any new neurological signs/symptoms need to be evaluated promptly. Spinal cord compression from either abscess or hematoma is a surgical emergency that requires immediate imaging confirmation, usually followed by emergency surgery for the best outcome.

Paddle/Open Surgical Spinal Stimulation

The frequency of neural injury from open surgical SCS implants has been examined in several large studies. As with percutaneous SCS, spinal cord injury (SCI) associated with paddle lead SCS is very rare with a reported frequency of between 0.19% and 1.71%. In Petraglia's study of over 2800 patients who received paddle leads, the incidence of SCI was 1.71%. Levy and colleagues analyzed the outcomes from over 44,000 cases and identified 111 cases of major motor deficit, 61 cases of minor motor deficit, and 46 cases of sensory deficit. The NACC guidelines for surgical paddle SCS leads are similar to the percutaneous guidelines (see [2, 3]).

Deep Brain and Motor Cortex Stimulation

The major neurologic injury risks due to deep brain stimulation (DBS) and motor cortex stimulation (MCS) result from hemorrhagic complications. Infection is another risk, and the frequency as well as management and risk mitigation is similar to other neuromodulation interventions (e.g., paddle and percutaneous SCS). The 2017 NACC reported the risk of hemorrhage to be approximately 1.8% from DBS and 3.1% with MCS. Seizures are the other major neurological risk concern, especially with MCS. They may occur during routine programming, so it is important for facilities performing MCS programming to have the equipment, staff, and expertise to manage this potential adverse event.

Lead-Related Fibrosis

Foreign body reactions to the lead material presenting as a spinal cord compression syndrome are very rare but have been reported and need to be in the differential diagnosis when a patient with an implanted device presents with a new pain or neurological complaint related to the device. For SCS devices new back pain and tenderness in the area of the spine where the lead tip is located and/or new sensory or motor symptoms concerning for spinal cord compression need to be evaluated immediately with a neurological exam and advanced imaging (MRI scan with contrast if the device is MRI conditionally "safe" or CT scan). Treatment of a device tip mass that is causing symptomatic spinal cord compression is device removal and decompression of the mass.

Dural Puncture

Dural puncture or dural rents can occur in the setting of percutaneous and paddle SCS lead placement. The frequency of symptomatic post-dural puncture (i.e., postural headache) for percutaneous SCS lead placement is reported to be between 0.2% and 3% and for paddle lead placement approximately 0.05%. The most common clinical concern is postural headache which can be especially problematic if this occurs during trial SCS lead placement as it will have an adverse effect on the patients' ability to be up and mobile during the trial period. There are rare reports of intracranial epidural hematoma occurring in the setting of low pressure CSF after dural puncture. Management options of a dural puncture in the setting of a percutaneous trial lead placement include expectant therapy (as not all patients will be symptomatic), prophylactic epidural blood patch, epidural blood patch only if symptomatic, or abandoning the trial and re-trialing at a later date.

The other potential complication associated with a dural puncture/leak is a CSF hygroma. If this occurs and exerts sufficient pressure on a fresh surgical wound, the wound could break down or dehisce. This of course is a significant infection concern. Management options depend on the severity and include expectant therapy, image-guided epidural blood patch, or fibrin glue patch, and rarely open surgical repair is needed.

Infection

Surgical site infections (SSIs) related to neuromodulation devices are reported to occur between 2% and 6%. The spectrum of infection complications ranges from superficial infections to more serious infections including the possibility of meningitis and epidural abscess. Several consensus guidelines have been published on this topic, and the implanting physician should be familiar with the details including updates. Most notable among these guidelines are the Neuromodulation Appropriateness Consensus Committee (NACC) recommendations for infection prevention and control [3] and the US Centers for Disease Control and Prevention (CDC) strategies to prevent surgical site infection. Table 78.2 summarizes the current recommendations for periprocedural infection prevention.

The three major categories of infection are superficial infection, deep infections around the implanted hardware,

Table 78.2 Recommendations for periprocedural infection prevention

Periprocedural
Optimize medical risk factors (smoking, DM, immune status, etc.)
R/O occult infection (UTI, skin, etc.)
Test/decolonize for MSSA or MSRA (mupirocin nasal ointment and chlorhexidine or bleach baths)
Immediate Presurgery
If shaving, use electric clippers
Administer weight-based preoperative antibiotic within an hour of incision
Chlorhexidine skin prep in accordance with the instructions
All the usual routine sterile surgical procedures: sterile drapes, sterile gowns for operative staff, face masks and cap or hood to cover all hair (including facial hair), and double glove with sterile gloves
Intraoperative
Use laminar flow or positive pressure operating rooms
Minimize in and out room traffic during case
Minimize surgical time
Careful tissue handling
Careful hemostasis (post-op hematoma increases wound infection risk)
Thorough wound irrigation prior to closure (controversial: saline vs antibiotic solution vs dilute povidone/iodine solution)
Meticulous wound closure
Controversial: intra-wound antibiotics (e.g.,vancomycin powder or antibiotic-impregnated pouch)
Postsurgical
Keep covered with a sterilely applied occlusive dressing for the first 24–48 hours
Dressing changes should be performed with sterile technique (wash hands, sterile dressing)
Patient and caregiver education regarding wound care and signs of possible infection

and spine/brain infection (epidural abscess, meningitis). Superficial infections, as the name implies, involve only the skin and/or subcutaneous tissues and, if caught early, can often be managed with appropriate antibiotics. These infections must be monitored carefully as they can progress to deep infection. Deep infections involve muscle and fascial layers and usually one or more components of the hardware. Deep infections most often require device removal and antibiotics for management. More serious infections including epidural abscess have been reported and are a medical urgency/emergency as they can rapidly lead to permanent neurologic injury if not caught and properly attended to early on.

The major principles of SSI reduction are to optimize preoperative medical risk factors, adhere to published procedural SSI risk mitigation guidelines, meticulous surgical technique, and appropriate follow-up after the procedure. The medial risk factors known to increase the risk of infection include smoking, poorly controlled diabetes, and immune system dysfunction which is most commonly due to the patients' use of immune-modulating drugs. Since neuromodulation implantation is an elective procedure, patients should be counseled to discontinue smoking prior to the procedure. Patients with diabetes should have their disease controlled, and most experts suggest a hemoglobin A1C level of 8.0 or less before proceeding with elective surgery.

Hardware-Related Complications

In terms of frequency, hardware-related issues are cited as the most common group of adverse events and complications. Table 78.3 lists the most common hardware-related adverse events. Historically, percutaneous SCS lead migration and peripheral nerve stimulator lead migration have been the most common complication in terms of frequency. During the early years of device implantation, published SCS lead migration rates as high as 15–20% were reported, and occipital nerve stimulator lead migration rates from 25 to 50-plus percent were reported. Fortunately, with newer lead anchors, adherence to published lead anchor guidelines, and improved surgical techniques, the lead migration rates have gone down significantly. In 2015 Gazelka and colleagues reported a lead migration rate of 2% in over 140 percutaneous SCS lead implants [5]. Additional lead-related issues include lead fracture and fibrosis and fluid collection (seroma) around the hardware. Lead fracture is in the differential diagnosis when the patient reports a sudden loss of stimulation or pain relief. Diagnosis is by system interrogation and noting high impedances in one or more of the lead contacts. X-ray imaging may or may not demonstrate the fracture as often the fracture is partial and within the lead casing such that it is not obvious by imaging. The treatment is lead revision.

Foreign body reactions to implanted hardware may occur in the form of localized sterile fluid collection (seroma) or as a fibrinous tissue deposition around the lead(s), anchors, or generator. Fibrous tissue reaction around the lead does occur and most commonly manifests as the need for more current/power to achieve stimulation. As mentioned previously, on very rare occasions the fibrous reaction can be significant enough to create a mass effect on the adjacent spinal cord.

Another significant hardware-related event is pain related to the implanted hardware. Pain can occur at the lead anchor site, in the area of lead tunneling, and most commonly over the generator. The incidence of generator site-related pain has been reported to be as high as 12%. Most of these cases

Table 78.3 Adverse events related to hardware

Lead migration with loss of pain relief
Lead fracture/malfunction
Hardware-related pain lead anchors and generator site are the most common
Tissue reaction including seromas and fibrosis around leads
Generator malfunction

can be managed conservatively, but occasionally, revision or even removal is necessary to successfully resolve the problem. The most common conservative management strategies include padding over the painful device area and the use of topical analgesia (gels, creams, or patches).

Aberrant Stimulation

With conventional spinal cord stimulation, one of the goals is for the device to create a paresthesia that is perceived by the patient and that the paresthesia closely covers as much of the area of the patients' pain as is possible. In order to do this, often the stimulation extends beyond the area of the desired target in order to cover as much of the pain area as possible. In some cases, this is merely a mild inconvenience, while at other times it can be unpleasant or even painful for the patient. In the case of an unpleasant or painful aberrant paresthesias, this often requires a compromise in the programming to capture as much of the painful area as possible while trying to minimize the aberrant stimulation. As the SCS lead position relative to the spinal cord can change with postural changes, one of the most common complaints from patients is posture change-related stimulation surges. Many of the newer stimulation platforms have addressed this issue of aberrant stimulation in different ways. Of course some of the paresthesia-free SCS waveforms eliminate this issue all together by eliminating the paresthesia. Hf10 stimulation (Nevro), DRG stimulation (Abbott), and Burst stimulation (Abbott) are paresthesia-free or nearly paresthesia-free techniques. Medtronic utilizes what they have termed "adaptive stimulation" in which an accelerometer built into the generator senses patient positional changes and adjusts the level of stimulation output. It should be noted that even the paresthesia-free SCS systems may have aberrant or "excessive" stimulation patterns though it may be harder to definitively diagnose in the paresthesia-less environment. Some of these newer platforms are associated with a much higher energy or charge delivery to the neural targets, and it appears that this too may in some cases be associated with patient discomfort.

Pearls

1. Preoperative cross-sectional imaging (MRI or if contraindicated, CT scan) should be available and personally reviewed by the implanting practitioner prior to proceeding with a stimulator trial or implant. Areas of significant stenosis or other potential structural impediments should be noted, and in the case of severe stenosis, SCS hardware should be avoided.
2. In a patient with an existing SCS implant, new neurological complaints and/or new back pain and tenderness in the area associated with the lead implants should be promptly investigated with an in-person examination and appropriate cross-sectional imaging to rule out nerve and/or spinal cord compression from the device, an infection, hemorrhage, or fibrous tissue reaction.
3. Periprocedural infection remains one of the most significant complications associated with neurostimulation due to the possibility of serious patient harm (paralysis, death) and the costs associated with treating an infected device. The implanting practitioner should thoroughly understand the risk factors and implement the risk mitigation steps outlined in Table 78.2.

Recommended Reading

1. Bendel MA, O'Brien T, Hoelzer BC, Deer TR, Pittelkow TP, et al. Spinal cord stimulator related infections: findings from a multicenter retrospective analysis of 2737 implants. Neuromodulation. 2017;20(6):553–7.
2. Deer TR, Lamer TJ, Pope JE, Falowski SM, Provenzano DA, Slavin K, et al. The neurostimulation appropriateness consensus committee (NACC) safety guidelines for the reduction of severe neurological injury. Neuromodulation. 2017a;20(1):15–30, Epub 2017.
3. Deer TR, Provenzano DA, Hanes M, Pope JE, Thomson SD, Russo MA, et al. Neurostimulation appropriateness consensus committee (NACC): recommendations for infection prevention and management. Neuromodulation. 2017b;20(1):31–50.
4. Fitzgibbon DR, Stephens LS, Posner KL, et al. Injury and liability associated with implantable devices for chronic pain. Anesthesiology. 2016;124:1384–93.
5. Gazelka HM, Freeman ED, Hooten WM, Eldrige JS, Lamer TJ. Incidence of clinically significant percutaneous spinal cord stimulator lead migration. Neuromodulation. 2015;18(2):123–5.
6. Hayek SM, Veizi E, Hanes M. Treatment-limiting complications of percutaneous spinal cord stimulator implants: a review of eight years of experience from an academic center database. Neuromodulation. 2015;18(7):603–8.
7. Levy R, Henderson J, Slavin K, et al. Incidence and avoidance of neurologic complications with paddle type spinal cord stimulation leads. Neuromodulation. 2011;14:412–22.
8. Narouze S, Benzon HT, Provenzano DA, Buvanendran A, De Andres J, Deer TR, et al. Interventional spine and pain procedures in patients on antiplatelet and anticoagulant medications: guidelines from the American Society of Regional Anesthesia and Pain Medicine, the European Society of Regional Anaesthesia and Pain Therapy, the American Academy of Pain Medicine, the International Neuromodulation Society, the North American Neuromodulation Society, and the World Institute of Pain. Reg Anesth Pain Med. 2015;40:182–212.
9. Neal JM, Barrington MJ, Brull R, Hadzic A, Hebl JR, Horlocker TT, et al. The second ASRA practice advisory on neurologic complications associated with regional anesthesia and pain medicine: executive summary 2015. Reg Anesth Pain Med. 2015;40:401–30.
10. Petraglia FW, Farber SH, Gramer R, Verla T, Wang F, Thomas S, et al. The incidence of spinal cord injury in implantation of percutaneous and paddle electrodes for spinal cord stimulation. Neuromodulation. 2016;19(1):85–90.
11. Shils JL, Arle JE. Intraoperative neurophysiologic methods for spinal cord stimulator placement under general anesthesia. Neuromodulation. 2012;15:560–71.

Part VII

Neuroaxial Therapies

Intrathecal Pharmacology

79

Lucas W. Campos

Introduction

With the experience of more than 300,000 implanted pumps, IT has been established as a safe and effective treatment for intractable spasticity, cancer, and noncancer pain. IT was typically considered as a salvage therapy when conservative medical management and invasive surgical therapies failed. IT was also considered when the side effects of systemic opioids, such as sedation, constipation, and urinary retention, were the limiting factors of an otherwise life-changing treatment regimen.

As the indications for IT grew, a number of issues limiting its use became apparent. These included which drug or drug combinations were best for treatment of neuropathic, nociceptive, or mixed pain states. Other issues included the appropriate dose and concentration of the intrathecal medicines, catheter placement, and infusion strategies such as continuous, timed bolus, or patient-activated bolus. This called for more research to be done on the dynamic forces present in the intrathecal space. Work began to elucidate effective solutions to these common questions. Based on new data, guidelines were created to improve patient safety by reducing variability in catheter placement, medications used, and patient pain types best treated using IT.

A subsequent comprehensive review of the existing data resulted in consensus guidelines for IT aimed at significantly reducing noncancer pain from failed back surgery syndrome and complex regional pain syndrome. Later research concluded that ITs were effective, cost neutral, and appropriate in a larger number of disease processes. While device-related complications such as catheter kinking or transection can occur, the main therapy-related safety issues are respiratory depression, inflammatory mass formation, dosing errors, and pump refilling errors where the medication is mistakenly delivered into the tissue surrounding the pump rather than into the pump itself. The formation of the PACC successfully addressed these safety concerns by analyzing all available high-quality research as well as individual provider experience and created guidelines regarding best practices, safe dosing, and contraindications for IT.

Background and Historical Perspective

The history of intrathecal (IT) drug delivery (IDD) therapy for chronic cancer and noncancer pain is rooted in experimentation with local anesthetics administered into the cerebrospinal fluid (CSF). As early as 1885, James Leonard Corning, a New York neurologist, experimented with cocaine-induced spinal anesthesia in dogs. When he administered cocaine into the CSF, paralysis and anesthesia of the hind legs followed. Almost 15 years later, in 1898, a German surgeon named August Karl Gustav Bier exploited Corning's finding and used a cocaine-induced, spinal anesthetic to facilitate lower limb surgery. The first experimentation using opioids in the CSF to treat postsurgical pain was in 1901. A Romanian surgeon, Nicolae Racoviceanu-Piteşti, presented his experience with IT opioid analgesia. The use of neuraxial opioids to treat acute pain was not pursued again for almost a century until experimentation with opiate-based epidural analgesia began.

These previous IT experiments all used single-shot techniques that would wear off in a matter of hours. This meant that the patient would have to receive repeated IT injections in order to prolong the analgesia. Multiple, IT single-shot treatments increased the incidence of severe spinal headaches. This was addressed by the surgeon Dr. William Leonard in 1940 when he demonstrated the benefits of continuous, spinal anesthesia by administering procaine as the primary anesthetic to nearly 200 patients.

This technique used a malleable needle surgically implanted in the lumbar spine. His technique was soon widely adopted by other surgeons for patient's thought to be too high a risk for inhaled anesthesia. The idea of a continu-

L. W. Campos (✉)
Interventional Pain Physicians, Chico, CA, USA

T. R. Deer et al. (eds.), *Deer's Treatment of Pain*, https://doi.org/10.1007/978-3-030-12281-2_79

ous intrathecal anesthetic infusion for surgery and post-op analgesia was further advanced in 1944 by Edward Tuohy. He used a 15-gauge spinal needle and passed a nylon catheter into the subarachnoid space to administer continuous, spinal anesthetic for postsurgical pain.

In addition to these local anesthetic-based techniques, the use of intrathecal opiate analgesia was re-explored after opioid receptors were identified in 1971. In 1973, multiple labs confirmed the presence of opioid receptors in neural tissue. In 1976, Yaksh and Rudy demonstrated that intrathecal opioids produced selective analgesia in rats with few motor, sensory, or autonomic side effects. In 1979, Wang, Nauss, and Thomas demonstrated pain relief in humans using IT administration of morphine.

Yaksh continued to pioneer the development of this technology and worked with neurosurgeon, Bert Onofrio, on continuous intrathecal administration of morphine in cancer patients using the implanted Infusaid model#400 (Shiley Infused Company of Massachusetts).

A year later, this work was reproduced by Greenberg and Taren at the University of Michigan in another cancer patient. In 1987, 43 patients experienced tremendous relief from intractable pain due to lumbar arachnoiditis, multiple sclerosis, and thoracic compression fractures using continuous IT using continuous infusion by external or implanted pumps. Medtronic Inc. received FDA approval for the first battery-powered, programmable pump for cancer-related pain in 1988 and later in 1991 for chronic pain (see Fig. 79.1).

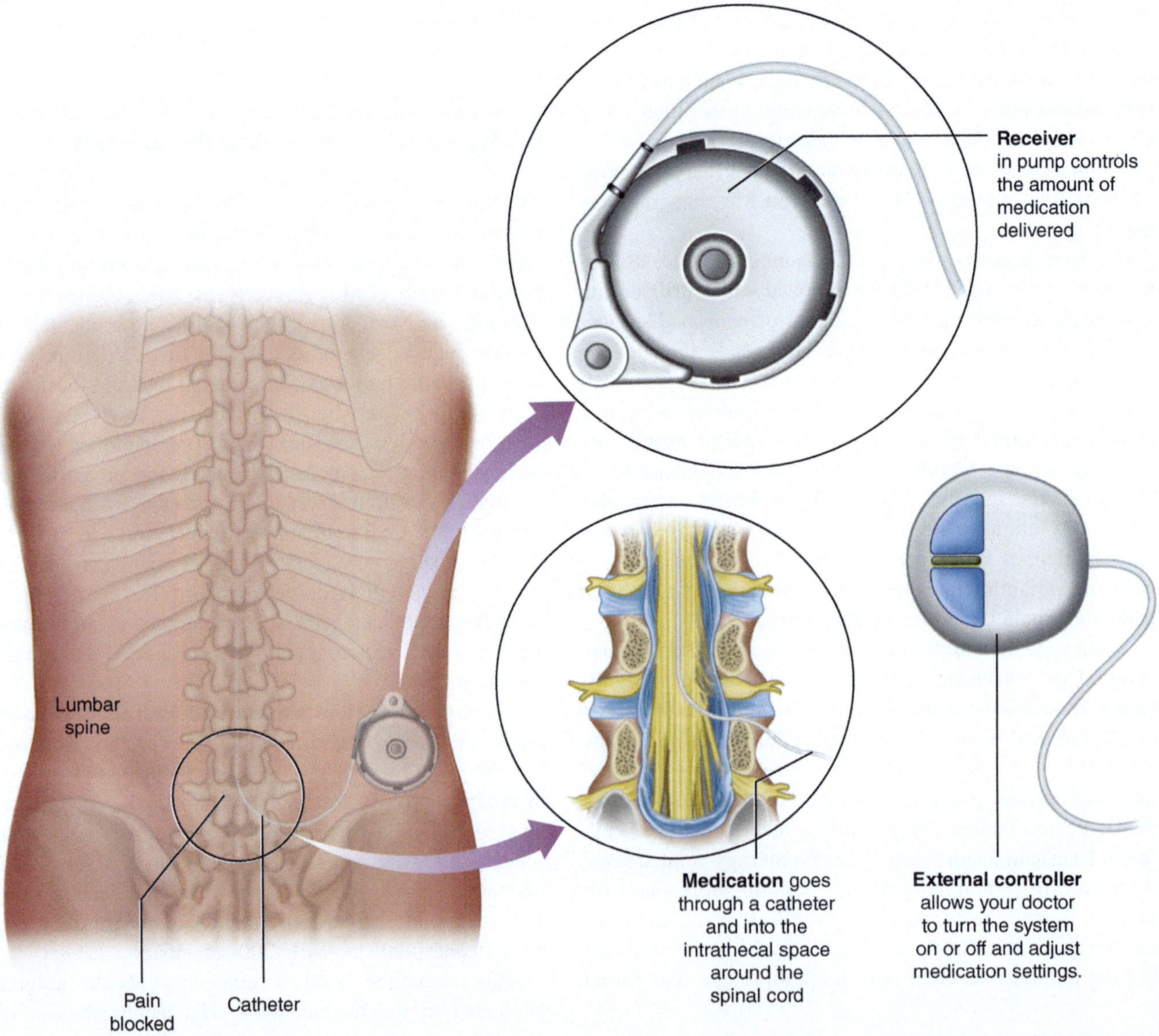

Fig. 79.1 Intrathecal drug delivery system implant

Uses and Indication

Patients can have nociceptive, neuropathic, or a mixture of these root causing chronic pain. Neuropathic pain is typically described as burning, gnawing, and lancinating, whereas nociceptive pain is commonly described as aching, mechanical, and sharp. Conservative therapies commonly include ultrasound or fluoroscopically guided injections; oral medications such as gabapentin, tricyclic antidepressants, and opiates; and systemic medication trials with IV lidocaine or ketamine. Chronic opioid therapy has not been found to be beneficial for long-term treatment of neuropathic pain and can actually worsen pain as found in opiate-based treatment of HIV peripheral neuropathy.

Failure of patients to respond to these conservative treatments means advanced therapies such as spinal cord stimulation (SCS) and IT should be the focus for effective treatment. For many chronic pain syndromes, SCS is used before IT as there is compelling data suggesting SCS is a safer option due to lack of risks including respiratory depression, psychosis, and endocrine suppression. Study patient populations shown to benefit from IT include those with failed back surgery syndrome (FBSS), vertebral compression fractures, nonoperative spondylolisthesis, and radiculopathy. IT has also been shown to be an effective treatment of visceral, pelvic, and abdominal pain in both cancer and noncancer patients. In order to be an IT trial candidate, the patient must meet both the disease indications and patient selection criteria shown to optimize successful outcomes. Patient selection criteria includes preoperative stabilization of medical comorbidities, capacity to understand the therapy, ability to be present for medication refills as well as scheduled visits, and stabilization of any psychiatric diagnoses such as depression, anxiety, or personality disorders.

Evidence for Efficacy

To best understand the evidence for efficacy of intrathecal medications, the physician must understand the dynamics of these medications in the intrathecal space. After delivery into the CSF, active molecules must diffuse across the pia mater and white matter of the spinal cord to reach target receptors in the gray matter or nerve rootlets. The pia mater, being only a single layer of cells without intercellular junctions, is very permeable to IT medications. For medications to enter the parenchyma of the spinal cord, fluid pathways paralleling the intraparenchymal vasculature can be used. In the spinal cord, white matter consists of myelinated axons making it hydrophobic, whereas the gray matter consists of cell bodies making this region hydrophilic. Continuous IT infusion results in stable CSF drug concentrations, establishing a gradient that drives drug diffusion into these central neural tissues.

A number of physicochemical factors intrinsic to the chosen IT medication determine the level of drug uptake. Of these, lipid solubility and molecular weight are the most important. Hydrophilic medications, such as morphine and hydromorphone, have a pharmacokinetic advantage in the CSF over hydrophobic agents, such as fentanyl and bupivacaine. In the CSF, hydrophilic molecules have longer half-lives because hydrophobic agents enter the vasculature and are readily cleared out of the subarachnoid space. Hydrophilic medications have smaller volumes of distribution, resulting in deeper spinal cord penetration and less rostral spread. Limited spread is an advantage of hydrophobic medications when precise, targeted delivery is desired.

Here are the most commonly used on- and off-label medications and the evidence for their efficacy:

Opioids

Presynaptic opioid receptor activation inhibits the release of the neurotransmitters substance P and calcitonin gene-related peptide. This is done by downstream inhibition of N-type, voltage-dependent, calcium channels which reduces calcium influx, thereby minimizing neurotransmitter release. Postsynaptically, activation of opioid receptors leads to inhibition of adenylate cyclase and the opening of potassium channels. Open potassium channels hyperpolarize cells, rendering the postsynaptic, second-order neurons less responsive.

The pharmacokinetics of intrathecal opioid administration is very complex, especially with low-volume infusions. The opioid receptors are concentrated in lamina II (substantia gelatinosa) of the dorsal horn. Early work in rabbit models showed that hydrophilic opioids administered into the CSF diffused further into the gray matter than hydrophobic opioids. Later, work using pig models showed hydrophobic opioids readily diffused across the dura and into the epidural fat, thereby failing to activate the opiate receptors contained within the gray matter. These findings demonstrated that the superior bioavailability of hydrophilic opioids is due to their longer presence in the CSF, allowing for greater penetrance and concentration into the hydrophilic dorsal horn gray matter. Morphine and hydromorphone leave the CSF by simple diffusion into the plasma where they are renally and hepatically cleared.

Common side effects of IT opioids include respiratory depression, the development of tolerance, hyperalgesia, urinary retention, constipation, pruritus, peripheral edema, and hypogonadism. Respiratory depression happens with rostral spread of opioids and is more likely with hydrophilic opioids such as morphine as opposed to hydrophobic opioids such as fentanyl. Respiratory depression most commonly results from an excessively rapid titration and accidental overdosing. Therefore, strict monitoring of a patient's respirations during trialing and ensuring proper infusion concentrations are vital. Tolerance to intrathecal opioids is most common in patients younger than 50 years old. Tolerance leads to dose escalation. Opioid tolerance can be attenuated using combination therapy with opioids and bupivacaine. Lowering a patient's oral opioid dose or weaning them off of opioids prior to trialing and implant has also been shown to limit dose escalation.

Another serious risk with opioid-based IT is the formation of a sterile, expanding inflammatory mass known as a granuloma at the tip of the spinal catheter. Development of a granuloma is one of the most serious risks of IT because of the potential for temporary or permanent neurological injury. The first report of granuloma formation was published in 1991, a decade after implantable pumps were introduced. A retrospective longitudinal study that included 56 patients on long-term IT therapy with morphine or diamorphine found granuloma development in four patients. Granuloma formulation has been found to have a significant positive correlation with opioid dose and yearly increase in opioid dose but not with flow rate or opioid concentration.

Morphine

Morphine and other opiates used in IT underwent preclinical safety examination in animals as measured by the neurotoxicity standardized assessments. In chronically catheterized, large animal models, the data shows that continuous infusions of morphine, hydromorphone, methadone, or fentanyl, for at least 28 days, cause no spinal tissue damage. Morphine monotherapy efficacy and clinical data continues to support its use as a first-line therapy. Results from several long-term studies support the efficacy of intrathecal morphine for treating patients with both cancer and noncancer pain. One retrospective study examined patients with chronic, malignant pain on long-term IT opioid therapy including morphine, hydromorphone, or sufentanil. They noted that the VASPI significantly decreased from baseline up to the time of first refill. These scores remained stable and significantly lower than baseline scores for 3 years.

Recent results from several long-term studies support the efficacy of intrathecal morphine. In a prospective, open-label study of IT morphine infusion, 110 patients with chronic pain were implanted and followed for 1 year. Pain relief was noted within 1 month and was sustained for the 12-month period. Another open-label study examined patients with intractable pain due to chronic pancreatitis. These results showed a reduction in pain scores from an average of 8.3 to an average of 0.75, sustained for 29 months.

For patients with vertebral fractures due to osteoporosis who do not respond to oral opiates, an open-label study of IT morphine was conducted. The mean VASPI scores decreased significantly from 8.7 cm before IT therapy to 1.9 cm after 1 year. They also saw improvements in quality of life, ambulation, and perception of health status. Interestingly, a retrospective study designed to identify characteristics of patients likely to benefit from IT morphine therapy found a greater than 50% decrease in pain in 73% of patients. The study included patients with multiple types of pain including cancer-related, nociceptive, or neuropathic. No differences in responder rates were noted regardless of pain type, patient age, or morphine dosage.

Expert consensus in the recent PACC 2016 recommends morphine as a first-line agent for neuropathic and nociceptive pain at starting doses of 0.1–0.5 mg/day, 20 mg/mL maximum concentration, and a 15 mg/day maximum dose.

Fentanyl

Fentanyl is an anilinopiperidine analog with limited rostral spread relative to morphine. With limited CSF distribution, precise catheter placement is required. The availability of fentanyl as a sterile, preservative-free injectable solutions has led to increased IT use for the management of refractory, chronic pain as reported in physician surveys. Although animal studies using fentanyl for a limited duration have demonstrated efficacy, high-quality, clinical evidence for effectiveness in treating neuropathic and nociceptive pain is lacking.

Intrathecally administered fentanyl rarely causes drug tolerance or the formation of granulomas. Studies examining neurotoxic effects of fentanyl showed no neural tissue damage at concentrations of 5000 mcg/mL. The 2016 PACC group suggests maximum concentrations of 10 mg/mL for fentanyl. The majority of 2016 PACC members agreed that in most clinical settings, patients will not benefit from daily doses higher than 1000 mcg of fentanyl.

Hydromorphone

Hydromorphone is a hydrophilic, semi-synthetic opioid, similar in structure to morphine but with greater potency. Hydromorphone is highly soluble in a compounded mixture up to 80 mg/mL. In a retrospective review of 24 patients with refractory, chronic, nonmalignant pain, 8 patients began IT hydromorphone at the time of pump placement and 16 changed to hydromorphone after failed epidural or IT morphine trials. No change in opioid-related side effects was reported. Although average pain scores were significantly lower at the 3-month follow-up, worst pain scores were unchanged. Despite a lack of controlled studies, hydromorphone is included in the algorithms for nociceptive and neuropathic pain as a first- and second-line agent, respectively. The recommended starting doses are 0.02–0.5 mg/day up to a maximum of 10 mg/day and with a maximum concentration of 15 mg/mL. The suggested maximum daily dose of IT hydromorphone is 10 mg/day.

Preclinical studies of IT hydromorphone in large animal models showed granuloma formation at higher concentrations. Two case reports described granuloma development in patients treated with IT hydromorphone. The first report described a patient who developed a granuloma using IT morphine. Nine months after removal of the first granuloma, the patient developed another granuloma 1 month after starting IT hydromorphone therapy. The second report described a 52-year-old man with a history of chronic, lumbar spine pain who developed a granuloma while receiving high-concentration IT hydromorphone (85 mg/mL) at a dose of 19.8 mg/day.

Ziconotide

Ziconotide is the only non-opioid IT option for the treatment of chronic, refractory pain. Ziconotide is a peptide synthesized from the venom of *Conus magus*, a marine snail (see Fig. 79.2). It reversibly binds N-type, voltage-gated, calcium channels in the central nervous system (CNS) and prevents the release of glutamate, calcitonin gene-related peptide, and substance P in the dorsal horn (Fig. 79.3). Ziconotide possesses linear pharmacokinetics within the CSF and is cleared by diffusion into the systemic circulation where it is metabolized by peptidases and proteases. Its safety and efficacy have been evaluated in several double-blinded, placebo-controlled RCTs in humans with malignant and nonmalignant pain. These trials showed a significant, yet small, decrease in visual analog scale of pain intensity (VASPI) scores when compared with placebo.

Respiratory depression, granuloma formation, and development of tolerance to the drug have not been found to occur. Intolerable effects are primarily neurologic and psychologic. The most common adverse neurologic reactions associated with ziconotide are dizziness, nystagmus, confusion, memory impairment, and nausea. Psychiatric side effects, such as increased risk of suicide in patients with a history of depression, happen with a fast titration rate and are more common in elderly patients. Discontinuation of ziconotide therapy due to intolerable side effects is generally low but have been reported to be as high as 61%. Creatine kinase (CK) levels also need to be checked at baseline and even intermittently during therapy with ziconotide. Clinical trials showed that

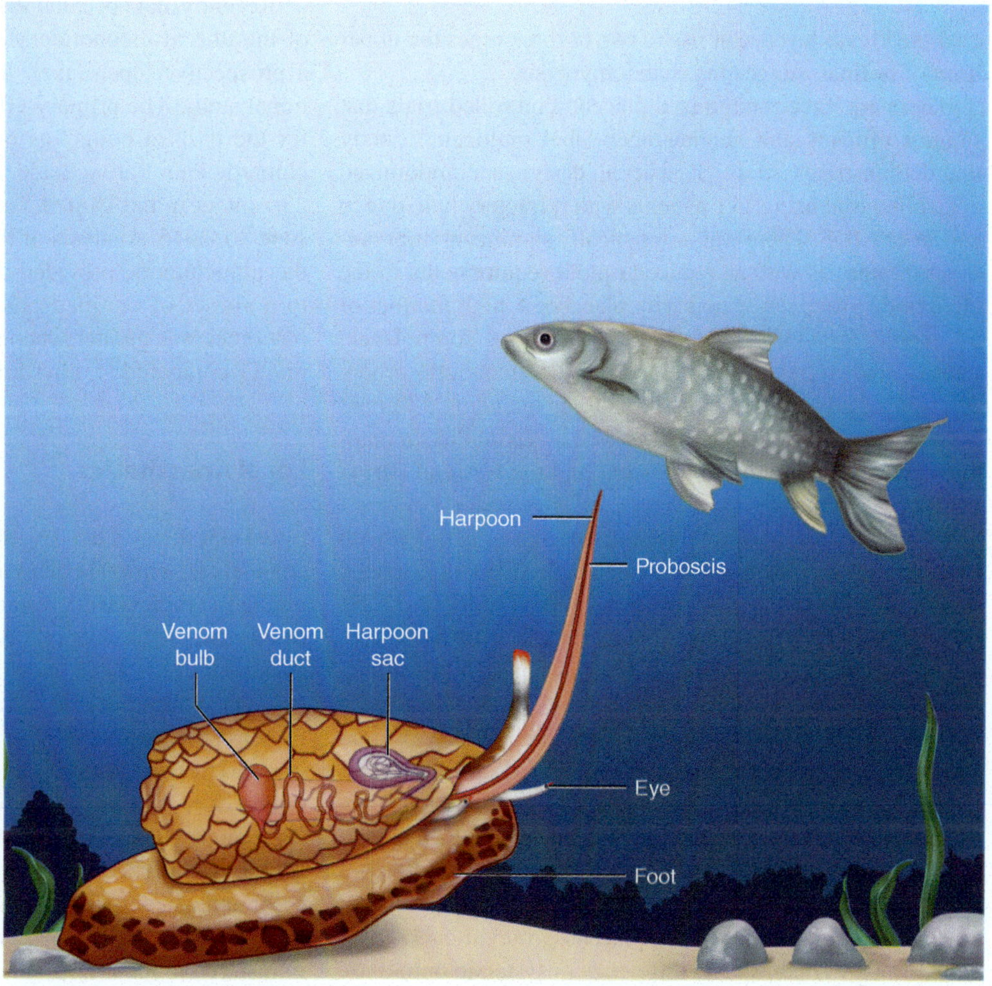

Fig. 79.2 Ziconotide is a conotoxin. Conotoxins are neurotoxic peptides isolated from the venom of the marine cone snail

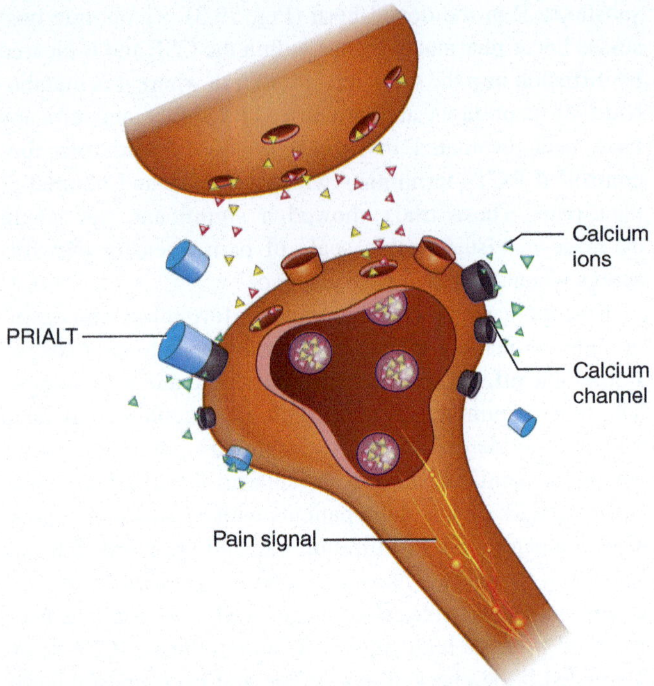

Fig. 79.3 Mechanism of action of ziconotide (Prialt)

creatine kinase levels can rise to two or three times the upper limit of normal, suggesting rhabdomyolysis.

There are three randomized placebo-controlled trials that suggest efficacy and another open-label multicenter study that demonstrates safety. Staats et al. designed a randomized controlled trial using 111 patients with refractory pain due to cancer or AIDS. There was a statistically significant improvement in pain, as well as reduced opioid requirements in the ziconotide group compared with placebo. A high number of adverse events (30.6%) including dizziness, somnolence, nausea, and nystagmus were seen in the ziconotide group. The study had several design limitations including a limited 2-week exposure to ziconotide as well as variability in management of the intrathecal infusions and the washout period prior to the RCT.

Wallace et al. repeated this study design in patients with severe chronic nonmalignant pain. Ziconotide-treated patients had a mean improvement in the VASPI of 31.2% compared with 6.0% improvement in the placebo group. Unlike Staats et al., there was no decrease in the concomitant use of pain medications. Twenty-four ziconotide-treated patients, and none of the patients receiving placebo, discontinued the study at the initial titration due to drug side effects.

Lastly, Rauck et al. performed a double-blind, placebo-controlled, randomized study of IT ziconotide in adults with severe chronic pain. The authors reported a 14.7% improvement in pain from baseline in the ziconotide group compared to a 7.2% improvement in the placebo group after 3 weeks of treatment. There was no difference in systemic opioid use between groups. Adverse events were reported in both the placebo and ziconotide groups, with central nervous system adverse events being reported more frequently using ziconotide.

Ziconotide has also been studied in combination therapy, meaning the combination of ziconotide with another intrathecal compound such as morphine or bupivacaine. In a phase 2, open-label study, the addition of intrathecal ziconotide was examined in 26 patients with suboptimal pain relief on IT morphine therapy. Ziconotide therapy began at a dosage of 0.6 mcg/day and was titrated to a maximum of 7.2 mcg/day. Reduction in VASPI scores was noted after 2 weeks of combination therapy, with a 14.5% mean VASPI score improvement by week 5. Notably, use of systemic opioids was reduced in these patients. A retrospective observational study of severe chronic pain of noncancer origin included 16 patients who had inadequate analgesia with intrathecal opioid therapy and had ziconotide added to their intrathecal regimen. Ziconotide therapy began at a dosage of 0.5 mcg/day and was titrated to a mean dosage of 2.64 mcg/day over the course of 12 weeks. At the end of this titration period, 20% of patients had 4-point decreases in their VAS scores and 20% reported increased functional capacity.

Recently, data became available from the Patient Registry of Intrathecal Ziconotide Management (PRIZM). PRIZM is a prospective, open-label, long-term, multicenter, observational study. The primary efficacy outcome is "average pain for the past 24 hours" as rated by patients on an 11-point Numeric Pain Rating Scale. Ninety three patients enrolled at 23 centers in the United States from September 5, 2013 to June 30, 2015. Analysis of the PRIZM data found that intrathecal ziconotide provided clinically meaningful pain relief to a subset of enrolled patients. Improvement on efficacy outcomes was greater when ziconotide was initiated as first-line IT compared to other first-line agents.

Local Anesthetics

Local anesthetics act by blocking the voltage-gated Na+ channels in neuronal cell membranes. They preferentially act on the fila radicularia given the large surface to volume ratio of these nerve rootlets relative to the dorsal horn cells. Local anesthetics have been shown to act synergistically with opioids when administered intrathecally in cancer pain studies. A retrospective review showed that coadministration of intrathecal bupivacaine with an opioid decreased the rate of opioid dose escalation by 65% over the first year in noncancer pain patients. However, a double-blind, crossover, multicenter randomized controlled trial (RCT) showed that the combination of opioids and bupivacaine had no additional analgesic efficacy. Nonetheless, bupivacaine is often coadministered to reduce opioid dose escalation.

The most concerning complication associated with intrathecal local anesthetic use is neurotoxicity. Other complications include extremity weakness, paresthesias, hypotension, and urinary retention. Bupivacaine is the only local anesthetic that is included in the PACC treatment algorithms and is considered first-line in combination with morphine for neuropathic pain and as a second-line agent in combination with morphine, hydromorphone, or fentanyl for nociceptive pain. Safety studies show no neurologic sequelae or toxicity at doses up to 30 mg/day.

Bupivacaine

Bupivacaine is an amide local anesthetic with high lipid solubility that is often used off-label for IT therapy. Several pharmacodynamic properties give it utility with spinal delivery:

1. Delivery of low bupivacaine concentrations alters sensory processing while sparing motor function.
2. There is synergy with other analgesic targets in animal and human models.
3. There is an absence of tachyphylaxis in patients with neuropathic or somatic pain.

Early rat studies using a continuous infusion of 0.5% bupivacaine showed modest increases in neuronal vacuolation. On autopsy, cancer patients who received a combination of intrathecal bupivacaine and morphine showed no significant histopathology of the examined spinal tissue.

A retrospective study of 109 patients who were initially given opioid-only treatment and then switched to combination therapy with bupivacaine and opioids found improved patient pain control and decreased oral opioid consumption. The average daily bupivacaine dose in that study was 10 mg. A small double-blind RCT of post-laminectomy syndrome patients suggested that the combination of bupivacaine and morphine or hydromorphone did not result in improved pain control. However, a large study in noncancer pain patients showed reduced opioid dose escalation when using combination therapy. The average bupivacaine daily dose in those patients was 9.8 mg 1 year post implant.

No formal studies have been performed to assess starting and maximal doses of bupivacaine for IT. In addition, there are no prospective studies of chronic intrathecal bupivacaine administration as a sole agent. The most recent PACC guidelines have suggested a maximal concentration of 30 mg/mL, a starting dose of 1–4 mg/day, and a maximal daily dose of 10 mg. Serious, cardiotoxic side effects can occur when significant amounts of bupivacaine reach the bloodstream, but this does not occur with intrathecal administration. Clearly, the limiting factor for bupivacaine infusions would be sensorimotor loss. Nevertheless, bupivacaine doses as high 5 mg/h and bolus doses as high as 7 mg in the high cervical space have been reported without complication. The most recent version of the PACC guidelines recommends combination bupivacaine/morphine therapy for treatment of neuropathic pain. Bupivacaine in combination with morphine, fentanyl, and hydromorphone is a second-line therapy when treating nociceptive pain.

Clonidine

This medication is an alpha2-receptor agonist. When delivered intrathecally, it is thought to provide pain relief by inhibiting the activation of NF-κB and p38 in glial cells. This causes inhibition of several pro-inflammatory cytokines that have been associated with neuropathic pain states. Like opioids, when delivered systemically, clonidine reduces presynaptic calcium entry and increases postsynaptic potassium influx, hyperpolarizing the neuron. Clonidine is typically combined with local anesthetics and morphine due to their synergistic actions for pain relief. Intrathecal clonidine has been shown to reduce the risk of morphine tolerance. Serious side effects include sedation, bradycardia, and hypotension. Sudden discontinuation of long-term IT may lead to rebound hypertension, panic attacks, and psychotic behavior.

The PACC 2012 categorized the use of clonidine for neuropathic pain as a second-line treatment when used in combination with hydromorphone or morphine. Clonidine is recommended as a third-line agent when used as a monotherapy or when combined with fentanyl. For nociceptive pain, it is categorized as a third-line agent when used in combination with an opioid and a fourth-line when combined with an opioid and bupivacaine. The recommended starting dose is 40–100 mcg/day, and the maximum recommended dose is 600 mcg/day.

Resiniferatoxin

Resiniferatoxin is an ultrapotent capsaicin analog, derived from a cactus-like plant called *Euphorbia resinifera.* It is an agonist of the transient receptor, vanilloid 1 (TRPV1) receptor. The TRPV1 receptor transduces noxious heat stimulus applied to peripheral C-fibers. Prolonged calcium influx induced by resiniferatoxin causes cytotoxicity and death of only those sensory neuronal cell bodies that express the TRPV1 ion channel in the dorsal root ganglia. Resiniferatoxin is considered a promising therapeutic target for analgesia. It is currently in a phase 1 study examining its safety and analgesic effect for advanced cancer patients. Brown et al. recently published a single-blind RCT in in companion dogs with bone cancer pain. IT resiniferatoxin (1.2 mg/kg) demonstrated improved analgesia and decreased lameness. The analgesic effect was documented in these dogs without any evidence of deafferentation pain syndrome that can be seen with some neurolytic therapies. For a more in-depth discussion of new molecules for IT use, see the chapter by Leong and Staats in this book.

Conclusion

Since the advent of IT, numerous advances have been made with regard to pump technology, pharmacology, and patient selection. Strong evidence exists for the use of IT in cancer pain. There is weak evidence supporting long-term efficacy in noncancer pain. In carefully selected patients, combination therapy appears to provide the ideal balance between efficacy and side effects. Areas most ripe for future investigation include identification of pain conditions most amenable to IT and the long-term efficacy of infusion therapy for noncancer pain. Studies delineating which drug combinations provide the best balance between efficacy and adverse effects are also needed.

Challenges limiting the increased use of IT include risks associated with the devices and medications. For example, combination therapy is complicated by the use of single-chamber pumps. In addition, all the work put into performing trials, placing implants, and refilling pumps is not well compensated. Poor reimbursement limits the development of advanced devices, novel dosing strategies, and alternative medications, which could offer improved analgesia and safety. The cost effectiveness of IT therapy has been demonstrated to be superior to conventional therapy, with high start-up costs being recovered within 28 months.

Unfortunately, despite the number of years IT therapy has been in use, there is a scarcity of rigorous evidence examining the long-term effectiveness of the agents being used. There are far more systematic reviews and narrative reviews than high-quality comparative studies of IT therapy vs. conventional treatment. Higher-quality evidence could lead to a wider adoption of this therapy due to improved and more consistent patient outcomes.

Recommended Reading

1. Abrahams M, Higgins P, Whyte P, Breen P, Muttu S, Gardiner J. Intact proprioception and control of labour pain during epidural analgesia. Acta Anaesthesiol Scand. 1999;43(1):46–50.
2. Åkerman B, Arweström E, Post C. Local anesthetics potentiate spinal morphine Antinociception. Anesthesia & Analgesia. 1988;67(10):943.
3. Allen JW, Horais KA, Tozier NA, Yaksh TL. Opiate pharmacology of intrathecal granulomas. Anesthesiology. 2006;105(3):590–8.
4. Artru AA. CSF dynamics, cerebral edema and intracranial pressure. In: Textbook of neuroanesthesia: with neurosurgical and neuroscience perspectives. New York: McGraw-Hill; 1997. p. 61–115.
5. Atli A, Theodore BR, Turk DC, Loeser JD. Intrathecal opioid therapy for chronic nonmalignant pain: a retrospective cohort study with 3-year follow-up. Pain Med. 2010;11(7):1010–6.
6. Balédent O, Henry-Feugeas MC, Idy-Peretti I. Cerebrospinal fluid dynamics and relation with blood flow: a magnetic resonance study with semiautomated cerebrospinal fluid segmentation. Invest Radiol. 2001;36(7):368–77.
7. Behar M, Magora F, Olshwang D, Davidson JT. Epidural morphine in treatment of pain. Lancet. 1979;1(8115):527–9.
8. Belverud S, Mogilner A, Schulder M. Intrathecal pumps. Neurotherapeutics. 2008;5(1):114–22.
9. Berg A, Barsa J, Deer T, et al. Efficacy of morphine sulfate infusion via the Prometra® intrathecal infusion pump. A prospective multicenter evaluation: 5th World Congress Institute of Pain; 2009.
10. Bernards CM. Understanding the physiology and pharmacology of epidural and intrathecal opioids. Best Pract Res Clin Anaesthesiol. 2002;16(4):489–505.
11. Bernards CM. Recent insights into the pharmacokinetics of spinal opioids and the relevance to opioid selection. Curr Opin Anaesthesiol. 2004;17(5):441–7.
12. Bernards CM. Cerebrospinal fluid and spinal cord distribution of baclofen and bupivacaine during slow intrathecal infusion in pigs. Anesthesiology. 2006;105(1):169–78.
13. Bhadelia RA, Bogdan AR, Kaplan RF, Wolpert SM. Cerebrospinal fluid pulsation amplitude and its quantitative relationship to cerebral blood flow pulsations: a phase-contrast MR flow imaging study. Neuroradiology. 1997;39(4):258–64.
14. Boswell MV, Iacono RP, Guthkelch AN. Sites of action of subarachnoid lidocaine and tetracaine: observations with evoked potential monitoring during spinal cord stimulator implantation. Reg Anesth. 1992;17(1):37–42.
15. Brill S, Gurman GM, Fisher A. A history of neuraxial administration of local analgesics and opioids. Eur J Anaesthesiol. 2003;20(9):682–9.
16. Brown DC, Agnello K, Iadarola MJ. Intrathecal resiniferatoxin in a dog model: efficacy in bone cancer pain. Pain. 2015;156(6):1018–24.
17. Calthorpe N. The history of spinal needles: getting to the point. Anaesthesia. 2004;59(12):1231–41.
18. Caterina MJ, Schumacher MA, Tominaga M, Rosen TA, Levine JD, Julius D. The capsaicin receptor: a heat-activated ion channel in the pain pathway. Nature. 1997;389(6653):816–24.
19. Coffey RJ, Owens ML, Broste SK, et al. Mortality associated with implantation and management of intrathecal opioid drug infusion systems to treat noncancer pain. Anesthesiology. 2009;111(4):881–91.
20. Coffey RJ, Owens ML, Broste SK, et al. Medical practice perspective: identification and mitigation of risk factors for mortality associated with intrathecal opioids for non-cancer pain. Pain Med. 2010;11(7):1001–9.
21. Cohen SP, Dragovich A. Intrathecal analgesia. Anesthesiol Clin. 2007;25(4):863–82, viii.
22. Corning JL. Local anaesthesia in general medicine and surgery. D. Appleton; 1886.
23. Covino BG. The pharmacology of local anesthetic agents. In: Stanley TH, Clayton Petty W, editors. Anesthesiology 1986. Developments in critical care medicine and anesthesiology: Springer Netherlands; 1986. p. 6–10.
24. Dahm P, Nitescu P, Appelgren L, Curelaru I. Efficacy and technical complications of long-term continuous intraspinal infusions of opioid and/or bupivacaine in refractory nonmalignant pain: a comparison between the epidural and the intrathecal approach with externalized or implanted catheters and infusion pumps. Clin J Pain. 1998;14(1):4–16.
25. Dahm PO, Nitescu PV, Appelgren LK, Curelaru I. Long-term intrathecal (i.t.) infusion of bupivacaine relieved intractable pain and spasticity in a patient with multiple sclerosis. Eur J Pain. 1998;2(1):81–5.
26. Deer TR. A critical time for practice change in the pain treatment continuum: we need to reconsider the role of pumps in the patient care algorithm. Pain Med. 2010;11(7):987–9.

27. Deer TR. History of intrathecal drug delivery. In: Atlas of implantable therapies for pain management. New York: Springer; 2011. p. 139–41.
28. Deer TR, Pope JE. Factors to consider in the choice of intrathecal drug in the treatment of neuropathic pain. Expert Rev Clin Pharmacol. 2015;8(5):507–10.
29. Deer TR, Serafini M, Buchser E, Ferrante FM, Hassenbusch SJ. Intrathecal bupivacaine for chronic pain: a review of current knowledge. Neuromodulation. 2002;5(4):196–207.
30. Deer TR, Caraway DL, Kim CK, Dempsey CD, Stewart CD, McNeil KF. Clinical experience with intrathecal bupivacaine in combination with opioid for the treatment of chronic pain related to failed back surgery syndrome and metastatic cancer pain of the spine. Spine J. 2002;2(4):274–8.
31. Deer TR, Kim C, Bowman R, Tolentino D, Stewart C, Tolentino W. Intrathecal ziconotide and opioid combination therapy for noncancer pain: an observational study. Pain Physician. 2009;12(4):E291–6.
32. Deer TR, Krames E, Levy RM, Hassenbusch SJ 3rd, Prager JP. Practice choices and challenges in the current intrathecal therapy environment: an online survey. Pain Med. 2009;10(2):304–9.
33. Deer TR, Smith HS, Cousins M, et al. Consensus guidelines for the selection and implantation of patients with noncancer pain for intrathecal drug delivery. Pain Physician. 2010;13(3):E175–213.
34. Deer TR, Prager J, Levy R, et al. Polyanalgesic consensus conference 2012: recommendations for the management of pain by intrathecal (intraspinal) drug delivery: report of an interdisciplinary expert panel. Neuromodulation. 2012;15(5):436–64; discussion 464–466.
35. Deer TR, Levy R, Prager J, et al. Polyanalgesic Consensus Conference--2012: recommendations to reduce morbidity and mortality in intrathecal drug delivery in the treatment of chronic pain. Neuromodulation. 2012;15(5):467–82; discussion 482.
36. van der Plas AA, Marinus J, Eldabe S, Buchser E, van Hilten JJ. The lack of efficacy of different infusion rates of intrathecal baclofen in complex regional pain syndrome: a randomized, double-blind, crossover study. Pain Med. 2011;12(3):459–65.
37. van Dongen RTM, Crul BJP, van Egmond J. Intrathecal Coadministration of Bupivacaine Diminishes Morphine Dose Progression During Long-term Intrathecal Infusion in Cancer Patients. Clin J Pain. 1999;15(3):166.
38. Du Pen S, Du Pen A, Hillyer J. Intrathecal hydromorphone for intractable nonmalignant pain: a retrospective study. Pain Med. 2006;7(1):10–5.
39. Duarte RV, Raphael JH, Southall JL, Baker C, Hanu-Cernat D. Intrathecal inflammatory masses: is the yearly opioid dose increase an early indicator? Neuromodulation. 2010;13(2): 109–13.
40. Feng X, Zhang F, Dong R, et al. Intrathecal administration of clonidine attenuates spinal neuroimmune activation in a rat model of neuropathic pain with existing hyperalgesia. Eur J Pharmacol. 2009;614(1-3):38–43.
41. Fukushima S, Takenami T, Yagishita S, Nara Y, Hoka S, Okamoto H. Neurotoxicity of intrathecally administered fentanyl in a rat spinal model. Pain Med. 2011;12(5):717–25.
42. Ghafoor VL, Epshteyn M, Carlson GH, Terhaar DM, Charry O, Phelps PK. Intrathecal drug therapy for long-term pain management. Am J Health Syst Pharm. 2007;64(23):2447–61.
43. Goldstein A, Lowney LI, Pal BK. Stereospecific and nonspecific interactions of the morphine congener levorphanol in subcellular fractions of mouse brain. Proc Natl Acad Sci U S A. 1971;68(8):1742–7.
44. Greenberg HS, Taren J, Ensminger WD, Doan K. Benefit from and tolerance to continuous intrathecal infusion of morphine for intractable cancer pain. J Neurosurg. 1982;57(3):360–4.
45. Grider JS, Harned ME, Etscheidt MA. Patient selection and outcomes using a low-dose intrathecal opioid trialing method for chronic nonmalignant pain. Pain Physician. 2011;14(4):343–51.
46. Hayek SM, Hanes MC. Intrathecal therapy for chronic pain: current trends and future needs. Curr Pain Headache Rep. 2014;18(1):388.
47. Hayek SM, Joseph PN, Mekhail NA. Pharmacology of intrathecally administered agents for treatment of spasticity and pain. Seminars in Pain Medicine. 2003;1(4):238–53.
48. Hayek SM, Deer TR, Pope JE, Panchal SJ, Patel VB. Intrathecal therapy for cancer and non-cancer pain. Pain Physician. 2011;14(3):219–48.
49. Hayek SM, Veizi IE, Narouze SN, Mekhail N. Age-dependent intrathecal opioid escalation in chronic noncancer pain patients. Pain Med. 2011;12(8):1179–89.
50. Herz A, Teschemacher HJ. Activities and sites of antinociceptive action of morphine-like analgesics and kinetics of distribution following intravenous, intracerebral and intraventricular application. Adv Drug Res. 1971;6:79–119.
51. Hildebrand KR, Elsberry DD, Deer TR. Stability, compatibility, and safety of intrathecal bupivacaine administered chronically via an implantable delivery system. Clin J Pain. 2001;17(3):239–44.
52. Hoederath P, Gautschi OP, Land M, Hildebrandt G, Fournier JY. Formation of two consecutive intrathecal catheter tip granulomas within nine months. Cent Eur Neurosurg. 2010;71(1):39–42.
53. Holzer P. The pharmacological challenge to tame the transient receptor potential vanilloid-1 (TRPV1) nocisensor. Br J Pharmacol. 2008;155(8):1145–62.
54. Hsu Y, Hettiarachchi HDM, Zhu DC, Linninger AA. The frequency and magnitude of cerebrospinal fluid pulsations influence intrathecal drug distribution: key factors for interpatient variability. Anesth Analg. 2012;115(2):386–94.
55. Johansen MJ, Satterfield WC, Baze WB, Hildebrand KR, Gradert TL, Hassenbusch SJ. Continuous intrathecal infusion of hydromorphone: safety in the sheep model and clinical implications. Pain Med. 2004;5(1):14–25.
56. Karai L, Brown DC, Mannes AJ, et al. Deletion of vanilloid receptor 1_expressing primary afferent neurons for pain control. J Clin Invest. 2004;113(9):1344–52.
57. Kongkam P, Wagner DL, Sherman S, et al. Intrathecal narcotic infusion pumps for intractable pain of chronic pancreatitis: a pilot series. Am J Gastroenterol. 2009;104(5):1249–55.
58. Krames ES. Intrathecal infusional therapies for intractable pain: patient management guidelines. J Pain Symptom Manage. 1993;8(1):36–46.
59. Krames ES, Olson K. Clinical realities and economic considerations: patient selection in intrathecal therapy. J Pain Symptom Manage. 1997;14(3 Suppl):S3–S13.
60. Krashin DL, Merrill JO, Trescot AM. Opioids in the management of HIV-related pain. Pain Physician. 2012;15(3 Suppl):ES157–68.
61. Kroin JS. Intrathecal drug administration. Clin Pharmacokinet. 1992;22(5):319–26.
62. Kumar K, Hunter G, Demeria DD. Treatment of chronic pain by using intrathecal drug therapy compared with conventional pain therapies: a cost-effectiveness analysis. J Neurosurg. 2002;97(4):803–10.
63. Kumar K, Bodani V, Bishop S, Tracey S. Use of intrathecal bupivacaine in refractory chronic nonmalignant pain. Pain Med. 2009;10(5):819–28.
64. Li DF, Bahar M, Cole G, Rosen M. Neurological toxicity of the subarachnoid infusion of bupivacaine, lignocaine or 2-chloroprocaine in the rat. Br J Anaesth. 1985;57(4):424–9.
65. Lundborg C, Dahm P, Nitescu P, Biber B. High intrathecal bupivacaine for severe pain in the head and neck. Acta Anaesthesiol Scand. 2009;53(7):908–13.

66. Mironer YE, Haasis JC, Chapple I, Brown C, Satterthwaite JR. Efficacy and safety of intrathecal opioid/bupivacaine mixture in chronic nonmalignant pain: a double blind, randomized, crossover, multicenter study by the National Forum of Independent Pain Clinicians (NFIPC). Neuromodulation Technol Neural Interface. 2002;5(4):208–13.
67. Netter FH. Atlas of human anatomy. Elsevier Health Sciences; 2010.
68. Nitescu P, Dahm P, Appelgren L, Curelaru I. Continuous infusion of opioid and bupivacaine by externalized intrathecal catheters in long-term treatment of" refractory" nonmalignant pain. Clin J Pain. 1998;14(1):17–28.
69. North RA. Drug receptors and the inhibition of nerve cells. Br J Pharmacol. 1989;98(1):13–28.
70. North RB, Cutchis PN, Epstein JA, Long DM. Spinal cord compression complicating subarachnoid infusion of morphine: case report and laboratory experience. Neurosurgery. 1991;29(5): 778–84.
71. Onofrio BM, Yaksh TL, Arnold PG. Continuous low-dose intrathecal morphine administration in the treatment of chronic pain of malignant origin. Mayo Clin Proc. 1981;56(8):516–20.
72. Papisov MI, Belov VV, Gannon KS. Physiology of the intrathecal bolus: the leptomeningeal route for macromolecule and particle delivery to CNS. Mol Pharm. 2013;10(5):1522–32.
73. Patel VB, Manchikanti L, Singh V, Schultz DM, Hayek SM, Smith HS. Systematic review of intrathecal infusion systems for long-term management of chronic non-cancer pain. Pain Physician. 2009;12(2):345–60.
74. Penn RD, Paice JA. Chronic intrathecal morphine for intractable pain. J Neurosurg. 1987;67(2):182–6.
75. Perruchoud C, Eldabe S, Durrer A, et al. Effects of flow rate modifications on reported analgesia and quality of life in chronic pain patients treated with continuous intrathecal drug therapy. Pain Med. 2011;12(4):571–6.
76. Pert CB, Snyder SH. Opiate receptor: demonstration in nervous tissue. Science. 1973;179(4077):1011–4.
77. Pope JE, Deer TR. Ziconotide: a clinical update and pharmacologic review. Expert Opin Pharmacother. 2013;14(7): 957–66.
78. Pope JE, Deer TR, Bruel BM, Falowski S. Clinical uses of intrathecal therapy and its placement in the pain care algorithm. Pain Pract. 2016; https://doi.org/10.1111/papr.12438.
79. Prager J, Deer T, Levy R, et al. Best practices for intrathecal drug delivery for pain. Neuromodulation. 2014;17(4):354–72; discussion 372.
80. Rainov NG, Heidecke V, Burkert W. Long-term intrathecal infusion of drug combinations for chronic back and leg pain. J Pain Symptom Manage. 2001;22(4):862–71.
81. Ramsey CN, Owen RD, Witt WO, Grider JS. Intrathecal granuloma in a patient receiving high dose hydromorphone. Pain Physician. 2008;11(3):369–73.
82. Rauck RL, Wallace MS, Leong MS, et al. A randomized, double-blind, placebo-controlled study of intrathecal ziconotide in adults with severe chronic pain. J Pain Symptom Manage. 2006;31(5):393–406.
83. Reig E, Abejón D. Continuous morphine infusion: a retrospective study of efficacy, safety, and demographic variables. Neuromodulation. 2009;12(2):122–9.
84. Rennels ML, Blaumanis OR, Grady PA. Rapid solute transport throughout the brain via paravascular fluid pathways. Adv Neurol. 1990;52:431–9.
85. Resiniferatoxin to Treat Severe Pain Associated with Advanced Cancer – Full Text View – ClinicalTrials.gov. https://clinicaltrials.gov/show/NCT00804154. Accessed 13 Sept 2017.
86. Saltari MR, Shaladi A, Piva B, et al. The management of pain from collapse of osteoporotic vertebrae with continuous intrathecal morphine infusion. Neuromodulation. 2007;10(2): 167–76.
87. Schmidtko A, Lötsch J, Freynhagen R, Geisslinger G. Ziconotide for treatment of severe chronic pain. Lancet. 2010;375(9725):1569–77.
88. Scott DB, McClure JH, Giasi RM, Seo J, Covino BG. Effects of concentration of local anaesthetic drugs in extradural block. Br J Anaesth. 1980;52(10):1033–7.
89. Sjoberg M, Nitescu P, Appelgren L, Curelaru L. Long-term intrathecal morphine and bupivacaine in patients with refractory cancer pain-results from a morphine-bupivacaine dose regimen of 0.5/4.75 mg/ml. Anesthesiology. 1994;80(2): 284–97.
90. Staats PS, Yearwood T, Charapata SG, et al. Intrathecal ziconotide in the treatment of refractory pain in patients with cancer or AIDS: a randomized controlled trial. JAMA. 2004;291(1): 63–70.
91. Stockman HW. Effect of anatomical fine structure on the flow of cerebrospinal fluid in the spinal subarachnoid space. J Biomech Eng. 2006;128(1):106–14.
92. Tobias G, Sands RP Jr, Bacon DR. Continuous spinal anesthesia: a continuous history? Reg Anesth Pain Med. 1999;24(5): 453–7.
93. Tuohy CEB. Costinuous spinal anesthesiaits usefitiisess and technic involved. Anesthesiology. 1944;5(2):142–8.
94. Uhle EI, Becker R, Gatscher S, Bertalanffy H. Continuous intrathecal clonidine administration for the treatment of neuropathic pain. Stereotact Funct Neurosurg. 2000;75(4): 167–75.
95. Ummenhofer WC, Arends RH, Shen DD, Bernards CM. Comparative spinal distribution and clearance kinetics of intrathecally administered morphine, fentanyl, alfentanil, and sufentanil. Anesthesiology. 2000;92(3):739–53.
96. Van Dongen RT, Crul BJ, De Bock M. Long-term intrathecal infusion of morphine and morphine/bupivacaine mixtures in the treatment of cancer pain: a retrospective analysis of 51 cases. Pain. 1993;55(1):119–23.
97. Veizi IE, Hayek SM, Narouze S, Pope JE, Mekhail N. Combination of intrathecal opioids with bupivacaine attenuates opioid dose escalation in chronic noncancer pain patients. Pain Med. 2011;12(10):1481–9.
98. Waara-Wolleat KL, Hildebrand KR, Stewart GR. A review of intrathecal fentanyl and Sufentanil for the treatment of chronic pain. Pain Med. 2006;7(3):251–9.
99. Wagemans MF, van der Valk P, Spoelder EM, Zuurmond WW, de Lange JJ. Neurohistopathological findings after continuous intrathecal administration of morphine or a morphine/bupivacaine mixture in cancer pain patients. Acta Anaesthesiol Scand. 1997;41(8):1033–8.
100. Wallace MS, Charapata SG, Fisher R, et al. Intrathecal ziconotide in the treatment of chronic nonmalignant pain: a randomized, double-blind, placebo-controlled clinical trial. Neuromodulation. 2006;9(2):75–86.
101. Wallace MS, Rauck R, Fisher R, et al. Intrathecal ziconotide for severe chronic pain: safety and tolerability results of an open-label, long-term trial. Anesth Analg. 2008;106(2):628–37, table of contents.
102. Wallace MS, Kosek PS, Staats P, Fisher R, Schultz DM, Leong M. Phase II, open-label, multicenter study of combined intrathecal morphine and ziconotide: addition of ziconotide in patients receiving intrathecal morphine for severe chronic pain. Pain Med. 2008;9(3):271–81.

103. Webster LR, Fakata KL, Charapata S, Fisher R, MineHart M. Open-label, multicenter study of combined intrathecal morphine and ziconotide: addition of morphine in patients receiving ziconotide for severe chronic pain. Pain Med. 2008;9(3):282–90.
104. Webster LR, Fisher R, Charapata S, Wallace MS. Long-term intrathecal ziconotide for chronic pain: an open-label study. J Pain Symptom Manage. 2009;37(3):363–72.
105. Wermeling DP. Ziconotide, an intrathecally administered N-type calcium channel antagonist for the treatment of chronic pain. Pharmacotherapy. 2005;25(8):1084–94.
106. Wermeling D, Drass M, Ellis D, et al. Pharmacokinetics and pharmacodynamics of intrathecal ziconotide in chronic pain patients. J Clin Pharmacol. 2003;43(6):624–36.
107. Yaksh TL, Rudy TA. Analgesia mediated by a direct spinal action of narcotics. Science. 1976;192(4246):1357–8.
108. Yaksh TL, Jessell TM, Gamse R, Mudge AW, Leeman SE. Intrathecal morphine inhibits substance P release from mammalian spinal cord in vivo. Nature. 1980;286(5769):155–7.
109. Yaksh TL, Horais KA, Tozier NA, et al. Chronically infused intrathecal morphine in dogs. Anesthesiology. 2003;99(1):174–87.

Patient Selection

80

Lucas W. Campos

Introduction

Success using intrathecal therapy (IT) is dependent on very careful patient selection. Evidence- and consensus-based recommendations regarding patient selection have been published in the literature recently with the new 2016 Polyanalgesic Consensus Conference (PACC). There have been numerous other reports suggesting best practice in patient selection which take into account complexity of chronic pain including underlying disease, patient characteristics, and IT medication used. As this chapter will demonstrate, there is a complex interplay between disease indications and patient selection. Proper screening and patient selection increase the likelihood of success with IT therapy. Screening should consider infection risk, BMI, OSA, psychological risk factors, pulmonary function, age, diabetes control, MRI compatibility, and coagulopathy or anticoagulant use; please refer to Tables 80.1 and 80.2.

Table 80.1 Key considerations for selection and implantation of patients with noncancer pain for intrathecal therapy

Contraindications for IT trial/implant
Immunocompromised patients at high risk for infection
Patients presenting with an active infection
Untreated addiction
Active psychosis
Uncontrolled or poorly treated depression/anxiety
Serious cognitive deficits such that their ability to understand how to use the technology is impaired
Inability to maintain insurance coverage or means to pay surgical implantation and ongoing medication refills
Inability to comply with medication refill schedule due to geographic limitations

Table 80.2 Indications for IT therapy

Chronic pain results in significant interference with ability to work, socialize, and enjoy hobbies
Severe diffuse joint pain
Visceral or somatic abdominal pain
Postherpetic neuralgia
Cancer pain due to tumor compression of neural or visceral structures
Effective analgesia with systemic opioids that cause intolerable side effects
Complex regional pain syndrome

Background and Historical Perspective

1898 marks the year August Bier applied cocaine, a newly discovered local anesthetic, to his own CSF as well as that of six patients. This technique was extremely effective in providing immediate, profound relief of pain in the lower half of the body. Later, Rudolph Matas demonstrated that morphine could reduce side effects seen with intrathecal cocaine including acute rise in arterial pressure and tachycardia. Continuous spinal analgesia came into use in the 1940s, but this therapy lacked scientific rationale for widespread use. With the discovery of opiate receptors in the spinal cord in 1973 work began to perfect continuous intrathecal infusion for cancer pain treatment. Wang et al. first reported the successful use of intrathecal morphine for the treatment of intractable cancer pain in 1977. Two years later, an implantable intrathecal drug delivery system (IDDS) was shown to improve function and quality of life. During the 1980s, IDDS allowed physicians to use lower doses of analgesics and minimize opiate side effects like sedation and constipation. In 1991, externally programmable, battery-powered IDDS pumps were introduced, allowing for noninvasive dose changes using an external programmer. Now it was easier to change a patient's analgesic level in response to the dynamic changes in pain.

L. W. Campos (✉)
Interventional Pain Physicians, Chico, CA, USA

T. R. Deer et al. (eds.), *Deer's Treatment of Pain*, https://doi.org/10.1007/978-3-030-12281-2_80

Infection Risk

Patients should be assessed preoperatively for an increased risk of infection. Comorbidities such as uncontrolled diabetes, immunosuppressive drugs for systemic diseases (e.g., rheumatoid arthritis), immunosuppression from malignancy or HIV, or a history of poor wound healing should be disqualifiers for IT. In patients with a history of methicillin-resistant *Staphylococcus aureus* (MRSA) infection or colonization, extra precautions are needed. Use of intranasal Bactroban ointment (mupirocin) for 5 days or greater, perianal Bactroban ointment for 5 days or more, chlorohexidine 4% bathing prior to surgery, and preoperative antibiotics that are consistent with coverage for that organism are imperative to avoid a devastating complication. Preoperative culturing of patients for intranasal MRSA will reduce the incidence of postoperative spinal infections with MRSA. One study evaluated multiple series of preoperative patients who tested positive for intranasal MRSA and were treated prior to surgery with mupirocin BID for 7 days. This regimen was accompanied by the application of a 2% CHG preparation on the skin. The overall number of surgical infections was decreased by 63%. Infections due to MRSA were diminished by 78%.

The use of preoperative antibiotics is well established and should be completed prior to incision. The choice of preoperative antibiotic administration should be based on local pathogens and sensitivity. The physician should consult with local infectious disease experts on bacterial antibiotic resistance in their facility. This may vary based on geographic location, institution, and patient populations.

Immunocompromised Patients

Studies have examined the safety and efficacy of IT therapy in the immunodeficient patient, including individuals with cancer and HIV. It is currently uncertain whether immune compromise independently increases the rate of IT therapy failure due to device infection because reported device infection rates are similar between immunocompromised and control patient populations using indirect comparative data. In the absence of conclusive data, the risks and benefits should be discussed, and vigilant postoperative wound examinations should take place regularly with cancer and HIV patient populations.

Diabetes Mellitus

Diabetes affects approximately 23.6 million individuals in the US population along. There are an estimated additional 57 million patients having blood glucose levels indicative of prediabetes. It is clear that poor wound healing and an increased rate of surgical site infections occur in this patient population. Wound infection is the most common device-related complication associated with IT therapy. There is also sound evidence that patients who undergo surgery with better long-term glycemic control, lower hemoglobin A1c levels immediately prior to surgery, have lower rates of surgical site infection. Diabetic patients must be counseled regarding the increased risk of surgical site infection. The potential consequence of severe infection post-surgery in this patient population must be carefully considered and discussed in terms of overall risk/benefit. This escalated risk of wound infection in diabetics also warrants increased vigilance for signs and symptoms of evolving wound infection after implantation.

Cardiac Disease

Limited data support the notion that dose-related cardiac abnormalities may occur when the N-type calcium channel antagonist ziconotide is used. In a randomized controlled safety and efficacy study of IT ziconotide, investigators noted that cardiovascular adverse effects, such as postural hypotension, occurred more frequently in patients in the active treatment group vs the placebo group (33.3% vs 10%, respectively). Notably, 32.3% of postural hypotension events occurred at doses greater than 0.1 μg/hour compared to 17.1% happening at doses less than or equal to 0.1 μg/hour 24 hours following opioid and non-opioid IT treatments. Using lower dosages, smaller dose increments, and increasing the time between dose titrations can reduce the frequency of adverse effects. Since there are no specific guidelines detailing the impact of cardiac abnormalities on IT therapy, all candidates with a history of cardiovascular disease should be evaluated using the risk stratification guidelines outlined by the American College of Cardiology (ACC) and the American Heart Association (AHA).

Obstruction Sleep Apnea

Obesity predisposes individuals to developing symptoms of obstructive sleep apnea (OSA) due to upper-airway obstruction during normal sleep, causing temporary apneic episodes. More than 18 million Americans have OSA, which can lead to pulmonary hypertension caused by carbon dioxide retention. OSA has also been associated with an increased sensitivity to the respiratory-depressant effects of opioids. An observational study by Webster et al. reported that sleep-disordered breathing was present in 75% of patients treated with chronic opioid therapy, with 39% of these individuals having OSA (n = 147). In that study, polysomnographies demonstrated opioids may have contributed to sleep-related apnea in chronic pain patients. Opioid therapy may still be permissible in individuals with chronic pain provided they are carefully monitored by prescribing physicians. IT therapy may potentially reduce the severity of both OSA and pain, particularly when utilizing combination therapy. Also, the use of IT ziconotide as monotherapy may offer advantages in this setting.

Chronic Lung Disease

Reactive airway disease, restrictive pulmonary disease, and chronic obstructive pulmonary disease (COPD) all experience significant retention of carbon dioxide and are more prone to respiratory depression and respiratory arrest with the administration of systemic opioids. A retrospective case-controlled analysis by Taylor et al. found that patients with COPD are most at risk for a respiratory event when administered opioids following surgery (odds ratio 5.09 within the 95% confidence interval), as compared with patients without chronic lung disease. Long-term risk of IT therapy in chronic lung disease patients is unknown, and it is likely that patients with COPD may be safely treated with IT opioids if dosed cautiously. Alternatively, this patient population may benefit from nonopioid IT agents or combination therapy. Thus, the panel recommends close monitoring in patients with chronic lung disease during any IT trial and postimplantation of a permanent system for 24 hours following either.

Psychological Factors

In a systematic review of the literature relating to presurgical somatization, depression, anxiety, and poor coping are predictors of a poor response to IT. Celestin et al. identified a positive relationship between 1 or more psychological factors and poor treatment outcomes in 92% of the 25 studies they reviewed. Although these data suggest a possible correlation between psychological status and the effect of pain-related treatment, current empiric research has yet to reveal a specific set of variables associated with positive or negative outcomes. A study by Doleys and Brown demonstrated that patients with mildly abnormal Minnesota Multiphasic Personality Inventory-2 (MMPI-2) personality profiles reported a higher percentage of improvement in pain after 4 years of IT therapy compared with patients with a more typical MMPI scores. Thus, patients should not be excluded based solely on such findings without first considering other aspects of the psychological evaluation.

The inability to have a specialist conduct the psychological consult is not an absolute contraindication to device implantation. The provider must become acquainted with the relevant psychosocial issues typically found in chronic pain patients and integrate into the evaluation and treatment of the patient. The psychological evaluation should also assess the need for any pretrial, preimplantation, or postimplantation targeted psychological and psychiatric interventions.

Device Limitations

There are a number of technical concerns that must be considered when selecting a patient for IT. Most notable are the size of the pump, the subcutaneous position of the pump, and the route that the tunneled catheter will take during surgical placement. The patient must clearly understand the size and location of the proposed pocket for the IT pump. Most devices are large, and the only region suitable for placement is the left- or right-lower quadrant of the abdomen. However, in patients with an overhanging panniculus, higher placement may be necessary. It is important to mark the pump location while the patient is in the sitting position for optimum placement. Avoid proximity to the anterior rib or iliac crest as this can cause painful contact of the pump with these structures even after complete healing of the surgical incisions. Depth of the implant site must have special consideration regarding accessibility for required refills. The pump may be implanted within the mid-fat plane of the lower quadrant of the abdomen or directly over the anterior fascia of the rectus abdominis muscle to accommodate for variation in body habitus of individual patients.

Economic Factors

These can greatly influence treatment choices and can potentially prevent the implementation of effective therapy. According to a 2009 survey of healthcare practitioners who actively utilize implantable drug devices, 40.5% of respondents identified the cost of pump implantation as the greatest economic barrier to providing IT therapy. Drug and refill fees were also an important deciding factor, which deterred 34.5% and 25% of respondents, respectively. In fact, 87.2% of those surveyed believed the cost of IT agents to be at least somewhat important during the patient selection process.

Previous Systemic Opioid Use

More patients are taking systemic opioid medications than ever before in the United States, with increasing mortality. Diversion and misuse contribute to the associated morbidity and mortality on society. The California State Medical Board has created guidelines for systemic opioids to be less than 80 morphine equivalents (MEs), while others advocate for less than 100 or 120 MEs. The CDC recently recommended chronic maintenance doses of systemic opioids of 50 MEs or less, with extra vigilance and risk assessment above 90 MEs. The history of systemic exposure is important when considering IT therapy, not just for calculating the total amount of systemic opioids but also for considering the impact of IT opioid dose escalation. Preclinical work has shown cross tolerance between IT and systemic morphine. In one IT opioid study of patients with chronic pain, during the washout period before randomization to another IT drug, the majority of patients were able to wean IT opioid medications but with average systemic supplementation of near 300 MEs per day. The patients had visual analogue scale of pain intensity (VASPI) scores of greater than 80 mm, suggesting failing IT therapy. If patients are maintained on large amounts of systemic opioids before starting IT therapy, the likelihood of monotherapy failure seems to be higher. This concept supports the approach of weaning or reducing systemic opioids prior to initiating IT therapy. This potency shift is not predictable based on previous models for systemic to IT conversion, and there are reports of tolerance reversal in as little as a week off IT agents. Veizi et al. reported a reduction of dose escalation of nearly three times when employing a local anesthetic. Many authors recommend weaning strategies.

Coagulopathies and Anticoagulant Therapy

Anticoagulant therapy is common in many disorders, including atherosclerotic coronary artery disease, atrial fibrillation, and deep vein thrombosis. Patients can receive long-term therapy with warfarin or an increasing array of potent platelet and factor X inhibitors. Patients receiving anticoagulants have an increased risk for the development of spinal epidural hematoma during catheter insertion or removal. Despite an estimated incidence of 1:220,000 and 1:150,000 following IT and epidural instrumentation, respectively, epidural hematomas comprise almost half of the reported spinal cord injuries associated with neuromodulation therapy. The elevated risk of bleeding associated with a wide array of anticoagulant and antiplatelet agents has been systematically reviewed by the American Society of Regional Anesthesia and Pain Medicine, and very specific recommendations exist for each prescribed anticoagulant medication.

Conclusions

Appropriate patient selection is vital to achieving successful outcomes with chronic IT therapy. Specific patient selection indications for implantation with an IT drug delivery system are not supported by rigorous, literature-based scientific data. The ultimate determination to proceed with IT therapy depends on the practitioner deciding who to conduct an IT trial and when to implant the device if the trial is successful. Consideration of a patient's physical, psychological, and social characteristics helps practitioners minimize the potential for treatment failure, adverse events, and mortality. Understanding a patient's possible psychological pathology and current mental state is crucial to the success of IT. Providers should have access to neurosurgical and neuroradiological expertise in case of epidural hematoma formation as this can quickly lead to permanent spinal cord damage if not treated in time.

Recommended Reading

1. Bernards CM. Cerebrospinal fluid and spinal cord distribution of baclofen and bupivacaine during slow intrathecal infusion in pigs. Anesthesiology. 2006;105(1):169–78.
2. Celestin J, Edwards RR, Jamison RN. Pretreatment psychosocial variables as predictors of outcomes following lumbar surgery and spinal cord stimulation: a systematic review and literature synthesis. Pain Med. 2009;10(4):639–53.
3. Chaney MA. Intrathecal and epidural anesthesia and analgesia for cardiac surgery. Anesth Analg. 2006;102(1):45–64.
4. Chou R, Turner JA, Devine EB, et al. The Effectiveness and Risks of Long-Term Opioid Therapy for Chronic Pain: A Systematic Review for National Institutes of Health Pathways to Prevention Workshop Effectiveness and Risks of Long-Term Opioid Therapy for Chronic Pain. Ann Intern Med. 2015;162(4):276–86.
5. Coffey RJ, Owens ML, Broste SK, et al. Medical practice perspective: identification and mitigation of risk factors for mortality associated with intrathecal opioids for non-cancer pain. Pain Med. 2010;11(7):1001–9.
6. Czernicki M, Sinovich G, Mihaylov I, et al. Intrathecal drug delivery for chronic pain management-scope, limitations and future. J Clin Monit Comput. 2015;29(2):241–9.
7. Deer TR, Pope JE. Factors to consider in the choice of intrathecal drug in the treatment of neuropathic pain. Expert Rev Clin Pharmacol. 2015;8(5):507–10.
8. Deer T, Krames ES, Hassenbusch S, et al. Future directions for intrathecal pain management: a review and update from the interdisciplinary polyanalgesic consensus conference 2007. Neuromodulation. 2008;11(2):92–7.
9. Deer T, Ranson M, Stewart D. Relevant anatomy for spinal delivery. Neuromodulation. New York: Elsevier; 2009a.
10. Deer TR, Krames E, Levy RM, Hassenbusch SJ 3rd, Prager JP. Practice choices and challenges in the current intrathecal therapy environment: an online survey. Pain Med. 2009b;10(2):304–9.
11. Deer TR, Smith HS, Burton AW, et al. Comprehensive consensus based guidelines on intrathecal drug delivery systems in the treatment of pain caused by cancer pain. Pain Physician. 2011;14(3):E283–312.
12. Deer TR, Prager J, Levy R, et al. Polyanalgesic Consensus Conference--2012: recommendations on trialing for intrathecal (intraspinal) drug delivery: report of an interdisciplinary expert panel. Neuromodulation. 2012;15(5):420–35; discussion 435.
13. Deer TR, Pope JE, Hayek SM, et al. The polyanalgesic consensus conference (PACC): recommendations on intrathecal drug infusion systems best practices and guidelines. Neuromodulation. 2017;20(2):96–132.
14. Department of Health and Human Services US. Centers for Disease Control and Prevention National diabetes fact sheet. at: www.cdc.gov/diabetes/pubs/ …. 2002.

15. DiPaola CP, Saravanja DD, Boriani L, Zhang H. Postoperative infection treatment score for the spine (PITSS): construction and validation of a predictive model to define need for single versus multiple irrigation and …. Spine J. 2012. http://www.sciencedirect.com/science/article/pii/S1529943012000939.
16. Doleys DM, Brown J. MMPI profile as an outcome "predictor" in the treatment of noncancer pain patients utilizing intraspinal opioid therapy. Neuromodulation. 2001;4(3):93–7.
17. Epstein NE. Preoperative, intraoperative, and postoperative measures to further reduce spinal infections. Surg Neurol Int. 2011;2:17.
18. Farney RJ, Walker JM, Cloward TV, Rhondeau S. Sleep-disordered breathing associated with long-term opioid therapy. Chest. 2003;123(2):632–9.
19. Fitzgibbon DR, Rathmell JP, Michna E, Stephens LS, Posner KL, Domino KB. Malpractice claims associated with medication management for chronic pain. Anesthesiology. 2010;112(4):948–56.
20. Flack SH, Bernards CM. Cerebrospinal fluid and spinal cord distribution of hyperbaric bupivacaine and baclofen during slow intrathecal infusion in pigs. Anesthesiology. 2010;112(1):165–73.
21. Fleisher LA, Fleischmann KE, Auerbach AD, et al. 2014 ACC/AHA guideline on perioperative cardiovascular evaluation and management of patients undergoing noncardiac surgery: executive summary: a report of the American College of Cardiology/American Heart Association Task Force on practice guidelines. Developed in collaboration with the American College of Surgeons, American Society of Anesthesiologists, American Society of Echocardiography, American Society of Nuclear Cardiology, Heart Rhythm Society, Society for Cardiovascular Angiography and Interventions, Society of Cardiovascular Anesthesiologists, and Society of Vascular Medicine Endorsed by the Society of Hospital Medicine. J Nucl Cardiol. 2015;22(1):162–215.
22. Follett KA, Burchiel K, Deer T, DuPen S. Prevention of intrathecal drug delivery catheter-related complications. Technology at the …. 2003. http://onlinelibrary.wiley.com/doi/10.1046/j.1525-1403.2003.03005.x/full.
23. Follett KA, Boortz-Marx RL, Drake JM, et al. Prevention and management of intrathecal drug delivery and spinal cord stimulation system infections. Anesthesiology. 2004;100(6):1582–94.
24. Friese S, Hamhaber U, Erb M, Kueker W, Klose U. The influence of pulse and respiration on spinal cerebrospinal fluid pulsation. Investig Radiol. 2004;39(2):120–30.
25. Ghafoor VL, Epshteyn M, Carlson GH, Terhaar DM, Charry O, Phelps PK. Intrathecal drug therapy for long-term pain management. Am J Health Syst Pharm. 2007;64(23):2447–61.
26. Greenhalgh DG. Wound healing and diabetes mellitus. Clin Plast Surg. 2003;30(1):37–45.
27. Grider JS, Harned ME, Etscheidt MA. Patient selection and outcomes using a low-dose intrathecal opioid trialing method for chronic nonmalignant pain. Pain Physician. 2011;14(4):343–51.
28. Hage FG, Venkataraman R, Zoghbi GJ, Perry GJ, DeMattos AM, Iskandrian AE. The scope of coronary heart disease in patients with chronic kidney disease. J Am Coll Cardiol. 2009;53(23): 2129–40.
29. Hayek SM, Deer TR, Pope JE, Panchal SJ, Patel VB. Intrathecal therapy for cancer and non-cancer pain. Pain Physician. 2011a;14(3):219–48.
30. Hayek SM, Veizi IE, Narouze SN, Mekhail N. Age-dependent intrathecal opioid escalation in chronic noncancer pain patients. Pain Med. 2011b;12(8):1179–89.
31. Horlocker TT, Wedel DJ, Benzon H, et al. Regional anesthesia in the anticoagulated patient: defining the risks (the second ASRA consensus conference on neuraxial anesthesia and anticoagulation). Reg Anesth Pain Med. 2003;28(3):172–97.
32. Knight KH, Brand FM, Mchaourab AS, Veneziano G. Implantable intrathecal pumps for chronic pain: highlights and updates. Croat Med J. 2007;48(1):22–34.
33. Manchikanti L. Evidence-based medicine, systematic reviews, and guidelines in interventional pain management, part I: introduction and general considerations. Pain Physician. 2008;11(2):161–86.
34. Maves TJ, Gebhart GF. Antinociceptive synergy between intrathecal morphine and lidocaine during visceral and somatic nociception in the rat. Anesthesiology. 1992;76(1):91–9.
35. Mekhail N, Mahboobi R, Farajzadeh Deroee A, et al. Factors that might impact intrathecal drug delivery (IDD) dose escalation: a longitudinal study. Pain Pract. 2014;14(4):301–8.
36. Nemeth TA, Beilman GJ, Hamlin CL, Chipman JG. Preoperative verification of timely antimicrobial prophylaxis does not improve compliance with guidelines. Surg Infect. 2010;11(4):387–91.
37. Ordia JI, Fischer E, Adamski E, Chagnon KG, Spatz EL. Continuous intrathecal baclofen infusion by a programmable pump in 131 consecutive patients with severe spasticity of spinal origin. Neuromodulation. 2002;5(1):16–24.
38. Patel VB, Manchikanti L, Singh V, Schultz DM, Hayek SM, Smith HS. Systematic review of intrathecal infusion systems for long-term management of chronic non-cancer pain. Pain Physician. 2009;12(2):345–60.
39. Penning JP, Yaksh TL. Interaction of intrathecal morphine with bupivacaine and lidocaine in the rat. Anesthesiology. 1992;77(6):1186–2000.
40. Pergolizzi J, Böger RH, Budd K, Dahan A. Opioids and the management of chronic severe pain in the elderly: consensus statement of an international expert panel with focus on the six clinically most often …. Pain. 2008. http://onlinelibrary.wiley.com/doi/10.1111/j.1533-2500.2008.00204.x/full.
41. Practice Guidelines for the Prevention, Detection, and Management of Respiratory Depression Associated with Neuraxial Opioid Administration. An Updated Report by the American Society of Anesthesiologists Task Force on Neuraxial Opioids and the American Society of Regional Anesthesia and Pain Medicine. Anesthesiology. 2016;124(3):535–52.
42. Prager J, Deer T, Levy R, et al. Best practices for intrathecal drug delivery for pain. Neuromodulation. 2014;17(4):354–72; discussion 372.
43. Rathmell JP, Lake T, Ramundo MB. Infectious risks of chronic pain treatments: injection therapy, surgical implants, and intradiscal techniques. Reg Anesth Pain Med. 2006;31(4):346–52.
44. Rauck RL, Wallace MS, Leong MS, et al. A randomized, double-blind, placebo-controlled study of intrathecal ziconotide in adults with severe chronic pain. J Pain Symptom Manag. 2006;31(5):393–406.
45. Smith HS, Deer TR. Safety and efficacy of intrathecal ziconotide in the management of severe chronic pain. Ther Clin Risk Manag. 2009;5(3):521–34.
46. Smith TJ, Staats PS, Deer T, et al. Randomized clinical trial of an implantable drug delivery system compared with comprehensive medical management for refractory cancer pain: impact on pain, drug-related toxicity, and survival. J Clin Oncol. 2002;20(19):4040–9.
47. Staats PS, Yearwood T, Charapata SG, et al. Intrathecal ziconotide in the treatment of refractory pain in patients with cancer or AIDS: a randomized controlled trial. JAMA. 2004;291(1):63–70.
48. Stearns L, Boortz-Marx R, Du Pen S, et al. Intrathecal drug delivery for the management of cancer pain: a multidisciplinary consensus of best clinical practices. J Support Oncol. 2005;3(6):399–408.
49. Taylor S, Kirton OC, Staff I, Kozol RA. Postoperative day one: a high risk period for respiratory events. Am J Surg. 2005;190(5):752–6.
50. Ummenhofer WC, Arends RH, Shen DD, Bernards CM. Comparative spinal distribution and clearance kinetics of intrathecally administered morphine, fentanyl, alfentanil, and sufentanil. Anesthesiology. 2000;92(3):739–53.
51. Van den Berghe G. How does blood glucose control with insulin save lives in intensive care? J Clin Invest. 2004;114(9):1187–95.

52. Veizi IE, Hayek SM, Narouze S, Pope JE, Mekhail N. Combination of intrathecal opioids with bupivacaine attenuates opioid dose escalation in chronic noncancer pain patients. Pain Med. 2011;12(10):1481–9.
53. Wang JK. Analgesic effect of intrathecally administered morphine. Reg Anesth Pain Med. 1977;2(3). journals.lww.com):3.
54. Webster LR, Choi Y, Desai H, Webster L, Grant BJB. Sleep-disordered breathing and chronic opioid therapy. Pain Med. 2008;9(4):425–32.
55. Yaksh TL, Fisher CJ, Hockman TM, Wiese AJ. Current and future issues in the development of spinal agents for the management of pain. Curr Neuropharmacol. 2017;15(2):232–59.
56. Young T, Peppard PE, Gottlieb DJ. Epidemiology of obstructive sleep apnea: a population health perspective. Am J Respir Crit Care Med. 2002;165(9):1217–39.

Intrathecal Device Considerations

81

Chong H. Kim

Introduction

Once careful patient selection is completed, the decision to proceed with implantation of the intrathecal (IT) system requires thoughtful planning, consideration, and technical skill. Implantation process requires knowledge and training. The use of intrathecal drug delivery system (IDDS) not only consists of a catheter and a programmable delivery device but also the skills of catheter placement, tunneling of the catheter, pocketing of the device, and connection and anchoring of the system.

The use of intrathecal drug delivery (IDD) started in the 1880s, when local anesthetics were administered neuraxially, with the first reported intraspinal morphine use in 1901. Since then, various developments, such as continuous catheter use, application of continuous spinal anesthesia, and use of implantable, programmable IT pumps, have occurred.

Since the early 1980s, when the first human clinical implant of an IT, programmable pump occurred, the use of IDD has been evolving to treat new conditions. Additionally, numerous advances in technology and safety have since expanded adoption.

All IDDS requires an implanted intrathecal catheter connected either to an implanted pump or to an external pump. There are four methods of delivering IT medications. Two methods include the use of an external pump, while the other two are fully implantable devices. The implantable pumps can be programmable or non-programmable. The use of an external pump offers the benefit of being less invasive. IDDS with an external pump can be used with a percutaneous catheter (tunneled or not tunneled) and is commonly considered in patients with a limited life expectancy. For patients with a short life expectancy, totally implanted catheters with a subcutaneous injection port connected to an external pump can be considered. These may also be used to conduct a prolonged trial.

One type of IDDS use a fully implanted fixed-rate (or constant flow) device, such as Codman 3000 (Codman and Shurtleff, Inc., Raynham, MA, USA). These devices are considered for long-term delivery of analgesia. Implanted fixed-rate devices, such as the Codman 3000, are based on the use of the patient's own body temperature to warm the propellant, which exerts a constant pressure on the bellows. This results in the drug to flow out of the inner chamber through a filter and flow restrictor then slowly out of the catheter. Fixed-rate delivery systems are less expensive than variable-rate delivery systems and do not require a battery to operate, thereby limiting the need for replacement due to end of battery life. However, due to the constant flow nature of the system, it lacks the flexibility to change medication delivery or allow for a patient-controlled bolus and is now less routinely used.

Another type of IDDS consists of a fully implanted programmable IDDS, such as the Medtronic SynchroMed II infusion system (Medtronic Inc., Minneapolis, MN, USA). These programmable devices deliver either an intermittent or continuous amount of medication intrathecally. Drug dosages can be changed without intervention such as the aspiration and refilling of a different medication concentration as seen in fixed-rate delivery systems. Programmable dose changes can be useful for conditions such as opioid tolerance or dynamic changes in pain requiring frequent dose alterations. The pump can be interrogated or deactivated without emptying the drug reservoir in cases of suspected malfunction. However, because the system is battery driven, the life span of a pump is typically 4–7 years and requires surgical revision. Recent advances to fully implantable programmable IDDS provide the option to self-administer a dose. The SynchroMed II system (Fig. 81.1) includes the patient therapy manager, a handheld device that a patient can use to self-administer a dose of drug intrathecally and thereby address breakthrough pain. The software includes additional features, such as registering the visual analog pain scale before and after a bolus. These numbers are stored and can be

C. H. Kim (✉)
MetroHealth/Case Western Reserve University, Department of PM&R, Cleveland, OH, USA
e-mail: ckim3@metrohealth.org

T. R. Deer et al. (eds.), *Deer's Treatment of Pain*, https://doi.org/10.1007/978-3-030-12281-2_81

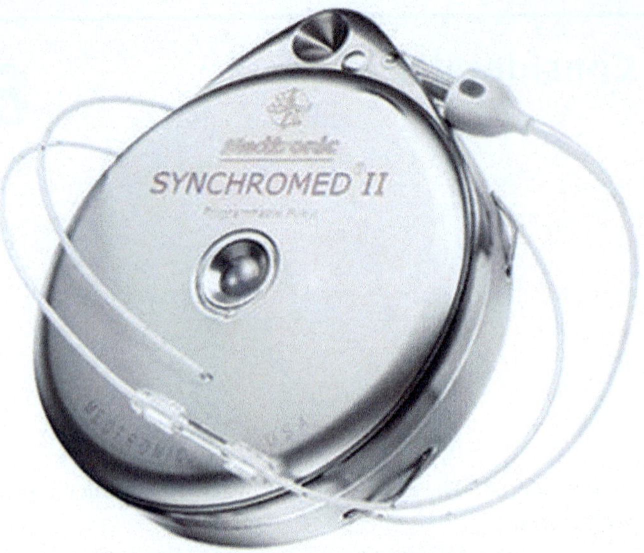

Fig. 81.1 Medtronic SynchroMed II. Implantable, programmable infusion system. (Image provided by Medtronic, Inc.)

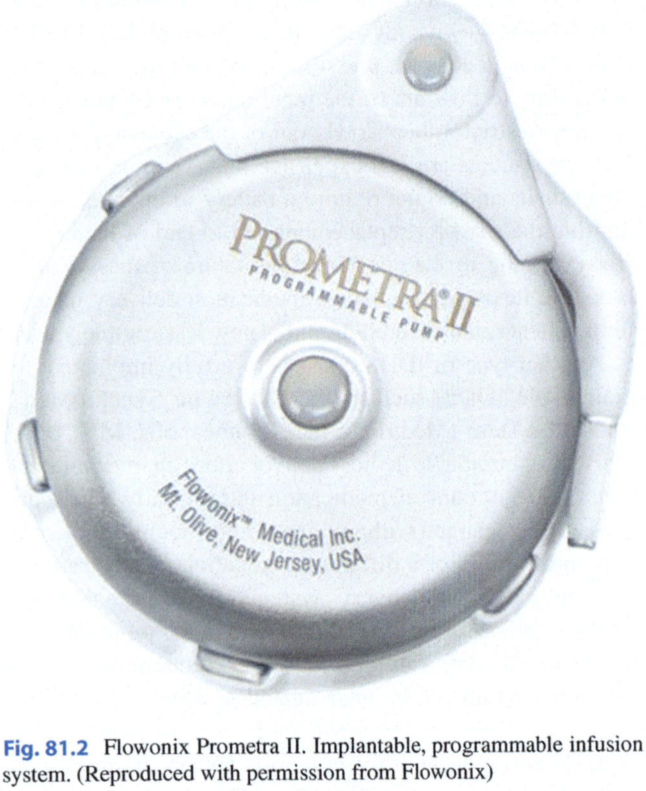

Fig. 81.2 Flowonix Prometra II. Implantable, programmable infusion system. (Reproduced with permission from Flowonix)

analyzed and used to reprogram the system for optimum dosing.

Flowonix Prometra II (Flowonix Medical Inc., Mount Olive, NJ, USA) is another fully implanted programmable IDDS. Prometra II (Fig. 81.2) pump uses a valve-gated dose regulation system rather than the typical peristaltic pump roller system found in the Medtronic SynchroMed II. The efficacy of this new system showed improved accuracy and longevity of use (at least 10 years) when compared with the Medtronic SynchroMed II. Both the SynchroMed II and Prometra pumps are magnetic resonance imaging (MRI) conditional.

Surgical Technique

The implantation of an IDDS includes needle and catheter placement, securing and anchoring the catheter, tunneling of the catheter, and pocketing for the IDDS, requiring two separate incisions. One incision is in the lower back for catheter insertion into the intrathecal space and the catheter anchoring device and another for the pump/reservoir into the abdominal region. Alternatively, the pump can be placed in the buttock region when abdominal pocket sites are unavailable (i.e., multiple ostomies). In general, several aspects must be considered when deciding where to place the pump reservoir. First, the pump should be placed away from bony landmarks such as the lower thoracic ribs or the iliac crest, to avoid irritation. The implanting physician should discuss whether or not the patient sleeps on his/her side. If so, then the pump should be placed on the contralateral side. In the majority of patients, the pump is surgically placed on either the left or right lower quadrant of the abdomen. Pre-planning and preparation is critical in the success of the IDDS implantation.

The most common position for IDDS implantation is the lateral decubitus, with flexion of the hips and spine. The patient should be positioned for the best possible placement of the needle and catheter. Fluoroscopic imaging is used and provides assessment of the bony structures and anatomy. Paramedian approach is recommended for needle placement, with entry one to two vertebral levels below the planned site or level of entry. Limiting multiple entries into the IT space will minimize loss of cerebrospinal fluid (CSF). A 30-degree entry is an ideal for needle entry, with the final needle tip positioned midline. Increased angle may be necessary, due to patients' body habitus; however greater angles (particularly over 60°) may lead to catheter failure due to excessive pressure. Once the needle is in the IT space, unobstructed flow and CSF should be visualized. The catheter can be advanced to the desired vertebral level, ideally midline, in the dorsal IT space. Upon verification of placement, a cutdown is made to the fascia and ligament. Fatty tissue can be debrided prior to placing an anchoring stitch and a purse string suture around the needle.

Catheter migration can lead to loss of efficacy, drug withdrawal, and need for surgical revision. Proper anchoring is crucial to minimizing the complication of catheter migration. Once the catheter is in place and the debridement is complete to visualize the fascia and ligament, a purse spring suture should be secured prior to needle removal. The purse string is

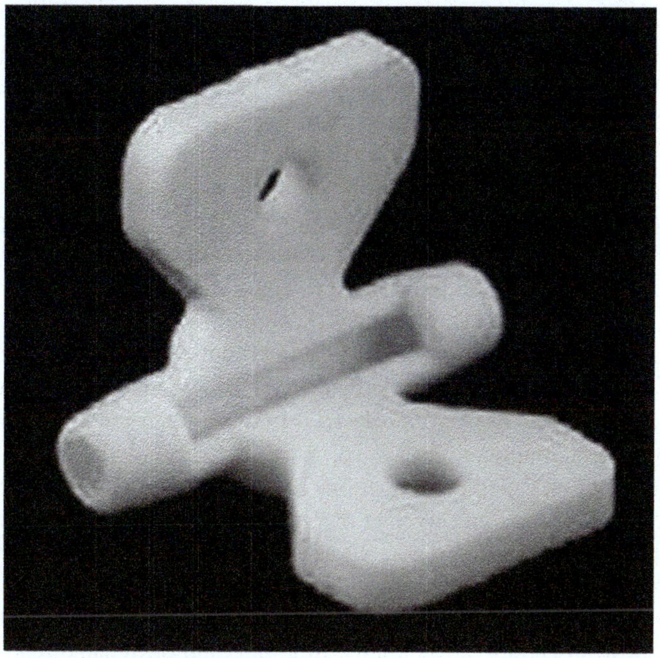

Fig. 81.3 "Butterfly" anchor

to secure the tissue around the catheter to reduce short-term risk of CSF leak around the catheter. It should be placed using a nonabsorbable suture around the catheter while the needle is still in place. This minimizes risk of catheter damage and occlusion. Some also prefer to use the purse string suture as the anchoring stitch, otherwise a suture should be placed into the fascia for the anchor. After the purse string placement, the needle and stylet for the catheter can be removed. Then the anchor can be placed on the catheter and tied to the suture. Various anchor types exist, though "butterfly" anchor (Fig. 81.3) is the most common. Once the catheter is anchored, strain relief loop should be created, and the catheter can be tunneled to the pocket location for the pump.

Once the catheter is placed and anchored, the catheter must be connected to the IT pump. As discussed earlier, the ideal location of the pump must be evaluated before the surgery. After adequate local anesthesia and sedation, the incision can be made for the pump pocket. Careful dissection and hemostasis are critical. Most commonly, the pocket is made at a depth of 1–3 cm, 110–120% of the total volume of the pump. If the pocket is too large, the pump may move or even flip, while too small of a pocket may lead to increased tissue pressure and patient discomfort or even tissue erosion. The pocket should be dissected, sized, and fit-tested with the pump. Nonabsorbable anchoring sutures are placed prior to catheter connection and final pump placement into the pocket.

After the best location of the pump is determined, the ideal path for the catheter can be assessed. Once again, the patient's anatomy and bony structures such as the iliac crest and rib margin must be considered. The tunneling path should be marked for local anesthetic placement. Once the patient is anesthetized, the tunneling device should be bent based on the contours of the patient's body and selected path. Palpation of the tunneling device during the entire process will ensure proper depth in the subcutaneous tissues, avoiding both the dermis and penetration of deep structures, such as bowel.

Proper trimming and confirmation of CSF flow need to be performed prior to connection of the catheter to the pump. A strain relief loop below the pump will minimize catheter migration and protect the catheter during closure and in the future.

Once the catheter is connected and the pump is placed and anchored to satisfaction, the pocket as well as the catheter insertion/anchoring site should be vigorously irrigated and closed with two to three layer suturing. Steri-Strips and abdominal binders can aid in reduction of postoperative pain and in seroma/hematoma formation.

Risks and Complications

Polyanalgesic Consensus Conference (PACC) guidelines have been published to improve efficacy and safety and to provide recommendations for IDD. PACC 2016 provides key safety-related aspects of IT therapy, including procedural and biologic challenges of trialing, implantation, maintenance, and explantation, and device-related complications and failures. Complications of IDD can be organized into several categories: procedural, pharmacologic, mechanical, refill-related, and patient-specific comorbidities.

Procedural or surgical complications include bleeding, infection, cerebrospinal fluid (CSF) leakage, seroma formation, neurological injury, shredded catheters, and malpositioned subcutaneous pockets.

Patients at increased risk for intra- and post-op bleeding should either undergo preoperative optimization, if possible. For patients on systemic anticoagulation therapy, the joint society guidelines on neuraxial pain procedures should be followed. Although bleeding is common, it is rarely clinically significant. However, undiagnosed and untreated epidural hematoma can be catastrophic. In any patients where an epidural hematoma is suspected, immediate imaging and surgical evaluation are warranted.

Some patients experience pain at the reservoir site due to tissue irritation or formation of a neuroma. Localized pump pocket irritation might be fever, chills, tenderness, edema, warmth, erythema, discharge, or induration along the incision or at the pump site. Laboratory studies can support clinical suspicion, including white blood cell count, erythrocyte sedimentation rate, or C-reactive protein levels. Sampling pocket fluid for culture can help distinguish infection from seroma.

Infection is rare, ranging from 2% to 5%, with most being superficial infections. Given the direct conduit to the central nervous system, any degree of infection can lead quickly to permanent neurological sequelae. Although most infections do not require removal of the device, deep infections including epidural abscess, discitis, and meningitis require immediate removal and intravenous antibiotics. While the most common agent is the *Staphylococcus* species, culture and sensitivity testing should guide antimicrobial therapy after the explanation. Fortunately, the rates of infection have decreased with improved training, strict sterile technique, preoperative antibiotics, and postoperative monitoring.

During the placement of the catheter into the IT space, persistent CSF leak can occur in as many as 20% of the patients, resulting in post-dural puncture headache. Most resolve without treatment, but severe symptoms may require an epidural blood patch or even surgical closure of the dural tear. Pericatheter CSF leaks have been described and can lead to low-pressure, post-dural puncture headaches. Persistent leaks can be treated similarly to post-dural puncture headaches of other antecedent etiologies, with a fluoroscopy-guided interlaminar epidural autologous blood patch. In the absence of the classic positional headache, the presence of clear fluid within the pocket can indicate pericatheter leaks. For recalcitrant cases, epidural injection of fibrin glue or even complete system explanation may be required.

Pharmacologic adverse effects are the most common complication associated with IDD. Serious pharmacologic complications of IDD can cause anaphylaxis, respiratory arrest, and meningitis from contaminated infusion. Specifically, IT opioids may cause centrally medicated respiratory depression, nausea, vomiting, sedation, pruritus, constipation, urinary retention, cognitive impairment, and headache. IT ziconotide may cause nausea, vomiting, dizziness, urinary retention, gait imbalance, nystagmus, and confusion. Psychosis, suicide, and rhabdomyolysis have also been seen, particularly at high doses. IT baclofen has been shown to potentially cause nausea, vomiting, dizziness, urinary retention, constipation, headaches, fatigue, hypotonia, and paresthesias. In cases of sudden discontinuation of baclofen, prompt oral supplementation, resumption of IT infusion with supportive care is required as life-threatening withdrawal can occur. IT clonidine can cause hypotension, bradycardia, and sedation. Paradoxical hypertension may be seen in sudden discontinuation. IT local anesthetics can cause autonomic dysfunction, motor impairment, sensory deficits and at higher doses, neurotoxicity, weakness, fatigue, somnolence, paresthesias, and urinary retention.

Mechanical complications can arise from the catheter to the pump. Catheter can become displaced or migrate, kink, fracture, or disconnect from the pump. The most common catheter-related malfunction is catheter migration. Catheter displacement, disconnection, and fracture can cause CSF leakage and leakage of the drug agent outside of the IT space and potentially cause a hygroma formation. Fractures are frequently seen at points of high stress, such as at the anchoring site and at the reservoir. Kinking can cause altered rate of drug delivery, typically underinfusion or even a motor stall. The pump can flip 180° within the abdomen, preventing access to the reservoir. In addition, complications from the pump device malfunction have been reported, particularly with off-label IT drug uses. The annual rate for mechanical complications requiring surgical intervention is ~10.5% with majority (6.5%) being catheter related. Recent advances in the catheter design and devices may improve mechanical-related complications.

Refill-related complications can occur during pump refill or reprogramming. Wrong medication or concentrations can be refilled, or the medication can be deposited outside the reservoir. Reprogramming with wrong rate can also occur. Systematic and standardized practices, including pre- and post-procedure verifications, time-out, and designated team members, can minimize refill-related complications.

Patient-specific complications can be varied in IDD. Hormonal fluctuations have been seen with opioid use. Levels of testosterone and other hormones have been found to decrease with IT opioid use, as sole agents or in combination. In patients with symptoms of fatigue, reduced libido, and sexual dysfunction, screening should be considered. Though titration of the opioid is an option, hormone replacement therapy may be more appropriate.

Finally, one of the most serious potential complications of IDD is an inflammatory mass. Also known as a granuloma, this inflammatory mass is a noninfectious collection of inflammatory cells located at the catheter tip. The major risk factor was high dose or concentration of opioid, especially morphine. No inflammatory masses have been reported with fentanyl or ziconotide. The etiology of this collection is unknown, but it can cause devastating consequences. Fortunately, mass formation is rare, 0.04% incidence at 1 year and 1.2% after 6 years. Mass formation has been consistently associated with opioids in the IT space, either alone or in combination. Most subjects reported decrease in efficacy, as well as new onset of pain or neurologic deficits. Signs of inflammatory masses include loss of analgesia, increasing pain, development of neurologic dysfunction (numbness, weakness, bowel or bladder incontinence), or permanent injury. In suspected patients, MRI with gadolinium contrast (CT myelogram if unable) is the gold standard. In confirmed cases without neurologic deficits, revision of the catheter inferiorly, reducing the drug concentration or dose, or switching to ziconotide or another agent can be considered as majority of granulomas regress when the offending agent is removed from the area. Neurosurgical evaluation is warranted in significant or progressive neurological deficits.

IDD with implantable, programmable, and continuous drug delivery systems can provide an effective means to treat refractory pain of malignant and nonmalignant origin. Understanding of the delivery devices, as well as the skills to effectively use the technology, is paramount for successful patient care.

Pearls and Pitfalls

- Pre-planning and preparation are critical in the success of the IDDS use and implantation.
- Limiting multiple entries into the IT space will minimize loss of cerebrospinal fluid.
- A 30-degree entry is an ideal for needle entry.
- Use purse string suture around the catheter to reduce short-term risk of CSF leak.
- In suspected patients with a catheter granuloma, MRI with contrast is the gold standard.

Recommended Reading

1. Deer T. Atlas if implantable therapies for pain management. New York: Springer Science Business Media; 2016.
2. Deer T, Hyaek S, Pope JE, Lamer TJ, Hamza M, Grider JS, Rosen S, Narouse S, Perruchoud C, Thompson S, Russo M, Grisby E, Doleys DM, Jacobs MS, Saulino M, Christo P, Kim P, Huntoon M, Krames E, Mekhail N. Polyanalgesic consensus conference guidelines for IT drug delivery: guidance for improving safety and mitigating risks. Neuromodulation. 2017;20(2):155–76.
3. Deer T, Hyaek S, Pope JE, Lamer TJ, Hamza M, Grider JS, Rosen S, Narouse S, Perruchoud C, Thompson S, Russo M, Grisby E, Doleys DM, Jacobs MS, Saulino M, Christo P, Kim P, Huntoon M, Krames E, Mekhail N. Polyanalgesic consensus conference (PACC) recommendations on intrathecal drug infusion systems best practices and guidelines. Neuromodulation. 2017;20(2):96–132.

Intrathecal Agents and Algorithms: Review of PACC 2012 and 2017 Guidelines and Beyond

82

Michael S. Leong, Lynn K. Ngai, and William A. Stuart

Intrathecal (IT) drug delivery has been increasingly utilized as an analgesic option for patients with chronic refractory pain since its origins in the 1980s. Since 2000, the Polyanalgesic Consensus Conference (PACC) has developed an IT drug selection algorithm and has continually updated consensus opinions on the safety and efficacy of IT based on best evidence, literature review, and expert opinion. Although there are newer technologies that have become available for pain control, specifically spinal cord stimulation with non-paresthesia systems (high frequency and burst), intrathecal therapy is still a reliable and durable method of delivering analgesia, especially for complex and multiple areas of pain.

Several indications for IT drug delivery have been studied, in cancer-related pain as well as noncancer-related pain, including failed back syndrome, abdominal/ pelvic pain, extremity pain, complex regional pain syndrome (CRPS), trunk pain, and pain in the setting of having intolerable side effects to systemic opioids. IT analgesia is generally thought to be a safe and efficacious treatment for both cancer and noncancer pain (see Table 82.1). IT in the past was viewed as salvage therapy, but updated evidence for neuromodulation therapy now calls for earlier consideration of IT therapy before a course of high-dose systemic opiates has been exhausted. Level I evidence exists for the utilization of intrathecal therapy with ziconotide for both cancer and noncancer-related pain, and for the utilization of opioids for cancer-related, but not noncancer-related, pain.

For noncancer-related pain, although IT opioids may have less mortality, morbidity, and diversion risks as compared to systemic opioids, IT therapy is only considered after non-pharmacological and non-opioid treatments as well as neuro-stimulation techniques have been explored (Fig. 82.1). Thus, IT therapy should be considered after neurostimulation if the noncancer-related pain is isolated and unlikely to spread. When IT therapy is considered, ziconotide should be the first drug selected in the population of noncancer pain, especially in nonpsychotic patients with >120 morphine equivalents or fast systemic dose escalation.

Table 82.1 Pain conditions likely responsive to intrathecal therapy

Global or widespread pain Cancer pain from either direct invasion or chemotherapyinduced Adequate opioid analgesia but with intolerable side effects (i.e. pruritus, opioid-induced hyperalgesia) Visceral pain syndromes or abdominal/ pelvic pain
Spine pain: Neck, thoracic, lumbosacral pain – especially in nonsurgical candidates for fusion or fixation Compression fractures Discogenic pain Spinal stenosis Spondylosis Failed multiple surgical syndrome (failed back surgery syndrome)
Neuropathic pain Complex regional pain syndromes (CRPS) types 1 and 2 Postherpetic neuralgia Post-thoracotomy syndromes

For cancer-related pain, one study demonstrated improvement in side effect profile and pain control with IT therapy compared to conservative medical management, and another showed pain improvement in one cancer population with IT ziconotide. PACC guidelines state Line 1A evidence (medications with level I evidence) for using ziconotide and morphine for localized neuropathic and nociceptive pain. Ziconotide monotherapy as well as opioid + bupivacaine has level I evidence for use in this cancer population.

It is important to keep in mind the possibility of respiratory depression with IT therapy, which depends on several factors including preexisting chronic opioid use, obstructive sleep apnea, advanced age, pulmonary disease, cardiac disease, and liver or kidney disorders.

The PACC guidelines and tables for cancer and noncancer pain are comprehensive and in some ways overwhelm-

M. S. Leong (✉)
Stanford Pain Management Center, Redwood City, CA, USA
e-mail: msleong@stanford.edu

L. K. Ngai
Stanford University, Stanford, CA, USA
e-mail: lkngai@stanford.edu

W. A. Stuart
Hartley Medical Center Pharmacy, Inc., Long Beach, CA, USA
e-mail: wstuart@hartleymedical.com

T. R. Deer et al. (eds.), *Deer's Treatment of Pain*, https://doi.org/10.1007/978-3-030-12281-2_82

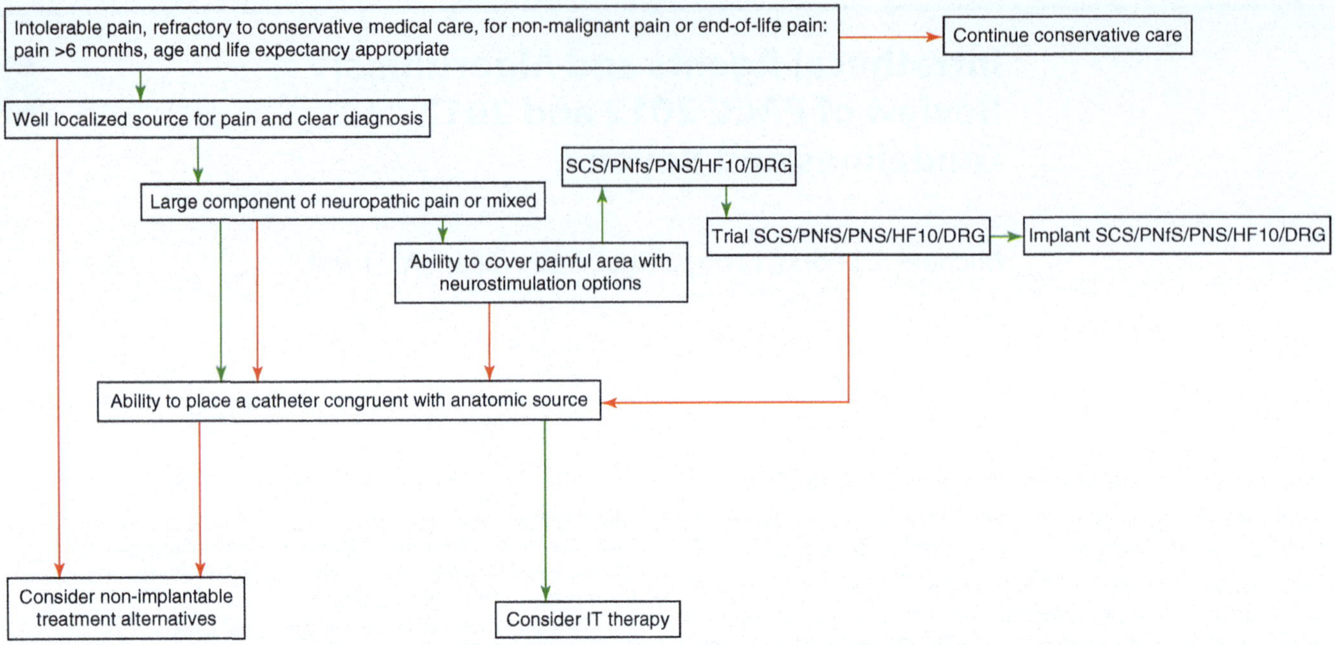

Fig. 82.1 Algorithm for placement within the pain care algorithm for noncancer or non-end-of-life pain. *DRG* dorsal root ganglion; *HF10* high-frequency stimulation; *PNfS* peripheral nerve field stimulation; *PNS* peripheral nerve stimulation; *SCS* spinal cord stimulation. Green arrows indicate affirmation or positive response; red arrows signify negative response. (Reproduced from Deer et al. The Polyanalgesic Consensus Conference (PACC): recommendations on intrathecal drug infusion systems best practices and guidelines. *Neuromodulation.* 2017;20:96–132. doi:10.1111/ner.12538. With permission from Robert M. Levy, Editor-in-Chief and Robert D. Foreman, Ph.D., Acting Editor-in-Chief. © International Neuromodulation Society)

ing. A simple way, particularly for the practitioner starting intrathecal therapy in his or her pain practice, is to assess whether the patient benefits from opioids for pain control or not. Currently, the FDA has only approved three intrathecal medications: morphine (pain), ziconotide (pain), and baclofen (spasticity). Ziconotide is the only non-opioid specifically approved for intrathecal administration for chronic intractable pain, especially in patients with neuropathic components. Ziconotide as a first-line agent may make sense to be trialed on all patients desiring intrathecal analgesia, since there is no oral compound that works with the same mechanism of action at N-type calcium channels. Opioids, which are currently being discussed in the popular press and on Capitol Hill due to the opioid crisis, are definitely effective for acute pain but may need to be modified for chronic pain, especially when used intrathecally. IT opioids may be more effective when a patient has an "opioid holiday" prior to their trial.

Over the last 10 years, there has been a growing cohort of providers studying the strategy of "microdosing." The basic premise involves tapering the oral opioid medications the patient is taking so that he or she has an opioid-free period prior to implantation; then, once the intrathecal drug delivery system is implanted, the doses of opioid medications delivered intrathecally will be started and kept as low as possible, typically in the microgram range. The purported benefits include reduction in tolerance to opioid medications and a decrease in opioid-induced hyperalgesia. There are retrospective studies that demonstrate a trend toward sustainability of low doses, with a reduction in patient-reported pain and improvement in patient functionality. There has not yet been agreement regarding a protocol for employing microdosing. The available studies describe varying strategies regarding weaning, duration of opioid-free interval, trialing (dosing, inpatient vs outpatient, epidural vs intrathecal, catheter vs single shot, definitions of trial failure vs success), anesthetic technique for implant surgery, intrathecal medication dose escalation/ changes, and use of concomitant oral and intrathecal opioids.

In a retrospective cohort of patients with chronic noncancer pain, one study found a sustained reduction in pain scores with relatively low doses of intrathecal opioids using a protocol involving a 6-week opioid-free period, followed by an inpatient intrathecal trial and implantation within 2 weeks of trial, if successful. It is also notable that none of the patients in this review was taking oral opioids at his or her 12-month follow-up. Hamza et al. demonstrate similar results in a prospective cohort of patients with chronic noncancer pain, specifically regarding pain score reduction and improved functional outcomes at 36 months. Their protocol involved a 1-week opioid-free period and an inpatient intrathecal trial that occurred halfway through the opioid taper. These studies provide the groundwork for future studies in this area.

The most common criticisms or open questions regarding the microdosing strategy surround whether or not patients actually need chronic opioid therapy following a successful tapering of their oral medications [via intrathecal or other delivery route] and trial methodology. The natural question following a successful opioid taper, and extended opioid-free period, is whether a patient benefits from opioids, or whether alternative treatment modalities would be more appropriate. Has the taper reset receptors so that opioids are not needed in the patient's pain control? Some suggest that if patients taper their oral opioids and their pain scores do not significantly change between opioid therapy and the opioid-free period, it may not be wise to reintroduce opioids, even intrathecally at low doses, as one reintroduces the risks of tolerance and opioid-induced hyperalgesia. Another concern is the number of patients who continue oral opioids in combination with intrathecal opioids. The lack of data and guidelines for practitioners presented with this common scenario can prove dangerous for patients in this situation. Although in the abovementioned studies few patients were taking oral opioids in combination with intrathecal opioids, this combination seems to be commonplace per many other providers. Future research areas should include head-to-head comparisons of intrathecal microdosing, to oral opioids, and to non-opioid therapy. Trial methodology encompasses a multitude of strategies, and ultimately yields the question of whether a trial is even necessary, as a provider cannot possibly trial every potential combination of medication and dose to the patient. As no single method has demonstrated itself superior, providers must decide whether to perform the trial as inpatients or outpatients; what the optimal timing should be; whether to use an epidural, intrathecal catheter, or as a single shot; which medication at which dose(s) should be used; and whether there will be a control medication (typically normal saline) or not. Future research areas should focus on establishing specific evidence-based guidelines for trial methodology to provide a generally accepted standard of care that providers can then adapt to individual patients.

Rational Initiation of Intrathecal Treatment

1. If the patient is on high-dose oral opioids (>120 MEDs): taper for microdosing or ziconotide trial.
2. If the patient is on moderate oral opioids (50–100 MEDs): ideally taper opioids and then opioid or ziconotide initiation.
3. If the patient cannot tolerate low oral opioids: microdosing or ziconotide.

For Patients Started on Intrathecal Therapy but with Diminishing Effectiveness

1. Consider an opioid rotation.
2. Add or substitute ziconotide.
3. Set a limit for opioid dosage and add adjuvants (bupivacaine, clonidine) depending on localized or diffuse pain.
4. Consider patient controlled intrathecal analgesia (PCITA) for continuous + bolus or bolus-only analgesia.

Ideally, monotherapy would be the easiest way to deliver intrathecal analgesia to monitor for efficacy, duration, and especially side effects. However, many patients require a combination of medications of one, two, and sometimes three or more agents to get the best effects. Physicians are dependent on compounding pharmacies to optimize their intrathecal combinations. Some principles for having compounded intrathecal therapies warrant review.

Intrathecal Agents: Pharmacology and Formulations

Overview

The infusion of intrathecal analgesics or other agents enables the optimal treatment of chronic pain and spasticity. For reference, an analgesic may be characterized as a drug which brings about the insensibility to pain without loss of consciousness. Intrathecal opioids exert their effect on specific mu, delta, and delta receptors located at the substantia gelatinosa region within the dorsal horn of the spinal cord. Numerous studies have indicated the delivery of certain pharmaceuticals intraspinally can deliver greater analgesia with fewer side effects than more conservative traditional medication therapy. This review will delve into the various aspects of intrathecal medication properties to obtain a greater understanding of their applications and benefits. Solubilities are expressed at room temperature (21π C) in water, and in some cases solubility of certain agents increases with temperature. The side effect of these agents include pruritic, nausea, vomiting, urinary retention, altered mental status, fatigue, lethargy, somnolence, and respiratory depression.

Morphine Sulfate

Morphine sulfate which was discovered in the early nineteenth century and derived from opium, *Papaver somniferum*, contains numerous alkaloids such as morphine, codeine, noscapine, and papaverine. It is often considered the gold standard of opioids for the treatment of pain due to its history of clinical applications. Morphine's analgesic effect is primarily via mu receptor agonist; however at higher doses, it can interact with kappa and delta receptors as well. Morphine is a hydrophilic substance with maximum solubility of 64 mg/ml (see Table 82.2).

Table 82.2 Opioid solubility table

Opioid	Lipid solubility	Equal analgesic conversion (mg)	Max. solubility at 21 °C	Receptors	Morphine equivalence
Morphine SO_4	1	1	64.0 mg/ml	μ,κ,δ	1
Hydromorphone HCl	1.4	0.25	250 mg/ml	μ	1:4
Fentanyl cit.	580	0.01	25.0 mg/ml	μ	1:50
Sufentanil cit.	1270	0.001	76.0 mg/ml	μ	1:500

Hydromorphone Hydrochloride (HCl)

Hydromorphone hydrogenated ketone of morphine sulfate, a semisynthetic opiate analgesic discovered in 1921. Similar to morphine, hydromorphone also produces its analgesia via the mu receptor. Hydromorphone is relatively more lipophilic compared to morphine with a solubility at 250 mg/ml. The relative potency compared to morphine ranges from 1:3 to 1:5.

Fentanyl Citrate and Sufentanil Citrate

Fentanyl was patented by Janssen Pharmaceuticals in 1963 and was developed as a unique modification of meperidine HCl. Fentanyl is a potent narcotic analgesic containing some of the highest binding affinity to isolated opiate receptors. Fentanyl is primarily used for spinal analgesia. The drug possesses a high solubility, with a maximum concentration of 25,000 mcg per milliliter. Fentanyl is extremely lipophilic and when administered intraspinally limits its spinal distribution, a factor which must be considered in the treatment of pain at the site of nociception. In published literature fentanyl is 100 times more potent than morphine sulfate for acute pain and 40–50 times more potent in chronic pain. Some clinicians have converted fentanyl, from a morphine dose using a ratio of 1:25. Conversions should be based upon literature, pharmacological properties, and extensive clinical experience. Sufentanil citrate is a congeners of fentanyl which is considered to be ten times more potent than fentanyl. It has an astonishing maximum solubility of 76,000 mcg/ml.

Non-opioid

Ziconotide

Ziconotide, or Prialt®, is the newest pain treatment drug approved by the FDA for intraspinal administration. A unique agent, the drug is a synthetic version of the conopeptide derived from a marine snail. Ziconotide is an N-type calcium channel blocker within the dorsal horn of the spinal cord. According to the literature, no cases of granuloma or meningitis have been reported.

Significant ziconotide degradation follows when combined with morphine, hydromorphone, and bupivacaine at concentrations exceeding conference recommendations or when combined with drugs within the pump for more than 4 weeks. Other studies show ziconotide to be very stable with baclofen and fentanyl. For patients treated with ziconotide, I suggest performing pump refills every 4 weeks to optimize therapy and maintain drug stability.

Bupivacaine HCl

Bupivacaine is an anesthetic which is structurally similar to lidocaine with the addition of amide group. Bupivacaine binds to the intracellular sodium channel inhibiting sodium influx, which prevents depolarization of nerve fibers. Bupivacaine is considered hydrophilic with a lipophilic amide group. It has a solubility of 40 mg/ml in water at room temperature. Side effects include paresthesias, motor blockade, numbness, and urinary retention.

Clonidine HCl

Synthesized in 1962 as a derivative of the known alpha sympathomimetic drug naphazoline, clonidine exerts to inhibit sympathetic tone on systemic blood vessels, thereby reducing mild-to-severe hypertension. Marketed under the brand name of Catapres®, it is classified as an "alpha 2 adrenergic agonist for the treatment of high blood pressure."

Clonidine was recently discovered to have analgesic properties when administered intraspinally (Polyanalgesic Consensus Conference 2012) and is currently administered for the treatment of chronic and neuropathic pain. Discontinuing treatment should be approached cautiously and a slow titration to avoid rebound hypertension. Clonidine has a solubility of 76.9 mg/ml at room temperature (20 °C). Side effects associated with clonidine are hypotension, drowsiness, and lethargy.

Ketamine HCl

Ketamine is a drug that has been around for many, many years. Classified as an "NMDA receptor antagonist," it can be administered orally, parenterally, epidurally, and intrathecally as a sedative but is used most often by clinicians as an intrathecal treatment for pain that remains unrelieved following use of traditional opioids. It has proven very effective in administration for cancer pain toward the end of life. The maximum solubility is 200 mg/ml.

Droperidol

Since its introduction to the US market in 1961, droperidol had been a popular choice for the prevention and treatment of postoperative nausea and vomiting (PONV) due to its clinical efficacy. Droperidol, a butyrophenone neuroleptic structurally similar to haloperidol, lends its antiemetic property to the antagonism of dopamine D_2-receptors in the chemoreceptor trigger zone (CTZ) of the brain.

There were case reports of torsades de pointes that prompted the FDA to issue a black box warning in 2001, despite the lack of evidence that low-dose droperidol may be responsible for cardiac dysrhythmias. One must also keep in mind that most of these case reports involved patients having been administered with much larger doses (25–600 mg IM/IV) than that recommended for PONV (0.625–1.25 mg IM/IV).

In addition to droperidol's use in PONV, there have been several studies pointing toward the use of intrathecal and epidural droperidol as an adjunct analgesic for potentiating analgesia in opioid-tolerant patients. However, it is unclear whether this potentiated analgesia is due to droperidol's sedative effect at the cerebral level rather than to the actual potentiation of opioid analgesia at the spinal level. Many clinicians utilize droperidol for treating nausea and vomiting secondary to chemotherapy or opioids. The chronic intrathecal administration of morphine and droperidol does not appear to exert any neurotoxicological effect based on a histopathological study looking at rat spinal cord. This may suggest the safety of long-term intrathecal droperidol use as an adjunct to opioid analgesics. There are limited studies with scope and depth as to the clinical intraspinal applications.

There are limited publications or studies of intraspinal ketamine and droperidol; therefore use of these agents should occur after careful consideration of risk versus benefit prior to treatment.

Stability of IT Drugs

Although not related to compounding of intrathecal agents, a clinician needs to consider the stability of pharmaceuticals infused with implantable devices. Over the last 30 years, there are small numbers of stability studies performed on single or combination intrathecal drugs. One could say drug stability of medications infused via implantable devices is based upon clinical experience which is anecdotal. Similarly the pharmacist who compounds the medications is assuming based on experience and interaction with the clinicians that there is a theoretical drug stability. On the contrary side, there is very limited information on drug instability in monotherapy or combination with intrathecal drugs. There are numerous published studies demonstrating degradation of ziconotide in combination with other IT medications. Most of the stability studies confirm what clinicians' suspect; long-term stability of each agent is sustainable.

Compounding Intrathecal Pharmaceuticals

Compounding involves a process by which a pharmacist or physician combines, mixes, or alters ingredients to create a customized medication for an individual patient. A compounded preparation consists of two or more elements whose composition is altered but remains stable in its new state. A drug compounded by a pharmacist, on order of a licensed practitioner, is not subject to FDA regulations and does not receive a national drug code (NDC). Such compounding of drugs is considered to be a part of the practice of "pharmacy/medicine." This chapter will emphasize the standards for compounding of intrathecal medications and less about the actual process.

Standards for Compounding

All sterile compounding follows general principles and guidelines. The conditions and procedures for compounding sterile medications have certain requirements to ensure that quality and accuracy are attained. The compounding of intrathecal medications requires a much higher standard than traditional sterile preparations for compounding medicines due to the nature of the subarachnoid space.

The current standards for sterile compounding have evolved significantly over the past 17 years. In 2004, the United States Pharmacopeia released Chapter 797, the most comprehensive set of enforceable guidelines for sterile compounding. This chapter was revised and published in 2008 with many changes aimed at further enhancing previous guidelines. The USP 797 standards have become integrated into pharmacy regulations across the United States.

Regulatory Considerations

The profession of pharmacies and pharmacists is regulated by each State Board of Pharmacy or similar licensing board related to health. Each state has established specific regulations governing the profession and the facilities in which the profession is practiced. From a legal perspective, the regulations governing the profession of pharmacists and pharmacies are developed by the State Boards of Pharmacy by each state. Individual state regulations have gradually developed new and stronger regulatory language affecting sterile compounding. Having stated this, the Food and Drug Administration has been aware of compounding pharmacies for over three decades, and in light of New England Compounding Center (NECC) tragedy, the FDA has applied greater attention to compounding pharmacies across the United States. According to the FDA, a pharmacy categorized as 503A can provide sterile compounded preparations pursuant to a patient-specific prescription. The 503B pharmacies must register with the FDA, be inspected, and practice under cGMP guidelines.

Compounding Pharmacy Considerations

The compounding of sterile IT preparations should be performed in a dedicated and separate control area, which minimizes airborne contamination. The square footage shall enable staff to freely move about the room without distractions or interruptions. The environment should be comfortable and well lighted. The facility should consist of at least two rooms, an anteroom, and buffer room that are separated by hard walls, doors, and pass-through windows.

The anteroom area will be utilized for storage of supplies, hand-washing, and gowning of compounding staff. The ceiling should contain an appropriate number of high efficiency particulate air (HEPA) filters and low-particulate shedding panels. The air quality of the anteroom shall be ISO 8.

The buffer room will contain similar features as the anteroom, including laminar air flow workbenches (LAFW) where the actual compounding will take place. The LAFW's air velocity shall be sufficient to remove particulates or bacteria from the direct compounding area. The buffer room shall be constructed in such a manner that prevents turbulent airflow introducing microbes or particulates into sterile compounding area. The buffer room shall have ISO 7 air quality with a temperature of 20 °C or cooler and a relative humidity 30–55%. Figure 82.2 provides a general compounding area layout.

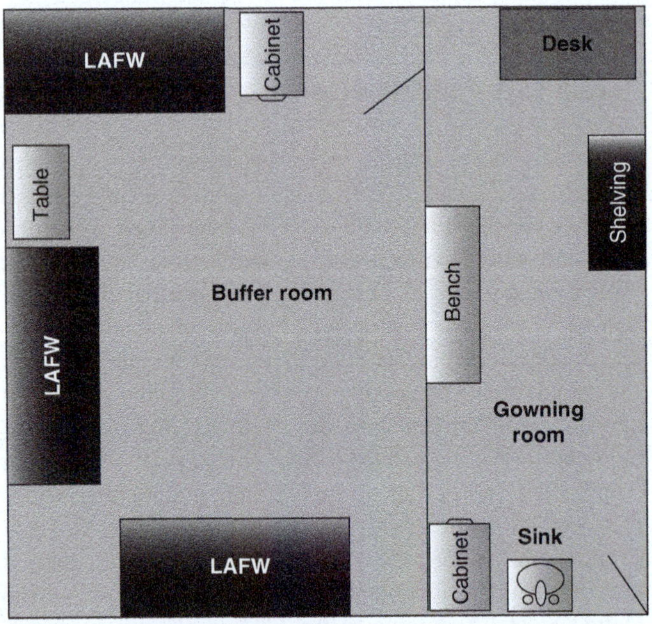

Fig. 82.2 provides a general compounding area layout

The interior of the sterile preparation area shall consist of floors, walls, ceiling panels, fixtures, counters, and storage cabinets, which surfaces must be smooth, impervious, and nonporous and will sustain continuous cleaning and disinfection treatments. The anteroom shall contain a fixed sink with hot and cold running water. The sink cannot be located in the buffer room under any circumstances. This area will require a dedicated HVAC system with advanced filtration devices to continuously remove particulates and bacteria. The buffer area must have a minimum 30 air changes per hour.

Equipment Standards

The compounding of sterile preparations shall be performed with specific equipment to provide ISO 5 or better air quality. This defined equipment is commonly referred to as the primary engineering control (PEC or LAFW). Within PEC is the direct compounding area.

The PEC is essentially a work surface that contains high efficiency particulate air (HEPA) filters to provide a superior air quality for safe sterile compounding. The HEPA filter removes both bacteria and particulates. The PEC must be located in the ISO 7, buffer room. The sterile compounding facility must employ a meticulous cleaning and disinfecting procedure for the sterile compounding area. The compounding personnel should be trained and responsible for cleaning and disinfecting the compounding facility.

Personnel Training and Gowning

USP chapter 797 provides specific guidance on the responsibility of compounding personnel. The personnel who prepare compounded preparations will receive skillful training by an expert. All staff involved with sterile compounding must have a dedicated, internal, training program which includes a didactic exam; review of current, sterile, compounding guidelines; and testing to verify aseptic technique. A significant portion of the training should also be focused on hand-washing, gowning, and the application of sterile gloves. The education of compounding staff is an important fundamental prior to the engagement of sterile compounding. Pharmacy staff involved in sterile compounding should follow a dedicated procedure for donning gowns (Fig. 82.3).

Provider Liability

Physicians share liability when working with a compounding pharmacy. In July 2013, a judge ruled that the victims and their families could sue medical providers who were

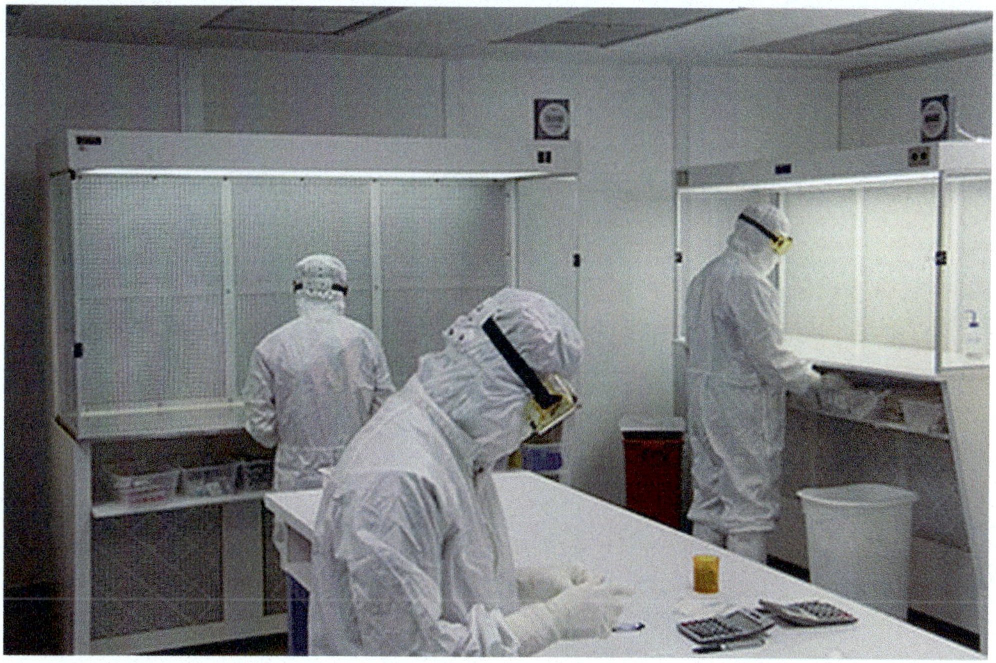

Fig. 82.3 Pharmacy staff involved in sterile compounding should follow a dedicated procedure for donning gowns

associated with the New England Compounding Center (NECC) pharmacy contamination accident. It is therefore important too that the physician ordering IT medications performs due diligence with their current or prospective compounding pharmacy.

Conclusion

Intrathecal analgesia can be highly effective in treating complex and multiple area intractable pain conditions. In light of the current opioid crisis, thoughtful initiation to minimize opioid exposure to patients dealing with chronic pain is warranted. Ziconotide as the only FDA-approved intrathecal analgesic for any chronic intractable pain is first-line therapy and might be a good starting place since there is no oral analogue. Intrathecal opioids may have improved efficacy with a prior "opioid holiday" and utilizing microdosing. Adding other intrathecal analgesics can be helpful in reducing side effects while maintaining analgesia but add complexity with compounding pharmaceuticals into one solution. Nevertheless, intrathecal analgesia is an effective method of pain control that is available when other conservative and specialized interventional pain methods, including spinal cord stimulation, have failed to relieve a patient's chronic pain.

Recommended Reading

1. Deer TR, Prager J, Levy R, et al. Polyanalgesic Consensus Conference 2012: recommendations for the management of pain by intrathecal (intraspinal) drug delivery: report of an interdisciplinary expert panel. Neuromodulation. 2012;15(5):436–66.
2. Grider JS, Harned ME, Etscheidt MA. Patient selection and outcomes using a low-dose intrathecal opioid trialing method for chronic nonmalignant pain. Pain Physician. 2011;14:343–51.
3. Pope JE, Deer TR. Intrathecal pharmacology update: novel dosing strategy for intrathecal monotherapy ziconotide on efficacy and sustainability. Neuromodulation. 2015;18:414–20.
4. Prager J, Deer T, Levy R, et al. Best practices for intrathecal drug delivery for pain. Neuromodulation. 2014;17:354–72; discussion 372.
5. Rauck RL, Wallace MS, Leong MS, et al. A randomized, double-blind, placebo controlled study of intrathecal ziconotide in adults with severe chronic pain. J Pain Symptom Manag. 2006;31: 393–406.
6. Smith TJ, Staats PS, Deer T, et al. Randomized clinical trial of an implantable drug delivery system compared with comprehensive medical management for refractory cancer pain: impact on pain, drug-related toxicity, and survival. J Clin Oncol. 2002;20: 4040–9.
7. Wallace MS, Charapata SG, Fisher R, et al. Intrathecal ziconotide in the treatment of chronic nonmalignant pain: a randomized, double-blind, placebo-controlled clinical trial. Neuromodulation. 2006;9:75–86.

Implantable Drug Delivery Systems for Cancer Pain and End of Life Care

83

Ann Cai Shah, Kenneth Ike, Lisa Stearns, and Lawrence R. Poree

Background and Historical Perspective

Each year, approximately 1.5 million people are diagnosed with cancer, with approximately 500,000 cancer deaths each year. Up to 90% of patients with advanced cancer have pain that significantly impacts their function, mood, and sleep. Since the World Health Organization (WHO) Step Ladder was established in 1984 for pain management, there has been significantly improved pain control for cancer patients, but there still remain 10–20% of patients who have pain refractory to intravenous or parenteral management. However, the WHO Step Ladder does not include any interventions; yet, intrathecal therapy has increasingly become an accepted alternative to comprehensive medical management for patients with severe cancer pain that is either refractory to conventional management or who are unable to tolerate the side effects of the medications. In fact, the 2015 National Comprehensive Cancer Network (NCCN) Practice Guidelines state, "The intrathecal route of opioid administration should be considered in patients with intolerable sedation, confusion and/or inadequate pain management with systemic opioid administration."

Systemic oral opioids are commonly associated with significant side effects, such as sedation, confusion, respiratory depression, drug dependence, opioid-induced hyperalgesia, nausea/vomiting, and constipation. Because intrathecal (IT) medications are targeted and delivered directly to the receptors around the spinal cord, significantly lower doses of intrathecal medications are required to produce equivalent or better analgesia compared with systemic medications. A seminal study by Smith et al. from 2002 showed that IT therapy had a better side effect profile and improved pain control compared with comprehensive medical management alone.

Uses and Indications

Cancer patients may particularly benefit from intrathecal therapy. They are often on high milligram morphine equivalents (MME), especially late in their disease progression, and often have poorly controlled pain, either due to inadequate analgesia or inability to tolerate side effects. By utilizing intrathecal therapy and potentially improving analgesia while decreasing side effects, patients may be able to improve their functioning and ambulation. Enhanced ambulation leads to decreased risks of vascular and pulmonary emboli and respiratory disease such as atelectasis or pneumonia, potentially leading to improved quality of life.

Polyanalgesic Consensus Conference (PACC) Guidelines

The Polyanalgesic Consensus Conference panel was initiated in 2000; since then, the guidelines have been updated several times. The aims of the PACC guidelines are to review existing research for intrathecal (IT) therapy, provide clinical management strategies, and identify best practices to limit morbidity and mortality. The PACC guidelines are discussed extensively throughout other chapters of this text; therefore, we will focus on specific cancer pain topics within the PACC guidelines.

A. C. Shah
Department of Anesthesia and Perioperative Care, Anesthesia and Pain Medicine, University of California at San Francisco, San Francisco, CA, USA
e-mail: Ann.Shah@ucsf.edu

K. Ike
Department of Anesthesia, Pain Management Clinic, Grady Hospital, Atlanta, GA, USA
e-mail: kenneth.ike@emory.edu

L. Stearns
Center for Pain and Supportive Care, Phoenix, AZ, USA
e-mail: lstearns@azcpsc.com

L. R. Poree (✉)
Department of Anesthesia and Perioperative Care, University of California at San Francisco, San Francisco, CA, USA
e-mail: Lawrence.Poree@ucsf.edu

T. R. Deer et al. (eds.), *Deer's Treatment of Pain*, https://doi.org/10.1007/978-3-030-12281-2_83

In the most recent version, the 2016 PACC guidelines identified level I evidence for treatment of active cancer-related pain with opioids or ziconotide. IT therapy may be considered if the anatomical area of pain can be covered with intrathecal therapy and can be considered prior to neurostimulation options if neurostimulation may not cover the painful areas or the cancer is expected to spread. Additionally, nociceptive/mechanical pain may be better addressed with intrathecal therapy compared with neurostimulation.

The PACC guidelines also advocate for categorization of cancer patients based on the severity of their illness. See Table 83.2. Category 1 patients should be considered palliative in nature; any barriers such as psychological evaluation or preimplantation trials should be avoided to minimize the time between evaluation and implantation. Category 2 patients should be considered for psychological screening and possible IT trial. Finally, Category 3 patients should be considered nearly equivalent to non-cancer pain patients and undergo standard psychological screening and preimplantation IT trial. The most recent data from the Surveillance, Epidemiology, and End Results (SEER) Cancer Statistics Review shows that 5-year survival rates for all cancer types have increased from approximately 49% in the 1970s to 69% in 2013. With an ever-increasing number of cancer survivors, the distinction between the three different categories (Table 83.2) becomes more important than ever, as patient selection for cancer pain potentially more mirrors that of chronic nonmalignant pain.

The PACC guidelines recommend ziconotide or morphine monotherapy as first-line therapy for cancer pain, whether localized or diffuse pain. Fentanyl alone, or bupivacaine with either morphine or fentanyl, is also first line for localized pain; for diffuse pain, hydromorphone alone, or bupivacaine with either morphine or hydromorphone, is also first line. For both diffuse and localized pain, preference is given to on-label use of monotherapy if patients are responsive for first-line therapy and are denoted as 1A. See Table 83.1 for complete PACC guidelines medication recommendations.

Cancer-Specific Considerations

While cancer patients are a heterogeneous population, there are some general considerations. Cancer patients are prone to breakthrough pain and may particularly benefit from the use of patient-controlled intrathecal analgesia (PCITA) both for the rapid onset and for the increased spread with bolus delivery as compared with basal rate infusion for the same daily dose. While there are no consensus guidelines on optimal programming for PCITA, this can be programmed to represent anywhere from 10% to 90% of the maximum daily dose. Another alternative for breakthrough pain is systemic immediate-release oral opioids; this may be beneficial for patients who have difficulty managing the PCITA or for patients who need analgesia at other locations not adequately covered by the spread of the intrathecal medications. However, the use of systemic oral opioids for breakthrough pain will subject patients to the same side effect and risk profiles such as sedation, nausea, constipation, respiratory depression, and potentially even opioid-induced hyperalgesia.

Table 83.1 PACC guidelines tiered medication recommendations. Medication options within a line are considered equivalent. Differences between localized and diffuse recommendations are highlighted in green and purple, respectively

	LOCALIZED nociceptive or neuropathic pain						DIFFUSE nociceptive or neuropathic pain					
Line 1A	Z	M					Z	M				
Line 1B	F	B + M/F					H	B+M/H				
Line 2	H	H+B	C+M/H/F	Z+ M/H/F			C+H/M	Z+M/H				
Line 3	B+C+ M/H/F	Z+B	Z+C	B+Z+ M/H/F	S		B+C+ M/H/F	Z+B	Z+C	B+Z+ M/H/F	S	
Line 4	S+Z	S+B	Ba	S+C	B+C+Z	B+C	S+Z	S+B	Ba	S+C	B+C+Z	B+C
Line 5	S+B+C						S+B+C	S+B+Z	S+C+Z			
Line 6	Opioid+B+C+adjuvants						Opioid+B+C+adjuvants					

Abbreviations: *B* bupivacaine, *Ba* baclofen, *F* fentanyl, *M* morphine, *H* hydromorphone, *C* clonidine, *S* sufentanil, *Opioid* all known intrathecal opioids, *Adjuvants* include midazolam, ketamine, octreotide

Back slashes indicate "or"; for example, M/H/F indicates morphine or hydromorphone or fentanyl

Table 83.2 Cancer patient classification

Cancer patient classification		
Category 1	Category 2	Category 3
Patient with imminent death or life expectancy relatively short, with *palliation primary objective*	Patient whose disease is stable or slowed, with *high likelihood of recurrence or progression*	Patient with cancer in partial remission or cured, with *residual chronic pain*

While it has been reported that only 11% of cancer patients undergo psychological evaluation (compared with 89% in non-cancer pain patients) prior to intrathecal pump implantation, psychological factors remain an important consideration for pain. Depression, anxiety, and other mood disturbances are known to have a profound impact on pain and vice versa. The requirement for psychological screening prior to implantation should be considered based on the cancer patient classification (see above, Table 83.2).

For patients at the end of life, consider utilizing higher concentrations of medication in order to minimize refills needed in hospice. Unfortunately, this may be limited due to decreased analgesia if this results in inadequate spread of the medication due to CSF kinetics. Not all hospices are comfortable with intrathecal therapy and may not accept patients with intrathecal pumps. Additionally, not all hospices have access to home infusion services that might help with pump refills or programming. The primary intrathecal pump manager may need to refill the pump immediately before hospice enrollment to ensure a smooth transition and/or work with the hospice physician to arrange further programming and/or pump refills.

Understanding the expected natural course of various cancer types, as well as expected side effects of chemotherapy or radiation therapy, may prove critical to intrathecal therapy. Patients often experience worsening pain with certain chemotherapeutic and/or immunotherapeutic agents or with new metastases or tumor growth. This may require more frequent adjustments with their pump programming during these time points. Brain metastases may present as altered mental status, which might be misinterpreted for an intrathecal medication side effect. Also, knowledge of the expected side effects of various different chemotherapy or immunotherapy regimens may be extremely helpful; intrathecal therapy and cancer treatments share known side effects such as nausea, sedation, fatigue, and edema. Therefore, even if common side effects of intrathecal therapy may present, it may not be a cause of the intrathecal therapy itself but possibly either a side effect of the cancer treatment or progression of the disease itself.

Additionally, while the PACC guidelines have specific maximum concentrations and dosages for intrathecal medications, the guidelines also state that these doses may be exceeded for cancer pain. While dose escalation of most intrathecal medications may result in problems such as intrathecal granulomas, given the typically shortened prognosis of cancer patients compared to non-cancer pain patients, the actual incidence of intrathecal granulomas is lower.

Cancer Pain

Cancer pain affects a large proportion of cancer patients and can have dramatic effects on their experience, quality of life, and function. There are many suspected mechanisms that lead to the development of cancer pain that involve changes in the microenvironments of involved viscera or somatic structures.

Visceral/Tumor Burden

Visceral pain is likely a consequence of pathology, organic, or functional that involves the viscera. Unfortunately, when viscera are affected, pain signals are often poorly localized and can present a challenge in terms of diagnosis and treatment. Pain signals from the viscera utilize sympathetic (thoracolumbar) and parasympathetic (sacral) pathways to relay pain signals back to the dorsal column. The convergence of visceral input at the level of the cord likely explains the poor pain localization. In addition, visceral pain is often associated with autonomic signs including changes in heart rate, blood pressure, sweating, pallor, and nausea. Oncologic processes can cause pain through a variety of mechanisms including direct invasion, obstruction with associated stretch, extension into the retroperitoneal space, and peritoneal spread. Cancers in the abdominal and pelvic cavity that produce visceral pain are amenable to treatment with intrathecal devices.

Somatic Tumor Pain

Tumor involvement of somatic structures (bones, muscles, connective tissues) is responsible for the development of somatic pain syndromes. Bone involvement in particular is the etiology of the most common cause of cancer pain. Metastasis from the lung, prostate, and breast is common. It typically produces a clinical picture of local pain at the involved site or may involve dermatomal distribution if nerve roots are involved. The pain is typically described as constant, steady, throbbing, intense, and achy and is disproportionate to the size of the metastasis. The pain, particularly when the axial skeleton is involved, is usually worsened with manipulation or stress on the spine. Because of the presence of Batson's plexus, a valveless network of veins that provide a conduit for pelvic metastases to travel superiorly to the vertebral column or even the brain, the vertebral column, and, particularly, the thoracic level is at high risk for metastasis. Also, bones of the pelvis, hip, and skull can be a target for metastasis. Either through direct extension or hematological spread, tumor metastasis interferes with bone physiology.

Derangement in bone physiology can ultimately lead to destabilization of bone structure resulting in compressive or deleterious processes that further increase nociceptive input. Epidural spread from vertebral body extension may cause neurologic compromise as tumor extends in the epidural space. Pain usually precedes neurologic compromise by weeks to months. Metastasis to bones of the hip, pelvis, or base of the skull may cause syndromes involving the bone directly or nearby structures.

Pain Due to Chemotherapy or Radiation

While chemotherapy is one of the mainstays of cancer treatment, it also has toxic effects on the body. Agents have drastic effects on all aspects of the cell cycle in an effort to disrupt the foundations of cellular replication and growth. These agents also have a dramatic effect on normal tissue types, and their destructive force can lead to the development of pain syndromes. Damage to bone, vasculature, and direct nerve injury all manifest as pain. Steroid therapy serves as a cornerstone for treatment in patients with cancer, but it also contributes to osteopenia. This weakness may lead to structural instability and eventually compression of the vertebral body which can manifest as severe pain at the level involved. Platinum agents (such as cisplatin) are directly toxic to peripheral nerves and can lead to the development of polyneuropathy. Chemotherapy-induced peripheral neuropathy is not an uncommon or inconsequential side effect of chemotherapy. A meta-analysis of 4000 chemotherapy-treated patients found that the prevalence of CIPN was 68.1% at 1 month, 60.0% at 3 months, and 30% at 6 months.

Radiation therapy has been utilized in palliative situations to help shrink tumors and improve pain. However, with patients living longer, there has been an increasing number of cases of radiation neuropathy causing pain. An example of this phenomena includes radiation brachial plexopathy. Inflammation and ischemia are two likely mechanisms leading to the damage of axons and support cells of the brachial plexus. Additionally, cranial nerves may also be involved. For example, we have direct experience with patients who developed painful neuropathy of the trigeminal nerve after repeated radiation treatments for a substantial head and neck cancer.

With improvements in cancer therapy, there are more cancer survivors with increased longevity, resulting in an increasing population of patients with chronic pain resulting from their cancer treatment.

Specific Cancer Types

When determining the need or potential efficacy for an intrathecal device, it is important to consider the expected course of the oncologic process. Certain cancer types may start locally and spread in an adjacent fashion either slowly or aggressively. Other cancer types may metastasize more widely and have diffuse involvement. Some tumors may require frequent surgical intervention but would be amenable to intrathecal therapy in the interim.

An example of a cancer that usually starts in a limited fashion and then spreads is osteosarcoma. It is the most common primary malignant bone cancer affecting children. In adults, it is rare and more likely arises secondarily to a primary insult. While local spread occurs, distal metastasis is also recognized at presentation in about 20% of patients. For example, Chai et al. published a case study of an intrathecal pump placed in a patient with high-grade upper thigh osteosarcoma who was deemed a candidate for intrathecal therapy. Despite the patient's localized disease, metastatic tumor burden was not evaluated prior to pump placement, and the patient was subsequently found to have thoracic cord compression secondary to osseous metastatic disease. This provides an example how expected localized disease can spread and have distal effects that may complicate the management and placement of intrathecal pumps. Preimplantation MRI of the spine may help identify potential complications.

Colorectal cancer is the third most common cancer in the United States and second most common in women worldwide. Surgical resection of a colonic lesion can be followed by multiple surgical interventions for either recurrence or revision of the primary surgery. This will complicate the decision of when and how to place intrathecal devices. Specific considerations will have to be made for where the pump will be placed (abdomen versus flank) and how the catheter will be tunneled.

Surgical Considerations

Infection

Cancer patients may have more infectious complications following intrathecal pump implantation because they are generally immunocompromised and may have leukopenia from the cancer itself, chemotherapy, or radiation, all of which can lead to increased infection. However, a 2013 retrospective review by Engle et al. showed no difference in infection rates between cancer and non-cancer patients. A discussion with the treating oncologist may prove critical to understanding expected time course from the cancer, chemotherapy, or radiation with regard to infection and coagulopathy risks. For example, the white blood cell count may be expected to recover between chemotherapy cycles.

Coagulopathy/Hypercoagulopathy

Cancer patients are typically prothrombotic, with increased risk of deep venous thromboses, for example. As a result, they may be on chronic anticoagulation, and PACC and the American Society of Regional Anesthesia and Pain

Medicine (ASRA) guidelines should be consulted for appropriate cessation of anticoagulants prior to implantation. Furthermore, they may be taking chemotherapeutic or immunotherapeutic agents with known coagulopathic effects. Of note, bevacizumab is known to cause coagulopathy up to 28 days, and implants should not take place within 28 days of the last dose.

Chemotherapy and Radiation Therapy

Cancer patients may also undergo radiation therapy or chemotherapy, both of which may lead to impaired wound healing. With either large doses of radiation therapy or when treatment occurs within 3 weeks of surgery, there is an increased risk of wound complications. Furthermore, wound healing is most impaired 6 months or more after radiation therapy due to dysfunctional fibroblasts; it can cause delayed/prolonged wound healing, wound necrosis, and infection. If possible, radiation therapy should be delayed at least 3 weeks after surgery to allow for adequate wound healing prior to radiation therapy.

Another important consideration is that if the field of radiation therapy directly overlies the pump, there may be resultant battery drain or electrical failure. Before implanting a pump, the possible locations of radiation therapy should be discussed with the medical and/or radiation oncologists to ensure that it will not be in the way. The location of the battery and electrical components is in the left side of the Flowonix and Prometra II and the top left of the Medtronic SynchroMed II (with the orientation of the catheter access port at the top). Refer to Figs. 83.1 and 83.2. In order to mitigate damage to the pump, it may need to be rotated to minimize the exposure of the electrical/battery components to the radiation field. If the pump is already in place and may potentially be exposed to radiation, the pump may need to be shielded with lead. Interrogation immediately after and potentially more frequent routine interrogation may be required after radiation.

Chemotherapeutic agents have been shown repeatedly to negatively impact wound healing in animal studies; however, in human studies, and especially at lower dose of chemotherapeutic agents, this has not been validated. One exception is Avastin (bevacizumab), which carries a black box warning that it should not be used for at least 28 days before or after surgery or until surgical wounds are fully healed. This is due to both its coagulopathic effects and detrimental effect on wound healing. A retrospective study by Erinjeri et al. identified 120 explants out of 1108 patients treated with bevacizumab due to wound complications and dehiscence, with the highest risk occurring when less than 14 days passed between treatment and port placement.

Additionally, particular attention to nutrition must be paid to cancer patients, since 40–80% of cancer patients may be malnourished, leading to increased risk of delayed wound healing. Optimizing nutrition by meeting calorie and macronutrient needs (carbohydrates, protein, fat) may help mitigate some of these wound healing deficiencies. Additionally, vitamin A, vitamin C, and zinc have shown benefit with wound healing in some patient studies.

Tumor Burden

The location of the tumor at the time of implant and the expected progression of the tumor are all critical to surgical planning. The catheter needs to be placed based on the primary tumor, as well as expectations of where the tumor may spread. For example, head and neck cancers may require placement at C1 and brachial plexus involvement at C4. For patients with cancers with significant liver metastases, their

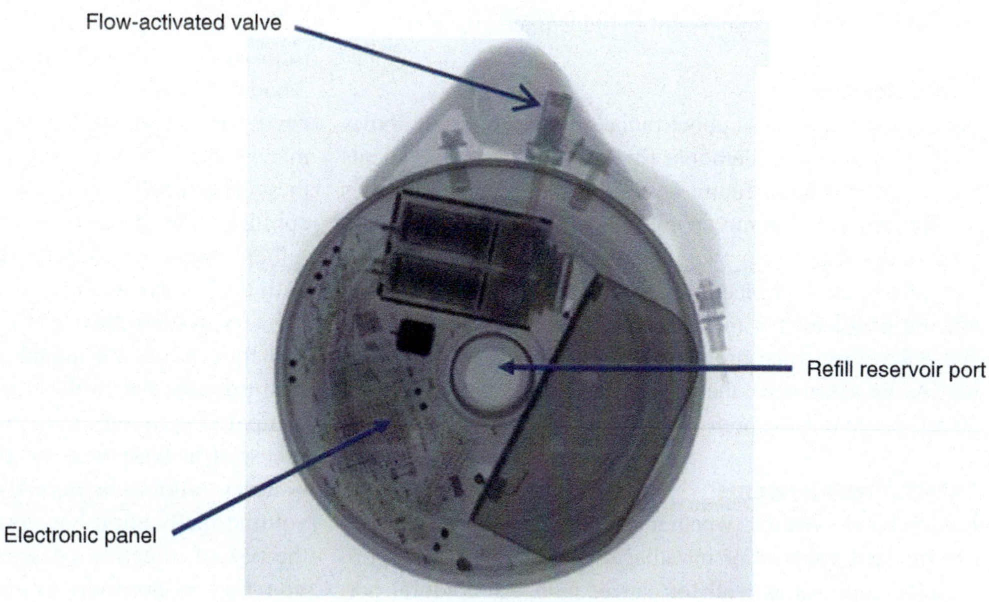

Fig. 83.1 Flowonix Prometra II pump

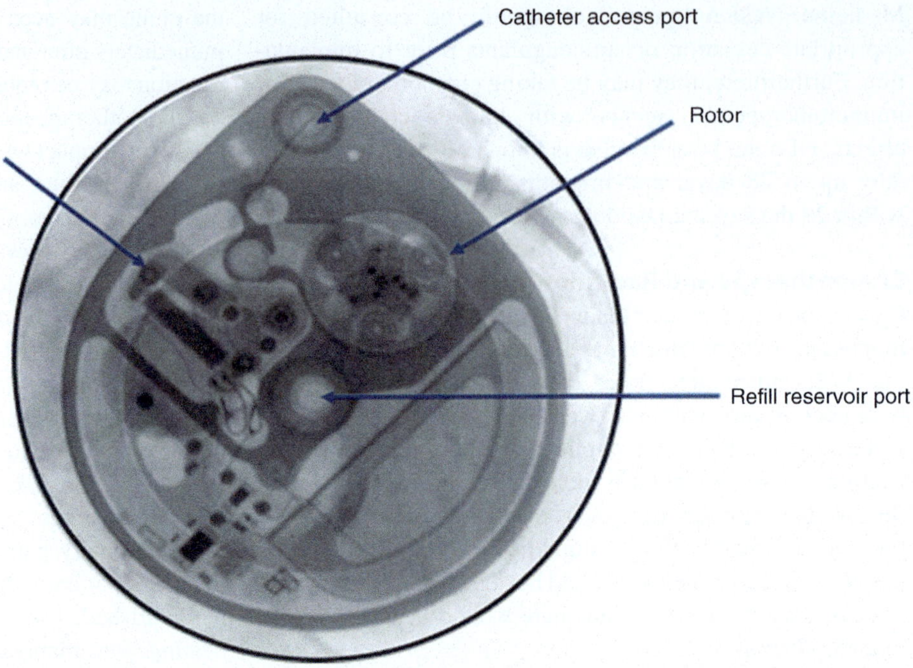

Fig. 83.2 Medtronic SynchroMed II pump

catheters may need to be placed significantly higher at C2 due to referred pain from the diaphragm. While the T8/9 dermatome is classically associated for epidural coverage of pancreatic cancer, the sympathetic innervations to the celiac plexus include the greater splanchnic nerve, which arises from T4-9; therefore, intrathecal catheters for pancreatic cancer may need to placed more cephalad at T4/5. Additionally, metastatic disease may involve the epidural space, leading to spinal stenosis. This may not only lead to technical difficulties with placing a catheter through the stenotic area but could even potentially seed the tumor further. Additionally, the tumor may infiltrate into the nerve roots as well, and intrathecal spread of medications may be limited around this area and may result in inadequate analgesia.

Pump Position

In addition to concerns about radiation therapy listed above, there are further considerations for the pump position. Patients may have existing or future ostomies, limiting potential sites for the intrathecal pump. While the buttock region is sometimes utilized to try to avoid the abdominal region, this is a particularly difficult place to refill a pump because of the significant positioning it may require to access the pump itself and may prove to be prohibitively challenging at the end of life. As an alternative, the pectoral area may be preferred. A 20 mL pump may be preferred for these alternative sites.

Externalized Systems

Externalized systems, whether through an epidural port or externalized epidural or intrathecal delivery without a port, are other options as well for cancer pain. An epidural port involves two incisions: one on the back for the epidural catheter entry site, similar to an intrathecal pump, and a second on the front, typically over a rib for the port pocket. An externalized epidural or intrathecal delivery system without a port is similar to those used for postsurgical epidurals or for intrathecal trials, with the catheter connected to an external delivery system such as an infusion pump.

There are multiple advantages as well as disadvantages to these different systems. On the one hand, externalized systems are most often considered for patients with limited prognosis of less than 3 months given the high upfront costs associated with intrathecal pump placement. On the other hand, the financial implications should not be the only concern given that intrathecal pumps may provide improved quality of life, even with limited prognosis. Another benefit of an externalized system is that there is no need for placement of the medication pump itself, and many cancer patients may be so severely debilitated that they cannot tolerate any surgical procedure. However, the epidural port placement also requires a second incision (albeit a smaller pocket is required for the port compared with the pump), and the externalized intrathecal or epidural delivery system may lead to more medication errors given that they might be mistaken for an intravenous infusion. Additionally, the epidural port is at higher risk of infection compared with intrathecal therapy because the port must be accessed at least weekly. External epidural or intrathecal systems without a port should be connected to a large volume medication bag (potentially up to 1 liter) because the risk of infection occurs with changing out the medication bag in non-port systems. Non-port systems can be inserted bedside and may not require the use of the operating room; however, fluoroscopy may help ensure that the catheter is placed at the correct level, potentially achieving improved analgesia. Non-port non-tunneled systems may be more prone to catheter migration, but if the patient's prognosis is days-weeks, this may be an appropriate option. An additional consideration is the patient's discharge plan. For patients who are leaving the hospital and going to either home or hospital hospice, coordination is critical. Some hospice programs may prefer to admit patients with an externalized system that does not require special expertise to refill a pump; others may prefer the intrathecal pump because it is more self-contained.

While typically, for non-cancer pain, adjustments are made slowly to increase analgesia due to concerns for side effects, and, in particular, respiratory compromise, in cancer patients, frequent uptitration may be required due to increasing pain, especially at the end of life.

Evidence for Efficacy

Healthcare expenditure has continued to grow year after year. According to the Centers for Medicare and Medicaid Services, in 2015 healthcare expenditure grew 5.8% to 3.2 trillion and accounted for 17.5% of the GDP. National health spending is projected to grow at an average rate of 5.6% per year from 2016 to 2025. Given the high upfront cost of intrathecal device therapy, many have raised questions about the cost and efficacy of intrathecal drug delivery systems (IDDS) compared to conservative or conventional medical therapy.

Multiple studies have demonstrated the efficacy of IDDS compared with comprehensive medical therapy (Table 83.3). Smith et al. completed a prospective, multicenter, randomized study that demonstrated IDDS improved clinical success in pain control, avoided drug toxicity, and improved survival in cancer patients. Rauck et al. completed a prospective open-label study with 119 patients and demonstrated that IDDs therapy resulted in a 50% improvement in pain and decrease in systemic opioid use and complications. Staats et al. demonstrated a 53.1% improvement in mean VASPI scores in patients with cancer or AIDS receiving intrathecal ziconotide.

Other studies have addressed the cost-effectiveness of IDDS as well (Table 83.4). Stearns et al. examined the cost of treating cancer pain with intrathecal delivery devices in 142 patients compared to 3188 patients who received conventional medical therapy and found lower medical utilization after 1 year in the intrathecal drug delivery group. The average payments for IDDS therapy were $3195 lower compared to the conventional medical management group. This study suggests that IDDS therapy may be cost-effective. Other studies have been used to quantify the real-world costs of IDDS therapy. Bolash et al. completed a study examining the real-world cost of intrathecal placement in 365 patients. With limitations, they were able to arrive at an estimate of $10.46 per day of therapy over a median of 5.4 years. Brogan et al. completed a study that demonstrated a cost-benefit for IDDS patients after 6 months compared to medical therapy for a subset of cancer patients. These findings show that we must continue to advocate for efficacious and cost-effective care and determine the role IDDS should play early in cancer pain treatment.

Pearls and Pitfalls

- Refer to the PACC guidelines for issues pertaining to medication management of intrathecal drug delivery systems.
- Determining drug dosage in the cancer population is best utilized with clinical discretion and an understanding that higher doses and/or patient-controlled intrathecal analgesia may be needed to achieve benefit.
- The natural history of various cancer types is pivotal to selecting appropriate dosing strategies.
- The expected spread patterns of specific cancer types are important for perioperative intrathecal device considerations.

Table 83.3 Comparison chart for studies evaluating cost-benefit of IDDS therapy

Author/year	Study type	N	Study comparison	Primary outcome	Results
Stearns et al./2016	Retrospective claims-data analysis	142 IDD 3188 CMM	Implantable intrathecal drug delivery (IDD) system versus conventional medical management (CMM)	Health services utilization and payments for cancer patients	IDDS patients incur lower medical utilization and payments over the first year post-implant
Bolash et al./2015	Retrospective analysis	365 patients	N/A	Cost determination IDDS therapy	Median pump longevity 5.4 years. Median system cost per day $10.46
Brogan et al./2013	A retrospective chart review	36 patients	Median daily cost of opioid medications pre-ITT to post-ITT	ITT cost-benefit	IDDS more cost effective versus patients with high-cost conventional opioid regimen at 6 months

Table 83.4 Comparison chart of multiple studies evaluating efficacy of IDD therapy

Author/year	Study type	N	Study comparison	Primary outcome	Results
Smith et al./2002	Prospective, multicenter, randomized	202 patients	Comprehensive medical management versus implantable intrathecal drug delivery	Pain control and change of toxicity	IDDS patients with better pain relief, lower drug side effects, improved survival
Rauck et al./2003	Prospective open-label study	119 patients	Patients with patient-activated intrathecal pump	Safety and efficacy of patient-activated delivery of intrathecal morphine boluses delivered by novel internalized intrathecal system	Greater than 50% reduction in pain in 83% at 1 month, 90% at 2 months, 85% at 3 months, and 91% at 4 months
Staats et al./2004	Prospective randomized trial	111 patients	Patients with intrathecal ziconotide	Mean percentage change in VASPI score from baseline to the end of the initial titration period	Mean VASPI scores improved 53.1% in the ziconotide group and 18.1% in the placebo group

- Cancer and chemotherapy affect surgical infection rates, wound healing, and predisposition for coagulopathy in the context of intrathecal device placement.
- Complications/disease progression from primary cancer disease may be mistaken for side effects/complications from intrathecal pumps.

Intrathecal drug delivery systems are cost-effective and efficacious; therefore, if intrathecal therapy is clinically indicated, earlier utilization is warranted and should not be delayed due to financial concerns.

Recommended Reading

1. Bentley JN, Viswanathan A, Rosenberg WS, Patil PG. Treatment of medically refractory cancer pain with a combination of intrathecal neuromodulation and neurosurgical ablation: case series and literature review. Pain Med. 2014;15(9):1488–95.
2. Bernards CM. Cerebrospinal fluid and spinal cord distribution of baclofen and bupivacaine during slow intrathecal infusion in pigs. Anesthesiology. 2006;105(1):169–78.
3. Bolash R, Udeh B, Saweris Y, Guirguis M, Dalton JE, Makarova N, Mekhail N. Longevity and cost of implantable intrathecal drug delivery systems for chronic pain management: a retrospective analysis of 365 patients. Neuromodulation. 2015;18(2):150–5.
4. Brogan SE, Winter NB, Abiodun A, Safarpour R. A cost utilization analysis of intrathecal therapy for refractory cancer pain: identifying factors associated with cost benefit. Pain Med. 2013;14(4):478–86.
5. Deer TR, Smith HS, Burton AW, Pope JE, Doleys DM, Levy RM, et al. Comprehensive consensus based guidelines on intrathecal drug delivery systems in the treatment of pain caused by cancer pain. Pain Physician. 2011;14(3):E283–312.
6. Deer TR, Pope JE, Hayek SM, Bux A, Buchser E, Eldabe S, et al. The Polyanalgesic Consensus Conference (PACC): recommendations on intrathecal drug infusion systems best practices and guidelines. Neuromodulation. 2017;20(2):96–132.
7. Deer TR, Pope JE, Hayek SM, Lamer TJ, Veizi IE, Erdek M, et al. The Polyanalgesic Consensus Conference (PACC): recommendations for intrathecal drug delivery: guidance for improving safety and mitigating risks: guidance for improving safety and mitigating risks. Neuromodulation. 2017;20(2):155–76.
8. Engle MP, Vinh BP, Harun N, Koyyalagunta D. Infectious complications related to intrathecal drug delivery system and spinal cord stimulator system implantations at a comprehensive cancer pain center. Pain Physician. 2013;16(3):251–7.
9. Mueller-Schwefe G, Hassenbusch SJ, Reig E. Cost effectiveness of intrathecal therapy for pain. Neuromodulation. 1999;2(2):77–87.
10. Payne WG, Naidu DK, Wheeler CK, Barkoe D, Mentis M, Salas RE, et al. Wound healing in patients with cancer. Eplasty. 2008;8:e9. Available from: https://www.ncbi.nlm.nih.gov/pmc/articles/PMC2206003/.
11. Seretny M, Currie GL, Sena ES. Incidence, prevalence, and predictors of chemotherapy- induced peripheral neuropathy: a systematic review and meta-analysis. Pain. 2014;155(12):2461–70.
12. Shaiova L. Difficult pain syndromes: bone pain, visceral pain, and neuropathic pain. Cancer J. 2006;12(5):330–40.
13. Smith TJ, Staats PS, Deer T, Sterns LJ, Boortz-Marx RL, Buchser E, Catala E, Bryce DA, Coyne PJ, Pool GE. Randomized clinical trial of an implantable drug delivery system compared with comprehensive medical management for refractory cancer pain: impact on pain, drug-related toxicity, and survival. J Clin Oncol. 2002;20(19):4040–9.
14. Stearns L, Boortz-Marx R, Du Pen S, Friehs G, Gordon M, Halyard M, et al. Intrathecal drug delivery for the management of cancer pain: a multidisciplinary consensus of best clinical practices. J Support Oncol. 2005;3(6):399–408.
15. Stearns LJ, Hinnenthal JA, Hammond K, Berryman E, Janjan NA. Health services utilization and payments in patients with cancer pain: a comparison of intrathecal drug delivery vs. conventional medical management. Neuromodulation. 2016;19(2):196–205.
16. Zheng S, He L, Yang X, Li X, Yang Z. Evaluation of intrathecal drug delivery system for intractable pain in advanced malignancies: a prospective cohort study. Medicine. 2017;96(11):e6354.

Intrathecal Drug Delivery Systems for Chronic Non-cancer Pain

84

Ankit Maheshwari and Elias Veizi

Introduction

Chronic non-cancer pain affects more than 100 million Americans. Infusion drug delivery systems (IDDS) has emerged over the last few decades as an effective therapy for severe intractable pain. This is generally reserved for a population of patients where spontaneous improvement of pain is highly unlikely and numerous other more conservative options have typically been exhausted. This patient population consistently reports a 25–50% improvement in pain as significant. This improvement may be enough to significantly affect the quality of life in this subset of patients and typically leads to very high patient satisfaction even though the actual pain improvement may be modest. The treatment has evolved over the last few decades with better mechanistic understanding and availability of multiple agents. In this chapter we will focus on important clinical considerations when treating patients with this modality with a focus on outcomes and safety. Patient selection, pharmacology of agents, and types of devices have been discussed in the previous chapters.

Background and Historical Perspective

Intrathecal analgesia for chronic pain bears its origin in the use of intrathecal medications for operative anesthesia. The discovery of opioid receptors in neural tissue in the early 1970s provided the impetus for the treatment of pain by injecting analgesic medications intrathecally. As the understanding of the physiological processes driving pain grew, it became apparent that targeting neuraxial structures could be a viable way of providing analgesia for chronic painful conditions. With advances in technology, it was possible to deliver continuous intrathecal analgesia; the first case of an implanted pump was reported in 1982. The initial trialing and implantation were largely left to clinician experience in the early days of this therapy. With rise in the popularity of this modality, patient selection guidelines, new pharmacological agents, varying device and catheter types, and new guidelines on catheter tip placement emerged. Overtime, literature regarding prognostic factors, outcomes, and complications is now available which helps guide clinical decision-making and improve outcomes.

As evidence for effectiveness became clearer, this therapy was FDA approved for the treatment of severe pain. This includes both cancer and non-cancer pain with two agents, morphine and ziconotide. However, it largely remains a common practice to utilize a combination of other drugs, specifically local anesthetics and other opioids, which may result in better analgesia as compared to morphine alone.

As the availability of interventional modalities to treat chronic pain grew over the last three decades, so did the widespread use of chronic systemic opioid therapy. Increasingly more experience showed the serious problems associated with chronic systemic opioid therapy including tolerance, hyperalgesia, dependence, and addiction. While the beginnings of IDD were in conjunction with systemic opioid therapy, it is now largely used to replace systemic opioid therapy as treatment for chronic intractable pain.

A. Maheshwari
Case Western Reserve University, Cleveland, OH, USA

University Hospitals of Cleveland, Cleveland, OH, USA
e-mail: Ankit.maheshwari@UHhospitals.org

E. Veizi (✉)
Case Western Reserve University, Cleveland, OH, USA

Louis Stokes VA Medical Center, Cleveland, OH, USA
e-mail: Elias.Veizi@VA.gov

T. R. Deer et al. (eds.), *Deer's Treatment of Pain*, https://doi.org/10.1007/978-3-030-12281-2_84

Important Factors Influencing the Success of the IT Therapy for CNCP

The Food and Drug Administration (FDA) has approved the use of intrathecal morphine and ziconotide for the treatment of chronic severe pain. Thus, no specific indications are defined for the use of this modality for chronic NCP. Based on clinical experience and review of literature, the common indications are listed in Table 84.1. Failed back surgery syndrome and vertebral compression fractures are by far the commonest indication (Fig. 84.1).

According to the 2009 Medtronic Product Performance Report released in 2010, 53% of 3786 patients were implanted with intrathecal pump for NCP. Of these 53% patients, 52% were implanted for failed back surgery syndrome.

Table 84.1 Uses and indications, NCP

Failed back surgery syndrome	Spinal cord injury-related pain
Compression fractures, osteoporosis	Multiple sclerosis
Chronic pancreatitis, other visceral pain	Postherpetic neuralgia
Chronic regional pain syndrome (CRPS)	Intractable peripheral neuropathy [HIV]
Arachnoiditis	Lumbosacral neuritis (other than surgical), plexopathy
Diabetic peripheral neuropathy	

Mechanism

Analgesia following intrathecal administration of medications is based on receptors/channels present in the dorsal horn of the spinal cord or dorsal root entry zone (bupivacaine). The action of these medications is agent specific based on the presence of specific receptors in the dorsal horn. Due to the flow dynamics of CSF, typically diffusion of medications is limited close to where the catheter tip is located. It is therefore recommended to place the catheter as close as possible to the affected dermatome/sclerotome/viscerotome. IDDS is typically a very successful therapy for nociceptive pain in contrast to mixed neuropathic and nociceptive pain and purely neuropathic pain. Neuromodulation has gained more popularity for the treatment of the latter. This mechanistic difference may exist because of the good results of spinal cord stimulation with neuropathic pain treatment of lower extremities and better evidence considering the multiple randomized clinical trials. With the evolution of neuromodulation for treatment of CNCP, the use of IDDS has decreased. There is no data on head-to-head comparison of the two modalities. However, according to the 2016 Polyanalgesic Consensus Conference, most panelists made a strong (>80% agreed) recommendation that IDDS should be considered after neurostimulation strategies to treat NCP if the pain is isolated and unlikely to spread. The consensus was moderate (40–79%) that IDDS should be considered within the same line as neurostimulation strategies for NCP. The evidence to support these statements is level III (USPSTF).

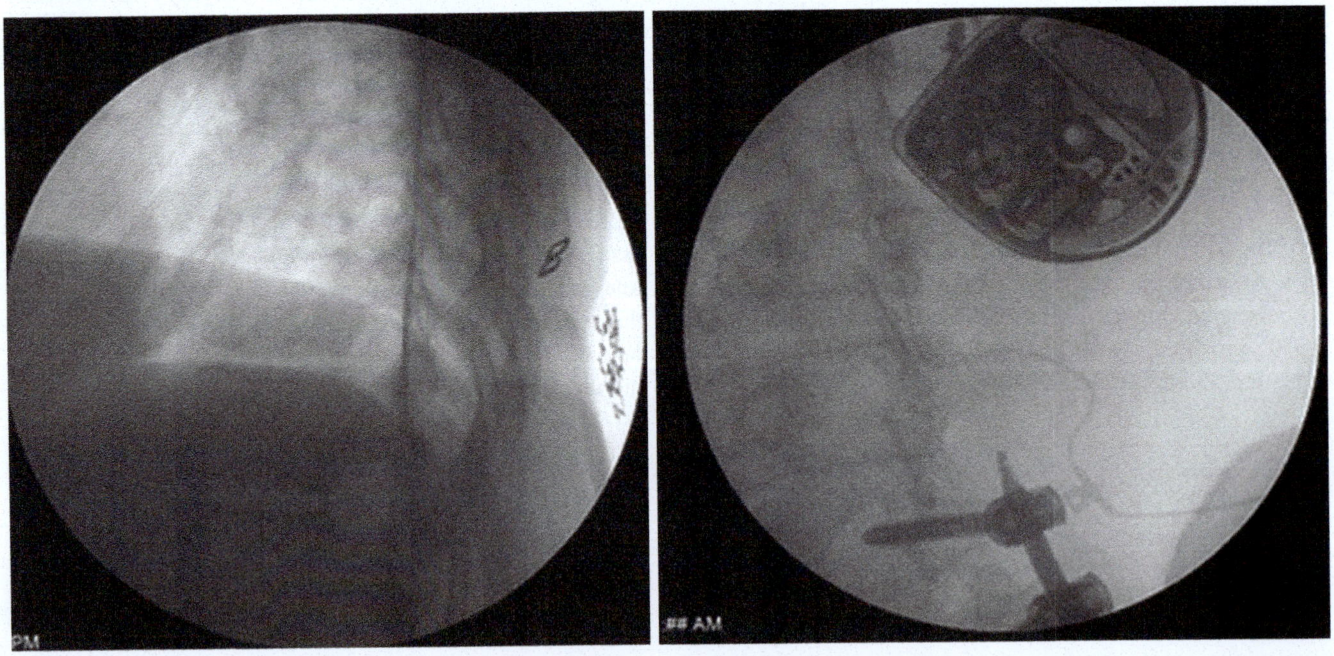

Fig. 84.1 Pumpogram. Posterior spread of the contrast injected into the intrathecal space

Patient Factors/Screening

This topic has been addressed in detail in prior chapters; however it is still important to discuss the specific relevance to NCP. In contrast to cancer pain, where patient selection may not play a big role, in NCP psychological factors are strong predictors of outcome of treatment with IDDS. Although there is no robust evidence for the routine use of screening tools such as Nelson's criteria and MMPI, there is definitely consensus about patient factors such as depression and PTSD that may predict worse treatment outcomes. The presence of psychological factors such as psychopathology, mood disorders, and somatization disorders reduces the chance of a successful treatment. Untreated addiction is an absolute contraindication for this form of therapy. Furthermore, significant emphasis has been placed on the oral opioid treatment dose prior to commencement of IT therapy. Weaning or significant decrease of the oral opioid dose could play a role on effectiveness of IT therapy or IT opioid escalation. Smoking like in other implantable device treatment is associated with higher incidence of infection as such smoking cessation is often required prior to consideration for IT implantable device placement.

Role of Trailing

Historically, trialing has been considered to be necessary as a determinant of effectiveness of intrathecal drug delivery prior to a surgical implant. Over the years, the prognostic value of trialing has come into question. The common types of intrathecal trialing are:

(a) Single bolus administration: A bolus administration of morphine is usually administered via intrathecal injection starting from small doses of 0.5 mg and progressing in consecutive injections with higher doses while assessing effectiveness or adverse effects after each dose.
(b) Continuous infusion via an intrathecal catheter. A single agent (morphine or hydromorphone) or a combination of agents (combination with bupivacaine) are infused in the intrathecal space started from a low dose and progressively increasing the flow (dose of agent/hour) to effectiveness or side effect whichever is reached first.

The utility of continuous delivery by catheter vs single-shot administration is unclear. However, one can envision that continuous intrathecal infusion allows for combination trialing (morphine or hydromorphone with bupivacaine), better placement of the intrathecal catheter, and targeting infusion and better mixing and spread of medication in CSF vs a single bolus injection.

Appropriate starting opioid dosages may vary according to the patient's baseline oral intake at the time IT therapy is initiated, and it is suggested that patients be stratified by cardiopulmonary risk factors. Conservative dosing and careful vigilance are recommended while titrating dose during the trial. The strongest recommendation for trialing is still for morphine and ziconotide. However, according to the PACC guidelines, other drugs/combinations that are commonplace include fentanyl, hydromorphone, and combinations of opioids with clonidine and bupivacaine.

Trialing as a predictor of outcome is highly questionable. There are many variables that differ between continuous IDDS and trialing even if it is done as an infusion over 1–2 days. It is well established that continuous IDDS requires several months establish dosing and concentrations that could achieve optimal effectiveness. This cannot be practically achieved during a brief trial. The volume injected via a single dose or continuous infusion is usually outside of the spectrum of volume/flow delivered by a pump. Additionally, the placebo effect of trialing has not been quantified. On the other hand, determining effective catheter location might be an advantage of trialing as the location of the catheter is an important determinant of IDDS.

Catheter Tip Location

The nature of CSF dynamics renders chronic infusion to slow, low volume, and low kinetic energy delivery of medications. Catheter placement should be congruent with the dermatomal area of pain, and placement of the catheter should be dorsal to the spinal cord. This allows for delivery of the medication closer to the dorsal elements of the spinal cord where the receptors are located. Several receptors and ion channels that are targets of intrathecal infusion therapy such as μ-opioid receptor, α2-adrenergic receptors and N-type chalcium channels are located at the central terminals of primary afferent (sensory) neurons that terminate in the dorsal horn of the spinal cord. Redistribution of CNS-active, IT-delivered drugs out of the IT space is the likely reason for respiratory effect.

Role of Bupivacaine in Admixtures of Intrathecal Infusion

A double-blind study by Mironer et al. found no added analgesia or improvement in quality of life in 24 patients with chronic non-cancer pain when bupivacaine was added to the infusion solution to deliver 4, 6, or 8 mg/day. However, Veizi et al. showed in a retrospective study that initiating bupivacaine along with an opioid (morphine or hydromorphone) from the onset of intrathecal therapy blunts opioid dose escalation. It is common practice to include admixtures of local anesthetics with opioids and other additives such as clonidine for intrathecal delivery to broaden the scope of receptor targets in the dorsal horn.

Other pharmacological agents have also been described as additives or sole ingredients of intrathecal therapy. There is insufficient and inconclusive evidence for the use of these adjuvants, namely, alpha-2 agonists, NMDA antagonists, and opioid antagonists.

The most studied and only FDA-approved alpha-2 agonist for IT use is clonidine. In a prospective, open-label study evaluating combination IT therapy for FBSS, Rainov et al. reported good results at 2-year follow-up in 73% of patients. Sixteen patients received clonidine as part of their IT therapy. Siddall et al. conducted a double-blind, placebo-controlled study assessing the efficacy of IT morphine or clonidine, alone or combined, for up to 6 days in 15 patients with central pain secondary to spinal cord injury. The authors found the combination of clonidine and morphine provided significantly better pain relief than saline (37% versus 0% reduction) or either drug alone (20% reduction for morphine, 17% for clonidine). No significant difference was noted in the incidence of side effects. However, this data is very limited to make any reasonable recommendation regarding the use of clonidine as an adjuvant in IDDS.

Intrathecal baclofen is the gold standard for spasticity and related pain. In a double-blind, placebo-controlled study by Herman conducted in patients with MS and SCI, the authors found significant reductions in dysesthetic and spasm-related pain, but no effect on evoked pain. Similarly, Taira et al. found that 9 of 14 patients with central pain secondary to stroke or SCI experienced significant reductions in spontaneous pain, allodynia, and hyperalgesia following an IT baclofen bolus. In contrast, Loubser and Akman found that while musculoskeletal pain decreased in a large majority of SCI patients 1 year after initiation of IT baclofen, only 22% experienced a significant decline in neurogenic pain. In addition to chronic pain associated with spasticity, IT baclofen has been reported to relieve neuropathic pain secondary to FBSS, amputation, and plexopathy.

The evidence for use of ketamine, a noncompetitive NMDA antagonist, as an additive to IT therapy is nearly nonexistent outside of cancer pain. GABA agonists and midazolam, a benzodiazepine, fall in the same category. Theoretically and anecdotally, these agents show promise, but data to support clinical effectiveness is lacking.

The effective dose ranges of these different agents have been discussed in earlier chapters.

Dose Escalation

Dose escalation is a phenomenon widely observed with intrathecal therapy. Few correlations with IT opioid escalation observed are young age (under 50 years old), indication for IT therapy (neuropathic pain), and prior high doses of oral opioids. Escalation of IT opioids has been seen particularly in patients with neuropathic, visceral, deafferentation, and mixed pain. According to the Polyanalgesic Consensus Committee 2016 recommendations, there is strong evidence to consider reducing or eliminating systemic opioids prior to the initiation of intrathecal therapy. Even if clinical circumstances do not allow for complete elimination of systemic opioids prior to implantation, this should be done shortly after thereafter. The rationale for doing so lies in decreasing the risk of systemic side effects specifically respiratory depression. Additionally, the other risks of systemic opioid therapy like abuse, dependence, and addiction make chronic opioid therapy undesirable in a lot of patients.

Microdosing (Low-Dose Intrathecal Therapy)

The concept of "microdosing" was introduced as a method of reversing or slowing opioid tolerance and hyperalgesia by significantly reducing or eliminating concomitant systemic opioid therapy. Although the low-dose concept is intriguing, it has not been studied in any large, multicenter, randomized, controlled prospective study. The PACC 2016 suggests replacing this term with "low-dose IT opioid therapy." The concept of low-dose IT opioid therapy describes a methodology of identifying, trialing, and maintaining subjects, who are largely opioid naïve or weaned prior to commencement of IT therapy and have chronic NCP, with the goal of using low IT opioids doses (0.5–1.4 mg of morphine as described by Hamza et al.) for treatment. Further research is needed to define the parameters and define a protocol for this treatment paradigm.

Patient-Controlled Bolus Option

Breakthrough pain in patients managed with an intrathecal delivery system historically required additional oral pain medication. IDDS now incorporates the ability to provide daily programmable additional doses. Typically each dose is 10–20% of the total daily dose and has been shown to provide relief of breakthrough pain, decrease oral opioid analgesia, and improve patient satisfaction. Continuous infusion, bolus administration, and continuous infusion + bolus administration are three types of medication delivery that have been used for improving outcomes of the IT therapy. While there are no clear benefits of one vs the other, infusion protocol future research will likely elucidate which subpopulation of patients would benefit more from one type of administration vs the other. Bolash et al. also demonstrated a cost-saving advantage to using bolus administration via patient therapy manager (PTM).

Evidence for Efficacy

The evidence supporting IT opioids in nonmalignant pain is less robust than for cancer pain. Studies have shown neuropathic pain to be less responsive than nociceptive pain to opioids. CNCP is largely neuropathic in nature as compared to cancer pain, which is generally a mix of nociceptive and neuropathic pain as mass effect is typically present.

Several studies have looked at the effectiveness of IDDS for chronic NCP. These are largely observational studies with variable end points, which limit the strength of recommendation in favor of this modality. Table 84.2 lists evidence for effectiveness from selected key studies with a sample size of at least over 50 patients.

Atli et al. demonstrated a two-point reduction in VAS pain scores along with over a threefold decrease in oral opioid consumption in their cohort of 57 patients over a 3-year follow-up period. Kumar et al. and Thimeneur et al. both reported improvements in pain, mood, and function as compared to baseline. Kumar et al. reported an average pain reduction after 6 months of 67.5% and 57.5% at follow-up range of 13–49 months. In a large, retrospective cohort study conducted in 109 patients with FBSS and metastatic cancer of the spine, Deer et al. reported that the combination of opioid and bupivacaine provided superior analgesia and greater patient satisfaction with overall lower opioid doses. Veizi et al. showed similar beneficial effects of adding a local anesthetic to opioids. One hundred twenty-six NCP patients were implanted with IDDS and initiated with an IT opioid as a single medication or an IT opioid + bupivacaine. Significant reduction in pain intensity was observed in both groups at 12-month post-implant averaging nearly two VAS points. The combination of opioids with bupivacaine from the start of IT infusion treatment resulted in a reduced progression of opioid dose escalation in comparison to patients started with opioids alone.

Table 84.2 Summary of evidence for effectiveness of IDDS for NCP

Author	N	Type of study	Outcomes	Results
Atli (2010)	43	Retrospective study	Three-year follow-up Self-reported pain levels Complications Opioid consumption	Average VAS pain reduction from 7.7 at baseline to 5.7 18% (9 patients) with >50% pain reduction and 37% (18 patients) with >30% pain reduction) Mean oral opioid dose at baseline 183.9 MEQ and 57.6 MEQ at 3 years
Hayek (2011)	135	Retrospective study	One-year post-implant Pain scores Opioid consumption stratified by age and gender	Mean NRS pain reduction from 7.21 to 5.8 Twenty-six patients (19%) reported over 50% pain reduction
Deer (2004)	136	Data from National Outcome Registry for Low back pain	NRS pain score ODI Patient satisfaction at 1-year post-implant	NRS reduction of 47% (8.2 at baseline to 4.4 at 1 year) for back pain and 31% (6.3 at baseline to 4.1 at 1 year) for leg pain ODI reduction in 65% of patients from severe disability to minimum/moderate disability range High patient satisfaction with 87% patients reporting they would undergo same treatment again
Roberts (2001)	88	Retrospective study	~Maximum of 3-year follow-up with 6-month data for at least 80% of the patients Global pain relief Physical activity levels Medication consumption Work status Patient satisfaction	Mean pain relief of 60% Seventy-four percent of patients reported increased physical activity No change in work status with 43 of the 50 working age patients not working High patient satisfaction of 88%
Rauck (2010)	110	Prospective Observational study	Six-month follow-up NRS ODI	Average NRS reduction from 7.5 at baseline to 5.5 at 6 months ODI reduction from 57.1 at baseline to 49.9 at 6 months
Veizi (2011)	126	Retrospective study with drug admixture	Up to 12-month post-implant Pain relief Oral opioid consumption	Average NRS reduction of two points from baseline. ~70% of the patients showed more than 30% pain reduction Significant reduction in oral opioid dose consumption

(continued)

Table 84.2 (continued)

Author	N	Type of study	Outcomes	Results
Hamza (2012)	58	Prospective study with low-dose intrathecal opioids	Three-year follow-up BPI	Average worst pain reduced from 8.91 to 4.02 and the average pain reduced from 7.47 to 3.41 at 36 months Improvement in physical function as determined by BPI changed from an average of 25.41 at baseline to 14.58 at 3 years. Similar sustained improvements were also seen in BPI behavior and BPI enjoyment The oral opioid doses remained extremely low during the study period
Winkelmueller (1996)	120 (Follow-up data on 82 patients)	Retrospective study	Mean follow-up period of 3.4 years Follow-up period varied throughout the cohort of patients studied	Average pain reduction at 6 months was 67.4% and at last follow-up 58.1% Ninety-two percent of the patients were satisfied with therapy, and 81% reported improvement in quality of life as determined by non-validated/standardized questioning
Thimineur MA (2004)	38 (Small N but prospectively collected data with control group)	Prospective study with control group	Three-year follow-up period SF36 BDI NRS Pain drawings McGill ODI	In pump recipients average VAS pain reduction was 8.4 at baseline to 6.1 McGill 40.4 to 33.4 All other domains showed modest improvements in the pump recipients, while practically no change was seen in the non-pump recipients with similar pathology

In a comprehensive review by the ECRI institute published in 2008, a summary of seven included studies showed consistent improvement in chronic NCP with IDDS; however the quality of evidence was weak due to the nature of included studies and sample size. The evidence for the use of IDDS for the treatment of NCP is limited however convincing for both short-term and long-term pain relief and functional improvement.

Economic Impact of IT Therapy

Kumar et al. compared cost-effectiveness of treatment with IDDS vs control in 2002 in 63 patients, 23 of whom were treated with IDDS for FBSS and followed for a 5-year period. The cost calculation showed that the initial high cost of IDDS was recovered in 28 months and the therapy was deemed more cost effective as compared to conservative management.

Recently Bolash and Mekhail et al. showed in a retrospective analysis of 365 patients that the median system cost per day was $10.46. The median cost per day of pumps explanted for end of battery life was $9.26 versus $44.59 for pumps explanted prematurely due to complications. They conclude that interventions aimed at reducing earlier explants, or revisions may significantly improve the cost-effectiveness of IDDS. Furthermore, in another retrospective analysis of 69 patients with IDDS followed for 65 months, the same group demonstrated a possible cost advantage of using IDDS with bolus dosing as compared to using modest doses of oral opioids for breakthrough pain. The break-even point for IDDS was determined to be only 9.5 months of continuous use.

Pearls and Pitfalls

- Patient selection criteria are important determinant of long-term success of the therapy. The presence of well-defined pathology rather than diffuse not well-characterized pain would be more responsive to IT therapy.
- Good surgical planning would result in reduced complication rates. Good planning should include not only imaging and screening for comorbidities but also smoking cessation, weaning, or reducing oral opioids. It is recommended that when starting intrathecal therapy, systemic opioids should be weaned and stopped if possible or at least reduced by 50% or more. IT therapy should be started with low doses, and escalation should be slow. After reaching a stable dose, per-episode dose increases should generally be limited to no more than 20% in stable patients with NCP.
- Patient education about the therapy, its uses, and combination with rehab approaches could increase the long-term success.
- Good surgical techniques include IT catheter placement in posterior intrathecal space and close to dermatome/viscerotome of presenting pain phenotype.

- The goal of fine-tuning the opioid dose is to reach the lowest efficacious dose to minimize side effects. Individual variations exist in patients' responses to opioids, no safe ceiling doses have been established, and the consequences of inappropriate dosing and rapid titration can be life-threatening.
  - The complication rates with IDDS for NCP are as high as 20%. This includes major and minor complications including death. Coffey et al. reported an IT opioid therapy mortality rate of 0.088% at 3 days after implantation, 0.39% at 1 month, and 3.89% at 1 year. The incidence of discontinuation of therapy is typically due to failure but sometimes also due to physician judgment that is about 8%.
  - IT therapy requires close monitoring even after successful initial implantation. Great care must be taken in selecting dosing regimens for IDDS. Detailed knowledge of intrathecal dose labeling and pharmacology for each drug filled in the pump is essential.
  - Long-term opioid therapy, whether systemic or intrathecal, profoundly alters neuroendocrine function, affecting two major hormonal systems: the hypothalamic-pituitary-adrenal axis and the hypothalamic-pituitary-gonadal axis. An endocrinological consultation in patients maintained on intrathecal opioid therapy is warranted.
  - Inflammatory mass or granuloma is a complication that is considered uncommon and can occur in 3% of patients; however estimates of this go as high as 50% in some studies. The diagnosis may either be too late (after paralysis) or oftentimes in asymptomatic patients. A high degree of suspicion is required since screening for granuloma formation on a routine basis is not recommended, as it is not cost effective. Typically, stopping the infusion and switching pharmacological agents lead to resolution of the inflammatory mass. Surgical treatment may be necessary to remove the mass when neurological impairment is severe.
  - There is also concern that drug mixing may increase permeability of medications into the pump rotor, resulting in corrosion and pump failure. Pump stalls/failures have been reported [Galicia et al.] with use of admixtures; however the exact etiology is not really understood.

Summary

Intrathecal therapy can be a successful option for the treatment of refractory chronic non-cancer pain of various etiologies including failed back surgery syndrome (FBSS), compression fractures, CRPS, and SCI pain. Considering the complexity of chronic pain, all patients should undergo a psychological evaluation prior to considering a trial for an implantable device. Ideally, patients would benefit from weaning from oral opioids. The benefits of total weaning versus reduction in daily dose to under 30 mg MEDD are not clear and require more research. Patients with clearly localized pain could benefit more from IT therapy with combined medication mixtures containing local anesthetic. When utilizing local anesthetic, the IT catheter tip localization becomes important in determining the success of the therapy since local anesthetics act at the dorsal root entry zone (DREZ). IDDS therapy should not be seen as a last resort but as a treatment modality in the rehabilitation continuum of a chronic pain patient.

Recommended Reading

1. Falco FJ, Patel VB, Hayek SM, Deer TR, Geffert S, Zhu J, Onyewu O, et al. Intrathecal infusion systems for long-term management of chronic non-cancer pain: an update of assessment of evidence. Pain Physician. 2013;16(2):185–216.
2. Prager J, Deer T, Levy R, Bruel B, Buchser E, Caraway D, et al. Best practices for intrathecal drug delivery for pain. Neuromodulation. 2014;17(4):354–72.
3. Ver Donck A, Vranken JH, Puylaert M, Hayek S, Mekhail N, Van Zundert J. Intrathecal drug administration in chronic pain syndromes. Pain Pract. 2014;14(5):461–76.

IDDS for Movement Disorders

85

Sadie E. Smith and Bunty J. Shah

Introduction

Oral baclofen therapy has long been used as a treatment option for spasticity resulting from a variety of disorders but has its limitations. Patients may develop intolerable side effects at high doses of oral baclofen that may preclude them from achieving clinically significant benefit from the medication. The advent of baclofen for intrathecal delivery via an implantable catheter pump system has brought with it the possibility of treatment of movement disorder-related spasticity that allows for targeted delivery of concentrated baclofen which can mitigate the variable bioavailability of oral baclofen, as well as its side effects. Continuous infusion of baclofen via an intrathecal drug delivery system has been studied in both adults and children alike. If left untreated, spasticity can lead to uncontrolled pain, persistent contractures, limb deformities, decubitus ulcers, falls, fractures, and even respiratory compromise.

This chapter will include an overview of the history of baclofen from its early use to treat spasticity via the oral route and the advent of intrathecal infusion of baclofen as a treatment modality for spasticity related to various different movement disorders. Patient selection and screening for potential permanent implantation of a programmable continuous intrathecal drug delivery system will be covered as an important means for determining the likelihood that a patient will respond to intrathecal baclofen. The potential complications and intrathecal baclofen infusion pump-specific considerations will be discussed as well as the evidence-based justification for the use of intrathecal baclofen for patients with an inadequate or subtherapeutic response to oral baclofen as a valuable therapy for patients suffering from movement disorder-related spasticity from various causes.

Background and Historical Perspective

Treatment of spasticity with oral baclofen has been used since the first clinical trials in the late 1960s and early 1970s. In 1974, a study found that the optimal therapeutic responses (i.e., significant spasticity reduction) in patients taking oral baclofen were found at variable plasma and CSF drug levels. This study also uncovered that spasticity as a consequence of spinal lesions, often had a therapeutic response at variable levels in the plasma and CSF; and decreased or no antispasmodic effects were seen in many patients with spasticity from cerebral lesions at the same plasma and CSF drug concentrations. The implications and findings in the study were very significant as this showed quantitative evidence that oral baclofen therapy for spasticity not only requires large oral doses to cross the blood-brain barrier, but the doses needed for a therapeutic response are unpredictable and variable. Oftentimes, the therapeutic dose of oral baclofen needed for spasticity reduction leads to undesirable side effects such as drowsiness, dizziness, and slurred speech. The other important take-home point from this study is that baclofen is more effective at treating spasticity of spinal origin, rather than cerebral origin.

In the early 1980s, animal studies showed reduced spinal reflexes after intrathecal baclofen administration. These previous studies led to the flagship case report in 1984 when baclofen was first injected into the lumbar subarachnoid space in two patients with mid-thoracic spinal cord injuries. Both patients in this study suffered from severe spasms and hypertonia in their lower extremities. An injection of 5–25 mcg of intrathecal baclofen given as a one-time dose was needed to reduced spasticity for 5–8 hours. Neither patient experienced adverse effects.

S. E. Smith
Department of Anesthesiology and Perioperative Medicine, Penn State Health/Penn State College of Medicine, Hershey, PA, USA
e-mail: ssmith38@pennstatehealth.psu.edu

B. J. Shah (✉)
Penn State Milton S. Hershey Medical Center, Hershey, PA, USA
e-mail: bshah@psu.edu

T. R. Deer et al. (eds.), *Deer's Treatment of Pain*, https://doi.org/10.1007/978-3-030-12281-2_85

Table 85.1 Etiology of spasticity and intrathecal baclofen treatment

Cerebral origin	Spinal origin	Acquired conditions	Neurodegenerative disease
Cerebral palsy Traumatic brain injury Stroke Multiple sclerosis Arteriovenous malformation Mass/tumor Anoxic encephalopathy Metabolic/toxic encephalopathy	Multiple sclerosis Spinal cord injury Tetanus Infectious transverse myelitis	Autoimmune conditions (Stiff-person syndrome) Reflex sympathetic dystrophy Dystonic sympathetic storm Segmental myoclonus	Hereditary spastic paraparesis Multiple system atrophy Spinal cerebellar ataxia Leukodystrophies (Krabbe disease) Pantothenate kinase-associated neurodegeneration Amyotrophic lateral sclerosis

Reproduced from Furr-Stimming E, Boyle AM, Schiess MC. Spasticity and intrathecal baclofen. *Semin Neurol* 2014; 34(1) with permission from Georg Thieme Verlag KG. © Georg Thieme Verlag KG

In 1987, Penn and Kroin published a study of long-term intrathecal baclofen administration in seven patients with severe spasticity. These patients underwent implantation of a programmable medication infusion pump connected to a lumbar subarachnoid catheter. Within days of initiation of the continuous intrathecal baclofen infusion, muscle tone was reduced in all patients. These patients were followed every 4 weeks for 2 years. Over the course of 2 years, some patients had a mild increase in spasms, and 6 out of the 7 patients required a gradual increase in the infusion dose. This study not only highlighted the success of continuous intrathecal baclofen at treating severe spasticity, but it also highlighted several complications associated with this mode of delivery; two patients in this study suffered baclofen overdoses due to a pump malfunction. These events lead to respiratory depression, unconsciousness, and hypotonia that required mechanical ventilatory support for 3 days prior to regaining strength and consciousness. Withdrawal from intrathecal baclofen was also observed in one patient who did not return for a pump refill on time. In this patient, rigidity gradually increased over a 3–4-day period.

Decades after the initiation of intrathecal baclofen treatment for spasticity by Penn and Kroin in 1984, numerous studies have been published regarding dose-response curves, patient selection, and optimal best practice techniques for intrathecal baclofen pump placement and management. Intrathecal baclofen pumps are now widely used for many patients with severe spasticity and hypertonia of various origins.

Uses and Indications

Spastic Hypertonia Pathophysiology

Spasticity is a pathological state of sustained and increased muscle tone. It is often characterized by hyperactive tendon and muscle stretch reflexes, abnormal spinal reflexes, and abnormal resistance to passive movement. It is classified as a disorder of the sensorimotor system and is also known as clasp-knife spasticity. It is the result of demyelination from a variety of disorders of both cerebral origin (i.e., cerebral palsy, traumatic brain injury, space-occupying lesions, stroke, encephalopathy, etc.) and spinal origin (i.e., spinal cord injury, multiple sclerosis, etc.). Cortical spasticity is characterized by dystonic posturing and hemiplegia, whereas spinal spasticity commonly involves antigravity muscles such as flexor upper extremity muscles and extensor lower extremity muscles. Multiple sclerosis is routinely grouped with spinal spasticity due to the location of lesions in the spinal cord, although they may also possess cortical lesions.

The progression of spasticity is variable based on the origin of the disease (hereditary vs. acquired). However, the pathogenesis of spasticity as a result of stroke or spinal cord injury has been well described and is split into an acute and chronic phase. Immediately following a lesion in the central nervous system, there is an interruption between upper motor neurons and lower motor neurons or their respective interneurons. Flaccid paralysis immediately follows along with the loss of tendon reflexes below the level of the lesion. This acute phase, also known as spinal shock, can last anywhere from a few days to a few weeks. The chronic phase is characterized by neurogenic and nonneurogenic components. The neurogenic component comprises the gradual development of exaggerated tendon reflexes, increased muscle tone, and involuntary muscle spasms that are a consequence of the absence of normal inhibitory control. The nonneurogenic component encompasses irreversible muscle fiber shortening that can lead to joint immobility and contractures. If left untreated, spasticity can lead to painful spasms, contractures, limb deformity, decubitus ulcers, falls, fractures, and even respiratory compromise (see Table 85.1).

Patient Selection

In 2016, a series of articles were published in neuromodulation from the Intrathecal Baclofen Therapy Best Practices Consensus Panel that sought to provide the best recommendations for patient selection, screening trials, chronic maintenance therapy, and troubleshooting to help optimize intrathecal baclofen therapy. The expert panel consisted of 21 multidisciplinary clinicians from physical medicine and rehabilitation, neurology, orthopedic surgery, neurosurgery, and advanced nursing practice. Prior to convening, this panel conducted a broad literature search of over 2980 related journal articles. Much of the information in the next few sections is referenced from the recommendations published by this panel.

In order to qualify for intrathecal baclofen (ITB) therapy patients must have significant impairment from spasticity of cortical or spinal origin that is unresponsive to conservative management. Conservative management includes oral antispasmodic medication, botulinum toxin injections, and physical therapy.

Traditionally, ITB therapy was limited to patients who had failed multiple conservative therapies, as well as had a delayed amount of time after initial upper motor neuron injury. More recently however, ITB therapy is considered earlier in the disease process, as there can be significant musculoskeletal consequences in delayed intervention (contractures, ankylosis, decubitus ulcers, etc.). Formally, intrathecal baclofen labeling requires a failure of oral medications prior to initiating ITB therapy; however there is no definition as to the duration of oral medication trial needed. The ITB Therapy Best Practices Expert Consensus Panel recommends that appropriately selected patients could proceed quickly to ITB therapy.

The only absolute contraindications to intrathecal baclofen therapy are allergy to baclofen (which is very rare) and active infection. Relative medical contraindications include untreated hydrocephalus, general medical instability, poorly controlled seizures, and/or severe depression that can be exacerbated by baclofen. Relative nonmedical contraindications include poor compliance with attending medical appointments, inadequate social support, and financial barriers. Prior abdominal surgery is quite common in this patient population and is not a contraindication for IT pump placement. Patients and families must be educated about the long-term commitment of intrathecal baclofen therapy which includes the cost of frequent clinic visits for dose adjustments and pump refills. Realistic expectations must be addressed with patients. For instance, intrathecal baclofen therapy is a treatment of a symptom (spasticity), but not the underlying disease. It may improve gait and some muscle function, but will not return patients to their pre-injury level of agility.

Screening Test

Once a patient has been labeled as a suitable candidate for intrathecal baclofen therapy, the next step is the screening test. This usually consists of a single lumbar intrathecal injection of baclofen and then observation of any reduction in spasticity or enhanced functionality. The screening test also allows for the physician to assess the patient/caregiver interest in proceeding with long-term intrathecal baclofen therapy.

The first step for intrathecal baclofen screening is setting reasonable and appropriate expectations for the patient. Long-term goals of intrathecal baclofen therapy will not be realized during the screening test. Also, given its brief nature, improvement in functionality is observed inconsistently. If a patient fails to demonstrate improvement in spasticity, enhanced functionality, or they have a decline in functionality, this does not preclude them from continuous intrathecal baclofen therapy. These patients will rather need careful titration of IT baclofen during an extended rehabilitation.

Since the goal of the screening test is to as accurately as possible predict patients' response to long-term ITB therapy with a single injection of IT baclofen, all oral antispasmodic drugs should be weaned prior to the screening test.

Contraindications for the baclofen screen test include confounding medical issues such as multiple sclerosis exacerbations, active urinary tract infections, and non-healing wounds. These problems may make the results of the screening test unreliable for comparison to long-term ITB treatment.

The screening test can be performed in the hospital, outpatient surgical center, or office setting as long as there are appropriate resources for patient safety and extending monitoring if needed. During the lumbar puncture, the opening pressure of the CSF should be measured. Should the opening pressure be higher than normal (even if the patient has no symptoms of hydrocephalus), the patient should have a CT or MRI of the brain to rule out ventriculomegaly. If ventriculomegaly is present, the patient should be referred to a neurosurgeon for possible ventriculoperitoneal shunt, as the hydrocephalus may increase the risk of CSF leaks after implantation of the intrathecal drug delivery system.

In most adult patients, a single bolus dose of 50mcg of intrathecal baclofen is all that is needed for the screening test. A smaller dose of 25mcg of IT baclofen may be all that is needed for very small pediatric patients to detect a change in spasticity. Vital signs should be monitored frequently during the first 2 hours postinjection and then as indicated.

Assessment of patient response to the screening test should be both objective and subjective. Objective measurements should include deep tendon reflexes, manual muscle test, and the use of well-established scales such as the Ashworth, Modified Ashworth, or the Tardieu scales (see Table 85.2). Subjective measures should include patients' self-assessment through logs of spasm frequency and intensity. Patients should be assessed by the provider preinjection, as well as at least two times in the first 4 hours postinjection. Reduction of hypertonia and spasticity for greater than 8 hours is considered a prolonged response. Some patients may exhibit hypotonia after the single IT baclofen bolus.

Table 85.2 Comparison of commonly used spasticity scales

Score	Ashworth scale (Ashworth, 1964)	Modified Ashworth scale (Bohannon & Smith, 1987)	Tardieu scale (Tardieu 1954)
	Muscle tone	Muscle tone	Muscle reaction
0	No increased tone	No increased tone	No resistance to passive ROM
1	Slight increase in tone causing a catch when the limb is moved in flexion or extension	Slight increase in tone causing a catch and release or minimal resistance at the end range of the joint in flexion or extension	Slight resistance to passive ROM
1+		Slight increase in tone, with a catch, followed by minimal resistance throughout the remainder (less than half) of the range of movement (ROM)	
2	Increased tone, with no difficulty moving the limb into flexion	Increased tone throughout most ROM Affected part is still easy to move	Catch followed by a release
3	Considerable increase in tone. Passive movement is difficult	Passive movement is difficult	Fatigable clonus (<10 s)
4	The limb is rigid in flexion or extension	Affected part is rigid in flexion or extension	Infatigable clonus (>10 s)

Reproduced from Boster AL, Bennett SE, Bilsky GS, Gudesblatt M, Koelbel SF, McManus M, Saulino M. Best practices for intrathecal baclofen therapy: screening test. *Neuromodulation* 2016 with permission from John Wiley and Sons
ROM range of motion

These patients should not be discharged until their baseline tone has returned.

If no response is detected in the patient after the single bolus dose, a higher dose (75 mcg) can be given, and then 100 mcg if no response is seen with the 75 mcg dose. Each intrathecal bolus should be at least 24 hours apart.

The most common adverse effects of the ITB screening test include nausea, vomiting, and sedation (2–8%). Other side effects that occur greater than 1% of the time include pharmacologic side effects from the baclofen. This includes hypotonia, dizziness, paresthesia, hypotension, and respiratory depression. Of course, there is always the risk of post-dural puncture headache after an intrathecal injection.

Therapy Initiation

Once a patient has had a successful screening test and has been deemed an appropriate candidate for implantation of an intrathecal drug delivery device for baclofen, surgery for implantation should be scheduled. It is recommended that the physician implanting the device should also be involved in the patient selection, as well as the evaluation of management of complications of the device. Patients who need intrathecal baclofen therapy will require frequent dose adjustments, so programmable pumps are preferred. Implantation of the intrathecal drug delivery pump will require general anesthesia. Therefore, medically complex patients should be evaluated by an anesthesiologist prior to the day of surgery.

The ideal location for the termination of the intrathecal catheter tip varies depending on the nature of the spasticity. The initial studies by Penn and Kroin described placing the catheter tip at the lumbar enlargement, around T10–T12. However, a later study by Kroin and associates found that if baclofen is infused in the lumbar region, the concentration required at that location is four times higher than the concentration of baclofen at the cervicomedullary junction. Therefore, if a patient suffers from upper and lower extremity spasticity, placement of the intrathecal catheter more cephalad in the spine will result in a greater baclofen concentration at the cervical enlargement and will likely result in improved spasticity relief in the upper extremity.

The pump should be filled and primed, and the drug delivery should be initiated at the time of surgery. Once implanted, a prime of the catheter should be performed. This allows for the medication to reach the tip of the catheter quickly and allows for therapy initiation under close medical surveillance.

There are three commercially available concentrations of intrathecal baclofen (500, 1000, and 2000mcg/ml). It is recommended to initiate therapy using the 500 mcg/ml concentration to allow for more flexibility with dosing in the lower range. The starting daily dose should be double the effective bolus dose during the screening test. Therefore, if the effective dose during the screening test was 50mcg, the starting daily dose should be 100 mcg/day of intrathecal baclofen. If the patient had a prolonged response during the screening test, the starting daily dose should be equal to the screening test dose.

Titration of intrathecal baclofen post-implant should ideally take place in the inpatient setting. This allows for rapid, daily drug titration and close monitoring, 24-hour rehabilitation nursing to address pump-related changes to bowel and bladder function, and close monitoring of postoperative complications (i.e., post-dural puncture headache, hematoma, infection, etc.). The inpatient setting is also ideal for rapid titration for patients that have barriers to clinic return and for patients with cognitive deficits, who cannot provide an accurate assessment to their response to therapy.

The daily dose increase in adults for cerebral spasticity should be 5–15% every 24 hours and 10–30% increase every 24 hours with patients with spasticity of spinal origin. Daily dose increases for pediatric patients should be 5–15% every 24 hours. Drug titration can also take place in the ambulatory setting. Dose adjustments should occur on a weekly or biweekly schedule. In some cases, the dose adjustment can occur every 24 hours depending on the patient's willingness to return to clinic every 24 hours. Regardless of the setting of titration, oral baclofen should be available as needed during the dose titration and after establishment of a stable dose for the management of ITB withdrawal.

Long-Term Maintenance

After every dose adjustment, subjective and objective assessments should be made (see screening test section for examples of these assessments). A therapeutic dose is achieved once a patient has been weaned from oral antispasmodics, and additional dose increases do not provide further benefit or lead to adverse side effects. Once the optimal dose is reached, it may be beneficial to switch to a more concentrated baclofen solution at the first pump refill in order to allow for a longer time interval between refills. Patients that frequently miss appointments should have their low-reservoir alarm volume increased (from 2 to 3 ml) and have their pump refills scheduled 1 week prior to their low-reservoir volume alarm date.

There are several different dosing options that a clinician can use for their patients. The most common dosing mode is the simple continuous mode. This delivers a consistent dose of the drug over a 24-hour period. Another commonly used dosing mode is known as "flex dosing." This programming mode allows for different doses of ITB to be delivered during the day based on the variable spasticity pattern and daily schedule of the patient. The need for the flex dosing program is most commonly seen in patients that have interrupted sleep due their spasticity. This can be seen as a dose increase before bedtime. On the other hand, a single bolus can be programmed before bedtime (or time of desired effect) while maintaining the same basal infusion over 24 hours. Boluses are usually delivered over 5 minutes. While most patients may benefit from the simple continuous mode, or the flex dosing mode, some patients may have limited response to ITB therapy despite dose escalation. In cases where the total daily dose has reached four to six times the screening test dose, and the patient has yet to have a similar clinical effect to that of the screening dose, they may benefit from periodic bolus dosing. The idea is that periodic bolus dose allows for better intrathecal spread. In these patients, the basal rate is reduced, and the total daily dose is maintained with the periodic boluses. The initial boluses should be 25–50% of the screening test dose. As mentioned above, subjective and objective assessments of the patient's spasticity should be made throughout the maintenance therapy to ensure optimal dosing.

Common Complications with IDDS for Baclofen

The majority of complications with the IDDS for baclofen occur in the first year of implantation. Surgical complications with the implantation of the intrathecal baclofen pump include catheter-related complications, CSF leakage, and infection. An external CSF leak through the incision is a surgical emergency. If the leak is within a few hours to a few days of surgery, then the wound can be oversewn, and an occlusive tissue adhesive should be applied to the wound. A leak that appears after that time should be considered a possible infection. If there is concern for a pump or catheter infection (as opposed to a superficial wound infection), cultures of the intrathecal cerebrospinal fluid (CSF) and peri-pump fluid should be examined. If both fluid samples are infected, the entire system should be explanted, and the patient should receive a 2-week course of intravenous (IV) antibiotics. If only the peri-pump fluid is infected, the patient should receive a 3-day course of IV antibiotics, and then the peri-pump fluid should be re-cultured. If the second culture is positive as well, then the hardware should be removed.

Non-infected, subcutaneous CSF accumulations are usually treated with bed rest and pressure dressings. The fluid should be aspirated and tested for β_2-transferrin (to see if fluid is actually CSF). If the leak persists, then a flat AP plate of the abdomen and lumbar and thoracic spine series should be conducted to visualize all tubing, connectors, and entrance of the catheter into the spinal canal. If there is no disconnection detected, then contrast dye should be injected via the side port of the pump under fluoroscopy to localize the source of the leak.

The most common complications related to IDDS for baclofen are intrathecal catheter-related complications. The incidence of catheter-related complications requiring surgical intervention has been quoted anywhere from 10% to 89% in the literature. Catheter complications include kinking, dislodgment, disconnections, breaks, tears, and occlusions of the catheter. An international, multicenter prospective study measuring safety and performance of the catheter system over the course of 9 months revealed that most catheter complications are related to the implantation technique, rather than the catheter itself. This study showed that catheter migration was the most common surgical complication (aside from infection) and that this was primarily due to failure to anchor the catheter to the underlying fascia during implantation.

Another less common complication is intrathecal baclofen overdose due to incorrect pump programming, or pump malfunction. Overdose occurs most commonly in the periodic bolus dosing mode. Patients that have an overdose on the periodic bolus mode should be switched to a simple continuous mode, as they are unlikely to have a baclofen overdose on this drug delivery mode.

If a system malfunction is ever considered, the pump should be interrogated. Interrogation can reveal any rotor stalls in a patient that may have had a temporary withdrawal from baclofen. For example, high magnetic fields (such as magnetic resonance imaging (MRI) scanners) can result in a temporary cessation of drug delivery in the Medtronic intrathecal delivery system; likewise, there may be cases of rotor stalls in the absence of exposure to MRI. During evaluation of a possible system malfunction, the reservoir volume should also be measured. This can reveal the presence of a rotor stall or kink in the catheter if the volume is too high; alternatively, this can reveal over-infusion if the volume is lower than expected. Another method to detect system under function is to deliver both a lumbar intrathecal bolus and a programed bolus through the pump, at different times. If a patient responds positively to the lumbar bolus, compared to the pump bolus, this may indicate microtears in the catheter in the absence of radiographic findings. An urgent pump replacement should be performed if unexplained rotor stalls, permanent rotor stalls, over-infusion, or low battery condition are detected.

If at any time ITB therapy is discontinued (i.e., due to removal of pump and catheter), large oral doses of baclofen should be given prophylactically *in the inpatient setting* (e.g., 20 mg every 4–6 hours) in order to prevent a life-threatening baclofen withdrawal. Oral baclofen may be insufficient if the dose of ITB therapy was high prior to the pump removal (such as >900 μcg/day). In these cases, a lumbar spinal catheter can be placed. This intrathecal catheter can be connected to an external microinfusion pump (although this is not FDA approved for this function) to deliver tapering doses of ITB until the oral baclofen is sufficient alone.

Evidence of Efficacy

Baclofen is a $GABA_B$ receptor agonist that signals an inhibitory cascade that leads to a decrease in excitatory neurotransmitter release through hyperpolarization of the neurons primarily in the superficial layers of the dorsal gray matter. This results in presynaptic inhibition at the spinal cord level. Although oral baclofen is rapidly absorbed by the gastrointestinal tract, it has limited ability to cross the blood-brain barrier due to its primarily hydrophilic nature. Animal and human studies have shown that baclofen, when given parenterally, will be distributed evenly between brain and spinal cord tissues. This has important implications because baclofen is a centrally acting drug; in other words, the depressive effects of baclofen are more profound with increased doses by oral administration. Other common side effects that can affect 10–20% of patients include dizziness, somnolence, and confusion. Less common but undoubtedly serious side effects include hallucinations, hypotonia, ataxia, and respiratory depression.

The hydrophilic nature of baclofen and its limited ability to cross the blood-brain barrier make it an ideal drug for intrathecal administration. This allows for localized administration of the drug close to the target site (the dorsal gray matter of the spinal cord); this makes it more efficacious and also significantly limits the systemic side effects that are often seen with large oral doses of baclofen. Intrathecal baclofen has a half-life of approximately 4 hours and is cleared at the same rate as CSF through bulk flow (approximately 30 ml/hr).

Baclofen Overdose

Excessive salivation, dizziness, nausea and vomiting, hypotonia, confusion, and somnolence are some early signs of baclofen overdose. Baclofen overdose can ultimately lead to respiratory depression, seizures, and coma. Treatment includes supportive care in the intensive care unit, including intubation and mechanical ventilation in some patients. Patients at risk for seizure development should be considered for anti-seizure prophylaxis. In addition to supportive care, ITB overdose should be treated by CSF drainage through both aspiration of the side port of the baclofen pump and sequential lumbar punctures and/or a lumbar drain. Rebound withdrawal should be monitored closely once the infusion is stopped.

Baclofen Withdrawal

Sudden cessation of ITB therapy can lead to withdrawal symptoms within a few to 48 hours. Baclofen withdrawal symptoms range from mild to severe; the severity of the symptoms are not consistently related to the dose of ITB prior to the withdrawal. One most common sign noted after baclofen cessation is the return of the patient's baseline hypertonia. Other signs include pruritus, seizures, hallucinations, and autonomic dysreflexia. Life-threatening signs of baclofen withdrawal are characterized by exaggerated/rebound spasticity, fever, hemodynamic instability, and altered mental status. These life-threatening signs are not unique to baclofen withdrawal; they also characterize other medical emergencies such as serotonin syndrome, neuroleptic malignant syndrome, and malignant hyperthermia. Therefore, undertreatment from ITB should not be immediately attributed to the above symptoms. The definitive treatment of baclofen withdrawal is the restoration of ITB therapy, beginning with bolus administration. If the patient has had a short withdrawal, then it would be reasonable to restore their previous ITB delivery dose. However, if withdrawal took place over days to weeks, then the ITB dose should be restarted at a reduced dose (30–50% of the previous dose). If the patient is unable to receive intrathecal administration, then oral baclofen should be used as a temporizing measure. Benzodiazepines may also work as adjuvant therapy for baclofen withdrawal as they help minimize symptoms of spasticity, rigidity, and hyperthermia. Cyproheptadine (a serotonin agonist) can also be used to help improve symptoms of spasticity, fever, hyperthermia, and pruritus.

Pearls and Pitfalls

- If left untreated, spasticity can lead to painful spasms, contractures, limb deformity, decubitus ulcers, falls, fractures, and even respiratory compromise.
- The ITB Therapy Best Practices Expert Consensus Panel recommends that appropriately selected patients could proceed quickly to ITB therapy.
- Relative medical contraindications include untreated hydrocephalus, general medical instability, poorly controlled seizures, and/or severe depression that can be exacerbated by baclofen.
- The goal of the screening test is to as accurately as possible predict patients' response to long-term ITB therapy with a single injection of IT baclofen.
- Titration of intrathecal baclofen post-implant should ideally take place in the inpatient setting.
- A therapeutic dose is achieved once a patient has been weaned from oral antispasmodics, and additional dose increase do not provide further benefit or lead to adverse side effects.
- The majority of complications with the IDDS for baclofen occur in the first year of implantation. The most common complications related to IDDS for baclofen are intrathecal catheter-related complications.
- If at any time ITB therapy is discontinued, large oral doses of baclofen should be given prophylactically, in order to prevent a life-threatening baclofen withdrawal. Life-threatening signs of baclofen withdrawal are characterized by exaggerated/rebound spasticity, fever, hemodynamic instability, and altered mental status.
- Excessive salivation, dizziness, nausea and vomiting, hypotonia, confusion, and somnolence are some early signs of baclofen overdose. Baclofen overdose can ultimately lead to respiratory depression, seizures, and coma.

Recommended Reading

1. Adams MM, Hicks AL. Spasticity after spinal cord injury. Spinal Cord. 2005;43:577–86.
2. Albright AL, Turner M, Pattisapu JV. Best- practice surgical techniques for intrathecal baclofen therapy. J Neurosurg Pediatr. 2006;104:233–9.
3. Booster AL, Bennet SE, Bilsky GS, Gudesblatt M, Koebel SF, McManus M, Saulino M. Best practices for Intrathecal Baclofen therapy: screening test. Neuromodulation. 2016;91:616–22.
4. Boster AL, Adair RL, Gooch JL, Nelson MES, Toomer A, Urquidez J, Saulino M. Best practices for Intrathecal Baclofen therapy: dosing and long-term management. Neuromodulation. 2016;19:623–31.
5. Follett KA, Naumann CP. A prospective study of catheter-related complications of Intrathecal Drug delivery systems. J Pain Symptom Manag. 2000;19:209–15.
6. Furr-Stimming E, Boyle A, Schiess M. Spasticity and Intrathecal Baclofen. Semin Neurol. 2014;34:591–6.
7. Hill DR, Bowery NG. H-baclofen and H-GABA bind to bicuculline-insensitive $GABA_B$ sites in rat brain. Nature. 1981;290:149–52.
8. Knutsson E, Lindoblom U, Martensson A. Plasma and cerebrospinal fluid levels of Baclofen (Lioresal) at optimal therapeutic responses in spastic paresis. J Neurol Sci. 1974;23:473–84.
9. Lewis KS, Mueller WM. Intrathecal Baclofen for severe spasticity secondary to spinal cord injury. Ann Pharmacother. 1993;27:767–73.
10. Penn RD, Kroin JS. Intrathecal Baclofen Alleviates spinal cord spasticity. Lancet. 1984;1(8385):1078.
11. Penn RD, Kroin JS. Long-term intrathecal baclofen infusion for treatment of spasticity. J Neurosurg. 1987;66:181–5.
12. Ridley B, Rawlins PK. Intrathecal Baclofen therapy: ten steps toward best practice. J Neurosci Nurs. 2006;38:72–82.
13. Saulino M, Anderson DJ, Doble J, Farid R, Gul F, Konrad P, Boster A. Best practices for Intrathecal Baclofen therapy: troubleshooting. Neuromodulation. 2016;19:632–41.
14. Saval A, Chiodo A. Intrathecal Baclofen for spasticity management: a comparative analysis of spasticity of spinal vs. cortical origin. J Spinal Cord Med. 2010;33:16–21.
15. Sheean G, McGuire JR. Spastic hypertonia and movement disorders: pathophysiology, clinical presentation, and quantification. PM R. 2009;1:827–33.

Ziconotide for Intrathecal Use

86

Corey W. Hunter and Dipan Patel

Introduction

Simply put, IDDS refers to the infusion of one or more drugs into the intrathecal space. IDDSs are frequently utilized for chronic, refractory pain depending on practitioner awareness of therapy and comfort of implementation. This particular therapy tends to be favored by pain physicians due to the long-term durability, reduction in overall healthcare cost, and consistent/sustained delivery of medication leading to improved pain relief. IDDS is an excellent option for patients with refractory pain syndromes like cancer and axial back pain as well as those intolerant to systemic opioid pharmacotherapy. Important determining factors for a potential medication regimen are tailored to the individual patient care plan.

While IDDS provides a therapeutic answer to a great many pain syndromes that would otherwise be left untreated, the use of intrathecal opioids carries several risks such as granuloma, respiratory depression, cognitive impairment, and even death. Ziconotide, the only non-opioid analgesic approved for intrathecal use in the United States, is an excellent alternative to opioids with IDDS with a safer profile. The purpose of this chapter will be to elucidate the current role of ziconotide for intrathecal use in the management of refractory chronic pain.

C. W. Hunter (✉)
Department of Rehabilitation Medicine, Icahn School of Medicine at Mount Sinai, New York, NY, USA

Ainsworth Institute of Pain Management, New York, NY, USA
e-mail: chunter@ainpain.com

D. Patel
Garden State Pain Control Center, Clifton, NJ, USA

Residents & Fellows Society, North American Neuromodulation Society (NANS), Jersey City, NJ, USA

Background and Historical Perspective

Intrathecal drug delivery (IDD) is well established in the literature as an effective treatment for chronic refractory pain. The IT space, also known as the subarachnoid space, refers to the area between the arachnoid mater and pia mater in which cerebrospinal fluid (CSF) circulates (refer to Chaps. 85, 86, 87, 88 and 89). IDD involves the direct delivery of medications directly into the IT, thus bypassing the digestive and circulatory system through the use of a catheter, to allow the drug(s) direct access within the central nervous system. And because these medications avoid the blood-brain barrier, smaller doses are required as compared with traditional routes (e.g., oral, IV, transdermal, and sublingual) as well as a more rapid and steady pharmacologic response.

The spinal cord is a key site for pain processing, and the dorsal horn of the spinal cord within the intrathecal space plays a crucial role as a target for IDD. There are several key receptors for pain regulation located within the spinal cord such as opioid (μ, κ, and δ), γ-aminobutyric acid, α-2, dopaminergic, N-methyl-D-aspartate (NMDA), and voltage-gated calcium channels.

Current intrathecal pharmacologic regimens are empirically derived on the basis of recommendations from literature reviews and the recently published by the Polyanalgesic Consensus Council (PACC). Although several drugs have been used for IT drug delivery, morphine is most commonly used. Morphine functions as an opioid agonist, resulting in analgesia mainly through μ-receptor activation. The mechanisms of analgesia for intrathecal opioids result from a direct spinal mechanism, which occurs once the opioid has diffused from the IT space to the substantia gelatinosa in the dorsal horn of the spinal cord. Analgesia is also the result of a supraspinal effect secondary to systemic absorption. The intrathecal concentration of hydrophilic opioids such as morphine is likely to remain elevated for a longer period of time compared with lipophilic opioids such as fentanyl; thus, morphine is more likely to cause delayed respiratory depression via an increased level of cephalad spread.

T. R. Deer et al. (eds.), *Deer's Treatment of Pain*, https://doi.org/10.1007/978-3-030-12281-2_86

Two other commonly used opioids for IDDS are fentanyl and hydromorphone:

- Fentanyl – more lipophilic than morphine, thus more likely to leave the intrathecal space and be systemically absorbed. **Lipophilic opioids cause less intrathecal spread (smaller area of analgesia) and carry a lower risk of respiratory depression.*
- Hydromorphone – another commonly used opioid for IT, has an intermediate lipid solubility.

As a general rule of practice, 1/300th of the total daily oral morphine dose or equivalent is used as a starting point (for epidural delivery it is 1/10th) – consequently, there is a small margin for error. The powerful analgesic properties of intrathecal morphine unfortunately come with the risk of a wide range of potential adverse side effects, even with the small doses utilized with IDD (see Table 86.1). Ideally, one would prefer to retain the advantages of IDD and discard the unwanted side effects and potential long-term complications inherent to the use of opioids.

Enter ziconotide – an FDA-approved IT medication for the treatment of chronic pain. Ziconotide is considered a first-line medication for IDD and, most importantly, is not an opioid. It is a synthetic of the ω-conotoxin peptide derived from the venom of the piscivorous marine snail, *Conus magus*. The name brand version is known as Prialt® (Jazz Pharmaceuticals, PLC) (Fig. 86.1) and is approved for use in the Medtronic SynchroMed® EL, SynchroMed® II Infusion System, and Cadd-Micro® ambulatory infusion pumps.

Although the mechanism of action of ziconotide has not been entirely established in humans, results in animal models suggest that ziconotide is a presynaptic N-type calcium channel blocker that is thought to bind to the N-type calcium channels located on the primary nociceptive (A-δ and C) afferent nerves in the superficial layers (Rexed laminae I and II) of the dorsal horn in the spinal cord resulting in analgesia. Results in animals suggest that its binding block N-type calcium channels leads to a decrease in excitatory neurotransmitter release (glutamate), CGRP, and substance P from the primary afferent nerve terminals resulting in pain relief (Fig. 86.2).

Of all complications that could potentially occur with IDDS, the most common is related to the pharmacologic nature of the drug within the pump. Given that ziconotide is not an opioid, the complications that could potentially occur with IT opioids (i.e., granuloma, respiratory depression, etc.) are not an issue. Moreover, ziconotide is easier to use in clinical practice than IT opioids:

- *Trialing* – ziconotide can be trialed in an outpatient setting with the patient discharged home the same day without any concerned for overdose or respiratory depression. Trialing with IT opioids requires vigilant monitoring for several hours after the procedure given the possibility of delayed-onset respiratory depression that can sometimes require overnight monitoring. With IT opioids, there is a 7.5-fold increase in mortality over the first 3 days after an IDDS procedure in patients with chronic nonmalignant pain.
- *Safety* – at the time of this publication, there has not been a single report of overdose or drug-related death with IT ziconotide.

Table 86.1 Potential adverse effects of opioid analgesics

Acute	Chronic
Allergic reaction	Tolerance
Constipation	Physical dependence
Dizziness	Delayed gastric emptying
Fatigue	Hyperalgesia
Mental clouding	Myoclonus
Nausea	Immunologic dysfunction
Pruritus	Addiction
Respiratory depression	
Sedation/somnolence	
Urinary retention	
Vomiting	

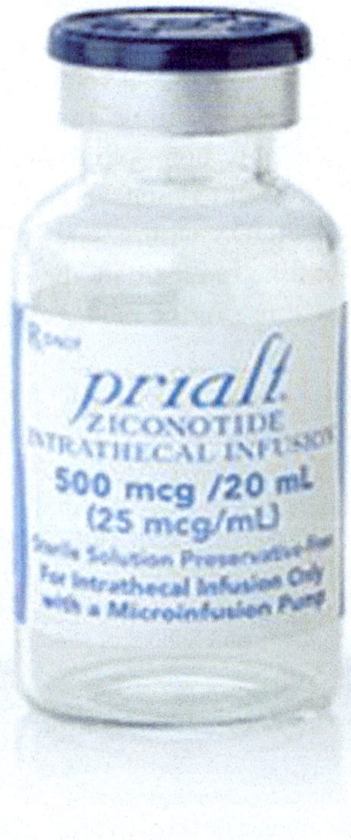

Fig. 86.1 Prialt (ziconotide)

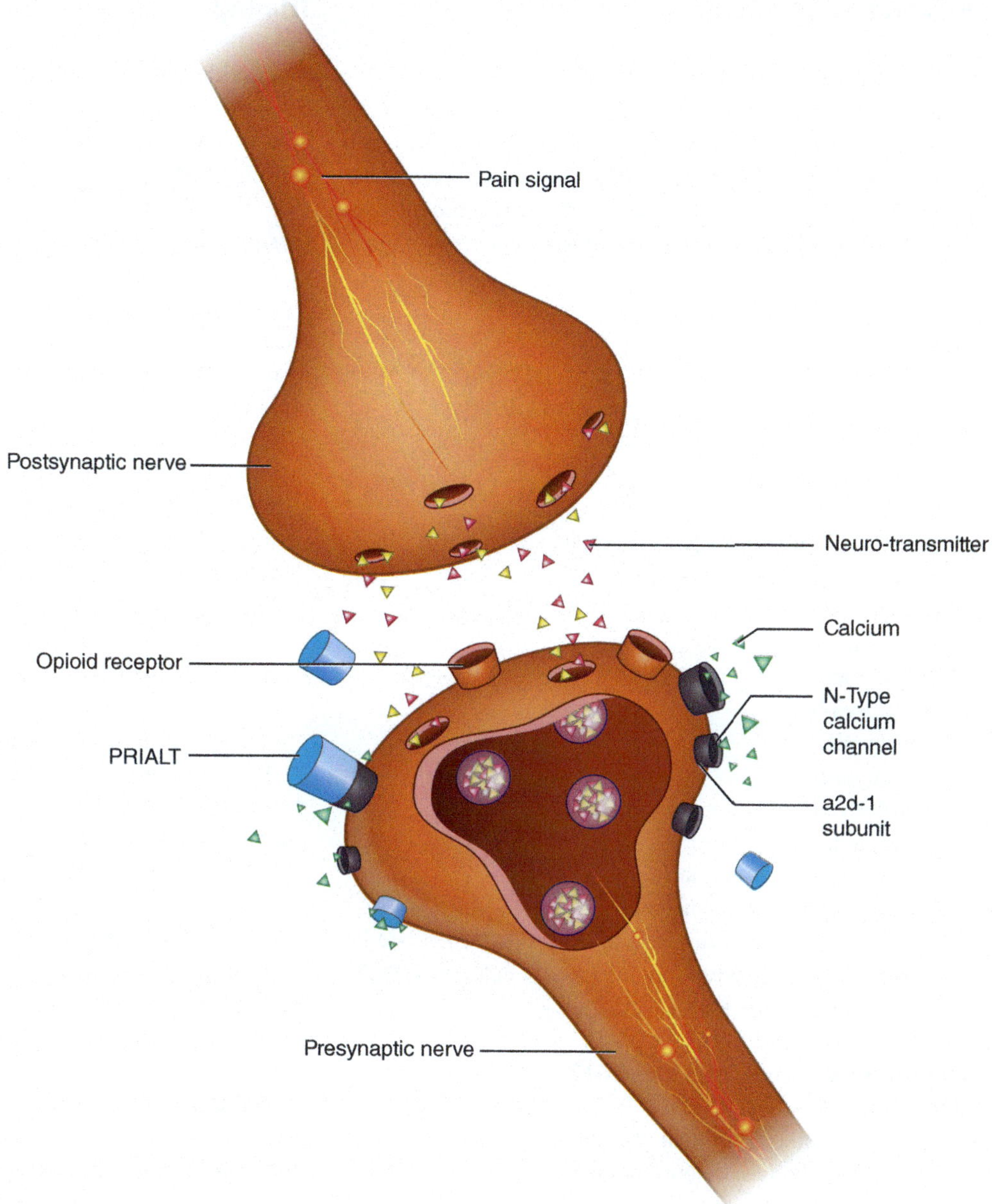

Fig. 86.2 Mechanism of action of intrathecal ziconotide

- *Refills* – ziconotide does not cross the blood-brain barrier. While an overdose with ziconotide has yet to be reported, if it were possible, overdose due to a pocket refill would not be a concern.
- *Reversible side effect profile* – confusion, memory impairment, sedation, urinary retention, and psychiatric symptoms (hallucinations, delirium, and psychosis) have been observed with IT ziconotide use. Discontinuation of therapy causes immediate cessation of symptomatology with no risk of drug withdrawal.

For a complete summary, refer to Table 86.2 for comparison of intrathecal opioids versus intrathecal ziconotide.

Table 86.2 Comparing the side effect profiles of IT opioids and IT ziconotide

Opioids	Ziconotide
Respiratory depression	No reports of respiratory depression
Overdose-related death	No reports of overdose-related deaths
Granuloma formation	No reports of granuloma formation
Overdose related to pocket refill	Limited ability to cross blood-brain barrier
Overnight monitoring recommended	In office trial and same day discharge
Potential for withdrawal	No reports of withdrawal
Combined with other medications (bupivacaine, clonidine, etc.)	Efficacy established as monotherapy
Tolerance	No reports of tolerance

Uses and Indications

Per the official labeling registered with the FDA:

PRIALT (ziconotide intrathecal infusion) is indicated for the management of severe chronic pain in patients for whom intrathecal (IT) therapy is warranted and who are intolerant of or refractory to other treatment, such as systemic analgesics, adjunctive therapies, or IT morphine.

Indications

- Axial neck or back pain; not a surgical candidate
  - Multiple compression fractures
  - Discogenic pain
  - Spinal stenosis
  - Diffuse multiple-level spondylosis
- Failed back surgery syndrome
- Abdominal/pelvic pain
  - Visceral
  - Somatic
- Extremity pain
  - Radicular pain
  - Joint pain
- Complex regional pain syndrome (CRPS)
- Trunk pain
  - Postherpetic neuralgia
  - Post-thoracotomy syndromes
- Cancer pain, direct invasion, and chemotherapy related
- Analgesic efficacy with systemic opioid delivery complicated by intolerable side effect

Recommendations from the 2017 PACC guidelines

- Cancer or other terminal condition-related pain with diffuse nociceptive or neuropathic pain.
  - Line 1A.
    - Ziconotide and morphine.
- Non-cancer-related pain with localized nociceptive or neuropathic pain.
  - Line 1A.
    - Ziconotide and morphine.
- Non-cancer-related pain with diffuse nociceptive or neuropathic pain.
  - Line 1A.
    - Morphine and ziconotide.
- Ziconotide should be the first choice in patients with >120 morphine equivalents (ME) or fast systemic dose escalation, in the absence of history of psychosis.

Patients with a positive trial (determined by a decrease in visual analog scale (VAS) and an improvement in function/quality of life) may benefit from permanent implantation of an IDDS with long-term maintenance infusion of ziconotide.

Trialing

Ziconotide, like most IT medications, may be trialed by two basic means: continuous infusion or IT bolus dosing. Since it does not cross the blood-brain barrier, epidural testing is not recommended.

- *Continuous infusion trialing* – a catheter is placed percutaneously into the IT and connected to an external infusion pump. The patient is then infused with progressively increasing doses of ziconotide while the patient is monitored for therapeutic effect. This is extremely time intensive and performed on an inpatient basis.
- *IT bolus dosing* – an IT injection of ziconotide is administered and the patient is monitored for several hours for safety and therapeutic effect. The generally accepted dosing is 2.4 mcg followed by a second injection of 4.8 mcg several hours later if the initial injection is ineffective. Due to the nonexistent risk of delayed-onset respiratory depression, this can be performed as an outpatient with the patient discharged home a few hours later after a cursory physical exam has been performed.

Trialing with ziconotide can be challenging because of the drug's narrow therapeutic window, and the side effect profile is more closely related to the rate of dosage increase. If not dosed appropriately, trialing can cause side effects, which may reject patients who might otherwise have benefited from IT ziconotide therapy. Early studies using ziconotide relied on continuous infusion as the primary trial method; however this method has multiple drawbacks including increased cost, patient burden, and safety concerns.

Bolus trialing methods among clinicians can vary. In 2013, Mohammed et al. described a technique for bolus injection trialing with IT ziconotide using multiple (2 to 3) single-shot bolus doses administered at least 1 week apart, with a starting dose of 2.5 mcg and subsequent doses of 2.5 mcg, 1.2 mcg, or 3.75 mcg, depending on the patient's response to the initial dose (neuromodulation). A successful trial was defined as one that provided a good analgesic response (≥30% reduction in visual analog scale rating of pain), with no significant side effects to two separate bolus doses. Overall, 55% of patients (11 of 20) had a good analgesic response to the bolus injection trial. Patient reports on the VAS indicated a 43% reduction in pain from pre-treatment. In another study, trialing involved an initial 2 mcg bolus dose of IT ziconotide injected with barbotage at L1-2, followed by 23 hours of observation. Patients who achieved ≥75% pain reduction without adverse effects received a second IT bolus injection using a similar method. Successful trial, defined as similar favorable responses (≥75% pain reduction without adverse effects) to both trial doses of ziconotide, identified patients as appropriate candidates for implantation of an IDDS using ziconotide. The 16 patients who met the criteria for trialing had successful trialing with IT ziconotide and received an implantable device, with IT ziconotide monotherapy initiated at the successful trial dose (2 mcg/day). These studies further supported intermittent multiple, single-shot bolus trial method for IT ziconotide.

Overall, trialing with IT ziconotide has been conducted and studied by means of single-shot bolus and continuous infusion methods. The current literature does not support the use of one trialing method over the other. Based on clinical findings, the advantages of single-shot bolus trialing appear to supersede the demands of a continuous infusion trial in most cases.

Pump Management

- The maximum recommended IT ziconotide dose is 19.2 mcg/day.
- Use only undiluted 25 mcg/mL formulation for naïve pump priming. Rinse the internal surfaces of the pump with 2 mL of ziconotide at 25 mcg/mL. Repeat twice for a total of three rinses.

Initial Pump Fill

- Use only the undiluted 25 mcg/mL formulation for the initial pump fill.
- Fill the naïve pump after priming with the appropriate volume of ziconotide 25 mcg/mL.
- Begin dosing at a delivery rate no higher than 2.4 mcg/day (0.1 mcg/hr).

How to Prime and Fill a Naïve Pump

In a naïve pump, ziconotide is lost due to two factors that do not occur upon subsequent refills: adsorption on internal device surfaces, such as titanium, and by dilution in the residual space of the device. Consequently, the pump reservoir should be refilled with ziconotide within 14 days of the initial fill to ensure appropriate dose administration.

- *Step 1: Prime*
  - The first time that the pump is used with ziconotide, it must be primed. Using a 5 mL syringe, remove 2 mL from the vial of undiluted 25 mcg/mL ziconotide.
  - Use only the undiluted ziconotide for naïve pump priming.
  - Set aside the remaining 18 mL in the vial.
- *Step 2: Rinse*
  - Attach the syringe to the catheter with a luer lock connector, and rinse the internal surfaces of the pump with the 2 mL of undiluted ziconotide.
  - Discard the used 2 mL solution after the rinse.
  - Repeat this rinse procedure two more times for a total of three rinses.
  - A naïve pump must be rinsed three times in order to prevent a reduction in the dose during the initial fill.
- *Step 3: Fill*
  - Using a 20 mL syringe, remove the remaining 14 mL of undiluted ziconotide from the vial.
  - Fill the pump with the 14 mL of ziconotide and set the appropriate dose and flow rate. Initiate dosing with ziconotide at a delivery rate no higher than 2.4 mcg per day or 0.1 mcg per hour.
  - On or before day 14: Refill
  - Discard the remaining ziconotide in the pump and perform the first pump refill.
  - The IT pump should be refilled using a new vial of ziconotide within 14 days of the initial pump fill to help ensure appropriate dose administration.

Pump Refills

- For subsequent pump refills, fill the pump at least every 40 days if ziconotide is used diluted. For undiluted ziconotide, fill the pump at least every 84 days.

Dosing and Titration

The generally accepted guideline for titrating ziconotide is to start low and titrate slowly to avoid side effects or adverse events. See Table 86.3 for the suggested titration guidelines.

Recommended Starting Dosage

- 0.5–1.2 mcg/day (to 2.4 mcg/day per product labeling)

Titration

- Increase by increments of ≤0.5 mcg/day on a weekly basis based on analgesia and tolerability. In light of the marked inter-patient variations in dosing observed in longer-term studies, individualized dosing regimens are important.

Maximum (as recommended by PACC 2012 and 2017)

- Daily dose: 19.2 mcg
- Concentration: 100 mcg/mL

Table 86.3 Recommendations for dosing of IT ziconotide continuous infusion

Recommendations for dosing of IT ziconotide continuous infusion	
Ziconotide prescribing information	Starting dose: <2.4 mcg/day Upward titration: <2.4 mcg/day (no more than 2–3 adjustments per week) Max dose: 19.2 mcg/day
Expert consensus	Starting dose: <0.5 mcg/day Upward titration: <0.5 mcg/day, no more than once per week
PACC guidelines	Starting dose: 0.5–2.4 mcg/day Max dose: 19.2 mcg/day

More aggressive IT dosing and titration schedules may be appropriate, if tolerable, in patients deemed to be short-term survivors (i.e., life expectancy ≤1 year) in order to address escalating pain and maintain quality of life.

Evidence exists that could expand ziconotide to include other dosing regimens beyond the traditional low volume/slow continuous infusion approach, such as PCA with the PTM system or bolus nocturnal flex dosing. These modalities could open new opportunities for further improving the management of chronic refractory pain with IT ziconotide.

Use of Patient-Controlled Analgesia with Intrathecal Ziconotide

This is a relatively newer technique with IDDS which allows for greater individualization of therapy and more aggressive management of challenging cancer-related pain. It is similar to patient-controlled analgesia (PCA), which is widely used in the intravenous administration of opioids and other analgesics, particularly for managing postoperative pain and cancer pain. As it pertains to patient-controlled bolus dosing with ziconotide, no evidence or formal studies exist to define proper assess efficacy, safety, and tolerability. As such, this should only be utilized if it is known how this patient in question responds to an IT bolus of ziconotide.

Flex Dosing of Intrathecal Ziconotide

This approach uses the flex-mode feature of the SynchroMed II® (Medtronic®) infusion pump to program delivery of IT medication at varying rates throughout the day or enables administration of scheduled bolus doses. To date, only a single publication exists describing this technique: larger investigations are needed to confirm the results of this proof-of-concept study and to determine the optimal times and intervals for administration of ziconotide bolus doses.

Warnings and Precautions

The most commonly reported side effects are cognitive and/or neuropsychiatric adverse reactions:

- Cognitive impairment, hallucinations, or changes in mood or consciousness.
- May cause or worsen depression, with the risk of suicide in susceptible patients.
- Severe psychiatric symptoms and neurological impairment may occur during treatment with ziconotide; therefore it is contraindicated in patients with a pre-existing history of psychosis.
- The safety and effectiveness in pediatric or pregnant patients has not yet been established. Additionally, it is not known whether ziconotide is excreted in human breast milk.
- There is a higher incidence of confusion in elderly patients; therefore one should exercise caution with dosing and low end of the typical dosing range.
- See Table 86.4 for a complete list of potential adverse reactions.

Table 86.4 Commonly reported adverse reactions

Common adverse events
Dizziness
Nausea
Asthenia
Diarrhea
Somnolence
Vomiting
Confusion
Abnormal gait
Ataxia
Headache
Nystagmus
Dysarthria
Memory impairment
Rigors
Tremor
Vertigo
Anorexia
Muscle spasms
Urinary retention

Fortunately, ziconotide therapy can be interrupted or discontinued abruptly without evidence of withdrawal effects in the event of serious neurological or psychiatric signs or symptoms. The cognitive effects of ziconotide are generally reversible within 2 weeks after drug discontinuation. Before resuming, a comprehensive evaluation must be performed on a case-by-case basis as well as potential reduction in dosing.

Contraindications

Ziconotide is contraindicated in patients with:

- A known hypersensitivity to ziconotide or any of its formulation components
- Any other concomitant treatment or medical condition that would render IT administration hazardous, such as the presence of infection at the microinfusion injection site, uncontrolled bleeding diathesis, and spinal canal obstruction that impairs circulation of cerebrospinal fluid (CSF)
- A pre-existing history of psychosis

Overdose/Toxicity

There is no known antidote to ziconotide. General medical supportive measures should be administered to patients who receive an overdose until the exaggerated pharmacological effects of the drug have resolved. Treatment for an overdose is hospitalization, when needed, and symptom-related supportive care.

Monitoring

In clinical trials, serum creatine kinase (CK) levels above the upper limit of normal (ULN) were reported in 40% of patients. Incidences were higher during the first 2 months of treatment. Therefore, serum CK levels should be monitored periodically. If CK levels remain elevated or continue to rise, reduce the dose or discontinue, altogether.

Evidence and Efficacy

A number of clinical trials have been published on ziconotide, thus establishing its place in the treatment of chronic, refractory pain for both malignant and nonmalignant settings.

- 2004 – Staats et al. published the results of a study on the safety and efficacy IT ziconotide in patients with pain refractory to conventional treatment (JAMA). The authors showed the mean Visual Analog Scale of Pain Intensity (VASPI) scores improved 53.1% in the ziconotide group versus 18.1 in the placebo group, with no loss of efficacy of ziconotide in the maintenance phase of infusion therapy.
- 2005 – Collins et al. performed a meta-analysis on the efficacy of ziconotide. The authors showed it provided significant pain relief relative to placebo for a number of etiologies, including neuropathic pain, myelopathy, radiculopathy, and failed back surgery syndrome.
- 2006 – Wallace et al. published a study showing similar results with mean percent reduction in VASPI score from baseline being 31.2% for ziconotide versus 6.0% in placebo treated patients, respectively (neuromodulation). These patients (169 ziconotide, 86 placebo) suffered from severe chronic nonmalignant pain unresponsive to conventional therapy and were treated over a 6-day period in an inpatient hospital setting.
- 2006 – Rauck et al. published the results of a randomized, double-blind, placebo-controlled study on the use of IT ziconotide. Patients were randomized to ziconotide ($n = 112$) or placebo ($n = 108$) and started IT infusion at 0.1 mcg/hour (2.4 mcg/day), increasing gradually (0.05–0.1 mcg/hour increments) over 3 weeks. Using a slow titration schedule, the ziconotide group showed a statistically significant reduction in VASPI at week 3 over the placebo group (14.7–7.2%) (J Pain Symptom Manage)
- 2009 – Rauck et al. conducted a review of IT ziconotide for the treatment of neuropathic pain. The authors collectively examined evidence from double-blinded, placebo-controlled trials, open-label studies, case series, and case studies which suggested that ziconotide, as either monotherapy or in combination with other IT drugs, is a viable therapeutic option for patients with refractory neuropathic pain (*Pain Practice*).
- 2017 – Deer et al. published the results of the PRIZM trial (Patient Registry of Intrathecal Ziconotide Management), an open-label, long-term, multicenter, observational study of adult patients with severe chronic pain, relying heavily on outpatient intrathecal single-shot bolus trial as the primary method. Overwhelming success of single-shot bolus injections for trial was observed in terms of analgesia and reduced side effect profile. The PRIZM registry displays direct analysis of ziconotide as the initial vs. noninitial intrathecal agent in IT pump therapy. Greater improvements in efficacy outcomes were observed when ziconotide was initiated as first-line intrathecal therapy versus non-first intrathecal agent (*Pain Practice*).

Pearls and Pitfalls

- Ziconotide should be considered a first-line drug for IDD.
- Combination of ziconotide with intrathecal opiates is not recommended.
- Due to a more favorable side effect profile as compared to opioids, ziconotide can be trialed as an outpatient via IT bolus injections.
- Granulomas, respiratory depression, and withdrawal have not been reported with ziconotide.
- FDA approved ziconotide for use with the Medtronic SynchroMed® II Infusion System (Minneapolis, MN, USA) or the CADD-Micro® Ambulatory Infusion Pump (Smiths Medical; St. Paul, MN, USA). Ziconotide has also been used off-label with the Prometra® Pump (Flowonix, Mt. Olive, NJ, USA).
- Due to its large molecular size and hydrophilic structure, ziconotide cannot cross the blood-brain barrier.
- Due to a narrow therapeutic window, a low starting dose is indicated, and a slow titration schedule should be utilized.
- A naïve pump should be emptied and refilled 14 days after the initial filling
- Meclizine treatment is sometimes used before IT ziconotide trials in clinical practice although there is insufficient evidence to support this approach. Proper hydration via intravenous (IV) infusion before trialing may limit the side effect of hypotension that can sometimes occur.
- Ziconotide should be kept refrigerated.

Recommended Readings

1. Ahmed S, Martin N, Chang Y. Patient selection and trial methods for Intraspinal drug delivery for chronic pain: a national survey. Neuromodulation. 2005;8(2):112–20.
2. Bhatia G, Lau M, Gulur P. Intrathecal Drug Delivery (ITDD) systems for cancer pain. F1000Research, 2013.
3. Burton A, Rajagopal A, Shah H, Mendoza T, Cleeland C, Hassenbusch S, Arens J. Epidural and Intrathecal Analgesia is effective in treating refractory cancer pain. Pain Med. 2004;5(3):239–47.
4. Burton AW, Deer TR, Wallace MS, Rauck RL, Grigsby E. Considerations and methodology for trialing ziconotide. Pain Physician. 2010;13:23–33.
5. Christo P, Bottros M. Current perspectives on intrathecal drug delivery. J Pain Res. 2014;7:615.
6. Collins R, Lieberburg I, Ludington E, Howard R. Effectiveness of intrathecal ziconotide in multiple pain etiologies: a meta-analysis of three controlled trials [abstract]. Pain Med. 2005;6:195.
7. Deer T, Caraway D, Wallace M. A definition of refractory pain to help determine suitability for device implantation. Neuromodulation. 2014;17(8):711–5.
8. Deer TR, et al. The Polyanalgesic Consensus Conference (PACC): recommendations for trialing of Intrathecal drug delivery infusion therapy. Neuromodulation. 2017;20:133–54. https://doi.org/10.1111/ner.12543.
9. Deer TR, et al. The Polyanalgesic Consensus Conference (PACC): recommendations for Intrathecal drug delivery: guidance for improving safety and mitigating risks. Neuromodulation. 2017;20:155–76. https://doi.org/10.1111/ner.12579.
10. Deer TR, et al. The Polyanalgesic Consensus Conference (PACC): recommendations on Intrathecal drug infusion systems best practices and guidelines. Neuromodulation. 2017;20:96–132. https://doi.org/10.1111/ner.12538.
11. Deer T, et al. Effectiveness and safety of Intrathecal Ziconotide: Interim analysis of the patient registry of Intrathecal Ziconotide Management (PRIZM). Pain Pract. 2017; https://doi.org/10.1111/papr.12599.
12. Deer T, Rauck R, Kim P, Saulino M, Wallace M, Grigsby E, Huang I, Mori F, Vanhove G, McDowell G. Effectiveness and safety of Intrathecal Ziconotide: Interim analysis of the patient registry of Intrathecal Ziconotide Management (PRIZM). Pain Pract. 2017;18:230.
13. Hayek S, Hanes M, Wang C, Veizi I. Ziconotide combination Intrathecal therapy for noncancer pain is limited secondary to delayed adverse effects: a case series with a 24-month follow-up. Neuromodulation. 2015;18(5):397–403.
14. Hunter C, Diwan S, Deer T. Neuroaugmentation by stimulation vs. Intrathecal drug delivery. In: Intrathecal pump delivery for pain and spasticity, vol. 2. Philadelphia: Elsevier; 2012.
15. Maeyaert J, Buchser E, Van Buyten J, Rainov N, Becker R. Patient-controlled Analgesia in Intrathecal therapy for chronic pain: safety and effective operation of the Model 8831 personal therapy manager with a pre-implanted synchromed infusion system. Neuromodulation. 2003;6(3):133–41.
16. McDowell GC. Use of the personal therapy manager with Prialt® (ziconotide) for patient-controlled analgesia: a case series highlighting techniques and outcomes. Las Vegas. Presented at the 14th Annual Meeting of the North American Neuromodulation Society, December 2–5, 2010. http://www.slideserve.com/uri/use-of-the-personal-therapy-manager-with-prialt-ziconotide-intrathecal-infusion-for-patient-controlled-analgesia-case. Accessed 28 Aug 2017.
17. McDowell GC, Pope JE. Intrathecal Ziconotide: dosing and administration strategies in patients with refractory chronic pain. Neuromodulation. 2016;19(5):522–32. https://doi.org/10.1111/ner.12392.
18. McGivern J. Ziconotide: a review of its pharmacology and use in the treatment of pain. Neuropsychiatr Dis Treat. 2007;3(1):69–85.
19. Patel D, Dang S, Weber G. Neuromodulation of cancer pain. Top Pain Manag. 2016;31(12):1–10.
20. Pope JE, Deer TR. Intrathecal ziconotide in the treatment of failed back surgery syndrome. Pain Med News Spec Ed. 2014:79–80.
21. Pope JE, Deer TR. Intrathecal pharmacology update: novel dosing strategy for intrathecal monotherapy ziconotide on efficacy and sustainability. Neuromodulation. 2015;18:414–20.
22. PRIALT [package insert] Jazz Pharmaceuticals: Palo Alto; 2013.
23. Rauck R, Wallace M, Leong M, Minehart M, Webster L, Charapata S, Abraham J, Buffington D, Ellis D, Kartzinel R. A randomized, double-blind, placebo-controlled study of Intrathecal Ziconotide in adults with severe chronic pain. J Pain Symptom Manag. 2006;31(5):393–406.
24. Rauck R, Wallace M, Burton A, Kapural L, North J. Intrathecal Ziconotide for neuropathic pain: a review. Pain Pract. 2009;9(5):327–37.
25. Sanford M. Intrathecal Ziconotide: a review of its use in patients with chronic pain refractory to other systemic or Intrathecal Analgesics. CNS Drugs. 2013;27(11):989–1002.
26. Saulino M, Kim P, Shaw E. Practical considerations and patient selection for intrathecal drug delivery in the management of chronic pain. J Pain Res. 2014:627.
27. Smith T, et al. Randomized clinical trial of an implantable drug delivery system compared with comprehensive medical management for refractory cancer pain: impact on pain, drug-related toxicity, and survival. J Clin Oncol. 2002;20(19):4040–9.
28. Staats P, Yearwood T, Charapata S, Presley R, Wallace M, Byas-Smith M, Fisher R, Bryce D, Mangieri E, Luther R, Mayo M, McGuire D, Ellis D. Intrathecal Ziconotide in the treatment of refractory pain in patients with cancer or AIDS. JAMA. 2004;291(1):63.
29. Stearns L, Boortz-Marx R, Du PS, et al. Intrathecal drug delivery for the management of cancer pain: a multidisciplinary consensus of best clinical practices. J Support Oncol. 2005;3:399–408.
30. Vos T, Flaxman AD, Naghavi M, et al. Years lived with disability (YLDs) for 1160 sequelae of 289 diseases and injuries 1990-2010: a systematic analysis for the Global Burden of Disease Study 2010. Lancet. 2012;380:2163–96.
31. Wallace M, Charapata S, Fisher R, Byas-Smith M, Staats P, Mayo M, McGuire D, Ellis D. Intrathecal Ziconotide in the treatment of chronic nonmalignant pain: a randomized, double-blind, Placebo-controlled clinical trial. Neuromodulation. 2006;9(2):75–86.
32. Webster L. The relationship between the mechanisms of action and safety profiles of Intrathecal Morphine and Ziconotide: a review of the literature. Pain Med. 2015;16(7):1265–77.

Part VIII

Regenerative Therapies for Chronic Pain

Scientific Bases of PRP Therapy

87

Corey W. Hunter and Ajax Yang

Introduction

In the simplest of terms, platelet-rich plasma (PRP) is defined as a volume of plasma containing a concentrate of platelets above the baseline of typical/healthy blood levels. While PRP therapy has received significant attention as of late from professional athletes, it has been utilized by physicians for over 30 years in dental and orthopedic surgeries to assist in healing. Its growing popularity with the general public stems from its ability to aid in the repair of soft tissue injuries that are reluctant to heal on their own (i.e., tendon, ligament, and muscle). Moreover, there is no fear of immunogenicity as the whole blood from which PRP is derived is autologous. Given the ever-growing applications and versatility of PRP therapy to facilitate healing in chronically inflamed tissues, it is important to understand and establish the role(s) of platelets as well as the mechanisms involved in normal repair and regeneration.

Microanatomy

Platelets (aka thrombocytes) range from 1 to 4 μm in diameter and are derived from the fragmentation of megakaryocyte lineage in the bone marrow. Platelets contain the following compounds contributing to the different phases of healing (Fig. 87.1).

C. W. Hunter (✉)
Department of Rehabilitation Medicine, Icahn School of Medicine at Mount Sinai, New York, NY, USA

Ainsworth Institute of Pain Management, New York, NY, USA
e-mail: chunter@ainpain.com

A. Yang
Department of Rehabilitation Medicine, Icahn School of Medicine at Mount Sinai, New York, NY, USA

Platelet Function and Tissue Healing

Regardless of the tissue type, the normal healing process relies on a combination of two main processes:

1. Regeneration – the replacement of damaged tissues by the surrounding healthy living tissues
2. Repair – scar tissue formation through granulation tissue maturation to substitute the diseased tissues

In order to ensure the PRP technology is applied safely and logically, it is important to understand the fundamentals of platelet function and normal tissue healing stages: hemostasis, inflammation, proliferation, and remodeling.

Immediately following trauma, the locally damaged blood vessels release blood plasma and other cell mediators into the surrounding areas to induce platelet aggregation to form a fibrin clot. This clot plug is the product of the collagen receptor glycoprotein (GPIb/IX/V) binding to the damaged endothelial wall to act as a base for additional aggregation factor, such as platelet integrin αIIbβ3, to adhere themselves to the area. Once the platelets aggregate, they become activated to chemotactically mobilize monocytes, neutrophils, and lymphocytes toward the clot. More importantly, platelet activation and degranulation release seven important growth factors:

- Platelet-derived growth factor (PDGF)
- Insulin growth factor one and two (IGF-1, IGF-2)
- Transforming growth factor-β1 (TGF-β1)
- Vascular endothelial growth factor (VEGF)
- Fibroblast growth factor (FGF)
- Keratinocyte growth factor (KGF)
- Connective tissue growth factor (CTGF)
- Epithelial growth factor (EGF)

Over 95% of the abovementioned growth factors are released within the first hour of injury and will continue to release growth factors for the next 7–10 days. Fibroblast

T. R. Deer et al. (eds.), *Deer's Treatment of Pain*, https://doi.org/10.1007/978-3-030-12281-2_87

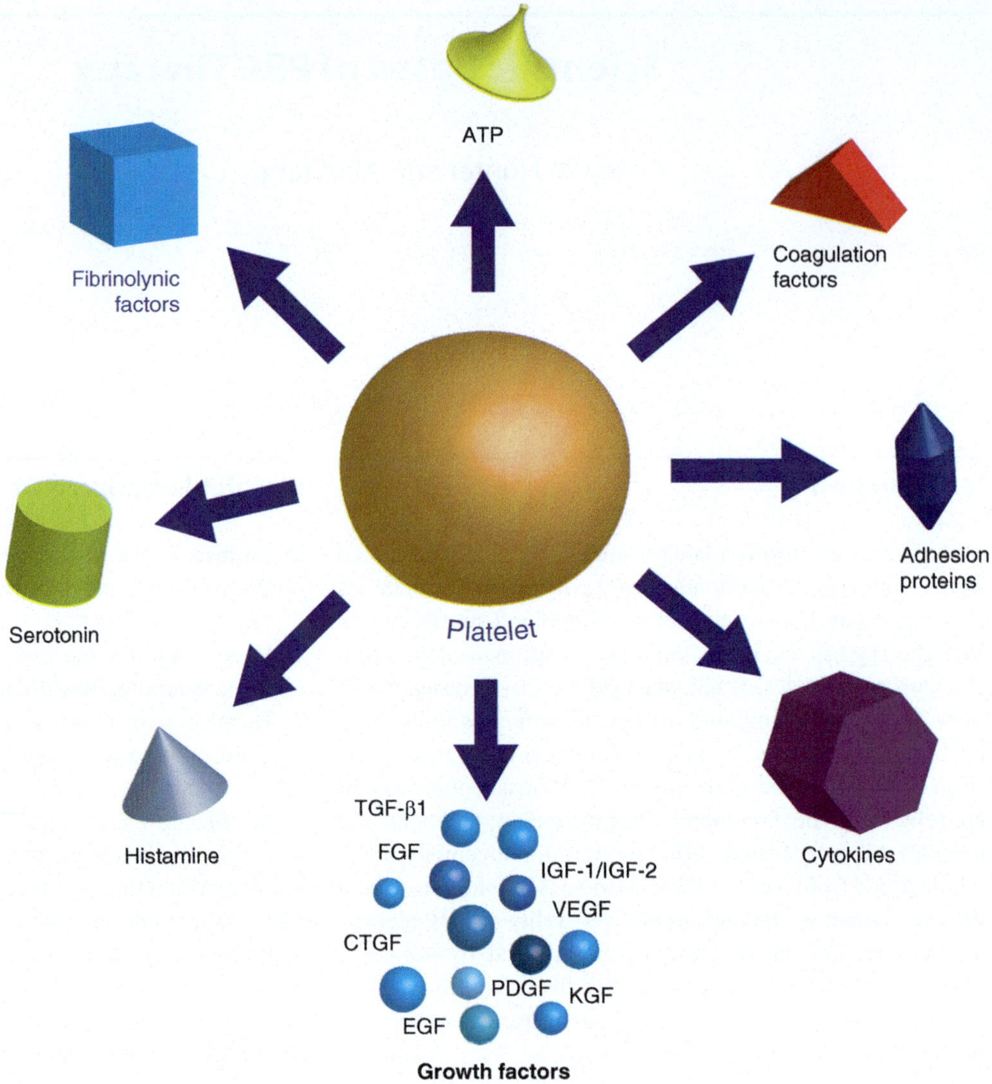

Fig. 87.1 Figure illustrating the different compounds contained within a platelet

stimulation promotes collagen production to replace the fibrin clot during the proliferative phase. Endothelial cells enhance angiogenesis to increase local cellular metabolism. In addition to the growth factors, PRP also contains other bioactive molecules that promote healing. Interleukin 8 (IL-8) promotes angiogenesis. Fibrin, fibronectin, and vitronectin are known cell adhesion molecules for osteoconduction, bone matrix, connective tissue, and epithelial migration during tissue repair.

It is obvious that adequate blood supply is crucial to proper tissue healing. Tendons, ligaments, joints, and certain segments of the muscle all have poor blood supply and are therefore prone to chronic inflammation following initial injury. Chronic inflammation results when acute inflammatory responses are inadequate to restore the prior physiological state. Due to poor blood supply and insufficient endogenous platelet activation/aggregation, macrophages, lymphocytes, fibroblasts, and plasma cells continue to linger at a low concentration without proper healing. Chronic inflammation causes persistent pain, tissue damage, neo-neurovascularization, tissue necrosis, and fibrosis. The exact mechanisms causing incomplete acute inflammation are unknown; however, overuse and repetitive microtrauma to a structure have been implicated.

The success and appropriateness of PRP therapy rely on meeting the following conditions:

1. Deliver the high concentration of growth factors to "jump-start" tissue healing in areas with suboptimal blood supply.
2. The target tissue must have the ability to undergo sufficient angiogenesis and accommodate vascularization – thus allowing the body to finish the job.

The rationale is that the high concentration of growth factors merely acts as a beacon to attract and activate endogenous healing molecules that govern protein transcription, cellular division/proliferation, extracellular matrix synthesis, and collagen formation to the injury site. Continued proliferation of epithelial cells, fibroblastic cells, osteoblastic cells, and mesenchymal stem cells must be sustained by sufficient blood circulation to allow healing to reach completion.

Background and Historical Perspective

By definition, any volume of plasma that contains supra-physiologic platelet count is considered "platelet rich." The characterization of PRP, historically, depended on the platelet concentration alone. However, the concentration and composition of PRP can range widely – this can be due to a number of variables including the physiological state of the patient from which the PRP is derived as well as the method of preparation. This focus on platelet concentration leads to every PRP kit manufacturer claiming their particular product yields the highest platelet counts and/or growth factor concentration. It is important to note that PRP is exempt from the traditional regulatory pathway (human and animal clinical trials) set forth by the Food and Drug Administration (FDA); therefore, any claims by the manufacturers are unverified. Additionally, the ideal platelet concentration is likely to differ depending on tissue type and disease state.

The use of PRP was first introduced in the 1980s in the field of cardiothoracic surgery as a method to conserve intraoperative use of the whole blood. In the 1990s, PRP showed promising results in promoting wound healing in extremity chronic ulcers. Since then, many surgical subspecialties such as maxillofacial, orthopedics, plastics, and podiatry had success of using PRP to achieve excellent outcomes.

The therapeutic effects of PRP rely on complex interactions of platelet-derived proteins, growth factors, cytokines, hormones, and white blood cells (WBC) to create an ideal microenvironment for cellular repair and regeneration at the site of injury. Similar to platelet concentration, WBC quantification has also been studied and used to categorize PRP into:

1. Pure PRP (low WBC, anti-coagulated)
2. Leukocyte-rich PRP (high WBC, anti-coagulated)
3. Pure platelet-rich fibrin (PRF) (low WBC, coagulated)
4. Leukocyte-rich PRF (high WBC, coagulated)

The inclusion of WBC-rich buffy coat has been debated as excessive WBC may cause pain and unwanted scarring. Different cell types cultured in the same PRP yielded different tissue responses. It has also been found that extreme platelet concentrations produced inferior bone regrowth, while moderate concentrations were more effective. Similarly, rotator cuff fibroblasts responded favorably to low and moderate concentrations compared to high concentration. Future research is needed to better define the ideal PRP compositions and concentrations that are disease specific.

Uses and Indications

With the biotechnological advancement in improving the precision and ease of PRP preparation, PRP therapy can be conveniently and safely administered in the office settings. While there are many potential indications and uses for PRP therapy, the most important step begins with patient selection. Physicians should carefully obtain a thorough history including history of injury, location, chronicity, intensity of pain, aggravating and alleviating factors, and prior treatments. Clinical presentation must be supported by imaging to confirm that underlying tissue damage is indeed the symptom/pain generator. After the diagnosis has been established, the standard treatment(s) should be tried first. Similar to rationales that govern regenerative medicine as a whole, PRP therapy candidates typically fall into one of the three groups:

1. Asymptomatic patients with high degeneration risks.
2. Symptomatic patients in the beginning phase of degeneration process.
3. Symptomatic patients in the late phase of degeneration process.

The therapeutic effects of PRP therapy are reduced in older individuals with obesity and advanced stages of degeneration. In contrast, younger patients with lower body indices and early stages of disease demonstrated a more favorable outcome with PRP treatment. Therefore, it is important to present the advantages and disadvantages to all patients considering pursuing PRP therapy:

Advantages:

1. Blood sample is easily and safely obtained from peripheral venipuncture.
2. PRP therapy can be performed in an office setting.
3. It is relatively inexpensive compared to other tissue regenerative options.
4. Since the blood sample is obtained directly from the patient, there is low risk of allergic reaction and infection.

Disadvantages:

1. Injection could be very painful as PRP creates an acute inflammatory reaction.
2. The patient is required to avoid NSAIDS days before and several weeks after PRP administration.

Tendinous and ligamentous injuries are the earliest and common conditions that PRP was used to treat and showed good outcomes. PRP is particularly effective in treating injured body parts with tenuous blood supply. As hemostasis of the inflammatory cascade is vascular dependent, poor blood supply impedes optimal delivery of endogenous platelets and growth factors to initiate the tissue healing process. Injections of PRP to these areas can essentially mitigate a decrease in vascular perfusion and "jump start" the healing cascade. The common musculoskeletal pathologies encountered by pain management physicians can be grouped into the following:

1. **Tendon/Ligamentous Injury**
   - *Medial/lateral epicondylopathy/epicondylitis*
   - *Medial/lateral collateral ligament injury*
   - *Anterior cruciate ligament injury*
   - *Patellar tendinopathy*
   - *Rotator cuff tendinopathy*
   - *Achilles tendinopathy*
2. **Cartilage Degeneration**
   - *Acetabular labral tear*
   - *Glenoid labral tear*
   - *Osteoarthritis (OA)*
3. **Muscle Injury**
4. **Degenerative Disc Disease**

Contraindications, relative and absolute, for the use of PRP are listed in Table 87.1.

Evidence for Efficacy

The evidence of PRP therapy is rapidly expanding. At the time of this chapter preparation, PRP search on Pumed.gov alone yielded nearly 4000 publications. The evidence supporting the use of PRP in treating musculoskeletal pathology will undoubtedly continue to grow. The highest level of available evidence with the corresponding musculoskeletal pathologies is tabulated in the order of empirical evidence strength (Table 87.2).

Table 87.1 Relative and absolute contraindications for PRP

Relative contraindications	Absolute contraindications
1. Oncological history 2. History of arthroplasty 3. Pregnancy 4. Smoking 5. Systemic disorder	1. Inflammatory arthritis, e.g., rheumatoid arthritis, gout, and ankylosing spondylitis 2. Active local and systemic infection, e.g., septic arthritis 3. Active malignancy 4. Immunodeficiency 5. Bleeding disorder or thrombocytopenia 6. Hypofibrinogenemia 7. Anemia (hemoglobin less than 11 g/dL) 8. Ongoing NSAID or steroid therapy 9. Complicated anatomy 10. Acute injury 11. Inability to obtain consent or follow post PRP therapy care plans

Table 87.2 PRP evidence table

Quality of evidence assessment	Musculoskeletal pathology
I: Evidence obtained from at least one properly randomized controlled trial	Lateral epicondylopathy/epicondylitis
	Hip OA and labral tear
	Knee pain OA and soft tissue injury
	Maxillofacial surgery
	Shoulder pathology including acromioclavicular joint and rotator cuff injuries
II-1: Evidence from well-designed controlled trials without randomization	Patellar tendinopathy
	Anterior cruciate and medial collateral Ligament repairs
II-2: Evidence from well-designed cohort (prospective or retrospective) or case-control studies, preferably from more than one research group	Achilles tendinopathy
	Plantar fasciitis
	Medial epicondylopathy/epicondylitis
	Lumbar facet joint arthropathy
II-3: Evidence obtained from comparisons between times or places with or without the intervention	Degenerative disc disease

Pearls and Pitfalls

- PRP is safe and effective to induce or accelerate healing and pain relief.
- Despite a lack of coverage by the current insurance system, there is good and growing evidence to support the use of PRP.
- Pain physicians should be familiar with the absolute and relative contraindications to ensure patient safety.
- NSAIDs should be held for at least 7 days and 10 days for steroid before initiating PRP therapy. Following PRP treatment, NSAIDS should not begin within 30 days.
- Multiple repeated PRP injections in the same location may be necessary in order to achieve an optimal clinical outcome.
- Future standardized studies are needed to delineate different tissue disease-specific PRP concentration and composition.

Recommended Reading

1. Al-Ajlouni J, Awidi A, Samara O, et al. Safety and efficacy of autologous intra-articular platelet lysates in early and intermediate knee osteoarthrosis in humans: a prospective open-label study. Clin J Sport Med. 2015;25(6):524–8.
2. Alsousou J, Ali A, Willett K, Harrison P. The role of platelet-rich plasma in tissue regeneration. Platelets. 2013;24(3):173–82.
3. Andia I, Maffulli N. Muscle and tendon injuries: the role of biological interventions to promote and assist healing and recovery. Arthroscopy. 2015;31(5):999–1015.
4. Anitua E, Andia I, Ardanza B, Nurden P, Nurden AT. Autologous platelets as a source of proteins for healing and tissue regeneration. Thromb Haemost. 2004;91(1):4–15.

5. Anitua E, Sánchez M, Zalduendo MM, et al. Fibroblastic response to treatment with different preparations rich in growth factors. Cell Prolif. 2009;42(2):162–70.
6. Assoian RK, Komoriya A, Meyers CA, Miller DM, Sporn MB. Transforming growth factor-beta in human platelets. Identification of a major storage site, purification, and characterization. J Biol Chem. 1983;258(11):7155–60.
7. Basso M, Cavagnaro L, Zanirato A, et al. What is the clinical evidence on regenerative medicine in intervertebral disc degeneration? Musculoskelet Surg [Internet] 2017; Available from: https://doi.org/10.1007/s12306-017-0462-3.
8. Bertrand H, Reeves KD, Bennett CJ, Bicknell S, Cheng A-L. Dextrose prolotherapy versus control injections in painful rotator cuff tendinopathy. Arch Phys Med Rehabil. 2016;97(1):17–25.
9. Boswell SG, Cole BJ, Sundman EA, Karas V, Fortier LA. Platelet-rich plasma: a milieu of bioactive factors. Arthroscopy. 2012;28(3):429–39.
10. Cavallo C, Filardo G, Mariani E, et al. Comparison of Platelet-Rich Plasma formulations for cartilage healing. J Bone Joint Surg Am. 2014;96(5):423–9.
11. Cerza F, Carnì S, Carcangiu A, et al. Comparison between hyaluronic acid and platelet-rich plasma, intra-articular infiltration in the treatment of gonarthrosis. Am J Sports Med. 2012;40(12):2822–7.
12. Chen W-H, Lo W-C, Lee J-J, et al. Tissue-engineered intervertebral disc and chondrogenesis using human nucleus pulposus regulated through TGF-β1 in platelet-rich plasma. J Cell Physiol. 2006;209(3):744–54.
13. Cole BJ, Seroyer ST, Filardo G, Bajaj S, Fortier LA. Platelet-rich plasma: where are we now and where are we going? Sports Health. 2010;2(3):203–10.
14. Crane D, Everts P. Platelet rich plasma (PRP) matrix grafts. Pract Pain Manag. 2008;8(1):11–26.
15. Diehl JW. Platelet-Rich plasma therapy in chronic Achilles Tendinopathy. Tech Foot Ankle Surg. 2011;10(1):2.
16. Ferrari M, Zia S, Valbonesi M, et al. A new technique for hemodilution, preparation of autologous platelet-rich plasma and intraoperative blood salvage in cardiac surgery. Int J Artif Organs. 1987;10(1):47–50.
17. Filardo G, Kon E, Della Villa S, Vincentelli F, Fornasari PM, Marcacci M. Use of platelet-rich plasma for the treatment of refractory jumper's knee. Int Orthop. 2010;34(6):909–15.
18. Foster TE, Puskas BL, Mandelbaum BR, Gerhardt MB, Rodeo SA. Platelet-rich plasma: from basic science to clinical applications. Am J Sports Med. 2009;37(11):2259–72.
19. Gallin JI, Goldstein IM, Snyderman R. Inflammation: basic principles and clinical correlates. Philadelphia: Lippincott Williams & Wilkins; 1999.
20. Ganio C, Tenewitz FE, Wilson RC, Moyles BG. The treatment of chronic nonhealing wounds using autologous platelet-derived growth factors. J Foot Ankle Surg. 1993;32(3):263–8.
21. Golebiewska EM, Poole AW. Platelet secretion: From haemostasis to wound healing and beyond. Blood Rev. 2015;29(3):153–62.
22. Gosens T, Peerbooms JC, van Laar W, den Oudsten BL. Ongoing positive effect of platelet-rich plasma versus corticosteroid injection in lateral epicondylitis: a double-blind randomized controlled trial with 2-year follow-up. Am J Sports Med. 2011;39(6):1200–8.
23. Gui K, Ren W, Yu Y, Li X, Dong J, Yin W. Inhibitory effects of platelet-rich plasma on intervertebral disc degeneration: a preclinical study in a rabbit model. Med Sci Monit. 2015;21:1368–75.
24. Gullung GB, Woodall JW, Tucci MA, James J, Black DA, McGuire RA. Platelet-rich plasma effects on degenerative disc disease: analysis of histology and imaging in an animal model. Evid Based Spine Care J. 2011;2(4):13–8.
25. Hamilton B, Tol JL, Knez W, Chalabi H. Exercise and the platelet activator calcium chloride both influence the growth factor content of platelet-rich plasma (PRP): overlooked biochemical factors that could influence PRP treatment. Br J Sports Med. 2015;49(14):957–60.
26. Heldin CH, Westermark B, Wasteson A. Platelet-derived growth factor. Isolation by a large-scale procedure and analysis of subunit composition. Biochem J. 1981;193(3):907–13.
27. Hohaus C, Ganey TM, Minkus Y, Meisel HJ. Cell transplantation in lumbar spine disc degeneration disease. Eur Spine J. 2008;17(Suppl 4):492–503.
28. Jang S-J, Kim J-D, Cha S-S. Platelet-rich plasma (PRP) injections as an effective treatment for early osteoarthritis. Eur J Orthop Surg Traumatol. 2013;23(5):573–80.
29. Karey KP, Sirbasku DA. Human platelet-derived mitogens. II. Subcellular localization of insulinlike growth factor I to the alpha-granule and release in response to thrombin. Blood. 1989;74(3):1093–100.
30. Kepler CK, Anderson DG, Tannoury C, Ponnappan RK. Intervertebral disk degeneration and emerging biologic treatments. J Am Acad Orthop Surg. 2011;19(9):543–53.
31. Kevy S, Jacobson M. Preparation of growth factors enriched autologous platelet gel (2001) Proceedings of the 27 th Annual Meeting of Service Biomaterials. April [Links].
32. Knighton DR, Ciresi K, Fiegel VD, Schumerth S, Butler E, Cerra F. Stimulation of repair in chronic, nonhealing, cutaneous ulcers using platelet-derived wound healing formula. Surg Gynecol Obstet. 1990;170(1):56–60.
33. Kon E, Mandelbaum B, Buda R, et al. Platelet-Rich plasma intra-articular injection versus hyaluronic acid viscosupplementation as treatments for cartilage pathology: from early degeneration to osteoarthritis. Arthroscopy. 2011;27(11):1490–501.
34. Li J, Chen J, Kirsner R. Pathophysiology of acute wound healing. Clin Dermatol. 2007;25(1):9–18.
35. Lind M. Growth factor stimulation of bone healing. Effects on osteoblasts, osteotomies, and implants fixation. Acta Orthop Scand Suppl. 1998;283:2–37.
36. Marx RE. Platelet-rich plasma: evidence to support its use. J Oral Maxillofac Surg. 2004;62(4):489–96.
37. Middleton KK, Barro V, Muller B, Terada S, Fu FH. Evaluation of the effects of platelet-rich plasma (PRP) therapy involved in the healing of sports-related soft tissue injuries. Iowa Orthop J. 2012;32:150–63.
38. Möhle R, Green D, Moore MAS, Nachman RL, Rafii S. Constitutive production and thrombin-induced release of vascular endothelial growth factor by human megakaryocytes and platelets. Proc Natl Acad Sci. 1997;94(2):663–8.
39. Nagae M, Ikeda T, Mikami Y, et al. Intervertebral disc regeneration using platelet-rich plasma and biodegradable gelatin hydrogel microspheres. Tissue Eng. 2007;13(1):147–58.
40. Nguyen RT, Borg-Stein J, McInnis K. Applications of platelet-rich plasma in musculoskeletal and sports medicine: an evidence-based approach. PM R. 2011;3(3):226–50.
41. Niemansburg SL, van Delden JJM, Oner FC, Dhert WJA, Bredenoord AL. Ethical implications of regenerative medicine in orthopedics: an empirical study with surgeons and scientists in the field. Spine J. 2014;14(6):1029–35.
42. Patel S, Dhillon MS, Aggarwal S, Marwaha N, Jain A. Treatment with platelet-rich plasma is more effective than placebo for knee osteoarthritis: a prospective, double-blind, randomized trial. Am J Sports Med. 2013;41(2):356–64.
43. Peebooms J, et al. Positive effect of an autologous platelet concentrate in lateral epicondylitis in a double-blind randomized controlled trial. Am J Sports Med. 2009;38(2):255–62.
44. Pourcho AM, Smith J, Wisniewski SJ, Sellon JL. Intraarticular platelet-rich plasma injection in the treatment of knee osteoarthritis: review and recommendations. Am J Phys Med Rehabil. 2014;93(11 Suppl 3):S108–21.

45. Ruggeri ZM. Platelets in atherothrombosis. Nat Med. 2002;8(11):1227–34.
46. Sadoghi P, Lohberger B, Aigner B, et al. Effect of platelet-rich plasma on the biologic activity of the human rotator-cuff fibroblasts: a controlled in vitro study. J Orthop Res. 2013;31(8):1249–53.
47. Sánchez M, Fiz N, Azofra J, et al. A randomized clinical trial evaluating plasma rich in growth factors (PRGF-Endoret) versus hyaluronic acid in the short-term treatment of symptomatic knee osteoarthritis. Arthroscopy. 2012;28(8):1070–8.
48. Sawamura K, Ikeda T, Nagae M, et al. Characterization of in vivo effects of platelet-rich plasma and biodegradable gelatin hydrogel microspheres on degenerated intervertebral discs. Tissue Eng Part A. 2009;15(12):3719–27.
49. Serhan CN, Ward PA, Gilroy DW. Fundamentals of inflammation: Cambridge University Press; 2010.
50. Sun Y, Feng Y, Zhang CQ, Chen SB, Cheng XG. The regenerative effect of platelet-rich plasma on healing in large osteochondral defects. Int Orthop. 2010;34(4):589–97.
51. Tetschke E, Rudolf M, Lohmann CH, Stärke C. Autologous proliferative therapies in recalcitrant lateral epicondylitis. Am J Phys Med Rehabil. 2015;94(9):696–706.
52. Thanasas C, Papadimitriou G, Charalambidis C, Paraskevopoulos I, Papanikolaou A. Platelet-rich plasma versus autologous whole blood for the treatment of chronic lateral elbow epicondylitis: a randomized controlled clinical trial. Am J Sports Med. 2011;39(10):2130–4.
53. Tinsley BA, Ferreira JV, Dukas AG, Mazzocca AD. Platelet-Rich plasma nonoperative injection therapy—a review of indications and evidence. Oper Tech Sports Med. 2012;20(2):192–200.
54. Tozum TF, Demiralp B. Platelet-rich plasma: a promising innovation in dentistry. J Can Dent Assoc. 2003;69(10):664–5.
55. Vora A, Borg-Stein J, Nguyen RT. Regenerative injection therapy for osteoarthritis: fundamental concepts and evidence-based review. PM R. 2012;4(5 Suppl):S104–9.
56. Walter JB, Israel MS. General Pathology. 6th ed. Edinburg: Churchill Livingstone; 1987. p. 151–3.
57. Weibrich G, Hansen T, Kleis W, Buch R, Hitzler WE. Effect of platelet concentration in platelet-rich plasma on peri-implant bone regeneration. Bone. 2004;34(4):665–71.
58. Whitman DH, Berry RL, Green DM. Platelet gel: an autologous alternative to fibrin glue with applications in oral and maxillofacial surgery. J Oral Maxillofac Surg. 1997;55(11):1294–9.
59. Wroblewski AP, Mejia HA, Wright VJ. Application of Platelet-Rich plasma to enhance tissue repair. Oper Tech Orthop 2010/6;20(2):98–105.
60. Wu J, Du Z, Lv Y, et al. A new technique for the treatment of Lumbar Facet joint syndrome using intra-articular injection with autologous Platelet Rich plasma. Pain Physician. 2016;19(8):617–25.

Scientific Basis for Stem Cell Therapy

88

Luke A. Law, Christine L. Hunt, and Wenchun Qu

Introduction

The body's ability to regenerate and heal damaged tissues is awe inspiring. Understandably, the mechanisms responsible for this regenerative capacity have garnered intense interest from the scientific community, with broad applications to multiple fields of medicine. The field of stem cell research is expanding rapidly in research and clinical practice, including for musculoskeletal and pain medicine. Current investigations have shown promise for many autoimmune diseases including rheumatoid arthritis, systemic lupus erythematosus, multiple sclerosis, systemic sclerosis, Crohn's disease, autoimmune cytopenias, and diabetes mellitus, among others. Stem cells have shown efficacy for multiple neurologic disorders such as amyotrophic lateral sclerosis, Parkinson's disease, spinal cord lesions, Huntington's disease, stroke, and vision loss. Chronic conditions including heart failure, cirrhosis, hair reconstitution, disorders of hematopoiesis, and muscular dystrophies also show promise as therapeutic targets. Of particular interest in the treatment of chronic pain are the applications of cell therapy to painful diseases such as critical limb ischemia, osteoarthritis and other bone and cartilage defects, neuropathic pain, discogenic pain, ligamentous and tendinous injuries, as well as nerve injury. Further, exciting opportunities occur at the intersection of bioengineering and stem cells. One example from 2008 was the successful in vitro growth and transplant of a new trachea using a decellularized trachea seeded with autologous mesenchymal stem cells (MSCs) or stromal cells. From more accurate and personalized drug testing platforms, improved developmental models, and both direct and indirect tissue repairs, stem cells have enormous potential to benefit the human condition and further medicine.

L. A. Law
Department of Anesthesiology, Mayo Clinic, Rochester, MN, USA

C. L. Hunt
Department of Physical Medicine and Rehabilitation, Mayo Clinic, Rochester, MN, USA

W. Qu (✉)
Department of Physical Medicine and Rehabilitation, Division of Pain Medicine, Spine Center, Mayo Clinic, Rochester, MN, USA
e-mail: qu.wenchun@mayo.edu

History and Background

Stem Cell Potency

A stem cell is a cell that consists of two basic characteristics: the ability to undergo self-renewal and the ability to differentiate into two or more cell lines. Self-renewal is the process by which stem cells divide without undergoing differentiation, with each of the daughter cells retaining their undifferentiated stem cell potential. When subject to the correct environmental factors, this undifferentiated stem cell can differentiate into the proper cell type, as is the second basic characteristic of stem cells. Not all stem cells possess equal potency in regard to the ability to differentiate, and this leads to a natural means of categorization. The most potent of all stem cells occurs with the fertilization of an egg by a sperm. The resultant cell is termed a zygote and is a cell capable of reproducing to form every cell, tissue type, and structure in the body. This cell is totipotent – the ability to become a total living organism – and the zygote is the sole example. Very quickly, cells start to lose the number of lineages into which they can differentiate. After only a few rounds of cell division, the zygote develops into the inner cell mass (ICM) and the trophoblast. The ICM cells are capable of dividing into all cells comprising an embryo, but cannot divide into the extraembryonic structures such as the placenta. ICMs are pluripotent, defined as able to differentiate into all embryonic tissues – in other words tissues of endoderm, mesoderm, or ectoderm lineage. Examples of pluripotent cells include ICM where embryonic stem cells (ESC) are derived from and induced pluripotent stem cells (iPSCs). Adult stem cells are comprised of multipotent, oligopotent, or unipotent cells.

T. R. Deer et al. (eds.), *Deer's Treatment of Pain*, https://doi.org/10.1007/978-3-030-12281-2_88

Table 88.1 Stem cell potency

Potency	Tissue source	Differentiates to	Example
Totipotent	Embryonic cells	All cell types including placenta	Zygote
Pluripotent	Embryonic stem cells	All endoderm, mesoderm, or ectoderm	ESC
	Adult cells	All endoderm, mesoderm, or ectoderm	iPSCs
Multipotent	Adult stem cells	More than one cell type, often closely related	HSC, NSC, MSC
Oligopotent	Adult stem cells	Several cell types in a tissue	CMP, CLP
Unipotent	Adult stem cells	One cell type	Satellite cell

ESC embryonic stem cell, *iPSC* induced pluripotent stem cell, *HSC* hematopoietic stem cell, *NSC* neural stem cell, *MSC* mesenchymal stem cell, *CMP* common myeloid progenitor, *CLP* common lymphoid progenitor

Multipotent stem cells are capable of dividing to form all lineages of a specific tissue/organ. Examples include hematopoietic stem cells (HSC) and neural stem cells (NSC). Oligopotent stem cells can produce several but not all of the lineages for a tissue/organ with examples including common myeloid progenitor (CMP) and common lymphoid progenitor (CLP) cells. The least potent stem cells are termed unipotent and are only capable of producing a single lineage of a tissue. An example is satellite cells which give rise to a single cell type, muscle cells. A summary of stem cell potency can be found in Table 88.1.

Embryonic Stem Cells

Broadly, stem cells may be categorized into two main groups: adult stem cells and embryonic stem cells (ESC). ESCs derive from the ICM and are not ordinarily present in the postnatal body. Martin Evans and Gail Martin independently established and described the first tissue culture of pluripotent ESCs in 1981 utilizing a mouse model. This allowed for the close study of developmental biology and hope for the discovery of many drugs; however, mouse biology proved to be sufficiently different from human biology to temper some of the initial enthusiasm. Many other cell lines were established from various species, but it wasn't until 1998 when James Thomson and colleagues were able to establish a line of human ESC. Thomson put forward three properties to define primate ESCs as (i) derived from the pre- or peri-implantation embryo, (ii) capable of prolonged proliferation without differentiation, and (iii) possessing developmental potential to produce all three germ layers even after many passes in culture. ESCs make ideal cells for regenerative medicine and hold significant promise for understanding developmental biology. However, there has been significant resistance for implementation and research due to ethical concerns related to their origin. In 1996 the Dickey-Wicker Amendment prohibited the use of federal funds for ESC research. This was followed by a period of political debate, until President Barack Obama's executive order in 2009 allowing for responsible research on the topic. This was challenged in court shortly after as a violation of the Dickey-Wicker Amendment but ultimately was upheld in 2011.

In the midst of this controversy (2006), Yamanaka and Takahashi described the induction of mouse somatic cells to dedifferentiate into a pluripotent state via the introduction of retroviral-mediated ectopic expression of four genes: *Oct3/4*, *Sox2*, *Klf4*, and *c-Myc*. Within a year Thomson and Yamanaka had reproduced the process in human cells, and by 2010 hundreds of papers had been published on the topic. The first clinical trial in humans utilizing iPSCs was in 2014 in one patient with macular degeneration. Skin fibroblasts were taken and transformed to autologous iPSCs, grown into sheets of retinal pigment epithelium cells, and then implanted resulting in "brightening" of the patient's vision and halting of her macular degeneration. The trial was quickly halted, however, due to the detection of DNA, copy number changes in the iPSCs of the second patient. The second patient additionally demonstrated a modest response to the more traditional anti-VEGF therapy and so did not undergo the iPSC procedure.

Adult Stem Cells

In contrast to ESCs, adult stem cells reside in many tissues of the body, though it remains unclear if every tissue contains a dedicated population of cells. As opposed to ESCs, adult stem cells remain in a quiescent state, also known as G_0, for the majority of their existence, and only upon sufficient stimulus will they activate to replenish and repair damaged tissues in a manner consistent with and to maintain homeostasis. A key function of this G_0 state is to preserve the ability to differentiate and maintain a population of cells ready to respond to injury, and recent data propose this is not a passive process but rather an actively maintained state. When adult stem cells do divide, they do so by asymmetrical division, where one of the daughter cells retains its "stemness" and the other differentiates to the appropriate cell. After a period of time, this differentiated daughter cell will die and be replaced by another cell which itself originated from a stem cell through asymmetrical division. In this manner the adult organism is maintained in homeostasis.

The first rigorous description of "stem cells" was pioneered by Ernest McCulloch and James Till in the 1960s using a mouse model. They were investigating regeneration within the blood system in vivo. They irradiated mice with a 250 rads X-ray, implanted nucleated bone marrow cells, and then re-irradiated the mice 4 hours later with 650 rads utilizing a cobalt-60 γ-ray source. After 11 days, the mice were sacrificed, the spleen was examined, and colonies of the transplanted cells were found. These cells had the interesting characteristics of self-replication and the ability to differentiate into three lines: erythrocyte, granulocytic, and megakaryocytic cells. These cells are known as hematopoietic stem cells (HSCs) and demonstrate the same capacity for multi-lineage differentiation and self-renewal as other adult stem cells. They are used clinically for treatment of various hematologic diseases and are harvested from primarily bone marrow, peripheral blood, and cord blood. HSC transplant is commonly used for treatment of loss of function of hematopoietic cells, whether from genetic or immunologic disease states, neoplasm, reconstitution of hematopoietic capacity following chemotherapy, induction of tolerance, or graft-versus-tumor disease. The use of HSCs for the treatment of pain is limited, and therefore this chapter will focus on MSCs and pluripotent cells (ESCs and iPSCs).

In the 1960s, Alexander Friedenstein began working with MSCs, demonstrating these cells had the capacity to differentiate into multiple mesenchymal tissues including osteoblasts, chondrocytes, and adipocytes. The classic paradigm posited that these cells would migrate to sites of injury and then engraft and differentiate to the appropriate tissue type to regenerate the tissue. This has been challenged, however, from observations which suggest far too few MSCs engraft and/or are not present for sufficient lengths of time to functionally replace the injured tissue. This led researches on a hunt to fully explain the observed therapeutic effects of MSCs. Newer evidence points toward the combined effects of paracrine activity, cell-cell interactions, and release of extracellular vesicles (EVs) along with direct engraftment as the primary mechanisms of action which will be described below. These mechanisms combine to decrease cell apoptosis, promote cell survival, and modulate the immune response. Each of these effects is beneficial to the pain management practitioner and can result in decreased inflammation and regeneration of damaged tissue with resolution of (or at least decrease in) the pain the tissue defects caused.

MSCs have been derived from multiple mesodermal tissues including dental pulp bone marrow, adipose tissue, synovial membrane, breast milk, umbilical cord, urine, peripheral blood, amniotic fluid, periodontal ligament, hair follicle, placenta, and endometrium. In clinical practice and research involving MSCs in the field of pain medicine, bone marrow and adipose tissue are the most commonly used sources due to the relative abundance of MSC concentration in these sources and ease of harvest and preparation. For more information regarding their application in discogenic back pain, please refer to Chap. 94.

Classification of Mesenchymal Stem Cells

MSCs are multipotent adult tissue progenitor cells that have attracted great attention in musculoskeletal medicine for their immunomodulatory and paracrine effects, particularly for management of degenerative joint and intervertebral disc conditions. They are defined by the International Society for Cellular Therapy to possess the characteristics of adherence to plastic, specific cell surface markers (CD44+, CD73+, CD90+, CD105+, CD271+, CD34−, CD45−, CD31−, Stro-1 +, HLA-DR-) and the ability to differentiate into adipocytic, chondrocytic, and osteogenic cell lines. MSCs may be classified according to preparation strategy, see Fig. 88.1 and Table 88.2. First generation (G1): tissue with MSCs can be extracted by processes that do not alter the relevant biological characteristics of cells or tissues for homologous use in the same surgical setting, meeting the FDA's criteria for "minimal manipulation." The most common sources of MSCs for office-based practices are bone marrow and adipose tissue. Second generation (G2): MSCs may be selected according to surface markers and undergo culture expansion yielding a significantly larger dosage concentration, overcoming one of the main limitations of first-generation MSCs. Additionally, the decreased heterogeneity and improved quality control are attractive for clinical use and research. The G2 culture-expanded MSCs have been the most prevalently studied in current clinical trials for application in neurologic, cardiac, renal, and MSK conditions. Third generation (G3): MSCs can be further lineage-directed by culturing in a cocktail of bioactive molecules, an approach that enhances the MSCs' target tissue specificity and efficacy. Fourth generation (G4): gene therapy and gene editing technology make it possible to change the MSCs' phenotype for intended effect, such as reducing inflammatory responses and increasing matrix content for degenerative MSK conditions. Fifth generation (G5): induced pluripotent stem cells (iPSCs) are reprogrammed adult cells that are pluripotent and similar to an embryonic stem cell. Unlike MSCs that may be present in target tissue after transplantation for only a limited duration, iPSCs are immortal and may provide a cell source for cartilage and disc repair by directly differentiating to and sustaining the tissue volume.

MSCs in Musculoskeletal Disease

MSCs are used in a myriad of musculoskeletal disorders, and many clinical trials and retrospective studies have been published investigating the safety and preliminary efficacy of MSCs. Current treatment options often include physical therapy, pain medication, steroid injections, and surgical intervention. These measures are palliative by nature, treating the symptoms and not addressing the cellular and

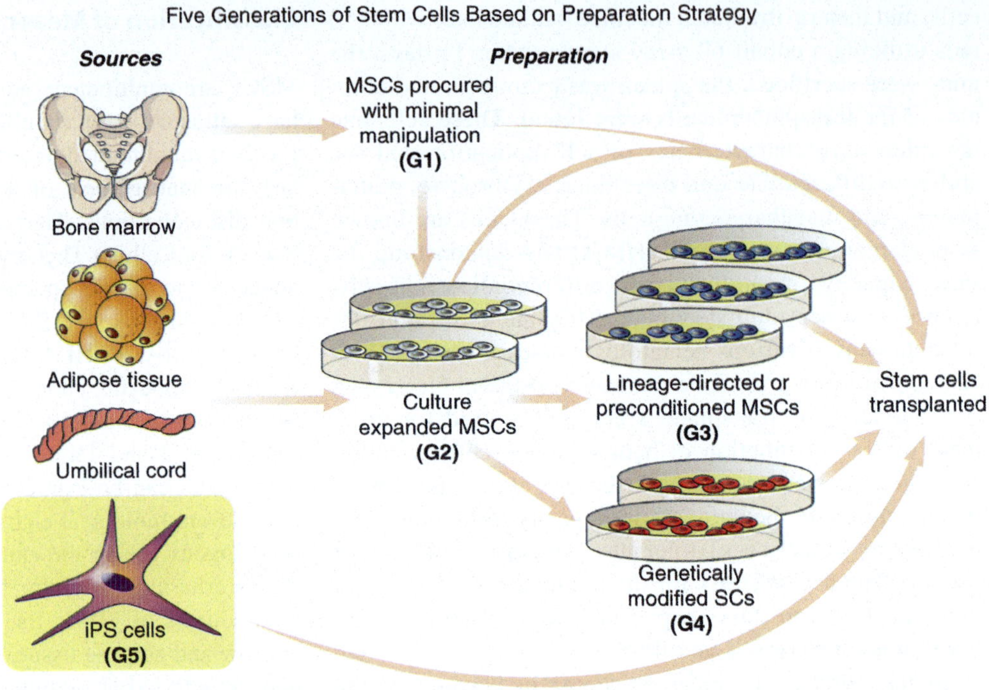

Fig. 88.1 Sources and means of production of mesenchymal stem cells. MSC, mesenchymal stem cells; iPS, induced pluripotent stem cells; G1, first generation; G2, second generation; G3, third generation; G4, fourth generation; G5, fifth generation

Table 88.2 Generations of MSCs

Generation	Preparation	Advantages	Notes
1	Minimal manipulation Enzymatic degradation is not G1	Meets criteria for surgical exemption for point-of-care application	Bone marrow aspirate and adipose graft are most commonly used
2	Culture expanded	Increased dose concentration	cGMP to ensure identity, strength, quality, and purity
3	Preconditioned MSCs Lineage-directed MSCs	Enhancement of desired properties	Preconditioned with growth factors/cytokines
4	Genetically modified	Targeted enhancement of desired properties	Technologies include viral modes of gene delivery and genetic editing technology
5	iPSCs	Immortal phenotype for tissue repair Pluripotent	Safety concerns

molecular processes that underlay these conditions. The immunomodulatory and trophic effects of MSCs offer a possible solution to actually correct these problems in addition to symptom management.

Eight studies utilizing first-generation (G1 – minimally manipulated) MSCs have been published for musculoskeletal (MSK) conditions. In 5 studies a total of 784 patients received bone marrow aspirate concentrate (BMAC), and 65 patients in 3 studies received peripheral blood-derived stem cells (PBSCs). No serious adverse events were reported, but nonserious adverse events included swelling at the injection site, transient and self-resolving pain, and warmth. The primary take-away from these studies is a strong safety signal across a variety of pathologies; however, they also demonstrated low-level evidence for improvement of pain and function. Three randomized controlled trials (RCTs) provided Level 2 evidence that BMAC injection in knee osteoarthritis improved pain and function (measured by clinical scores), with corresponding improvement in assessment by MRI. Other studies investigated the use of BMAC for degenerative disc disease (DDD), chronic patellar tendinopathy, and femoral head osteonecrosis. Again no serious adverse events were reported, and positive clinical outcomes were seen; no definitive conclusions are drawn given small study sizes.

Second-generation MSCs (G2) have significantly more studies conducted that established safety of a cell dosage between 2 and 50 × 10^6 for intra-articular knee injection. A systematic review of clinical trials investigating the use of MSCs for the treatment of painful degenerative disc disease (DDD) identified six studies involving human subjects, five of which were phase I studies that found culturally expanded MSCs to be generally safe and well-tolerated with no serious adverse events. This review also highlighted three ongoing phase II studies looking at MSCs for treatment of DDD and one ongoing phase III study investigating DDD.

The majority of human trials utilizing MSCs are phase I studies. A larger phase II trial for DDD with culturally expanded MSCs (G2) found significant improvement in pain and function in patients who received MSC injection as compared to controls. The initial research has proved promising; however, further research is required. There has been no report in the application of lineage-directed (G3) or genetically modified MSCs (G4) for treatment of MSK conditions.

MSCs in Neuropathic Pain

Neuropathic pain is characterized by pain following lesion or disease of the nervous system with the common symptoms of spontaneous and evoked types of pain and is present in about 3–9% of the population. The pathophysiology of neuropathic pain is complex and includes alterations in the function, structure, and local environment of the nervous system resulting in altered sensorium and aberrant response to stimuli. In the periphery, the production of multiple mediators including cytokines and growth factors, alterations in Na^+ and Ca^{++} channel density/activity, and proliferation of nerve endings result in upregulated pain signals reaching the central nervous system. In the central nervous system, stimulation of the N-methyl-D-aspartate (NMDA) receptor, increased production of growth factors, and brain-derived neurotrophic factor along with altered inhibitory signals propagate and reinforce neuronal hyperexcitability. Traditional therapy includes opioids, anticonvulsants, antidepressants, NMDA antagonists, and topical agents. Unfortunately, neuropathic pain can be highly refractory to treatment with significant impairment of quality of life.

Neuropathic pain occurs with central nervous system as well as peripheral nerve conditions and injuries. After suffering a spinal cord injury (SCI), the majority of patients suffer from some degree of chronic neuropathic pain. Multiple preclinical trials have demonstrated promising results for the potential role of MSCs in functional recovery following SCI. More recently, Yousefifard et al. demonstrated not only functional improvement but improvement in neuropathic pain as well. Using a compression model of SCI in rats, Yousefifard et al. transplanted one million cells of either bone marrow- or umbilical cord-derived MSCs and showed improvement in functional recovery, allodynia, and hyperalgesia. Cheng et al. have shown in a chronic constriction injury model of the sciatic nerve in rats that both intravenous and intrathecal transplantations of MSCs significantly decreased the rats' neuropathic pain. No significant difference was found between intravenous and intrathecal injection, and no signs of toxicity were found.

In humans, two recent small studies have shown positive response to MSC injections. The first from Vickers et al. recruited ten subjects with trigeminal neuralgia. They obtained autologous stromal vascular fraction MSCs (lipoaspirate, digested with collagenase, not cultured) and injected this in a perineural fashion. The total cell count of injectate was 33–162 million cells with a viability of 62–91%. The results were a significant decrease in mean standard numerical pain scale from 7.5 to 4.3 with a concordant significant decrease in neuropathic pain medication use at 6 months. The second study from Venturi et al. recruited 15 females with pudendal neuralgia not responsive to medical therapy. Autologous lipoaspirate was injected. Significant improvement of VAS scores, SF-36 scores, and trend toward improvement in pudendal nerve motor terminal latency (PNMTL) at 12 months was reported. While these results are promising, they are both small non-randomized studies, and more research is warranted. No adverse effects related to treatment were reported.

Mechanism of Action

The mechanism of action of MSCs is complex and multifactorial. MSCs utilize a combination of mechanisms to influence native tissues with immunomodulation, paracrine, direct cell-to-cell, and extracellular vesicle activities. Additionally, iPSCs (G5) are expected to engraft, produce these active molecules continuously, and directly repair tissue. The end result of these mechanisms includes reduction of inflammatory activities, promotion of native cell survival, decreased apoptosis, and ultimately tissue repair.

Immunomodulation

The immune modulation component of the therapeutic mechanism of action of MSCs is thought to be caused by T-cell inhibition via both non-apoptotic and apoptotic pathways as well as modulation of macrophage and B-cell activity. Multiple studies have demonstrated marked inhibition of inflammatory T cells using mixed lymphocyte reaction (MLR) assays in a histocompatibility complex independent and non-apoptotic fashion. The soluble factors responsible for this T-cell inhibition include transforming growth factor beta (TGF-β), hepatocyte growth factor (HGF), and prostaglandin E2 (PGE2) that ultimately upregulate the anti-inflammatory cytokine interleukin IL-10 and reducing secretion of the pro-inflammatory TNFα and IL-2. The net result is a predilection for the anti-inflammatory T helper (T_H) 2 subtype over the T_H1 pro-inflammatory subtype and suppression of inflammation.

MSCs also induce apoptosis of T cells via the Fas-Fas ligand interaction which then stimulates native T cells to differentiate toward (T_{reg}) cells. This is helped by T-cell debris stimulation of activated phagocytes to secrete TGF-β. Additionally, MSC expression of indoleamine-2,3-dioxygenase (IDO) catalyzes the tryptophan to kynurenine reaction. This is significant as kynurenine also inhibits T-cell proliferation. Nitrous oxide (NO) also seems to play a role, but the extent of this role is not well defined. The net result is a decrease in the inflammatory cascade from T cells and an upregulation of the anti-inflammatory T_{reg} cells which promotes tissue healing and decreased pain.

MSCs also temper the activity of macrophages, decreasing their secretion of inflammatory factors (TNFα, IL1β, IL6) in response to stimulus. In the presence of TNFα, MSCs are stimulated to produce TNFα-stimulated gene protein (TSG)6 which then inhibits macrophage release of TNFα by activation at the CD44 receptor and downstream inhibition of NFkB. This is a direct negative feedback loop. Additionally, in response to TNFα, MSCs also secrete PGE2. This induces macrophages to upregulate the anti-inflammatory IL10 which strengthens the negative feedback loop from TSG6. Further, MSCs by both paracrine and direct action decrease activity and proliferation of B cells.

In summary, particularly in response to stress or activated immune cells, MSCs secrete biologically active factors or directly stimulate immune cells to reduce inflammation and temper pro-inflammatory immune activation.

Trophic Effects: Enhancing Native Cell Survival

MSCs promote cell survival in healthy tissue as well as promote injury repair and regeneration in stressed tissues. They may even rescue injured cells that would otherwise die. MSCs secrete a vast array of paracrine factors, known as a secretome, which includes factors that enhance native cell survival. These so-called trophic factors are comprised of a large number of cytokines and growth factors which collectively serve to create a microenvironment conducive to survival of HSCs, repair of tissue damage and areas of ischemia, inhibition of fibrosis and apoptosis, promotion of angiogenesis, and stimulation of already present progenitor cells to increase their own regenerative potential. Thus, MSCs should not be thought of as directly replacing tissue, rather creating a supportive microenvironment and inducing native tissue repair mechanisms. The effects of this paracrine action last considerably longer than the life of transplanted MSCs, do not require long-term engraftment, and can be influential even at large distances. For example, following IV injection, the majority of MSCs will be sequestered in the lung vasculature but appear to have effects at distant targets. Further, MSCs have demonstrated preclinical efficacy as anti-fibrotic agents likely from their immunomodulating properties, inhibition of fibroblasts, and reduction of oxidative stress. This has significant implications for treatment of inflammatory conditions and musculoskeletal diseases which are one of the most common pain generators.

MSCs can also transfer mitochondria to neighboring cells by means of tunneling nanotubes (TNTs) rescuing cells from oxidative stress. RNA, other organelles, and proteins are also transferred by MSCs in this fashion. When co-cultured with epithelial cells deficient of functional mitochondria, MSCs were able to restore the epithelial cells' aerobic respiration by this mechanism. This oxidative repair ability becomes more pronounced when the receiving cells are under stress. This effect has also been demonstrated in vivo in eye and lung models, and it has been shown that the TNTs do not require strict cell-cell contact and can be steered toward the stressed recipient cell. The transfer of mitochondria is also an attractive option being investigated as a vector for the transfer of genetic information.

Extracellular Vesicles: Exosomes and Microvesicles

The paracrine effects of MSCs may in large part be due to packaging of bioactive factors into small membrane bound vesicles known as extracellular vesicles (EVs). EVs include 1–5 μm apoptotic bodies, endocytic 30–100 nm exosomes, and non-endocytic 50–1000 nms microvesicles (MVs). EVs are exceedingly common and are secreted by nearly all somatic cell lineages. The workhorse of this system for MSCs appears to be MVs and exosomes. Hundreds of different active molecules have been recovered from MVs secreted from MSCs. The mechanism of MV packaging and composition is not fully understood; however, they have been demonstrated to contain lipids, protein, microRNAs, precursor microRNAs, mRNAs, transfer RNA, and myriad trophic factors, growth factors, and cytokines. MVs in preclinical trials have shown the ability to reduce apoptosis following ischemic injury in multiple tissues, reduce inflammation, and increase cell proliferation supporting tissue repair. The specific factors that have the protective and immunomodulating effects require further research and remain an exciting area of investigation. MVs represent an attractive therapeutic option as they may capture much of the paracrine function of MSCs without the corresponding concerns of engraftment, immune reactions, or development of ectopic tissue. They could also be mass-producible to develop an "off-the-shelf" allogeneic product and circumvent the need to develop a proprietary preparation for each patient.

Mesenchymal Stem Cell Survival

MSCs were long thought to be completely immune privileged – able to survive immunocompatibility-mismatched allogeneic and even xenogeneic transplants. The mechanism for these observations seem to be threefold: (1) MSCs are hypoimmunogenic, (2) modulation of T-cell phenotype, and (3) local immunosuppression. This could allow for a universal donor and centralized cell lines for large-scale treatment. However, recently some evidence challenging the status of complete immune privilege has emerged, which shows that in certain circumstances, MSCs can be rejected, although this happens significantly slower than would be expected with other allogeneic cell types. Strategies to prolong MSC survival are being investigated, often borrowing from solid organ transplant models. Additionally, genetic engineering of MSCs to reduce immunogenicity (by permanently suppressing MHC class I, e.g.) is also being investigated.

The Future of Pluripotent Stem Cells: Induced and Embryonic

Induced pluripotent stem cells (iPSCs) were first described in 2006 through the use of the four factors OCT4, SOX2, KLF4, and MYC (OSKM). Within a year in 2007, human iPSCs had been described following a similar protocol. This has resulted in the promise of significant progress in the fields of disease modeling, drug discovery, and regenerative medicine.

The first uses for iPSCs were the modeling of diseases in the petri dish and drug discovery. The promise of personalized medicine drives this field, with one end goal being the development of real-time patient specific in vitro disease and target models to test response to different drugs and the discovery of side effects prior to drug administration. A second exciting field is the investigation of disease models, with the expectation being humans cell models should be superior to the current animal models. This holds true so long as the iPSCs can be reliably induced to demonstrate the characteristics of the desired cell types. iPSCs have also garnered significant interest in the field of regenerative medicine for ease of collection and regenerative capacity of embryological tissues.

The mechanism of OSKM action is complex and is thought to involve a positive feedback loop of waves of transcription resulting in activation of an entire network of pluripotency genes and inhibition of pro-differentiation genes. The resulting cascade of epigenetic changes involves genome-wide modifications to histone and DNA methylation, preceding phenotypic changes. Unfortunately, this process is often incomplete. Aberrations are found in the product iPSCs making safety a major concern in their adoption for clinical use. The use of CRISPR-Cas9 technology and future technologies which increase the specificity of genetic engineering is improving and helps address these concerns. However, significant challenges remain including the very high cost of research and development as well as continued difficulty with off-target effects. Further, the very properties which make these cells so attractive, namely, pluripotency and endless self-renewal, are the same properties that raise concerns regarding tumorigenesis. An ESC study from Geron for spinal cord injury was suspended in 2009 when mice in the dose escalation arm developed cysts at the regenerating tissue sites. Five patients were treated before the trial was suspended, and at their 3-year follow-up, no serious adverse events were reported. Both ocular tumors and neural overgrowths have been shown in mouse-based models, as well as in primate models. ESCs have shown tumorigenicity in humans as well, including a young boy transplanted with fetal ESCs for ataxia telangiectasia. No tumors have been seen with iPSCs in humans; however significant caution is warranted, especially as the induction process causes widespread epigenetic changes. Multiple strategies for diminishing the risk of tumorigenicity are being investigated, including vector delivery methods such as non-integrating vectors including plasmids and epichromosomal viruses or excisable vectors such as flanking of vectors by loxP sites. Other attractive options include dispensing with c-MYC and replacing the viral vectors with small molecules.

The clinical potential for human iPSC therapy to regenerate damaged tissues directly or instigate endogenous regenerative capacity has garnered considerable interest from the scientific community. Many of the current studies using ESCs and iPSCs are for macular degeneration or are in preclinical stages. One interesting report from 2016 was a total quadriplegic patient treated with ESCs who had successful recovery of motor function in the upper extremities at 2 months as part of the SCiStar study (www.scistar-study.com). As described above only one clinical trial has used iPSCs with only one patient treated before being suspended – though that patient experienced no adverse events and improvement in her macular degeneration. iPSCs can escape the immunosuppression required for ESCs, particularly when developed autologously; however, this is expensive and slow, limiting clinical utility. If the immunogenicity problems of allogeneic iPSCs can be solved and the long validation time and quality assurance for the cell lines are circumvented, many common and acute problems such as myocardial infarctions and stroke become more practical therapeutic targets.

Further research is beginning to investigate the creation of organoids or structures which resemble entire organs. These represent an exciting avenue for more thorough drug testing systems and as possible future candidates for transplantation of virtually any tissue. For example, Koo and Huch et al. have recently developed a protocol for growing stomach, liver, pancreas, and small intestine organoids, and these could in the short term improve drug modeling and physiological assays and, in the long term, play a significant role in regeneration of these tissues. Given the possibilities, iPSCs continue to generate intense interest.

Main Points

- Stem cells are an established field of research with many current and exciting possibilities and a well-established safety profile.
- MSCs in clinical use today have demonstrated efficacy in treating musculoskeletal and neuropathic pain. They also offer a potential cure via repair and regeneration in the case of degeneration or injury. Their beneficial effects include immunomodulatory, trophic, anti-apoptotic, and pro-survival effects. These effects are moderated by paracrine, cell-cell interactions, direct engraftment, and extracellular vesicles.
- iPSCs represent an exciting future for regenerative medicine; however, their safety profile has not been well established in humans.

Recommended Reading

1. Aggarwal S, Pittenger MF. Human mesenchymal stem cells modulate allogeneic immune cell responses. Blood. 2005;105(4):1815–22.
2. Ahmad KA, Ibrahim YA, Saber NZ, Darwish BA. MR cartilage imaging in assessment of the regenerative power of autologous peripheral blood stem cell injection in knee osteoarthritis. Egypt J Radiol Nucl Med. 2014;45(3):787–94.
3. Akiyama K, Chen C, Wang D, Xu X, Qu C, Yamaza T, et al. Mesenchymal-stem-cell-induced immunoregulation involves FAS-ligand-/FAS-mediated T cell apoptosis. Cell Stem Cell. 2012;10(5):544–55.
4. Ankrum JA, Ong JF, Karp JM. Mesenchymal stem cells: immune evasive, not immune privileged. Nat Biotechnol. 2014;32(3):252–60.
5. Aoyama T, Goto K, Kakinoki R, Ikeguchi R, Ueda M, Kasai Y, et al. An exploratory clinical trial for idiopathic osteonecrosis of femoral head by cultured autologous multipotent mesenchymal stromal cells augmented with vascularized bone grafts. Tissue Eng Part B Rev. 2014;20(4):233–42.
6. Asari S, Itakura S, Ferreri K, Liu CP, Kuroda Y, Kandeel F, et al. Mesenchymal stem cells suppress B-cell terminal differentiation. Exp Hematol. 2009;37(5):604–15.
7. Atoui R, Chiu RC. Concise review: immunomodulatory properties of mesenchymal stem cells in cellular transplantation: update, controversies, and unknowns. Stem Cells Transl Med. 2012;1(3):200–5.
8. Bae HW, Amirdelfan K, Coric D, McJunkin TL, Pettine KA, Hong HJ, et al. A phase II study demonstrating efficacy and safety of mesenchymal precursor cells in low back pain due to disc degeneration. Spine J. 2014;14(11):S31–S2.
9. Bartholomew A, Sturgeon C, Siatskas M, Ferrer K, McIntosh K, Patil S, et al. Mesenchymal stem cells suppress lymphocyte proliferation in vitro and prolong skin graft survival in vivo. Exp Hematol. 2002;30(1):42–8.
10. Becker AJ, Mc CE, Till JE. Cytological demonstration of the clonal nature of spleen colonies derived from transplanted mouse marrow cells. Nature. 1963;197:452–4.
11. Brix J, Zhou Y, Luo Y. The epigenetic reprogramming roadmap in generation of iPSCs from somatic cells. J Genet Genomics. 2015;42(12):661–70.
12. Broutier L, Andersson-Rolf A, Hindley CJ, Boj SF, Clevers H, Koo BK, et al. Culture and establishment of self-renewing human and mouse adult liver and pancreas 3D organoids and their genetic manipulation. Nat Protoc. 2016;11(9):1724–43.
13. Capelli C, Gotti E, Morigi M, Rota C, Weng L, Dazzi F, et al. Minimally manipulated whole human umbilical cord is a rich source of clinical-grade human mesenchymal stromal cells expanded in human platelet lysate. Cytotherapy. 2011;13(7):786–801.
14. Caplan AI, Dennis JE. Mesenchymal stem cells as trophic mediators. J Cell Biochem. 2006;98(5):1076–84.
15. Caplan A, et al. Mesenchymal stem cells. J Orthop Res. 1991;9:641–50.
16. Cassinotti A, Annaloro C, Ardizzone S, Onida F, Della Volpe A, Clerici M, et al. Autologous haematopoietic stem cell transplantation without CD34+ cell selection in refractory Crohn's disease. Gut. 2008;57(2):211–7.
17. Centeno CJ. Clinical challenges and opportunities of mesenchymal stem cells in musculoskeletal medicine. PM R. 2014;6(1):70–7.
18. Centeno CJ, Busse D, Kisiday J, Keohan C, Freeman M, Karli D. Regeneration of meniscus cartilage in a knee treated with percutaneously implanted autologous mesenchymal stem cells. Med Hypotheses. 2008;71(6):900–8.
19. Centeno C, Pitts J, Al-Sayegh H, Freeman M. Efficacy of autologous bone marrow concentrate for knee osteoarthritis with and without adipose graft. Biomed Res Int. 2014;2014:370621.
20. Chakravarthy K, Chen Y, He C, Christo PJ. Stem cell therapy for chronic pain management: review of uses, advances, and adverse effects. Pain Physician. 2017;20(4):293–305.
21. Chinnery HR, Pearlman E, McMenamin PG. Cutting edge: membrane nanotubes in vivo: a feature of MHC class II+ cells in the mouse cornea. J Immunol. 2008;180(9):5779–83.
22. Choi H, Lee RH, Bazhanov N, Oh JY, Prockop DJ. Anti-inflammatory protein TSG-6 secreted by activated MSCs attenuates zymosan-induced mouse peritonitis by decreasing TLR2/NF-kappaB signaling in resident macrophages. Blood. 2011;118(2):330–8.
23. Colombo M, Raposo G, Thery C. Biogenesis, secretion, and intercellular interactions of exosomes and other extracellular vesicles. Annu Rev Cell Dev Biol. 2014;30:255–89.
24. Corcione A, Benvenuto F, Ferretti E, Giunti D, Cappiello V, Cazzanti F, et al. Human mesenchymal stem cells modulate B-cell functions. Blood. 2006;107(1):367–72.
25. Dai W, Hale SL, Martin BJ, Kuang JQ, Dow JS, Wold LE, et al. Allogeneic mesenchymal stem cell transplantation in postinfarcted rat myocardium: short- and long-term effects. Circulation. 2005;112(2):214–23.
26. de Almeida PE, Meyer EH, Kooreman NG, Diecke S, Dey D, Sanchez-Freire V, et al. Transplanted terminally differentiated induced pluripotent stem cells are accepted by immune mechanisms similar to self-tolerance. Nat Commun. 2014;5:3903.
27. Dermanovic Dobrota V, Hrabac P, Skegro D, Smiljanic R, Dobrota S, Prkacin I, et al. The impact of neuropathic pain and other comorbidities on the quality of life in patients with diabetes. Health Qual Life Outcomes. 2014;12:171.
28. Desponts C, Ding S. Using small molecules to improve generation of induced pluripotent stem cells from somatic cells. Methods Mol Biol. 2010;636:207–18.
29. Dexter TM, Spooncer E. Growth and differentiation in the hemopoietic system. Annu Rev Cell Biol. 1987;3:423–41.

30. Dexter TM, Wright EG, Krizsa F, Lajtha LG. Regulation of haemopoietic stem cell proliferation in long term bone marrow cultures. Biomedicine. 1977;27(9–10):344–9.
31. Dexter TM, Spooncer E, Toksoz D, Lajtha LG. The role of cells and their products in the regulation of in vitro stem cell proliferation and granulocyte development. J Supramol Struct. 1980;13(4):513–24.
32. Di Nicola M, Carlo-Stella C, Magni M, Milanesi M, Longoni PD, Matteucci P, et al. Human bone marrow stromal cells suppress T-lymphocyte proliferation induced by cellular or nonspecific mitogenic stimuli. Blood. 2002;99(10):3838–43.
33. Dominici M, Le Blanc K, Mueller I, Slaper-Cortenbach I, Marini F, Krause D, et al. Minimal criteria for defining multipotent mesenchymal stromal cells. The International Society for Cellular Therapy position statement. Cytotherapy. 2006;8(4):315–7.
34. Dominici M, Horwitz EM, et al. Minimal criteria for defining multipotent mesenchymal stromal cells. Cytotherapy. 2006;8:315–7.
35. Elabd C, Centeno CJ, Schultz JR, Lutz G, Ichim T, Silva FJ. Intradiscal injection of autologous, hypoxic cultured bone marrow-derived mesenchymal stem cells in five patients with chronic lower back pain: a long-term safety and feasibility study. J Transl Med. 2016;14:253.
36. Evans MJ, Kaufman MH. Establishment in culture of pluripotential cells from mouse embryos. Nature. 1981;292(5819):154–6.
37. Fischer UM, Harting MT, Jimenez F, Monzon-Posadas WO, Xue H, Savitz SI, et al. Pulmonary passage is a major obstacle for intravenous stem cell delivery: the pulmonary first-pass effect. Stem Cells Dev. 2009;18(5):683–92.
38. Franquesa M, Hoogduijn MJ, Bestard O, Grinyo JM. Immunomodulatory effect of mesenchymal stem cells on B cells. Front Immunol. 2012;3:212.
39. Friedenstein AJ. Precursor cells of mechanocytes. Int Rev Cytol. 1976;47:327–59.
40. Friedenstein AJ, Piatetzky S II, Petrakova KV. Osteogenesis in transplants of bone marrow cells. J Embryol Exp Morphol. 1966;16(3):381–90.
41. Friedenstein AJ, Chailakhjan RK, Lalykina KS. The development of fibroblast colonies in monolayer cultures of Guinea-pig bone marrow and spleen cells. Cell Tissue Kinet. 1970;3(4):393–403.
42. Friedenstein AJ, Gorskaja JF, Kulagina NN. Fibroblast precursors in normal and irradiated mouse hematopoietic organs. Exp Hematol. 1976;4(5):267–74.
43. Friedenstein AJ, Ivanov-Smolenski AA, Chajlakjan RK, Gorskaya UF, Kuralesova AI, Latzinik NW, et al. Origin of bone marrow stromal mechanocytes in radiochimeras and heterotopic transplants. Exp Hematol. 1978;6(5):440–4.
44. Gnecchi M, He H, Liang OD, Melo LG, Morello F, Mu H, et al. Paracrine action accounts for marked protection of ischemic heart by Akt-modified mesenchymal stem cells. Nat Med. 2005;11(4):367–8.
45. Goldblatt F, Isenberg DA. New therapies for systemic lupus erythematosus. Clin Exp Immunol. 2005;140(2):205–12.
46. Hassiotou F, Beltran A, Chetwynd E, Stuebe AM, Twigger AJ, Metzger P, et al. Breastmilk is a novel source of stem cells with multilineage differentiation potential. Stem Cells. 2012;30(10):2164–74.
47. Hera YF, Hunt CL, Law LA, Bydon M, Nassr A, Smith J, et al. Five generations of cell preparation: a translational framework for categorizing regenerative stem cell therapies. J Am Acad Regen Med. 2017.
48. Hindley CJ, Cordero-Espinoza L, Huch M. Organoids from adult liver and pancreas: stem cell biology and biomedical utility. Dev Biol. 2016;420(2):251–61.
49. Hiyama A, Watanabe M, Katoh H, Sato M, Sakai D, Mochida J. Evaluation of quality of life and neuropathic pain in patients with low back pain using the Japanese Orthopedic Association Back pain evaluation questionnaire. Eur Spine J. 2015;24(3):503–12.
50. Hofstetter CP, Schwarz EJ, Hess D, Widenfalk J, El Manira A, Prockop DJ, et al. Marrow stromal cells form guiding strands in the injured spinal cord and promote recovery. Proc Natl Acad Sci U S A. 2002;99(4):2199–204.
51. Hotta A, Yamanaka S. From genomics to gene therapy: induced pluripotent stem cells meet genome editing. Annu Rev Genet. 2015;49:47–70.
52. Hu C, Cao H, Pan X, Li J, He J, Pan Q, et al. Adipogenic placenta-derived mesenchymal stem cells are not lineage restricted by withdrawing extrinsic factors: developing a novel visual angle in stem cell biology. Cell Death Dis. 2016;7:e2141.
53. Hunt CL, Shen S, Nassr A, van Wijnen AJ, Larson AN, Eldrige JS, et al. Current understanding of safety and efficacy of stem cell therapy for discogenic pain— a systematic review of human studies. Tech Reg Anesth Pain Manag. 2015;19(1):32–7.
54. Hwu P, Du MX, Lapointe R, Do M, Taylor MW, Young HA. Indoleamine 2,3-dioxygenase production by human dendritic cells results in the inhibition of T cell proliferation. J Immunol. 2000;164(7):3596–9.
55. Islam MN, Das SR, Emin MT, Wei M, Sun L, Westphalen K, et al. Mitochondrial transfer from bone-marrow-derived stromal cells to pulmonary alveoli protects against acute lung injury. Nat Med. 2012;18(5):759–65.
56. Iso Y, Spees JL, Serrano C, Bakondi B, Pochampally R, Song YH, et al. Multipotent human stromal cells improve cardiac function after myocardial infarction in mice without long-term engraftment. Biochem Biophys Res Commun. 2007;354(3):700–6.
57. Kabu S, Gao Y, Kwon BK, Labhasetwar V. Drug delivery, cell-based therapies, and tissue engineering approaches for spinal cord injury. J Control Release. 2015;219:141–54.
58. Khubutiya MS, Vagabov AV, Temnov AA, Sklifas AN. Paracrine mechanisms of proliferative, anti-apoptotic and anti-inflammatory effects of mesenchymal stromal cells in models of acute organ injury. Cytotherapy. 2014;16(5):579–85.
59. Koerner J, Nesic D, Romero JD, Brehm W, Mainil-Varlet P, Grogan SP. Equine peripheral blood-derived progenitors in comparison to bone marrow-derived mesenchymal stem cells. Stem Cells. 2006;24(6):1613–9.
60. Kota DJ, Wiggins LL, Yoon N, Lee RH. TSG-6 produced by hMSCs delays the onset of autoimmune diabetes by suppressing Th1 development and enhancing tolerogenicity. Diabetes. 2013;62(6):2048–58.
61. Lai RC, Arslan F, Lee MM, Sze NS, Choo A, Chen TS, et al. Exosome secreted by MSC reduces myocardial ischemia/reperfusion injury. Stem Cell Res. 2010;4(3):214–22.
62. Lai RC, Chen TS, Lim SK. Mesenchymal stem cell exosome: a novel stem cell-based therapy for cardiovascular disease. Regen Med. 2011;6(4):481–92.
63. Lai RC, Tan SS, Teh BJ, Sze SK, Arslan F, de Kleijn DP, et al. Proteolytic potential of the MSC exosome proteome: implications for an exosome-mediated delivery of therapeutic proteasome. Int J Proteomics. 2012;2012:971907.
64. Lai RC, Tan SS, Yeo RW, Choo AB, Reiner AT, Su Y, et al. MSC secretes at least 3 EV types each with a unique permutation of membrane lipid, protein and RNA. J Extracell Vesicles. 2016;5:29828.
65. Lancaster MA, Knoblich JA. Organogenesis in a dish: modeling development and disease using organoid technologies. Science. 2014;345(6194):1247125.
66. Le Blanc K, Tammik L, Sundberg B, Haynesworth SE, Ringden O. Mesenchymal stem cells inhibit and stimulate mixed lymphocyte cultures and mitogenic responses independently of the major histocompatibility complex. Scand J Immunol. 2003;57(1):11–20.
67. Lee RH, Pulin AA, Seo MJ, Kota DJ, Ylostalo J, Larson BL, et al. Intravenous hMSCs improve myocardial infarction in mice because cells embolized in lung are activated to secrete the anti-inflammatory protein TSG-6. Cell Stem Cell. 2009;5(1):54–63.

68. Lee C, Mitsialis SA, Aslam M, Vitali SH, Vergadi E, Konstantinou G, et al. Exosomes mediate the cytoprotective action of mesenchymal stromal cells on hypoxia-induced pulmonary hypertension. Circulation. 2012;126(22):2601–11.
69. Lee AS, Tang C, Rao MS, Weissman IL, Wu JC. Tumorigenicity as a clinical hurdle for pluripotent stem cell therapies. Nat Med. 2013;19(8):998–1004.
70. Liu K, Ji K, Guo L, Wu W, Lu H, Shan P, et al. Mesenchymal stem cells rescue injured endothelial cells in an in vitro ischemia-reperfusion model via tunneling nanotube like structure-mediated mitochondrial transfer. Microvasc Res. 2014;92:10–8.
71. Liu L, Hua Z, Shen J, Yin Y, Yang J, Cheng K, et al. Comparative efficacy of multiple variables of mesenchymal stem cell transplantation for the treatment of neuropathic pain in rats. Mil Med. 2017;182(S1):175–84.
72. Lodi D, Iannitti T, Palmieri B. Stem cells in clinical practice: applications and warnings. J Exp Clin Cancer Res. 2011;30:9.
73. Macchiarini P, Jungebluth P, Go T, Asnaghi MA, Rees LE, Cogan TA, et al. Clinical transplantation of a tissue-engineered airway. Lancet. 2008;372(9655):2023–30.
74. Mahla RS. Stem cells applications in regenerative medicine and disease therapeutics. Int J Cell Biol. 2016;2016:6940283.
75. Majore I, Moretti P, Stahl F, Hass R, Kasper C. Growth and differentiation properties of mesenchymal stromal cell populations derived from whole human umbilical cord. Stem Cell Rev. 2011;7(1):17–31.
76. Mandai M, Watanabe A, Kurimoto Y, Hirami Y, Morinaga C, Daimon T, et al. Autologous induced stem-cell-derived retinal cells for macular degeneration. N Engl J Med. 2017;376(11):1038–46.
77. Mao Q, Wang W, Xu T, Zhang S, Xiao L, Chen D, et al. Combination treatment of biomechanical support and targeted intra-arterial infusion of peripheral blood stem cells mobilized by granulocyte-colony stimulating factor for the osteonecrosis of the femoral head: a randomized controlled clinical trial. J Bone Miner Res. 2015;30(4):647–56.
78. Martin GR. Isolation of a pluripotent cell line from early mouse embryos cultured in medium conditioned by teratocarcinoma stem cells. Proc Natl Acad Sci U S A. 1981;78(12):7634–8.
79. Meisel R, Zibert A, Laryea M, Gobel U, Daubener W, Dilloo D. Human bone marrow stromal cells inhibit allogeneic T-cell responses by indoleamine 2,3-dioxygenase-mediated tryptophan degradation. Blood. 2004;103(12):4619–21.
80. Mellor AL, Munn DH. Tryptophan catabolism and T-cell tolerance: immunosuppression by starvation? Immunol Today. 1999;20(10):469–73.
81. Mellor AL, Munn DH. IDO expression by dendritic cells: tolerance and tryptophan catabolism. Nat Rev Immunol. 2004;4(10):762–74.
82. Mirotsou M, Zhang Z, Deb A, Zhang L, Gnecchi M, Noiseux N, et al. Secreted frizzled related protein 2 (Sfrp2) is the key Akt-mesenchymal stem cell-released paracrine factor mediating myocardial survival and repair. Proc Natl Acad Sci U S A. 2007;104(5):1643–8.
83. Mosaad YM. Hematopoietic stem cells: an overview. Transfus Apher Sci. 2014;51(3):68–82.
84. Muraro PA, Martin R, Mancardi GL, Nicholas R, Sormani MP, Saccardi R. Autologous haematopoietic stem cell transplantation for treatment of multiple sclerosis. Nat Rev Neurol. 2017;13(7):391–405.
85. Murata D, Miyakoshi D, Hatazoe T, Miura N, Tokunaga S, Fujiki M, et al. Multipotency of equine mesenchymal stem cells derived from synovial fluid. Vet J. 2014;202(1):53–61.
86. Mutlu L, Hufnagel D, Taylor HS. The endometrium as a source of mesenchymal stem cells for regenerative medicine. Biol Reprod. 2015;92(6):138.
87. Nagoshi N, Kaneko S, Fujiyoshi K, Takemitsu M, Yagi M, Iizuka S, et al. Characteristics of neuropathic pain and its relationship with quality of life in 72 patients with spinal cord injury. Spinal Cord. 2016;54(9):656–61.
88. Najar M, Raicevic G, Fayyad-Kazan H, Bron D, Toungouz M, Lagneaux L. Mesenchymal stromal cells and immunomodulation: a gathering of regulatory immune cells. Cytotherapy. 2016;18(2):160–71.
89. Nakajima-Takagi Y, Osawa M, Iwama A. Manipulation of hematopoietic stem cells for regenerative medicine. Anat Rec (Hoboken). 2014;297(1):111–20.
90. Nauta AJ, Fibbe WE. Immunomodulatory properties of mesenchymal stromal cells. Blood. 2007;110(10):3499–506.
91. Noiseux N, Gnecchi M, Lopez-Ilasaca M, Zhang L, Solomon SD, Deb A, et al. Mesenchymal stem cells overexpressing Akt dramatically repair infarcted myocardium and improve cardiac function despite infrequent cellular fusion or differentiation. Mol Ther. 2006;14(6):840–50.
92. Nombela-Arrieta C, Ritz J, Silberstein L. The elusive nature and function of mesenchymal stem cells. Nat Rev Mol Cell Biol. 2011;12:126.
93. Nomura Y, Ishikawa M, Yashiro Y, Sanggarnjanavanich S, Yamaguchi T, Arai C, et al. Human periodontal ligament fibroblasts are the optimal cell source for induced pluripotent stem cells. Histochem Cell Biol. 2012;137(6):719–32.
94. Park HW, Shin JS, Kim CW. Proteome of mesenchymal stem cells. Proteomics. 2007;7(16):2881–94.
95. Pascual-Garrido C, Rolon A, Makino A. Treatment of chronic patellar tendinopathy with autologous bone marrow stem cells: a 5-year-followup. Stem Cells Int. 2012;2012:953510.
96. Pearl JI, Kean LS, Davis MM, Wu JC. Pluripotent stem cells: immune to the immune system? Sci Transl Med. 2012;4(164):164ps25.
97. Pers YM, Rackwitz L, Ferreira R, Pullig O, Delfour C, Barry F, et al. Adipose mesenchymal stromal cell-based therapy for severe osteoarthritis of the knee: a phase I dose-escalation trial. Stem Cells Transl Med. 2016;5(7):847–56.
98. Pettine KA, Murphy MB, Suzuki RK, Sand TT. Percutaneous injection of autologous bone marrow concentrate cells significantly reduces lumbar discogenic pain through 12 months. Stem Cells. 2015;33(1):146–56.
99. Phinney DG, Hill K, Michelson C, DuTreil M, Hughes C, Humphries S, et al. Biological activities encoded by the murine mesenchymal stem cell transcriptome provide a basis for their developmental potential and broad therapeutic efficacy. Stem Cells. 2006;24(1):186–98.
100. Pierdomenico L, Bonsi L, Calvitti M, Rondelli D, Arpinati M, Chirumbolo G, et al. Multipotent mesenchymal stem cells with immunosuppressive activity can be easily isolated from dental pulp. Transplantation. 2005;80(6):836–42.
101. Plotnikov EY, Khryapenkova TG, Vasileva AK, Marey MV, Galkina SI, Isaev NK, et al. Cell-to-cell cross-talk between mesenchymal stem cells and cardiomyocytes in co-culture. J Cell Mol Med. 2008;12(5A):1622–31.
102. Plotnikov EY, Silachev DN, Popkov VA, Zorova LD, Pevzner IB, Zorov SD, et al. Intercellular signalling cross-talk: to kill, to heal and to rejuvenate. Heart Lung Circ. 2017;26(7):648–59.
103. Polo JM, Anderssen E, Walsh RM, Schwarz BA, Nefzger CM, Lim SM, et al. A molecular roadmap of reprogramming somatic cells into iPS cells. Cell. 2012;151(7):1617–32.
104. Raposo G, Stoorvogel W. Extracellular vesicles: exosomes, microvesicles, and friends. J Cell Biol. 2013;200(4):373–83.
105. Reis FJ, Lopes D, Rodrigues J, Gosling AP, Gomes MK. Psychological distress and quality of life in leprosy patients with neuropathic pain. Lepr Rev. 2014;85(3):186–93.

106. Roegiers F, Jan YN. Asymmetric cell division. Curr Opin Cell Biol. 2004;16(2):195–205.
107. Rosado MM, Bernardo ME, Scarsella M, Conforti A, Giorda E, Biagini S, et al. Inhibition of B-cell proliferation and antibody production by mesenchymal stromal cells is mediated by T cells. Stem Cells Dev. 2015;24(1):93–103.
108. Rumman M, Dhawan J, Kassem M. Concise review: quiescence in adult stem cells: biological significance and relevance to tissue regeneration. Stem Cells. 2015;33(10):2903–12.
109. Sacchetti B, Funari A, Michienzi S, Di Cesare S, Piersanti S, Saggio I, et al. Self-renewing osteoprogenitors in bone marrow sinusoids can organize a hematopoietic microenvironment. Cell. 2007;131(2):324–36.
110. Sahni V, Kessler JA. Stem cell therapies for spinal cord injury. Nat Rev Neurol. 2010;6(7):363–72.
111. Sato K, Ozaki K, Oh I, Meguro A, Hatanaka K, Nagai T, et al. Nitric oxide plays a critical role in suppression of T-cell proliferation by mesenchymal stem cells. Blood. 2007;109(1):228–34.
112. Schinkothe T, Bloch W, Schmidt A. In vitro secreting profile of human mesenchymal stem cells. Stem Cells Dev. 2008;17(1):199–206.
113. Schmidt D, Achermann J, Odermatt B, Genoni M, Zund G, Hoerstrup SP. Cryopreserved amniotic fluid-derived cells: a lifelong autologous fetal stem cell source for heart valve tissue engineering. J Heart Valve Dis. 2008;17(4):446–55; discussion 55
114. Schrepfer S, Deuse T, Reichenspurner H, Fischbein MP, Robbins RC, Pelletier MP. Stem cell transplantation: the lung barrier. Transplant Proc. 2007;39(2):573–6.
115. Scott CT, Magnus D. Wrongful termination: lessons from the Geron clinical trial. Stem Cells Transl Med. 2014;3(12):1398–401.
116. Seyed-Razavi Y, Hickey MJ, Kuffova L, McMenamin PG, Chinnery HR. Membrane nanotubes in myeloid cells in the adult mouse cornea represent a novel mode of immune cell interaction. Immunol Cell Biol. 2013;91(1):89–95.
117. Shi Y, Inoue H, Wu JC, Yamanaka S. Induced pluripotent stem cell technology: a decade of progress. Nat Rev Drug Discov. 2017;16(2):115–30.
118. Siminovitch L, McCulloch EA, Till JE. The distribution of colony-forming cells among spleen colonies. J Cell Comp Physiol. 1963;62:327–36.
119. Sinha P, Islam MN, Bhattacharya S, Bhattacharya J. Intercellular mitochondrial transfer: bioenergetic crosstalk between cells. Curr Opin Genet Dev. 2016;38:97–101.
120. Snowden JA, Passweg J, Moore JJ, Milliken S, Cannell P, Van Laar J, et al. Autologous hemopoietic stem cell transplantation in severe rheumatoid arthritis: a report from the EBMT and ABMTR. J Rheumatol. 2004;31(3):482–8.
121. Spees JL, Olson SD, Whitney MJ, Prockop DJ. Mitochondrial transfer between cells can rescue aerobic respiration. Proc Natl Acad Sci U S A. 2006;103(5):1283–8.
122. Spees JL, Lee RH, Gregory CA. Mechanisms of mesenchymal stem/stromal cell function. Stem Cell Res Ther. 2016;7(1):125.
123. Takahashi K, Tanabe K, Ohnuki M, Narita M, Ichisaka T, Tomoda K, et al. Induction of pluripotent stem cells from adult human fibroblasts by defined factors. Cell. 2007;131(5):861–72.
124. Tate DG, Forchheimer MB, Karana-Zebari D, Chiodo AE, Kendall Thomas JY. Depression and pain among inpatients with spinal cord injury and spinal cord disease: differences in symptoms and neurological function. Disabil Rehabil. 2013;35(14):1204–12.
125. Thomson JA, Itskovitz-Eldor J, Shapiro SS, Waknitz MA, Swiergiel JJ, Marshall VS, et al. Embryonic stem cell lines derived from human blastocysts. Science. 1998;282(5391):1145–7.
126. Toh WS, Lai RC, Hui JHP, Lim SK. MSC exosome as a cell-free MSC therapy for cartilage regeneration: implications for osteoarthritis treatment. Semin Cell Dev Biol. 2017;67:56–64.
127. Tse WT, Pendleton JD, Beyer WM, Egalka MC, Guinan EC. Suppression of allogeneic T-cell proliferation by human marrow stromal cells: implications in transplantation. Transplantation. 2003;75(3):389–97.
128. Usunier B, Benderitter M, Tamarat R, Chapel A. Management of fibrosis: the mesenchymal stromal cells breakthrough. Stem Cells Int. 2014;2014:340257.
129. Vickers ER, Karsten E, Flood J, Lilischkis R. A preliminary report on stem cell therapy for neuropathic pain in humans. J Pain Res. 2014;7:255–63.
130. Vignais ML, Caicedo A, Brondello JM, Jorgensen C. Cell connections by tunneling nanotubes: effects of mitochondrial trafficking on target cell metabolism, homeostasis, and response to therapy. Stem Cells Int. 2017;2017:6917941.
131. Vlassov AV, Magdaleno S, Setterquist R, Conrad R. Exosomes: current knowledge of their composition, biological functions, and diagnostic and therapeutic potentials. Biochim Biophys Acta. 2012;1820(7):940–8.
132. Vranken JH. Elucidation of pathophysiology and treatment of neuropathic pain. Cent Nerv Syst Agents Med Chem. 2012;12(4):304–14.
133. Wagner B, Henschler R. Fate of intravenously injected mesenchymal stem cells and significance for clinical application. Adv Biochem Eng Biotechnol. 2013;130:19–37.
134. Wang Y, Liu J, Tan X, Li G, Gao Y, Liu X, et al. Induced pluripotent stem cells from human hair follicle mesenchymal stem cells. Stem Cell Rev. 2013;9(4):451–60.
135. Waterman RS, Tomchuck SL, Henkle SL, Betancourt AM. A new mesenchymal stem cell (MSC) paradigm: polarization into a pro-inflammatory MSC1 or an immunosuppressive MSC2 phenotype. PLoS One. 2010;5(4):e10088.
136. Xin H, Li Y, Cui Y, Yang JJ, Zhang ZG, Chopp M. Systemic administration of exosomes released from mesenchymal stromal cells promote functional recovery and neurovascular plasticity after stroke in rats. J Cereb Blood Flow Metab. 2013;33(11):1711–5.
137. Yan D, Chen L, Li Z, Guo W, Sun W. Autologous mesenchymal stem cell implantation in the management of osteonecrosis of the femoral head. Current Orthop Pract. 2015;26(3):265–8.
138. Yawn BP, Wollan PC, Weingarten TN, Watson JC, Hooten WM, Melton LJ 3rd. The prevalence of neuropathic pain: clinical evaluation compared with screening tools in a community population. Pain Med. 2009;10(3):586–93.
139. Yousefifard M, Nasirinezhad F, Shardi Manaheji H, Janzadeh A, Hosseini M, Keshavarz M. Human bone marrow-derived and umbilical cord-derived mesenchymal stem cells for alleviating neuropathic pain in a spinal cord injury model. Stem Cell Res Ther. 2016;7:36.
140. Yu C, Liu Y, Ma T, Liu K, Xu S, Zhang Y, et al. Small molecules enhance CRISPR genome editing in pluripotent stem cells. Cell Stem Cell. 2015;16(2):142–7.
141. Zappia E, Casazza S, Pedemonte E, Benvenuto F, Bonanni I, Gerdoni E, et al. Mesenchymal stem cells ameliorate experimental autoimmune encephalomyelitis inducing T-cell anergy. Blood. 2005;106(5):1755–61.
142. Zhang Y, McNeill E, Tian H, Soker S, Andersson KE, Yoo JJ, et al. Urine derived cells are a potential source for urological tissue reconstruction. J Urol. 2008;180(5):2226–33.

143. Zhang B, Wang M, Gong A, Zhang X, Wu X, Zhu Y, et al. HucMSC-exosome mediated-Wnt4 signaling is required for cutaneous wound healing. Stem Cells. 2015;33(7):2158–68.
144. Zhang Y, Chopp M, Zhang ZG, Katakowski M, Xin H, Qu C, et al. Systemic administration of cell-free exosomes generated by human bone marrow derived mesenchymal stem cells cultured under 2D and 3D conditions improves functional recovery in rats after traumatic brain injury. Neurochem Int. 2016.
145. Zhao T, Zhang ZN, Westenskow PD, Todorova D, Hu Z, Lin T, et al. Humanized mice reveal differential immunogenicity of cells derived from autologous induced pluripotent stem cells. Cell Stem Cell. 2015;17(3):353–9.
146. Zuk PA, Zhu M, Ashjian P, De Ugarte DA, Huang JI, Mizuno H, et al. Human adipose tissue is a source of multipotent stem cells. Mol Biol Cell. 2002;13(12):4279–95.

Stem Cells

89

Ajax Yang, Corey W. Hunter, Tory L. McJunkin,
Paul J. Lynch, and Edward L. Swing

Introduction

Stem cell engineering is emerging as a promising therapy option in regenerative medicine because of its capability to differentiate into cells of the target tissue (regeneration) and modulate via growth factors to initiate a cascade of healing responses (repair) in the host tissue. When deposited into neuronal, osseous, cartilaginous, and tendinous tissues or muscular defects, stem cells have shown excellent restorative properties through angiogenic, anti-inflammatory, immunomodulatory, antiapoptotic, and antifibrotic mechanisms. While embryonic and induced pluripotent stem cells have unlimited potential to differentiate into various tissues types, the ethical, political, and tumorigenic concerns have limited embryonic and induced pluripotent stem cell engineering, respectively. Furthermore, embryonic stems are fragile and difficult to manipulate. These limitations paved the way for the development of adult mesenchymal stem cell (MSC) technology where MSCs can be harvested from individual patients in abundance and injected into the patient without ethical conflicts and with reduced immunogenic and reduced oncological concerns.

Background and Historical Perspective

The present-day routine bone marrow transplant to treat leukemia began in the 1960s when Mathé demonstrated improved long-term survival in patients with leukemia treated with hematopoietic stem cell treatment. Friedenstein et al. was the first group to observe small deposits of bone- and cartilage-like tissues cultured from MSCs isolated from guinea pig bone marrow and spleen cells in the 1970s. Regardless of where the MSCs are obtained, stem cell regenerations are governed by four fundamental components: viable stem cells, growth factors, scaffolds, and mechanical stimulation of the local environment.

A. Yang (✉)
Department of Rehabilitation Medicine, Icahn School of Medicine at Mount Sinai, New York, NY, USA

C. W. Hunter
Department of Rehabilitation Medicine, Icahn School of Medicine at Mount Sinai, New York, NY, USA

Ainsworth Institute of Pain Management, New York, NY, USA
e-mail: chunter@ainpain.com

T. L. McJunkin · P. J. Lynch · E. L. Swing
Arizona Pain Specialists, Scottsdale, AZ, USA

Adult-Derived Mesenchymal Stem Cells

MSCs are adult stem cells that are capable of differentiating into multiple lineages to cause clonal expansion. MSCs are commonly isolated from bone marrow or adipose cells. One of the most well-studied MSCs, also known as stromal stem cells, was first derived from bone marrow. Since the time when MSCs were identified in the bone marrow aspirate, MSC have been harvested ubiquitously throughout the body.

Due to the heterogeneity the cells and their surface markers found in the specimen, International Society for Cellular Therapy defines MSCs as a heterogeneous population of progenitor cells expressing a pattern of characteristic surface markers including:

- CD73, CD90, and CD105 in greater than 95%
- Lacking the expression of hematopoietic markers CD34, CD45, CD14 or CD11, CD79a or CD19, and HLA class II in greater than 95% of the culture

For practical purposes, the three main sources of stem cells are:

- Autologous bone marrow aspirate concentrate (BMAC)
- Autologous stromal vascular fraction (SVF) of adipose tissues
- Allogenic stem cells (e.g., Mesoblast Ltd.) from sources such as bone marrow or adipose cells

T. R. Deer et al. (eds.), *Deer's Treatment of Pain*, https://doi.org/10.1007/978-3-030-12281-2_89

Each stem cell source possesses unique properties (see Table 89.1). Collectively, the number of endogenous MSCs obtained may depend on the individual's age, medical comorbidities, and tissue donor site. MSCs obtained from different tissue types display varied ability to differentiate into specific target tissues. Therefore, the ideal source and number of MSCs needed to promote optimal tissue regeneration is yet under investigation.

Table 89.1 Differences among bone marrow-derived MSC, adipose-derived MSC, and allogenic MSC

Bone marrow-derived MSCs (BM-MSC)	Adipose-derived MSCs (AD-MSC)
Advantages	**Advantages**
Harvest is easy to perform	Cellular expansion is not required to improve efficacy
Minimal processing is required	May be used in conjunction with PRP for a combined effect·
BM-MSC are hypoimmunogenic; therefore, immunosuppression is not required for allogenic transplantations	AD-MSC are hypoimmunogenic; therefore, immunosuppression is not required for allogenic transplantations
Disadvantages	**Disadvantages**
Greater lineage differentiation potential	Harvest is technically challenging and requires tumescent liposuction and other additional equipment
Cellular expansion prohibited under US FDA regulation. If manipulated (e.g., through in vitro expansion), the cells cannot be injected back into the donor	Requires a lengthy multistep processing, including enzymatic digestion, washes, and cellular cultures
May differentiate uncontrollably into an undesired lineage (i.e., fibroblasts to cause scarring)	The amount of adipose tissue that can be harvested and processed is contingent upon the patient's size and body fat content
	Lower differentiation potential into desired osteogenic and chondrogenic lineages, instead, preferentially differentiating into adipocytes
Allogenic MSC	
Advantages	
Potentially painful harvesting procedure is eliminated	
Off-the-shelf" pre-expanded and preprocessed cell lines are readily for use with a constant supply	
Hypoimmunogenic	
No preferential cellular lineage differentiations	
Decreased processing requirements reduce infection risks	
Mesenchyme precursor cells (MPC-06-ID) by Mesoblast Ltd. shows promising results during intradiscal clinical trials	
Disadvantages	
Still in clinical trial (phase 3)	

Allogeneic bone marrow stromal cells have been the most extensively studied. Animal studies demonstrated survival and replication up to 48 weeks after transplantation and restored disc height and proteoglycan content, 6 months after single injection. Restored disc height and improved symptomatology following allogeneic stem cells injection have also been reported in humans. Currently, "off-the-shelf" bone marrow-derived allogenic stem cells are undergoing phase 3 clinical trial (Mesoblast Ltd.) and are showing promising potential in the treatment of degenerative disc disease (Table 89.2).

Growth Factors

MSCs induce direct cellular interactions and signaling via growth factors and anti-inflammatory cytokine secretions to activate endogenous progenitor cells in the pathologic tissues that were previously dormant. These growth factors contribute significantly to the angiogenic and healing properties of stem cells. This results in tissue regeneration with reduction in pain and inflammatory response at the affected area. Some of the growth factor examples are the following:

- Transforming growth factor-β1 (TGF-β1)
  - Regulate cellular proliferation and differentiation
- Vascular endothelial growth factor (VEGF)
  - Stimulate neovascularization
- Placental growth factor (PGF)
  - Promote angiogenesis
- Hepatocyte growth factor (HGF)
  - Responsible to wound healing and organ regeneration
- Stromal-derived factor-1 (SDF-1)
  - Homing factor: recruit and retain progenitor cells to the injury site via chemotaxis
- Fibroblast growth factor (FGF-2)
  - Facilitate angiogenesis and wound healing

Scaffolds

The biocompatible scaffolds serve as a three-dimensional interface to allow the MSCs to undergo proliferation, maturation, and matrix deposition. Examples of injectable scaffold materials are:

- Fibrin glue
- Platelet-rich plasma
- Hyaluronic acid
- Platelet lysate
- Collagen-rich extracellular matrix derived from dermis and small intestine submucosa

Table 89.2 Evidence for efficacy table

Reference	Study design	Size	Indication	MSC source	Outcomes
Degenerative joint disease					
Centeno (2008)	Case report	1	Knee OA	Bone marrow	Increased meniscus and cartilage volume on MRI Increased knee range of motion 95% pain reduction
Davatchi (2011)	Case series	4	Knee OA	Bone marrow	Mild improvement in pain and gait
Centeno (2011)	Case series	339	Multiple joints	Bone marrow	Most improvements seen in patients with knee OA
Richter (2013)	Case series	25	Foot/ankle chondral defect	Bone marrow	Improved pain and disability scores
Vagsness (2014)	Randomized clinical trial	55	Knee meniscal tear	Bone marrow	Partial meniscectomy with MSC injection group experienced a greater pain reduction than meniscectomy alone group
Centeno (2014)	Case series	196	Hip OA	Bone marrow	Most improvement seen in ≤55 age group. 6.4 points improvement on Oxford Hip Scale (OHS) 1.2-point reduction on numeric pain scale (NPS)
Vega (2015)	Randomized clinical trial	30	Knee OA	Bone marrow	MSC group reported significant pain and functional mobility improvement compared to hyaluronic acid group
Koh (2016)	Randomized clinical trial	80	Knee OA	Adipose	Mircrofracture with MSC and fibrin glue group demonstrated improved pain and functional mobility scores than microfracture alone group
Tendinopathy					
Connell (2009)	Case Series	12	Lateral epicondylopathy	Dermal fibroblast	Improved in clinical scores and ultrasound imaging
Clark (2011)	Randomized clinical trial	46	Chronic patella tendinopathy	Tenocyte-like cells	Faster healing response seen on ultrasound imaging Improved clinical response
Hernigou (2014)	Case controlled	45	Rotator cuff tear	Bone marrow	MSC group had a low rate or re-injury compared to control following rotator cuff repair
Centeno (2015)	Case series	102	Shoulder OA and rotator cuff tear	Bone marrow	MSC therapy improved upper extremity function and reduced shoulder pain
Degenerative disc disease					
Meisel (2007)	Randomized clinical Trial	28	Degenerative disc disease	Disc chondrocytes	Improved pain and disability scores sustained at 24 months
Yoshikawa (2010)	Case series	2	Degenerative disc disease	Bone marrow	Clinical and radiographic improvements recorded
Orozco (2011)	Case series	10	Degenerative disc disease	Bone marrow	Increased disc hydration on MRI. Rapid pain and disability improvement
Pang (2014)	Case series	2	Degenerative disc disease	Umbilical cord blood	Improved pain and disability scores
Mochida (2015)	Case series	9	Degenerative disc disease	Autologous nucleus pulposus with marrow-derived MSC	Minimally efficacious
Pettine (2016)	Case series	26	Degenerative disc disease	Bone marrow	Improved pain and disability scores sustained over 24 months
Neuropathic pain					
Vickers (2014)	Case series	10	Trigeminal neuralgia	Adipose	Improved pain and disability scores sustained at 6 months
Venturi (2015)	Case series	15	Pudendal neuralgia	Adipose	Improved pain and disability scores sustained at 12 months

Mechanical Stimulation

Studies have shown that in addition to cytokines and growth factors, mechanical forces also play an important role in MSCs differentiation such as:

- Weight-bearing exercises provide mechanical stimulation for axial bone and muscle mass development and maintenance.
- Under tensile stress (stretching), MSCs have shown to preferentially undergo osteogenesis and tenogenesis in vitro.
- Similarly, hydrostatic pressure, compressive loading, and hypoxic environment induce chondrogenesis.

These findings translated to using fixators and continuous passive machines to enhance bone and knee joint healing, respectively. While the importance of mechanical stimulation is appreciated in regulating MSCs, incorporating this knowledge into regenerative and rehabilitation medicine protocols remains a complex issue.

Uses and Indications

Musculoskeletal conditions that are commonly treated with stem cell technology include:

- Knee/hip/ankle osteoarthritis and rheumatoid arthritis
- Tendinopathy
- Partial ligament or meniscal tear
- Hip or shoulder labral tear
- Degenerative intervertebral disc disease

Despite broad regenerative therapy indications, physicians must comply with the regulations set forth by the US Food and Drug Administration (FDA). The FDA mandates that in order for cell and tissue product to be exempt from pre-marketing approval, the biologics must meet the following criteria:

- Minimally manipulated. Minimal manipulation is defined as:
  - Structural tissues: processing that does not alter the original relevant characteristics of the tissue relating to the tissue's utility for reconstruction, repair, or replacement.
  - Cells or nonstructural tissues: processing that does not alter the relevant biological characteristics of cells or tissues. For example, the use of collagenase is considered more than "minimally manipulated" by current good manufacturing practice requirements. However, nonenzymatic isolation methods using mechanical protocols are deemed less than minimally manipulated.
- Homologous use.
- Cell numbers cannot be expanded.
- Not mixed with other substances for the purpose of preservation, sterilization, or storage.
- Does not exert systemic or metabolic influence.
- Limited to autologous or administering in first- or second-degree relatives.

Contraindications to stem cell therapy in musculoskeletal conditions:

- Complete ligament or tendon rupture
- Intra-articular loose body
- Active local or systemic infections
- Uncontrolled cardiovascular disease
- Bleeding disorders

Stem Cells Source and Harvesting Technique #1: Bone Marrow Aspirate Concentrate (BMAC)

- Position the patient prone on a procedure table, and target the marrow extraction sites around the posterior superior iliac spine (PSIS) as bone marrow can be easily aspirated from this thick portion of the iliac crest.
- Prepare and drape the intended site using strict sterile technique.
- Use ample amount of local anesthetics to anesthetize the skin (e.g., 10–15 cc of 1% lidocaine or 0.25% ropivacaine). Lidocaine is cytotoxic; therefore, it must not come in contact with the bone marrow aspirate.
- Ensure sufficient time and anesthetics are allocated to allow the skin and soft tissue to be effectively anesthetized.
- Unless otherwise indicated by the instructions of the kit, fill the draw syringes with 1000 units of heparin per cc of aspirant to be drawn.
- Fill a 30 cc and a 5 cc syringe with 30,000 units and 5000 of heparin per syringe, respectively.
- Under direct ultrasound or fluoroscopic guidance, insert the needle until the tip is in direct contact with the bone cortex and then sequentially advance the guidewire, stylet/trocar. Maintain a forward pressure while turning the trocar clock- and counterclockwise until 5–10 mm of the trocar tip is seated in the cortex.
- Gently twist the trocar to ensure the trocar-bone cortex is securely snug.
- Remove the stylet from the trocar, and recheck if firmly implanted in the cortex by performing a second wiggle test. If not, then advance the trocar until firm, not exceeding approximately 1 cm in depth.
- Secure the 5 cc syringe with the 5000 units of heparin to the trocar, and inject approximately 500–750 units of heparin into the marrow space immediately on entry into the cortex. It is crucial to prevent the marrow sample from clotting as this renders MSC unusable. Repeat this step for each target aspiration site.
- Remove the 5 cc syringe and attach the draw syringe to the trocar. Match the aspiration speed to the patient's tolerance.
- Drawing a large volume (over 20 cc) from a single bone site reduces MSC yield. We recommend drawing small volumes (5–15 cc) from many sites to increase yield.
- Gently agitate the syringe to mix the heparin and the initial bone marrow aspirate. Once thoroughly mixed, only draw 5–15 cc of bone mineral aspirate per site.
- Move the trocar tip to a new cortex for aspiration without retrieving the trocar from the skin.

- Draw volumes are decided based on the patient weight and the dimension of the treatment area. Use the following guidelines:
  - Females <105 pounds: do not draw more than 50 cc.
  - Female patients between 105 and 120 pounds: the upper acceptable volume limit is 60 cc.
  - Patients of either sex between 120 and 180 pounds: the upper acceptable volume limit is 90 cc.
  - Male patients >180 pounds: up to 120 cc can be collected.

BMAC Preparation and MSC Quantification

Bone marrow aspirate concentrate can be processed with various automated commercial kits or prepared manually inside a biosafety cabinet. Regardless of which method is used, the end goal is to isolate the buffy coat. At this time, there are limited data comparing the MSC outputs of various concentration devices.

Quantification can be accomplished by using the following methods:

- Flow cytometry – This technique uses fluorescent antibodies to bind the specific cell surface markers. Surface markers stained with various colored antibodies intact differently with a laser beam, which enables the amount of BMCs to be measured. This method requires expertise to interpret the results, and it is often cost inhibitive for routine clinic uses.
- Colony-forming unit (CFU) assay – BMC is cultured and incubated until colonies of MSCs form. These MSCs are counted. This method of estimating MSC in BMC is mostly used in the lab and not at the bedside.
- Total nucleated cell count (TNC) – A manual hemocytometer or a commercial automated counting system can be used to indirectly estimate the MSC amount in a BMC sample.
- A higher CFU or TNC is associated with better clinical outcome.

Stem Cell Source and Harvesting Technique #2: Adipose Tissue SCF via Lipoaspiration

Tumescent Fluid Preparation and Dosing

Tumescent mixture is the standard anesthetic solution used for liposuction procedures. The solution is infiltrated into the subcutaneous tissues to provide local anesthesia during the procedure.

The tumescent fluid amount required is determined by:

1. The patient's weight: the maximum lidocaine dosage is 4.5 mg/kg or 7 mg/kg when combined with epinephrine. The standard recommended tumescent lidocaine is 3.5 mg/kg (27).
2. The amount of adipose to be harvested.
   - For small amounts of adipose tissue (60–120 cc), 0.1% tumescent solution may be used. 0.1% tumescent solution can be prepared in a 1000 ml bag of 0.9% sodium chloride by mixing the following:
     - 50 ml 2% lidocaine
     - 1 ml 1:1000 epinephrine
     - 10 ml 8.4% sodium bicarbonate
   - For larger amounts of adipose tissue (>120 cc), 0.05% tumescent solution may be used. Similarly, 0.05% tumescent solution can be prepared in a 1000 ml bag of 0.9% sodium chloride by mixing the following:
     - 25 ml 2% lidocaine
     - 1 ml 1:1000 epinephrine
     - 8 ml 8.4% sodium bicarbonate
3. The tumescent solution should be mixed on the same day as the procedure, and the epinephrine should be added immediately prior to use. The bag should be clearly identified and dated.

Infiltration of Tumescent Anesthetic Fluid

- The patient is positioned supine for abdominal adipose harvesting and lateral decubitus for flank or hip adipose harvesting.
- Vital sign monitoring is placed.
- Drape and clean the lipoaspiration site while adhering to strict sterile technique.
- If harvesting adipose tissue from the abdomen, the intended port site(s) should be placed in line with the bilateral anterior axillary line, at the level of the anterior iliac spine. If the second port site is needed, it should be staggered to the first site.
- Anesthetize the skin over the marked target port sites.
- Use a number 11 scalpel to make a 3 mm incision.
- Insert a 14G garden spray infiltration needle to saturate area of lipoaspiration with the tumescent fluid.
- The tumescent fluid IV bag maybe pressurized with a pressure bag in conjunction with gravitational assist. Another method is to deliver the tumescent fluid via a 60 cc syringe.
- Regardless of the delivery method, tumescent fluid infiltration should be deposited slowly and evenly throughout the subcutaneous tissue.

- Maintain the infiltration needle parallel with the abdominal wall to prevent any unintentional transabdominal or peritoneal perforation injury.
- The skin over the abdomen may appear firm with demarcating blanching following sufficient tumescent fluid with epinephrine infiltration. At this time, the physician may begin lipoaspiration.

Lipoaspiration Technique

- Attach a Mercedes Lipo Cannula (3 mm × 25 cm) to a 60 cc Toomey syringe.
- After the needle is held subcutaneously, the syringe plunger is pulled back to create roughly 18 inches of Hg vacuum. A snap lock or Johnnie snap will keep the plunger in the retracted position to maintain a negative pressure inside the syringe.
- Maneuver the needle back and forth in a fan-shaped fashion throughout the subcutaneous tissue as the negative pressure pulls the lipoaspirate into the syringe.
- The physician should place the non-dominant hand on the patient's abdomen to ensure that the needle tip remains at the safe distance from the superficial skin and the needle does not extend beyond the intended treatment area.
- We recommend sequentially aspirate the deeper layers followed by more superficial regions.
- Avoid removing excess adipose tissue from any one area as this results in skin dimpling.
- Continue to suction the aspirate until the syringe is full.
- Place the syringe right on a rack to allow the fat to rise above the supernatant fluid.
- Discard any supernatant fluid into a sterile stainless steel basin, and repeat this step until the desired volume of fat has been obtained.
- Cap the syringe before transporting to the processing area.

Post-Lipoaspiration Procedures

- Gently express any excess tumescent fluid through the port site(s).
- Approximate the skin edges, and secure the puncture wound with steri-strips before dressing the area with an ABD pad.
- Following an abdominal adipose tissue harvest, an elastic abdominal binder will generally be sufficient to provide comfort, minimize bruising, and improve skin aesthetics. Similarly, a compression body suit may be useful when adipose tissue is extracted from thigh or hip subcutaneously.
- The patient should wear the compression device continuously for the first 72 hours followed by minimal interruptions for the next 3–4 days.
- Continue to monitor the patient's vital signs until the patient is stable to be discharged.

Adipose SVF Processing

- SVF from adipose tissue can be safely processed either by mechanical or enzymatic means.
- Mechanical separation method is preferred when extracting SVF from a lower adipose tissue amount because mechanical processing is more economical and requires a shorter processing turnaround time. However, the mechanical method yields fewer progenitor cells and a higher mononuclear cell count.
- Enzymatic processing is expensive, but it has been shown to provide a more consistent and reliable way of breaking down extracellular matrix. The authors advocate the enzymatic isolation.
  - Enzymatic isolation of the SVF
    - All specimens should be clearly marked with patient identifiers.
    - We recommend that all tissue handling outside of the sterile procedure suite occur under a Class 100 HEPA-Filtered Laminar Flow Biological Cabinet using aseptic technique.
    - The basic steps universally utilized to isolate adipose stem cells involve a cell wash, collagenase digestion, followed by centrifugal separation and filtration to isolate the single cell stromal vascular fraction from the primary adipocytes.
    - There are several commercially available, single-use kits that offer proprietary formulas and unique prepackaged digestive enzymes.
    - SVF is resuspended in a carrier solution for final treatment. The carrier solutions include autologous platelet-rich plasma (PRP) and preservative-free normal saline. Autologous PRP is the authors' recommended scaffold solution for musculoskeletal, intrathecal, or intravascular therapeutic applications. The total resuspension volume may range from 2 to 10 cc depending on the site of treatment.

Uses and Indications

Intradiscal Application

Preprocedure Considerations

- Other sources, such as facet- and/or sacroiliac joint-mediated low back pain, must be ruled out.

- Magnetic resonance imaging (MRI) must demonstrate mild disc degeneration: less than 50% disc height loss and no more than grade 1 listhesis at the targeted level.
- As previously stated, allogenic stem cells are demonstrating excellent clinical outcomes during phase 3 clinical trial at the time of this chapter writing. Mesoblast may soon be available for clinical use.

Technical Aspects

- Posterolateral intradiscal approach
  - Patient is placed in a prone position on the fluoroscopy table.
  - The skin over the lumbar area is carefully cleaned and draped using strict sterile techniques.
  - AP view of the lumbar spine is centered on the target disc with the vertebral endplates clearly focused and aligned.
  - C-arm is obliqued contralaterally to the uninvolved side to produce the trajectory view.
  - Safe needle advancement is performed under direct fluoroscopic visualization using lateral views.
  - We recommend using the two-needle technique (a smaller gauge needle is inserted through the larger gauge needle) so that the needle that pierces the annulus does not first contact the skin to minimize infection risk.
  - Needle(s) is (are) advanced into Kambin's triangle under intermittent fluoroscopic guidance.
  - Do not use contrast dye during this procedure because contrast material may impede with cell regenerative functions.
  - Cellular injectate is slowly deposited with the needle tip properly positioned inside the disc.
  - A minute amount (0.5 cc) of preservative-free normal saline can be flushed into the disc before withdrawing the needle. This minimizes the risk of stem cells tracking into the epidural space during needle retraction.
  - Instruct the patient to avoid rigorous activities for 1–2 days as a general precaution.
  - Apply sterile dressing to needle entry site.

Intra-articular Application

Lumbar Facet Joint

- The patient lies prone with a pillow under the abdomen for comfort.
- Direct the C-arm beam parallel to the facet joint to allow direct visualization of the open facet joint space.
- Mark the skin where the beam is projected, and clean the area using strict sterile technique.
- Anesthetize the skin and superficial soft tissues using a 27G needle and 1–2% lidocaine.
- Insert a 21G, 3.5 inch spinal needle under fluoroscopic visualization.
- 0.1–0.2 ml nonionic contrast material can be injected into the joint space to confirm intra-articular needle placement.
- Slowly inject 0.5 ml of stem cell suspension with low pressure to prevent capsule rupture.

Knee Joint Injection

- Place the patient supine with the treatment knee slightly flexed (place a pillow or a bolster under the treatment knee for support), and close to the side of the table where the physician will be standing.
- Place the ultrasound probe in long axis to bring the patella, the femur, and the joint recess in view.
- While keeping the knee joint recess in the center of the screen, turn the probe 180° to examine the anterior knee in the short-axis view.
- Ensure the joint recess can be clearly visualized.
- The needle entry point and depth can be determined in the short-axis view.
- Clean the skin using strict sterile technique and mark the skin.
- A sterile sheath-covered ultrasound probe is reapplied to obtain short-axis view.
- A 22G, 1.5 inch needle is advanced under direct in-plane visualization toward the joint recess.
- Aspirate to monitor for blood before injecting.
- Once the needle tip enters the joint recess, the injectate should be advanced into the joint space without resistance.
- Inject the stem cell suspension while moving the needle in a fenestrating-fan fashion.
- Carefully withdraw the needle and apply a sterile dressing.

Hip Joint Injection

- Place the patient supine with the treatment hip close to the side of the table where the physician will be standing.
- Place the ultrasound probe in long axis to the femoral neck to identify the femoral head, neck, and anterior recess. Because of the femoral neck angle, the probe orientation will be in the oblique sagittal plane.
- Hip vasculatures, medial to the hip joint, can be further delineated using the power Doppler function. The acetabular labrum appears hyperechoic and extends from the margins of the acetabulum.

- Clean the skin using strict sterile technique, and mark the skin 2–3 cm lateral to the vascular bundle in line with the femoral neck.
- Anesthetize the skin and superficial soft tissues using a 27G needle and 1–2% lidocaine.
- A sterile sheath-covered ultrasound probe is reapplied to obtain view.
- A 22G, 3.5 inch needle is advanced under direct visualization toward the femoral neck.
- Aspirate to monitor for blood before injecting.
- Once the needle tip is inside the hip capsule, inject the stem cell suspension while moving the needle in a fenestrating-fan fashion.
- Carefully withdraw the needle and apply a sterile dressing.

Glenohumeral Joint Injection

- The patient is seated with the arm in internal rotation to rest the hand on the ipsilateral hip. This position facilitates the opening of the posterior joint space.
- Place the transducer parallel the scapular spine, and move inferiorly until infraspinatus and teres minor are identified. The probe is then turned long axis to examine the posterior labrum (hyperechoic triangularly shaped).
- Lower frequency may provide a better visualization of deeper structures in large or athletic shoulders.
- Identify the position of the labrum in the middle of the computer screen.
- Mark the needle entry point with a surgical marker.
- Carefully clean the skin with chlorhexidine or betadine or 70% isopropyl alcohol using sterile technique.
- 3–5 cc of 1–2% lidocaine is used to anesthetize the skin and superficial soft tissues.
- Position the sterile sheath-covered ultrasound probe to center the image of the lesion on the computer screen.
- A 22G, 3.5 inch needle is placed 1 cm lateral to the lateral edge of the transducer and advanced using "in-plane technique" medially toward the glenohumeral joint space.
- Maintain constant visualization of the needle tip to avoid penetrating the labrum.
- Slowly deliver the injectate while moving the needle in a fenestrating-fan fashion.
- Carefully withdraw the needle and apply a sterile dressing.

Tendinous Application

Supraspinatus and Subscapularis Injection: Anterior Approach to Rotator Cuff Interval

- Supraspinatus and subscapularis tendinopathies are best addressed using this technique.
- Supraspinatus: the patient is seated with the hand placed on the ipsilateral hip area and with the elbow pointed posteriorly while maintaining shoulder external rotation (modified Crass position).
- Subscapularis: the patient is seated with forearm in supination and shoulder external rotation.
- The ultrasound probe is placed in short axis on the anterior shoulder just superior to the greater and lesser tuberosity.
- The biceps tendon is visualized between the supraspinatus and subscapularis tendons.
- Identify the lesion, and position the image of the lesion in the middle of the computer screen. Tears are most often found in the distal 1/4 of the tendon in the transverse direction.
- Mark the needle entry point with a surgical marker.
- Carefully clean the skin with chlorhexidine or betadine or 70% isopropyl alcohol using sterile technique.
- 3–5 cc of 1–2% lidocaine is used to anesthetize the skin and superficial soft tissues.
- Position the sterile sheath-covered ultrasound probe to center the image of the lesion on the computer screen.
- A 20 or 22 gauge, 3.5 inch needle is advanced using "in-plane technique" toward the space just lateral to the coracoid process at the humeral head.
- The needle is advanced into the rotator cuff interval toward the supraspinatus tendon for supraspinatus injection.
- The area caudal to the coracoid process is the target for the subscapularis injection.
- Slowly inject the stem cell suspension while moving the needle in a fenestrating-fan fashion to immerse the damaged area.
- Carefully withdraw the needle and apply a sterile dressing.

Infraspinatus and Teres Minor Injection: Posterior Approach

- The patient is seated with the arm by the side and the hand resting on the ipsilateral thigh. This position facilitates the opening of the posterior joint space.
- Place the transducer angled obliquely and superiorly toward the humeral head and parallel to the scapular spine inferiorly.
- Identify the lesion, and position the image of the lesion in the middle of the computer screen.
- Mark the needle entry point with a surgical marker.
- Carefully clean the skin with chlorhexidine or betadine or 70% isopropyl alcohol using sterile technique.
- 3–5 cc of 1–2% lidocaine is used to anesthetize the skin and superficial soft tissues.

- Position the sterile sheath-covered ultrasound probe to center the image of the lesion on the computer screen.
- A 20 or 22G, 3.5 inch needle with an approximately 30-degree tip curvature is advanced using "in-plane technique" medially toward the glenohumeral joint space.
- Slowly inject the stem cell suspension while moving the needle in a fenestrating-fan fashion to immerse the damaged area.
- Carefully withdraw the needle and apply a sterile dressing.

Clinical Pearls and Pitfalls

- Universal precautions should be followed strictly by all personnel involved in handling patient specimens.
- When permissible, medications such as statins, corticosteroids, NSAIDs, and ACE inhibitors should be held for at least 2–4 weeks following MSC therapy because of their MSC inhibitory effects.
- Continuous monitoring of vital signs with airway resuscitative equipment and crash cart in reach is recommended as there have been transient rise in blood pressure, headache, and vasovagal response following parenteral administration of regenerative injectate.
- Refrain from using antibiotics and radio-opaque material, as they have been reported to be cytotoxic.
- Do not use needles less than 22 gauge to introduce the stem cell matrix into the patient. Smaller needles will affect the structural integrity of stem cells.
- Select appropriate injectate volume to match the volume which the target body part is able to accommodate.
- As with any injection therapy, correctly identifying the pain generator will render highest chance for a successful treatment.
- The recommended site to harvest bone MSC is the iliac crest.
- Provide ample local anesthesia from the skin and deep tissues down to the periosteum to prevent intense pain and poor patient experience.
- Only use 0.25% or less of ropivacaine. All other local anesthetics are cytotoxic regardless of anesthetics concentration.
- Allow sufficient time for local anesthesia to provide coverage.
- When collecting bone marrow, use multiple smaller syringes to optimize a higher specimen yield.
- Heparin is preferred over anticoagulant citrate dextrose (ACD) to prevent clotting of bone marrow aspirate inside the draw syringe (i.e., minimize the risk of cell count loss inside the syringe). Heparin must also be used at the cannulation site on the bone which will also prevent clotting.
- Recommended rehabilitation protocol:
  - 0–2 weeks: isometric exercises without range of motion.
  - 3–5 weeks: range of motion exercises, isotonic exercises with low-level resistance.
  - >6 weeks: eccentric exercises can be added as tolerated. Full physical activity can be resumed at 8–10 weeks.

Recommended Reading

1. Centeno CJ, Busse D, Kisiday J, Keohan C, Freeman M, Karli D. Increased knee cartilage volume in degenerative joint disease using percutaneously implanted, autologous mesenchymal stem cells. Pain Physician. 2008;11(3):343–53.
2. Centeno CJ, Schultz JR, Cheever M, et al. Safety and complications reporting update on the re-implantation of culture-expanded mesenchymal stem cells using autologous platelet lysate technique. Curr Stem Cell Res Ther. 2011;6(4):368–78.
3. Centeno CJ, Pitts JA, Al-Sayegh H, Freeman MD. Efficacy and safety of bone marrow concentrate for osteoarthritis of the hip; treatment registry results for 196 patients. J Stem Cell Res Ther. 2014;4(242):2.
4. Dragoo JL, Carlson G, McCormick F, et al. Healing full-thickness cartilage defects using adipose-derived stem cells. Tissue Eng. 2007;13(7):1615–21.
5. Hernigou P, Flouzat Lachaniette CH, Delambre J, et al. Biologic augmentation of rotator cuff repair with mesenchymal stem cells during arthroscopy improves healing and prevents further tears: a case-controlled study. Int Orthop. 2014;38(9):1811–8.
6. Karahuseyinoglu S, Cinar O, Kilic E, et al. Biology of stem cells in human umbilical cord stroma: in situ and in vitro surveys. Stem Cells. 2007;25(2):319–31.
7. Mishra A, Tummala P, King A, et al. Buffered platelet-rich plasma enhances mesenchymal stem cell proliferation and chondrogenic differentiation. Tissue Eng Part C Methods. 2009;15(3):431–5.
8. Mochida J, Sakai D, Nakamura Y, Watanabe T, Yamamoto Y, Kato S. Intervertebral disc repair with activated nucleus pulposus cell transplantation: a three-year, prospective clinical study of its safety. Eur Cell Mater. 2015;29:202–12; discussion 212
9. Nelson L, Fairclough J, Archer CW. Use of stem cells in the biological repair of articular cartilage. Expert Opin Biol Ther. 2010;10(1):43–55.
10. Orozco L, Soler R, Morera C, Alberca M, Sánchez A, García-Sancho J. Intervertebral disc repair by autologous mesenchymal bone marrow cells: a pilot study. Transplantation. 2011;92(7):822–8.
11. Pang X, Yang H, Peng B. Human umbilical cord mesenchymal stem cell transplantation for the treatment of chronic discogenic low back pain. Pain Physician. 2014;17(4):E525–30.
12. Pantalone A, Antonucci I, Guelfi M, et al. Amniotic fluid stem cells: an ideal resource for therapeutic application in bone tissue engineering. Eur Rev Med Pharmacol Sci. 2016;20(13):2884–90.
13. Petrie Aronin CE, Tuan RS. Therapeutic potential of the immunomodulatory activities of adult mesenchymal stem cells. Birth Defects Res C Embryo Today. 2010;90(1):67–74.
14. Pettine K, Suzuki R, Sand T, Murphy M. Treatment of discogenic back pain with autologous bone marrow concentrate injection with minimum two year follow-up. Int Orthop. 2016;40(1):135–40.

15. Richter M, Zech S. Matrix-associated stem cell transplantation (MAST) in chondral defects of foot and ankle is effective. Foot Ankle Surg. 2013;19(2):84–90.
16. Sakai D, Mochida J, Iwashina T, et al. Regenerative effects of transplanting mesenchymal stem cells embedded in atelocollagen to the degenerated intervertebral disc. Biomaterials. 2006;27(3):335–45.
17. Sen B, Xie Z, Case N, Ma M, Rubin C, Rubin J. Mechanical strain inhibits adipogenesis in mesenchymal stem cells by stimulating a durable beta-catenin signal. Endocrinology. 2008;149(12):6065–75.
18. Stanco D, Viganò M, Perucca Orfei C, et al. Multidifferentiation potential of human mesenchymal stem cells from adipose tissue and hamstring tendons for musculoskeletal cell-based therapy. Regen Med. 2015;10(6):729–43.
19. Tremolada C, Beltrami G, Magri A, et al. Adipose mesenchymal stem cells and "regenerative adipose tissue graft"(Lipogems®) for musculoskeletal regeneration. Eur J Musculoskelet Dis. 2014;3(2):57–67.
20. Vangsness CT Jr, Farr J 2nd, Boyd J, Dellaero DT, Mills CR, LeRoux-Williams M. Adult human mesenchymal stem cells delivered via intra-articular injection to the knee following partial medial meniscectomy: a randomized, double-blind, controlled study. J Bone Joint Surg Am. 2014;96(2):90–8.
21. Vega A, Martín-Ferrero MA, Del Canto F, et al. Treatment of Knee Osteoarthritis With Allogeneic Bone Marrow Mesenchymal Stem Cells: A Randomized Controlled Trial. Transplantation. 2015;99(8):1681–90.
22. Voleti PB, Buckley MR, Soslowsky LJ. Tendon healing: repair and regeneration. Annu Rev Biomed Eng. 2012;14:47–71.
23. Vora A, Borg-Stein J, Nguyen RT. Regenerative injection therapy for osteoarthritis: fundamental concepts and evidence-based review. PM R. 2012;4(5 Suppl):S104–9.
24. Westminster CO, Westminister CO, Vail CO, Busse D. Increased knee cartilage volume in degenerative joint disease using percutaneously implanted, autologous mesenchymal stem cells. Pain Physician. 2008;11(3):343–53.

Regenerative Therapies for Chronic Intradiscal Pain

90

Christine L. Hunt, Luke A. Law, and Wenchun Qu

Introduction

Pain originating from the intervertebral disc (IVD) is a common pain complaint and is the source of discomfort in up to 40% of patients with axial low back pain (LBP). Estimates of the annual prevalence of LBP range from 15% to 45%, and patients frequently experience relapse and recurrence for which they seek subspecialty care. LBP carries significant morbidity and is the leading global cause of disability. A recent population-based study estimated the incidence of IVD disc degeneration to be 31.6% in men and 44.7% in women, with a positive correlation observed with aging.

Discogenic pain tends to occur more commonly in the younger population (age < 45 years), and disc abnormalities on MRI occur commonly in the asymptomatic population, making appropriate diagnostic evaluation paramount in guiding treatment decisions. As the driving force behind degenerative LBP, lumbar disc degeneration begins at approximately 13.3 years of age in humans and degenerates on average at a rate of 0.034 disc per year. As the population continues to age, degenerative spine conditions are expected to increase accordingly, representing a substantial increase in total health-care utilization costs. The use of interventional spine procedures increased 54% in the Medicare population from 2000 to 2014, with an annual increase of 3.1%.

The IVD is composed of a central nucleus pulposus (NP), the surrounding annulus fibrosus (AF), and the end plates at the cranial and caudal end. The NP is comprised of chondrocyte-like NP cells and an extracellular matrix (ECM) made up of a large amount of proteoglycan, type II collagen fibers, and other fibers such as elastin. The NP is highly hydrated due to the large amount of negative charge in glycosaminoglycan (GAG) that attracts water molecules. The annulus fibrosus (AF) is comprised of type I and III collagen fibers organized in 15–25 concentric layers that encase the NP and resist tensile forces. The end plate has a hyaline cartilage and an osseous component that together prevent the NP from penetrating to the vertebral body and allow nutrients to permeate from the trabecular space to the avascular IVD through the marrow contact channels.

The pathophysiology of IVD degeneration involves three intricately related processes: a cellular process related to loss of NP cells, a pro-inflammatory process characterized by the increase of pro-inflammatory cytokines and chemokines, and a molecular process resulting in net loss of extracellular matrix (ECM). Subsequent changes of neovascularization and neoinnnervation are also part of the pathology that is related to clinical manifestations as pain. Aging, genetic propensity, and abnormal mechanical loading are associated with accelerated disc degeneration [13]. Subsequently, the loss of disc height and resultant altered biomechanical features can also exacerbate damage to associated motion segments.

Throughout the human lifespan, the NP contains three types of cells: notochordal cells (disappear around age 10), chondrocyte-like cells (dominate after age 10), and progenitor cells that are capable of disc repair. The degenerated IVD is characterized by decreased NP cell number and an increased proportion of cells in the "senescent" state. As humans reach skeletal maturity, NP cell density decreases to approximately 4000 cells/mm^3 and continues to go through apoptosis. The proportion of senescent cells increases with time. Shortened DNA telomeres lead to reduced cellular replication and increased senescent cell density.

The ECM of the NP undergoes a dynamic balance of synthesis and degradation. NP cells produce ECM molecules, and their capacity of production is affected by loss of cell

C. L. Hunt
Department of Physical Medicine and Rehabilitation, Mayo Clinic, Rochester, MN, USA

L. A. Law
Department of Anesthesiology, Mayo Clinic, Rochester, MN, USA

W. Qu (✉)
Department of Physical Medicine and Rehabilitation, Division of Pain Medicine, Spine Center, Mayo Clinic, Rochester, MN, USA
e-mail: qu.wenchun@mayo.edu

T. R. Deer et al. (eds.), *Deer's Treatment of Pain*, https://doi.org/10.1007/978-3-030-12281-2_90

population due to apoptosis. Pro-inflammatory factors, on the other hand, upregulate catabolic mediators, including ADAMTS-4, ADAMTS-5, MMP-1, MMP-2, MMP-3, MMP-13, and MMP-14. Degenerated IVDs are in a chronic inflammatory state, with increased expression of multiple pro-inflammation cytokines including interleukin 1 (IL-1), matrix metalloproteinase 10 (MMP10), IL-8, tumor necrosis factor-α (TNF-α), IL-2, IL-4, IL-17, monocyte chemotactic protein-1 (MCP- 1), and prostaglandin E2 (PGE2). These cytokines are derived from either IVD cells or invaded immune cells.

The growth of nerve and blood vessels into the typically avascular and aneural IVD, observed in zones of granulation tissue extending from the NP through the AF in DDD, permits migration of macrophages and mast cells that produce pro-inflammatory cytokines and also causes pain.

Stem cells may offer a renewable source of replacement of cells and tissues to treat conditions including macular degeneration, stroke, heart disease, osteoarthritis, and painful degenerative disc disease (DDD). Stem cells are characterized by the capacity for self-renewal through cell division and multilineage differentiation under certain physiologic or experimental conditions. Stem cells in regenerative medicine may be subcategorized based on potency. Pluripotent stem cells are either derived from an embryo or genetically reprogramed specialized adult cells called induced pluripotent stem cells (iPSCs). Multipotent stem cells can be derived from a tissue or organ as they function to maintain or repair the tissue in which they are found. These multipotent stem cells are called adult stem cells or mesenchymal stem cells (MSCs). Concerns over their tumorigenicity and ethical controversies have largely precluded the use of embryonic stem cells in regenerative medicine in the United States. Research on MSCs, however, has attracted a great deal of attention and has been the main focus of clinical trials.

Regenerative therapy for DDD largely depends on MSC's immunomodulatory effects that reduce pain and trophic effects that activate the endogenous NP cells. MSCs are defined by characteristics according to the International Society for Cellular Therapy, including adherence to plastic, specific cell surface markers (CD44+, CD73+, CD90+, CD105+, CD271+, CD34−, CD45−, CD31−, Stro-1 +, HLA-DR-), and tripotency (potential to differentiate toward adipocytic, chondrocytic, or osteogenic lineages). MSCs can be obtained from a variety of tissue sources. In musculoskeletal applications, they are most commonly obtained from bone marrow or adipose tissue. The number of clinical trials devoted to regenerative medicine in the application of bone and cartilage disease is steadily increasing, with clinical trials of all three phases being conducted. Herein we will discuss the background and rationale for intradiscal regenerative therapies for the treatment of painful DDD, describe their clinical use today, and discuss ongoing research investigating the safety and efficacy of such procedures.

Background and Historical Perspective

Diagnosis of Discogenic Pain

There is considerable heterogeneity with respect to the approach to diagnosis and treatment of pain originating from the IVD. Diagnosing the IVD as the source of LBP requires a conscientious approach in terms of history, physical examination, and decisions on further testing. Patients typically report axial, midline, or immediately paraspinal LBP, sometimes with radiation to flanks or buttocks either unilaterally or bilaterally. The pain is normally worsened with axial loading, sitting, or lumbar flexion, and it is improved with standing, extension, or lying flat. The physical examination is an important part of the evaluation for identifying patients for potential discogenic pain. The reliability of exam maneuvers is poor in accurately diagnosing discogenic pain, and it is not performed as often as might be indicated. A report showed that 43% of patient visits for LBP involve no focused inspection and almost 20% do not involve palpation.

Discogenic pain, facetogenic pain, and non-specific low back pain often share similar clinical features, and further workup ranging from simple radiograph to interventional procedures is necessary for appropriately evaluating suspected discogenic pain based on clinical findings. Imaging studies and discography are indicated when intradiscal intervention or surgery is considered. Some MRI findings have been found to be indicative of a painful disc, such as a high-intensity zone (HIZ) in combination with a disc protrusion, or Modic vertebral end plate and marrow changes of type I or type II involving greater than 25% of the vertebral body, which reflects an increased amount of pro-inflammatory cytokines (IL-8, IL-6, TNF-α). On the contrary, normal T2 nuclear signal virtually rules out a painful disc. In most instances, however, those findings would need further confirmation due to lack of specificity in imaging studies. While there is no gold standard test for discogenic pain, the current reference standard is provocative discography. A systematic review of the literature suggests that current evidence supports lumbar provocation discography as a useful tool. This is supported by multiple professional societies including the International Association for the Study of Pain (IASP), the Spine Intervention Society (SIS), and the North American Spine Society (NASS). Caution should be exercised as discography may accelerate the degenerative process in patients who undergo this procedure, and its use should be limited to cases where an accurate diagnosis will make a clear difference in management and should be performed by well-trained operators. In addition, the IVD as the largest avascular organ poses a heightened infection risk, and practitioners should utilize strict sterile technique.

Treatment of Discogenic Pain

A number of treatments for discogenic LBP have been proposed and trialed. Definitive efficacious treatment remains elusive, with many patients trialing a variety of approaches ranging from conservative measures to surgery. Physical therapy and the establishment of targeted home exercise programs are an important first step in the treatment of discogenic low neck pain. Nonsteroidal anti-inflammatory drugs (NSAIDs) may be moderately effective in the treatment of non-specific chronic LBP, although long-term consequences in safety remain controversial, and the supporting evidence is not particularly robust. Tramadol used in combination with NSAIDs may ameliorate the risk for transition of acute LBP to chronic LBP, but their potential interactions with other medications are myriad, and its potency is variable based on each patient's cytochrome p450 metabolism. Opioids are the most commonly prescribed medication for LBP, but evidence for their efficacy is scant. This is particularly true in chronic LBP, with a high risk of developing tolerance and hyperalgesia with long-term opioid use. Potential complications also include addiction and overdose-related mortality. As a result, the risk-benefit ratio is not optimal, and the Centers for Disease Control cautions strongly against the routine use of opioid analgesics for treatment of chronic LBP.

A variety of intradiscal interventional procedures have been proposed to target discogenic pain that fails to respond to conservative management, including intradiscal injection, nucleoplasty, intradiscal electrothermal therapy (IDET), and biacuplasty. A systematic review of non-operative interventional management of discogenic LBP provides Level 2A evidence indicating intradiscal methylene blue injection may be clinically effective for treatment of intradiscal pain. Neither traction therapy nor epidural steroid injections have demonstrated efficacy for intradiscal pain, and support for ablative therapy has been mixed but largely considered to be inadequate. Corticosteroid injected into the IVD has been attempted to treat inflammation contributing to discogenic pain. Level 1B evidence suggests intradiscal steroid injection may be efficacious for only short-term relief of LBP associated with "active discopathy" on MRI, but not for improvement of function or other health-related quality of life measures. Nucleoplasty is a minimally invasive procedure to decompress herniated discs that has been shown to have only moderate clinical relevance for pain or function in cervical disc herniation, without definitive evidence supporting its efficacy in relief of lumbar discogenic pain. Thermal annular procedures including biacuplasty and IDET propose to involve thermocoagulation of nociceptors and nerve ingrowth of the AF but have also failed to demonstrate definitive clinical efficacy [60, 68, 69]. Patients who have failed conservative treatments are sometimes offered surgery for intractable discogenic pain. Level 1A evidence exists to suggest that there is no significant difference in functional improvement between patients who have undergone fusion surgery for discogenic LBP compared to nonsurgical interventional treatment 2 years after the surgery.

Similarly, lumbar disc replacement surgery has shown short-term improved pain relief, function, and patient satisfaction. Older patients, who comprise a large proportion of patients with DDD, may fare worse than younger patients postoperatively in terms of pain and functional improvement. In short, well-studied therapeutic options for chronic LBP associated with DDD or discogenic pain have not been shown to consistently display long-term efficacy in pain relief or functional improvement in discogenic back pain. Furthermore, none of the traditional management strategies including manual therapies, interventional procedures, or surgery result in reconstruction of the damaged or painful IVD.

Regenerative Medicine in Discogenic Pain

The use of regenerative medicine including stem cell therapies and platelet-rich plasma (PRP) for the management of chronic pain is drawing increasing interest. Discogenic pain has been the most studied in painful degenerative spine conditions. Current evidence examining the use of MSCs has been encouraging in terms of safety and feasibility, and high-quality randomized clinical trials (RCTs) are being conducted. This is the first time biologics have been used to help address the underlying pathophysiology in painful DDD. These have shown promising preliminary results, with larger studies needed to further examine efficacy and long-term safety.

The Mechanism of MSCs in Regenerative Medicine

MSCs are thought to exert their beneficial effects in the IVD through a variety of mechanisms including decreasing cell loss in the NP, decreasing pro-inflammatory cytokine activities, improving cellular matrix, and subsequently improving nuclear hydration (see Fig. 90.1).

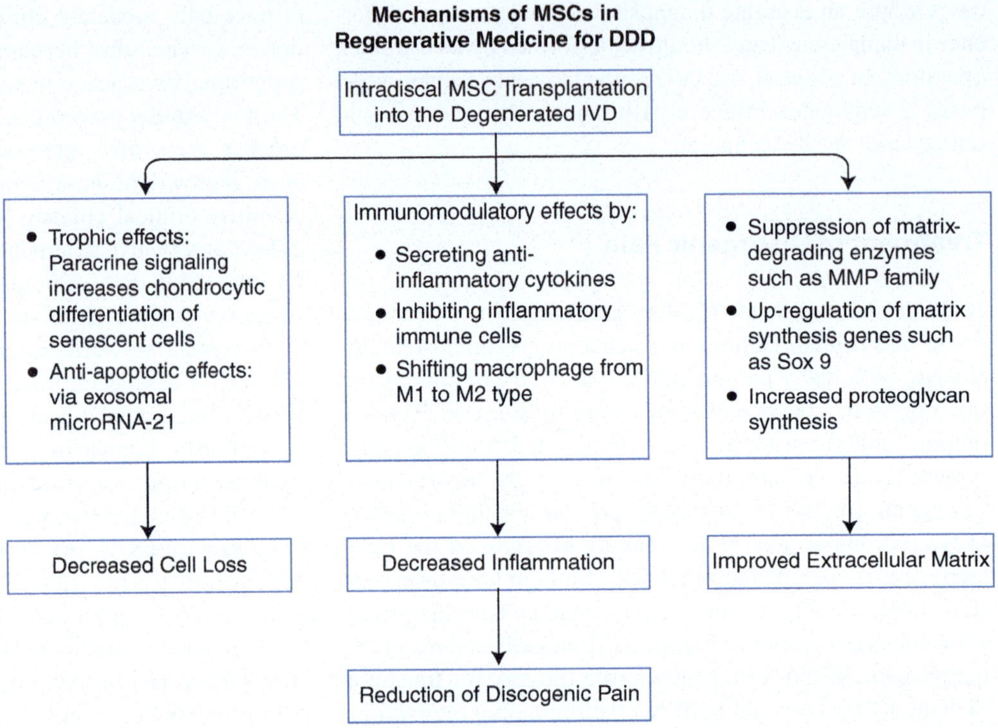

Fig. 90.1 Mechanisms of MSCs in regenerative medicine

Decreased Cell Loss

MSCs co-cultured with degenerated NP cells from the human IVD have been shown to stimulate matrix synthesis and cell proliferation of the degenerated NP cells in vitro. MSC interaction with vascular endothelial cells enhances the chondrocytic lineage potential via activation of the AKT signaling pathway. This interaction is thought to be a paracrine signaling mechanism that may increase chondrocytic differentiation of senescent cells in the degenerated IVD. This is likely particularly important in the NP, an avascular niche with little access to blood supply other than in the periphery of the AF. Recently, in vitro studies have demonstrated that the anti-apoptotic effects of MSC may be mediated via exosomal microRNA-21. When transplanted into the IVD, MSC exosomes containing miR-21 were taken up and internalized by NP cells and exerted a protective effect against TNF-α-induced apoptosis.

Decreased Inflammation

MSCs secrete bioactive mediators such as cytokines and growth factors that not only aid in the reparative process but also decrease inflammation. Bone marrow-derived MSCs have been shown to inhibit T lymphocyte proliferation via soluble effector molecules, decreasing inflammation. In addition to their redifferentiation capacity, MSCs also exist endogenously as perivascular cell "pericytes" that have beneficial immunomodulatory effects and help establish an anti-inflammatory, pro-reparative microenvironment. They are capable of responding to local environmental stimuli with several beneficial interventions. Endogenous pericytes, residing on blood vessels, are stimulated by soluble growth factors and chemokines to become activated MSCs that respond to the microenvironment by secreting trophic (mitogenic, angiogenic, or anti-apoptic), immunomodulatory, or antimicrobial factors.

Improvement in Extracellular Matrix

Decreased cell loss and decreased inflammation provide the opportunity for improvement in the degraded ECM of the degenerated IVD. Intradiscal MSC transplantation has been shown to suppress matrix metalloproteinase (MMP)-related genes and inflammatory cytokines, promoting expression of type II collagen by endogenous NP cells and increasing disc height and T2 signal intensity on MRI. What is perhaps more remarkable than the activity of MSCs with NP cells in vitro is their robustness in the harsh microenvironment of the IVD. MSCs have demonstrated their engraftment capability and viability in the IVD, although high acidity in more degenerated discs likely continues to pose a threat to undifferentiated MSCs. Co-cultured NP cells in contact with MSCs lead to increased NP marker genes in MSCs as well as increased type II collagen expression in both MSCs and NP cells, suggesting that intradiscal MSC transplantation into the NP may induce differentiation and matrix gene expression of the transplanted MSCs. MSC transplantation has been shown to halt or significantly decelerate ECM loss via increased type II collagen expression, promotion of proteoglycan synthesis preserving IVD water content, and preservation of the NP via differentiation of MSCs toward the NP phenotype.

Intradiscal MSCs and PRP in Preclinical Models

Stem cell transplantation in preclinical models has been shown to be associated with significantly increased type II collagen expression, T2-weighted MRI signal intensity, disc height, and significantly reduced histologic disc degenerative grade, suggesting that stem cells may halt the degenerative process in DDD and promote IVD regeneration. This regenerative capacity was hypothesized to be due to the trophic, immunomodulatory, and matrix producing ability of stem cells induced by the local microenvironment after transplantation. These findings in animal studies have provided a foundation for testing the effects of stem cells in human subjects.

Intradiscal injection of platelet-rich plasma (PRP) for degenerative disc animal models has also shown regenerative activities demonstrated by increased water content, disc height, and induced cell proliferation. The mechanism is based on the role of platelets in wound healing, where growth factors of platelets such as PDGF, IGF-1, TGF- β, and VEGF act to promote tissue proliferation. In addition, PRP is hypothesized to influence local inflammatory processes by its antibacterial and bactericidal proteins.

Advances in Technology

Cell leakage is a concern in discs with complete annular fissures, but advancements in delivery including hydrogels and collagen scaffolds may ameliorate the risk of MSCs escaping the intended therapeutic target site. Discography should also exclude the presence of complete annular tears with epidural leakage prior to intradiscal transplantation of MSCs.

Regenerative medicine possesses the unique niche of holding promise for possible IVD regeneration in painful DDD, particularly with technological advances with genetically modified stem cells and induced pluripotent stem cells.

Uses and Indications

Intradiscal Mesenchymal Stem Cells

MSCs are increasingly being offered as treatment for pain in the clinical and research setting across the United States, with significant enthusiasm for their potential as a therapeutic option for patients who have failed other treatment. MSCs have been most commonly procured from two main sources for treatment of degenerative disc-related conditions: bone marrow or adipose tissue. Culture-expanded cells of both types are being studied in clinical trials. Bone marrow aspirate concentrate (BMAC) and minimally processed adipose harvest are used in point-of-care settings. There are no head-to-head comparisons of the quality of MSCs among different sources. However, the general understanding is that adipose tissue has a larger number of MSCs per unit volume of tissue, while bone marrow MSCs are easier to isolate under point-of-care settings. This is because BMAC can be separated via simple centrifugation, and historically common digestion methods for lipoaspirate including enzymatic degradation and ultrasound separation have been deemed noncompliant with US Food and Drug Administration (FDA) guidelines because they are considered beyond minimal manipulation.

Patients with a clinical diagnosis of discogenic pain with corresponding imaging findings and confirmed with provocative discography may be treatment candidates. Most clinical trials investigating intradiscal MSC transplantation have studied subjects with discogenic pain associated with mild to moderate IVD degeneration. In clinics, patients with more advanced DDD should be considered as well. Indeed, the therapeutic benefit of MSCs may actually be enhanced in later stages of degeneration. Firm contraindications to intradiscal MSC transplantation generally include patients with active cancer within the past 5 years, except for noninvasive skin cancers.

Periprocedural planning may proceed with thoughtful consideration given to medications, activity restrictions, and rehabilitation. The use of NSAIDs may theoretically impair the chondrogenesis of MSCs and influence the exogenous MSCs to differentiate and stimulate cartilage repair; therefore, it is recommended that patients do not take NSAIDs periprocedurally. Low-dose aspirin has been reported to promote MSC growth and inhibit apoptosis and thus can be continued. Corticosteroids are known to inhibit the regenerative capacity of MSCs and reduce their viability, and exogenous administration should be avoided periprocedurally if at all possible. General periprocedural considerations with respect to interventional procedures should apply in regenerative therapy cases, including anticoagulation, bleeding diathesis, pregnancy (in the case of fluoroscopy use), infection, allergies, and anatomic derangement that may render the intradiscal procedure technically challenging.

In today's clinical setting, stem cells are often transplanted at point-of-care using autologous BMAC. Bone marrow is typically harvested from the iliac crests using either an anterior or posterior approach. The yield of bone marrow mononuclear cells is higher when harvested from the iliac crest compared to the tibia or calcaneus and carries less morbidity such as post-procedural pain. This may be performed using ultrasound assistance or under fluoroscopic guidance to identify the bone marrow needle entry point or trajectory;

some practitioners may use landmark palpation to identify proposed entry points. After harvest of bone marrow, the aspirate undergoes centrifugation to prepare BMAC. Depending on the available space within the painful index disc, injectate greater than 2 ml may be very painful and lead to several days of LBP symptoms following the injection.

A centrifuge with higher concentration capability is particularly helpful in the case of intradiscal injections, in order to maximize the yield of MSCs per ml of prepared BMAC and minimize the total amount of injectate. For BMAC, at a rate of 0.001–0.005% of colony forming unit-fibroblasts (CFU-F) and 1–30 × 10^6 bone marrow mononuclear cells per ml of bone marrow aspirate, 60 ml of bone marrow aspirate is estimated to yield 30,000–150,000 CFU-F per prepared BMAC. Certainly these numbers may vary by technique, site of aspiration, and bone density of the patient; the degree to which such factors substantially impact cell yield and clinical outcomes is a subject of study still underway. Compared to other sources of MSCs, CFU-F yield is greatest in bone marrow and adipose, making these tissue sources particularly attractive for application in regenerative medicine.

There is some evidence that MSCs show a preference for differentiating toward their tissue of origin, for example, bone marrow-derived MSCs may have superior osteogenesis compared to adipose-derived MSCs. However, this has not been shown to have a definitively significant impact on their safety or efficacy in clinical applications. Adipose-derived MSC yield is greater than from BMAC; the frequency of stromal progenitors in lipoaspirate ranges from 1 to 10% related to the total nucleated cell population, yielding approximately 300,000 CFU-F per aspiration of adipose.

As described in Chap. 92, research on stem cells in regenerative medicine is ongoing in a number of areas including in the IVD, with a focus on phase II and III clinical trials. Randomized controlled trials (RCTs) investigating MSC transplantation into the IVD primarily involve transplanted culture-expanded stem cells, rather than "minimally manipulated" cells such as BMAC or lipoaspirate. Culture expansion may only be performed in laboratories that meet the strictest standards for good manufacturing practices (GMP), to minimize the risk of infection. The product is deemed as more than minimally manipulated. Future areas of research on MSC transplantation in the IVD will likely include culture expansion and may also involve lineage-directed or genetically modified MSCs, as well as human-induced pluripotent stem cells. For now, preclinical studies on transplantation of these "later generation" MSCs into the IVD continue to establish their safety in animal disc models. (For more on this topic, please see Chap. 92.)

Intradiscal Platelet-Rich Plasma

Platelet-rich plasma (PRP) is a non-cell regenerative therapy that is increasingly used in the clinical setting for the treatment of musculoskeletal pain. The high concentration of platelets in PRP releases growth factors (PDGF, IGF-1, TGF-β, VEGF, bFGF, EGF, and CTGF) and cytokines that may stimulate endogenous stem cells (or co-transplanted MSCs) to proliferate, reduce inflammation, upregulate collagen production, encourage proteoglycan synthesis of fibroblasts and chondrocytes, and stimulate extracellular matrix synthesis. The benefits from these growth factors on the IVD and its associated microenvironment have been demonstrated both in vitro and in vivo in animal models.

Preclinical studies investigating intradiscal PRP are encouraging. NP cells cultured with PRP demonstrate 7–11-fold increased proliferation and upregulated proteoglycan synthesis, and PRP leads to downregulation of pro-inflammatory cytokines and upregulated synthesis of proteoglycans, collagen, extracellular matrix, and proliferation of AF cells. Animal models have demonstrated improved preservation of disc morphology and improved fluid content, although study design has been noted to be heterogenous, and thus consistent conclusions are somewhat limited.

As the efficacy of PRP lies in its ability to activate native and transplanted stem cells, co-transplantation with MSCs for the treatment of painful DDD may be a reasonable treatment to pursue in patients whose endogenous intradiscal stem cells are likely decreased in number and more senescent than in a non-degenerated IVD. One published study (see Table 90.1) has examined such an application, and injection of autologous PRP with MSCs for eligible candidates is commonly employed in regenerative practices for performing such procedures if there is not a contraindication to MSC transplantation.

Evidence for Safety and Efficacy

A systematic review included a total of 167 subjects in six studies who received intradiscal stem cell injection and did not experience any serious adverse events related to treatment. Improvement in pain, function, and water content of the IVD were observed, suggesting that such treatment holds promise to help improve pain and restore function. Four of the six studies were cohort studies; thus, there is good (Level 2A) evidence to suggest that intradiscal MSC injection is safe and well-tolerated. Three of these studies compared MRI pre- and posttreatment, and 24/43 patients demonstrated improvement in water content of the treated IVD. All studies reported significant improvement in pain and function among treatment groups. However, as most of these studies were small and did not include control groups, the efficacy of intradiscal MSC transplantation is not yet proven. To demonstrate the efficacy of such treatments, well-designed RCTs with larger numbers of subjects are needed. Currently active clinical trials focus on establishing safety, tolerability, and efficacy with respect to injected MSCs for discogenic pain.

There is Level 1B evidence that intradiscal PRP for the treatment of painful degenerative disc disease is safe and effective, with no adverse events reported. A subsequent phase I study has provided Level 4 evidence that intradiscal transplantation of PRP releasate in subjects with chronic LBP and mild to moderate degenerative disc disease is safe and feasible, with the only adverse events reported being transient leg numbness in two patients at 1 and 6 months following injection that resolved within 7 days without intervention.

Published literature to date summarizing the clinical data which exists in support of intradiscal regenerative therapy for the treatment of degenerative disc disease is presented in Table 90.1 below. This includes all studies in which intradiscal injection of MSCs and/or PRP for treatment of painful DDD without concomitant surgical intervention. Completed studies include 136 human subjects and examine the safety and efficacy of intradiscally injected MSCs with or without PRP in the treatment of discogenic pain. These studies reported no serious adverse events related to the procedure or treatment. Side effects were mild and self-limited, resolving with either conservative care or without specific intervention. Improvement in pain, function, and water content in the nucleus pulposus were reported. Intradiscal transplantation of MSCs at dosage levels up to 100 million cells has

Table 90.1 Currently published evidence for treatment of discogenic pain with MSCs or PRP

Author (year) # of cases	Design	Injectate	Dosage	Adverse events	Observed clinical outcomes	Follow-up
Orozco et al. (2011) [120] $N = 10$	Open label, single arm	Autologous BMSC, culture-expanded	18–28 M	None reported	Pain and disability were significantly improved by 3 months. Disc height did not improve, but there was improvement in the water content of the disc at 12 months	12 months
Pang et al. (2014) [121] $N = 2$	Case study	Allogeneic HUC-MSCs, culture-expanded	100 M	None reported	Both subjects reported improvement in pain and function. One patient demonstrated higher T2 signal intensity on MRI at the treated disc at 2 years	24 months
Pettine et al. (2016) [122] $N = 26$	Open label, 2 arms (13 patients received single-level injection, 13 patients received 2-level injections)	Autologous BMAC	5404–8106 CFU-F per injected IVD	None reported	Improvement in pain and function were observed at all time points but statistically significant at 3 and 6 months. On average, 77% improvement was observed among patients that received >2000 CFU-F/ml, and 64% improvement was observed in patients that received <2000 CFU-F/ml concentration. 8/20 patients at 12 months improved by 1 Pfirrmann grade, the rest did not change. 5 patients went on to surgery	24 months
Comella et al. (2017) [123] $N = 15$	Open label, single arm	SVF with PRP	30–60 M cells in 1–3 cc of PRP	SAEs: None. AEs: soreness at harvest site, injection site (resolved within 10 days without intervention)	Positive trends were observed in lumbar range of motion and pain relief. Moderate improvement in ODI was observed	12 months
Levi et al. (2016) [124] $N = 22$	Open label, single arm	Neutrophil-rich PRP	1.5 ml	None reported	47% reported at least 50% improvement in VAS and 30% improvement in ODI	6 months
Tuakli-Wosornu et al. (2016) [118] $N = 47$	Prospective, double-blind RCT (2:1 treatment to control)	PRP	1–2 ml	None reported	Statistically significant improvement in FRI and NRS best pain score in treatment group compared to control	2 months
Akeda et al. (2017) [119] $N = 14$	Open label, single arm	PRP (mean platelet count 3.7 times greater than whole blood, mean WBC count 1/230 of whole blood)	2 ml	2 patients reported leg numbness (at 1 month and at 6 months), which disappeared within 7 days without intervention. The 2 subjects who worsened after initial improvement returned to baseline but did not worsen further	71% reported >50% pain reduction within 4 weeks after injection (LBP returned in 2 subjects), and 79% reported >50% improvement in physical disability within 4 weeks (this worsened again in the same 2 subjects who experienced recurrent LBP). No changes in disc height or T2 signal intensity were observed on X-ray or MRI	10 months

been demonstrated to be safe in human subjects with painful degenerative disc disease, with preliminary evidence of their efficacy supported by improvements in pain and functional scores. Nevertheless, due to low numbers of subjects and most of the studies being non-randomized, the quality of evidence with respect to the efficacy of intradiscal regenerative therapies remains low to moderate. To obtain adequate numbers of subjects for well-powered, high-quality RCTs, multicenter studies are needed in collaboration with GMP facilities. Biostatistical support plays an important role to ensure appropriate analysis and interpretation of results. One such trial, sponsored by industry, is investigating intradiscal injection of 6 million mesenchymal precursor cells for the treatment of chronic discogenic LBP and endeavors to recruit 360 subjects (https://clinicaltrials.gov/show/NCT02412735). The results of a previously phase II trial involved 200 subjects and appeared to be promising in terms of safety and efficacy but did not undergo peer review and formal publication. We are currently leading a phase I clinical trial investigating the safety and feasibility of intradiscal injection of autologous, culture-expanded adipose-derived MSCs for the treatment of discogenic low back pain.

Main Points

- LBP is the most common disabling pain complaint among patients presenting to primary care physicians and subspecialty providers. Discogenic pain is an important differential diagnoses for back and neck pain, and it requires conscientious diagnosis and management. Diagnostic testing including advanced neuroimaging and discography should be considered when they are likely to significantly influence treatment decisions.
- Treatment options for intractable discogenic pain are limited, with poor to moderate evidence for traditional treatment approaches. Many procedures that initially held promise for relief of pain and improvement in function have met with challenges in long-term effectiveness, including surgery.
- MSCs in clinical use today for intradiscal pain exert their beneficial effects through immunomodulatory and trophic effects. The most common sources for MSCs include bone marrow and adipose tissue.
- Intradiscal PRP injections are being used alone and in conjunction with MSCs for treatment of discogenic back pain.
- There is moderate to good evidence that intradiscal regenerative therapies for the treatment of discogenic pain are safe. Evidence for their efficacy is still being studied, and proper investigation will require well-powered RCTs.

Recommended Reading

1. DePalma MJ, Ketchum JM, Saullo T. What is the source of chronic low back pain and does age play a role? Pain Med. 2011;12(2):224–33.
2. Manchikanti L, Singh V, Falco FJ, Benyamin RM, Hirsch JA. Epidemiology of low back pain in adults. Neuromodulation. 2014;17(Suppl 2):3–10.
3. Billis E, Koutsojannis C, Matzaroglou C, et al. Association of low back pain on physical, sociodemographic and lifestyle factors across a general population sample within Greece. J Back Musculoskelet Rehabil. 2017;30(2):279–90.
4. Hoy D, March L, Brooks P, et al. The global burden of low back pain: estimates from the global burden of disease 2010 study. Ann Rheum Dis. 2014;73(6):968–74.
5. Teraguchi M, Yoshimura N, Hashizume H, et al. Progression, incidence, and risk factors for intervertebral disc degeneration in a longitudinal population-based cohort: the Wakayama spine study. Osteoarthr Cartil. 2017;25(7):1122–31.
6. Paajanen H, Erkintalo M, Kuusela T, Dahlstrom S, Kormano M. Magnetic resonance study of disc degeneration in young low-back pain patients. Spine. 1989;14(9):982–5.
7. Zheng C-J, Chen J. Disc degeneration implies low back pain. Theor Biol Med Model. 2015;12(1):24.
8. Global Burden of Disease Study 2013 Collaborators. Global, regional, and national incidence, prevalence, and years lived with disability for 301 acute and chronic diseases and injuries in 188 countries, 1990-2013: a systematic analysis for the global burden of disease study 2013. Lancet. 2015;386(9995):743–800.
9. Manchikanti L, Pampati V, Hirsch JA. Utilization of interventional techniques in managing chronic pain in medicare population from 2000 to 2014: an analysis of patterns of utilization. Pain Physician. 2016;19(4):E531–46.
10. Farshad-Amacker NA, Hughes A, Herzog RJ, Seifert B, Farshad M. The intervertebral disc, the endplates and the vertebral bone marrow as a unit in the process of degeneration. Eur Radiol. 2017;27(6):2507–20.
11. Moore RJ. The vertebral endplate: disc degeneration, disc regeneration. Eur Spine J. 2006;15(Suppl 3):S333–7.
12. Taylor JR. Growth of human intervertebral discs and vertebral bodies. J Anat. 1975;120(Pt 1):49–68.
13. Wang F, Cai F, Shi R, Wang XH, Wu XT. Aging and age related stresses: a senescence mechanism of intervertebral disc degeneration. Osteoarthr Cartil. 2016;24(3):398–408.
14. Freemont AJ. The cellular pathobiology of the degenerate intervertebral disc and discogenic back pain. Rheumatology (Oxford). 2009;48(1):5–10.
15. Trout JJ, Buckwalter JA, Moore KC. Ultrastructure of the human intervertebral disc: II. Cells of the nucleus pulposus. Anat Rec. 1982;204(4):307–14.
16. Johnson WE, Caterson B, Eisenstein SM, Hynds DL, Snow DM, Roberts S. Human intervertebral disc aggrecan inhibits nerve growth in vitro. Arthritis Rheum. 2002;46(10):2658–64.
17. Johnson WE, Caterson B, Eisenstein SM, Roberts S. Human intervertebral disc aggrecan inhibits endothelial cell adhesion and cell migration in vitro. Spine. 2005;30(10):1139–47.
18. Wang D, Hu Z, Hao J, et al. SIRT1 inhibits apoptosis of degenerative human disc nucleus pulposus cells through activation of Akt pathway. Age (Dordr). 2013;35(5):1741–53.
19. Wang J, Markova D, Anderson DG, Zheng Z, Shapiro IM, Risbud MV. TNF-alpha and IL-1beta promote a disintegrin-like and metalloprotease with thrombospondin type I motif-5-mediated aggrecan degradation through syndecan-4 in intervertebral disc. J Biol Chem. 2011;286(46):39738–49.

20. Tian Y, Yuan W, Fujita N, et al. Inflammatory cytokines associated with degenerative disc disease control aggrecanase-1 (ADAMTS-4) expression in nucleus pulposus cells through MAPK and NF-kappaB. Am J Pathol. 2013;182(6):2310–21.
21. Richardson SM, Doyle P, Minogue BM, Gnanalingham K, Hoyland JA. Increased expression of matrix metalloproteinase-10, nerve growth factor and substance P in the painful degenerate intervertebral disc. Arthritis Res Ther. 2009;11(4):R126.
22. Igarashi T, Kikuchi S, Shubayev V, Myers RR. 2000 Volvo Award winner in basic science studies: exogenous tumor necrosis factor-alpha mimics nucleus pulposus-induced neuropathology. Molecular, histologic, and behavioral comparisons in rats. Spine. 2000;25(23):2975–80.
23. Ahn SH, Cho YW, Ahn MW, Jang SH, Sohn YK, Kim HS. mRNA expression of cytokines and chemokines in herniated lumbar intervertebral discs. Spine. 2002;27(9):911–7.
24. O'Donnell JL, O'Donnell AL. Prostaglandin E2 content in herniated lumbar disc disease. Spine. 1996;21(14):1653–5.. discussion 1655-1656
25. Shamji MF, Setton LA, Jarvis W, et al. Proinflammatory cytokine expression profile in degenerated and herniated human intervertebral disc tissues. Arthritis Rheum. 2010;62(7):1974–82.
26. Abe Y, Akeda K, An HS, et al. Proinflammatory cytokines stimulate the expression of nerve growth factor by human intervertebral disc cells. Spine. 2007;32(6):635–42.
27. Peng B, Wu W, Hou S, Li P, Zhang C, Yang Y. The pathogenesis of discogenic low back pain. J Bone Joint Surg. 2005;87(1):62–7.
28. Murphy MB, Moncivais K, Caplan AI. Mesenchymal stem cells: environmentally responsive therapeutics for regenerative medicine. Exp Mol Med. 2013;45:e54.
29. Doorn J, Moll G, Le Blanc K, van Blitterswijk C, de Boer J. Therapeutic applications of mesenchymal stromal cells: paracrine effects and potential improvements. Tissue Eng Part B Rev. 2012;18(2):101–15.
30. Strassburg S, Hodson NW, Hill PI, Richardson SM, Hoyland JA. Bi-directional exchange of membrane components occurs during co-culture of mesenchymal stem cells and nucleus pulposus cells. PLoS One. 2012;7(3):e33739.
31. Niu CC, Yuan LJ, Lin SS, Chen LH, Chen WJ. Mesenchymal stem cell and nucleus pulposus cell coculture modulates cell profile. Clin Orthop Relat Res. 2009;467(12):3263–72.
32. Dominici M, Le Blanc K, Mueller I, et al. Minimal criteria for defining multipotent mesenchymal stromal cells. The International Society for Cellular Therapy position statement. Cytotherapy. 2006;8(4):315–7.
33. Mahla RS. Stem cells applications in regenerative medicine and disease therapeutics. Int J Cell Biol. 2016;2016:6940283.
34. Squillaro T, Peluso G, Galderisi U. Clinical trials with mesenchymal stem cells: an update. Cell Transplant. 2016;25(5):829–48.
35. Simon J, McAuliffe M, Shamim F, Vuong N, Tahaei A. Discogenic low back pain. Phys Med Rehabil Clin N Am. 2014;25(2):305–17.
36. Schwarzer AC, Aprill CN, Derby R, Fortin J, Kine G, Bogduk N. The prevalence and clinical features of internal disc disruption in patients with chronic low back pain. Spine. 1995;20(17):1878–83.
37. Press J, Liem B, Walega D, Garfin S. Survey of inspection and palpation rates among spine providers: evaluation of physician performance of the physical examination for patients with low back pain. Spine. 2013;38(20):1779–84.
38. Manchikanti L, Abdi S, Atluri S, et al. An update of comprehensive evidence-based guidelines for interventional techniques in chronic spinal pain. Part II: guidance and recommendations. Pain Physician. 2013;16(2 Suppl):S49–283.
39. Burke J, Watson R, McCormack D, Fitzpatrick J, Stack J, Walsh M. MR endplate changes are associated with increased disc inflammatory mediator production. J Bone Joint Surg Br. 2003;85-B(SUPP II):164.
40. Maus TP, Aprill CN. Lumbar diskogenic pain, provocation diskography, and imaging correlates. Radiol Clin N Am. 2012;50(4):681–704.
41. Teichtahl AJ, Urquhart DM, Wang Y, et al. Lumbar disc degeneration is associated with modic change and high paraspinal fat content - a 3.0T magnetic resonance imaging study. BMC Musculoskelet Disord. 2016;17(1):439.
42. Jha SC, Higashino K, Sakai T, et al. Clinical significance of high-intensity zone for discogenic low back pain: a review. J Med Investig. 2016;63(1-2):1–7.
43. Manchikanti L, Glaser SE, Wolfer L, Derby R, Cohen SP. Systematic review of lumbar discography as a diagnostic test for chronic low back pain. Pain Physician. 2009;12(3):541–59.
44. Manchikanti L, Dunbar EE, Wargo BW, Shah RV, Derby R, Cohen SP. Systematic review of cervical discography as a diagnostic test for chronic spinal pain. Pain Physician. 2009;12(2):305–21.
45. Shah RV, Everett CR, McKenzie-Brown AM, Sehgal N. Discography as a diagnostic test for spinal pain: a systematic and narrative review. Pain Physician. 2005;8(2):187–209.
46. Manchikanti L, Benyamin RM, Singh V, et al. An update of the systematic appraisal of the accuracy and utility of lumbar discography in chronic low back pain. Pain Physician. 2013;16(2 Suppl):Se55–95.
47. Cuellar JM, Stauff MP, Herzog RJ, Carrino JA, Baker GA, Carragee EJ. Does provocative discography cause clinically important injury to the lumbar intervertebral disc? a 10-year matched cohort study. Spine J. 2016;16(3):273–80.
48. Fraser RD, Osti OL, Vernon-Roberts B. Discitis after discography. J Bone Joint Surg. 1987;69(1):26–35.
49. Sarig-Bahat H. Evidence for exercise therapy in mechanical neck disorders. Man Ther. 2003;8(1):10–20.
50. Madigan L, Vaccaro AR, Spector LR, Milam RA. Management of symptomatic lumbar degenerative disk disease. J Am Acad Orthop Surg. 2009;17(2):102–11.
51. Jandric S, Antic B. Low back pain and degenerative disc disease. Med Pregl. 2006;59(9-10):456–61.
52. Enthoven WT, Roelofs PD, Deyo RA, van Tulder MW, Koes BW. Non-steroidal anti-inflammatory drugs for chronic low back pain. Cochrane Database Syst Rev. 2016;2:Cd012087.
53. Inage K, Orita S, Yamauchi K, et al. Low-dose tramadol and non-steroidal anti-inflammatory drug combination therapy prevents the transition to chronic low back pain. Asian Spine J. 2016;10(4):685–9.
54. Miotto K, Cho AK, Khalil MA, Blanco K, Sasaki JD, Rawson R. Trends in tramadol: pharmacology, metabolism, and misuse. Anesth Analg. 2017;124(1):44–51.
55. Park SH, Wackernah RC, Stimmel GL. Serotonin syndrome: is it a reason to avoid the use of tramadol with antidepressants? J Pharm Pract. 2014;27(1):71–8.
56. Deyo RA, Von Korff M, Duhrkoop D. Opioids for low back pain. BMJ. 2015;350:g6380.
57. Abdel Shaheed C, Maher CG, Williams KA, Day R, McLachlan AJ. Efficacy, tolerability, and dose-dependent effects of opioid analgesics for low back pain: a systematic review and meta-analysis. JAMA Intern Med. 2016;176(7):958–68.
58. Dowell D, Haegerich TM, Chou R. CDC guideline for prescribing opioids for chronic pain--United States, 2016. JAMA. 2016;315(15):1624–45.
59. Lu Y, Guzman JZ, Purmessur D, et al. Nonoperative management of discogenic back pain: a systematic review. Spine. 2014;39(16):1314–24.
60. Helm Ii S, Deer TR, Manchikanti L, et al. Effectiveness of thermal annular procedures in treating discogenic low back pain. Pain Physician. 2012;15(3):E279–304.

61. Freeman BJ, Mehdian R. Intradiscal electrothermal therapy, percutaneous discectomy, and nucleoplasty: what is the current evidence? Curr Pain Headache Rep. 2008;12(1):14–21.
62. Macario A, Pergolizzi JV. Systematic literature review of spinal decompression via motorized traction for chronic discogenic low back pain. Pain Pract. 2006;6(3):171–8.
63. Nguyen C, Boutron I, Baron G, et al. Intradiscal glucocorticoid injection for patients with chronic low back pain associated with active discopathy: a randomized trial. Ann Intern Med. 2017;166(8):547–56.
64. Wullems JA, Halim W, van der Weegen W. Current evidence of percutaneous nucleoplasty for the cervical herniated disk: a systematic review. Pain Pract. 2014;14(6):559–69.
65. Manchikanti L, Falco FJ, Benyamin RM, et al. An update of the systematic assessment of mechanical lumbar disc decompression with nucleoplasty. Pain Physician. 2013;16(2 Suppl):Se25–54.
66. Streitparth F, Disch AC. Interventions on the intervertebral discs. Indications, techniques and evidence levels. Radiologe. 2015;55(10):868–77.
67. Ong D, Chua NH, Vissers K. Percutaneous disc decompression for lumbar radicular pain: a review article. Pain Pract. 2016;16(1):111–26.
68. Freeman BJ. IDET: a critical appraisal of the evidence. Eur Spine J. 2006;15(Suppl 3):S448–57.
69. Helm S, Hayek SM, Benyamin RM, Manchikanti L. Systematic review of the effectiveness of thermal annular procedures in treating discogenic low back pain. Pain Physician. 2009;12(1):207–32.
70. Wang X, Wanyan P, Tian JH, Hu L. Meta-analysis of randomized trials comparing fusion surgery to non-surgical treatment for discogenic chronic low back pain. J Back Musculoskelet Rehabil. 2015;28(4):621–7.
71. Bydon M, De la Garza-Ramos R, Macki M, Baker A, Gokaslan AK, Bydon A. Lumbar fusion versus nonoperative management for treatment of discogenic low back pain: a systematic review and meta-analysis of randomized controlled trials. J Spinal Disord Tech. 2014;27(5):297–304.
72. Jacobs WC, van der Gaag NA, Kruyt MC, et al. Total disc replacement for chronic discogenic low back pain: a Cochrane review. Spine. 2013;38(1):24–36.
73. Gautschi OP, Smoll NR, Joswig H, et al. Influence of age on pain intensity, functional impairment and health-related quality of life before and after surgery for lumbar degenerative disc disease. Clin Neurol Neurosurg. 2016;150:33–9.
74. Chakravarthy K, Chen Y, He C, Christo PJ. Stem cell therapy for chronic pain management: review of uses, advances, and adverse effects. Pain Physician. 2017;20(4):293–305.
75. Sainoh T, Orita S, Miyagi M, et al. Single intradiscal injection of the interleukin-6 receptor antibody tocilizumab provides short-term relief of discogenic low back pain; prospective comparative cohort study. J Orthop Sci. 2016;21(1):2–6.
76. Sainoh T, Orita S, Miyagi M, et al. Single Intradiscal administration of the tumor necrosis factor-alpha inhibitor, Etanercept, for patients with discogenic low back pain. Pain Med. 2016;17(1):40–5.
77. Song K, Gu T, Shuang F, et al. Adipose-derived stem cells improve the viability of nucleus pulposus cells in degenerated intervertebral discs. Mol Med Rep. 2015;12(3):4664–8.
78. Tsai TL, Wang B, Squire MW, Guo LW, Li WJ. Endothelial cells direct human mesenchymal stem cells for osteo- and chondro-lineage differentiation through endothelin-1 and AKT signaling. Stem Cell Res Ther. 2015;6:88.
79. Cheng X, Zhang G, Zhang L, et al. Mesenchymal stem cells deliver exogenous miR-21 via exosomes to inhibit nucleus pulposus cell apoptosis and reduce intervertebral disc degeneration. J Cell Mol Med. 2017;22:261.
80. Caplan AI, Dennis JE. Mesenchymal stem cells as trophic mediators. J Cell Biochem. 2006;98(5):1076–84.
81. Iyer SS, Rojas M. Anti-inflammatory effects of mesenchymal stem cells: novel concept for future therapies. Expert Opin Biol Ther. 2008;8(5):569–81.
82. Caplan AI, Correa D. The MSC: an injury drugstore. Cell Stem Cell. 2011;9(1):11–5.
83. Miyamoto T, Muneta T, Tabuchi T, et al. Intradiscal transplantation of synovial mesenchymal stem cells prevents intervertebral disc degeneration through suppression of matrix metalloproteinase-related genes in nucleus pulposus cells in rabbits. Arthritis Res Ther. 2010;12(6):R206.
84. Crevensten G, Walsh AJ, Ananthakrishnan D, et al. Intervertebral disc cell therapy for regeneration: mesenchymal stem cell implantation in rat intervertebral discs. Ann Biomed Eng. 2004;32(3):430–4.
85. Wuertz K, Godburn K, Iatridis JC. MSC response to pH levels found in degenerating intervertebral discs. Biochem Biophys Res Commun. 2009;379(4):824–9.
86. Wuertz K, Godburn K, Neidlinger-Wilke C, Urban J, Iatridis JC. Behavior of mesenchymal stem cells in the chemical microenvironment of the intervertebral disc. Spine. 2008;33(17):1843–9.
87. Richardson SM, Walker RV, Parker S, et al. Intervertebral disc cell-mediated mesenchymal stem cell differentiation. Stem Cells. 2006;24(3):707–16.
88. Watanabe T, Sakai D, Yamamoto Y, et al. Human nucleus pulposus cells significantly enhanced biological properties in a coculture system with direct cell-to-cell contact with autologous mesenchymal stem cells. J Orthop Res. 2010;28(5):623–30.
89. Vadala G, Studer RK, Sowa G, et al. Coculture of bone marrow mesenchymal stem cells and nucleus pulposus cells modulate gene expression profile without cell fusion. Spine. 2008;33(8):870–6.
90. Wang Z, Perez-Terzic CM, Smith J, et al. Efficacy of intervertebral disc regeneration with stem cells - a systematic review and meta-analysis of animal controlled trials. Gene. 2015;564(1):1–8.
91. Gou S, Oxentenko SC, Eldrige JS, et al. Stem cell therapy for intervertebral disk regeneration. Am J Phys Med Rehabil. 2014;93(11 Suppl 3):S122–31.
92. Oehme D, Ghosh P, Goldschlager T, et al. Reconstitution of degenerated ovine lumbar discs by STRO-3-positive allogeneic mesenchymal precursor cells combined with pentosan polysulfate. J Neurosurg Spine. 2016;24(5):715–26.
93. Gullung GB, Woodall JW, Tucci MA, James J, Black DA, McGuire RA. Platelet-rich plasma effects on degenerative disc disease: analysis of histology and imaging in an animal model. Evid Based Spine Care J. 2011;2(4):13–8.
94. Obata S, Akeda K, Morimoto R, et al. Intradiscal injection of autologous platelet-rich plasma-serum induces the restoration of disc height in the rabbit anular needle puncture model: 12. Paper presented at: Spine Journal Meeting Abstracts 2010.
95. Obata S, Akeda K, Imanishi T, et al. Effect of autologous platelet-rich plasma-releasate on intervertebral disc degeneration in the rabbit anular puncture model: a preclinical study. Arthritis Res Ther. 2012;14(6):R241.
96. Frechette JP, Martineau I, Gagnon G. Platelet-rich plasmas: growth factor content and roles in wound healing. J Dent Res. 2005;84(5):434–9.
97. Wan S, Borland S, Richardson SM, Merry CL, Saiani A, Gough JE. Self-assembling peptide hydrogel for intervertebral disc tissue engineering. Acta Biomater. 2016;46:29–40.
98. Li YY, Diao HJ, Chik TK, et al. Delivering mesenchymal stem cells in collagen microsphere carriers to rabbit degenerative disc: reduced risk of osteophyte formation. Tissue Eng Part A. 2014;20(9-10):1379–91.
99. Tong W, Lu Z, Qin L, et al. Cell therapy for the degenerating intervertebral disc. Transl Res. 2017;181:49–58.

100. Hunt CL, Her YF, Law LA, et al. Five generations of cell preparation: a translational framework for categorizing regenerative stem cell therapies. 2017;1(1).
101. Bowen JE. Technical issues in harvesting and concentrating stem cells (bone marrow and adipose). PM R. 2015;7(4 Suppl):S8–18.
102. Ho G, Leung VY, Cheung KM, Chan D. Effect of severity of intervertebral disc injury on mesenchymal stem cell-based regeneration. Connect Tissue Res. 2008;49(1):15–21.
103. Salem O, Wang HT, Alaseem AM, et al. Naproxen affects osteogenesis of human mesenchymal stem cells via regulation of Indian hedgehog signaling molecules. Arthritis Res Ther. 2014;16(4):R152.
104. Almaawi A, Wang HT, Ciobanu O, et al. Effect of acetaminophen and nonsteroidal anti-inflammatory drugs on gene expression of mesenchymal stem cells. Tissue Eng Part A. 2013;19(7-8):1039–46.
105. Du M, Pan W, Yang P, Ge S. [Effect of aspirin on cell biological activities in murine bone marrow stromal cells]. *Zhonghua kou qiang yi xue za zhi = Zhonghua kouqiang yixue zazhi =*. Chin J Stomatol. 2016;51(3):160–5.
106. Wyles CC, Houdek MT, Wyles SP, Wagner ER, Behfar A, Sierra RJ. Differential cytotoxicity of corticosteroids on human mesenchymal stem cells. Clin Orthop Relat Res. 2015;473(3):1155–64.
107. Narouze S, Benzon HT, Provenzano DA, et al. Interventional spine and pain procedures in patients on antiplatelet and anticoagulant medications: guidelines from the American Society of Regional Anesthesia and Pain Medicine, the European Society of Regional Anaesthesia and Pain Therapy, the American Academy of Pain Medicine, the International Neuromodulation Society, the North American Neuromodulation Society, and the World Institute of Pain. Reg Anesth Pain Med. 2015;40(3):182–212.
108. Kitchel SH, Wang MY, Lauryssen CL. Techniques for aspirating bone marrow for use in spinal surgery. Neurosurgery. 2005;57(4 Suppl):286–9; discussion 286-289.
109. Hyer CF, Berlet GC, Bussewitz BW, Hankins T, Ziegler HL, Philbin TM. Quantitative assessment of the yield of osteoblastic connective tissue progenitors in bone marrow aspirate from the iliac crest, tibia, and calcaneus. J Bone Joint Surg Am. 2013;95(14):1312–6.
110. Jones EA, Kinsey SE, English A, et al. Isolation and characterization of bone marrow multipotential mesenchymal progenitor cells. Arthritis Rheum. 2002;46(12):3349–60.
111. Galotto M, Berisso G, Delfino L, et al. Stromal damage as consequence of high-dose chemo/radiotherapy in bone marrow transplant recipients. Exp Hematol. 1999;27(9):1460–6.
112. Liao HT, Chen CT. Osteogenic potential: comparison between bone marrow and adipose-derived mesenchymal stem cells. World J Stem Cells. 2014;6(3):288–95.
113. Guneta V, Tan NS, Chan SK, et al. Comparative study of adipose-derived stem cells and bone marrow-derived stem cells in similar microenvironmental conditions. Exp Cell Res. 2016;348(2):155–64.
114. Bourin P, Bunnell BA, Casteilla L, et al. Stromal cells from the adipose tissue-derived stromal vascular fraction and culture expanded adipose tissue-derived stromal/stem cells: a joint statement of the International Federation for Adipose Therapeutics and Science (IFATS) and the International Society for Cellular Therapy (ISCT). Cytotherapy. 2013;15(6):641–8.
115. Wang SZ, Rui YF, Tan Q, Wang C. Enhancing intervertebral disc repair and regeneration through biology: platelet-rich plasma as an alternative strategy. Arthritis Res Ther. 2013;15(5):220.
116. Monfett M, Harrison J, Boachie-Adjei K, Lutz G. Intradiscal platelet-rich plasma (PRP) injections for discogenic low back pain: an update. Int Orthop. 2016;40(6):1321–8.
117. Hunt CL, Shen S, Nassr A, et al. Current understanding of safety and efficacy of stem cell therapy for discogenic pain—a systematic review of human studies. Tech Reg Anesth Pain Manag. 2015;19(1-2):32–7.
118. Tuakli-Wosornu YA, Terry A, Boachie-Adjei K, et al. Lumbar Intradiskal Platelet-Rich Plasma (PRP) injections: a prospective, double-blind, randomized controlled study. PM R. 2016;8(1):1–10; quiz 10
119. Akeda K, Ohishi K, Masuda K, et al. Intradiscal injection of autologous platelet-rich plasma releasate to treat discogenic low back pain: a preliminary clinical trial. Asian Spine J. 2017;11(3):380–9.
120. Orozco L, Soler R, Morera C, Alberca M, Sanchez A, Garcia-Sancho J. Intervertebral disc repair by autologous mesenchymal bone marrow cells: a pilot study. Transplantation. 2011;92(7):822–8.
121. Pang X, Yang H, Peng B. Human umbilical cord mesenchymal stem cell transplantation for the treatment of chronic discogenic low back pain. Pain Physician. 2014;17(4):E525–30.
122. Pettine K, Suzuki R, Sand T, Murphy M. Treatment of discogenic back pain with autologous bone marrow concentrate injection with minimum two year follow-up. Int Orthop. 2016;40(1):135–40.
123. Comella K, Silbert R, Parlo M. Effects of the intradiscal implantation of stromal vascular fraction plus platelet rich plasma in patients with degenerative disc disease. J Transl Med. 2017;15(1):12.
124. Levi D, Horn S, Tyszko S, Levin J, Hecht-Leavitt C, Walko E. Intradiscal platelet-rich plasma injection for chronic discogenic low back pain: preliminary results from a prospective trial. Pain Med. 2016;17(6):1010–22.

PRP Therapies (Tendons, Joints, Spine) 91

Ajax Yang, Corey W. Hunter, and Tory L. McJunkin

Introduction

Musculoskeletal disorders affect people of all ages and ethnicities and are the most common causes of chronic pain and disability worldwide. In the last decade, musculoskeletal-related disabilities increased by 45% around the world. In the United States, as the population continues to age, the incidence and the burden to address musculoskeletal pathologies will rise steadily. Tendinous injuries are often associated with significant disability and reduced quality of life. Furthermore, poor healing results in fibrosis, diminished structural integrity and propensity for reinjury, and development of chronic pain. Similarly, the ability for intra-articular cartilage and meniscus to heal is virtually nonexistent. Fundamentally, the body is poorly designed with respect to regeneration in these particular regions due to a particularly sparse blood supply; the body simply cannot heal these areas because it cannot get the building blocks needed for repair to the injury site. At the present time, the majority treatment strategies are limited to symptomatic management rather than curative. Consequently, there is a dire need to develop definitive therapies to revert the consequences of these disease processes due to the high frequency of injury to the musculoskeletal system.

Great strides have been made in the field pain management to focus on PRP therapy and regenerative medicine as a whole. The fundamental purpose of PRP is to "force" the body to heal a structure it normally would not or cannot. Administering PRP to an area of injury will serve two general purposes: (1) artificially deliver concentrated amounts of healing elements to initiate repair and (2) create an inflammatory alarm in that area for the body to respond to in kind by delivering more blood and consequently even more healing elements. As mentioned above, joints and local connective tissue are notoriously difficult to heal – PRP serves this need by circumventing the body's poor blood supply in those areas and hand delivering the building blocks needed to repair the injury.

A. Yang (✉)
Department of Rehabilitation Medicine, Icahn School of Medicine at Mount Sinai, New York, NY, USA

C. W. Hunter
Department of Rehabilitation Medicine, Icahn School of Medicine at Mount Sinai, New York, NY, USA

Ainsworth Institute of Pain Management, New York, NY, USA
e-mail: chunter@ainpain.com

T. L. McJunkin
Arizona Pain Specialists, Scottsdale, AZ, USA

Background and Historical Perspective

Platelets are naturally packed with a variety growth factors and are directly involved in tissue healing; therefore, the rationale behind PRP therapy is to target and deposit a high concentration of these healing particles into an injured area to accelerate tissue restoration. Historically, PRP was the final product derived from centrifuging the whole blood specimen from the patient in the lab and extracting the platelet-rich layer. At the present day, a plethora of commercially available kits with each product promise to deliver more competitive PRP consistency, precision, denser platelets, and higher growth factor concentration yield.

The platelets achieve their primary function of tissue healing and repair through the actions of growth factors. The main growth factors include the following (Fig. 91.1):

- Fibroblast growth factor (FGF)
- Granulocyte colony-stimulating growth factor (G-CSF)
- Transforming growth factor beta (TGF-β)
- Basic fibroblast growth factor (BFGF)
- Platelet-derived growth factor (PDGF a-b)
- Epidermal growth factor (EGF)
- Vascular endothelial growth factor (VEGF)
- Insulin growth factor (IGF-1)
- Interleukin-8 (IL-8)

T. R. Deer et al. (eds.), *Deer's Treatment of Pain*, https://doi.org/10.1007/978-3-030-12281-2_91

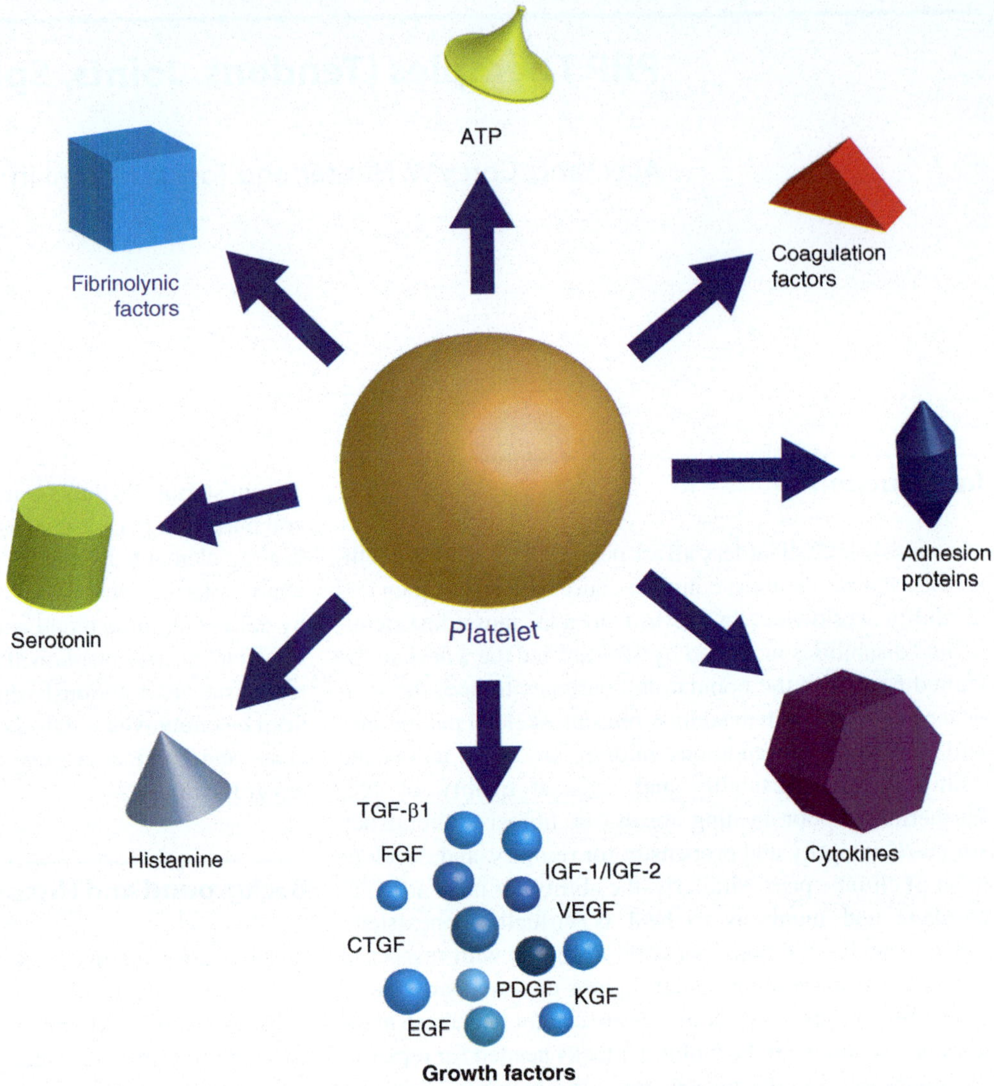

Fig. 91.1 Platelet-derived growth factors and other chemical signaling mediators

Soon following tissue injury, platelets are activated and growth factors are released into the area of damaged tissues. Growth factors initiate the inflammatory cascade that lasts 72 hours in duration. This is followed by proliferation and maturation. The detailed cellular mechanisms of tissue repair and inflammation are described extensively in Chap. 86.

Uses and Indications

PRP is a safe and minimally invasive procedure with. While its efficacy and application are supported by good evidence, the current insurance model and payment system consider it to be "investigational." Given that patients will pay out of pocket, physicians should provide patients with careful considerations and explanations of the conventional treatment methods, e.g., conservative vs. surgery, in conjunction with PRP and regenerative strategies.

Some basic concerns for PRP include:

- Inflammatory arthritis, e.g., rheumatoid arthritis, gout, and ankylosing spondylitis.
- Immunocompromised patients are potentially at high risk for infection.
- Oncological history: Patients with an active cancer, history of cancer, or suspicion of cancer should consult with their oncologist prior and obtain clearance.
- Patients may have thrombocytopenia or bleeding disorders.

Contraindications for PRP include:

- Active local and systemic infection, e.g., septic arthritis
- Patients on long-term and/or constant nonsteroidal anti-inflammatory drugs (NSAIDs) therapy or steroid therapy
- Inability to obtain consent or follow post PRP therapy care plans

Preoperative Considerations

- Provide a proper explanation of all potential benefit, risks, and alternatives prior to obtaining patient's informed consent.
- Anticoagulation poses a lower risk in PRP than for a neuraxial procedure; however, excessive bleeding and hemarthrosis can still occur.
- Carefully inspect injection site and surrounding areas for evidence of infection, skin ulceration or necrosis, and extent of disease.
- Advise the patient to refrain from taking NSAIDs (e.g., aspirin, ibuprofen, naproxen, etc.) and steroids (e.g., prednisone, medrol dose packs, cortisone, cortisone injections, etc.) for at least 7 and 10 days, respectively, prior to the procedure.
- The patient should be free of systemic infections for a minimum of 1 week (e.g., common cold, sore throat, cough, etc.). Any antibiotics should be completed prior to the procedure.
- When drawing blood, one must carefully match the blood volume needed to the size (e.g., elbow vs. hip) and or the number of target joint(s) (e.g., unilateral vs. bilateral). Many vendors provide kits in 30 cc and 60 cc denominations to suit this consideration.
- PRP injections can be easily performed via palpation of surface anatomy; however, given that PRP injectate volume is small, incorporating radiographic imaging guidance, e.g., ultrasound, is strongly recommended to optimize targeted delivery of PRP in the necessary area.
- Ultrasound – the literature suggests ultrasound guidance can offer improved accuracy for injection as compared to fluoroscopy. When injecting into tendons, ligaments, and other soft tissue, one can directly visualize in real time the target area, position of the needle tip, and spread of the injectate, thus making ultrasound a must for these types of PRP injections.

Post-Procedure Considerations

- Hold NSAIDs and/or steroids for 1 month after the procedure.
- Injuries to soft tissues such as tendons and ligaments may respond positively within the first week of injection, while joint pathologies may take as long as 6 weeks to show improvement.
- Depending on the severity of the injury or pathology, added treatments may be necessary. To date, there are no published studies that have established a paradigm for the number of treatments or amount of PRP needed to treat different conditions.

PRP Preparation Technique

Currently there are two general methods for obtaining PRP:

1. Conventional: This method uses the traditional laboratory equipment and methods for blood collection and preparation (e.g., conical vials, vacutainer, needles, etc.). The blood is prepared according to one of several accepted protocols (e.g., Anitua, Landesberg, etc.). We advocate using the double-spin method described by Landesberg. This protocol has shown consistently reproducible platelet concentrations and growth factors as oppose to the single-spin technique where the platelet concentrations are unclear in studies that reported favorable outcomes.

   Sample equipment needed to harvest 4–6 mL of PRP from 30 cc of blood is as follows:
   - Centrifuge
   - 20 mL conical vial (2)
   - 18G blunt tip needle (2)
   - 20 mL syringe
   - 10 mL syringe
   - Venous blood collection tubes (3) *(contents of vial varies depending on protocol)*
     - Landsberg: 5 mL vials with 0.5 mL of 0.129 mol/L sodium citrate (Becton Dickinson, Franklin Lackes, NJ)
     - Landsberg: 10 mL vials 1.0 mL of ACD Solution B (Becton Dickinson, Franklin Lackes, NJ)
     - Ethylenediaminetetraacetic acid (EDTA) may damage the platelets, so it should therefore be avoided.
   - 21G butterfly blood collection set (larger gauge needles are preferred to prevent premature mechanical platelet activation)
   - Tourniquet
2. Device or Prepackaged Kits: There are an abundance of commercially available kits with specially designed collection receptacles and modified centrifuges to process PRP from whole blood. These kits are designed for convenience and claim to produce higher platelet counts than conventional harvesting methods and their competitors. Each device offers options to achieve desired platelet, white blood cell, and growth factor concentration.

Whether to include the "buffy coat" into the injectate has been debated. The buffy coat is a yellowish-brown layer found in between the plasma and packed red cells following centrifugation of whole blood. It is rich in white blood cells and platelets. Therefore, some advocates for its inclusion to decreased infection risk from the presence of white blood cells to enhance the inflammatory cascade and promote healing. Our standpoint to exclude buffy coat is supported by others that the buffy coat increases pain and discomfort after the injection. Furthermore, excesses white blood cells create a detrimental inflammatory process that can result in excessive fibrosis and scarring instead of tissue regeneration.

The benefit of PRP activation has also been contended. Some argue that platelet activation, e.g., via calcium chloride, further encourages tissue healing by platelet degranulation to release growth factors to recruit osteoblasts, epidermal cells, stem cells, and fibrin matrix formation However, some evidence indicated that there are potent endogenous biological substrate (thromboplastin) found at the injury site to activate the platelets. We, the authors, leave it to the physician's discretion to determine if activation would optimize PRP's regenerative properties.

Equipment needed for injecting PRP:

- 18G 1.5-inch needle
- 27G 1.5-inch needle
- 3.5-inch spinal needle, 20G (shoulder)/22G (hip labrum)/25G (rotator cuff tendon)
- 1.5-inch needle, 20G (lateral epicondyles)/22G (medial and lateral collateral ligaments)
- 3 cc or 5 cc syringe – for local anesthetic
- 10 cc syringe – for collecting PRP from concentrating receptacle if not included in the kit
- 1% or 2% lidocaine
- Sterile fenestrated drape or utility drapes
- Chlorhexidine gluconate 2% or povidone-iodine
- PRP harvesting/processing kit
- Surgical marker
- Ultrasound
- Sterile sheath for ultrasound probe

Injection Techniques

Lateral Epicondylopathy

- The patient is seated comfortably with the painful elbow supported on the procedure table.
- The elbow is flexed at 45 degrees, with the wrist in a neutral position.
- The ultrasound probe is placed in parallel with the common extensor tendon to allow a long-axis view of the musculotendinous junction.
- Once the lesion is identified, align the center notch of the probe over the center of the lesion. The lesion is visualized in the middle of the computer screen.
- Mark the needle entry point roughly 1 cm away from the ultrasound probe to set up the long-axis view of the needle.
- Carefully clean the skin with chlorhexidine or betadine or 70% isopropyl alcohol using sterile technique.
- 3–5 cc of 1–2% lidocaine is used to anesthetize the skin and superficial soft tissues.
- Position the sterile sheath-covered ultrasound probe to center the image of the lesion on the computer screen.
- A 20 or 22G, 1.5-inch needle is advanced using "in-plane technique" toward to the tendinous defect.
- Roughly 0.5 cc of PRP is used to demonstrate good injectate spread.
- The remaining PRP (3.5 cc) is delivered while moving the needle in a fenestrating-fan fashion to immerse the damaged area with PRP.
- Carefully withdraw the needle and apply sterile dressing.

Supraspinatus and Subscapularis Tendinopathy: Anterior Approach to Rotator Cuff Interval

- Supraspinatus and subscapularis tendinopathies are best addressed using this technique.
- Supraspinatus: The patient is seated with the hand placed on the ipsilateral hip area with the elbow pointed posteriorly while maintaining shoulder external rotation (modified Crass position).
- Subscapularis: The patient is seated with forearm in supination and shoulder external rotation.
- The ultrasound probe is placed in short axis on the anterior shoulder just superior to the greater and lesser tuberosity.
- The biceps tendon is visualized between the supraspinatus and subscapularis tendons.
- Identify the lesion and position the image of the lesion in the middle of the computer screen. Tears are most often found in the distal 1/4th of the tendon in the transverse direction.
- Mark the needle entry point with a surgical marker.
- Carefully clean the skin with chlorhexidine or betadine or 70% isopropyl alcohol using sterile technique.
- 3–5 cc of 1–2% lidocaine is used to anesthetize the skin and superficial soft tissues.
- Position the sterile sheath-covered ultrasound probe to center the image of the lesion on the computer screen.
- A 20 or 22 gauge, 3.5 inch needle is advanced using "in-plane technique" toward the space just lateral to the coracoid process at the humeral head.
- The needle is advanced into the rotator cuff interval toward the supraspinatus tendon for supraspinatus injection.
- Area caudal to the coracoid process is the target for the subscapularis injection.
- Roughly 0.5 cc of PRP is used to demonstrate good injectate spread.

- The remaining PRP (3.5 cc) is delivered while moving the needle in a fenestrating-fan fashion to immerse the damaged area with PRP.
- Carefully withdraw the needle and apply sterile dressing.

Infraspinatus and Teres Minor Tendinopathy: Posterior Approach

- The patient is seated with the arm by the side and the hand resting on the ipsilateral thigh. This position facilitates the opening of the posterior joint space.
- Place the transducer angled obliquely and superiorly toward the humeral head and parallel the scapular spine inferiorly.
- Identify the lesion and position the image of the lesion in the middle of the computer screen.
- Mark the needle entry point with a surgical marker.
- Carefully clean the skin with chlorhexidine or betadine or 70% isopropyl alcohol using sterile technique.
- 3–5 cc of 1–2% lidocaine is used to anesthetize the skin and superficial soft tissues.
- Position the sterile sheath-covered ultrasound probe to center the image of the lesion on the computer screen.
- A 20 or 22G, 3.5-inch needle with an approximately 30-degree tip curvature is advanced using "in-plane technique" medially toward the glenohumeral joint space.
- Roughly 0.5 cc of PRP is used to demonstrate good injectate spread.
- The remaining PRP (3.5 cc) is delivered while moving the needle in a fenestrating-fan fashion to immerse the damaged area with PRP.
- Carefully withdraw the needle and apply sterile dressing.

Glenoid Labral Injury

- The patient is seated with the arm in internal rotation to rest the hand on the ipsilateral hip or the pati. This position facilitates the opening of the posterior joint space.
- Place the transducer parallel the scapular spine, and move inferiorly until infraspinatus and teres minor are identified. The probe is then turned long axis to exam the posterior labrum (hyperechoic triangularly shaped).
- Lower frequency may provide a better visualization of deeper structures in large or athletic shoulders.
- Identify the position the labrum in the middle of the computer screen.
- Mark the needle entry point with a surgical marker.
- Carefully clean the skin with chlorhexidine or betadine or 70% isopropyl alcohol using sterile technique.
- 3–5 cc of 1–2% lidocaine is used to anesthetize the skin and superficial soft tissues.
- Position the sterile sheath-covered ultrasound probe to center the image of the lesion on the computer screen.
- A 20 or 22 gauge, 3.5-inch needle is placed 1 cm lateral to the lateral edge of the transducer and advanced using "in-plane technique" medially toward the glenohumeral joint space.
- Maintain constant visualization of the needle tip to avoid penetrating the labrum. Once the humeral head is contacted, the needle should be redirected anterior toward the glenoid labrum.
- Roughly 0.5 cc of PRP is used to demonstrate good injectate spread.
- The remaining PRP (4 cc) is delivered while moving the needle in a fenestrating-fan fashion to immerse the damaged area with PRP.
- Carefully withdraw the needle and apply sterile dressing.

Knee Ligamentous Injuries

Medial Collateral Ligament

- Patient is lying in the lateral decubitus position with the affected limb on the table.
- Place the treatment leg in extension at the knee and slight flexion at the hip to allow the treatment limb to be anterior to the non-treated limb.
- Identify and mark the area of maximal tenderness by palpating from the superior portion of the MCL, the femoral condyle, and moving inferiorly toward its insertion on the medial condyle of the tibia.
- Anesthetize the skin and superficial soft tissues using a 27G needle and 1–2% lidocaine.
- A sterile sheath-covered ultrasound probe is used to scan the MCL
- Because MCL is relatively flat, it is important to obtain the short-axis view to assess the entire anterior and posterior portions.
- A 22G, 1.5-inch needle is inserted under direction visualization in the short-axis view toward the ligamentous defect.
- Once the needle tip is in close proximity to the lesion, 0.5 cc of PRP is administered to produce satisfactory spreading visualized on ultrasound imaging.
- The remaining PRP (2.5–3.0 cc) is delivered while moving the needle in a fenestrating-fan fashion to immerse the damaged area with PRP.
- Carefully withdraw the needle and apply sterile dressing.

Lateral Collateral Ligament

- The patient is supine with the treatment knee in extension
- Identify and mark the area of maximal tenderness by palpating from the superior portion of the LCL at the femoral condyle and moving inferiorly toward its insertion on the lateral condyle of the tibia.
- Anesthetize the skin and superficial soft tissues using a 27G needle and 1–2% lidocaine.
- A sterile sheath-covered ultrasound probe is used to scan the LCL.
- Because LCL is also a relatively flat structure, it is important to obtain the short-axis view to assess the entire anterior and posterior portions.
- A 22G, 1.5-inch needle is inserted under direction visualization in the short-axis view toward the ligamentous defect.
- Once the needle tip is in close proximity to the lesion, 0.5 cc of PRP is administered produce satisfactory spreading visualized on ultrasound imaging.
- The remaining PRP (2.5–3.0 cc) is delivered while moving the needle in a fenestrating-fan fashion to immerse the damaged area with PRP.
- Carefully withdraw the needle and apply sterile dressing.

Acetabular Labral Injury

- Place the patient supine with the treatment hip close to the side of the table where the physician will be standing.
- Place the ultrasound probe in long axis to the femoral neck to identify the femoral head, neck, and anterior recess. Because of the femoral neck angle, the probe orientation will be in the oblique-sagittal plane.
- Hip vasculatures, medial to the hip joint, can be further delineated using the power Doppler function. The acetabular labrum appears hyperechoic and extends from the margins of the acetabulum.
- Clean the skin using strict sterile technique, and mark the skin 2–3 cm lateral to the vascular bundle in line with the femoral neck.
- Anesthetize the skin and superficial soft tissues using a 27G needle and 1–2% lidocaine.
- A sterile sheath-covered ultrasound probe is reapplied to obtain view.
- A 22G, 3.5-inch needle is advanced under direct visualization toward the femoral neck.
- Aspirate to monitor for blood before injecting.
- Once the needle tip is inside the hip capsule, inject 5–7.5 cc of PRP while moving the needle in a fenestrating-fan fashion to immerse the damaged area with PRP.
- Carefully withdraw the needle and apply sterile dressing.

Facet Joint Arthropathy

- Although lumbar facet joint injection could be performed under ultrasound guidance, the traditional fluoroscopic method will be described here.
- The patient lies prone with a pillow under the abdomen for comfort.
- Position the C-arm in position such that the beam parallels the facet joint to allow direct visualization of the open facet joint space.
- Mark the skin where the beam is projected, and clean the area using strict sterile technique.
- Anesthetize the skin and superficial soft tissues using a 27G needle and 1–2% lidocaine.
- Insert a 21G, 3.5-inch spinal needle under fluoroscopic visualization.
- 0.1–0.2 ml nonionic contrast material can be injected into the joint space to confirm intra-articular needle placement.
- 0.5 ml of PRP is then injected slowly with low pressure to prevent capsule rupture.

Evidence for Efficacy (Table 91.1)

Clinical Pearls and Pitfalls

- Based on the current available evidence, PRP has been shown to be most efficacious in treating lateral epicondylopathy, knee osteoarthritis/hip, and shoulder pain.
- All PRP injections should be performed under radiographic guidance to maximize injection accuracy and safety.
- Diagnostic blocks can be used to identify pain generator(s) as a confirming step prior to PRP injection.
- Careful attention and sterility should be maintained to minimize infection risks. As with any medical or surgical procedure, there is always a risk of potential complication – even with the use of autologous-derived blood as the injectate.
- It is important to inform patients that it is normal to experience localized soreness or discomfort from the injection itself for up to 10 days postinjection. In many cases this can be due to the body intentionally creating some inflammation in and around the area where the PRP was injected. This inflammation is the body's response to the introduction of PRP into an injured area and attempting to offer additional assistance by luring growth factors and inflammatory markers.
- Graft rejection is a theoretical possibility in the event that PRP derived from one patient is accidentally injected into

Table 91.1 Evidence for efficacy

Reference	Study design	Size	Indication	PRP property	Outcomes
Peerbooms (2011)	Prospective and randomized	51	Medial and/or lateral epicondylopathy	Double centrifuged, GPS with buffy coat	At 1 year, PRP group had significant clinical improvements vs. control (corticosteroid)
Gosens (2011)	Controlled and randomized	26	Lateral epicondylopathy	Double centrifuged, GPS with buffy coat	At 2 years, PRP group had significant clinical improvements vs. control (corticosteroid)
Rha (2013)	Prospective, randomized, and controlled	26	Medial and/or lateral epicondylopathy	Single spin with Prosys PRP system	At 6 months, PRP group had significant clinical improvements vs. control (corticosteroid)
Vogrin (2010)	Prospective and randomized	25	Anterior cruciate ligament	Single centrifuged, Magellan ASP with buffy coat and autologous thrombin	At 6 months, PRP group had significant clinical improvements vs. control
Cerza (2012)	Prospective, randomized, and controlled	60	Knee OA	Single spin, without buffy coat	Significant short-term improvement noted
Sanchez (2012)	Multicentered, prospective, randomized, double blinded	176	Knee OA	Single-spin PRGF with buffy coat	PRP group showed superior short-term results when compared to hyaluronic acid group
Patel (2013)	Prospective, randomized, double blinded	156	Knee OA	Single-spin PRGF without buffy coat	PRP group showed superior short-term results when compared to saline group
Filardo (2011)	Case series	43	Chronic patellar tendinopathy	Double spin	Medium-long term improvements noted following repeated (3 injections, 2 weeks apart) PRP injections
Radice (2010)	Case control	22	Anterior cruciate ligament rupture	GPS, single spin with buffy-coat	PRP group showed improved ACL healing on MRI compared to control group following arthroscopic ACL reconstruction
Wu (2016)	Prospective case series	19	Lumbar facet joint arthropathy	Double spin	Significant improvement in pain and functional score maintained at 3 months

another. One should either carefully label each sample and perform "time-out" procedures before commencing with the injection, or prepare samples one at a time to avoid this possibility.

- It is important to inform patients that PRP therapy may require several weeks for improvement to take place. Furthermore, patients may experience temporary worsening of symptoms ranging from 5 to 7 days following their injection.
- Intradiscal PRP injection can be very painful and may induce autonomic nervous system instability. We recommend continuous vital signs monitoring and resuscitation preparedness.
- A larger gauge needle is preferred during venipuncture to avoid platelet shearing and premature activation.
- Buffy coat contains mostly white blood cells and, therefore, will increase the risk of unintended inflammation and pain.
- More importantly, PRP therapy is far from being a panacea, and the patients should be made aware of its limitations.
- Conditions such as significant partial tendon ruptures, calcific tendinopathies, or chronic tendon injuries may require multiple PRP injections (with 4–6-week follow-up between injections).
- We advise to hold nonsteroidal anti-inflammatory drugs (NSAIDS) for 7 days and glucocorticoids for 10 days prior to PRP therapy, respectively. Both medication types should be held for 6 weeks following PRP injection.
- Sonographic evidence may not be visible for several weeks following PRP injection to the tendons or ligaments.
- Recommended general rehab protocol following PRP injection.
  - Patients are encouraged to resume normal activities with no extra exercise for the first 48 hours.
  - After 10–12 days, start light exercise without stressful activity for 6 weeks. Returning to stressful activity before 6 weeks will result in incomplete healing of the treated tissue.

Recommended Reading

1. Anitua E. Plasma rich in growth factors: preliminary results of use in the preparation of future sites for implants. Int J Oral Maxillofac Implants. 1999;14(4):529–35.
2. Anitua E. The use of plasma-rich growth factors (PRGF) in oral surgery. Pract Proced Aesthet Dent. 2001;13(6):487–93.. quiz 487–93
3. Brooks PM. The burden of musculoskeletal disease—a global perspective. Clin Rheumatol. 2006;25(6):778–81.

4. Cavallo C, Filardo G, Mariani E, et al. Comparison of platelet-rich plasma formulations for cartilage healing. J Bone Joint Surg Am. 2014;96(5):423–9.
5. Cavallo C, Roffi A, Grigolo B, et al. Platelet-rich plasma: the choice of activation method affects the release of bioactive molecules. Biomed Res Int. 2016;2016:6591717.
6. Creaney L, Wallace A, Curtis M, Connell D. Growth factor-based therapies provide additional benefit beyond physical therapy in resistant elbow tendinopathy: a prospective, single-blind, randomised trial of autologous blood injections versus platelet-rich plasma injections. Br J Sports Med. 2011;45:966; bjsports82503
7. de Vos RJ, Weir A, van Schie HTM, et al. Platelet-rich plasma injection for chronic Achilles tendinopathy: a randomized controlled trial. JAMA. 2010;303(2):144–9.
8. Eby BW. Platelet-rich plasma: harvesting with a single-spin centrifuge. J Oral Implantol. 2002;28(6):297–301.
9. Finnoff JT, Fowler SP, Lai JK, et al. Treatment of chronic tendinopathy with ultrasound-guided needle tenotomy and platelet-rich plasma injection. PM R. 2011;3(10):900–11.
10. Fullerton BD, Reeves KD. Ultrasonography in regenerative injection (prolotherapy) using dextrose, platelet-rich plasma, and other injectants. Phys Med Rehabil Clin N Am. 2010;21(3):585–605.
11. Jang S-J, Kim J-D, Cha S-S. Platelet-rich plasma (PRP) injections as an effective treatment for early osteoarthritis. Eur J Orthop Surg Traumatol. 2013;23(5):573–80.
12. Kumar V, Fausto N, Abbas A. Pathologic basis of disease. 7th ed: WB Saunders; 2005.
13. Landesberg R, Roy M, Glickman RS. Quantification of growth factor levels using a simplified method of platelet-rich plasma gel preparation. J Oral Maxillofac Surg. 2000;58(3):297–300; discussion 300–1.
14. Marx RE. Platelet-rich plasma: evidence to support its use. J Oral Maxillofac Surg. 2004;62(4):489–96.
15. McShane JM, Shah VN, Nazarian LN. Sonographically guided percutaneous needle tenotomy for treatment of common extensor tendinosis in the elbow. J Ultrasound Med. 2008;27(8):1137–44.
16. Mishra A, Pavelko T. Treatment of chronic elbow tendinosis with buffered platelet-rich plasma. Am J Sports Med. 2006;34(11):1774–8.
17. Mody GM, Brooks PM. Improving musculoskeletal health: global issues. Best Pract Res Clin Rheumatol. 2012;26(2):237–49.
18. Narouze SN. Atlas of ultrasound-guided procedures in interventional pain management: Springer; 2010.
19. Peerbooms JC, Sluimer J, Bruijn DJ, Gosens T. Positive effect of an autologous platelet concentrate in lateral epicondylitis in a double-blind randomized controlled trial. Am J Sports Med. 2010;38(2):255–62.
20. Rabago D, Best TM, Zgierska AE, Zeisig E, Ryan M, Crane D. A systematic review of four injection therapies for lateral epicondylosis: prolotherapy, polidocanol, whole blood and platelet-rich plasma. Br J Sports Med. 2009;43(7):471–81.
21. Schilephake H. Bone growth factors in maxillofacial skeletal reconstruction. Int J Oral Maxillofac Surg. 2002;31(5):469–84.
22. Storheim K, Zwart J-A. Musculoskeletal disorders and the Global Burden of Disease study. Ann Rheum Dis. 2014;73(6):949–50.
23. Vora A, Borg-Stein J, Nguyen RT. Regenerative injection therapy for osteoarthritis: fundamental concepts and evidence-based review. PM R. 2012;4(5 Suppl):S104–9.
24. WHO Scientific Group on the Burden of Musculoskeletal Conditions at the Start of the New Millennium. The burden of musculoskeletal conditions at the start of the new millennium. World Health Organ Tech Rep Ser. 2003;919:i – x, 1–218, back cover.
25. Wu J, Du Z, Lv Y, et al. A new technique for the treatment of lumbar facet joint syndrome using intra-articular injection with autologous platelet rich plasma. Pain Physician. 2016;19(8):617–25.

Part IX

Intradiscal and Minimally Invasive Structural Surgeries

Discography

92

Bunty J. Shah

Introduction

Discography, commonly referred to as provocative discography, is a procedure that is used to diagnose a specific disc as being a potentially pain-producing structure. The rationale for performing discography is to ascertain whether or not injection of contrast media under pressure into a disc thought to be contributing to a patient's pain is capable of reproducing a patient's pain. If so, this pain is said to be concordant. In other words, the pain being produced intentionally by discography is similar in quality and possibly in intensity to that pain which the patient typically feels. Perhaps just as important is the concept of the negative control disc. In the context of discography, a negative control disc is a disc that is thought to be devoid of pathology that is capable of producing the patient's pain. Injection of at least one or more of such discs should not lead the reproduction of the patient's pain. As will be discussed later in this chapter, the criterion of a negative control disc is essential to validating the results of an otherwise seemingly positive discogram.

Once contrast medium is injected into the disc, the pattern of contrast spread is noted and interpreted. In Guyer et al.'s description of the appearance of contrast in a normal-appearing disc, the contrast is maintained completely in the disc and appears similar in shape to a "cotton ball." When the contrast spread diverges from this archetypal pattern, it may be reflective of pathology in the annulus fibrosus. The Dallas Classification has traditionally been utilized to assess the degree of internal disc disruption. (See Fig. 92.1). Schellhas et al. are responsible for the Modified Dallas Classification, which grades annular tears from 0 to 1 based on characteristics including the degree of extension of an annular tear, as well as the degree of extension circumferentially into the annulus with contrast administration, and whether or not the contrast medium exits the disc through an annular tear that reaches the outside of the disc. Sachs et al. created the original Dallas Classification, and Aprill and Bogduk later added grade 4 to this classification.

A number of practitioners of provocative discography advocate the use of postinjection computed tomography (CT) to assess the spread of contrast in or through a disc with axial images. In fact, Guyer et al., in their Position Statement from the NASS (North American Spine Society) Diagnostic and Therapeutic Committee, describe CT discography as the best means to assess the capability of a disc to retain liquid internally under pressure.

Background and Historical Perspective

Discography was first employed in the diagnosis of pain thought to be originating from the intervertebral disc in the 1940s. In Lindblom's paper, the early adopter of discography describes the injection of "red lead" into the nucleus pulposus of the lower lumbar discs, which led to passage of this material to the surface of the discs, spreading to the outer layer of the annulus fibrosus along the "nerves and other structures." Even in the 1940s, it was recognized that injection of the disc with some sort of contrast medium might be diagnostically helpful. The process was, of course, refined over the years. In fact, Lindblom's paper in 1948 described the utility of discography in the diagnosis of "sciatica," and not axial low back pain due to discogenic causes – its primary indication today. He posited in this paper that the radial tears in the annulus led to spinal nerve compression and symptoms consistent with what we call, in modern terms, lumbar radiculopathy. The utility of this test, in his opinion, was to ascertain which disc was responsible for the patient's radicular symptoms.

Since provocative discography was adopted, imaging modalities, including magnetic resonance imaging (MRI) and computed tomography (CT), have been employed to evaluate structural abnormalities in the annulus and disc in combination with low-pressure provocative discography.

B. J. Shah (✉)
Penn State Milton S. Hershey Medical Center, Hershey, PA, USA
e-mail: bshah@psu.edu

T. R. Deer et al. (eds.), *Deer's Treatment of Pain*, https://doi.org/10.1007/978-3-030-12281-2_92

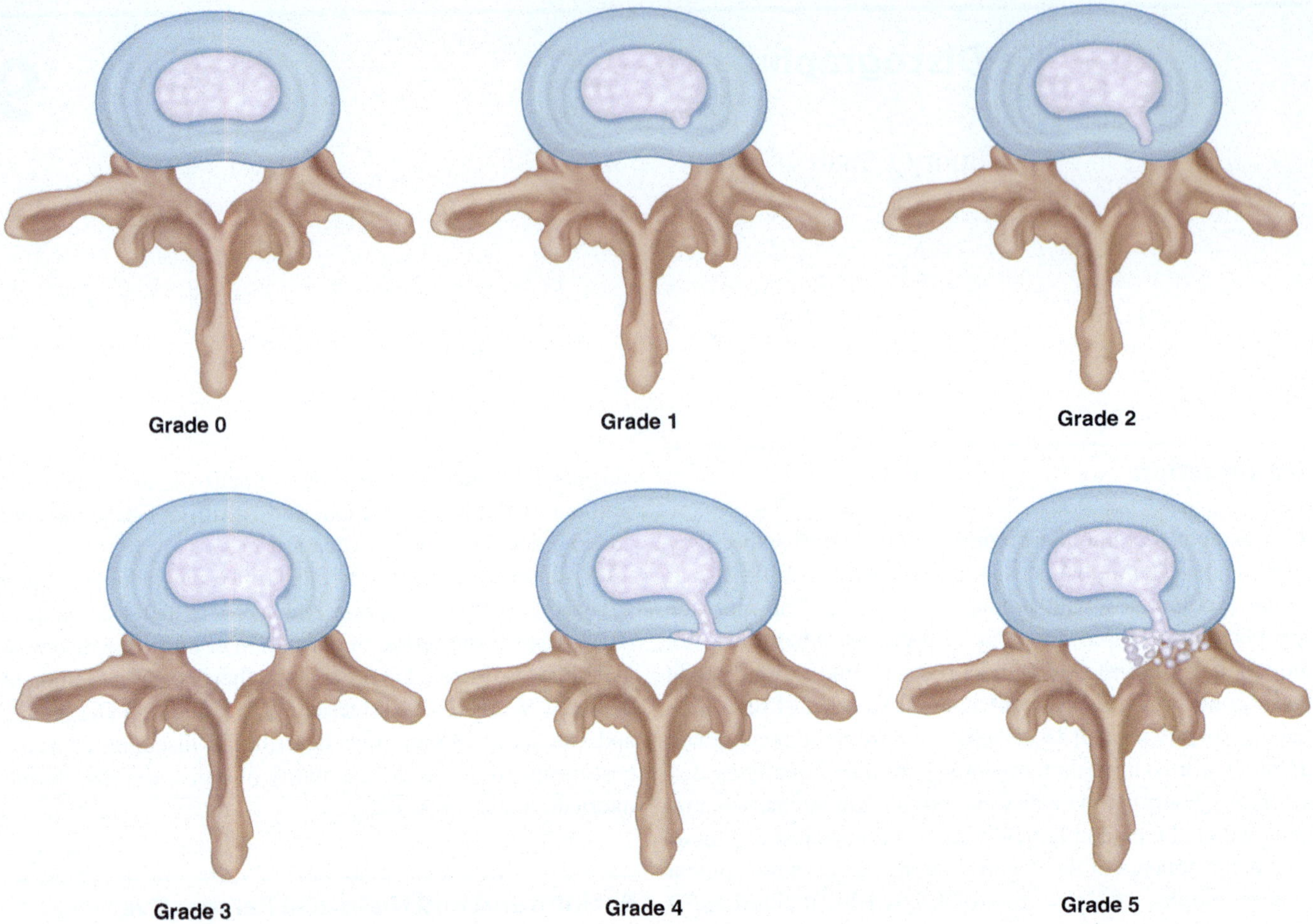

Fig. 92.1 Grade 0: normal-appearing annulus. Grade 1: annular tear reaches inner $\frac{1}{3}$ of annulus. Grade 2: annular tear reaches middle 1/3rd of annulus. Grade 3: annular tear reaches outer $\frac{1}{3}$ of annulus, but <30° annular circumference. Grade 4: annular tear reaches outer $\frac{1}{3}$ of annulus, >30° annular circumference. Grade 5: annular tear reaching the outer annulus with extension of contrast material outside the annulus

These imaging modalities, however, are not in and of themselves helpful in determining the relative contribution of a damaged or abnormal-appearing disc, as various studies have shown that imaging abnormalities on MRI are present even in asymptomatic individuals. Furthermore, it was advised that MRI abnormalities be correlated with clinical findings and interpreted in the context of patient age prior to consideration of surgical management for these findings.

Uses and Indications

Provocative discography is used when a patient's clinical history and physical examination raise a high suspicion that the patient's pain generator is an intervertebral disc. Typically, patients with discogenic back pain have midline back pain without radiation characteristic of radiculopathy. The pain is typically exacerbated by forward flexion of the spine at the hip, in the case of lumbar discogenic pain. Since, as mentioned previously, advanced imaging studies in and of themselves have limited utility in establishing a particular disc as a definitive pain generator on the basis of structural changes, provocative discography may be helpful in determining whether or not a particular disc is responsible for a patient's pain.

The majority of provocation discography procedures are performed at lumbar levels, but they can also be performed at presumed symptomatic discs in the cervical and thoracic spinal levels. The needle trajectory and access points vary based on the particular spinal level to be targeted based on anatomic features and the presence of intervening structures which should be avoided.

No discussion of a procedure is complete without a discussion about contraindications to the procedure. As with any procedure, patient refusal is an absolute contraindication. Due to the risk of discitis with introduction of a needle into the disc, local or systemic infection is also a contraindication to the discography. Fortunately, as stated by Bogduk et al., the prevalence of discitis is low, and there is no conclusive evidence to support the use of prophylactic intradiscal antibiotics. Nevertheless, many providers continue to do so out of an abundance of caution. The presence of a coagulopathy or other condition rendering the patient unable to achieve normal hemostasis is also a contraindication, as there is a theoretical risk of violation of the epidural space with potential hematoma formation. Pregnancy is a contraindication to discography as radiation from fluoroscopy or computed tomography can be detrimental to the developing fetus. Allergy to contrast media or local anesthetics is also a contraindication to the procedure. The patient must also be able to communicate the presence or absence of concordant pain in some way to the operator. Significant psychological distress may also confound the patient's response to provocative discography. A study by Block et al. examining 72 patients undergoing CT/discography at the three lowest lumbar levels was performed. Thirty-four patients reported a "discordant positive pain response," which is a painful response to injection of a "non-disrupted disc." The 38 other patients did not report painful injection of similarly "non-disrupted" discs. Statistical analysis of their MMPI (Minnesota Multiphasic Personality Inventory) scores, which were obtained prior to the procedures, showed that patients with MMPI scores >70 had an increased likelihood of reporting a positive discordant pain response compared with patients who had scores of 70 or less. The particular scales that were being evaluated in this study were those pertaining specifically to depression, hysteria, and hypochondriasis. Bogduk et al. interpret this study as a warning to physicians to consider that patients with MMPI scores >70 may have exaggerated responses to pain but emphasize that the procedure is not contraindicated in these patients solely on this basis.

If the patient is hearing impaired or if there exists a language barrier, accommodations should be made for an interpreter. All of the above contraindications, or situations regarding special attention, should be effectively identified using pre-procedure screening and a "time-out," process prior to the procedure (See Table 92.1). An ideal candidate for provocative discography has relatively localized disc degeneration rather than diffuse disc disease, so that control discs are available to provide a context with which to interpret provocation discography of the target disc.

Table 92.1 Discography contraindications

Contraindications to discography
Patient refusal
Local or systemic infection
Bleeding diatheses, abnormalities in hemostasis, decreased platelet count, coagulopathy
Pregnancy
Allergy to contrast medium to be injected
Inability to communicate pain to operator

Since the entire test depends upon the patient's response, sedation should be omitted or limited so as not to render the patient sedate to the point where he or she is not able to provide meaningful feedback.

During the entire procedure, strict sterile technique should be employed to minimize the risk of infection – namely, discitis. This should include donning a surgical cap, mask, gown, and sterile gloves. Sterile preparation and drape for the patient and imaging apparatus should also be utilized to maintain the sterility of the procedural field and equipment. The use of pre-procedural antibiotics should be strongly considered by the proceduralist.

Discography is usually performed with fluoroscopic (or CT) guidance to aid guide and assess needle placement continuously and anteroposterior (AP) and lateral views. The desired level is identified with image guidance, and the image intensifier should be oriented cephalocaudally to optimize end plate alignment for ease of needle entry into the desired intervertebral disc. Obliquity of the image intensifier is increased to one side to optimize lateral entry into the disc. Care should be taken to remain as close to the facet (superior articular process) as possible to avoid inadvertent contact with the spinal nerve, which could result in a significant amount of patient discomfort and movement. Typically, a 22-gauge spinal needle with or without a bent tip is utilized for this purpose. The bent tip can be employed to enhance needle steering and minimize the need to repeatedly withdraw the needle for reorientation. One to two additional discs should be identified adjacent to the disc in question to serve as control discs. It is important that the disc being provoked at any point in time is not divulged as a control or target disc when performing the study so as not to compromise the results by introducing patient bias in terms of response. A double-needle technique is often utilized by some operators, as it allows for a smaller gauge needle to be passed into the disc through a larger needle as a conduit, theoretically reducing the risk of infection.

Once imaging confirmation suggests that the needle is placed within the nucleus pulposus, the opening pressure is measured and noted. Water-soluble contrast medium is injected, and the volume at which a painful response in the patient is noted and documented, as is the contrast distribution and disc morphology. The volume injected is documented, and the disc is pressurized until a painful response is elicited at greater than 15 pounds per square inch (PSI) above the opening pressure or less than or equal to 50 PSI. No more than 3 mL of contrast should be injected (See Figs. 92.2 and 92.3). The contrast may be mixed with an antibiotic at the discretion of the operator in hopes of further reducing the risk of infection (discitis). The characteristics of the patient's pain, including quality and intensity, should be ascertained and documented, as

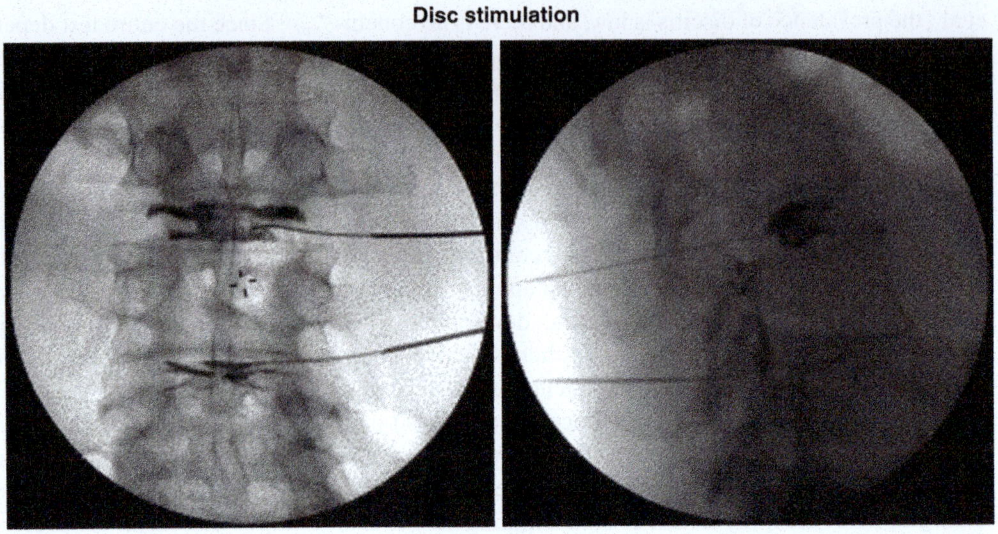

Fig. 92.2 Discogram fluoroscopic image of a Modified Dallas Classification grade 5 annular fissure. Note the extravasation of contrast posteriorly into the ventral epidural space. (Image courtesy of Yakov Vorobeychik, MD, Ph.D.)

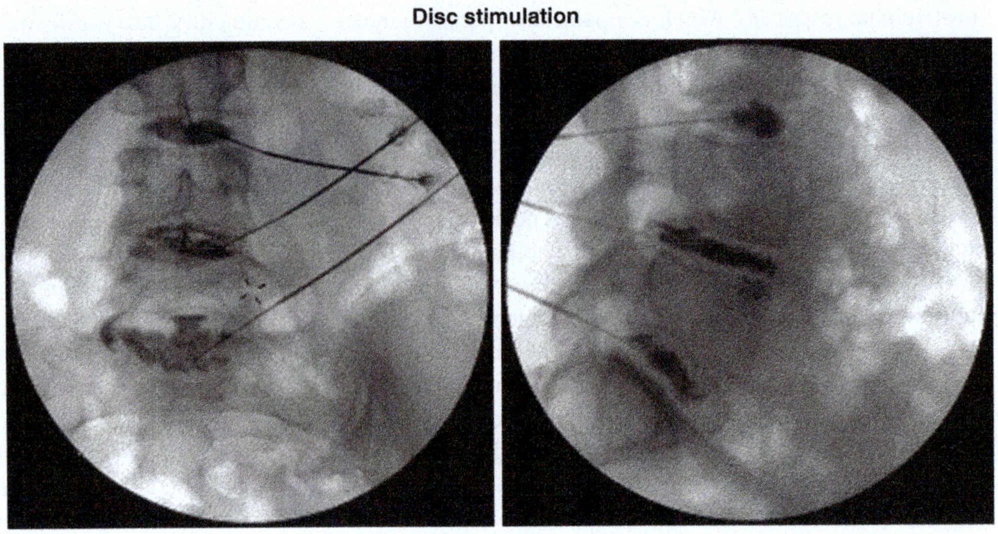

Fig. 92.3 Discogram fluoroscopic image of a Modified Dallas Classification grade 4 annular fissure. (Image courtesy of Yakov Vorobeychik, MD, Ph.D.)

should its concordance with the patient's usual pain. Videographic monitoring of the patient's response can be helpful to confirm the patient's response to injection after the procedure is completed.

The Spine Intervention Society Practice Guidelines for Spinal Diagnostic and Treatment Procedures include extensive guidelines for the interpretation of provocative discography data. At minimum, for the diagnosis of discogenic pain, stimulation of the index disc must produce concordant pain with a numeric rating scale pain score between 6 and 10. Another, equivalent scale may be used instead of the numeric rating scale. This concordant pain should be reproduced at less than 50 PSI or at less than 15 PSI above opening pressure. If provocative discography is performed on one adjacent disc, that disc should be painless or elicit non-concordant pain at greater than 15 PSI above opening pressure. If two adjacent control discs are utilized, the guidelines dictate that either both control discs are painless when stimulated or, if one disc is painful, that pain be non-concordant and reproduced at greater than 15 PSI above opening pressure.

Potential complications of discography include skin and soft tissue infection, discitis, nerve root injury (if the nerve root is contacted during needle placement or advancement), epidural hematoma, allergic reaction to contrast media, post-dural puncture headache if inadvertent dural puncture occurs. If care is not taken to suspend anticoagulant or antiplatelet medications for an appropriate length of time prior to the procedure and the epidural space is violated, epidural hematoma may ensue with neurologic sequelae. If sterile technique is not properly observed, infection in the epidural space may also result in epidural abscess.

Evidence for Efficacy

Multiple studies have been performed to evaluate the utility and diagnostic accuracy of provocation discography, yielding conclusions both supportive of and against the use of discography as a diagnostic tool.

An early study by Holt et al. in the 1960s examined 30 volunteer inmates with no history of back pain or radiculopathy, negative physical examinations suggestive of back pain, and x-ray images with no abnormalities (with the exception of two patients with asymptomatic spondylolisthesis). These patients were subjected over the course of 3 days to discography with sodium diatrizoate, an irritating contrast medium, which the authors acknowledged was "quite capable of irritating tissue." Furthermore, there were no strict operational criteria used including manometry, and the patient population consisted completely of young men. Holt et al. quoted a false-positive rate as high as 37%, based on this study.

In a recent philosophical essay and discourse with literature reference published by Bogduk et al., the authors emphasize the very fact that there is an anatomical basis for a disc to be painful as one of the requisite reasons to consider discogenic pain as a possible entity. Furthermore, they establish internal disc disruption (IDD) as a major etiology to discogenic pain and reference previous studies in which provocation of discs under local anesthesia with a blunt probe or hypertonic saline reproduced patients' back pain symptoms.

The authors make the very important point of emphasizing that the assessment of the validity of discography as a diagnostic test, however, is complicated by the very fact that there is no "physical reference standard," to which a painful disc can be compared. That is to say that analysis of a tissue sample or imaging study alone cannot be used to confirm a disc as being painful. They do, however, support the notion that discs not being painful in asymptomatic individuals be considered as a reference standard.

Carragee et al. performed a prospective study seeking to ascertain the validity of a positive discography test result for the diagnosis of discogenic low back pain. Thirty-two patients with isthmic spondylolisthesis (grade I or II) at L4–L5 or L5–S1 were matched with 30 patients with previous positive single-level provocative discography. Patients in both cohorts had previously failed conservative therapy. Both cohorts of patients underwent single-level lumbar fusion. Data from 2-year follow-up was used to calculate positive predictive value (PPV). The best-case PPV was for discography which was found to be between 55 and 57%. 91% of patients in the spondylolisthesis cohort achieved a minimally acceptable outcome, whereas 43% of patients in the discography cohort achieved a minimally acceptable outcome, thereby leading the authors to conclude that, despite application of strict test criteria, positive discography is not highly accurate in identifying "discogenic pain."

Wolfer et al. performed a systematic review and meta-analysis, the purpose of which was twofold. First, they sought to perform a systematic review to determine the false-positive rate of discography in asymptomatic individuals. Second, the authors sought to investigate the specificity of discography through a meta-analysis. They provided conclusions that were based on adjustments made to previous studies with Spine Intervention Society/IASP criteria applied. They concluded that an all-inclusive meta-analysis of studies of patients who were asymptomatic and receiving discography yielded a specificity of 0.94 (95% confidence interval 0.89–0.98) and a false-positive rate of only 6%. The authors of this review and analysis emphasize the importance of understanding the fact that a high pretest probability, also known as prevalence, of a condition or disease is correlated with a higher positive predictive value. Based on this paper, it seems that an adequately low false-positive rate is present with discography, when it is combined with physical examination and patient history findings suggestive of discogenic pain.

Carragee et al. recruited 26 volunteer subjects who did not suffer from back pain-related symptoms. Of these subjects, ten had no pain complaints whatsoever, ten had a history of chronic neck and arm pain after cervical discectomy and/or fusion, and ten had primary somatization disorders. The objective of the study was to determine the relative pain response and "pain-related behavior" in patients who were asymptomatic from a low back pain standpoint, on the basis that a previous study performed by Walsh et al. looked at patients who were asymptomatic from a low back pain standpoint, but did not represent a population that Carragee et al. felt closely resembled the typical chronic pain population. That is to say that the patients in Walsh et al.'s study numbered only ten were all young men and paid for their participation in the study, among other differences.

In this study, Carragee et al. found that a painful response was observed in 10% of the pain-free group, 40% of the group with chronic neck and arm pain after cervical spine surgery, and 83% of the group with a history of primary somatization disorder. On the basis of these results, the authors concluded that the strict application of positive discography criteria coupled with normal psychometric profiles in patients without chronic pain syndromes could yield relatively low false-positive rates. Additionally, the authors concluded that the presence of annular disruption and chronic pain or abnormal psychometric profiles was associated with higher rates of painful injection. This study was, however, criticized on the basis that discography would never practically be offered to asymptomatic patients and on the basis that a specific pressure threshold was not applied for a discography result to be considered positive.

Regarding specific pressure thresholds for interpretation of discography results, Derby et al. published a study which examined the prevalence of positive responses to discography in asymptomatic individuals (volunteers) controlling for both injection pressure and response intensity. Their findings supported the concept that discs in asymptomatic individuals could be made to hurt with intradiscal injection. However, this required high pressures and when made to hurt, only resulted in mildly intense pain (2–3/10). A receiver-operator curve based on these data resulted in a calculation of a false-positive rate of 0 or less than 10%. It is notable, in this study, that there was no identified correlation between the appearance of a disc on MRI and its tendency to provoke pain. Lower lumbar discs (L4–L5 and L5–S1) were found to be more likely to be painful upon stimulation than their more cephalad counterparts (L1–L2 or L3–L4).

Perhaps the more important question about the utility of provocative discography is whether or not it is associated with improved treatment outcomes. Knox et al. performed a retrospective study of 22 patients who underwent anterior lumbar interbody fusion after positive concordant discography. Results were recorded as poor in all patients who received two-level fusions, and in patients who received a single-level fusion, results were recorded as poor in 47% of patients.

A prospective, observational study by Wetzel et al. examined the success rate of lumbar arthrodesis in patient with positive discography and found that, although 48% of patients were found to have a solid arthrodesis, only 46% of patients were found to have a clinically satisfactory outcome at final follow-up.

Madan et al. performed a study of 73 patients who underwent posterolateral interbody and posterior spinal arthrodesis, 41 of whom did not undergo presurgical discography and 32 of whom did with successful pain reproduction during disc stimulation. The results of this study indicated that, with a minimum follow-up period of 2 years, 75.6% of the group not having presurgical discography versus 81.2% of those patients having had presurgical discography had satisfactory outcomes. This difference was not deemed to be statistically significant, and the authors concluded that presurgical discography did not improve outcomes in these patients.

A prospective study by Colhoun et al., on the other hand, reviewed the records of 195 patients at a minimum of 2 years post surgery including anterior and posterior fusions and laminectomies, which were deemed to be technically successful. Of 137 patients who had a positive discography result, 89% achieved significant and sustained clinical benefit, whereas of the 25 patients with morphological abnormality identified on discography, but negative discography, only 52% achieved this outcome. The results were hailed as being supportive of lumbar discography as being reflective of potential successful surgical outcomes by the authors.

The question of whether or not provocative discography causes acceleration of disc degeneration has been raised. Cuellar et al. performed a 10-year matched-cohort study with 71 discography subjects matched with 72 control subjects. At 10-year follow-up, the data for 57 discography subjects and 53 control subjects were available and were analyzed. The incidence of lumbar surgery (16 surgeries in the discography group versus 4 in the control group), imaging studies, work loss, and prolonged back pain episodes were all reported to be more frequent in the discography group compared to controls. The authors of the study acknowledged loss to follow-up as a potential downfall of this study as well as the fact that patients were chosen from a pool of patients who were independently at higher risk for the development of disc degeneration than most other individuals but emphasized that the risk of accelerated disc degeneration should be considered when making the decision to offer this procedure to a patient and should be included as a potential risk when discussing and consenting the patient for the procedure.

Pearls and Pitfalls

- Discography is a controversial procedure during which a thin, small gauge needle is used to puncture an intervertebral disc in an attempt to determine whether or not a particular disc is the source of a patient's axial back pain.
- Discography (more accurately described as provocative discography) is not intended to be an isolated test but rather used in combination with the patient's clinical history and available imaging studies. It has traditionally been used to confirm the diagnosis of discogenic pain.
- The procedure/study is intended not only as a means of eliciting a patient's pain but also gives important details about disc integrity and structure, which may lead to further intervention including intradiscal therapies and potentially surgical options, including fusion surgery.
- The key to the study is eliciting pain that is concordant with the patient's typical pain. The study is only truly positive if this is obtained with at least one negative control disc.
- Without the application of stringent criteria, there exists the theoretical potential for false-positive tests.

Recommended Reading

1. Aprill C, Bogduk N. High-intensity zone: a diagnostic sign of painful lumbar disc on magnetic resonance imaging. Br J Radiol. 1992;65(773):361–9.
2. Block AR, Vanharanta H, Ohnmeiss DD, Guyer RD. Discographic pain report: influence of psychological factors. Spine. 1996;21(3):334–8.

3. Boden SD, Davis DO, Dina TS, Patronas NJ, Wiesel SW. Abnormal magnetic-resonance scans of the lumbar spine in asymptomatic subjects. A prospective investigation. J Bone Joint Surg Am. 1990;72(3):403–8.
4. Bogduk N. Lumbar disc stimulation. In: Bogduk N, editor. Practice guidelines for spinal diagnostic and treatment procedures. San Francisco: International Spine Intervention Society; 2013.
5. Bogduk N, Aprill C, Derby R. Lumbar discogenic pain: state-of-the-art review. Pain Med. 2013;14(6):813–36.
6. Carragee EJ, Tanner CM, Khurana S, Hayward C, Welsh J, Date E, Truong T, Rossi M, Hagle C. The rates of false-positive lumbar discography in select patients without low back symptoms. Spine. 2000;25(11):1373–81.
7. Carragee EJ, Lincoln T, Parmar VS, Alamin T. A gold standard evaluation of the "discogenic pain" diagnosis as determined by provocative discography. Spine. 2006;31(18):2115–23.
8. Colhoun E, McCall IW, Williams L, Pullicino VC. Provocation discography as a guide to planning operations on the spine. Bone Joint J. 1988;70(2):267–71.
9. Cuellar JM, Stauff MP, Herzog RJ, Carrino JA, Baker GA, Carragee EJ. Does provocative discography cause clinically important injury to the lumbar intervertebral disc? A 10-year matched cohort study. Spine J. 2016;16(3):273–80.
10. Daly City CA, Daly City CA, Center SK, Wolfer L. Systematic review of lumbar provocation discography in asymptomatic subjects with a meta-analysis of false-positive rates. Pain Physician. 2008;11(4):513–38.
11. Derby R, Lee SH, Kim BJ, Chen Y, Aprill C, Bogduk N. Pressure-controlled lumbar discography in volunteers without low back symptoms. Pain Med. 2005;6(3):213–21.
12. Guarino AH. Discography: a review. Curr Rev Pain. 1999; 3(6):473–80.
13. Guyer RD, Ohnmeiss DD. Lumbar discography. Position statement from the North American Spine Society Diagnostic and Therapeutic Committee. Spine. 1995;20(18):2048–59.
14. Holt EP Jr. The question of lumbar discography. J Bone Joint Surg Am. 1968;50(4):720–6.
15. Knox BD, Chapman TM. Anterior lumbar interbody fusion for discogram concordant pain. J Spinal Disord. 1993;6(3):242–4.
16. Lindblom K. Diagnostic puncture of intervertebral disks in sciatica. Clin Orthop Relat Res. 1969;67:6–8.
17. Madan S, Gundanna M, Harley JM, Boeree NR, Sampson M. Does provocative discography screening of discogenic back pain improve surgical outcome? Clin Spine Surg. 2002;15(3):245–51.
18. Provenzano DA. Diagnostic discography: what is the clinical utility? Curr Pain Headache Rep. 2012;16(1):26–34.
19. Sachs BL, Vanharanta HE, Spivey MA, Guyer RD, Videman TA, Rashbaum RF, Johnson RG, Hochschuler SH, Mooney VE. Dallas discogram description. A new classification of CT/discography in low-back disorders. Spine. 1987;12(3):287–94.
20. Schellhas KP, Pollei SR, Gundry CR, Heithoff KB. Lumbar disc high-intensity zone: correlation of magnetic resonance imaging and discography. Spine. 1996;21(1):79–86.
21. Walsh TR, Weinstein JN, Spratt KF, Lehmann TR, Aprill C, Sayre H. Lumbar discography in normal subjects. A controlled, prospective study. J Bone Joint Surg Am. 1990;72(7):1081–8.
22. Wetzel FT, LaRocca SH, Lowery GL, Aprill CN. The treatment of lumbar spinal pain syndromes diagnosed by discography. Lumbar Arthrodesis Spine. 1994;19(7):792–800.
23. Wetzel FT, Carragee EJ, Tanner CM, Khurana S, Hayward C, Welsh J, Date E, Truong T, Rossi M, Hagle C. Point of view. Response to: the rates of false-positive lumbar discography in select patients without low back symptoms. Spine. 2000;25(11):1373–81.

Endoscopic Discectomy

93

Jonathan D. Carlson, Abram H. Burgher, and Gabriel P. Jasper

Introduction

Pain originating in the spine, including the back and neck, is by far the most common form of chronic pain and disability, affecting an estimated two-thirds of people at some point in their life. Spinal pain includes a number of distinct etiologies, including lumbar facet syndrome, disc prolapse, degenerative disc disease, spinal stenosis, acute/subacute strain, and vertebral fracture. Disc prolapse (including protrusion, herniation, or extrusion of the disc) can produce pain, numbness, and/or weakness in the back or legs, known as lumbar radiculitis or sciatica. Estimates of the prevalence of sciatica vary from study to study, with a range from 1.2% to 43% making it one of the most common spinal pain etiologies.

Treatments for sciatica include conservative care, including rest and anti-inflammatory medications, interventional procedures (e.g., epidural steroid injection), and surgical procedures (e.g., discectomy). Though clinical trials demonstrate the efficacy of discectomy in rapidly relieving pain and disability, it carries additional risks beyond those of conservative care, such as infection, nerve injury, dural tear (which can lead to spinal headache), the formation of scar tissue in the spine, lumbar post-laminectomy syndrome, and the high possibility of patients getting worse after surgery. Further, there is a recovery period for patients undergoing discectomy. In light of these risks and recovery period, endoscopic techniques have been developed to allow for minimally invasive discectomies with the potential for lower complication rates and quicker recoveries than previous, more invasive discectomy methods. These endoscopic techniques can be divided into those involving an interlaminar approach and two types of transforaminal approaches ("inside-out" or "outside-in").

J. D. Carlson (✉)
Hawaii Pain & Spine, Kailua, HI, USA

Midwestern Medical School, Glendale, AZ, USA

Hawaii Pain & Spine, Arizona Pain, Kailua, HI, USA

A. H. Burgher
The Pain Center of Arizona, Peoria, AZ, USA
e-mail: ABurgher@ThePainCenter.com

G. P. Jasper
Jasper Spine Institute, Brick, NJ, USA

Jasper Spine Learning Institution, Jersey Shore University, Neptune, NJ, USA

Background and Historical Perspective

From ancient times and even into the 1900s, chronic pain conditions such as lumbar radiculopathy were often attributed to supernatural causes, though some ancient Greeks and Egyptians suspected a link between lumbar spinal pathology and leg pain. This idea was further developed in the late 1700s by Cotugno and Kocher, who differentiated arthritic hip pain from nerve-related sciatica. By the late 1800s and early 1900s, early spinal surgeries were being performed to treat spinal "enchondromas," though these were most likely disc herniations.

The original modern discectomy is usually attributed to Mixter and Barr in the 1930s. During the 1930s, the idea that herniation of the nucleus pulposus, rather than a tumor in the spine, was responsible for radicular symptoms gained widespread acceptance. Mixter and Barr advocated surgical treatment, eventually publishing a case series of 19 cases of "ruptured" discs. In 1938, Love described an intralaminar extradural approach to discectomy that included the removal of flavum and minimal removal of bone. The modern open approach is a modification of Love's technique.

By the 1970s, smaller, specialized instruments allowed discectomies to be performed with smaller incisions. In the early 1980s, techniques described by Caspar and Kambin, including a microscope to allow visualization of the herniated disc, allowed for a less invasive approach to discectomy. Though still an open surgical procedure, these microdiscectomies involve a relatively small incision (e.g., a few centimeters). As of the mid-1990s, more than 200,000 discectomies were performed each year in the USA alone. Though these discectomies were not as invasive as historical

T. R. Deer et al. (eds.), *Deer's Treatment of Pain*, https://doi.org/10.1007/978-3-030-12281-2_93

techniques, interest remained in even less invasive methods of discectomy. This led to the development of the endoscopic discectomy.

In 1993, Mayer and Brock reported the results of a randomized trial comparing percutaneous endoscopic discectomy with microdiscectomy. Endoscopic discectomy involved an automated high-power suction shaver and cutter system inserted percutaneously, with visualization provided by an endoscope coupled with a television and video unit. The use of endoscopic discectomy was initially limited to contained herniations. Subsequent systems have been developed, such as the microendoscopic discectomy (MED) system, which incorporated a tubular retractor, introduced by Foley and Smith in 1996. Instrumentation and techniques for endoscopic discectomy have continued to progress, allowing safer and more effective treatments.

Uses and Indications

Endoscopic discectomy procedures include the intralaminar approach, the transforaminal "inside-out" approach (see Figs. 93.1, 93.2, 93.3 and 93.4), and the transforaminal "outside-in" approach (see Figs. 93.5, 93.6, 93.7, 93.8 and 93.9). Patients may be positioned in either a lateral or prone position, depending on the nature of the disc prolapse and symptoms. For unilateral symptoms resulting from paracentral protrusions or extrusions, lateral decubitus positioning may be preferred. Benefits of the lateral patient position include: (1) gravity drops the dura out of position, thus decreasing chance of dural tear; (2) decrease intraabdominal pressure, thus decreasing intraabdominal pressure potentially leading to less venous congestion and bleeding; (3) optimizes needle/trocar placement for the procedure (i.e., "gun-barrel approach"); (4) easier access to airway for anesthesia provider; and (5) patient comfort.

The patient is positioned with the target side up, with lateral decubitus leading traversing nerves to fall away from the disc. Myelogram may be used at the level above the targeted disc to allow fluoroscopic guidance. This can improve visualization of the thecal sac, reducing the risk of nerve injury or dural tear. Patients with bilateral symptoms and/or protrusions or extrusions crossing the midline may be treated in the prone position.

Evidence for Efficacy

Discectomy has demonstrated superiority to non-operative treatment for patients with lumbar disc herniations, including in long-term follow-up. A multicenter, randomized trial compared discectomy and non-operative treatment in 501 patients across 13 centers for 4–8 years. Lumbar discectomy patients demonstrated significantly decreased pain and disability, relative to non-operatively treated patients. There has been some debate about the benefits of endoscopic discectomy compared with open discectomy. A meta-analysis of 837 patients across 6 randomized controlled trials (RCTs) comparing minimally invasive discectomy (primarily endoscopic) to open discectomy found both procedures to show equivalent efficacy and overall complication rates. Both open and endoscopic microdiscectomies appear to be effective for treating lumbar disc herniations. A more recent meta-analysis of 1092 patients in 9 RCTs found that endoscopic discectomy

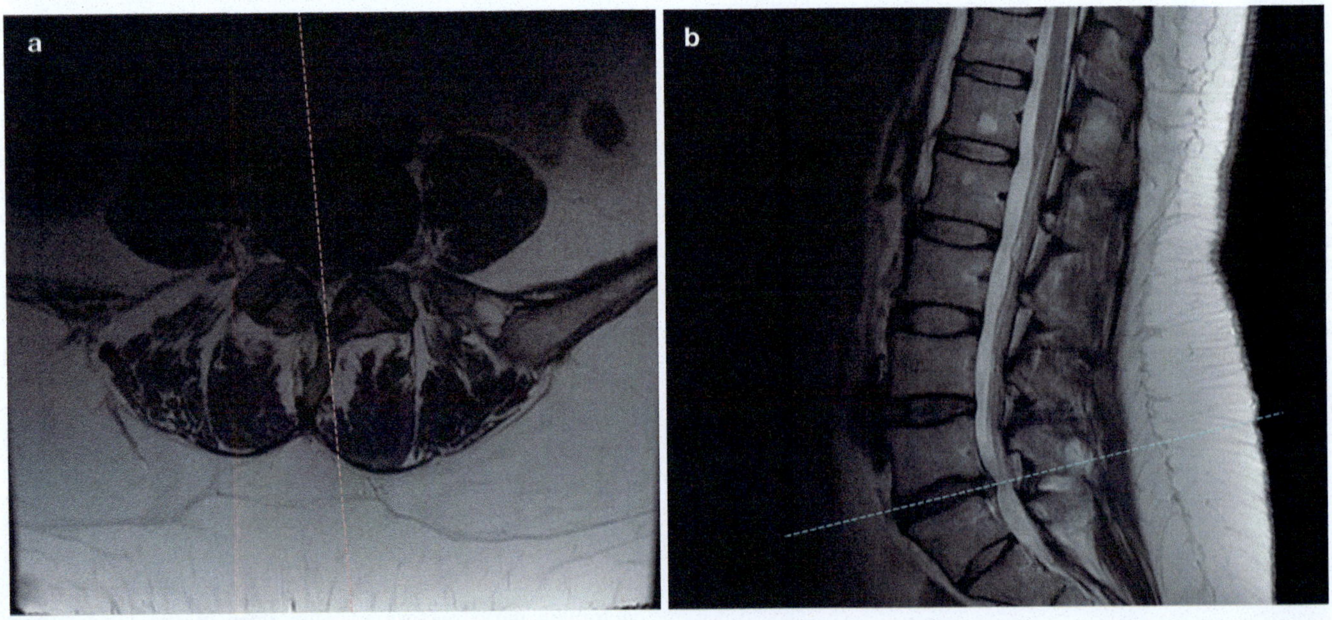

Fig. 93.1 (**a**) (axial) and (**b**) (sagittal) T2-weighted MRI of right L4/L5 paracentral disc protrusion

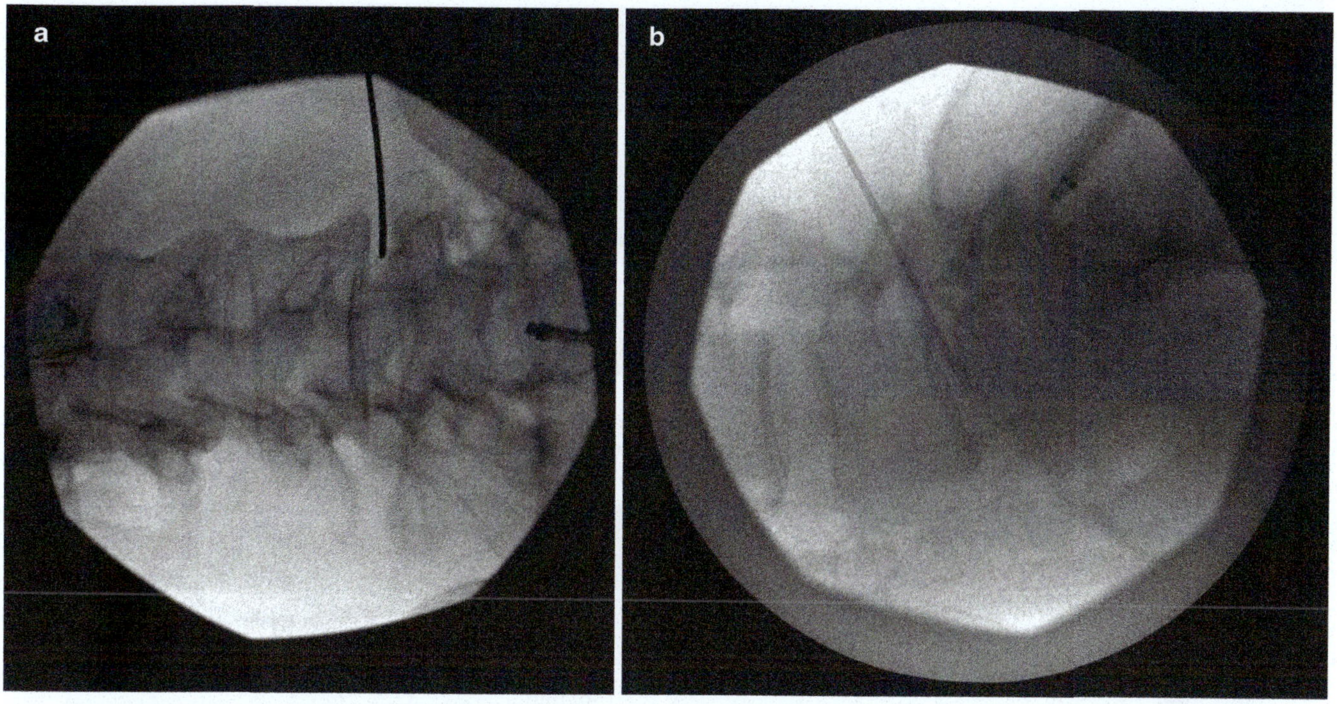

Fig. 93.2 (**a**) (oblique) and (**b**) (lateral) fluoroscopy depicting needle placement in the right dorsolateral quarter of the disc. The distal tip of the needle is in the vicinity of the nuclear-annular interface, anterior to the disc protrusion. The epiduroscope, passing from caudal to rostral, is also visible

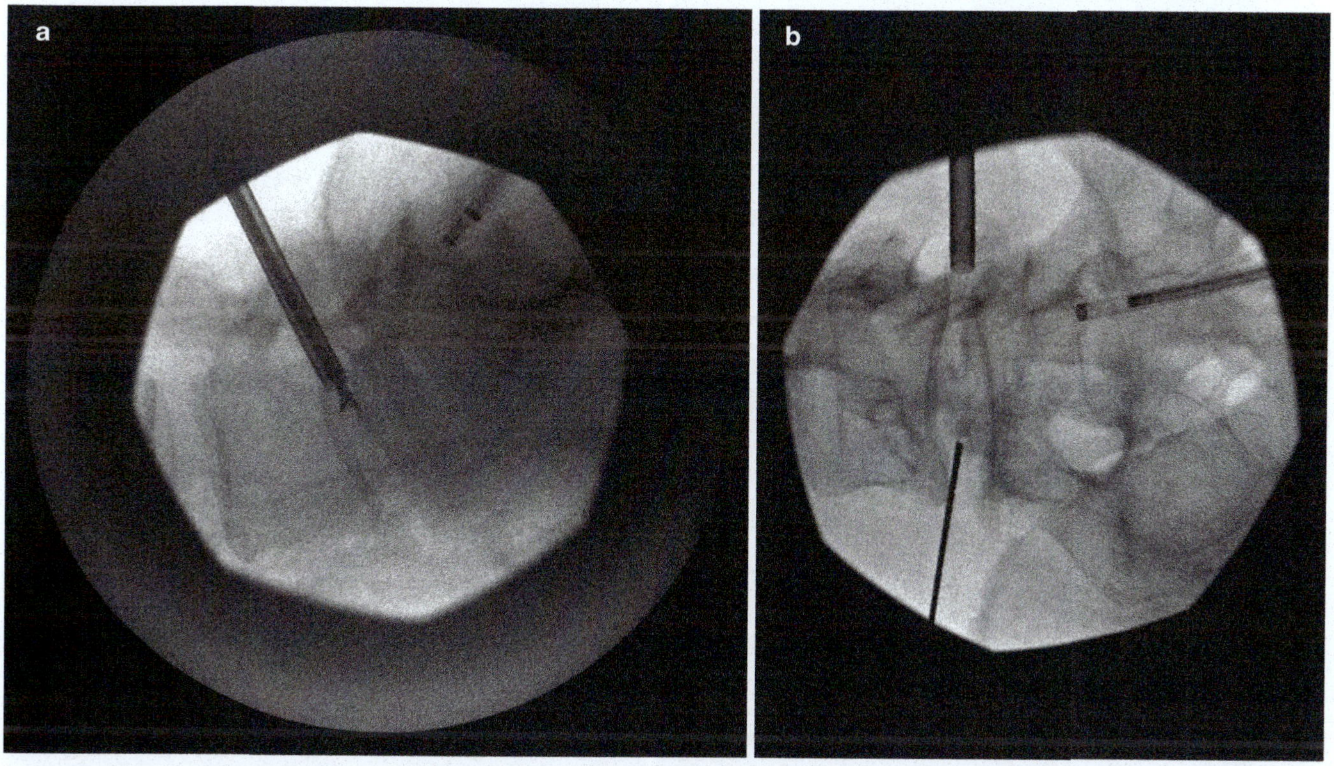

Fig. 93.3 (**a–b**) A series of dilators are placed using the Seldinger technique. The size of the dilator used varies based on the size of the targeted protrusion (final dilators are typically 4–8 mm). The dilator shown here has an internal diameter of 6 mm. A cavity is created beneath the protrusion using forceps. The amount of nuclear and internal annular tissue excised may range from 0.5 g for small protrusions to 1.0 g for large protrusions. For protrusions close to/crossing the midline, contralateral needle placement may be used, as in (**b**)

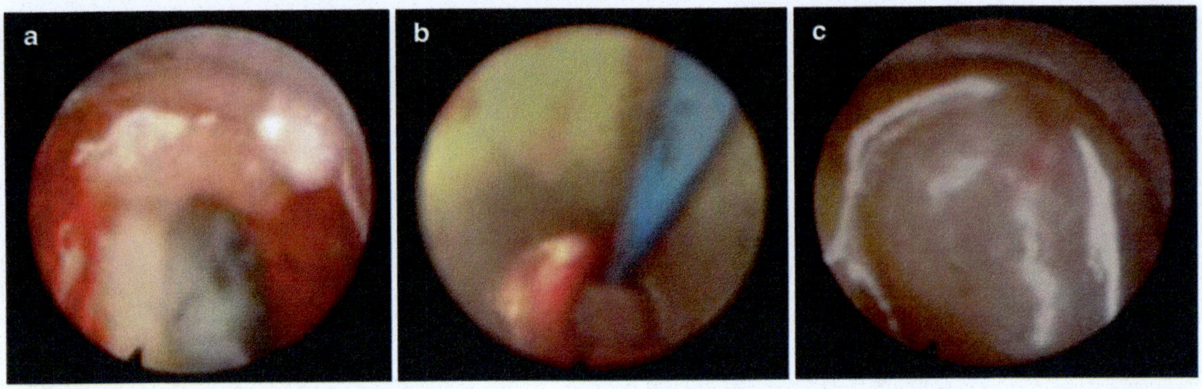

Fig. 93.4 (a–c) Endoscopic views of thulium laser cautery being used to collapse the cavity beneath the protrusion, reducing the protrusion while keeping most of the annulus intact. The surface of the disc as the dilator is withdrawn is depicted in (c)

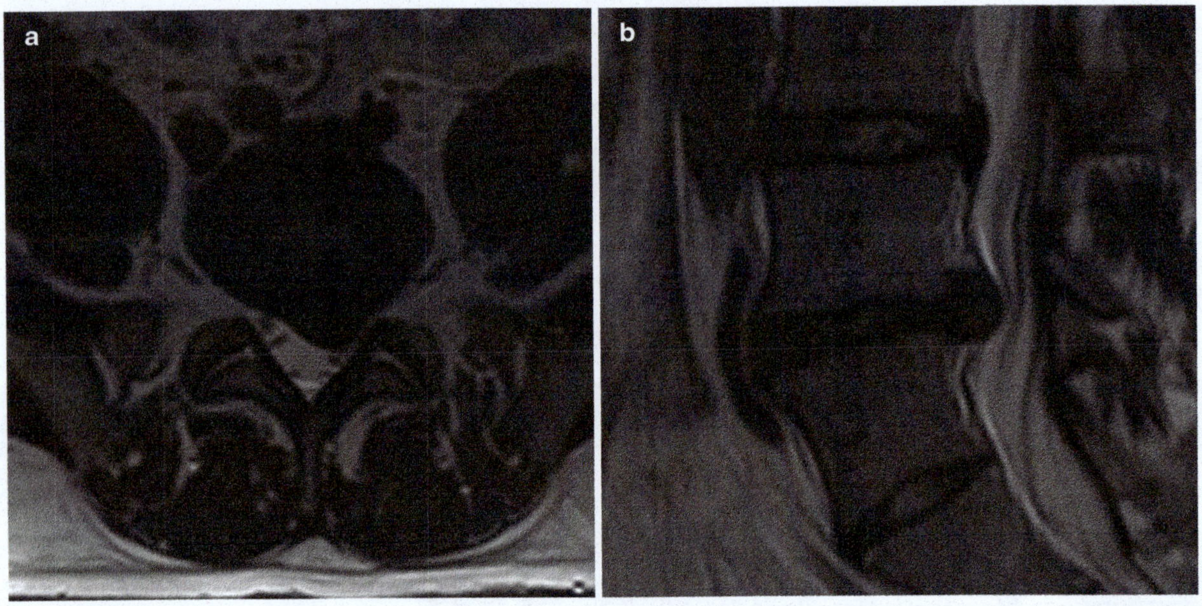

Fig. 93.5 (a) (axial) and (b) (sagittal) T2-weighted MRI of the left L5/S1 paracentral extrusion. This extrusion is severely narrowing the lateral recess and displacing the S1 nerve root

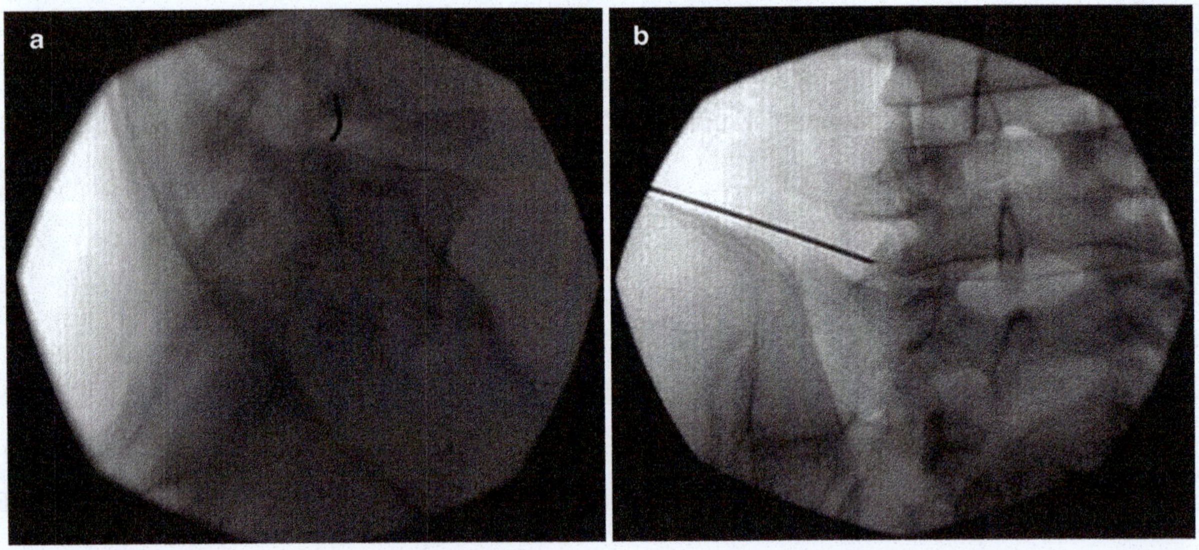

Fig. 93.6 (a, b) A needle is positioned at the S1 superior articular facet to engaging the annulus or disc (for discogram to help guide the discectomy). A flexible guidewire with sequential dilators may be inserted using the Seldinger technique

was associated with greater patient satisfaction, less intraoperative blood loss, and shorter hospital stays. Obtaining adequate decompression, regardless of discectomy method, appears to be the critical factor in determining procedure success.

Pearls and Pitfalls

- Discectomy may utilize either conscious sedation or general anesthesia. With general anesthesia, continuous neuromonitoring is recommended to avoid neural injury.
- For awake patients in the lateral decubitus position, the straight leg raise test may be used intraoperatively to determine whether decompression is sufficient.
- Patient habitus and instrument compatibility should be considered, particularly for the transforaminal "outside-in" approach. Larger or obese patients will require longer instrumentation.
- Transforaminal endoscopic discectomy targeting the L5/S1 disc level may be contraindicated if the patient's iliac crest obstructs access.
- Disc extrusions tend to require a steeper approach (cephalocaudad or caudocephalad).

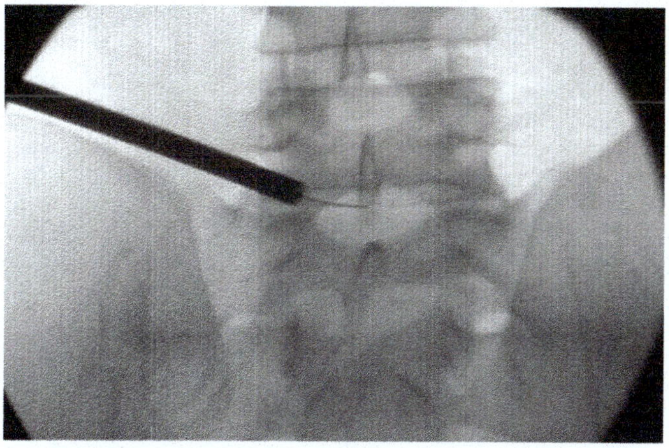

Fig. 93.7 If necessary, foraminotomy using sequential bone reamers can be done under fluoroscopic guidance. In order to avoid the exiting or transiting nerves, it is critical to keep instruments in the posterior of the foramen along the facet. Reaming should be limited to the medial pedicular line. During this process attention should be paid to patient-reported neurological signs or neuromonitoring

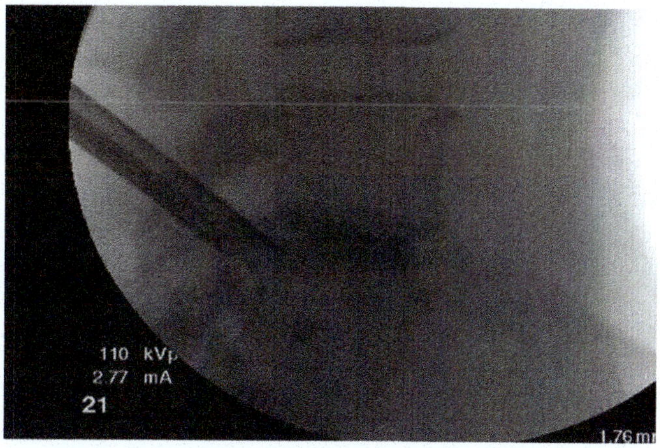

Fig. 93.9 A steeper cephalocaudad approach used to reach a migrated extrusion in a different patient. The working tube and articulating instrument are controlled via joystick manipulation

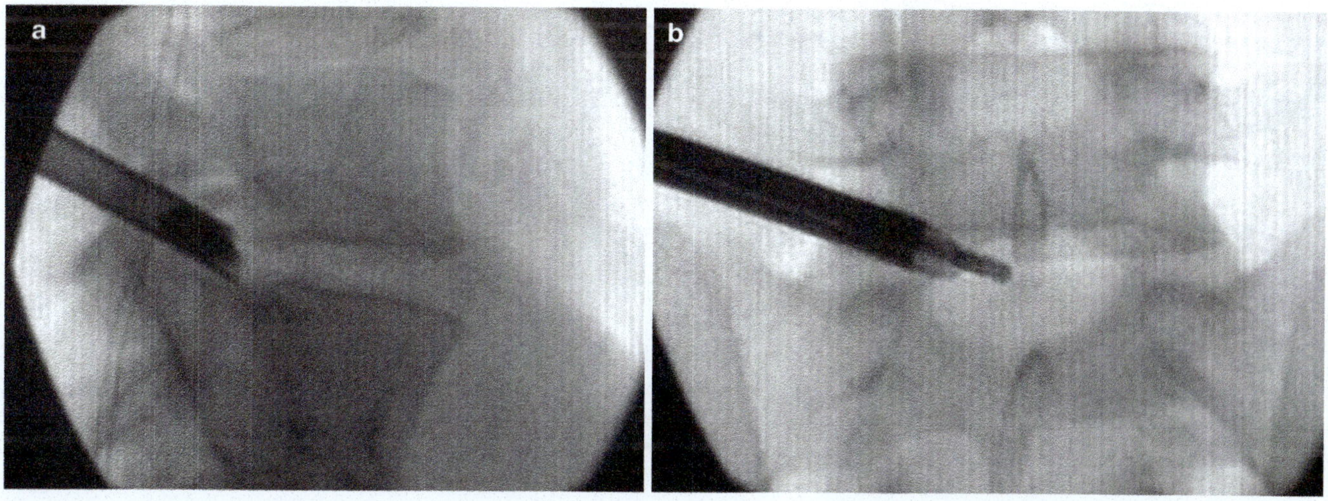

Fig. 93.8 (**a**, **b**) The beveled working tube is inserted over the largest dilator. The dilator pictured here has an outer diameter of 8 mm. Lateral fluoroscopy should be used to confirm placement posterior to the disc. AP fluoroscopy should be used to confirm placement relative to disc herniation on pre-surgical MRI/CT imaging

- A more lateral approach from midline should be taken for central disc herniations compared with paracentral or lateral herniations.
- Fluoroscopy can be used to identify the triangular working zone (or Kambin's triangle), the posterolateral annular surface near the spinal canal.
- Techniques for identifying the surgical site include (1) using a Steinman pin or long needle on the skin over the target disc under AP/lateral fluoroscopy to draw index lines or (2) in-line tunnel or gun-barrel view, involving lateral fluoroscopy with the angle reduced until the targeted superior articular process is lined up with the location of the posterior disc herniation based on pre-surgical MRI or CT imaging.

Recommended Readings

1. Cong L, Zhu Y, Tu G. A meta-analysis of endoscopic discectomy versus open discectomy for symptomatic lumbar disk herniation. Eur Spine J. 2016;25:134–43.
2. Dasenbrock HH, Juraschek SP, Schultz LR, et al. The efficacy of minimally invasive discectomy compared with open discectomy: a meta-analysis of prospective randomized controlled trials. J Neurosurg Spine. 2012;16:452–62.
3. Jasper GP, Francisco GM, Telfeian A. Outpatient, awake, ultra-minimally invasive endoscopic treatment of lumbar disc herniations. R I Med J. 2014;97:47–9.
4. Mayer HM, Brock M. Percutaneous endoscopic discectomy: surgical technique and preliminary results compared to microsurgical discectomy. J Neurosurg. 1993;78:216–25.
5. Truumees E. A history of lumbar disc herniation from Hippocrates to the 1990s. Clin Orthop Relat Res. 2015;473:1885–95.
6. Yong A, Lee SH, Park WM, Lee HY, Shin SW, Kang HY. Percutaneous endoscopic lumbar discectomy for recurrent disc herniation: surgical technique, outcome, and prognostic factors of 43 consecutive cases. Spine. 2004;29:E326–32.

94 Vertebral Augmentation for Painful Vertebral Compression Fractures

Tory L. McJunkin, Paul J. Lynch, and Edward L. Swing

Introduction

As people age, conditions of low bone density become increasingly common. More than 10 million Americans suffer from osteoporosis. This is particularly common among women, who represent 80% of these cases. Another 30 million Americans have osteopenia, a less severe condition of decreased bone density. Decreased bone density can lead to serious health problems, including vertebral compression fractures. In 85% of detected vertebral compression fractures (VCFs), patients experience moderate to severe pain – though this finding is more difficult to interpret because non-painful vertebral fractures often go undetected. This typically lasts 6–9 months but can last much longer. VCFs can lead to permanent reductions in height. Additionally, the pain often leads to restrictions in daily activities, which cause further decreases in bone density and numerous other health problems. Painful vertebral fractures can be treated with the injection of medical cement into the fractured vertebral body, a type of procedure known as vertebral augmentation.

Background and Historical Perspective

Osteoporotic vertebral compression fractures are the most common type of VCF, affecting 25% of postmenopausal women. The prevalence rises to 40% of women age 80 and older. An estimated 4 percent of patients presenting to primary care practices with low back pain are suffering from a VCF. Typically, osteoporosis leads to porous bones that are more prone to breaking. Among osteoporotic patients, a vertebral fracture often results from minor movements during regular daily activities, such as stepping out of a vehicle, sneezing, or lifting light objects. Though it is less common, in some cases non-osteoporotic patients may suffer a fracture after a more severe trauma, such as a motor vehicle accident, sports injury, or another type of hard fall. VCFs can also be caused by metastatic cancer, which can affect the spine and cause the vertebral body to fracture. Regardless of the cause, once a vertebral fracture has occurred, the patient often begins to experience back pain. This pain typically lasts 6–9 months, though in some cases it can last much longer.

In addition to the pain caused by VCFs, they can lead to a downward trend in activity level and overall health known as the vertebral compression fracture spiral. Pain leads many patients to reduce their ambulation, reducing their exercise tolerance and in turn leading to a reduction in bone density. This often results in further vertebral compression fractures, as well as other health problems including rib crowding, decreased lung capacity, and pulmonary function. It can lead to pneumonia, deep vein thrombosis, and even death. A study found that the mortality rate among Medicare patients with VCFs is approximately twice that of matched controls.

The first vertebral augmentation procedure was performed by Deramond and Galibert in France in 1984 for a patient with a painful hemangioma of the cervical spine. Initially this procedure was performed only for pain related to metastatic cancer, but this was soon expanded to osteoporotic vertebral compression fractures – a more common cause of VCFs. The procedure was first performed in the USA in the early 1990s using the technique pioneered by Deramond. The frequency of vertebral augmentation in the USA increased into the early 2000s, but between 2004 and 2014, the rate of vertebral augmentation procedures decreased 32% among Medicare patients.

Uses and Indications

Indications for vertebral augmentation include VCFs resulting from osteoporosis, metastatic cancer, or trauma, with osteoporotic VCFs being the most common of these indications. There are two widely used types of vertebral augmentation procedures: vertebroplasty and kyphoplasty.

T. L. McJunkin · P. J. Lynch · E. L. Swing (✉)
Arizona Pain Specialists, Scottsdale, AZ, USA
e-mail: DrMcJunkin@PainDoctor.com; DrLynch@PainDoctor.com; TedS@PainDoctor.com

T. R. Deer et al. (eds.), *Deer's Treatment of Pain*, https://doi.org/10.1007/978-3-030-12281-2_94

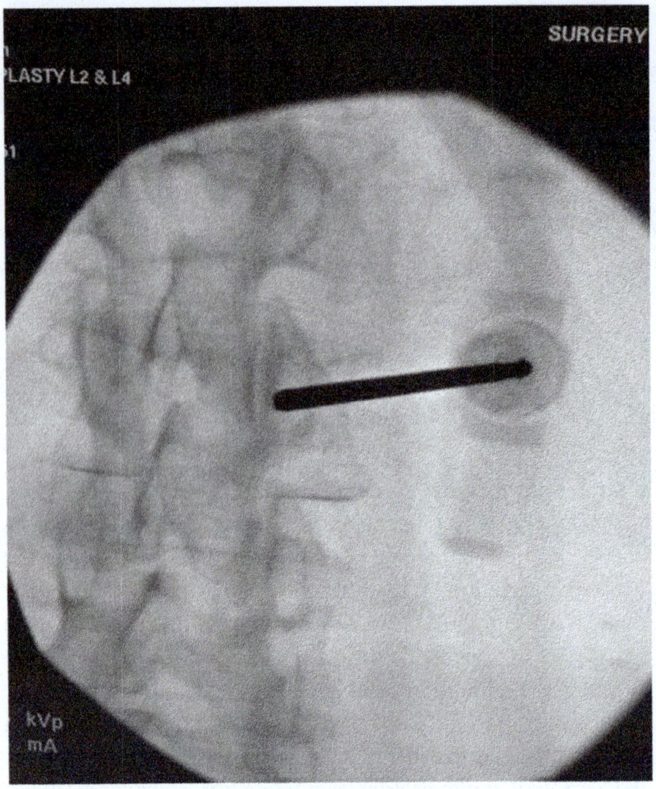

Fig. 94.1 The tip of the needle should be aligned with the lateral and superior aspect of the pedicle of the target vertebra. A lateral image can confirm that the tip of the needle is placed on the posterior wall of the pedicle and verify the trajectory of the needle. (Courtesy of Wayne Olan, MD)

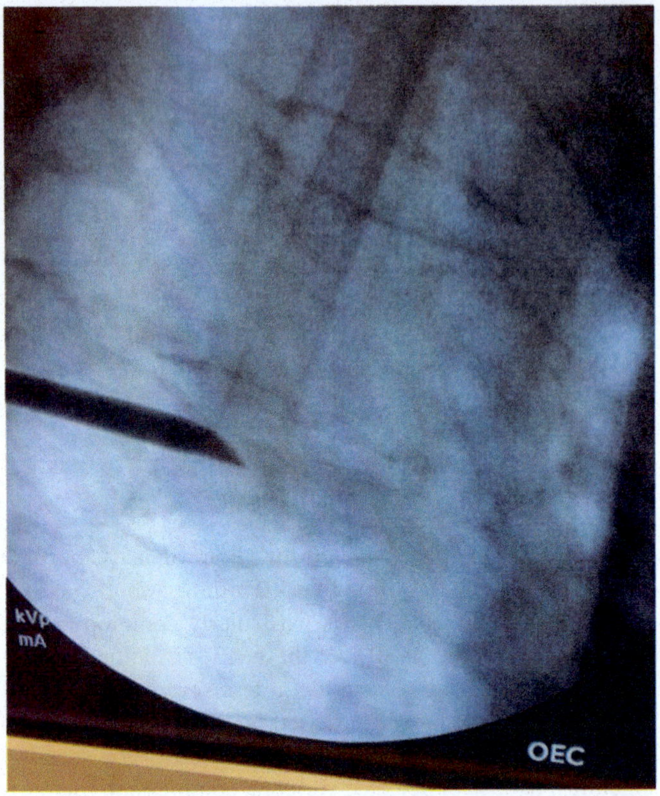

Fig. 94.2 When the needle tip reaches the medial border of the pedicle, verify on lateral view that it has entered the vertebral body. The needle should then be advanced approximately 4 mm past the posterior cortical wall. (Courtesy of Wayne Olan, MD)

Vertebroplasty involves the percutaneous insertion of a needle into the fractured vertebral body (see Fig. 94.1). Medical cement is then injected into the vertebra and the needle removed. The cement quickly hardens and most patients (80–90%) experience pain relief immediately.

Kyphoplasty involves the insertion of a needle into the fractured vertebral body (see Fig. 94.2). A small balloon is inflated from the end of this needle, creating a pocket of space within the vertebra (Figs. 94.3 and 94.4). The balloon is then deflated and removed (Figs. 94.5, 94.6 and 94.7), and medical cement is injected into the pocket of space (Fig. 94.8). The additional step of inflating the balloon within the fractures vertebra has the potential advantage of restoring the height lost from the fractured vertebra.

Evidence for Efficacy

Dozens of studies have examined the efficacy of vertebroplasty and kyphoplasty. The vast majority of studies, particularly older studies, were nonrandomized. Though these studies showed a high level of relief after treatment (87% for vertebroplasty, 92% for kyphoplasty), the scarcity of randomized controlled trials (RCTs) prior to the last 10 years led to debate about the efficacy of vertebral augmentation procedures. Two RCTs, both published in 2009, did not detect a beneficial effect for vertebral augmentation (one of vertebroplasty, one of kyphoplasty). This led some to conclude that vertebral augmentation patients did not perform better than control patients.

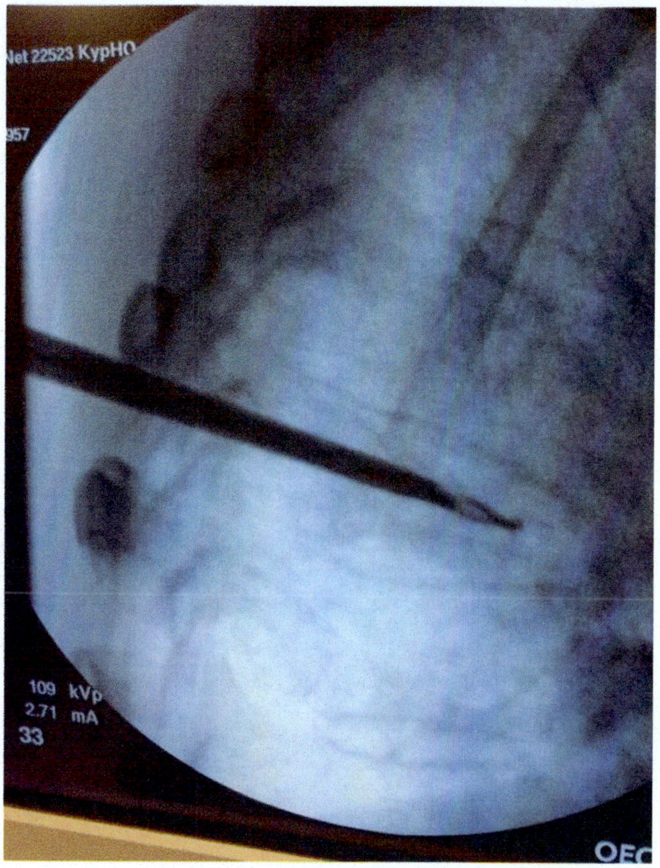

Fig. 94.3 Channel(s) for the balloon(s) should be created by drilling. (Courtesy of Wayne Olan, MD)

In the past several years, however, numerous additional randomized controlled trials have been published allowing for meta-analytic reviews to provide a more definitive assessment of the efficacy of vertebral augmentation. For example, a recent meta-analysis combined the results of 2046 patients from 16 RCTs. Compared with patients

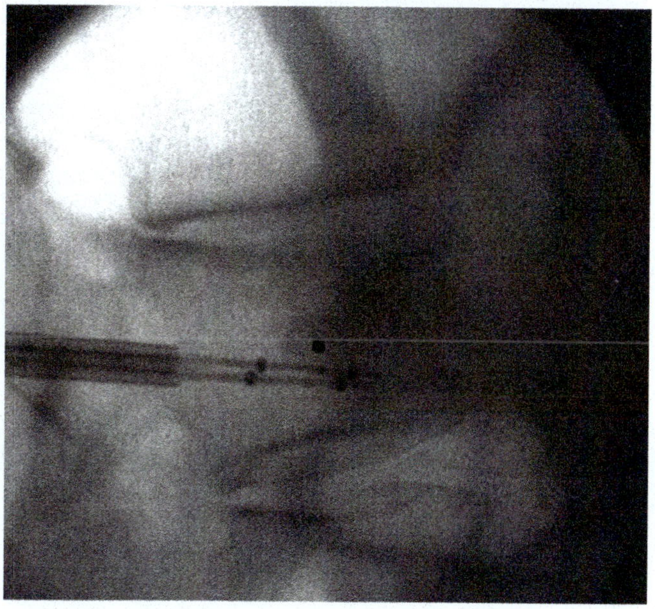

Fig. 94.4 The balloon(s) should be inserted through the needle. (Courtesy of Wayne Olan, MD)

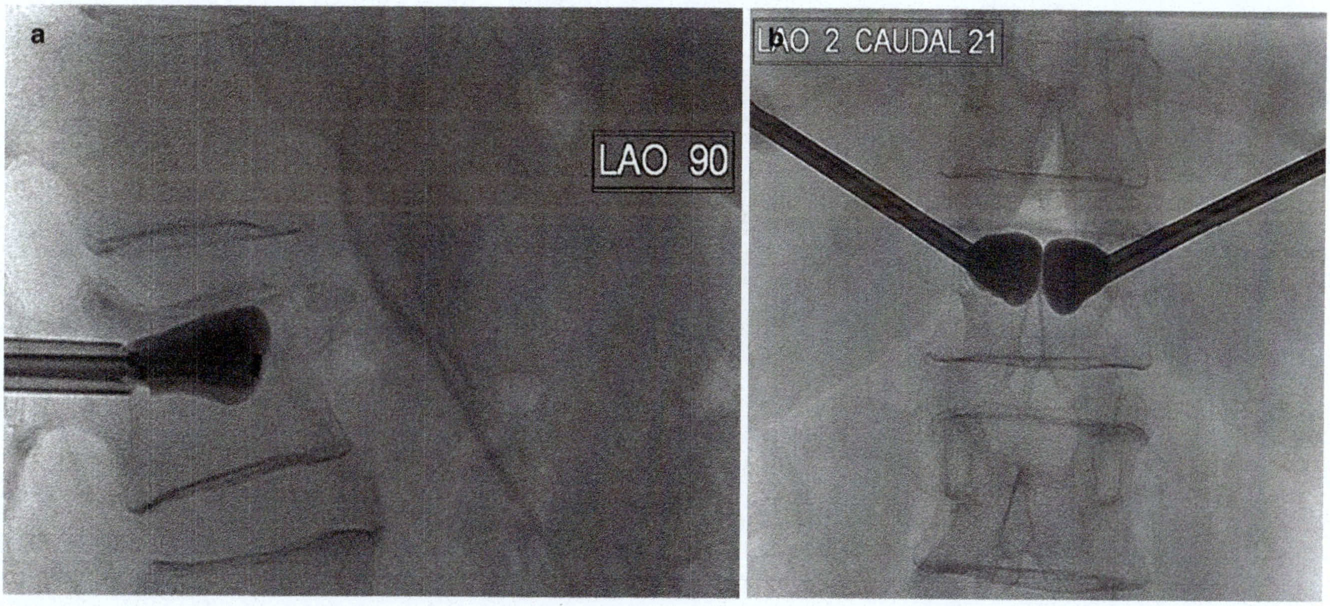

Fig. 94.5 (**a**, **b**) The balloon(s) should be inflated. (Courtesy of Wayne Olan, MD)

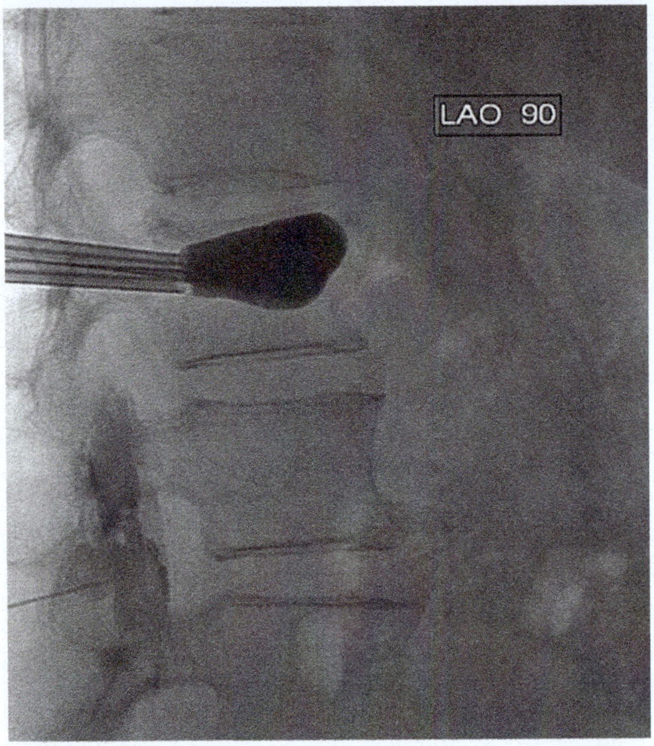

Fig. 94.6 Balloon(s) should be inflated until they reach their maximum safe distension. (Courtesy of Wayne Olan, MD)

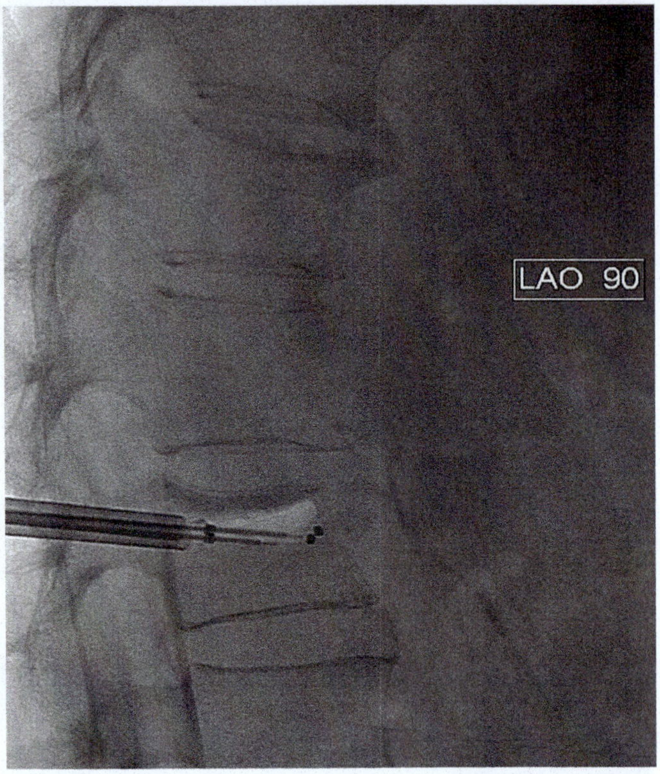

Fig. 94.7 Balloon(s) should be deflated and removed. (Courtesy of Wayne Olan, MD)

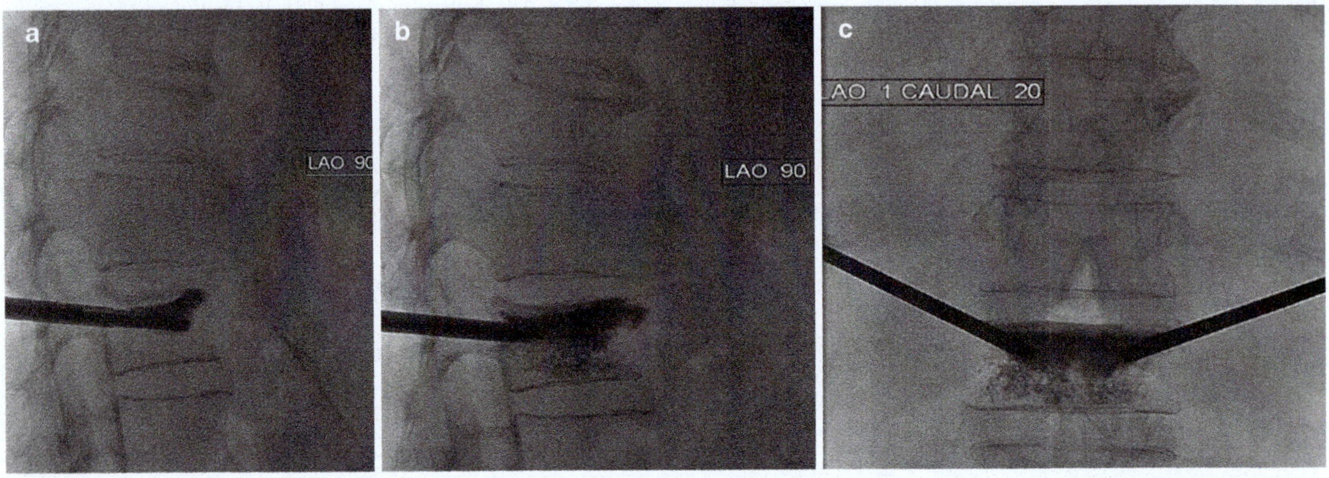

Fig. 94.8 (**a–c**) Cement is injected into the cavity produced by the balloon(s). The volume of cement will tend to vary by vertebral level, with smaller volumes in the high thoracic spine and larger volumes in the lower lumbar spine. Volumes typically range from 1 to 4 cc. (Courtesy of Wayne Olan, MD)

receiving conservative care, those undergoing vertebroplasty showed improved pain relief, daily function, and quality of life. Kyphoplasty had similar results to vertebroplasty. Compared to vertebroplasty, patients undergoing kyphoplasty showed slightly weaker evidence of pain relief but greater evidence of reduced chance of fracture and improved daily functioning and quality of life. A separate meta-analysis has also revealed that kyphoplasty results in a lower incidence of cement extravasation compared with vertebroplasty.

Pearls and Pitfalls

- Painful acute and subacute fractures seem to be the most responsive to vertebral augmentation.
- Aseptic sterile technique should be followed to prevent infection as this is an implant.
- Quality imaging is a must as precise trocar placement and angles are a necessity to prevent neurological compromise.
- Preoperative review and understanding of imaging and pathology is imperative.
- Trocar gauge sizes should be chosen based on the patient's anatomy and specifically the pedicle diameter.
- Most importantly, the trocar should not breach the medial border of the pedicle until it has entered the posterior vertebral body as per lateral image (this prevents intraspinal trocar placement).
- PMMA (bone cement) or biologic (Cortoss) should be injected slowly with frequent AP and lateral views compared to saved preinjection images to prevent extra-vertebral spread.

Recommended Reading

1. Galibert P, Deramond H, Rosat P, Le Gars D. Preliminary note on the treatment of vertebral angioma by percutaneous acrylic vertebroplasty. Neuro-Chirurgie. 1987;33:166–8.
2. Garfin SR, Yuan HA, Reiley MA. New technologies in spine: Kyphoplasty and vertebroplasty for the treatment of painful osteoporotic compression fractures. Spine. 2001;26:1511–5.
3. Hulme PA, Krebs J, Ferguson SJ, Berlemann U. Vertebroplasty and kyphoplasty: a systematic review of 69 clinical studies. Spine. 2006;31:1983–2001.
4. Zhang Y, Shi L, Tang P, Zhang L. Comparison of the efficacy between two micro-operative therapies of old patients with osteoporotic vertebral compression fracture: a network meta-analysis. J Cell Biochem. 2017;118:3205–12.
5. Zhao S, Xu CY, Zhu AR, Ye L, Lv LL, Chen L, Huang Q, Niu F. Comparison of the efficacy and safety of 3 treatments for patients with osteoporotic vertebral compression fractures. Medicine. 2017;96(26):e7328.

Vertebroplasty and Other Methods of Vertebral Augmentation

95

Julian Maingard, Nicole S. Carter, Hamed Asadi, Lee-Anne Slater, Thabele Leslie-Mazwi, Joshua A. Hirsch, and Ronil V. Chandra

Introduction

One in two women and one in five men over the age of 50 years will suffer a fracture due to osteoporosis. Vertebral compression fractures (VCFs) are the most common type of osteoporotic fracture, with 1.4 million new VCFs occurring worldwide every year. Some of these fractures are asymptomatic or result in tolerable symptoms, with only one-third of patients with a new fracture seeking medical attention. Acute back pain symptoms for most mildly symptomatic VCFs will generally subside over 6–8 weeks as the fracture heals. Patients with severe pain resulting in significant disability are a subset of patients with osteoporosis who may benefit from vertebroplasty.

Vertebroplasty is a minimally invasive, image-guided procedure that involves the injection of cement into the VCF (Fig. 95.1). The primary goal is reduction of back pain and disability. Vertebroplasty is also used for pathological fractures, particularly those caused by multiple myeloma or spinal metastasis. The spine is affected by osteolytic or osteopenic bone disease in 70% of those with multiple myeloma, with 30% of patients sustaining a VCF during the disease. Similarly, osteolytic metastases weaken bone integrity, leading to elevated VCF risk. Around one in eight patients who die of cancer has symptomatic spinal lesions during their illness. Vertebroplasty is used for pain relief for cancer patients with symptomatic pathological VCFs refractory to medical therapy. More recently, there is interest in combining vertebroplasty with adjunct procedures such as radiofrequency ablation and cryoablation to provide local tumor control.

This chapter will outline the background, uses and indications, evidence for efficacy and safety, and clinical pearls of the vertebroplasty procedure. Kyphoplasty and other methods of vertebral augmentation are reviewed in Chap. 99.

Background and Historical Perspective

Conservative Medical Therapy for Vertebral Compression Fractures

The key goals of conservative medical therapies are pain relief and improvement of mobility and function. For most

J. Maingard
Interventional Neuroradiology Service – Department of Radiology, Austin Hospital, Melbourne, Australia

School of Medicine – Faculty of Health, Deakin University, Waurn Ponds, Australia
e-mail: julian.maingard@austin.org.au

N. S. Carter
Faculty of Medicine, Nursing and Health Sciences, Monash University, Melbourne, Australia
e-mail: nscar6@student.monash.edu

H. Asadi
Interventional Neuroradiology Service – Department of Radiology, Austin Hospital, Melbourne, Australia

School of Medicine – Faculty of Health, Deakin University, Waurn Ponds, Australia

Interventional Neuroradiology Unit, Monash Imaging, Monash Health, Melbourne, Australia

L.-A. Slater · R. V. Chandra (✉)
Faculty of Medicine, Nursing and Health Sciences, Monash University, Melbourne, Australia

Interventional Neuroradiology Unit, Monash Imaging, Monash Health, Melbourne, Australia
e-mail: LeeAnne.Slater@monashhealth.org; ronil.chandra@monash.edu

T. Leslie-Mazwi · J. A. Hirsch
Neuroendovascular Program, Massachusetts General Hospital, Boston, MA, USA

Harvard Medical School, Boston, MA, USA
e-mail: tleslie-mazwi@mgh.harvard.edu; JAHIRSCH@mgh.harvard.edu

T. R. Deer et al. (eds.), *Deer's Treatment of Pain*, https://doi.org/10.1007/978-3-030-12281-2_95

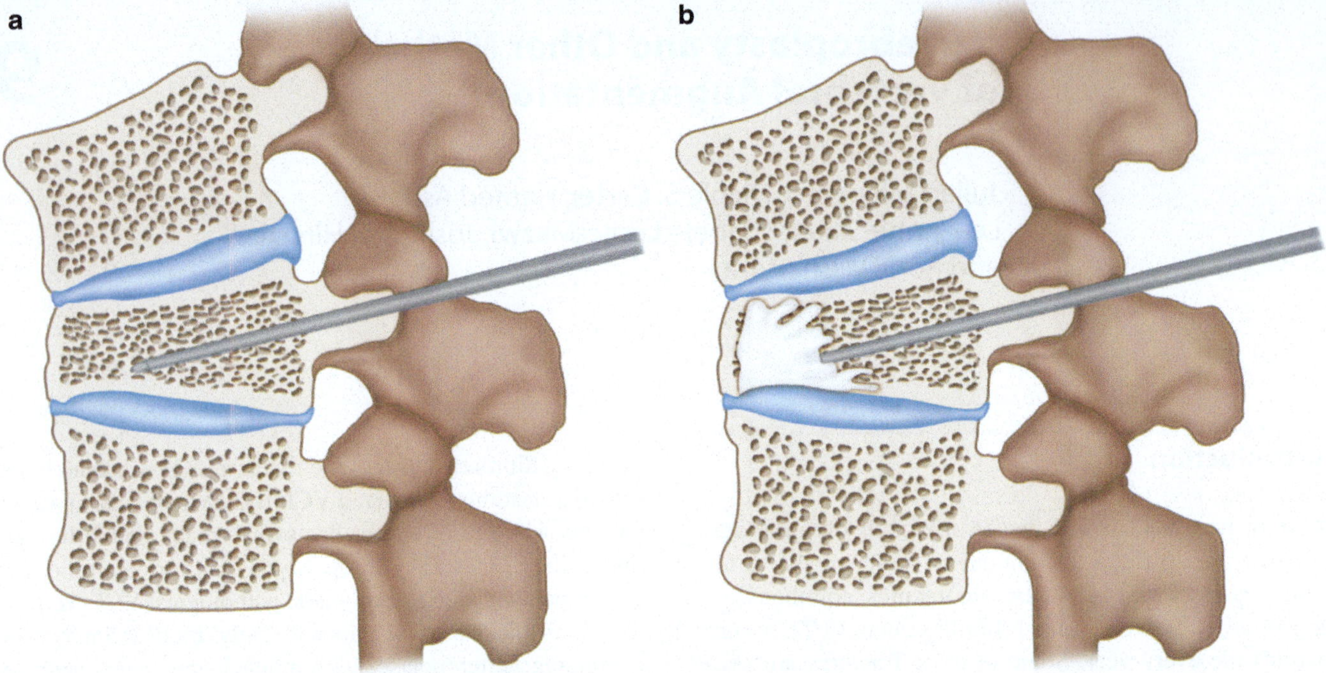

Fig. 95.1 The vertebroplasty procedure. (a) The initial steps of the vertebroplasty procedure involve the percutaneous insertion of a needle into the fractured vertebral body. (b) Cement is subsequently injected into the fractured vertebra

VCFs, medical management with combinations of analgesics, bed rest, orthosis, and physical therapy is the mainstay of treatment. For those with milder pain and no limitation of function, these measures may be sufficient. However, conservative treatment of those with more severe pain is not benign. In this cohort, medical management often involves a prolonged period of bed rest, which may result in loss of bone mass and muscle strength. Bone loss occurs at an estimated rate of 2% per week, while loss of muscle mass occurs at a rate of 10–15% per week. Furthermore, immobilization leads to an elevated risk of venous thromboembolic disease and decubitus ulceration. The addition of narcotic analgesia, and its associated side effects of sedation, confusion, addiction, and constipation, further complicates management and prolongs recovery. These ill effects are most pronounced in elderly patients.

Historical Perspective

Vertebroplasty was first described in literature in 1987 by Galibert et al., for the treatment of a vertebral hemangioma. Following this, vertebroplasty was introduced to the United States in 1993 by Dion and colleagues. In 1997, they published their treatment results from 29 patients with 47 painful osteoporotic VCFs. Almost all (90%) patients reported improvement of both pain and mobility within 24 hours. Since these early experiences, larger observational series, prospective open-label randomized controlled trials, and double-blind multicenter randomized controlled trials have followed further examining the efficacy and safety of vertebroplasty.

Use and Indications

The decision to proceed with vertebroplasty should be based on a thorough pre-procedural workup, involving history, examination, imaging, and appropriate laboratory investigations. Evaluation of potential candidates should identify those most likely to benefit and assess for contraindications.

Indications

- Acute (<6 weeks) symptomatic VCFs causing severe pain.
- Symptomatic osteoporotic VCFs not responsive to medical therapy.
- Symptomatic VCFs due to spinal neoplasia, not responsive to medical therapy.
- Failure of medical therapy is variably defined but may be considered when pain persists at a level that severely compromises mobility and function despite analgesic therapy or when undesirable side effects (e.g., sedation, confusion, or constipation) occur due to analgesic medications.

Absolute Contraindications

- Systemic sepsis or spinal infection
- Known allergy to polymethylmethacrylate (PMMA) bone cement
- Uncorrectable coagulopathy
- Myelopathy from fracture retropulsion or epidural tumor extension
- Inability to tolerate procedural sedation or anesthesia due to cardiopulmonary risk

Relative Contraindications (Best Performed by Experienced Operators)

- Vertebroplasty above T5 level
- More than 75% vertebral height loss or vertebra plana
- Disruption to the posterior vertebral body cortex
- Marked tumor destruction of vertebral body walls
- Epidural tumor extension into the central spinal canal or neural exit foramina

History and Examination

- The classic symptom of a VCF is deep midline pain. In osteoporotic or pathological bone, this may occur with minimal or no trauma.
- The pain is typically exacerbated on weight-bearing and motion (particularly flexion) and at least partially relieved by recumbency.
- Failure of conventional medical therapy should be documented, along with standardized pain and disability scores and current analgesic use. A reasonable trial of conservative management is 2–4 weeks, but it is reasonable to consider earlier treatment for those requiring narcotic analgesia, analgesic infusions, or hospitalization due to severe pain.
- Physical examination generally reveals midline tenderness at the fractured vertebra. Lower extremity neurologic examination should be performed to screen for myelopathy.

Imaging

Imaging of the spine is performed in all cases to identify the fracture level, assess acuity of fracture, and determine contraindications to treatment or potential technical difficulties. Plain frontal and lateral radiographs or computed tomography (CT) scans are often performed as the initial imaging modality but have limited capability for assessing fracture acuity. Magnetic resonance imaging (MRI) is the investigation of choice and is generally obtained if there are no contraindications. On short-tau inversion recovery (STIR) or fat-suppressed fast spin-echo T2 sequences, unhealed fractures show as T2 hyperintense signals consistent with bone marrow edema. MRI may identify other fracture levels that may not be evident on plain radiograph. It also allows for assessment of the posterior cortex, spinal canal, and neural exit foramina and determines the degree of fracture retropulsion and/or epidural tumor extension. CT is a useful adjunct for pre-procedural planning, particularly to evaluate the integrity of the posterior cortex.

In those with contraindications to MRI (such as a pacemaker), nuclear scintigraphic bone scan is the alternative investigation of choice. It allows the identification of unhealed fractures, which will take up injected tracer in higher concentrations than unhealed fractures. This can be particularly helpful when combined with CT-SPECT imaging to obtain three-dimensional imaging (Fig. 95.2).

Laboratory Investigation

Routine pre-procedural laboratory tests should screen for infection, coagulopathy, and major metabolic abnormality. The use of further tests, such as electrocardiography or chest radiography, is dictated by practitioner discretion and patient history.

The Vertebroplasty Procedure

Sedation

In the majority of patients, analgesia is achieved using a combination of moderate conscious sedation (intravenous fentanyl and midazolam) and local anesthesia (e.g., lidocaine). This approach is desirable as it allows feedback from the patient (e.g., worsening pain and changing neurological status) that can alert the operator to potential complications. However, general anesthesia may be required in some cases, particularly in those with high pre-procedure narcotic analgesic requirements. All patients receive continuous monitoring of pulse oximetry, blood pressure, and electrocardiography.

Patient Positioning

Patients are ideally positioned in the prone position for vertebroplasty procedures. In practical terms, an amount of freedom is allowed for patients to place themselves in a prone oblique position should this promote greater comfort during the procedure; this may introduce 10–15 degrees of

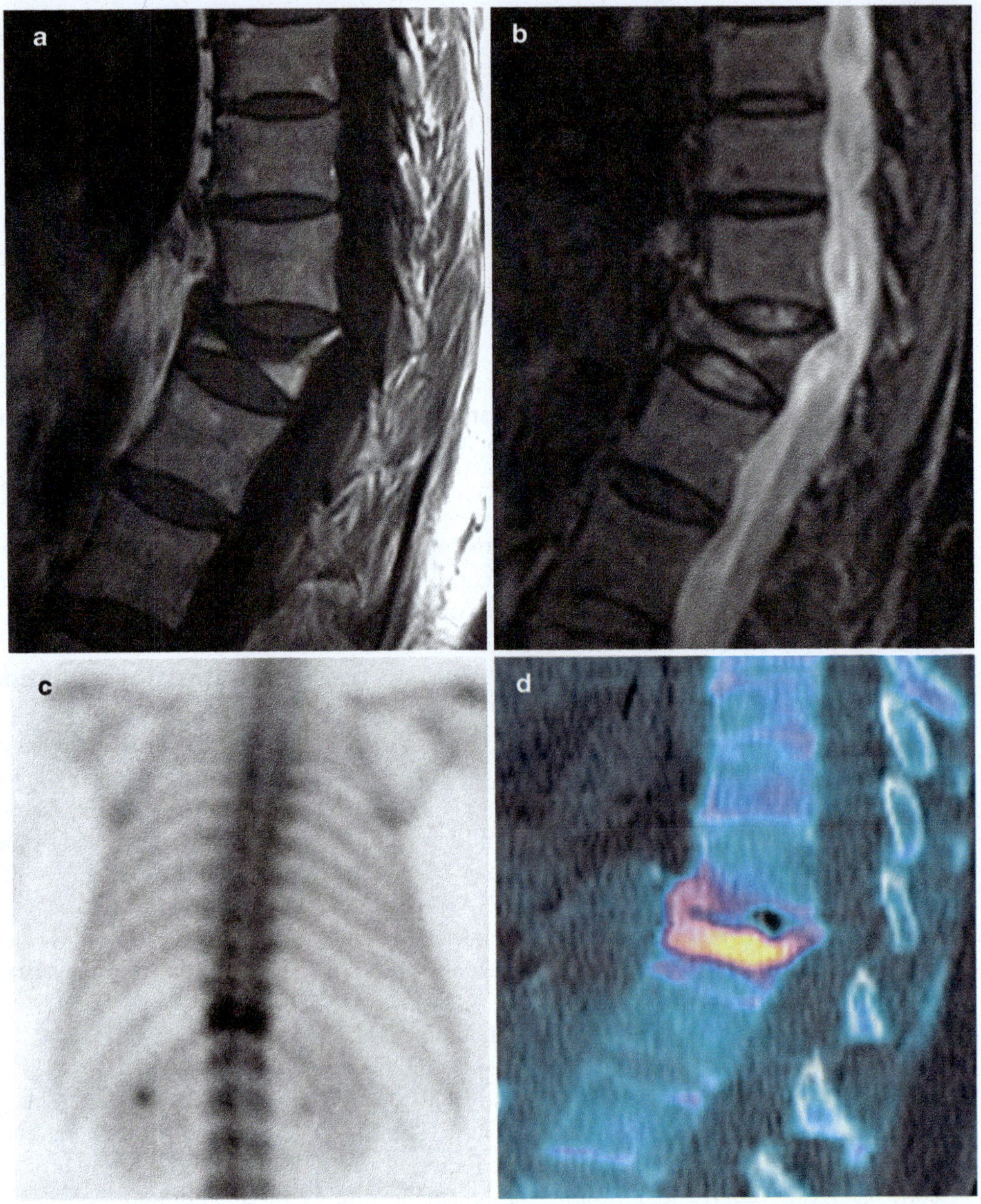

Fig. 95.2 Use of advanced imaging with MRI and bone scan with CT-SPECT to assess the fracture and select patients likely to respond to vertebroplasty. (**a**) Sagittal T1-weighted MRI image. Reduced T1 signal intensity at the T12 vertebral body from marrow edema. (**b**) Short-tau inversion recovery (STIR) MRI image. There is only mildly increased STIR signal intensity in the T12 vertebra. (**c**) Whole body delayed bone scan image. There is increased uptake in the T12 vertebral body. (**d**) Sagittal CT-SPECT image. There is significantly increased uptake that is clearly localized in the fractured vertebral body. The patient had significant pain reduction within 1 week of the vertebroplasty procedure

obliquity. Prone positioning, with proper cushion support under the upper chest and lower abdomen, maximizes extension of the fractured vertebral body, thus promoting reduction of kyphosis. The patient's arms should be placed toward the head, out of the path of the fluoroscope. Analgesia should be considered prior to positioning on the table, as transfer from the bed to the procedure table may be painful. Care should be taken in positioning the elderly and those with advanced osteoporosis, to avoid new fractures of the rib, extremities, or vertebra.

Antibiotic Prophylaxis and Skin Preparation

Infection risk is minimized by following standard guidelines for sterile skin preparation, draping, and operator scrubbing. No randomized controlled data currently support or oppose antibiotic administration, but there are reports of post-procedure spinal infections, and the use of PMMA can make these infections difficult to treat. Antibiotic prophylaxis is thus routinely used. Typical regimens include intravenous cefazolin (2 g) or clindamycin (600–900 mg, if penicillin allergy).

Needle Placement

In vertebroplasty, a needle is inserted through a small skin incision in the back, through the subcutaneous tissues and into the fractured vertebra. The key aspect of needle placement is to maintain the needle trajectory lateral to the medial cortex of the pedicle and superior to the inferior cortex. This prevents entry of the needle into the spinal canal or neural foramen. Ideally, the final needle position should be as close to the midline as possible. The trajectory taken may be transpedicular or parapedicular (Fig. 95.3). The transpedicular approach takes the needle from the posterior surface of the pedicle, through the entire length of the pedicle and into the vertebral body. However, the pedicle configuration may limit the ability to place the needle tip near the midline. A parapedicular approach takes the needle along the lateral surface of the pedicle, penetrating the pedicle along its path or penetrating the vertebral body at its junction with the pedicle. This may permit a more medial placement of the needle tip, which is particularly useful when treating anatomically smaller pedicles, such as in the thoracic spine.

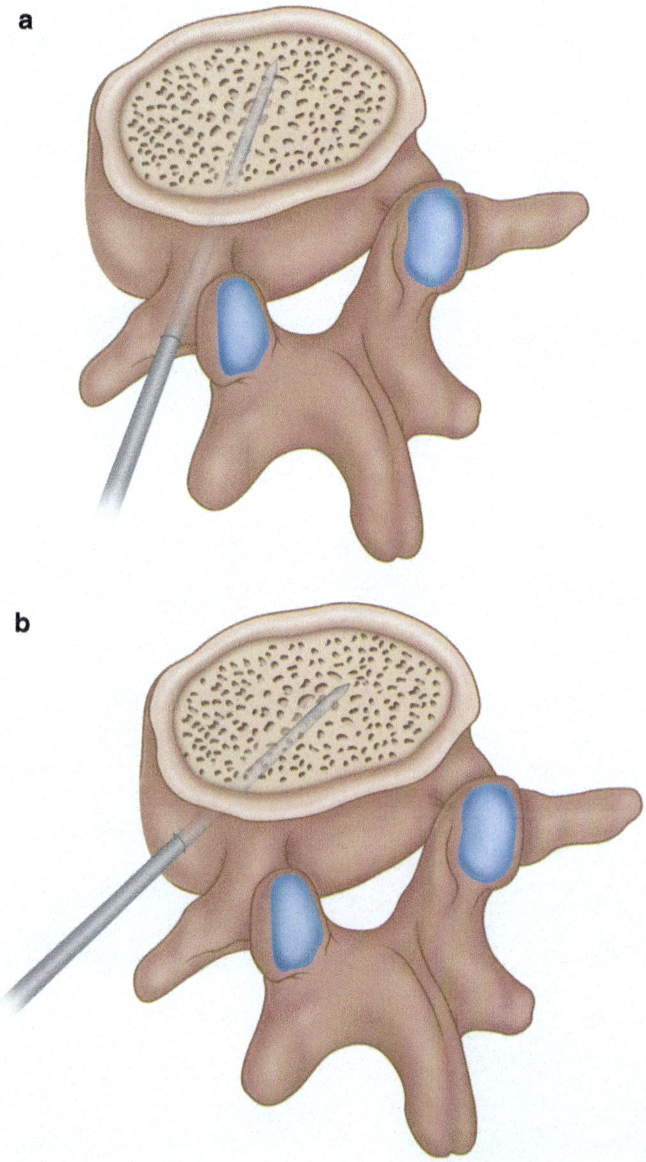

Fig. 95.3 Transpedicular compared to parapedicular approaches. (**a**) The transpedicular approach takes the needle from the posterior surface of the pedicle, through the entire length of the pedicle and into the vertebral body. (**b**) The parapedicular approach takes the needle along the lateral surface of the pedicle, penetrating the pedicle along its path or penetrating the vertebral body at its junction with the pedicle. This may permit a more medial placement of the needle tip, particularly when treating anatomically smaller pedicles

Vertebroplasty

- The trocar trajectory is planned. For a transpedicular approach, its entry position should be at the 3 o'clock position of the right pedicle or the 9 o'clock position of the left pedicle. For a parapedicular approach, an entry position just lateral to the 3 or 9 o'clock position of the pedicular cortex is optimal. 15 degrees of obliquity during planning may help facilitate unilateral trocar trajectories to achieve midline position (Fig. 95.4).
- The skin and periosteum are anesthetized with lidocaine or bupivacaine.
- A small vertical incision is made to the skin, and an 11- or 13-gauge diamond-tip stylet, sheathed in a cannula, is placed.
- In the bone, the needle is advanced by carefully tapping the handle of the needle with an orthopedic hammer.
- The needle must remain lateral to the medial cortex of the pedicle until it has traversed the entire pedicle. After this point, the diamond-tip needle may be replaced with a bevel-tip for improved maneuverability. The needle is then advanced further, to the anterior one-third of the vertebral body.
- The needle stylet is removed and the injecting system connected.
- The PMMA cement is prepared. Working time varies from 10 to 20 minutes, depending on temperature and the specific formulation. PMMA is slowly injected under continuous biplane fluoroscopic guidance. The optimal volume of cement remains a matter of debate. Ideally, cement will extend across midline from one pedicle to the opposite pedicle by the end of injection (Fig. 95.5).

Adjunct Procedures

For neoplasm-related fractures, vertebroplasty may be combined with the adjunct procedures of radiofrequency ablation (RFA) or cryoablation. In RFA, a high-frequency current is applied through an insulated needle prior to the injection of cement. The thermal energy produced at the tip of the needle may ablate pain-sensitive fibers and thus reduce transmission of pain signals from the periosteum. In addition, this may also provide local tumor control. Cryoablation is a similar procedure that applies extreme cold rather than current. Liquid nitrogen or high-pressure argon gas is administered through an applicator known as a cryoprobe, producing intense cold that may disrupt pain-sensitive fibers and ablate neoplastic tissue. Some of these ablative techniques are off-label and performed at operator discretion.

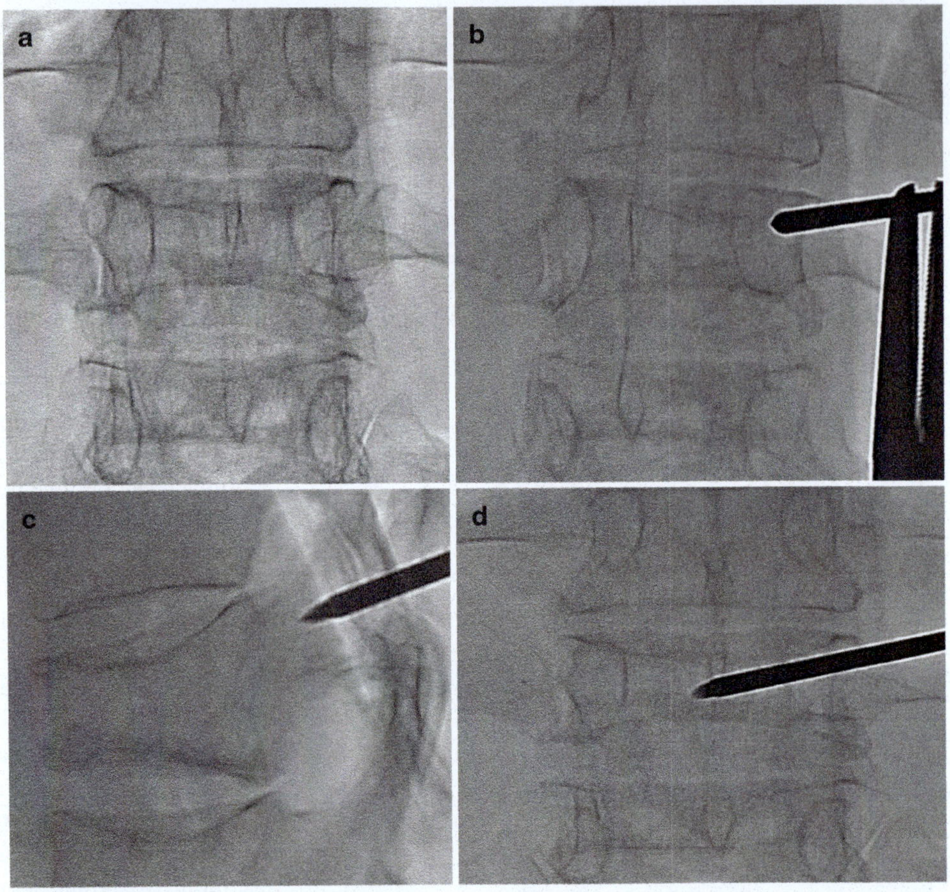

Fig. 95.4 Needle trajectory for unilateral approach. (**a**) Anteroposterior (AP) fluoroscopic image. The image intensifier is rotated to the AP position by aligning the spinous process midway between the pedicles (vertical dotted line), and adjustments are made in the craniocaudal angulation until the pedicles and anterior vertebral body endplates are within the midportion of the vertebral body (horizontal dotted lines). (**b**). AP fluoroscopic image. The image intensifier has been rotated 15 degrees oblique, and the needle tip has been placed approximately at the 3 o'clock position for pedicle entry. (**c**) Lateral fluoroscopic image. The entire needle trajectory is extrapolated during the initial planning and needle entry to optimize final needle position (solid line). (**d**) Midline needle position achieved via unilateral transpedicular approach

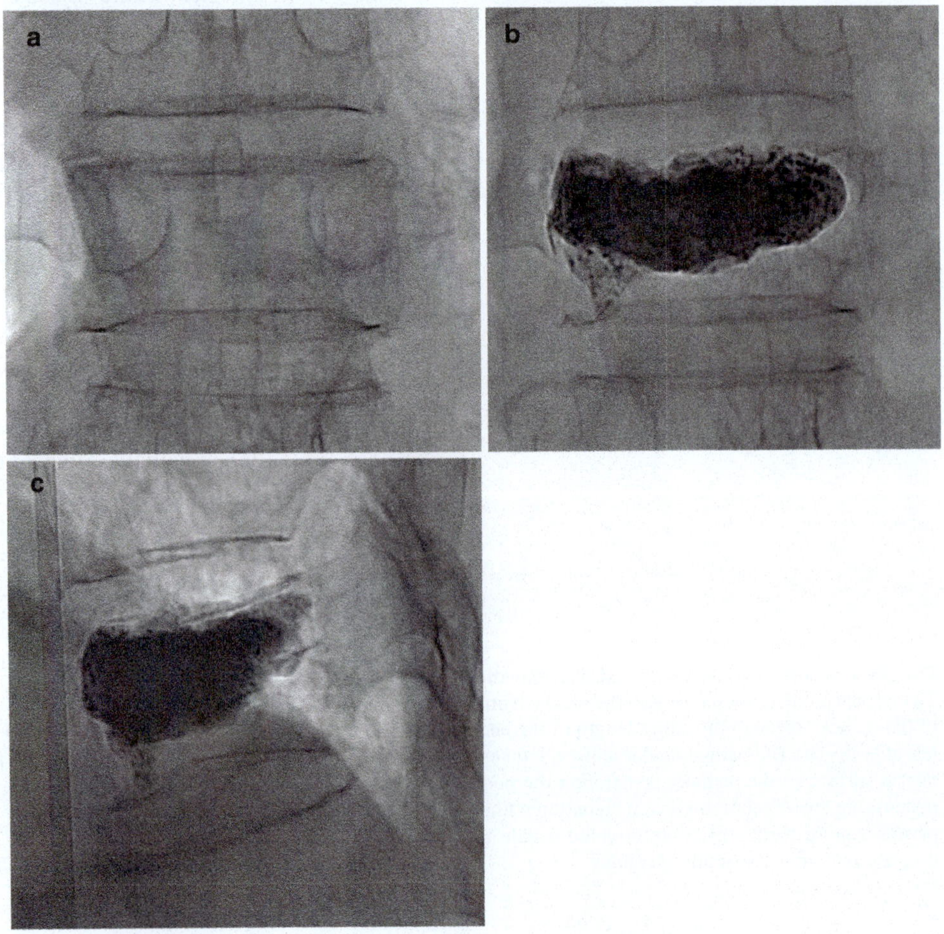

Fig. 95.5 Cement fill within the vertebral fracture. (**a**) Anteroposterior (AP) fluoroscopic image of the fractured vertebral body prior to vertebroplasty. (**b**). AP fluoroscopic image after unipedicular vertebroplasty. Note the cement has been deposited in the vertebral body across the midline. (**c**) Lateral fluoroscopic image. There is no cement extending into the spinal canal or pedicles

Post-procedure Care

Immediately following the procedure, manual compression is applied over needle access sides to prevent hematoma formation. The patient should remain supine and flat in bed for 2 hours post-procedure, followed by a further hour with the head of the best inclined at 30 degrees. Most patients may be discharged later in the same day, though more fragile patients may require an overnight stay for observation. Procedure-related pain is typically treated with nonsteroidal anti-inflammatory medications, or occasionally muscle relaxants or short-term narcotics, and generally resolves over a period of 24–72 hours.

Post-procedure review of the patient's progress should occur a few weeks after the procedure, to assess pain and mobility levels. The patient should be counseled to report any acute increase in back pain, or new back pain, as this may indicate a new fracture. Imaging should be performed, although it is important to note that normal MRI findings following vertebroplasty include persistent bone marrow edema at the treated level which may persist for many months post-procedure.

Evidence for Efficacy

The predominant mechanism for vertebroplasty reducing pain is thought to relate to reduced motion at the fracture site by PMMA interdigitating through the fracture and trabecular bone. There also is a direct thermal effect on the intraosseous nerves. To date, evidence for the efficacy of vertebroplasty in VCFs remains mixed. Initial enthusiasm was driven by positive results from meta-analyses and observational data. However, this was dampened by the 2009 publication of two highly publicized randomized controlled trials (RCTs) in the *New England Journal of Medicine (NEJM)* that found no improved pain outcomes from vertebroplasty. Since that time, several large prospective trials have focused on more stringent patient selection and provided further high-quality evidence. Discussion of the NEJM and subsequent randomized controlled trials are summarized below and in Table 95.1.

NEJM Trials

In 2009, two large double-blinded RCTs comparing vertebroplasty to a sham procedure in osteoporotic VCFs were published in the *New England Journal of Medicine (NEJM)*. The INVEST trial (Investigational Vertebroplasty Safety and Efficacy Trial) included patients aged ≥50 years, with moderate-to-severe back pain (≥3/10 on numerical rating scale (NRS)) and fracture age < 1-year duration. Fracture acuity was confirmed by plain radiography, with MRI performed if fracture age was uncertain. A total of 131 patients were randomized to receive vertebroplasty (N = 68) or a sham procedure (N = 63). At 1-month follow-up, there was

Table 95.1 Major prospective randomized trials evaluating the efficacy of vertebroplasty for osteoporotic fractures

	INVEST	Buchbinder et al.	VERTOS II	VAPOUR
Publication year	2009	2009	2010	2016
Total enrolment (n)	131	78	202	120
Comparator	Sham procedure: periosteal lidocaine	Sham procedure: periosteal lidocaine	Medical management	Sham procedure: subcutaneous lidocaine
Age (years) threshold	≥50	None	≥50	≥60
Mean (SD) age (years)	73.8 (9.4)	76.6 (12.1)	75.2 (9.8)	80.5 (7)
Pain score threshold	NRS ≥3/10	None	VAS ≥5/10	NRS ≥7/10
Mean (SD) baseline pain score (0–10 scale)	7.0 (1.9)	7.3 (2.2)	7.8 (1.5)	8.6
Number (percent) with severe pain (0–10 scale)	61 (47%) NRS ≥8	38 (49%) NRS ≥8	NR	120 (100%) NRS ≥7
Fracture age (weeks) threshold	<52	<52	<6	<6
Mean (SD) fracture age (weeks)	22.5 (16.3)	11.7 (11.1)	5.6	2.6
Number (percent) with fractures < 6 weeks	26 (20%)	31 (40%)	202 (100%)	120 (100%)
Advanced imaging (MRI, SPECT) required?	No	Yes	Yes	Yes
Mean (SD) PMMA volume (mL)	NR	2.8 (1.2)	4.1 (1.5)	7.5 (2.8)
Primary endpoint	Mean NRS pain and RDQ at 1 month	Mean NRS pain at 3 months	Mean VAS pain at 1 month	Percent NRS pain <4/10 at 2 weeks
Primary outcome	No difference	No difference	Vertebroplasty superior	Vertebroplasty superior
Notable secondary endpoints	Quality of life (EQ-5D) at 1 month	Disability (RDQ), quality of life, QUALEFFO, EQ-5D)	Disability (RDQ), quality of life (QUALEFFO)	Disability (RDQ), quality of life (QUALEFFO), analgesic use
Secondary outcomes	No difference	No difference	Vertebroplasty superior	Vertebroplasty superior

no difference between groups in back pain NRS ($p = 0.19$) or disability ($p = 0.49$) measured by Roland-Morris Disability Questionnaire (RDQ). Limitations included the inclusion of fractures up to 12 months old (one-third had fractures of >6-month duration), the lack of MRI as an inclusion requirement, and the use of a controlled intervention (periosteal local anesthetic infiltration) rather than a true sham procedure.

An Australian multicenter blinded RCT of vertebroplasty for osteoporotic fracture was also published in the *NEJM* in 2009, by Buchbinder and colleagues. Inclusion criteria were back pain of <1-year duration and fracture confirmed on MRI. A total of 78 patients were given vertebroplasty ($N = 38$) or sham procedure ($N = 40$). No significant differences in pain scores were observed at 1 week, 3 months, or 6 months. There was also no difference between groups in disability and quality of life measures. Key limitations included the lack of a minimum pain score for inclusion in the study, the lack of physical examination component, and, as with the INVEST trial, the inclusion of fractures up to 12 months old (only 32% of patients had fractures <6 weeks old).

The 2010 VERTOS II trial was a prospective open-label RCT comparing vertebroplasty with medical management for osteoporotic fractures. Patients were included if there was severe back pain (score < 5 on visual analogue scale (VAS)) of <6-week duration, focal tenderness on clinical examination, and bone edema on MRI (thus addressing some limitations from the 2009 trials). A total of 202 patients received vertebroplasty ($N = 101$) or medical therapy ($N = 101$). At 1 month, vertebroplasty resulted in significantly improved pain relief. The mean reduction of VAS was 2.6 greater in the vertebroplasty group than conservative management, and this difference between groups was sustained at 1 year. The vertebroplasty group also demonstrated greater improvements in quality of life (as determined by several standardized questionnaires), earlier significant (VAS reduction >3 points) pain relief (30 days vs 116 days, $P < 0.0001$), and gain of 120 pain-free days. The major limitation of this trial was the lack of blinding, which may have led to overestimation of treatment effect.

Multiple further small prospective RCTs comparing vertebroplasty with medical management for osteoporotic fractures have been subsequently published demonstrating benefit in acute (<6 weeks), subacute (6–12 weeks), and chronic (>12 weeks) old fractures. The hallmarks of these positive RCTs were inclusion of patients with moderate or severe pain with advanced imaging selection, mainly MRI edema. A large multicenter case series of 3320 patients treated with vertebroplasty for osteoporotic fractures also demonstrated significant reduction in pain 48 hours after vertebroplasty. However, over the course of these studies, there remained ongoing concern regarding the potential impact of the placebo effect from these open-label RCTs.

In 2016, the VAPOUR trial (Vertebroplasty for Acute Painful Osteoporotic fractURes) was published in *The Lancet*, comparing vertebroplasty with a placebo procedure. Patients were older than previously studied (inclusion criteria of >60 years), all had severe pain (≥7/10), and all fractures were < 6 weeks in duration (mean fracture age 2.6 weeks). Fractures were confirmed with MRI or SPECT. In total, 120 patients were randomized to vertebroplasty ($N = 61$) or placebo ($N = 59$). At 2 weeks, a significantly higher proportion of patients in the vertebroplasty arm had pain scores of 4 or less, compared to the placebo arm, meeting the primary outcome. This benefit was sustained at 1 and 6 months. Notable secondary outcomes observed in the vertebroplasty group included reduced disability, improved quality of life questionnaire scores, reduced analgesic use, and median reduction of 5.5 hospital inpatient days.

There is less high-quality data available for vertebroplasty for neoplastic vertebral fractures. A systematic review that included 987 patients with spinal metastasis and myeloma across 30 studies revealed pain reduction of 20–79% 1 month after vertebroplasty. At 6 months, pain reduction ranged from 47% to 87%. There was no association between cement volume and pain reduction. A subsequent large pooled analysis of vertebral augmentation in 923 myeloma patients (60% received vertebroplasty) also demonstrated significant and sustained pain reduction up to 1 year posttreatment; both vertebroplasty and kyphoplasty were equally effective at reducing pain.

The combination of vertebroplasty with local adjunctive therapies such as radiofrequency ablation and cryotherapy does not seem to achieve superior pain reduction to vertebroplasty alone. However, the use of these adjunctive therapies may be promising for local tumor control. In a recent small study of 49 patients with painful vertebral metastases who underwent combined vertebroplasty and RFA, apart from reduction in pain and disability scores by 2–4 weeks, short-term post-ablation MRI demonstrated reduced tumor bulk, and posttreatment FDG-PET showed either reduced or absent metabolic activity.

Evidence for Safety

Overall, the rates of major complications from vertebroplasty are low. Major complication rates are <1% for patients with osteoporotic fracture and < 5% of those treated for neoplastic fractures. Potential serious complications that have been reported in literature include permanent neurologic deficits resulting from nerve or spinal cord injury; fractures of the rib, sternum, or pedicle; symptomatic cement leakage; allergic or idiosyncratic reactions; infection; pulmonary embolus; hemothorax or pneumothorax; local vascular injury; or death from cardiac or pulmonary cement embolism or anaphylaxis.

Analysis of major RCTs reveals low rates of serious complication from vertebroplasty for osteoporotic fractures, with no procedure-related mortality reported. In the VERTOS II trial, the only symptomatic complication referable to vertebroplasty was one urinary tract infection. The INVEST study reported a single thecal sac injury, while the INVEST study reported one case of osteomyelitis in a patient who did not receive antibiotics. In the VAPOUR trial, one patient had a respiratory arrest after administration of sedation before starting the procedure. This patient was treated uneventfully 48 hours later. Another patient sustained a humeral fracture during transfer onto the procedure table. In contrast, two patients in the control group had interval vertebral collapse with spinal cord compression; one remained paraplegic.

For neoplastic fractures, the risk of serious complications is higher. A previous systematic review of vertebroplasty in 987 patients for neoplastic fracture revealed a serious complication rate of 2%. In a larger multicenter series of 4547 patients with a total of 13,437 treated vertebrae (73% osteoporotic fractures), no major neurological complications occurred. Rates of pulmonary embolism, hematoma, or infection were < 1%.

Asymptomatic cement leakage outside the vertebra is common when assessed with CT scanning (72% in the VERTOS II trial; 34% in VAPOUR). Leakage is more likely in cases with cortical disruption, fracture clefts, low-viscosity cement, and high-volume injections. Symptomatic cement leak is rare, with secondary cement embolization exceedingly rare. Although rates of cement leak are reduced by use of kyphoplasty compared to vertebroplasty, there is no difference in rates of pain or disability reduction.

Pearls and Pitfalls

- The optimal threshold of cement infusion volume remains controversial, with some operators advocating injecting cement to fill the vertebral body and others recommending injecting lower volumes of cement to maximize safety. However, there has been no clear data to suggest improved pain outcomes with higher cement volumes. Moreover, there is increased risk of cement extravasation from higher injected cement volume. The current evidence favors a more cautious approach to the injected cement volume to maximize safety.
- Consistency and viscosity vary between cement preparations with variable working times. Higher viscosity generally requires injection of cement at higher pressure and typically has shorter working time than low-viscosity cement, and thus less total volume of cement may be injected. However, use of higher-viscosity cement reduces the rates of cement leak, with data suggesting comparable pain outcomes. A drip test can be used to test cement viscosity—The cement should ball up at the end of the needle and not drip downward, resulting in a consistency slightly more viscous than toothpaste.
- Vertebroplasty can be performed with placement of a single unilateral approach or bilateral approach. Key benefits of a unipedicular approach include reduced procedure time and less risk of pedicular breach or adjacent tissue injury. The key advantage of a bipedicular approach is the likelihood to inject a greater cement volume. Importantly, there is no difference between the two approaches with regard to pain relief, anatomic outcomes, or quality of life measures. Use of a unilateral approach is sufficient in most cases and may be converted to bilateral if midline position is difficult to achieve due to vertebral or fracture morphology.
- Treating >3 fractures in a single session remains controversial, with concerns regarding prolonged prone positioning, excessive sedation, post-procedure discomfort resulting from multiple needles, and PMMA toxicity. While some studies have demonstrated the safety of vertebroplasty independent of the number of levels treated per session, previously published data have highlighted concerns regarding PMMA reactions including hypotension and death when multiple levels are treated in one setting. This may relate to the increased risk of systemic emboli with treatment of multiple levels. Thus, a more cautious approach would be to treat up to three levels in a single session.
- Optimize spatial resolution and magnification during fluoroscopy while performing vertebroplasty. Patients may have marked osteopenia or focal bony lysis from neoplasm making bony landmarks challenging to identify. This can be partially overcome by optimizing radiation dose and using appropriate magnification. Use of biplane fluoroscopy is particularly helpful to facilitate continuous monitoring during cement injection.
- When performing vertebroplasty in the setting of posterior wall osteolysis or epidural tumor extension, there should be awareness of the neurologic risks from epidural extension of cement or posterior displacement of the tumor by the cement. Certain safeguards should be considered, including biplane fluoroscopy, more modest cement injection, using thicker cement, limiting cement to anterior two-thirds of the vertebral body, and use of conscious sedation (to facilitate assessment of lower limb neurological status or development of new pain during the procedure).
- Needles used during vertebroplasty are typically straight. However, curved needle systems are available that may enable better maneuverability and the ability to target the

flow of PMMA within a quadrant of the vertebral body. This may allow one to reach a more desired radiographic endpoint, such as targeting of focal neoplasm or achieving final needle position beyond midline from a unilateral approach.

Recommended Reading

1. Buchbinder R, Osborne RH, Ebeling PR, Wark JD, Mitchell P, Wriedt C, et al. A randomized trial of vertebroplasty for painful osteoporotic vertebral fractures. N Engl J Med. 2009;361(6):557–68.
2. Chandra RV, Meyers PM, Hirsch JA, Abruzzo T, Eskey CJ, Hussain MS, et al. Vertebral augmentation: report of the Standards and Guidelines Committee of the Society of NeuroInterventional Surgery. J Neurointerv Surg. 2014;6:7–15.
3. Chew C, Craig L, Edwards R, Moss J, O'Dwyer PJ. Safety and efficacy of percutaneous vertebroplasty in malignancy: a systematic review. Clin Radiol. 2011;66:63–72.
4. Clark W, Bird P, Gonski P, Diamond TH, Smerdely P, McNeil HP, et al. Safety and efficacy of vertebroplasty for acute painful osteoporotic fractures (VAPOUR): a multicentre, randomised, double-blind, placebo-controlled trial. The Lancet. 2016;388(10052):1408–16.
5. Kallmes DF, Comstock BA, Heagerty PJ, Turner JA, Wilson DJ, Diamond TH, et al. A randomized trial of vertebroplasty for osteoporotic spinal fractures. N Engl J Med. 2009;361(6):569–79.
6. Klazen CAH, Lohle PNM, de Vries J, Jansen FH, Tielbeek AV, Blonk MC, et al. Vertebroplasty versus conservative treatment in acute osteoporotic vertebral compression fractures (Vertos II): an open-label randomized trial. The Lancet. 2010;376(9746):1085–92.
7. Tsoumakidou G, Too CW, Koch G, Caudrelier J, Cazzato RL, Garnon J, et al. CIRSE Guidelines on Percutaneous Vertebral Augmentation. Cardiovasc Intervent Radiol. 2017;40(3):331–4.

Minimally Invasive Lumbar Decompression

96

Sean Li

Introduction

Degenerative lumbar spinal stenosis (LSS) is the most common form of acquired spinal stenosis caused by biomechanical narrowing of the spinal canal and the associated neuroforamen which eventually lead to compression of neural fibers resulting in pain and disability. LSS is anatomically categorized as central, lateral, and foraminal. Neurogenic claudication and intermittent low back or lower extremity pain with prolonged standing or sitting that is alleviated with sitting and leaning forward are hallmark symptoms of LSS. This was first described by Verbiest in the 1950s; neurogenic claudication can affect up to 94% of patient with LSS.

LSS is a progressive, age-related degenerative process that causes narrowing of the lumbar spinal canal. More than 1.2 million patients in the USA are diagnosed with spinal stenosis each year (Longitudinal Medicare Database, Quorum Consulting). MILD is an image-guided minimally invasive lumbar decompression procedure that allows for the debulking of pathologic hypertrophied ligamentum flavum through a limited percutaneous laminotomy.

Equipment Used

The MILD kit (Vertos Medical, Inc., Aliso Viejo, CA, USA) consists of sterile, single-use instruments designed to perform the necessary percutaneous laminotomy and debulking of the hypertrophied ligamentum flavum. See Fig. 96.1.

S. Li (✉)
Premier Pain Centers, An Affiliate of National Spine and Pain Centers, Shrewsbury, NJ, USA
e-mail: Sli@treatingpain.com

MILD Procedure

Prior to the procedure, the surgeon must review the pertinent MRI (or CT) images to familiarize with the exact nature of the patient's stenosis. The patient is placed in a prone position with adequate bolstering to minimize the lumbar lordosis. C-arm fluorography is used to obtain surface anatomy including the targeted level(s) of the procedure, medial pedicle lines, and access point for the necessary epidurogram. The surgical skin prep is performed. Once appropriate level of sedation is achieved, infiltration of local anesthetic and the procedure is initiated with obtaining an epidurogram preferably at the level of scheduled decompression. Confirm radiopaque contrast within the epidural space with fluoroscopic imaging. Obtain contralateral oblique view, and assess the degree of stenosis and angulation of the surrounding lamina. In order to gain maximal access to the interlaminar space, the final trocar trajectory should be parallel to the lamina. The trocar insertion site is 1 to 1.5 lumbar segments inferior at the midpoint between the spinous process and the pedicle line. The skin is infiltrated with local anesthetic. A small 5 mm stab incision is made with a #11 blade. Under direct fluoroscopic visualization, the trocar is advanced in a paramedian approach toward the superior lamina of the targeted level. One should keep attention to both fluoroscopic AP and lateral views while having awareness of the trocar position in relation to the surface anatomy. The inner cutting trocar tip is removed. The depth guide and stabilization plate are placed. Make sure that the plate does not interfere with the epidural needle causing loss of access for injection of contrast. To begin the decompression, the bone sculpter rongeur is advanced via the port cannula, and the depth guide is adjusted to gain access to the interlaminar space. The bone sculpter can be engaged both forehand and backhand to the superior and inferior surfaces of the lamina. Only under direct fluoroscopic guidance, small bites of bone and ligament are removed. This tool is single action and must be withdrawn from the access port each time a piece of tissue is dissected. This step allows access for the tissue sculpter to debulk the

T. R. Deer et al. (eds.), *Deer's Treatment of Pain*, https://doi.org/10.1007/978-3-030-12281-2_96

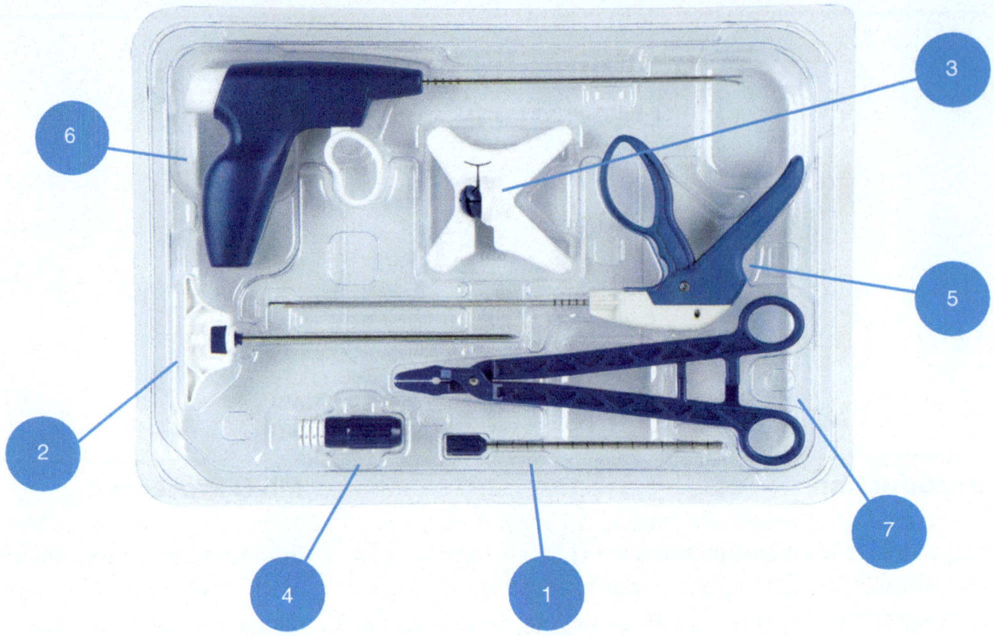

Fig. 96.1 MILD instrument kit. (1) 6-gauge, 15.9 cm cannula port, (2) 7-gauge, 16.8 cm trocar and locking handle, (3) Port stabilizer base, (4) Depth guide, (5) 7-gauge, 21.6 cm bone sculpter (rongeur) with 9.4 mm cutting area, (6) 8.5-gauge, 21.59 cm tissue sculpter, (7) Accessory surgical clamp. (Image courtesy of Vertos Medical, Inc.)

posterior aspect of the hypertrophied ligamentum flavum. The tissue sculpter is a multi-action device that will trap the dissected tissue in its jaws. It can only be used in a forward fashion. Direct fluoroscopic visualization of the tool during dissection is recommended. After 3–4 successful passes, the tissue sculpter is removed from the port to allow for removal of the retained ligament from the device with the push rod plunger. Periodically, the epidurogram is refreshed with 1–2 ml of contrast. During each pass of the bone or tissue sculpter, one must be aware of the its relationship to the posterior epidurogram and the epidural needle. The decompression is completed once the contrast fill defect is restored indicating successful debulking of excess ligament. These steps are repeated on the contralateral side if indicated. The importance of the epidurogram in the contralateral oblique view may necessitate the replacement of the epidural needle to the other side. At the completion of this procedure, it is optional to inject the epidural space with a mixture of local anesthetic and steroid for postoperative analgesia. The trocar and needle are removed. The port sites are closed with skin glue or a single suture (optional).

Link to procedure animation: https://youtu.be/fE8BJMJmjM0

Clinical Evidence

There have been 13 clinical trials and over 20 peer-reviewed journal articles supporting the efficacy of the MILD procedure for the treatment of symptomatic LSS. Table 96.1 shows the various prospective clinical trials that have been reported on MILD.

Pearls and Pitfalls

Patient selection is key. To ensure successful results from MILD, one must rule out other causes of back and leg pain. The patient must present with neurogenic claudication that is resolved with sitting and leaning forward. This clinical finding should also correlate with MRI findings of central spinal canal stenosis associated with ligamentum flavum hypertrophy. Additional factors such as scoliosis and low-grade spondylolisthesis are considered relative contraindications. The physician must review the MRI in addition to the radiological report. The location of the hypertrophied ligamentum flavum in relation to the adjacent lamina will provide crucial information in planning a successful operation. The most important step in the MILD procedure consists of obtaining an adequate epidurogram. A clear visualization of the epidurogram in the contralateral oblique view delineates the boundaries of the dissection. If severe central stenosis prevents the insertion of an epidural needle at the same level of planned MILD procedure, alternative option includes placement of two epidural needles above and below to create an epidurogram. Placement of a catheter from the caudal space has also been described. During the dissection portion of this procedure, one must be mindful that sufficient decompression is determined by the restoration of the epidurogram and not the physical amount of removed bone and ligament.

Billing and Coding

The MILD procedure has been approved for the indication of lumbar spinal stenosis ICD-10: M48.06. Under AMA

Table 96.1 Prospective clinical studies of MILD

Author (year)	Study design	Number of patients	Severe adverse effects	Outcome measures and conclusions
MiDAS I (2010)	Prospective, multicenter, 14 sites, 6 and 12 weeks	78	None	Statistically significant reduction in VAS (3.7 pts), ZCQ, and SF-12
Basu (2011)	Prospective, single center, 6 months	27	None	Improvement of VAS (5.2 pts) and ODI (24.0 pts)
Deer (2012)	Prospective, single center, 12 months	46	None	Improvement of VAS (2.9 pts), ODI (17.4 pts), and ZCQ
Mekhail (2012)	Single-center prospective, 12 months	40	None	Improvement of VAS (3.5 pts), standing time (8–56 min), and walking distance (246′ to 3956)
Mekhail (2012)	Prospective, multicenter, 11 sites, 12 months	58	None	Improvement of VAS (2.9 pts), ODI (11.9 pts)
Brown (2012)	Prospective, double-blind, single center, 12 weeks	38	None	MILD cohort showed improvement of VAS (2.9 pts) and ODI (18.6 pts)
Wong (2012)	Prospective, single center, 12 months	17	None	Improvement of VAS(5.4 pts), ODI (26.6 pts)
Chopko (2013)	Prospective, multicenter, 11 sites, 24 months	45	None	Improvement of VAS (3.8 pts) and ODI (11.6 pts)
MiDAS ENCORE (2016)	Prospective, multicenter, 26 sites, 12, 24 months	302	None	Statistical improvement of MILD versus ESI in ODI, NPRS, ZCQ

See Recommended Reading [1–5, 8, 9, 13]

(American Medical Association) CPT (Current of Procedural Terminology), the MILD procedure CPT 0275T is classified as a temporary code under the category III for being an emerging technology. As of March, 2017, CMS (Centers for Medicare and Medicaid Services) has regained reimbursement coverage through a Coverage with Evidence Development Program. Medicare patients with symptomatic neurogenic claudication due to ligamentum flavum hypertrophy are eligible for coverage of the MILD procedure through a claims-analysis study (NCT03072927).

Recommended Reading

1. Basu S. *mild*® procedure: Single-site experience prospective IRB study. Clin J Pain. 2012;28(3):254–8. https://doi.org/10.1097/AJP.0b013e31822bb344.
2. Benyamin RM, et al. *mild*® is an effective treatment for lumbar spinal stenosis with neurogenic claudication: MiDAS ENCORE Randomized Controlled Trial. Pain Physician. 2016;19:229–42.
3. Brown LL. A double-blind, randomized, prospective study of epidural steroid injection vs. the *mild*® procedure in patients with symptomatic lumbar spinal stenosis. Pain Pract. 2012;12(5):333–41.
4. Chopko BW, et al. MiDAS I (*mild*® Decompression Alternative to Open Surgery): a preliminary report of a prospective, multi-center clinical study. Pain Physician. 2010;13(4):369–78.
5. Deer T, et al. Study of percutaneous lumbar decompression and treatment algorithm for patients suffering from neurogenic claudication. Pain Physician. 2012;15(6):451–60.
6. Hall S, et al. Lumbar spinal stenosis. Clinical features, diagnostic procedures, and results of surgical treatment in 68 patients. Ann Intern Med. 1985;103(2):271–5.
7. https://clinicaltrials.gov/ct2/show/NCT03072927.
8. Lee SY, Kim T, Oh JK, Lee SJ, Park MS. Lumbar stenosis: a recent update by review of literature. Asian Spine J. 2015;9(5):818–28.
9. Mekhail N, et al. Functional and patient-reported outcomes in symptomatic lumbar spinal stenosis following percutaneous decompression. Pain Pract. 2012;12(6):417–25.
10. Mekhail N, et al. Long-term results of percutaneous lumbar decompression *mild*® for spinal stenosis. Pain Pract. 2012;12(3):184–93.
11. Staats P, et al. Long-term safety and efficacy of minimally invasive lumbar decompression procedure for the treatment of lumbar spinal stenosis with neurogenic claudication: 2-year results of MiDAS ENCORE. RAPAM. 2018;43:789–94.
12. Verbiest H. A radicular syndrome from developmental narrowing of the lumbar vertebral canal. J Bone Joint Surg Br. 1954;36:230–7.
13. Wong WH. *mild*® Interlaminar decompression for the treatment of lumbar spinal stenosis: procedure description and case series with 1-year follow-up. Clin J Pain. 2012;28(6):534–8.

Interspinous Process Spacers for Indirect Lumbar Decompression

97

Jonathan D. Carlson, W. Porter McRoberts, and Jeffery Rowe

Introduction

Narrowing of the spinal canal in the lower back, known as lumbar spinal stenosis (LSS), occurs as a result of one or more age-related, pathological changes, such as thickening of the ligamentum flavum, spondylolisthesis, facet arthropathy, or loss of disc height among others. LSS can lead to neurogenic intermittent claudication (NIC) – a pattern of pain, weakness, and/or numbness of the lower back and legs. These symptoms are typically exacerbated by standing or walking and may be relieved by sitting or bending forward. NIC impairs the ability to walk and causes both substantial disability and societal cost and burden. LSS is particularly common in older adults, representing the most common cause of spinal surgery among patients age 65 or older.[1] Approximately 40% of those suffering with LSS will require spine surgery in the following 10 years after diagnosis.[2]

Patients with mild to moderate LSS are typically treated with conservative methods, such as orthotics, physical therapy, medications, and epidural steroid injections. These treatments are limited in the extent to which they address the mechanical compression involved in LSS, and systematic review concludes there lacks sufficient evidence to recommend any specific type of nonsurgical treatment.[3] This is particularly problematic as the compression becomes more severe and morbidity increases.

The standard of care for patients with severe LSS is open lumbar laminectomy. Laminectomy is clearly indicated for many patients with severe LSS or cauda equina syndrome. However, patients with mild to moderate LSS may experience no relief or only partial relief from conservative care but be unable or unwilling to pursue traditional laminectomy due to the risks of invasive spine surgery. Depending on comorbidities, complications from open lumbar laminectomy can occur in 10–24% of patients.[4] Older adult patients, who are disproportionately represented among those with LSS, also tend to have more of these comorbidities. This high rate of complications has led to substantial interest in less invasive treatments for LSS.

This gap in the treatment algorithm for mild to moderate LSS between conservative treatments and open lumbar laminectomy can potentially be filled by interspinous process spacers. Interspinous process spacers are an implanted device designed to achieve indirect spinal decompression. These devices have the advantage of being minimally invasive, involving a relatively small incision compared with open laminectomy and involve implantation under fluoroscopic

[1]Deyo RA, Treatment of lumbar spinal stenosis: a balancing act. Spine J. 2010; 10(7):625–7.

[2]Atlas SJ, Keller RB, Wu YA, Deyo RA, Singer DE. Long-term outcomes of surgical and nonsurgical management of lumbar spinal stenosis: 8 to 10 year results from the maine lumbar spine study. Spine (Phila Pa 1976). 2005;30(8):936–943.

[3]Lurie J, Tomkins-Lane C. Management of lumbar spinal stenosis. BMJ. 2016; 352:h6234. https://doi.org/10.1136/bmj.h6234

[4]Zaina F, Tomkins-Lane C, Carragee E, Negrini S. Surgical versus nonsurgical treatment for lumbar spinal stenosis. Cochrane Database Syst Rev. 2016;(1):CD010264. https://doi.org/10.1002/14651858.CD010264.pub2.

J. D. Carlson (✉)
Hawaii Pain & Spine, Kailua, HI, USA

Midwestern Medical School, Glendale, AZ, USA

Hawaii Pain & Spine, Arizona Pain, Kailua, HI, USA

W. P. McRoberts
FAAPMR ABPMR ABA/Pain, University of Miami School of Medicine, Miami, FL, USA

J. Rowe
Main Line Spine & Main Line Spine Surgery Center, King of Prussia, PA, USA

T. R. Deer et al. (eds.), *Deer's Treatment of Pain*, https://doi.org/10.1007/978-3-030-12281-2_97

guidance. In most cases, these devices can be implanted as an outpatient procedure. Additionally, the implantation is reversible, with some spacers designed to be safely removed in a similarly noninvasive procedure.

Background and Historical Perspective

Lumbar spinal stenosis is one of the most common spinal pathologies, symptoms including pain, numbness, and weakness, particularly during extension. First designed in the 1950s by Fred Knowles, the potential for a mechanical implant located between the interspinous processes to prevent these symptoms has been recognized for decades, but he reported little success with these devices, due to initial problems of device displacement.

Further development of interspinous process devices continued with Abbott Spine's Wallis device, developed in 1984. The Wallis device was a titanium spacer placed between the spinous processes. It was tested for various conditions including recurrent disc herniation, though it was also used for treating spinal stenosis.

Subsequent spinal spacers included flexible devices, such as the Minns device, a soft, dumbbell-shaped silicone implant intended to correct sagittal plane instability. The results of implantation with this device were initially published in 1997 but not further tested or commercialized. Other similar devices include the Device for Intervertebral Assisted Motion (DIAM), from Medtronic, an H-shaped silicone interspinous spacer secured by two ligatures, and the coflex device, from Paradigm Spine, a U-shaped, interlaminar stabilization device first developed in 1994. The coflex is additionally compressible, allowing for some extension movement. This device compared favorably with posterolateral fusion for treating lumbar spinal stenosis and received FDA approval in 2012.

Recent commercialized interspinous process spacer devices for treating symptomatic LSS include the X-STOP and the Superion. Medtronic's X-STOP was an interspinous process device that limits pathologic extension but allows flexion and rotation. It was approved by the FDA in 2005, making it the first implantable device approved for treating NIC caused by LSS, but was withdrawn from the market in April of 2015. The Superion, developed by VertiFlex and FDA approved in 2015, was developed to present an even less invasive implantation procedure compared with the X-STOP. At 3-year follow-up, the Superion showed better results on a composite measure of pain and function than the X-STOP (See Figs. 97.1 and 97.2).

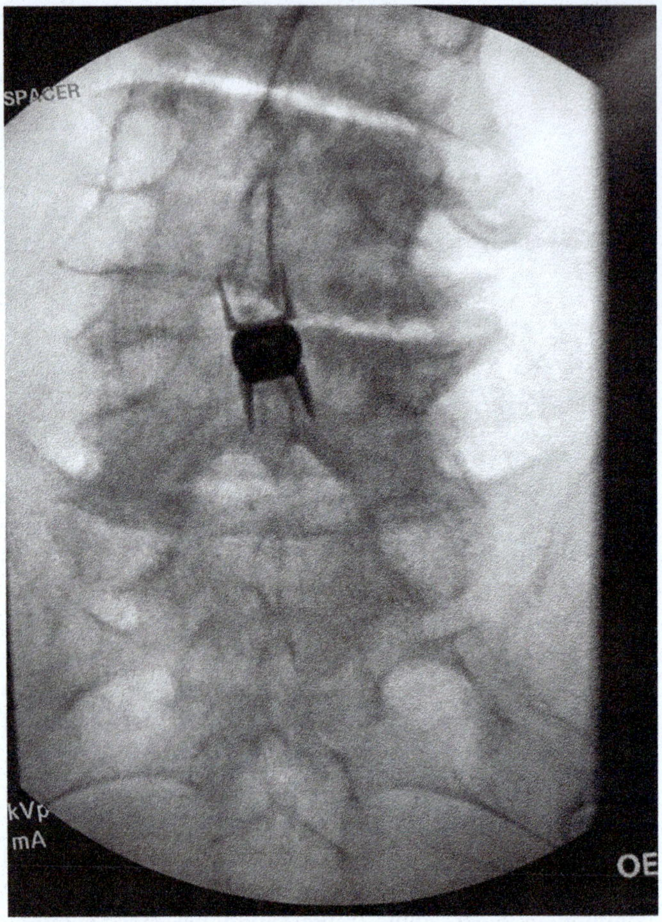

Fig. 97.1 AP fluoroscopic image of a L4/L5 Superion spacer

Uses and Indications

Interspinous process spacers, such as the VertiFlex Superion Indirect Decompression System (see Figs. 97.1, 97.2, and 97.3), are indicated for patients who meet the following criteria:

- Patients experiencing neurogenic intermittent claudication (NIC) as a result of lumbar spinal stenosis
- Pain in the legs and/or buttocks that is alleviated by flexion
- Moderate to severe impairment of physical function
- Moderate LSS (25–50% reduction in the area of the spinal canal at the target level, compared with adjacent levels), confirmed by radiograph
- LSS diagnosed in the central, lateral, and/or foraminal portions of the spinal canal

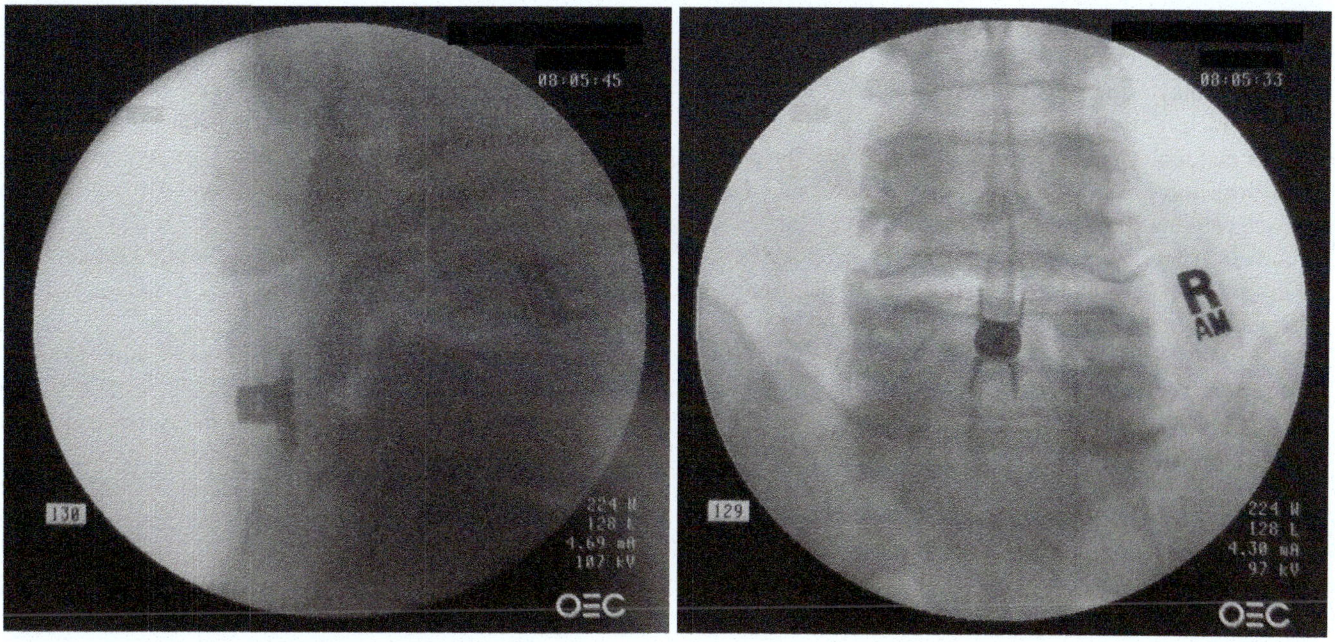

Fig. 97.2 Lateral fluoroscopic image of a L4/L5 Superion spacer

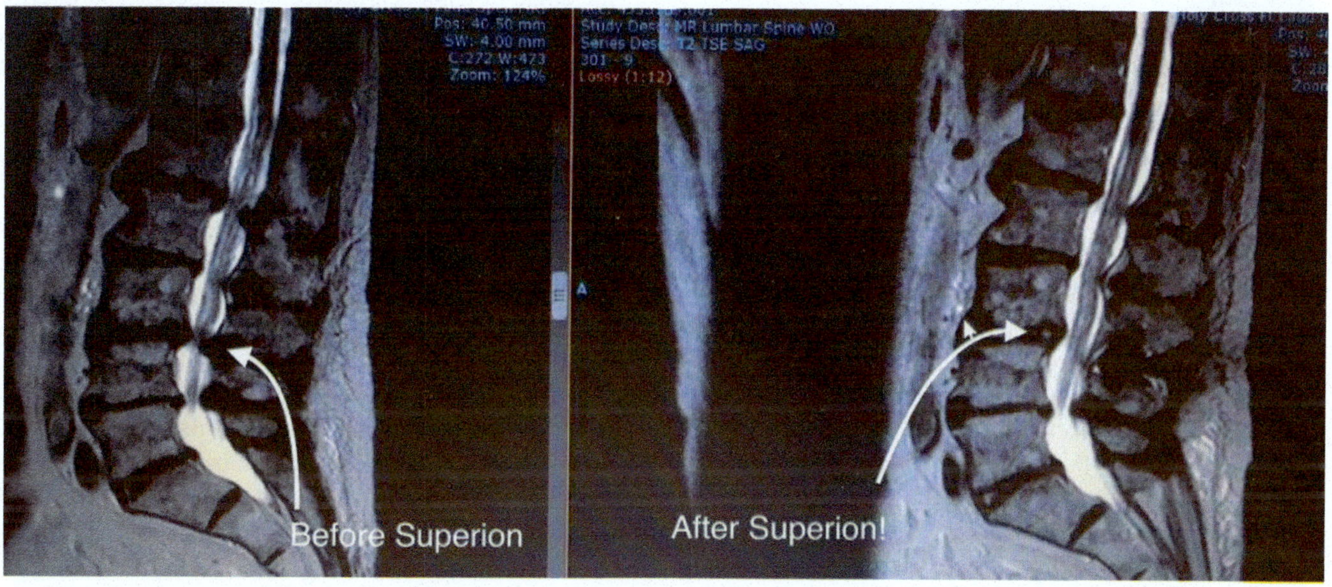

Fig. 97.3 Before and after spacer implant MR images

- Completed at least 6 months of conservative care for NIC symptoms
- Skeletally mature male or female
- LSS affecting one or two levels between L1 and L5

Contraindications to the Indirect Decompression System include:

- Constant pain of the legs and/or buttocks not alleviated by forward flexion
- Lower back pain that is primarily axial
- Moderate or severe spondylolisthesis (grade > 1.0)
- Dynamic instability of the lumbar spine (translation of ≥3 mm or ≥ 5^0 angulation during flexion/extension)
- Scoliotic changes at the target level (lateral curvature >10^0)
- Pathologic fracture or multiple fracture of the vertebrae and/or hips
- Baastrup's disease: spine degeneration causing spinous processes to be in close approximation
- Allergy to titanium or titanium alloys
- Any disease or spinal anatomy that prevents device implantation of the device or would cause instability of the device,

including lumbar spine instability due to isthmic spondylolisthesis or degenerative spondylolisthesis (grade > 1, from 1 to 4), ankylosing spondylitis at target level, spinous process fracture, pars interarticularis fracture, laminae fracture, and scoliosis with a Cobb angle >10^0

- Neurogenic bladder or bowel dysfunction secondary to cauda equina syndrome
- Severe osteoporosis of the hips or spine (DEXA scan greater than 2.5 standard deviations below adult normal)
- Infection at the implant site or an active systemic infection
- Previous decompression or fusion procedure at the target level
- Morbid obesity (body mass index greater than 40)

Relative contraindications include:

- Neurologic deficits secondary to severe spinal stenosis
- Symptomatic LSS at more than two levels
- Other previous lumbar surgery at target level(s)
- Vertebral metastases or Paget's disease

Evidence for Efficacy

Several interspinous process spacers have been evaluated in high-quality clinical trials, including randomized trials providing evidence of efficacy. A prospective randomized, multicenter study compared the X-STOP interspinous process spacer to non-operative treatments (e.g., NSAIDs, analgesics, physical therapy, epidural steroid injections). A total of 191 patients were randomized (100 to X-STOP, 91 to the control group) at 9 sites in the United States. At 2-year follow-up, X-STOP patients reported 45.4% improvement in symptom severity and a 44.3% physical function, compared to a 7.4% and −0.4% reductions among control patients, respectively.

Another study of interspinous process spacers comes from a randomized, multicenter trial of the VertiFlex Superion spacer compared to the X-STOP spacer group. This study included 391 patients with NIC secondary to moderate LSS, who were randomized at 29 sites. In both groups, 70% of patients reported significantly decreased severity of their mean pain as reported by visual analogue scale (VAS), and 65% had significantly reduced disability at 2 years. A 5-year follow-up of a subset of these patients found that 75% Superion patients continued to experience improved symptom severity and 81% continued to have improved physical function. (See Fig. 97.3.)

Pearls and Pitfalls

- Successful implantation of interspinous process spacers depends on patient selection. The two most important criteria are (a) neurogenic claudication (i.e., leg pain, weakness, or heaviness when walking) and (b) relief from symptoms during flexion.
- One or two levels can be treated (excluding L5/S1).
- Review the patient's imaging (MRI, CT, x-rays) to identify any potential contraindications.
- Proper patient positioning for the procedure involves exaggerated lumbar flexion, for example, with a Wilson frame or similar. This maximizes the interspinous space at the target level.
- Ideal body mass index (BMI) is less than 35. BMI greater than 35 is possible, but it may affect visualization of the spinal structures in a lateral fluoroscopic view.
- Use lateral fluoroscopic view when advancing cannulas. Never advance the cannulas past the intralaminar junction, as this could lead to dural injury.
- Frequent AP and lateral x-rays should be used to guide the angle of approach between the superior and inferior spinous processes of the target level. If the cannula is placed obliquely to the side of midline, this can make deployment of the spacer difficult or impossible.
- There is a risk of spinous process fracture during implantation. Risks for fracture are associated with thin/gracile spinous processes (<20 mm in superior-inferior dimension), degenerative spondylolisthesis, osteoporosis, kissing spinous processes (in contact or very close approximation), or shallow/dorsal placement of spacer (ensure deep/anterior placement of implant, verified with lateral fluoroscopy).
- Preventive precautions for sterility should be taken similar to those used in spinal cord stimulator implantation. This includes limited room traffic, preoperative antibiotics, double gloving, irrigation of the wound, full wound closure, and postoperative antibiotics.

Recommended Reading

1. Kim DH, Albert TJ. Interspinous process spacers. J Am Acad Orthop Surg. 2007;15:200–7.
2. Kondrashov DG, Hannibal M, Hsu KY, Zucherman JF. Interspinous process decompression with the X-STOP device for lumbar spinal stenosis: A 4-year follow-up study. J Spinal Disord Tech. 2006;19:323–7.
3. Nunley PD, Patel VV, Orndorff DG, Lavelle WF, Block JE, Geisler FH. Five-year durability of stand-alone interspinous process

decompression for lumbar spinal stenosis. Clin Interv Aging. 2017;12:1409–17.
4. Patel VV, Whang PG, Haley TR, Bradley WD, Nunley PD, Davis RP, Miller LE, Block JE, Geisler FH. Superion interspinous process spacer for intermittent neurogenic claudication secondary to moderate lumbar spinal stenosis: Two-year results from a randomized controlled FDA-IDE pivotal trial. Spine. 2015;40:275–82.
5. Tapp SJ, Martin BI, Tosteson TD, Lurie JD, Weinstein MC, Deyo RA, Mirza SK, Tosteson ANA. Understanding the value of minimally invasive procedures for the treatment of lumbar spinal stenosis: The case of interspinous spacer devices. Spine J. 2018;18:584–92. https://doi.org/10.1016/j.spinee.2017.08.246.
6. Zucherman JF, Hsu KY, Hartjen CA, Mehalic TF, Implicito DA, Martin MJ, et al. A multicenter, prospective, randomized trial evaluating the X STOP interspinous process decompression system for the treatment of neurogenic intermittent claudication. Spine. 2005;30:1351–8.

Part X

Rehabilitation and Adjuvant Therapies for Pain

Physical Therapy

98

Shamard Charles, Alexios G. Carayannopoulos, and Amanda Markow

Introduction

Insufficient pain education has been problematic across the healthcare spectrum. Although a number of psychological approaches to the treatment of chronic pain have demonstrated important success over the last few decades, the field of pain management has identified the need for additional and vigorous treatment options. Recent educational advancements have been made to combat deficits in this area. Growing awareness of the limitations of currently available pharmacological pain treatment makes physical therapy an attractive component of pain management. These advancements seek to ensure that healthcare professionals are proficient in the adequate assessment and management of pain. The field of physical therapy is one of the areas where advancements have been most robust. In fact, physical therapy is not only highly sought after but is now considered a first-line treatment in the management of many chronic pain syndromes.

Research has shown that pain is associated with many different symptoms and clinical manifestations. Properly identifying and understanding these manifestations helps in evaluation judgment, clinical reasoning, treatment, and prognosis of patients with pain. However, in order for physical therapists and clinicians to choose the most appropriate and specific treatment, one needs to have sufficient scientific and practical acumen. Using what we know about the unique neurophysiological mechanisms that cause pain can help physical therapists to tailor specific treatments which have the greatest clinical applicability. It is important to determine predominant pain mechanisms for physical therapy to be more effective. In addition, it is essential that physical therapists identify biopsychosocial factors that might provoke or contribute to pain as well as pain perception.

Mechanisms and theories have been proposed to explain the effects of physical therapy on pain control and handling. These involve local peripheral tissues, neurophysiological and psychophysiological mechanisms, and the placebo effect. They are currently based on pain processing stages in the nervous system and on neuroplasticity changes. In this chapter, we will discuss the common pain conditions treated most efficaciously with physical therapy (i.e., LBP), the action of physical therapy on pain modulation and perception, and physical therapy action techniques and mechanisms as well as their role in the context of psychophysiological effects.

Background and Historical Perspective

The history of physical therapy (PT) dates to the time of Hippocrates. For thousands of years, people with illnesses and disabilities were treated with various methods, making use of movement (with or without the aid of mechanical devices). In fact, massage and hydrotherapy were the treatments of choice. Eventually, this informal practice became a profession. In 1894, England created the Chartered Society of Physiotherapy. Soon after, the profession reached the

S. Charles (✉)
Harvard T.H. Chan School of Public Health, NBC News Group, New York, NY, USA
e-mail: Shamard_charles@alumni.brown.edu; Shamard.Charles@nbcuni.com

A. G. Carayannopoulos
Department of Physical Medicine and Rehabilitation, Rhode Island Hospital, Providence, RI, USA

Comprehensive Spine Center: Rhode Island Hospital, Providence, RI, USA

Newport Hospital, Newport, RI, USA

Warren Alpert Medical School, Brown University, Providence, RI, USA

American Society of Interventional Pain Physicians, Rhode Island Chapter, Paducah, KY, USA
e-mail: acarayannopoulos@lifespan.org

A. Markow
New York Presbyterian Brooklyn Methodist Hospital, New York, NY, USA

T. R. Deer et al. (eds.), *Deer's Treatment of Pain*, https://doi.org/10.1007/978-3-030-12281-2_98

United States, and the first graduate class of physical therapists from Portland, Oregon, received the title of "Reconstruction Aid" in 1914. Seven years later, the first professional association of physical therapists was formed. This was entitled "The American Women's Physical Therapy Association," led by Mary McMillian.

Until 1950, the field centered around two major historical events: the poliomyelitis epidemics and the ravages of war. The passage of the "Hill Burton Act," more formally known as the Hospital Survey and Construction Act of 1946, led to an increase in hospital-based practice for physical therapists. During this time, many states enacted licensure laws and required successful completion of competency exams to legally practice. The role of the physical therapist progressed increasingly in the 1950s from that of a technician to a professional practitioner; and physical therapists slowly moved their practice out of the hospital and into a wide variety of settings with the addition of "outpatient physical therapy" in amendments made to the Social Security Act (SSA) in 1967. PT specialization occurred in the United States by 1974. By the 1990s and 2000s, technological advances improved the APTA's ability to efficiently conduct research and to incorporate evidence-based practice into patient care. Today, a PT can specialize in many areas, ranging from manual orthopedic physical therapy or geriatrics to neurology and sports medicine.

The specialization of physical therapy has provided a viable alternative in the treatment of many challenging conditions. In 2010, the College of Physicians and Surgeons of Ontario stated that opioids are an important arsenal for treating chronic non-cancer pain but also noted that clear guidance on the prescribing of opioids was needed and the National Opioid Use Guideline Group developed the Canadian Guideline for Safe and Effective Use of Opioids for Chronic Non-Cancer Pain. The guideline noted that "not enough is known about the long-term benefits, risks, and side effects of opioid therapy" and that "more research is needed in these areas." The proposed guidelines addressed only one modality (pharmacology) for managing chronic non-cancer pain and did not discuss or provide guidance about other options. Of most significance, the guidelines noted that "although opioid therapy can be an adjunct therapy for chronic non-cancer pain, other therapeutic options need to be implemented before resorting to opioids." This major development shifted the traditional chronic pain treatment paradigm to include nonsurgical and non-pharmacological modalities as first-line management options.

Chronic knee, hip, and low back pain are the most common causes of chronic pain, which last for 3 months or longer. Increasingly sedentary lifestyles further exacerbate pain, preventing people from pursuing an active, healthier way of life. Osteoarthritis, the wearing away of the soft tissue between two bones, is the most frequent culprit for these pains followed by muscle or tendon injury, ligament sprains, and "pinched" nerves. For this reason, we will single out low back pain and take a deeper look into its epidemiology, clinical manifestation, and nonsurgical treatment options.

The lifetime prevalence of lower back pain is about 70% and increases between the peak ages of 35–55 years of age. Back pain also accounts for 2–5% of all physician visits, and about 25% of adults report low back pain lasting at least 1 day in the past 3 months. According to a 2016 report released by the Institute for Health Metrics and Evaluation, healthcare costs for LBP in the United States were approximately $87.4 billion in 2016 and have been increasing faster than overall healthcare spending.

Additionally, research conducted by Fritz, Brennan, and Hunter published in the journal *Health Services Research* found that initial treatment costs for patients with low back pain were 50% lower when the primary care consultation was followed by a physical therapy referral rather than an advanced imaging referral. Furthermore, average subsequent costs over the next year were nearly 72% lower for patients who began with a physical therapy referral--$1871, compared with $6664 for the imaging group over the same time period.[5] These findings note the importance of introducing physical therapy as an option earlier in treatment as a cost-effective alternative to surgery.

Uses and Indications

Physical therapy is used to target and alleviate sources of chronic pain diseases, including (but not limited to) lower back pain, osteoarthritis, fibromyalgia, chronic headache, rheumatoid arthritis, and neuropathic pain.

Lack of movement is commonly associated with chronic pain and further worsening of symptoms. Therefore, one of the goals of physical therapy is to help patients become stronger by identifying the biopsychosocial factors (sensory, emotional, and behavioral) that contribute to pain perception and to incorporate routine exercise and movement into a patient's daily life.

Physical therapy can alleviate chronic pain by teaching people how to move safely and functionally in ways that they might not have been able to previously.

Many different modalities are used in the treatment of common pain disorders including:

- Massage
- Manual manipulation of joints and bones
- Manual therapy using hands or tools on soft tissue
- Cold laser therapy to alleviate inflammation and pain

- Microcurrent stimulation, which emits alpha waves into the brain and increases serotonin and dopamine to alleviate pain naturally
- Movement therapy and exercise

It is not uncommon for multiple modalities to be combined and that a baseline physical assessment is taken at the initial evaluation. A physical activity plan is then created and tailors to the patient's pain level and physical ability.

Research has shown that exercising for just 30 minutes a day, 3–4 days a week, can help with chronic pain management by increasing:

- Strength in the muscles
- Endurance
- Stability in the joints
- Flexibility in the muscles and joints

Also, regular therapeutic exercise can help patients maintain the ability to move and function physically, rather than becoming disabled by their chronic pain; therefore, many physical therapists and doctors suggest that patients keep a consistent exercise routine to help control their pain. Manipulation and massage can treat inflammation and stiffness by boosting the body's production of natural-pain-relieving chemicals. The duality that exists in physical therapy increases its effectiveness.

While physical therapy and its multimodal approach can be extremely effective against chronic pain, it is important to emphasize that physical therapy is part of a combination approach method in pain management. To maximize recovery, the help of a multimodal pain management team consisting of a medical doctor, clinical psychologist, and pharmacist is essential in the formulation of an applicable personalized care plan.

Evidence for Efficacy

Exercise is one of the most frequently used modalities by physical therapists in the treatment of patients with chronic low back pain. Physical therapists utilize modalities such as exercise to assist patients in performing their normal life activities without pain and discomfort. Proprioceptive neuromuscular facilitation (PNF) exercises are designed to enhance the response of neuromuscular mechanisms by stimulating proprioceptors. Two commonly used forms of PNF exercises are rhythmic stabilization training (RST) and combination of isotonic exercises (COI).[7]

A study performed by Kofotolis and Kellis (2006) supports efficacy of PNF exercise as a modality by reducing chronic pain in patients with low back pain. Two experimental groups (RST group and COI group) participated in a 4-week-long exercise program aimed at developing strength, endurance, and lumbar mobility to improve overall body control. The study demonstrated improved overall pain intensity, increased muscle endurance, and decreased functional disability. It is suggested that continuation of exercise may produce better results when working with patients who experience chronic low back pain.

Main Points

- Pain education is an essential part of the recovery process.
- Research has shown that a lack of movement often leads to more reported pain symptoms. The implementation of a safe, therapeutic activity and exercise plan helps patients learn how to accommodate or even decrease their pain, increasing their ability to function independently.
- Recent observational studies report early physical therapy is associated with lower costs and reduced risk of invasive procedures when compared with delayed referral.
- The most effective chronic pain treatment plans are put forth by a pain management team that consists of physical therapists, clinical psychologists, and medical doctors.
- Exercise, in the context of rhythmic stabilization and combination isotonic exercise, has been shown to significantly reduce lower back pain, and routine exercise, in general, has been associated with less reported chronic pain symptoms.
- Studies have shown that other physical therapy modalities such as massage and manual manipulation are not as effective as exercise in the treatment of chronic pain particularly in the context of low back pain, one of the most reported sources of chronic pain.

Recommended Reading

Deyo RA, Mirza SK, Martin BI. Back pain prevalence and visit rates: estimates from US national surveys, 2002. Spine (Phila Pa 1976). 2006;31(23):2724–7.

Dieleman JL, Baral R, Birger M, Bui AL, Bulchis A, Chapin A, et al. US Spending on Personal Health Care and Public Health, 1996–2013. JAMA. 2016;316(24):2627. https://doi.org/10.1001/jama.2016.16885.

Finestone HM, Juurlink DN, Power B, Gomes T, Pimlott N. Opioid prescribing is a surrogate for inadequate pain management resources. Can Fam Physician. 2016;62(6):465–8.

Fritz JM, Brennan GP, Hunter SJ. Physical Therapy or Advanced Imaging as First Management Strategy Following a New Consultation for Low Back Pain in Primary Care: Associations with Future Health Care Utilization and Charges. Health Serv Res. 2015;50(6):1927–40.

Kofotolis N, Kellis E. Effects of Two 4-Week Proprioceptive Neuromuscular Facilitation Programs on Muscle Endurance, Flexibility, and Functional Performance in Women With Chronic Low Back Pain. Phys Ther. 2006;86:1001–12.

Licciardone JC. The epidemiology and medical management of low back pain during ambulatory medical care visits in the United States. Osteopat Med Prim Care. 2008;2:11.

Licht S. History. In: Licht S, editor. Therapeutic Exercise. 2nd ed. Baltimore, MD: Waverly Press; 1965. p. 426–71.

Louw A, Puentedura E. Therapeutic Neuroscience Education: Teaching Patient about Pain; A Clinicians Guide. 1st ed: International Spine and Pain Institute; 2013. ISBN: 978–0985718640

Moller AR. PAIN Its Anatomy, Physiology and Treatment. 2nd ed. CreateSpace Independent Publishing Platform; 2011. ISBN: 978-1466395107.

Sluka KA. Mechanisms and Management of Pain for the Physical Therapist. 1st ed. International Association for the Study of Pain; 2009. ISBN: 978-0931092770.

Acupuncture

99

Tony Y. Chon

Introduction

In its simplest form, acupuncture involves the insertion of fine metallic needles in specific and strategic points on the body known as acupuncture points. According to traditional Chinese medicine (TCM) philosophy, all living and nonliving things possess a circulating inner energy that is described as *Qi* (pronounced *chee*). The circulation of *Qi* is stated to occur in distinct meridians or channels on the body. Acupuncture points are described to be points on the body where the flow of *Qi* rises closer to the surface of the body where the flow can be manipulated by using acupuncture needles (Fig. 99.1). In TCM paradigm, balanced flow of *Qi* is paramount to optimal health. Therefore, the main purpose of an acupuncture therapy is restoring the balance, strengthening, and focusing the flow of *Qi* that may be interrupted along the meridians. Disease and illness are thought to result from the imbalance in the flow of *Qi*. Although there may be emphasis on the maintenance of health with classical acupuncture therapy, in its current clinical application, it is readily used to mitigate the symptoms of certain health conditions including pain.

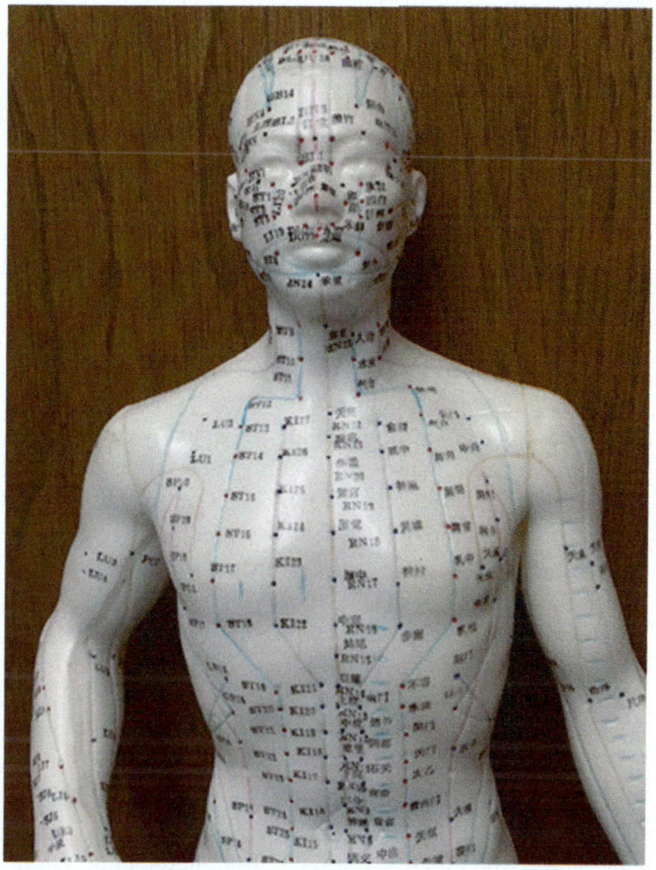

Fig. 99.1 Acupuncture mannequin depicting acupuncture points situated within various meridians

Background and Historical Perspective

By some estimates, acupuncture developed over 4000 years ago in China. Early practitioners used what was available locally to manufacture acupuncture "needles." Stones, rocks, bamboo, animal bones, and different metals were fashioned into sharp instruments to puncture areas along the body for healing purposes. Earliest available documented mention of acupuncture-like therapy is described in *Yellow Emperor's Classic of Internal Medicine* written around circa 200 BC.

During the rule of the Qing Dynasty (1644–1912), the practice of acupuncture was banned as it was viewed as being substandard to medical therapies introduced by Western cultures. Despite its ban, the practice of acupuncture was popular and widespread within Chinese society from the common people to the well-educated. During the early seventeenth century, Jesuit missionaries returning from China first introduced acupuncture to Europe. From France, the knowledge of acupuncture spread to the rest of Europe and Western world.

T. Y. Chon (✉)
Division of General Internal Medicine, Mayo Clinic, Rochester, MN, USA
e-mail: chon.tony@mayo.edu

T. R. Deer et al. (eds.), *Deer's Treatment of Pain*, https://doi.org/10.1007/978-3-030-12281-2_99

Acupuncture likely arrived in the United States by Chinese doctors who immigrated here as early as the 1800s. This is long before acupuncture gained public attention in 1971 when a *New York Times* reporter James Reston wrote about his first experience with acupuncture after undergoing emergent appendectomy while covering President Nixon's Secretary of State, Henry Kissinger's visit to China. James Reston experienced significant postoperative pain and bloating after undergoing successful surgery. Acupuncture was provided as a treatment modality where he soon experienced significant relief of his discomfort. Upon returning home, James Reston documented his story on the front page article of the *New York Times* revealing acupuncture to the millions of Americans for the first time.

By the 1990s, the practice of acupuncture had grown substantially. Millions of Americans were utilizing acupuncture for management of various health conditions including pain. The practice of acupuncture was even more widespread in the rest of the world. By 1997, the National Institute of Health (NIH) organized a 2.5-day conference to evaluate the scientific data on acupuncture therapy for variety of health conditions. This was in part to provide patients and medical professionals a responsible assessment of the use and effectiveness of acupuncture. Based on the scientific evidence presented, the panel representing multiple disciplines in healthcare was able to conclude that there exists ample evidence supporting the use of acupuncture for adult postoperative and chemotherapy-associated nausea and vomiting and for postoperative dental pain. However, other health conditions were identified in which acupuncture may be useful as an adjunct treatment or acceptable alternative or included in a comprehensive treatment plan such as headache, fibromyalgia, myofascial pain, osteoarthritis, and low back pain.

Uses and Indications

In China, the utilization of acupuncture continues to be very versatile, ranging from preventive therapy and maintenance of health to the treatment of many health conditions. In the United States, the utilization has been traditionally reserved as an adjunctive or a stand-alone therapy for management of health conditions that are closely associated with pain. Examples include the use of acupuncture for musculoskeletal conditions such as acute and chronic back pain, shoulder pain, hip pain, and knee pain related to osteoarthritis. It has also gained popularity in the use of acupuncture for myofascial pain related to fibromyalgia, pain management in the postoperative setting, cancer-associated pain, and neurologic conditions such as headaches. However, the scope of acupuncture continues to expand to include other non-pain-related health conditions, as there are more literature reports to support its use.

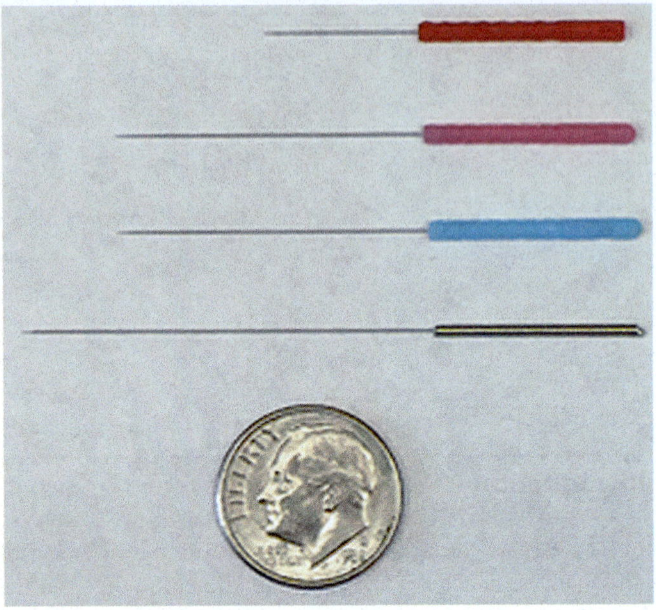

Fig. 99.2 Example of various acupuncture needles. Coin provided as reference for needle size

In the United States, nonphysician licensed acupuncturists continue to provide the bulk of acupuncture therapy. However, other healthcare providers offering acupuncture include physicians, dentists, and chiropractors. These providers may utilize acupuncture as an adjunctive therapy along with conventional therapy to help mitigate symptoms associated with certain health conditions.

Acupuncture needles utilized today are disposable, single-use needles, made from surgical stainless steel. They are solid, flexible needles with a non-cutting tapered tip designed to penetrate tissue without much noticeable adverse symptoms (Fig. 99.2). Patients are able to easily tolerate the insertion of many acupuncture needles without much difficulty. Patients commonly experience minimal or no discomfort with acupuncture needle insertion. Because of its sterile packaging techniques, the rate of infection or cross-contamination associated with acupuncture needles is low. Minor adverse events such as soreness and minor bleeding at the insertion site may occur. Acupuncture is also generally considered safe for patients with an underlying bleeding disorder or patients who are currently utilizing anticoagulant medications. Major adverse events such as organ puncture have been reported but usually associated with practitioner negligence.

Patients may experience improvement of their symptoms even with their first acupuncture treatment, but many patients require series of treatments to achieve their therapeutic goal. Patients may require 6–10 sessions of initial treatment with subsequent intermittent treatments to maintain its therapeutic benefit.

As the evidence of its therapeutic benefit grows, many commercial insurance providers in the United States now cover acupuncture as a viable treatment modality for many health conditions. However, limitations of coverage may still be applicable. Insurers may pose limits on the number of treatments per timeframe, health conditions covered, necessity for a referral from a healthcare provider, and possible out-of-pocket costs. Medicare continues not to cover acupuncture services. Coverage from Medicaid continues to be dependent on the individual state.

Evidence of Efficacy (Include a Table)

No single mechanism is able to explain how acupuncture is able to influence physiologic function observed in clinical practice. Multiple theories have been proposed to explain the physiologic effects of acupuncture. Some of the theories are able to explain the acute physiologic benefits seen with acupuncture but unable to explain the subacute and chronic benefits observed in clinical practice. One of the more popular theories includes the gate control theory of pain where acupuncture needles are able to inhibit the transmission of pain signals to the brain via the spinal cord. Other theories include the endorphin model where acupuncture needles are able to trigger the release endogenous opioids in the central nervous system to mitigate pain and the neurotransmitter model where acupuncture needles can alter the release of certain neurotransmitters in the central nervous system resulting in physiologic effects. Current research is able to observe the physiologic changes seen with acupuncture via imaging studies such as functional MRI scans and able to measure changes in the endogenous opioid levels following acupuncture therapy. In addition, there are distinct differences in the electrical conductivity of the tissue that have been observed between acupuncture points and adjacent tissue that may help to explain how the body is able to communicate with itself.

Decades of acupuncture research has been able to demonstrate its efficacy for pain related and non-pain-related health conditions. Although there continues to be methodologic challenges in conducting randomized controlled trials with acupuncture (e.g., lack of double-blinded trials as the acupuncture provider knows which patient is receiving true vs. sham-acupuncture), there is ample evidence in literature to support its use in clinical practice. Table 99.1 helps to summarize health conditions where literature has been able to support its efficacy of use.

Pearls and Pitfalls (in Bullet Points)

- Many commercial insurance providers now cover acupuncture services.
- Medicare does not cover acupuncture services.

Table 99.1 Acupuncture may be a useful adjunctive or a stand-alone therapy for management of health conditions associated with pain

Indication	Health condition
Musculoskeletal	Fibromyalgia Osteoarthritis (knee) Back/neck pain Hip pain
Neurologic	Migraine Tension headache Carpal tunnel syndrome
Hematology/oncology	Cancer-associated pain
Surgery	Preoperative anxiety Postoperative pain Postoperative dental pain Postoperative ileus
Gastrointestinal	Nausea and vomiting IBS Constipation
Gynecologic	Hot flashes PMS

IBS irritable bowel syndrome, *PMS* premenstrual syndrome

- Medicaid coverage for acupuncture services depends on the individual state.
- According to TCM paradigm, acupuncture therapy helps to restore the balanced flow of *Qi*.
- Acupuncture is used by many as an adjunctive therapy to conventional methods or as a stand-alone therapy for the management of pain and non-pain-related health conditions.
- Acupuncture is generally considered safe with minimal side effects or adverse events.
- Non-physician licensed acupuncturists provide the bulk of acupuncture therapy; however, other healthcare providers including chiropractors, dentists, and physicians may provide acupuncture services.
- Patients may experience improvement in symptoms even with their first acupuncture treatment, but many patients require series of treatments to achieve their goal.

Recommended Reading

1. A Manual of Acupuncture by Peter Deadman and Mazin Al-Khafaji with Kevin Baker.
2. Between Heaven and Earth: A Guide to Chinese Medicine by Harriet Beinfield and Efrem Korngold.
3. Clinical Introduction to Medical Acupuncture by Steven Aung and William Chen.
4. Li X, et al. Acupuncture for Myofascial Pain Syndrome: A Network Meta-Analysis of 33 Randomized Controlled Trials. Pain Physician. 2017;20:E883–902.
5. The Practice of Chinese Medicine: The Treatment of Diseases With Acupuncture and Chinese Herbs by Giovanni Maciocia.
6. The Web That Has No Weaver: Understanding Chinese Medicineby Ted Kaptchuk.

Part XI

Administrative Considerations

Cybersecurity of Medical Devices: Past, Present, and Future

100

Nameer Haider, Christopher Gates, Vikram Sengupta, and Sascha Qian

Introduction

In today's healthcare industry, the technological infrastructure is built on an outdated bedrock of software and hardware known. Designed in an era predating large-scale hacking and cyberterrorism, the current bedrock is rife with cybersecurity vulnerabilities. These vulnerabilities are further exposed as medical devices are adapted for connectivity in an increasingly interconnected world. Many of these devices were never intended to be connected to the Internet, to each other, or to the cloud. This issue is further complicated by their incorporation into human beings to form a network. As vulnerabilities are identified and exploited, snippets of code known as patches can be written to rectify them. However, the impact of a security patch on an older device can be incomplete, variable, and unpredictable.

Leo Scanlon, the deputy chief information security officer at the United States Department of Health and Human Services, has stated that the "healthcare sector is particularly sensitive to cyberattacks upon the 'Internet of things' (IOT), because many healthcare-related devices were not developed with the intention of being on the Internet. It was never intended they would be able to talk to other devices, yet they are." Here, the Internet of things are defined as the network of electronic devices and physical objects embedded with sensors and actuators, which are linked through wired and wireless networks; examples include roadways, pacemakers, and remote cameras (see Fig. 100.1). An extension of this concept is the "Internet of bodies," which is comprised of the devices that are attached to or implanted into the human body. Due to development and expansion of "Internet of bodies," medical device cybersecurity vulnerabilities pose an unprecedented and growing threat to human beings and their health.

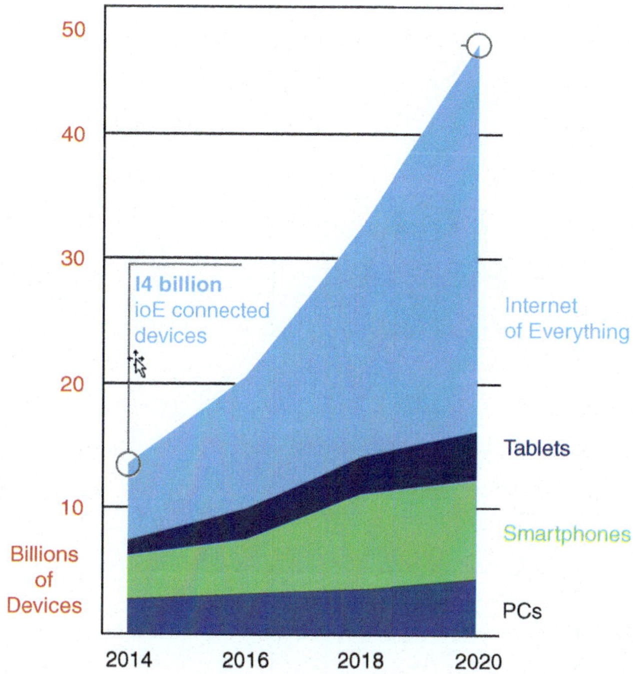

Fig. 100.1 Internet of things from 2014 to projected 2020. Proliferation of Internet of things-driven devices shows exponential growth

The fear of hacking medical devices has been present for years (see Fig. 100.2). Former United States Vice President Dick Cheney famously had the Wi-Fi on his cardiac pacemaker turned off in 2007 to preempt hacking and cyberattack. Indeed, from a cybersecurity standpoint, medical devices are largely built upon older, outdated, "legacy" technology and therefore cannot be easily updated with cybersecurity software. Consequently, to ensure compatibility with modern cybersecurity technology, most medical devices must either undergo core hardware and software redesign or be discarded entirely. Delays in the passage of federal legislative mandates to secure medical devices magnify the problem of legacy incompatibility daily.

N. Haider (✉) · V. Sengupta · S. Qian
Spinal & Skeletal Pain Medicine, Utica, NY, USA
e-mail: drhaider@killpain.com; drsengupta@killpain.com; drqian@killpain.com

C. Gates
Velentium LLC, Katy, TX, USA
e-mail: chris.gates@velentium.com

T. R. Deer et al. (eds.), *Deer's Treatment of Pain*, https://doi.org/10.1007/978-3-030-12281-2_100

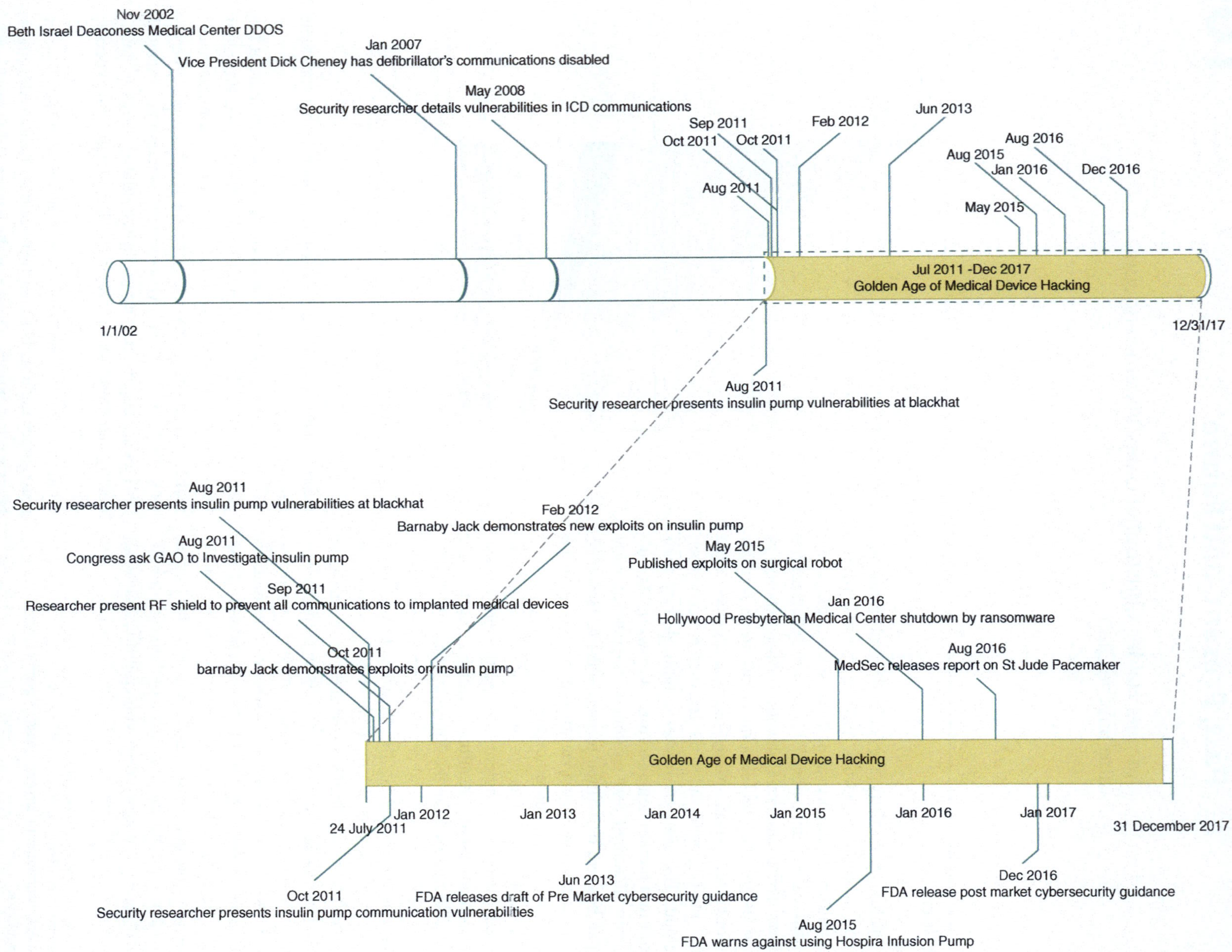

Fig. 100.2 Timeline of medical device security concerns and hacking from 2002 to 2017. The sentinel event was Beth Israel Deaconess Medical Center distributed denial-of-service (DDOS) attack in 2002. In 2007, Vice President Dick Cheney has his defibrillator's communications disabled preemptively. In May 2008, British and Belgian security researchers detail vulnerabilities in implantable cardiac defibrillator (ICD) communications. The Golden Age of medical device hacking then occurred between July 2011 and December 2017; this period included revelation of insulin pump vulnerabilities prompting the Government Accountability Office (GAO) investigations in addition to the shutdown of Hollywood Presbyterian Hospital by ransomware

In the Cybersecurity Act of 2015, Congress established the Healthcare Industry Cybersecurity Task Force to address the challenges the healthcare industry faces when securing and protecting itself against cybersecurity threats. In June 2017, this task force published a report entitled "Improving Cybersecurity in the Healthcare Industry"—one significant resolution was that the healthcare industry should "dramatically reduce the use of less defensible legacy and unsupported products and more effectively reduce risk in future products through robust development and support strategies." The report further elaborated by stating that in their present state, many healthcare organizations will be unable to identify or act upon potential threats as they do not have the resources nor experience to address the emerging security threats. Furthermore, these healthcare organizations may not even recognize the attack in time.

The cybersecurity of medical devices that are "embedded" in patients (henceforth referred to as "embedded medical devices") typically involves many more complexities than those that arise in the domain of management information systems and information technology (MIS/IT). Due to the age, evolution, and inherent nature of the Internet, the domain of MIS/IT is viewed by cybersecurity specialists as a "naturally occurring object," to which security mitigations are added as an afterthought. While the common security topics of confidentiality, integrity, and availability can be applied to both the MIS/IT and embedded medical devices, each applies to each in an entirely unique manner.

Physical Security

In the MIS/IT domain, physical security is achieved by keeping unauthorized personnel away from a server through the use of physical barriers, the simplest manifestation being a locked door. However, an embedded medical device must travel from place to place with its human host and therefore cannot be secured in such a simple manner. Therefore, a number of alternative mechanisms must to be designed and deployed into medical devices to enforce the confidentiality of sensitive information and integrity of executable programs. Examples include patient data utilized in device communication and storage of these valuable device assets.

While advances that increase remote connectivity of medical devices often enhance the quality of patient care, each modification introduces new security risks that must also be carefully assessed and minimized. In 2013, the FDA issued guidance on the use of radiofrequency for wireless medical devices, including a recommendation for authentication and encryption protocols as measures to reduce patient safety and security risks.

Available Resources

Inherent differences in resource utilization and availability lead to distinct cybersecurity issues in the information security and embedded medical device domains. Network servers tend to occupy a fixed location and can be physically augmented to fit their computational needs. Therefore, they can theoretically consume an unlimited supply of power and computational resources, including central processing unit throughput, memory, and time. In contrast, embedded medical devices are miniaturized, physically discrete, and battery powered. They cannot exploit an unlimited and flexible supply of energy, memory, and computational power for core and security operations. Consideration of these unique challenges must be made for the design and implementation of effective medical device security mechanisms.

Highly Fractured Landscape of Standards

MIS/IT utilize international communication standards to ensure interoperability on the Internet. These original standards focused on ensuring Internet communications seamlessly occur, with security being an afterthought, in addition to securing data that is being communicated while ignoring security of data.

The Cybersecurity Act of 2015 Congress established the Healthcare Industry Cybersecurity Task Force to address the challenges faced when securing and protecting against intentional or unintentional cybersecurity incidents.

Agencies involved in formulating medical device standards include the Food and Drug Administration (FDA), Health Insurance Portability and Accountability Act of 1996 (HIPAA), Center for Devices and Radiological Health (CDRH), National Institute of Standards and Technology (NIST), National Cybersecurity Center of Excellence (NCCoE), Information Sharing and Analysis Organizations (ISAOs), Health Information Trust Alliance (HITRUST), Department of Health and Human Services (HHS), and Department of Homeland Security (DHS).

The FDA, in conjunction with the Center for Devices and Radiological Health (CDRH), established a cybersecurity risk management program, making cybersecurity paramount and creating a trusted environment for information sharing. With very few exceptions, the FDA has facilitated implementation of cybersecurity into medical devices by not requiring premarket review or recall of software updates for cybersecurity. A vulnerability disclosure policy and coordinated disclosure are critical to improving security; however, the FDA will not be prescriptive with risk analyses and instead will evaluate the well-being of community as a whole.

In October 2016, the FDA entered into a new memorandum of understanding with the National Health Information Sharing and Analysis Center (NH-ISAC) and the Medical Device Innovation, Safety and Security Consortium (MDISS). The NH-ISAC is a nonprofit organization that coordinates cybersecurity incidence response by providing member organizations with actionable information on cybersecurity. The MDISS is a nonprofit organization that develops best practices in cybersecurity. The final FDA guidance, released on December 2016, recommends structured and comprehensive management of post-market cybersecurity vulnerabilities for medical devices throughout their product life cycle. In January 2017, the FDA held a webinar on the guidance: Postmarket Management of Cybersecurity in Medical Devices. In May 2017, the FDA partnered with the National Science Foundation (NSF) and the Department of Homeland Security Science and Technology to hold a public workshop "Cybersecurity of Medical Devices: A Regulatory Science Gap Analysis," with the goal of strengthening medical device cybersecurity.

HIPAA includes both privacy and security standards. The HIPAA security rule includes the Security Standards for the Protection of Electronic Protected Health Information (the Security Rule) and establishes a national set of security standards for protecting electronic health information.

National Institute of Standards and Technology (NIST), through the National Cybersecurity Center of Excellence (NCCoE), works to secure networked medical devices from risks such as malware, hacking, and access control. The NCCoE works with industry, academic, and government experts to find practical solutions for businesses cybersecurity needs. Mitre Corporation, awarded a contract to support NCCoE as the first federally funded research and development center dedicated to cybersecurity, works to support relationships and collaboration between government sponsors, industry, and academia.

Nongovernmental organizations such as the Information Sharing Analysis Standards Organization (ISAO) work with federal entities responsible for conducting cybersecurity and related activities to create national networks with automated mechanisms for information sharing. Presidential Executive Order 13691 encourages the development of the Information Sharing Analysis Standards Organization (ISAO) to serve as focal points for cybersecurity information sharing. MedISAO, an organization composed of members of the medical device community, is a registered ISAO providing compliance with the FDA's recommendation in the post-market management of cybersecurity in medical devices.

The Health Information Trust Alliance (HITRUST) is a privately held company located in the United States that, in collaboration with technology, healthcare, and information security leaders, has established a Common Security Framework (CSF) which may be used by organizations that create, access, store, or exchange sensitive or regulated data. Common Security Framework (CSF) includes a prescriptive set of controls which seek to harmonize the requirements of multiple regulations and standards—this helps organizations by providing an efficient and prescriptive framework for managing the security requirements of HIPAA. In a sense, this creates a voluntary industry-managed approach to meeting the HIPAA security rule requirements. Using globally recognized standards such as the HIPAA, the HITRUST provides clear updated actionable guidelines consistent with the latest healthcare industry and government regulations.

What Are the Risks?

Medical device security risks are shared across all domains, including medical device manufacturers, hospitals, clinics, healthcare providers, research institutions, software companies, public and private insurance carriers, and patients. Digital connectivity is required for the healthcare system to deliver safe and effective care. A connected but insecure healthcare system could cause unnecessary risk and jeopardize patient safety.

Medical device manufacturers have the luxury of creating medical devices with unique methods of storage and proprietary communication protocols, without regard to worldwide standards. Unfortunately, device manufacturers have not employed such methods thus far, since the security risks have been largely unrecognized or intentionally disregarded. Making the decision to prioritize cybersecurity within the medical device industry requires a critical shift in cognitive framework from corporate leadership.

Frequent cases of ransomware, identity theft, and targeted nation-state hacking remind and show us that our healthcare data is vulnerable. Data collected to treat patients can be used for nefarious purposes such as fraud, identity theft, supply chain disruptions, intellectual property theft, and stock manipulation. Most importantly, cybersecurity attacks disrupt patient care. For example, ransomware is typically a malicious software that either threatens to publish patient data or blocks access unless a ransom is paid.

Most medical device manufacturers face significant resource constraints as operating margins can be very low, and cybersecurity infrastructure is a very small portion of their overall budget. Due to previously believing that their cybersecurity vulnerability was low and lack of qualified and experienced staff, manufacturers often lack the ability to identify, track, analyze, audit, and translate threat data into actionable information. Given the increasing frequency of system compromises by ransomware, the reality of cybersecurity vulnerability can no longer be avoided. In light of such recent events, medical device manufacturers thus have increased their own education and awareness as it has been made clearly evident that risk mitigation can save money, prevent litigation, and protect against damages to the corporate reputation.

Patient Safety

The most obvious and serious risk of inadequate device security is to patient safety. The hacking of a medical device is extremely difficult to ascertain unless the attacker publicly admits to it. This may in fact have some bearing upon why we are as of yet unaware of anyone dying from a hacked medical device.

A recent report from security firm WhiteScope analyzed seven different pacemaker programmers from four different manufacturers and found more than 8600 flaws in pacemaker systems and the third-party libraries that power various components of the devices. Outdated libraries in pacemaker programmer software set therapy parameters and monitor device function. Problems found included lack of encryption and authentication, bugs in the code, and poor design that can put patient lives at risk. These design flaws highlight the need for a complete overhaul of basic medical device design.

In 2015, Hospira and an independent researcher confirmed the possibility of accessing the Symbiq Infusion System remotely through a hospital's network. In May 2015, the FDA issued a Safety Communication on vulnerabilities of Hospira LifeCare PCA3 and PCA5 Infusion Pump Systems after an independent researcher released information about these vulnerabilities.

In January 2017, the FDA issued a Safety Communication confirming vulnerabilities in St. Jude Medical's implantable cardiac devices and Merlin@home Transmitter. Subsequently in April 2017, the FDA sent a warning letter to Abbott charging the medical device manufacturer with failing to reveal a deadly defect with defibrillators marketed by St. Jude Medical, which was acquired by Abbott. The main issue was that St. Jude downplayed battery failure in its cardiac defibrillators and continued to ship devices despite evidence of rapid battery depletion. These issues led to a patient death which St. Jude failed to disclose this death to the FDA. Following a second warning letter from the FDA, the company recalled the remaining devices in question.

Thereafter, in August 29, 2017, the FDA issued a Safety Communication informing patients and healthcare providers about the release of a firmware update to address cybersecurity vulnerabilities. Abbott has told patients with affected defibrillators to register with St. Jude's MerlinHome Monitoring System, which itself had significant cybersecurity flaws. The FDA is urging all heart transplant patients who have received a St. Jude pacemaker to contact their healthcare provider and receive a software update to protect their device from being hacked which could drain battery power or administer inappropriate pacing. If the company doesn't correct the violations, the FDA could serve the company with an injunction, seizure, or monetary fine.

The Smiths Medical Medfusion 4000 device was recently found to have serious hackable flaws, which would allow a remote attacker to gain unauthorized access and impact the operation of the pump. The Department of Homeland Security (DHS) identified eight vulnerabilities in three versions of the device and cited issues which can allow a cybercriminal to execute a dangerous code and cause an overdose of medication administered.

Exposure of Patient Protected Health Information

Medical information can be used to defraud individuals and organizations, including identity theft and secondary attacks against patients. Such theft can have negative consequences on hospitals, clinics, and healthcare providers in the form of fines from the Department of Health and Human Services (HHS) and crippling legal actions from the Federal Trade Commission. In one recent incidence, actual unencrypted data that included Social Security numbers, names, and medical and patient data of a well-known hospital on the east coast was left exposed on a pacemaker programmer. With about 112 million records stolen in 2015, the medical information of nearly half all Americans is already on the dark web.

The Office for Civil Rights in the US Department of Health and Human Services issued guidance, via "HHS Fact Sheet," to help healthcare entities understand and respond to ransomware attacks. According to the HHS Fact Sheet, there had been 4000 daily ransomware attacks since early 2016. According to a 2017 report from Aite Group/Trend Micro, the black market value of a stolen credit card number with CVV is about $1 and a username and password on Amazon or Uber $2–$4, and a stolen medical record is valued at between $20 and $50.

Denial of Service

Denial of service attacks may prevent the operation of a device or all devices in a hospital until a ransom has been paid. This has recently become quite popular due to the ease of accomplishing this and the low risk being taken by the attacker. This can be devastating to a hospital, clinic, healthcare provider, and patient who may need the uninterrupted use of a medical device. It is predicted that future attacks will come through preplanted malware.

Exposure of Intellectual Property

Medical devices are physical implementations of concepts and algorithms. These algorithms require years of clinical study and analysis to derive and thus have value to the manufacturer's competitors. Exposure of these algorithms by attacking a single device to extract the program code is frequently performed and usually trivial in nature. However, this attack can also be the first in a series of attacks if the analysis of the exposed software discovers additional vulnerabilities that can be exploited.

Negative Public Relations and Loss of Public Confidence

Widespread public condemnation about handling of medical device hacks may negatively affect future medical device sales and corporate stock prices due to loss of consumer confidence. Such lapses in ability to adequately secure patient safety may ultimately lead to regulatory and consumer concerns affecting hospitals, clinics, vendors, and healthcare professionals. In one recent example, St. Jude Medical (STJ) corporation shares lost value and jeopardized the planned acquisition by Abbott Corporation due to allegations by the Carson Block's research firm Muddy Waters that STJ would lose more than half of its revenue due to device recalls.

Manufacturer Liability

Medical devices with cybersecurity lapses may expose manufacturers to significant liability. A bipartisan group of US senators have introduced legislation to address cybersecurity vulnerabilities in computing devices. Such future legislation may create liability for medical device manufacturers and their Board of Directors created by their vulnerable devices. The FDA has stated that manufacturers are legally required to comply with all applicable regulations and are subject to pre- and post-market cybersecurity guidance that articulates a comprehensive, structured, and systematic cybersecurity risk management program.

What Can We Learn from the Past?

Inception of medical device hacking is relatively recent, with the majority of events occurring since 2011 (see Fig. 100.2). Thereafter, significant progress has been achieved in securing new medical devices, which have been demonstrated in a more regulated environment.

Due to the long life span of the average medical device, it may be years before an older insecure medical devices are replaced by newer secure medical devices. Several proposals have been suggested to accelerate the replacement process, such as "cash for clunkers," where the government buys back older insecure medical devices. This is obviously not the concept of choice for surgically implanted medical devices. The FDA's 2017 recall of 465,000 Abbott Laboratories pacemakers alerted all medical device manufacturers that they should take cybersecurity issues more seriously and be more proactive in development and introduction of security updates.

What Are the Current Best Practices to Mitigate Risk Today?

Unfortunately, in the majority of medical device development life cycles, if security of the finished product is even considered, it is addressed in an unstructured approach. This typically manifest itself as someone during the design phase making a short and incomplete list of known security exploits, which are usually too vague to be traced throughout the development life cycle and so very little is done during the design and implementation portions of the project. After device development and testing have been completed, the device is sent out to independent third party for penetration testing where a "hacker for hire" documents all the methods used to subvert the security on the device. Since this information is arriving very late in the medical device development cycle, when schedules and budgets are typically exhausted, there is usually nothing to be done about such discovered vulnerabilities. Such a process has led to the current state of insecurity.

Where Do We Want to Be Tomorrow?

Currently, thought leaders in the medical device industry are following a more structured approach integrating security into their normal software development life cycle (see Fig. 100.3). Most of the added activities are new work items to be performed by regular development teams, with potential assistance in product security subject matter by security experts and consultants. The work is auditable and repeatable and focuses on the root cause of all actual and potential vulnerabilities in the end product, including software description, hazards, requirements, design specifications, traceability, development environment, verification, validation, revision history, unresolved anomalies, and documentation such as even premarket submissions for software contained in medical devices.

Medical device manufacturers must consider and plan for cybersecurity at medical design inception rather than add

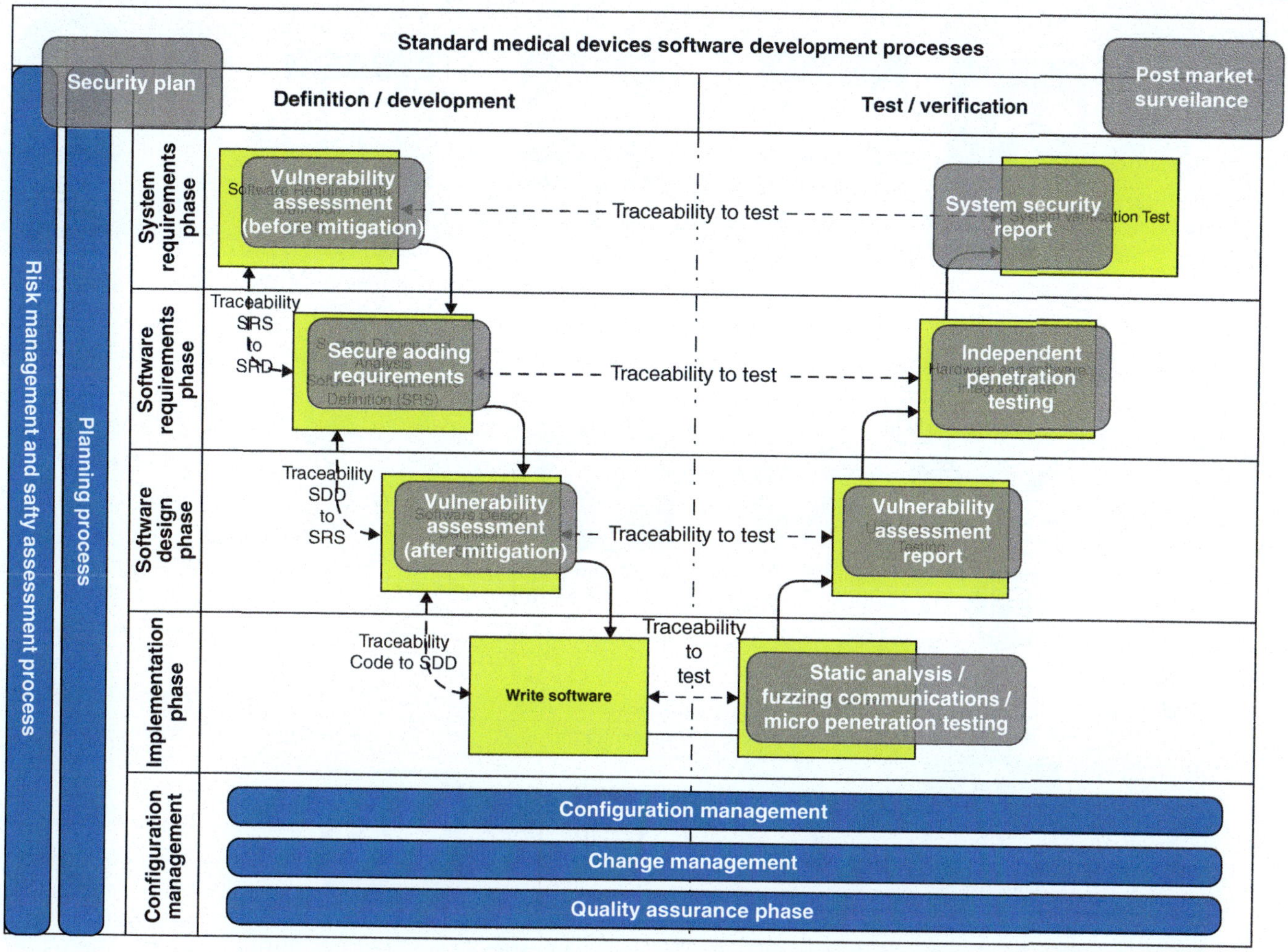

Fig. 100.3 Standard medical device software development process revolves around repeatable work and the root cause of all actual and potential vulnerabilities in the end product, including software description, hazards, requirements, design specifications, traceability, development environment, verification, validation, revision history, unresolved anomalies, and documentation such as even premarket submissions for software contained in medical devices

security to a device as an afterthought after the design process has been completed. Medical device manufacturers should adopt policies of good cybersecurity with risk mitigation occurring during the total product life cycle from conception to obsolescence. Integration and information sharing are imperative with all stakeholders identifying, protecting, detecting, and responding to cyber threats.

Vulnerabilities

Vulnerabilities can be created at the three following distinct points when a new device is being developed: (1) design, (2) implementation, and (3) post-market discovery in software libraries. Breaking out the activities in the Secure Development Lifecycle based upon these three areas of weakness details the activities to be performed (see Fig. 100.4)

Communications Infrastructure

The Internet was not originally designed as a robust and secure structure for communications. The exposure of databases on the Internet is partially the fault of this old aging infrastructure. What is needed is an "end-to-end" solution for securing data from its point of inception through multiple forms of communications and storage, including an end user who is authenticated to see only the proper data that has been aggregated (see Fig. 100.5). We are only now seeing tools for achieving this level of control of the data, as opposed to the control of the communications. This is happening at a time, which the latest available electronics for medical devices has been scaled up to support world-class cryptographic capabilities used for this type of data control.

Blockchain technology, an ingenious invention that allows digital information to be distributed but not copied, has recently been touted as the holy grail of cybersecurity.

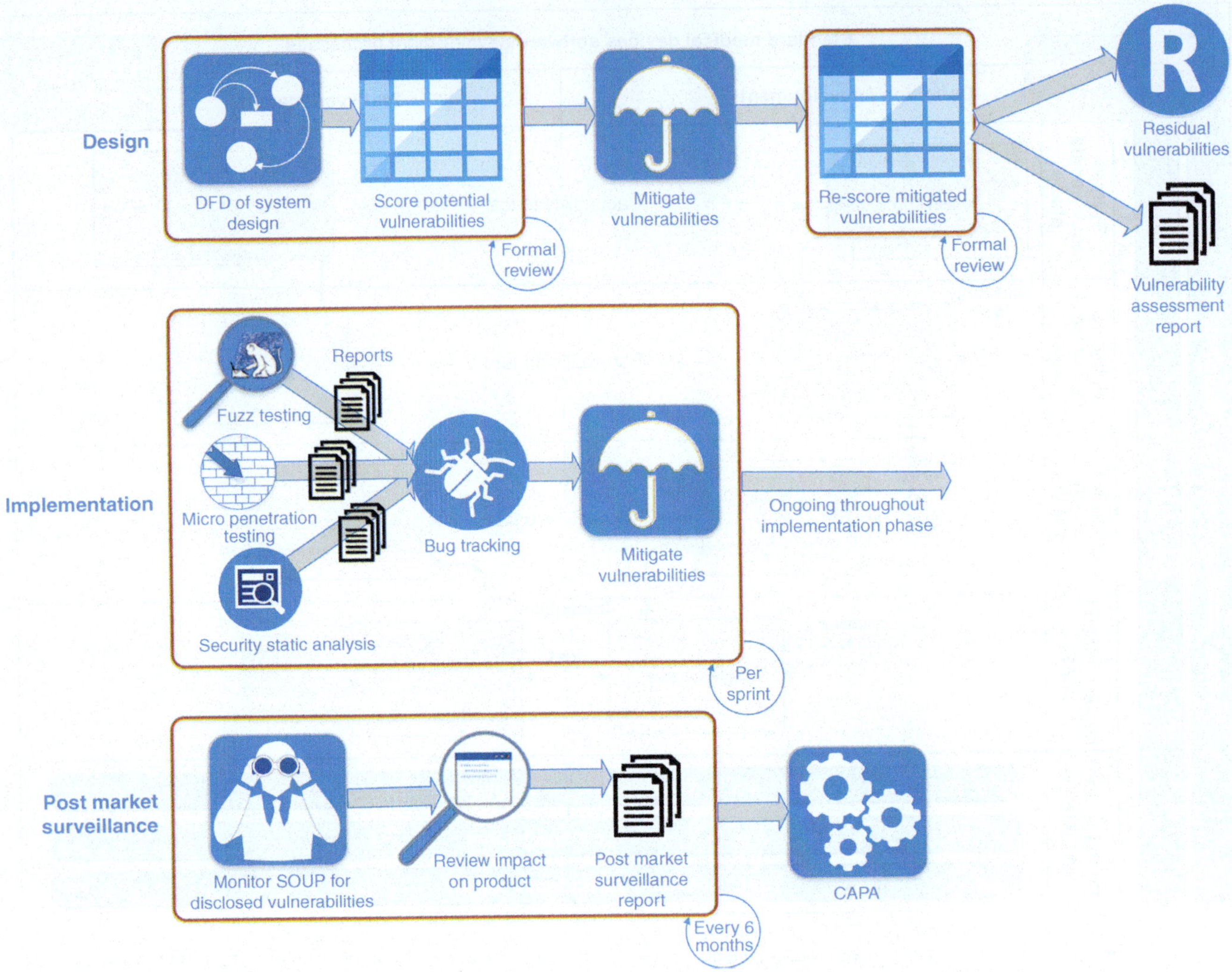

Fig. 100.4 Design, implementation, and post-market discovery are distinct points of vulnerability when a new device is being developed

Blockchain's original mandate was solely to prevent double payments on Bitcoin but has since evolved into a more generalizable security product. Unfortunately, because blockchain is still focused on encryption as the solution, the functionality is somewhat heavyweight. As encryption is only a subcomponent of cybersecurity, it would be impossible for the healthcare industry to discard existing systems and re-implement new systems on a blockchain architecture.

To date, cybersecurity has focused on securing infrastructure including security of hardware, networks, applications, devices, and identities. Perimeter security, the classic moat around the castle approach, is provided to computer networks. The network moat includes firewalls, sniffers, vulnerability scanning, and intrusion detection systems. Once the moat is breached, the network is hopelessly vulnerable. Data loss prevention (DLP) systems track sensitive data exiting or traversing corporate networks, and digital rights management (DRM) systems restrict access to proprietary information, but they do not track all data or data in transit across domains.

Secure File Transfer Protocol (FTP) tracks and manages the transfer of files between networks but uses unencrypted and unauthenticated transmission control protocol connections, creating the ability to eavesdrop, steal passwords, and hijack connections. Secure document vaults protect content in heavily regulated industries like healthcare and financial services but are vulnerable to hacking.

Mobile devices are quickly becoming the primary communications and computing platform for businesses. Mobile device management (MDM) solutions enforce policies for corporate smartphones and tablets but are vulnerable to password theft and unsecured Wi-Fi networks.

Cloud access security brokers (CASBs) are software systems that manage security between an organization's onsite network infrastructure and the cloud to create safe

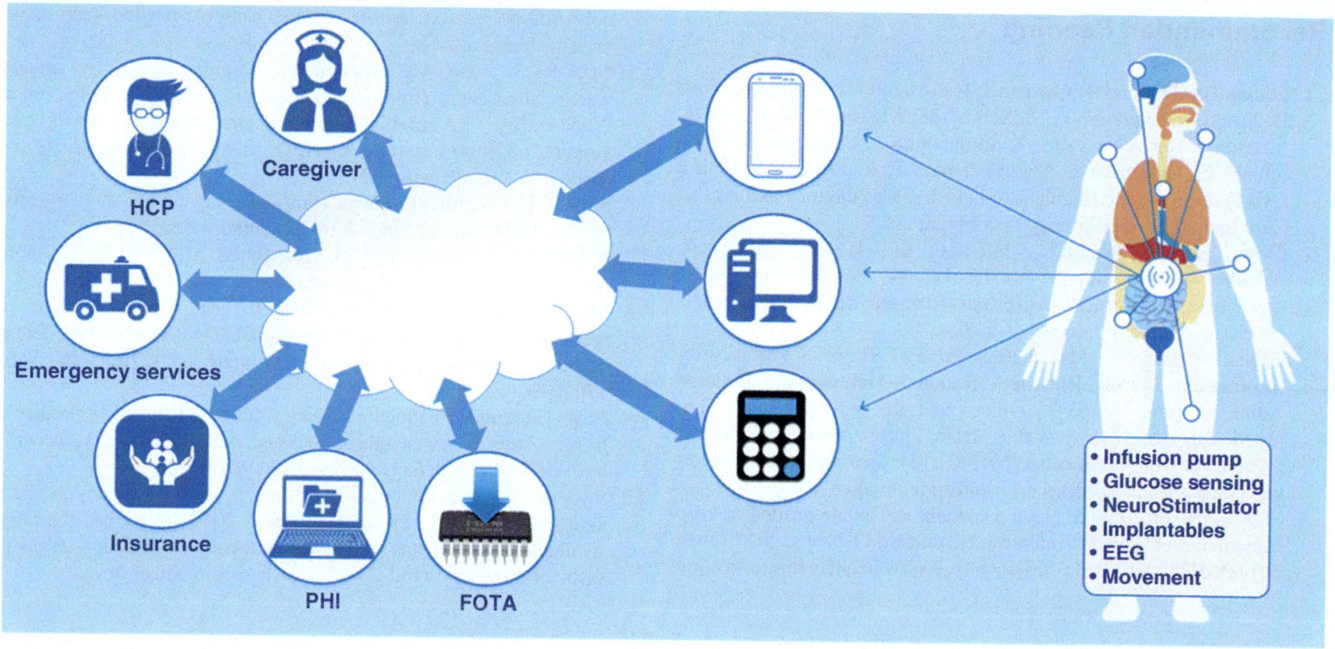

Fig. 100.5 "End-to-end" solution for securing data from its point of inception through multiple forms of communications and storage includes an end user who is authenticated to see only the proper data

environments for exchanging and sharing information. Cloud access security brokers (CASBs) are entirely cloud based or cloud solution only. They are not intended as a network product nor a hybrid product. CASBs data must be stored in the cloud, and data granularity within the CASB is limited to "software as a service" applications within the cloud. Once the cloud security perimeter has been breached, however, the data is still vulnerable.

Data encryption with zero-knowledge privacy means that not only are devices using data encryption but also that only authorized users can access data from a medical device. Identity management must require biometric and other multifactor identification tokens to ensure user true identity and access rights. Behavior analytics must include systems that learn and monitor user behavior patterns, alerting and reacting to any or all unusual activity. Secure and safe medical device connectivity requires Internet security without boundaries across all domains including server, cloud, mobile, and medical devices. Medical devices should have the ability to enforce rules that travel with data including the ability to recall data and access from any system. A secure system should provide tamper-proof granular activity audit reports clearly displaying who is accessing medical device data and how they are using it.

Ransomware protection is also necessary to protect valuable data from ransomware and prevent phishing or social engineering attacks. The medical device manufacturer should utilize a cybersecurity system certified by a recognized organization using industry standards, enabling the medical device to meet multiple regulatory requirements.

True medical device cybersecurity will involve securing the ecosystem's entire infrastructure, including applications, devices, networks, and identities. This can only be truly accomplished by securing the sensitive data itself through its entire life cycle.

To accomplish this, multiple defenses must be implemented including data encryption, identity management, behavioral analytics, data access and recall, granular reporting and audit, and ransomware protection, all while fulfilling regulatory requirements that are continually updated.

Summary

The future seems bright for new product security, with the confluence of new tools and technology available; the potential for attenuating this looming problem looks good. New regulations are required and will be forthcoming to mandate manufacturers to disclose and correct vulnerabilities in their medical devices. This will enable hospitals, clinics, and healthcare professionals to make informed decisions about where to spend their budgets when acquiring new medical devices.

Of course, the "legacy products" will continue to be a problem until they are removed from service. Today, the only way to protect medical devices and secure data is with an ecosystem that spans all domains, allowing the management of data security as if it were on your own domain, including your own medical device. The future of cybersecurity rests in the ability to protect data itself, while at rest, as well as in transit, anywhere in the cyber ecosystem.

Recommended Reading

1. Csulak E, Meadows T, Corman J, DeCesare G, Fernando A, Finn D, Jarrett M, Laybourn L, McNeil M, McWhorter D, Mellinger R, Monson J, Ramadoss, Rice T, Sardanopoli V, Suarez R, Stine K, Sublett C, Thompson L, Ting D, Trotter F. Report on Improving Cybersecurity in the Health Care Industry. Washington, DC: Health Care Industry Cybersecurity Task Force; 2017.
2. Cyber Risk Thursday: Internet of Bodies [Internet]. Atlantic Council. [cited 2017Dec13]. Available from: http://www.atlanticcouncil.org/events/upcoming-events/detail/cyber-risk-thursday-internet-of-bodies.
3. Executive Order – Promoting Private Sector Cybersecurity Information Sharing [Internet]. National Archives and Records Administration. National Archives and Records Administration; [cited 2017Dec13]. Available from: https://obamawhitehouse.archives.gov/the-press-office/2015/02/13/executive-order-promoting-private-sector-cybersecurity-information-shari.
4. FDA to patients with St. Jude pacemakers: Update needed to keep hackers out of devices [Internet]. Healthcare IT News. 2017 [cited 2017Dec13]. Available from: http://www.healthcareitnews.com/news/fda-patients-st-jude-pacemakers-update-needed-keep-hackers-out-devices.
5. Graf R. St. jude (stj) stock down despite response to muddy waters allegations [Internet]. TheStreet. TheStreet; 2016 [cited 2017Dec13]. Available from: https://www.thestreet.com/story/13687004/1/st-jude-stj-stock-down-despite-response-to-muddy-waters-allegations.html.
6. http://www.healthcareitnews.com/news/pacemaker-device-security-audit-finds-8600-flaws-some-potentially-deadly.
7. ICS-CERT Advisories I ICS-CERT. [cited 2017Dec13]. Available from: https://ics-cert.us-cert.gov/advisories/ICSMA-17-250-02.
8. Modern Healthcare [Internet]. Abbott recall signals new era in medical-device cybersecurity. [cited 2017Dec13]. Available from: http://www.modernhealthcare.com/article/20170901/NEWS/170909986.
9. News [Internet]. Healthcare IT News. [cited 2017Dec13]. Available from: https://www.healthcareitnews.com/news/device-maker-was-hush-defibrillator-defect-killed-patients-fda-says.
10. Sweeney E. Cash for clunkers: Could it work for legacy medical devices? [Internet]. FierceHealthcare. 2017 [cited 2017Dec13]. Available from: https://www.fiercehealthcare.com/privacy-security/cash-for-clunkers-could-it-work-for-legacy-medical-devices.

Coding and Billing

101

Tina Rivenbark and Jeffrey Peterson

Introduction

The promotion of patient-centered care offers many advantages in the healthcare process seemingly for all stakeholders: patients, providers, and payors. When patients are encouraged to take a more active role in their own care, they report increased satisfaction both with their providers and the services received. Additionally, treatment quality tends to increase and outcomes often improve.

Despite careful consideration and collaboration between the patient and provider, health plans often derail the thoughtful plans for care that are arrived upon with utilization management programs such as prior authorization and step therapy. These cost-cutting measures imposed by payors often result in delays of necessary treatment and can negatively impact treatment outcomes. In this age of technology when we can answer any question in the world with the smartphone we hold in a hand, it is clear payors are using the continued burdensome task of obtaining a prior authorization manually to further delay the payment process.

The integrity of the prior authorization process has become increasingly challenging in recent years. Clinical determinations are not always based upon the most current scientific data, but rather are more frequently cost driven. Exceptions to standard treatment protocols frequently go unaddressed or are not addressed in a timely fashion. Even after maneuvering the pitfalls of the prior authorization system, providers undoubtedly get the "escape clause" recited stating the authorization is not a guarantee of payment after all. To improve this process for both patients and providers, the process should be automated, appeals to denials should be fair and timely, and coverage once authorized should be guaranteed if services are performed within a stated time period.

Recently the third largest insurance provider in the country came under heated scrutiny when Dr. Jay Ken Iinuma, the Aetna medical director for the state of California, testified under oath in the presence of the insurance commissioner that he never once reviewed a patient chart.

If payors were vested in improving the process, there are a number of options that could be explored. To make quality and timely patient care a priority, payors could offer providers a physician-driven, clinically based alternative to the prior authorization process. Perhaps a "preferred provider" program or attestation to use of clinical decision support systems or clinical pathways could offer providers options for meeting treatment goals while avoiding the laborious current requirements. Additionally, providers who contract with payors in financial risk-sharing programs such as ACOs should be exempt from prior authorizations and step therapy requirements since they are already incentivized to contain costs.

Once a provider has moved beyond the authorization process, the battle is only half won. There are a number of keys to coding that providers must consider to help ensure an optimal revenue cycle. This starts with the provider as accurate documentation is the foundation for a successful, clean claim. Few physicians enjoy the increasingly burdensome tasks of charting. Electronic health record (EHR) templates can ease these burdens somewhat by making population of repetitive information a bit easier. High producers in their field find they experienced increased productivity and reduced frustration when they invest the time and resources on the front-end customizing templates for the needs of their processes. The increased efficiency enjoyed by using these templates does not allow providers to evade customized notes for each encounter.

T. Rivenbark (✉)
Advanced Practice Solutions, Wilmington, NC, USA
e-mail: tina@theapsllc.com

J. Peterson
COO, Center for Pain Relief, Inc. & The Spine and Nerve Centers of the Virginias, Charleston, WV, USA
e-mail: jpeterson@centerforpainrelief.com

T. R. Deer et al. (eds.), *Deer's Treatment of Pain*, https://doi.org/10.1007/978-3-030-12281-2_101

The Authorization Process

Authorization staff must ask specific questions regarding approval to the patient's insurer. General questioning increases the likelihood of error, including a retroactive denial of service or denial of payment from the carrier. All discussions with the insurer should be carefully documented, including, time, date, and names of representatives with whom the conversation has occurred. It may be helpful for the practice to develop an authorization checklist to ensure that all items have been discussed. On appropriate approval, the patient may then be scheduled for the procedure.

With the rise in Recovery Audit Contractor (RAC) and private payor audits, it has never been more important to ensure chart documentation is not only thorough but also accurate. Well-educated coders who know anatomy and understand procedures performed by interventional practitioners are paramount. These skilled administrative staff should understand the payors' expectations, recognize errors, and be proficient in extracting information from the note and assigning the correct code. Certified professional coders (CPC) should be kept current through continuing medical education and timely updates of changes by payors. Communication between providers and coders on corrections, changes, and updates helps to ensure integrity throughout the process. Finally, providers shouldn't discount the value of external chart audits. These valuable tools not only help to identify charting deficiencies that could prove to be costly if the practice should face a payor audit; external audits may also shed light on under-coding potentially giving the practice the opportunity to recover reduced or omitted revenue opportunity.

The Importance of Documentation of Neurostimulation

Appropriate documentation and coding for neurostimulation procedures are not only imperative for maintaining chart integrity but also to ensure reimbursement and mitigate financial and legal liability risk. Because of regionally diverse payor- and carrier-related issues, this chapter presents an overview of coding and billing topics.

It is also important to note that regulations pertaining to coding and billing changes are updated routinely; all readers are strongly encouraged to refer to their local carrier policies for the latest information. Although codes and reimbursement policies will certainly continue to change, proper documentation as a measure of practice health and stability remains a staple of practice management that demands daily attention.

Proper Documentation and Medical Necessity

Medical necessity should be documented in the office notes or operative preamble. This documentation should include the disease state, pain characteristics, functional limitations, and degree of suffering. Additional documentation should include failed treatments such as physical therapy, medications, injections, and previous surgical efforts. Any current options should be addressed, and a decision to move forward with the device should be noted. The surgical documentation should not only represent justification for necessity but should contain complete, concise data that support what the practitioner billed and why. An example of this documentation would be "Before this spinal cord trial the patient underwent medical management with oral medications from different classes (list classes), injections (list injections), physical medicine, and other (list other options). The patient had no acceptable surgical options and wished to move forward. Informed consent was obtained, and the patient was taken to the procedure area."

Spinal Cord Stimulation

All patients must meet clinical criteria, and medical necessity should be documented extensively in the patient record. Note that billing for removal of the trial percutaneous leads is not appropriate if no surgical incision and no surgical anchoring were performed in the initial placement. These codes were created specifically for trial leads that were placed using the "cutdown" technique. The global period for the listed surgical codes is 10 days. Wound checks and physical examinations are not typically billable for the first 10 days after placement of the spinal cord stimulation (SCS) system.

Peripheral Nerve Stimulation

To bill these codes, the patient should meet clinical criteria, and medical necessity should be well documented in the record. Please note that it is inappropriate to bill for the removal of the percutaneous electrode leads placed for the trial that are removed in the office setting. The removal codes are intended for leads that have been placed by surgical cutdown and require open surgical removal. Remember that it is appropriate for the physician to bill for the array, not the electrodes. Therefore, if two arrays are tunneled separately to provide stimulation to dual areas, the practitioner can attach either the 51 (multiple procedures) or 59 (distinct procedural service) modifiers, per carrier requirements. The surgical codes listed in the table fall under the 10-day global period. As with SCS, this period applies to wound checks, examinations, and other areas of management regarding the peripheral nerve stimulation system. In some cases, insurers do not understand the procedure being performed with peripheral nerve stimulation. This had led to some denials based on an "experimental therapies" designation. Peripheral nerve stimulation is not experimental; it has been done for many years, and clinical evidence supports its use. It is important for the implanter to educate the medical director of the insurance company about this therapy.

Tools for Billing Compliance

When billing more than one procedure, always refer to the Correct Coding Initiative (CCI) edits updated quarterly on the Centers for Medicare and Medicaid Services (CMS) website. If the code combinations are bundled, it may not be appropriate to bill the codes together; however, the appropriate use of modifiers may allow for the coding combinations selected by the physician. Many Medicare intermediaries have local coverage determination (LCD) guidelines in effect for their various states. The carrier in the local jurisdiction of the practice has those policies available for review. In the absence of local policy, check the CMS website for national coverage determination (NCD) policy. The NCD for electrical nerve stimulators for back or leg pain includes "surgery" as a required modality that must have been attempted (and failed) before implantation. If the patient was not a surgical candidate, it should be documented that surgery was considered and was not pursued because:

- No surgical lesions existed.
- The patient is contraindicated for surgery.
- The patient does not wish to pursue surgery.

If the clinician's medical record does not indicate to the satisfaction of the insurer why surgery was not selected as a treatment for this patient, the claim may be denied for medical necessity. If the patient's clinical picture does not meet the clinical criteria in a manner of certainty, the patient may be asked to take financial responsibility. Most commercial insurance carriers have individual policy regarding coverage of the neurostimulation procedure. Check with the individual carrier regarding those requirements before the service. The physician may want to consider generating a letter of predetermination. Document the medical condition of the patient and the procedures believed to be beneficial and why. List patient history, failed therapies and treatments, medications and adverse reactions, and the patient's functional ability in a detailed, comprehensive report. The insurer does not know the patient or his or her condition; thus, the more relevant documentation that can be provided, the better. Keep in mind that a service that has been precertified or preauthorized by an insurance company is still not a guarantee of payment.

Setting

In many circumstances the neurostimulation procedure is not billable at an office location; these services are usually billed in a hospital or ambulatory surgery center facility setting. Some payors do allow the procedures to be performed in the office setting, with a payment differential provided to the physician providing the services. The amount of reimbursement based on the trial or permanent implant stage varies. The implanter and the staff should ensure that the insurance company understands both the setting and the equipment required to achieve the implant.

Facility Billing

Medicare part B pays the facility fee to certified ambulatory surgical centers (ASCs) for services listed on the Medicare coverage list. Approximately 2400 surgical procedures are paid under "Groupers." If multiple procedures are done at the same setting, expect a reduction of 50% for the additional service. The higher grouper will be paid at 100%. "Add-on" codes are usually reduced 50% as well, although some private payors only pay one facility fee, no matter how many levels the physician treats. The device would be billed separately by the facility or ASC. Hospital facility or part A billing typically submits medical claims under revenue codes. As with an ASC, the devices are billed separately. The device codes used by CMS are listed in the *Healthcare Common Procedure Coding System (HCPCS), National Level II Medicare Codes* book. It is important to remember that not all commercial carriers use this same coding system for the devices as Medicare uses. Checking with each carrier before billing for the devices regarding the codes they accept and pay is necessary. As with all procedure codes, check coding resource books each year for possible changes in either the code or code description. Remember that facility and physician billing are very different. When a physician submits his claim with a single code for the lead or "array" (63650), the facility can submit the claims per electrode.

Common Errors in Billing

The most common billing errors made for these procedures are lack of supporting documentation to establish medical necessity and failure to predetermine if the insurance will cover the service. Costs are present at the time of implant and also going forward. There is typically a lifetime commitment to follow-up care, which includes analysis, reprogramming, and adjustments. Therefore, it is imperative that each aspect of these procedures be addressed.

Conclusion

The advent of patient-centered care planning offers the opportunity for an improved experience for both patients and providers as well as improved patient outcomes. However, utilization management programs such as prior authorization requirements and step therapy put the patient-centered model at risk of diminished success and may even result in negative outcomes as a result of delays in optimal therapy. Lack of integrity in the authorization process has caused increased friction between patients and their providers and the insurance companies they rely on to cover their necessary care. Proper documentation and coding are imperative to proper payment, compliance, and adherence to payor-specific requirements. Performing procedures for which the practitioner may not be paid appropriately or not paid at all is a financial and legal risk indicator for the pain practice. A successful practice must focus on excellent patient care as a primary goal, but the factors discussed in this chapter are critical for long-term viability of the practice.

Key Points

- The authorization process is a critical first step in the procedural scheduling process.
- Appropriate documentation is important not only for authorization but to mitigate legal and financial challenges from payors and auditors.
- Local coverage determinations (LCD) and national coverage determinations (NCD) should guide the clinician in decision-making for procedural considerations.
- Patient care is paramount, but proper documentation should be a key consideration in care delivery.

Recommended Reading

1. https://www.ama-assn.org/sites/default/files/media-browser/principles-with-signatory-page-for-slsc.pdf.
2. https://www.beckersasc.com/asc-coding-billing-and-collections/pain-management-in-2017-tips-for-thriving-despite-the-challenges.html.
3. https://www.cnn.com/2018/02/11/health/aetna-california-investigation/index.html.

Medicare Payment Quality Measures

102

Mehul J. Desai and Michael S. Leong

Key Points

- MACRA and its components MIPS and APM represent a fluid change in reimbursement in its transition from fee for service to quality.
- Interventional pain physicians and those that provide chronic pain services often practice in small groups; these clinicians should be aware of specifics or MACRA as they pertain to them as well as exceptions that exist.
- Moving forward performance will likely be gauged by compliance with quality, cost, advancing care information (ACI), and improvement activities.

The Medicare Access and CHIP Reauthorization Act of 2015 (MACRA) replaced the Medicare Sustainable Growth Rate (SGR) formula. SGR was a source of considerable physician anxiety and hand-wringing on an annual basis when dissension in Congress threatened to result in a failure to reauthorize SGR potentially resulting in a 20% reimbursement reduction, a potentially catastrophic blow to physician practices. MACRA initiated a new structure for physician payment based on pay for performance focused on quality outcomes rather than volume-based payments. Reimbursement under MACRA is divided into two groups, merit-based incentive payment systems (MIPS) and advanced alternative payments models (APMs).

The majority of community or private practice pain medicine physicians will fall into MIPS. Those physicians with access to APMs will be limited to those in multispecialty groups, academic centers, managed healthcare systems, and other members of accountable care organizations (ACOs). Expert estimation suggests that >95% of pain medicine physicians will participate under MIPS. A composite performance score based on four weighted performance categories will score physicians under MIPS. These include quality, resource use, clinical practice improvement activities, and meaningful use of certified EHR technology. Advanced APMs will have similar requirements to MIPS.

Physician Quality Reporting Initiative (PQRI) began in 2006 as a component of the Tax Relief and Healthcare Act. Originally consisting of a 179 quality measures, PQRI was a voluntarily quality reporting program for eligible professionals who care for Medicare patients. Originally conceived, as a means to link Medicare provider payments to quality, the expectation was an evolution toward mandatory, value-based purchasing or pay-for-performance program. Over the course of several years, the number of quality measures changed in number. This system eventually came to be known as Physician Quality Reporting System (PQRS) and will form the backbone of quality reporting under MIPS beginning in 2018.

On November 2, 2017, the 2018 Centers for Medicare and Medicaid Services (CMS) Quality Payment Program Final Rule was issued with comment for the 2nd year of the Quality Payment Program (calendar year 2018).

Several key elements include:

- Excluding individual MIPS-eligible clinicians or groups less than or equal to $90,000 in Part B allowed charges or less than or equal to 200 Part B beneficiaries.
- Extreme and unusual circumstances such as hurricanes and other natural disasters for both the transition year and the 2018 MIPS performance period are addressed.
- Included virtual groups as another participation option for Year 2.
- Made it easier for clinicians to qualify for incentive payments by participating in Advanced APMs that begin or end in the middle of a year.

M. J. Desai
International Spine, Pain & Performance Center, Washington, DC, USA

George Washington University, School of Medicine, Washington, DC, USA

M. S. Leong (✉)
Stanford Pain Management Center, Redwood City, CA, USA
e-mail: msleong@stanford.edu

T. R. Deer et al. (eds.), *Deer's Treatment of Pain*, https://doi.org/10.1007/978-3-030-12281-2_102

Additional options for small practices (those <15 clinicians):

- Excluding individual MIPS-eligible clinicians or groups with less than or equal to $90,000 in Part B allowed charges or less than or equal to 200 Part B beneficiaries
- Adding five bonus points to the final scores of small practices
- Giving solo practitioners and small practices the choice to form or join a virtual group to participate with other practices
- Continuing to award small practices three points for measures in the quality performance category that don't meet data completeness requirements
- Adding a new hardship exception for the advancing care information performance category for small practices

Quality

Quality represents 60% of the total composite score in 2017 and 50% in 2018 and requires the reporting of 6 measures, with each measure worth up to 10 points for a total of 60 points depending on actual performance, including one outcome measure or high-priority measure if one outcome measure is not applicable and reporting each of 50% of eligible Medicare and non-Medicare patients/visits for a minimum of 90 days.

Quality Payment Program Year 2: MIPS Highlights

Some minor changes include:

- Raising the performance threshold to 15 points in Year 2 (from 3 points in the transition year)
- Allowing the use of 2014 Edition and/or 2015 Edition of Certified Electronic Health Record Technology (CEHRT) in Year 2 and giving you a bonus for using only 2015 CEHRT
- Giving up to five bonus points on your final score for treatment of complex patients
- Automatically weighting the quality, advancing care information, and improvement activity performance categories at 0% of the final score for clinicians impacted by hurricanes Irma, Harvey, and Maria and other natural disasters
- Adding five bonus points to the final scores of small practices (Table 102.1)

Four new quality measures accepted and approved for 2018 include:

- AQI56: Use of neuraxial techniques and/or peripheral nerve blocks for total knee arthroplasty (TKA)
- AQI57: Safe opioid-prescribing practices
- AQI58: Infection control practices for open interventional pain procedures
- AQI59: Multimodal pain management

Table 102.1 Quality measures for chronic pain

Quality ID	Measure name	Measure type	Data submission method
021[a]	Perioperative care: Selection of prophylactic antibiotic – first- *or* second-generation cephalosporin	Process	Claims, registry
039	Screening for osteoporosis for women aged 65–85 years	Process	Claims, registry
047[a]	Care plan	Process	Claims, registry
109[a]	Osteoarthritis (OA): Function and pain assessment	Process	Claims, registry
128[b]	Care and screening: Body mass index (BMI) screening and follow-up plan	Process	Claims, EHR, CMS Web Interface, registry
130[a]	Documentation of current medications in the medical record	Process	Claims, EHR, registry
131[a]	Pain assessment and follow-up	Process	Claims, registry
134	Preventive care and screening: Screening for clinical depression and follow-up plan	Process	Claims, EHR, CMS Web Interface, registry
145[a]	Radiology: Exposure dose or time reported for procedures using fluoroscopy	Process	Claims, registry
154[a]	Falls: Risk assessment	Process	Claims, registry
155[a]	Falls: Plan of care	Process	Claims, registry
182[a]	Functional outcome assessment	Process	Claims, registry
220[a]	Functional status change for patients with lumbar impairments	Outcome	Registry
226[b]	Preventive care and screening: Tobacco use – screening and cessation intervention	Process	Claims, EHR, CMS Web Interface, registry
238[a]	Use of high-risk medications in the elderly	Process	Registry
276	Sleep apnea: Assessment of sleep symptoms	Process	Registry
318[a]	Falls: Screening for future fall risk	Process	EHR, CMS Web Interface
342[a]	Pain brought under control within 48 hours	Outcome	Registry
357[a]	Surgical site infection (SSI)	Outcome	Registry
374[a, b]	Closing the referral loop: Receipt of specialist report	Process	Registry, EHR
408	Opioid therapy follow-up evaluation	Process	Registry
412	Documentation of signed opioid treatment agreement	Process	Registry
414	Evaluation or interview for risk of opioid misuse	Process	Registry
435[a]	Quality of life assessment for patients with primary headache disorders	Outcome	Claims, registry

[a]"High-priority" measures

[b]Measure has substantive modifications in 2018. Clinicians reporting this measure should check measure specifications

Advancing Care Information

Advancing care information (ACI) represents 25% of total composite score in 2017 and will remain the same in 2018 (Figs. 102.1, 102.2, 102.3 and 102.4). ACI replaces the Medicare EHR Incentive Program also known as Meaningful Use. A minimum of the following base measures is required if reporting this category:

- Conduct security risk analysis.
- e-Prescribe.
- Provide patient electronic access.
- Send a care summary.
- Receive/accept a summary of care. (Table 102.2)

Clinical Practice Improvement Activities

Improvement activities represent 25% of the total composite score in 2017 and will be reduced to 15% in 2018. Physicians must attest to completing up to 2 high-weighted (20 points each) activities or 4 medium-weighted (10 points each) activities for a minimum of 90 days. In groups with fewer than 15 participants (majority of pain medicine physicians) or if you are in a rural or health professional shortage area, physicians must attest that they have completed one high-weighted or two medium-weighted activities for a minimum of 90 days. There are >90 possible measures to choose from; the following are suggestions for consideration:

- Collection and use of patient experience and satisfaction data on access (medium-weighted).
- Annual registration in the Prescription Drug Monitoring Program (PDMP) (medium-weighted).
- Engagement of new Medicaid patients and follow-up (high-weighted).
- Engage patients and families to guide improvement in the system of care (medium-weighted).
- Implementation of documentation improvements for practice/process improvements (medium-weighted).
- Implementation of improvements that contribute to more timely communication of test results (medium-weighted). (Table 102.3)

Cost

Unlike the first year of MIPS, Medicare will assess clinicians on cost performance beginning in 2018. Physicians report no cost data; instead, Medicare will calculate the clinician's cost performance on two cost efficiency mea-

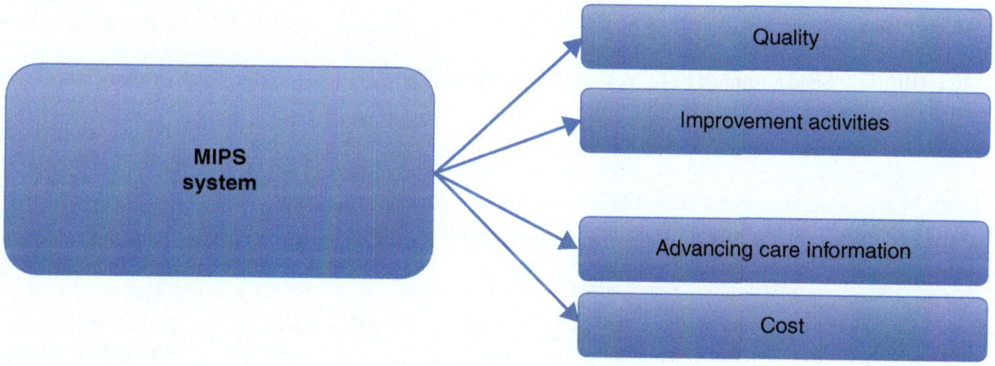

Fig. 102.1 Performance categories of the merit-based incentive payment system (MIPS)

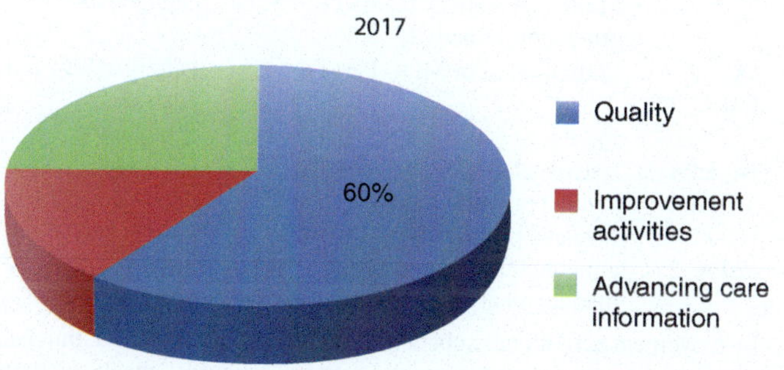

Fig. 102.2 MIPS total performance score weights by performance category 2017

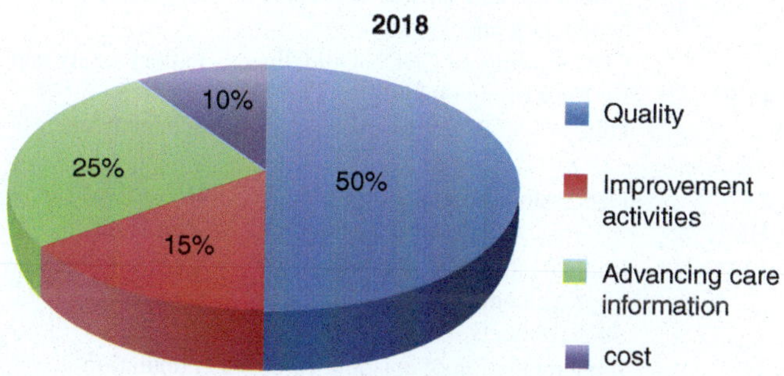

Fig. 102.3 MIPS total performance score weights by performance category 2018

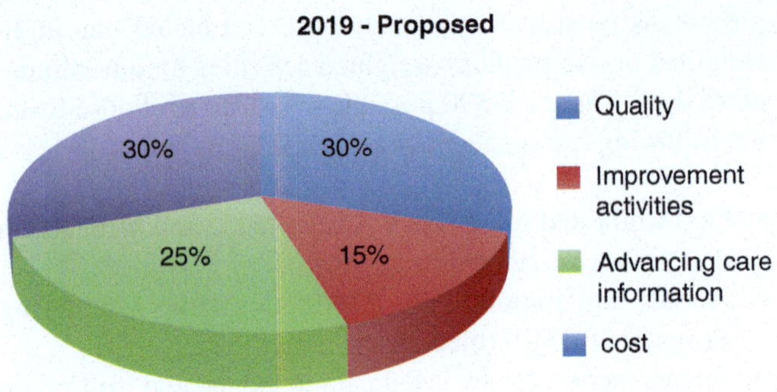

Fig. 102.4 MIPS total performance score weights by performance category 2019

Table 102.2 Advancing care information measures

Measure ID	Measure name	Required for base score	Performance score weight
ACI_PHCDRR_5	Clinical data registry reporting	No	0
ACI_PEA_2	Patient-specific education	No	Up to 10%
ACI_CCTPE_2	Secure messaging	No	Up to 10%
ACI_HIE_3	Clinical information reconciliation	No	Up to 10%
ACI_CCTPE_3	Patient-generated health data	No	Up to 10%
ACI_EP_1	e-Prescribing	Yes	0
ACI_PEA_1	Provide patient access	Yes	Up to 10%
ACI_PPHI_1	Security risk analysis	Yes	0
ACI_HIE_1	Send a summary of care record	Yes	Up to 10%

Table 102.3 Clinical practice improvement activities

Activity ID	Activity name	Subcategory name
High		
IA_PSPA_6	Consultation of the Prescription Drug Monitoring Program	Patient safety and practice engagement
IA_BE_6	Collection and follow-up on patient experience and satisfaction data on beneficiary engagement	Beneficiary engagement
IA_PSPA_22	CDC training on CDC's Guideline for Prescribing Opioids for Chronic Pain	Patient safety and practice engagement
Medium		
IA_BMH_4	Depression screening	Behavioral and mental health
IA_CC_8	Implementation of documentation improvements for practice/process improvements	Care coordination
IA_PM_15	Implementation of episodic care management practice improvements	Population management
IA_BMH_2	Tobacco use	Behavioral and mental health
IA_PSPA_21	Implementation of fall screening and assessment programs	Patient safety and practice engagement
IA_PSPA_5	Annual registration in the Prescription Drug Monitoring Program	Patient safety and practice engagement
IA_PSPA_10	Completion of training and receipt of approved waiver for provision opioid medication-assisted treatments	Patient safety and practice engagement
IA_PSPA_27	Invasive procedure or surgery anticoagulation medication management	Beneficiary engagement
IA_BE_14	Engage patients and families to guide improvement in the system of care	Beneficiary engagement
IA_BE_16	Evidence-based techniques to promote self-management into usual care	Beneficiary engagement
IA_BE_20	Implementation of condition-specific chronic disease self-management support programs	Beneficiary engagement
IA_CC_2	Implementation of improvements that contribute to more timely communication of test results	Care coordination
IA_BE_21[a]	Improved practices that disseminate appropriate self-management materials	Beneficiary engagement
IA_PSPA_18[a]	Measurement and improvement at the practice and panel level	Patient safety and practice engagement
IA_BE_13	Regularly assess the patient experience of care through surveys, advisory councils, and/or other mechanisms	Beneficiary engagement
IA_BE_1	Use of certified EHR to capture patient-reported outcomes	Beneficiary engagement
IA_EPA_3	Collection and use of patient experience and satisfaction data on access	Expanded practice access
IA_PM_16	Implementation of medication management practice improvements	Population management
IA_PSPA_3[a]	Participate in IHI Training/Forum Event: National Academy of Medicine, AHRQ TeamSTEPPS, or other similar activity	Patient safety and practice engagement
IA_PSPA_2[a]	Participation in MOC Part IV	Patient safety and practice engagement
IA_EPA_2	Use of telehealth services that expand practice access	Expanded practice access
IA_PSPA_27	Invasive procedure or surgery anticoagulation medication management	Patient safety and practice engagement

[a]Improvement activity has substantive modifications in 2018. Clinicians attesting to this improvement activity should check activity specifications

sures using claims data. Only certain clinicians will receive MIPS cost performance scores; "non-patient-facing" clinicians will not be assessed. MIPS will not penalize physicians if Medicare does not assign them a cost performance score in 2018. Medicare plans to provide informal feedback to clinicians during 2018 regarding their cost performance. Cost represents 10% of a clinician's MIPS total performance score in 2018 but may represent between 10 and 30% in 2019.

Qualified Registries

A qualified clinical data registry (QCDR) is a reporting mechanism for satisfactory MIPS participation, which:

- Offers an easy way to submit quality data to CMS for the MIPS for both individual physicians and physician group practices
- Allows users to submit non-CMS measures to meet their quality reporting requirements
- Provides direct assistance with compiling the needed data for quality improvement
- Provides feedback to registry participants at least quarterly and on-demand via a registry user dashboard
- Is a vehicle to attest **all** Quality Payment Program requirements:
  - Quality
  - Improvement activities
  - Advancing care information

The American Academy of Physical Medicine and Rehabilitation (AAPM&R) and the American Society of Anesthesiologists (ASA) in conjunction with the American Society of Regional Anesthesia and Pain Medicine (ASRA) currently sponsor QCDRs.

Gradual Implementation

CMS is continuing many of its transition year policies while introducing modest changes. These policies were finalized to ensure that clinicians are ready for full implementation in Year 3.

- Weighting the MIPS cost performance category to 10% of your total MIPS final score. The Medicare Spending per Beneficiary (MSPB) and total per capital cost measures to calculate your cost performance category score for the 2018 MIPS performance period. These two measures are carried over from the value modifier program and are currently being used to provide feedback for the MIPS transition year. CMS will calculate cost measure performance; no action is required from clinicians.
- Increasing the performance threshold to 15 points in Year 2 (from 3 points in the transition year).
- Continuing a phased approach to public reporting Quality Payment Program performance information on Physician Compare.

Twenty-First Century Cures Act

Enacted in 2016, the twenty-first Century Cures Act contains provisions affecting the advancing care information performance category for the Quality Payment Program's current transition year and future years. The twenty-first Century Cures Act was enacted after the publication of the Quality Payment Program Year 1 Final Rule. In this final rule with the comment period, CMS is implementing these provisions in the twenty-first Century Cures Act, some of which will apply to the MIPS transition year including:

- Reweighting the advancing care information performance category to 0% of the final score for ambulatory surgical center (ASC)-based MIPS-eligible clinicians
- Using the twenty-first Century Cures Act authority for significant hardship exceptions and hospital-based MIPS-eligible clinicians to reweight the advancing care information performance category to 0% of the final score

Virtual Groups

Another participation option for Year 2 is the inclusion of virtual groups. A virtual group is a combination of two or more taxpayer identification numbers (TINs) made up of solo practitioners and groups of ten or fewer eligible clinicians who come together "virtually" (no matter specialty or location) to participate in MIPS for a performance period of a year. CMS has developed a virtual groups toolkit with more information including the election process to become a virtual group.

Quality Payment Program Year 2: APM Highlights

New policies further encourage and reward participation in APMs in Medicare. Also incentives for clinicians who participate in APMs offered by payers other than Medicare starting in 2019 are detailed.

Better Coordination and Promoting Alignment

The final rule more closely aligns the standards that apply to Medicare and Other Payer Advanced APMs. Specific policies include:

- Establishing a generally applicable revenue-based nominal amount standard for Other Payer Advanced APMs. This standard allows a non-Medicare payment arrangement to meet the financial risk criterion to qualify as an Other Payer Advanced APM if participants are required to bear total risk of at least 8% of their revenues from a given payer.

Increasing APM Participation: Taking Steps to Increase APM Participation

This year's rule includes provisions to make it easier for eligible clinicians to participate in select APMs (known as Advanced APMs), which may allow them to qualify for incentive payments. Specific policies include:

- Extending the 8% generally applicable revenue-based nominal amount standard that allows APMs to qualify as Advanced APM for two additional years, through performance year 2020
- Exempting Round 1 Comprehensive Primary Care Plus participants or certain currently participating clinicians from the 50-clinician limit on organizations that can earn incentive payments by participating in medical home models
- Changing the requirement for medical home models so that the minimum required amount of total financial risk increases more slowly
- Making it easier for clinicians to qualify for incentive payments by participating in Advanced APMs that begin or end in the middle of the year

Reducing Complexity

CMS is continuing to establish policies through this year's rule that will further reduce burden and simplify the program. They have worked to provide clarity and additional details on many aspects of the program including the APM scoring standard and the All-Payer Combination Option. Specific policies include:

- More detail is provided on how eligible clinicians participating in selected APMs (known as MIPS APMs) will be assessed under the APM scoring standard. This special standard reduces the burden for MIPS APM participants who do not qualify as qualifying APM participants (QPs) and are therefore subject to MIPS.
- We elaborated on how the All-Payer Combination Option will be implemented. This option allows clinicians to become QPs through a combination of Medicare participation in Advanced APMs and participation in Other Payer Advanced APMs. Where possible, additional flexibilities and pathways were created to allow clinicians to be successful under the All Payer Combination Option. This option will be available beginning in performance year 2019.

Payments

Fee schedule updates from 2016 to 2019 will include a 0.5% increase annually capping in 2020 with no further increases. The MIPS program will begin with 4% bonus in 2019, 5% in 2020, and 7% in 2021. From 2022 onward, up to a 9% bonus is possible; certainly this would be reserved for those compliant with MIPS reporting measures, and the incentive pool would come from those paying penalties, as this is a revenue-neutral program. Those participating in APMs would be excluded from MIPS and receive a 5% incentive payment from 2019 onward.

The consequences of quality programs particularly on pain medicine and interventional pain medicine are not yet clear. What is apparent is that increasingly the value of treatments and therapies will be emphasized over pure efficacy. Therefore, the lens of cost will be applied to most if not all therapies moving forward. Pain medicine is particularly vulnerable in this setting; we often practice in small solo or group practices, and our treatment options have been under assault for years due to limited data for their support.

Already as a result of the opioid crisis, pain medicine utilization is under attack. From opioid prescriptions to various interventions including spinal cord stimulation treatment options face greater barriers.

Recommended Reading

1. www.aapmr.org
2. www.asahq.org
3. www.asra.com
4. www.qpp.cms.gov

Index

T. R. Deer et al. (eds.), *Deer's Treatment of Pain*, https://doi.org/10.1007/978-3-030-12281-2

D

E

F

N

O

The manufacturer's authorised representative in the EU is Springer Nature Customer Service Centre GmbH, Europaplatz 3, 69115 Heidelberg, Germany. If you have any concerns regarding our products, please contact ProductSafety@springernature.com

Printed and bound by CPI Group (UK) Ltd, Croydon, CR0 4YY
26/09/2026
02222871-0005